Pediatric Nephrology

Pediatric Nephrology

Seventh Edition

Editors

Arvind Bagga
MD DSc FAMS FIAP FISN
Director, Department of Pediatrics
Indraprastha Apollo Hospitals, New Delhi
Professor Emeritus
All India Institute of Medical Sciences
New Delhi, India

RN Srivastava
FRCP (Ed) FAMS FIAP FISN
Emeritus Consultant
Department of Pediatrics
Indraprastha Apollo Hospitals
New Delhi, India

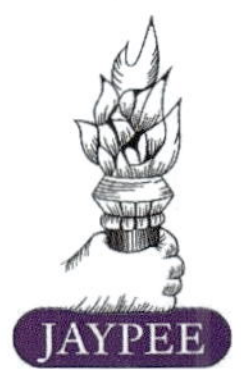

JAYPEE BROTHERS MEDICAL PUBLISHERS
The Health Sciences Publisher
New Delhi | London

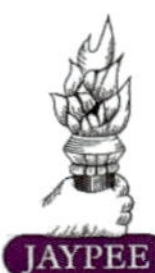

JAYPEE **Jaypee Brothers Medical Publishers (P) Ltd**

Headquarters

Jaypee Brothers Medical Publishers (P) Ltd
EMCA House, 23/23-B
Ansari Road, Daryaganj
New Delhi 110 002, India
Landline: +91-11-23272143, +91-11-23272703
+91-11-23282021, +91-11-23245672
Email: jaypee@jaypeebrothers.com

Corporate Office

Jaypee Brothers Medical Publishers (P) Ltd
4838/24, Ansari Road, Daryaganj
New Delhi 110 002, India
Phone: +91-11-43574357
Fax: +91-11-43574314
Email: jaypee@jaypeebrothers.com

Overseas Office

JP Medical Ltd.
83, Victoria Street, London
SW1H 0HW (UK)
Phone: +44 20 3170 8910
Fax: +44 (0)20 3008 6180
Email: info@jpmedpub.com

Website: www.jaypeebrothers.com
Website: www.jaypeedigital.com

Inquiries for bulk sales may be solicited at: jaypee@jaypeebrothers.com

Pediatric Nephrology

First Edition: 1994
Second Edition: 1997
Third Edition: 2001
Fourth Edition: 2005
Fifth Edition: 2011
Sixth Edition: 2016
Seventh Edition: **2025**

ISBN: 978-93-5696-706-9

Printed at: Samrat Offset Pvt. Ltd.

Dedicated to

Our patients for the opportunity to learn and serve

Our families for their patience and unstinted support

Contributors

Aditi Sinha MD (Pediatrics) DNB PhD
Additional Professor
Department of Pediatrics
Division of Nephrology
All India Institute of Medical Sciences
New Delhi, India

Amit Gupta MD
Research Consultant
Department of Radiodiagnosis
All India Institute of Medical Sciences
New Delhi, India

Amita Sharma MD
Assistant Professor
Harvard Medical School
Clinical Director
Division of Pediatric Nephrology
Massachusetts General Hospital
Boston, MA, USA

Arun Kumar Gupta MD
Former Professor and Head
Department of Radiodiagnosis and Interventional Radiology
All India Institute of Medical Sciences
New Delhi, India

Arvind Bagga MD DSc FAMS FIAP FISN
Director, Department of Pediatrics
Indraprastha Apollo Hospitals
New Delhi
Professor Emeritus
All India Institute of Medical Sciences
New Delhi, India

Asha Moudgil MD FASN FAST
Associate Chief of Pediatric Nephrology
Medical Director, Kidney Transplant Program
Children National Health System
Professor of Pediatrics
George Washington University School of Medicine
Washington, DC, USA

Ashima Gulati MD PhD FASN
Attending Nephrologist
Children's National Hospital
Washington, DC, USA

Ashley A Sharma BS MHS
Research Associate
Department of Pediatric Global Health
Massachusetts General Hospital
Boston, MA, USA

Geetika Singh MD (Pathology)
Professor
Department of Pathology
All India Institute of Medical Sciences
New Delhi, India

Georgie Mathew MD DM
Associate Professor
Department of Pediatric Nephrology
Christian Medical College and Hospital
Vellore, Tamil Nadu, India

Helen Liapis MD
Professor Emeritus of Nephrology
Ludwig Maximilian University
Munich, Germany

Jitendra Meena MD DM
Assistant Professor
Department of Pediatrics
All India Institute of Medical Sciences
New Delhi, India

Jyoti Sharma MD DNB (Pediatrics)
Senior Consultant, Pediatric Nephrology
Renal Unit
Department of Medicine
King Edward Memorial Hospital
Pune, Maharashtra, India

M Srinivas MS MCh (Ped. Surgery)
Director
All India Institute of Medical Sciences
New Delhi, India

Madhuri Kanitkar MD DNB (Pediatrics)
Vice Chancellor
Maharashtra University of Health Sciences
Nashik, Maharashtra, India

Manisha Jana MD DNB FRCR
Professor
Department of Radiodiagnosis and Interventional Radiology
All India Institute of Medical Sciences
New Delhi, India

Marie McGourty MD
University of Massachusetts Chan School of Medicine
Worcester, MA, USA

Mini Michael MD FRACP Mmed
Associate Professor
Baylor College of Medicine/Texas Children's Hospital
Houston, TX, USA

Nishikant Avinash Damle MD
Additional Professor
Department of Nuclear Medicine
All India Institute of Medical Sciences
New Delhi, India

Pankaj Hari MD FIAP FAMS
Professor
Department of Pediatrics
All India Institute of Medical Sciences
New Delhi, India

Paul Winyard BM BCh MA PhD
Professor of Pediatrics
UCL GOS Institute of Child Health
London, UK

Priyanka Khandelwal MD DM
Department of Pediatric Nephrology
Great Ormond Street Hospital for Children
London, UK

Ranjeet Wishram Thergaonkar MD PhD
Professor and Head
Department of Pediatrics
Command Hospital (Eastern Command)
Kolkata, West Bengal, India

RN Srivastava FRCP (Ed) FAMS FIAP FISN
Emeritus Consultant
Department of Pediatrics
Indraprastha Apollo Hospitals
New Delhi, India

Rukshana Shroff MD FRCPCH PhD
Professor
Department of Pediatric Nephrology and Dialysis
UCL GOS Institute of Child Health
London, UK

Shina Menon MD FASN
Associate Professor
Division of Pediatric Nephrology
Department of Pediatrics
Stanford University
Palo Alto, CA, USA

Soumita Bagchi MD DM (Nephrology)
Professor
Department of Nephrology
All India Institute of Medical Sciences
New Delhi, India

Srinivasavaradan Govindarajan MD DM
Assistant Professor
Department of Pediatrics
VMMC and Safdarjung Hospital
New Delhi, India

Stanley C Jordan MD FASN FAST
Distinguished Professor
Departments of Pediatrics and Medicine
UCLA School of Medicine
Cedars-Sinai Medical Center
Los Angeles, CA, USA

Sudarsan Krishnasamy MD DNB DM (Pediatric Nephrology)
Assistant Professor
Department of Pediatrics
Jawaharlal Institute of Postgraduate Medical Education and Research
Puducherry, India

Yogita Khandelwal MD
Senior Resident
Department of Nuclear Medicine
All India Institute of Medical Sciences
New Delhi, India

Preface to the Seventh Edition

We are happy to present the seventh edition of *Pediatric Nephrology*. This book was first published in 1994, and the last revision was in 2016.

The initial editions aimed to fulfill the need for a short text to help pediatricians in Asia manage children with disorders of kidney and urinary tract, and orient those with greater commitment towards the field of nephrology. These editions were received with enthusiasm and led to gradual expansion of its contents. Thus, over three decades, the 'handbook' has grown from 229 pages to its present size of approximately 850 pages.

Over the past two decades the scientific basis and the practice of pediatric nephrology have grown rapidly. Major progress has been made towards clarifying the mechanisms of diseases particularly the genetic, immunological and molecular aspects. The present edition continues to address these mechanistic issues, but the emphasis remains on clinical diagnosis and therapies. Wherever available, the contributors and editors have tried to incorporate contemporary clinical practice guidelines, proposed by pediatric and adult nephrology organizations.

We welcome new authors: Mini Michael, Jyoti Sharma, Priyanka Khandelwal, Soumita Bagchi, Nishikant Avinash Damle, Jitendra Meena, Srinivasavaradan Govindarajan, Sudarsan Krishnasamy and Georgie Mathew. Chapters on congenital anomalies of the kidneys and urinary tract, fluid and electrolyte disorders, nephrotic syndrome, hematuria and proteinuria, glomerulonephritis, acute kidney injury, thrombotic microangiopathy, urinary tract infection, tubular and tubulointerstitial diseases, chronic kidney disease, kidney support therapy and transplantation have been rewritten. The annexures are updated. Normative clinic and ambulatory blood pressure data, and gene lists for important kidney and urological diseases are provided as dynamic annexures through QR codes. We are grateful to all contributors for their scholarly work and ensuring that the chapters continue to provide updated information that meets the learning needs of the readers.

We appreciate the support of Geetika Singh and Adarsh Barwad (Nephropathology, All India Institute of Medical Sciences) for providing high quality photomicrographs and Jyoti Singhal for the illustrations. The editors gratefully acknowledge Aditi Sinha's association with the last two editions of this book, her erudite writings and meticulous proofreading.

The book should continue to meet the requirements of pediatricians and pediatric nephrologists, postgraduate and DM trainees, and urologists. We hope that at whatever stage of your career, the seventh edition of *Pediatric Nephrology* serves your needs to provide the best care for your patients and their families. They deserve nothing less.

January 2025

Arvind Bagga
RN Srivastava

Preface to the First Edition

The need for a short practical text on disorders of the kidney and urinary tract in children has been long-felt.

Rapid advances have taken place in the diagnosis and management of various renal disorders in children. Antenatal diagnosis of congenital anomalies of the kidney and urinary tract is being increasingly made with ultrasonography. Computerized scanning, magnetic resonance and radionuclide imaging can provide definitive diagnostic information and enable continued evaluation of conditions such as vesicoureteric reflux and renal scarring, growth of a solitary kidney and renovascular lesions. New insights have been gained into the management of acute glomerulonephritis, nephrotic syndrome, urinary tract infections and chronic renal failure. The efficacy and feasibility of renal replacement therapy and renal transplantation in children have been well established.

Pediatricians and other first contact physicians bear a heavy responsibility of making a prompt diagnosis, carrying out initial therapy and preventing complications. A large proportion of renal disorders are recurrent or chronic and require long-term care and surveillance. Psychoemotional and socioeconomic factors are very important in such cases and need to be tackled adequately for the optimal management of the child. Such patients need to be jointly cared for by the family pediatrician and the pediatric nephrologists.

In developing countries the efforts must be directed toward appropriate therapy, cost-effectiveness and preventive nephrology. Unnecessary laboratory investigations and therapeutic modalities of unproven measures and recommendations should be followed.

The present text emphasizes the diagnostic evaluation and the management of children with renal and urinary tract disorders. Detailed considerations of renal pathophysiology and the mechanisms of diseases are not included for which pediatric nephrology textbooks and other sources may be consulted. We have attempted to give clear guidelines. Uncommon conditions have been very briefly referred to. Only a short introduction to chronic dialysis and renal transplantation is given and those deciding to use these modalities will need detailed information.

We thank Prof UN Bhuyan for providing renal histology illustrations. The secretarial help of Mr Surest Sahni is gratefully acknowledged. We are extremely grateful to Mr Harish Chawla, Director, Cipla Limited, for a generous contribution towards publication of this book. We are indebted to Mr Rajesh Sardana of Cambridge Press for his help and guidance.

January 1994

RN Srivastava
Arvind Bagga

Contents

Renal Anatomy and Physiology

Arvind Bagga, Srinivasavaradan Govindarajan

Kidneys are two bean-shaped organs lying retroperitoneally on each side of the vertebral column. The kidney is anatomically complex and consists of highly specialized cells. The functional units of the kidney are called nephrons, which are tightly packed to form renal parenchyma. Each nephron consists of a glomerulus and a long tubule.

On cut surface, the pale outer cortex and a dark, inner medulla can be easily distinguished **(Fig. 1.1)**. The medulla consists of 8–12 conical masses, the pyramids. The base of a pyramid is at the corticomedullary junction and the apex toward the renal pelvis, forming a papilla. Each papilla contains 10–25 small openings that represent the distal ends of the collecting ducts. In the adult kidney, the cortex is about 1 cm thick and covers the base of the renal pyramids and extends between individual pyramids to form the columns of Bertini. From the base of the pyramid, at the corticomedullary junction, longitudinal medullary rays, consisting of collecting ducts and the straight segments of the proximal and distal tubules, extend into the cortex. The renal pelvis forms two or three major calyces, and from each of these several minor

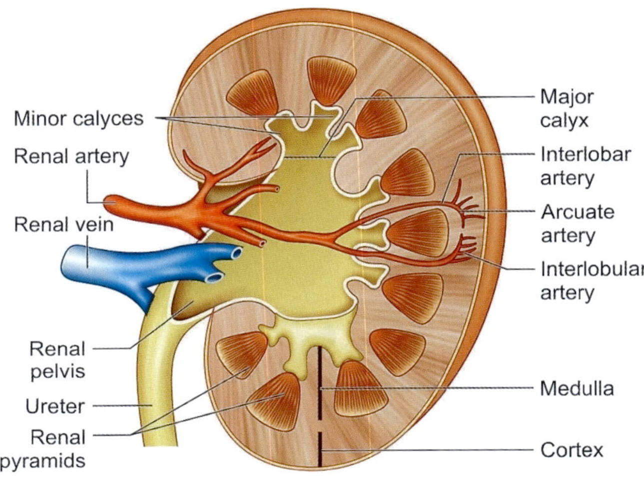

Fig. 1.1: Sagittal section of the kidney

calyces extend outward. The ureter begins at the lower portion of the pelvis, at the pelviureteric junction and descends to open into the fundus of the bladder. Peristaltic activity of these structures propels the urine toward the bladder.

NEPHRON

Each kidney contains about one million nephrons. A nephron consists of the glomerulus, proximal tubule, the thin limbs, the distal tubule, and the connecting segment.

Glomerulus

The structure of the glomerulus is depicted in **Figure 1.2**. The glomerulus is made up of a tuft of capillaries and a central region of mesangium containing cells and matrix. The capillaries arise from an afferent arteriole and eventually join to form an efferent arteriole, the entry and exit being at the vascular pole of the glomerulus. The capillary wall consists of a fenestrated endothelium, basement membrane, and specialized epithelial cells (podocytes). The glomerulus is surrounded by the Bowman's capsule lined by the parietal

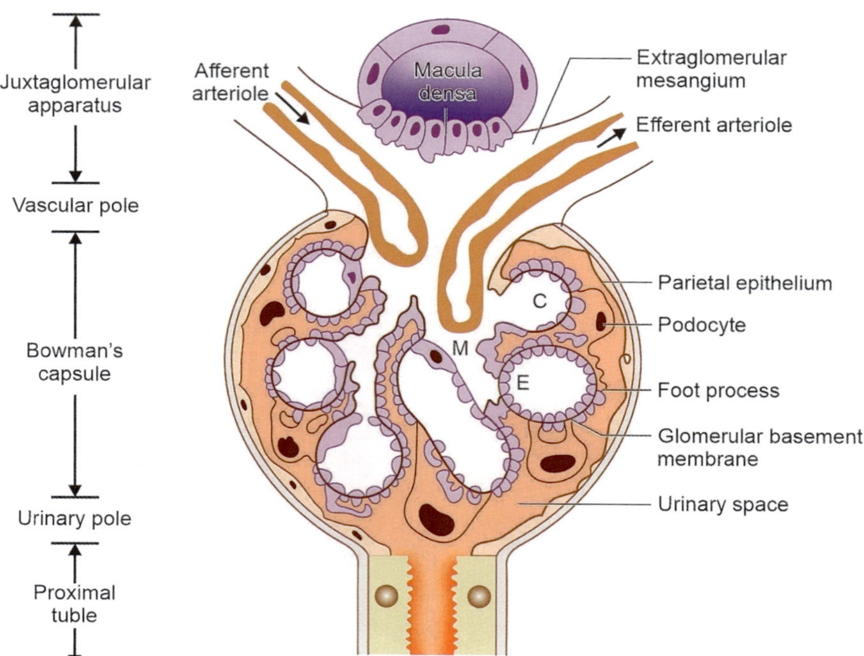

Fig. 1.2: Cross-section of glomerulus. C: capillary lumen; E: endothelium; M: mesangium

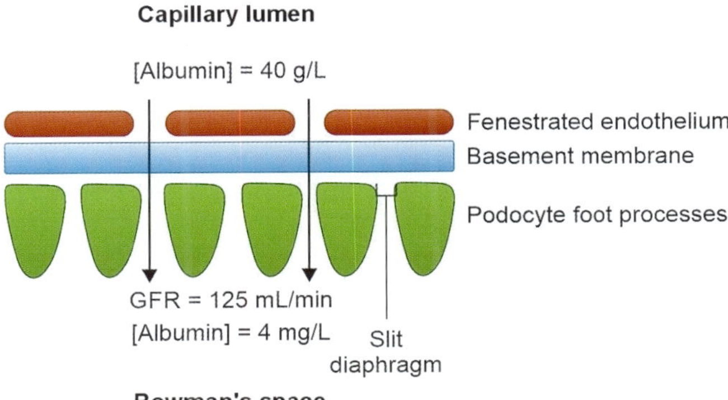

Fig. 1.3: Ultrastructure of glomerular basement membrane. Arrows indicate direction of flow of the filtrate

epithelium that is continuous with the visceral epithelium at the vascular pole. The Bowman's space leads into the proximal tubule.

The capillary endothelium contains pores of 70–100 nm diameter. The basement membrane consists of a central dense layer, the lamina densa, lamina rara interna, and lamina rara externa. The podocytes have long cytoplasmic foot processes (pedicels) that extend from the main cell body and interdigitate and come in contact with the lamina rara externa. The gap between individual pedicel is about 25–60 nm and is bridged by a thin slit diaphragm **(Fig. 1.3)**. All three components of the capillary wall contain negatively charged sites because of the presence of a polyanionic surface glycoprotein, podocalyxin.

Tubule

The proximal tubule starts at the urinary pole of the glomerulus and consists of an initial convoluted portion and a straight segment **(Fig. 1.4)**, which are contained in the cortex along with the glomerulus. The straight segment leads to the loop of Henle, which dips into the medulla. The descending limb and the initial part of ascending loop of Henle are thin walled. The rest of the ascending limb has thick walls like that of the proximal tubule, and in the cortex, it ends in the distal convoluted tubule. Within the cortex, up to eight distal tubules join to form the cortical collecting duct that passes downward into the medulla (where it is called "outer medullary collecting duct"). Several collecting ducts join to make increasingly large inner medullary collecting ducts, which eventually enter the renal pelvis through the tip of the papilla. Papillae are conical projections of the medulla protruding into renal calyces. Each kidney has about 250 large collecting ducts, each of which drains about 4,000 nephrons.

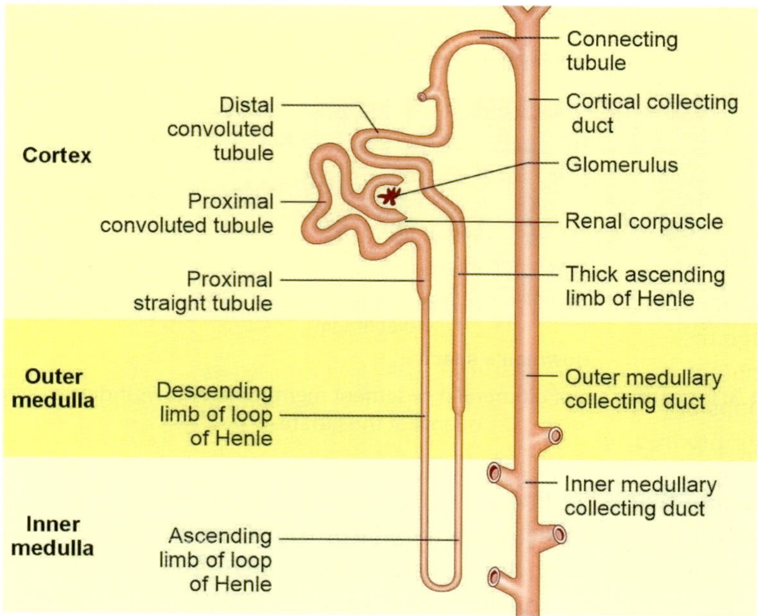

Fig. 1.4: Nephron showing glomerulus and renal tubule

Juxtamedullary Nephrons

About 20% nephrons have their glomeruli in the deeper parts of cortex and have very long loops of Henle that descend all the way to the papillary tips. These are called juxtamedullary nephrons. The nephrons in the superficial cortex have short loops of Henle that bend at the junction between the inner and outer medulla.

Juxtaglomerular Apparatus

The early part of the distal tubule in its ascent from the medulla to the cortex lies near the glomerulus of the same nephron. The cells of the tubule in the part that comes in contact with the afferent arteriole of the glomerulus are denser than the cells in the rest of the tubule, and are called macula densa **(Fig. 1.2)**. The smooth muscle cells of the afferent arterioles that approximate the macula densa contain prominent secretory cytoplasmic granules, which are the site of renin activity. The juxtaglomerular apparatus is composed of the afferent and efferent arterioles, the macula densa, and lacis cells located in the triangular space in between these structures. It is involved in systemic blood pressure regulation, electrolyte homeostasis, and tubuloglomerular feedback mechanisms.

Renal Vasculature

The renal artery divides into five segmental arteries. The latter divide into the interlobar arteries, which branch into arcuate arteries near the junction of the cortex and the medulla. Interlobular arteries arise at right angles from the arcuate arteries and pierce into the cortex **(Fig. 1.1)**. These provide the afferent arterioles for the glomeruli. The glomerular capillaries join to form the efferent arterioles that leave the glomerulus and form an extensive network of peritubular capillaries that surround the tubules, mostly in the cortex. After tubular reabsorption, enormous amounts of filtrate pass through these capillaries. From the deeper portions of these capillaries, long branching capillary loops (vasa recta) extend into the medulla adjacent to the loops of Henle. Thereafter, these vasa recta loop back toward the cortex and empty into the cortical veins. Only 1–2% of the total renal blood flow is through the vasa recti. The vasa recti along with the loops of Henle are responsible for the urinary concentration.

RENAL FUNCTION

The kidneys receive the greatest blood flow in proportion to weight. At rest, 20–25% of cardiac output goes to the kidneys. The chief elements of renal function are glomerular ultrafiltration, tubular reabsorption, and tubular secretion.

Glomerular Filtration

The glomerular capillary hydrostatic pressure forces a virtually protein-free filtrate into the Bowman space. The special structure of these capillaries makes them highly permeable, more than several times than ordinary capillaries. Despite that, the capillaries restrict proteins even of relatively low molecular weight (e.g., albumin, molecular weight 69,000 Da). Crystalloids and low molecular weight substances such as urea, glucose, and amino acids are freely filtered. The restriction of albumin is chiefly due to the anionic charge of the glomerular basement membrane, imparted by the presence of complex proteoglycans, and the integrity of the podocyte slit diaphragm. Genetic or acquired abnormalities of the podocyte are an important cause of proteinuria.

The glomerular filtrate has almost the same composition as that of plasma. It has no red blood cells and only 0.03 g/dL of protein. The normal glomerular filtration rate (GFR) is about 125 mL/min/1.73 m^2. Since the normal plasma flow through the kidneys is 650 mL/min, only about 20% is filtered. This proportion is termed the *filtration fraction.*

Factors Affecting the Glomerular Filtration Rate

The GFR is chiefly determined by the degree of constriction of afferent and efferent arterioles. Other factors, including plasma colloid osmotic pressure and the pressure in Bowman's capsule, also play a role. Afferent arteriolar vasoconstriction decreases the rate of blood flow into glomerular filtration. Constriction of the efferent arteriole increases the resistance to the outflow from the glomeruli, thereby increasing the glomerular pressure and glomerular filtration. Angiotensin II causes a preferential constriction of efferent arterioles.

Autoregulation of Renal Blood Flow and Glomerular Filtration Rate

Despite wide changes in systemic arterial pressure, the renal blood flow and the GFR are kept relatively constant. This phenomenon is termed autoregulation and probably mediated through tubuloglomerular feedback. A marked fall in GFR results in excessive reabsorption of Na^+ and Cl^- in the ascending loop of Henle, thus reducing their concentration at macula densa. This stimulates the juxtaglomerular cells to release renin, leading to increased angiotensin II formation, which constricts efferent arterioles. The resultant rise in glomerular pressure increases the GFR restoring the normal status. Additional mechanisms may be involved in the process of autoregulation **(Flowchart 1.1)**.

Flowchart 1.1: Tubuloglomerular feedback pathway

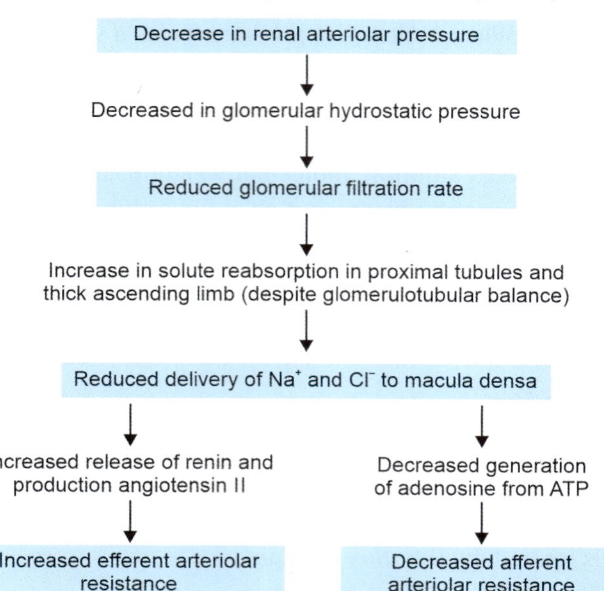

Tubular Reabsorption and Secretion

The glomerular filtrate undergoes a series of modifications before becoming final urine. Absorption, the movement of solute or water from the tubular lumen to blood, is the predominant process in renal handling of sodium, chloride, water, bicarbonate, glucose, amino acids, protein, phosphate, calcium, magnesium, urea, and uric acid. Secretion, the movement of solute from blood into the tubular lumen, is important in the renal handling of hydrogen, potassium, ammonium ions and organic acids and bases. Movement of ions and other substances occurs either by the transcellular pathway that requires traversing the luminal and the basolateral cell membranes, or by the paracellular pathway between cells.

Structure of Tubular Segments

The structure of various segments of the tubules is different and related to their characteristic absorptive and secretary function. The epithelial cells of proximal tubule, thick ascending limb of Henle, and the first part of the distal tubule have large number of mitochondria. The proximal tubular cells have a huge surface area, provided by the brush border for transfer of substances across the cell membrane. The thin segment of the loop of Henle has thin walls, few mitochondria, and no brush border. The epithelial cells of the collecting ducts are cuboidal with few mitochondria and without a brush border.

General Characteristics of Tubular Reabsorption

The proximal tubule reabsorbs a large amount of the filtrate. The descending limb of loop of Henle is highly permeable to water and moderately permeable to urea, sodium, and other ions. It is the site of simple diffusion of substances. The thick ascending limb is almost impermeable to both water and urea, which are retained in the lumen, as various ions are actively reabsorbed. At the end of the ascending limb, the tubular fluid is very dilute but has a high urea content. The first part of the distal tubule (cortical diluting segment), like the thick ascending limb of Henle, is also impermeable to urea and water. Thus, it further dilutes the tubular fluid. The latter part of distal tubule (also impermeable to urea) is involved in aldosterone-controlled sodium reabsorption and potassium secretion. The secretion of potassium in this segment is responsible for maintaining the potassium concentration in the extracellular fluid (ECF). The late distal tubule and the cortical collecting duct contain specialized epithelial cells (intercalated cells) that actively secrete hydrogen ions against a concentration gradient even as high as 1,000 to 1. This has a vital role in maximum urinary acidification. The late distal tubule and cortical collecting duct are permeable to water in the presence of antidiuretic hormone (ADH). The medullary collecting duct can also secrete hydrogen ions against a very high gradient. They are permeable to water in response to ADH and slightly permeable to urea. This segment is responsible for maximum urinary concentration.

Under usual circumstances, 65% of the glomerular filtrate (water) is reabsorbed in the proximal tubule, 15% in the loop of Henle, 10% in the distal tubule, and 9% in the collecting duct. Thus, only 1% of glomerular filtrate is excreted as urine.

Tubular Maximum

Substances such as glucose and amino acids that are actively reabsorbed (and others that are actively secreted) require specific transport systems mediated by enzymes. Each system has a saturation point at which the particular product can be transported at a maximum (Tm for that substance).

In adults, the tubular maximum (Tm) for glucose is 320 mg/min. A greater tubular load (plasma glucose × GFR) than that results in excretion of excess glucose in urine. Since under normal situations, the tubular load is only 125 mg/min, all the filtered glucose is reabsorbed.

REABSORPTION OF SPECIFIC SUBSTANCES

Sodium

On usual dietary intake, 99% of the filtered sodium is reabsorbed, including 67% in the proximal tubule and 33% in the loop of Henle, distal tubule or collecting duct **(Fig. 1.5)**. Sodium reabsorption in the distal tubule and the collecting duct is highly variable and controlled by the concentration of aldosterone. The basic mechanism for sodium reabsorption involves its active transport. On the basal and lateral surfaces of tubular epithelial cell, Na^+ is extruded from the cell through the Na^+-K^+ ATPase system. Three Na^+ ions are pumped out and two K^+ ions pumped inside the cell. This action reduces the Na^+ concentration within the cells and also makes the cell interior electronegative because of which Na^+ ions passively diffuse from the tubular lumen into the cell.

In the proximal tubule, sodium reabsorption is controlled by glomerulotubular balance (the amount reabsorbed is directly proportional to the amount filtered) and the state of intravascular volume. Expansion of intravascular volume decreases sodium reabsorption and its contraction increases it, irrespective of its serum level.

Much of sodium reabsorption in the proximal tubule results from active cotransport with organic solutes such as glucose and amino acids, or through the Na–hydrogen exchanger. The primary mediator of sodium uptake in the thick ascending limb of Henle is the frusemide sensitive Na^+-K^+-$2Cl^-$ (NKCC2)

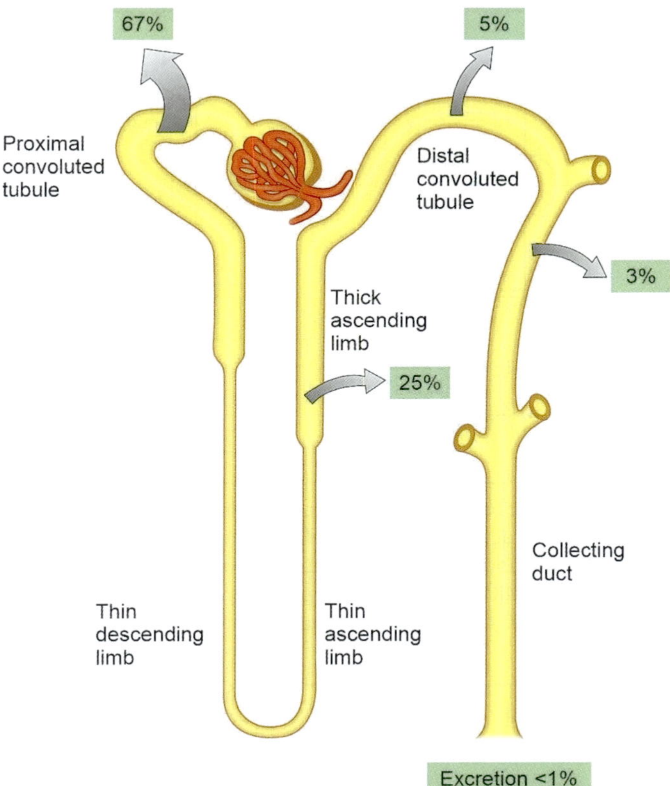

Fig. 1.5: Pathways and mediators involved in sodium (Na^+) reabsorption. Almost 67% of filtered Na^+ is reabsorbed in the proximal tubule. The distal portions of the nephron reabsorb the remainder

cotransporter **(Fig. 1.6)**. The levels of K^+ in the lumen of the loop of Henle are much lower than Na^+ and Cl^-. Therefore, K^+ entering the tubular cell from the lumen must be recycled to permit sustained NKCC2 activity. The renal outer medullary K^+ channel (ROMK) is an ATP-sensitive channel that "recycles" reabsorbed K^+ back into the tubular lumen ensuring efficient Na^+ and Cl^- uptake by NKCC2. The Cl^- channel, ClC-Kb, allows Cl^- reabsorption from the tubular cell into the bloodstream.

In the distal convoluted tubule, the thiazide-sensitive apical Na^+/Cl^- cotransporter (NCCT) is the principal mediator of Na^+ and Cl^- reabsorption **(Fig. 1.7)**. The amiloride-sensitive epithelial sodium channels (ENaC) mediate its reabsorption in collecting tubules and collecting ducts **(Fig. 1.8)**. The mineralocorticoid hormone aldosterone regulates Na^+/K^+ balance in the distal nephron chiefly through its effect on the activity of ENaC. In the distal tubule, Na^+ is reabsorbed in presence of aldosterone; in its absence, almost all is excreted.

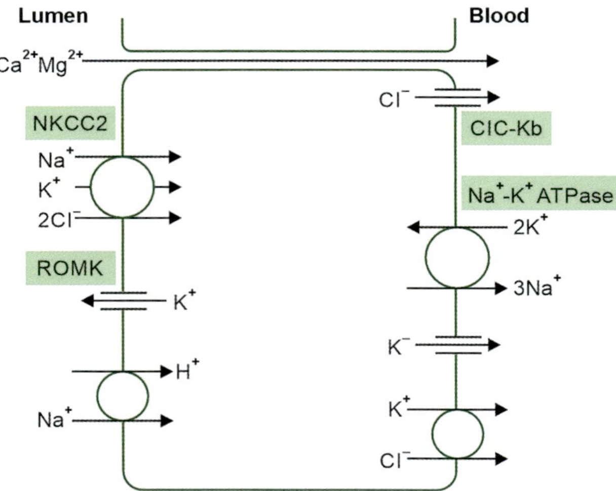

Fig. 1.6: Electrolyte transport in the thick ascending limb (TAL) of loop of Henle. Na^+, K^+, and Cl^- are absorbed across the apical cell membrane by the sodium potassium chloride (NKCC2) cotransporter. This transporter is driven by the renal outer medullary potassium channel (ROMK) on the luminal surface, and the Na^+-K^+ ATPase pump, Cl^- channel (ClC-Kb), and K^+ channels on the basolateral surface

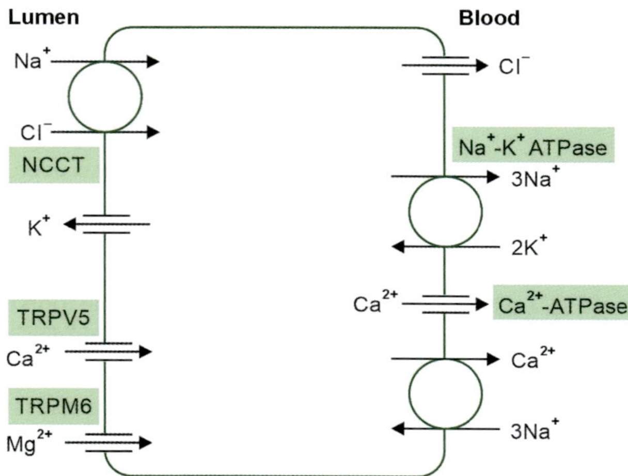

Fig. 1.7: Electrolyte transport in the distal convoluted tubule. Na^+ and Cl^- are reabsorbed across the apical membrane by the thiazide-sensitive NCCT cotransporter and leave the cell through the Cl^- channel and the Na^+-K^+ ATPase pump. Calcium enters the cell through the calcium channels and exits *via* the Na^+-Ca^{++} exchanger and Ca^{2+} ATPase

Aldosterone secretion is stimulated by angiotensin II, ECF volume contraction, and decreased ECF sodium concentration. A decrease in ECF volume reduces arterial pressure and increases sympathetic activity. The renal perfusion is reduced by stimulating the renin-angiotensin-II-aldosterone mechanism and increasing sodium reabsorption.

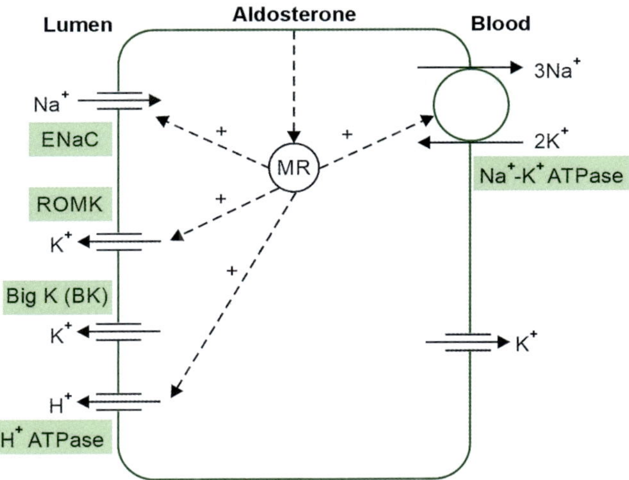

Fig. 1.8: Solute reabsorption in the principal cell of the collecting tubule. Na^+ is reabsorbed across the amiloride-sensitive epithelial Na^+ channel (ENaC). Na^+ uptake is coupled to K^+ and H^+ secretion. Aldosterone binds to the nuclear mineralocorticoid receptor (MR) and upregulates ENaC, ROMK, H^+ATPase and Na^+-K^+ ATPase. This increases Na^+ reabsorption and K^+ and H^+ secretion, resulting in hypokalemic alkalosis

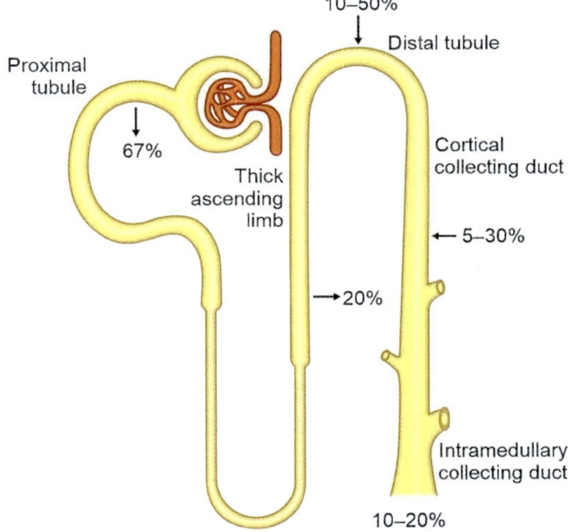

Fig. 1.9: Renal handling of potassium. Almost 65–70% of the filtered (K^+) is reabsorbed in the proximal tubule and a variable secretion occurs at the collecting duct

Potassium

Potassium is freely filtered at the glomerulus with 65–70% passively reabsorbed in the proximal tubule. Another 20% is reabsorbed in the thick ascending loop of Henle through the action of Na^+-K^+-2Cl cotransporter so that <10% reaches the distal part of the nephron **(Fig. 1.9)**. The greater part of regulation occurs in the distal tubule and collecting duct. The fractional excretion of potassium, under normal conditions, is 10–20%. In the cortical collecting duct, the most important cell that secretes K^+ into the tubular lumen is the principal cell. Potassium accumulates within the principal cell under the influence of Na^+-K^+-ATPase, located at the basolateral membrane, and escapes into the tubular lumen by passive diffusion along the electrochemical gradient. Potassium movement occurs through selective apical K^+ channels including the renal outer medullary potassium (ROMK) channels and the high conductance 'big' potassium (BK) channels. The latter are activated in response to increased urinary flow rate. The major determinants for potassium secretion by the principal cell are aldosterone, urinary flow and distal Na^+ delivery, the serum K^+ level, and functioning apical K^+ channels.

Regulation of Plasma Potassium

The primary regulation of plasma potassium occurs via the influence of aldosterone, mainly in the principal cells of the cortical and medullary collecting ducts. Decreased effective circulating volume or an increase in the potassium concentration leads to increased aldosterone production and increased potassium secretion in exchange for sodium. Increased effective circulating volume or decreased potassium leads to decreased aldosterone production. Aldosterone stimulates Na^+ reabsorption and, thus, increases the electrochemical gradient for K^+ diffusion into the tubular lumen. Aldosterone also increases the activity of Na^+-K^+ ATPase that helps K^+ accumulation within the tubular cells. Metabolic as well as respiratory acid–base alterations affect K^+ secretion by collecting duct cells; the secretion is decreased by acute acidosis and increased by alkalosis. The secretion of potassium is also dependent on adequate tubular flow in the distal nephron. Decreased ECF volume leads not only to increased aldosterone production but also to decreased distal flow rate, allowing plasma potassium to remain in a relatively normal range, barring additional factors. Conversely, increased ECF volume leads to not only a decrease in aldosterone production but also an increased distal flow rate, allowing plasma potassium to remain normal. With severe hypokalemia, the urinary concentration of K^+ is very low. This is achieved through the reabsorption of K^+ by intercalated A and B cells present in the collecting tubules.

Calcium

Calcium is the most abundant cation in the body. Calcium exists in three forms in plasma. The biologically active form termed "ionized calcium" constitutes 50%; 45% is bound to plasma proteins (chiefly albumin) and 5% is complexed to anions such as phosphate and citrate. The ionized fraction is physiologically active and, therefore, tightly regulated in a narrow range (4.5–5.1 mg/dL). Decreased total plasma calcium concentration is found in hypoalbuminemia without changes in the ionized calcium level. In general, for every 1.0 g/dL decrement in plasma albumin, there is a 0.8 mg/dL decline in the total plasma calcium level. Metabolic acidosis reduces protein binding and increases ionized calcium levels. The extracellular concentration of calcium is very closely regulated by parathyroid hormone (PTH), $1,25(OH)_2D$ (calcitriol), and calcitonin. PTH increases renal calcium reabsorption and its resorption from bone. It also enhances renal conversion of $25(OH)D_3$ to $1,25(OH)_2D$; the latter stimulates gastrointestinal calcium absorption.

The average diet contains 1000–1200 mg of calcium, mainly from dairy products. Of this, 20–40% is absorbed in the small intestine. A small amount of calcium is also secreted back into the colon (200 mg/day). Every day, 200–500 mg of calcium enters the ECF from the skeleton and the same amount is deposited back as a result of ongoing skeletal remodeling. The amount of calcium entering the ECF from the gut is excreted by the kidney, keeping the body in a net equal balance.

Tubular Handling

The nonprotein bound calcium is freely filtered and about 99% is reabsorbed. Proximal tubule reabsorbs 50–55% and the loop of Henle 20–30%, being linked to sodium reabsorption. Distal tubular and collecting duct reabsorption (about 10–15% and 2–8% respectively) is independent of sodium transport.

Regulation of Plasma Calcium

Plasma ionized calcium is regulated by an interplay of PTH and calcitriol in intestine, bone, and kidney. Parathyroid cells and renal tubules express a cell-surface calcium-sensing receptor (CaSR) that enables these cells to detect small changes in the extracellular calcium concentration. CaSR is also expressed in other tissues related to calcium homeostasis such as thyroid C-cells, intestines, and bones. An increase in extracellular calcium concentration activates CaSR, which decreases PTH secretion and inhibits renal calcium reabsorption, whereas a decrease in extracellular calcium has the opposite effect.

The PTH, in the presence of calcitriol, stimulates bone resorption by increasing osteoclast number and activity. In the intestine, PTH simulates calcium and phosphorus absorption by promoting calcitriol formation. In the kidneys, it enhances tubular reabsorption of calcium, stimulates the generation of calcitriol in the proximal tubule, and decreases proximal tubular reabsorption of phosphate.

Calcitriol is formed in the proximal tubule from 1-α hydroxylation of calcidiol. The main role of calcitriol is to improve the availability of calcium and phosphate. In the intestine and kidney, calcitriol stimulates calcium absorption. In bone, calcitriol complements the actions of PTH, stimulating osteoclastic bone resorption. Calcitriol acts directly on the parathyroid gland to inhibit both PTH synthesis and secretion **(Fig. 1.10)**.

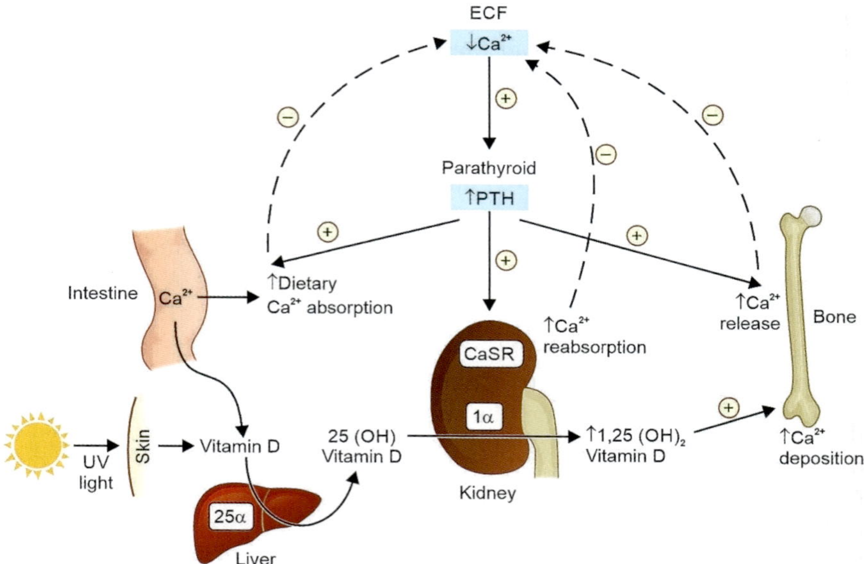

Fig. 1.10: Calcium regulation. Dotted lines denote inhibition. CaSR: calcium sensing receptor; ECF: extracellular fluid; PTH: parathyroid hormone

Phosphorus

The plasma concentration of inorganic phosphate is chiefly regulated by renal tubular reabsorption of filtered phosphate, which is decreased by PTH and enhanced by $1,25(OH)_2D_3$. The latter increases renal and intestinal reabsorption of phosphate. Plasma phosphate levels are influenced by dietary intake of phosphate, age, and sex. Normally, >85% of filtered phosphate is reabsorbed, 60–70% proximally and the remainder in distal segments, but this may approach 100% during phosphate deprivation. Factors that influence plasma phosphate concentration are outlined below.

PTH: In the kidney, phosphate is reabsorbed primarily in the proximal tubule (80%), where it is cotransported across the luminal membrane with sodium. PTH inhibits this reabsorption, lowering the plasma phosphate level. PTH acts directly on bone to increase phosphate entry into the ECF and indirectly on the intestine by stimulating the synthesis of calcitriol.

Calcitriol: Vitamin D increases plasma phosphate due to enhanced intestinal phosphorus absorption by increasing sodium-phosphate cotransport across the apical brush border membrane.

Plasma phosphate concentration: Elevated phosphorus level itself decreases proximal reabsorption in the renal tubule.

Insulin: Insulin lowers plasma phosphorus by shifting phosphate into cells.

Fibroblast growth factor (FGF): FGF-23 belongs to a group of phosphatonins. Their main effect is to promote renal excretion of phosphate and lower plasma phosphorus levels.

Magnesium

Only 1% of the total body magnesium is extracellular. Of the serum magnesium, 20% is protein bound and the remainder is freely filtered. Normally, >95% is reabsorbed, 20–30% proximally and the rest in the loop of Henle, particularly in the thick ascending limb.

Amino Acids

The plasma concentration of amino acids is maintained within 2.5–3.5 mM/L through several mechanisms. Digestion of dietary proteins and absorption of the fragments adds to the amino acid pool, whereas their deamination and formation of urea and ammonia subtract from the pool. Proximal tubular reabsorption of amino acids is almost total, with negligible amounts excreted in the urine. Groups of amino acids share a common transport mechanism. One cotransporter reabsorbs lysine, arginine, cystine and ornithine, and another glutamic and aspartic acids.

Protein

Despite electrostatic hindrance imparted by the glomerular capillaries, significant amounts of low molecular weight proteins are filtered. These are almost totally reabsorbed in the proximal tubule through the brush border by pinocytosis. Within the cell, the protein molecule is digested into its amino acid components, which diffuse across the basolateral membranes into the interstitial fluid and the peritubular capillaries.

Urea

Usually, 40–60% of filtered urea appears in the urine. As a rule, reabsorption of urea is by passive diffusion and parallels the movement of water. A recirculation mechanism of urea through the loop of Henle, the distal tubule, and the collecting duct is responsible for the high urea concentration in the urine.

Creatinine

Creatinine is not reabsorbed except in premature infants. There is an actual secretion of small amounts of creatinine by the proximal tubule.

URINARY ACIDIFICATION

The role of the kidney is to maintain plasma bicarbonate at a level of 22–24 mEq/L. The respiratory system maintains the plasma carbonic acid at

1.3–1.4 mEq/L. The concentrations of these two determine the pH of the plasma and interstitial fluid and indirectly, the intracellular pH.

The bicarbonate filtered is largely (80–85%) reabsorbed in the proximal tubule and the remainder in the initial part of distal tubule. The maximum urinary acidification is achieved distally, through the processes of titratable acid and ammonia excretion. The basic mechanism is an exchange of filtered sodium for hydrogen ion along the entire length of the nephron and is dependent upon the enzyme carbonic anhydrase. Titratable acid is formed by the buffering of hydrogen ions by phosphate in the tubular fluid. Ammonia is formed within the tubular cells and diffuses into the lumen where it combines with hydrogen ions to form ammonium that is trapped in the lumen. In the collecting duct, bicarbonate is almost completely removed from the tubular lumen. During maximal stimulation, the urine pH can be lowered below 5.3.

WATER REABSORPTION

The tonicity of the body fluid is maintained constant, between 280 and 290 mOsm/kg, through renal handling of water. The integrity of hypothalamus–posterior pituitary–ADH system and the adequacy of nephron structure and function are necessary for maintaining normal tonicity.

Water is passively reabsorbed in the proximal tubule and thin descending limb of the loop of Henle. The ascending limb of the loop of Henle and the distal convoluted tubule are impermeable to water. Epithelial cells of the collecting tubules and ducts are permeable to water in the presence of the ADH arginine vasopressin. The aquaporins (AQP) are a family of membrane channel proteins that serve as selective pores through which water crosses cell membranes **(Fig. 1.11)**.

Regulation of ADH Secretion

Antidiuretic hormone is synthesized in the neurons of supraoptic and paraventricular nuclei of the anterior hypothalamus and then transported down to the nerve endings in the posterior pituitary gland. ADH accumulates in large secretory granules and is released when appropriate stimuli are received.

The chief function of ADH is to increase the permeability of the collecting ducts to water. This results from the insertion of water channels in apical membranes of principal cells in the collecting ducts. ADH also causes arteriolar constriction and a rise in arterial blood pressure, but the physiological significance of this effect is not important.

Changes in the osmolality of ECF are sensed by osmoreceptors, which are a group of cells situated close to the cells that synthesize ADH. An increase in the ECF osmolality leads to a rise in the blood levels of ADH resulting in increased reabsorption of water **(Flowchart 1.2)**. During maximum urinary

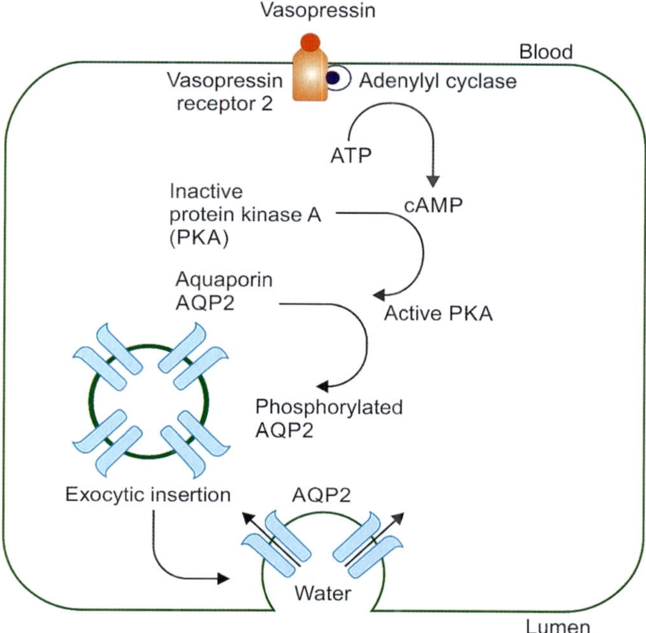

Fig. 1.11: Antidiuretic hormone (vasopressin) mediated water reabsorption in the distal tubule. Binding of vasopressin to the vasopressin receptor leads to activation of adenylyl cyclase with increased intracellular levels of cyclic AMP. Activation of cAMP-dependent protein kinase A (PKA) mediates protein phosphorylation that triggers exocytic insertion of AQP2 channels into the apical membrane. These channels increase the water permeability of the apical membrane, facilitating water transport. AQP: aquaporins; ATP: adenosine triphosphate; cAMP: cyclic adenosine monophosphate

Flowchart 1.2: Hypothalamus–posterior pituitary–antidiuretic hormone system

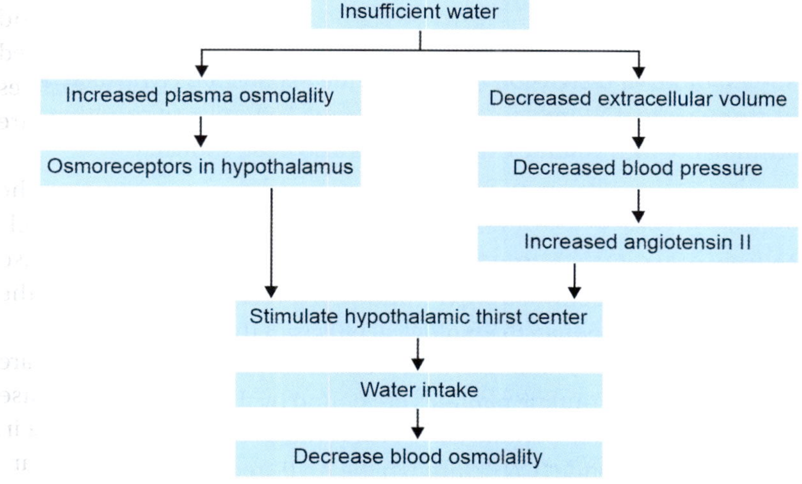

concentration, the urinary osmolality is about 1,000–1,400 mOsm/kg. Osmoreceptors are extremely sensitive to small variations in ECF osmolality, and just a 2% increase in the latter can cause maximum secretion of ADH. At plasma osmolality below 280 mOsm/kg, plasma ADH levels are almost undetectable.

Nonosmotic factors also affect ADH release; of these, hypovolemia and hypotension are most important. These act through baroreceptors in the carotid sinuses, aortic arch, and cardiac atria. Dehydration is the most common cause of hypovolemia and ADH release. Relatively larger changes in plasma volume are necessary to affect baroreceptor-mediated ADH release, and at small variations in plasma volume, the osmotic stimulus mediates ADH release. With severe contraction of the plasma volume, the baroreceptor mechanism stimulates ADH release, irrespective of the plasma osmolality.

The AQP2, exclusively present in the luminal side of principal cells of the collecting tubules and ducts, is the chief ADH regulated water channel involved in water reabsorption along with AQP3 and AQP4 present in the basolateral membrane of collecting tubules that are involved in movement of water from intracellular to hypertonic interstitium.

Thirst and Body Water

Thirst and oral fluid intake play a crucial role in the regulation of body fluid volume. The thirst center is located in the hypothalamus in close proximity to osmoreceptors. Intracellular dehydration is the chief factor for stimulating the thirst center and inducing a desire to drink. The most common cause of intracellular dehydration is depletion of ECF and a rise in ECF tonicity. Thirst center is also stimulated by hemorrhage and a low cardiac output.

Atrial Natriuretic Peptide

The predominant signal for atrial natriuretic peptide (ANP) release is atrial wall stretch or atrial distension due to volume expansion. Hypoxia is also a potent stimulus to ANP release, and enhanced ANP release resulting from hyperosmolality with volume expansion has also been shown.

Physiologic Effects of ANP

The ANP exerts its effects by binding to specific membrane-bound receptors; three receptors are identified. ANP_A and ANP_B receptors have guanylate cyclase activity and mediate the biological effects of the natriuretic peptides. ANP_C receptor functions mainly as a clearance receptor removing ANP from the circulation. All natriuretic peptides are bound by the ANP_C receptor. ANP and the brain natriuretic peptide (BNP) act through the ANP_A receptor, and C-type natriuretic peptide (CNP) through the ANP_B receptor.

The main targets of ANP are kidneys and vascular smooth muscle. It decreases blood pressure due to a direct relaxation of vascular smooth muscle. In addition, it acts on the collecting ducts to cause sodium and water diuresis, thus increasing salt and water excretion, enhances capillary permeability, and inhibits the release or action of several hormones, such as aldosterone, angiotensin II, endothelin, renin, and vasopressin. The natriuretic effect results from a direct inhibition of sodium absorption in the renal collecting duct, increased glomerular filtration, and inhibited aldosterone production and secretion. ANP, therefore, counteracts the renin–angiotensin–aldosterone system.

BIBLIOGRAPHY

1. Cuzzo B, Padala SA, Lappin SL. (2023) Physiology, Vasopressin. Available from https://www.ncbi.nlm.nih.gov/books/NBK526069/. [Last accessed June, 2024] PMID 30252325
2. Devuyst O, Zennaro MC, Vargas-Poussou R, et al. Inherited disorders of sodium and potassium handling. In: Emma F, Goldstein S, Bagga A, Bates CM, Shroff R (Eds). Pediatric Nephrology, 8th edition. New York: Springer Nature; 2022, pp. 987-1032.
3. Kettritz R, Loffing J. Potassium homeostasis: Physiology and pharmacology in a clinical context. Pharmacol Ther. 2023;249:108489.
4. Kriz W, Elgar M. Renal anatomy. In: Johnson RJ, Feehally J (Eds). Comprehensive Clinical Nephrology. London: Mosby; 2000, pp.1.1-1.10.
5. Moritz ML. Sodium and water disorders. In: Emma F, Goldstein S, Bagga A, Bates CM, Shroff R (Eds). Pediatric Nephrology, 8th edition. New York: Springer Nature; 2022, pp. 1108-20.
6. Murray SL, Wolf M. Calcium and phosphate disorders: Core curriculum 2024. Am J Kidney Dis. 2024;83:241-56.
7. Palmer BF, Clegg DJ. Physiology and pathophysiology of potassium homeostasis: Core curriculum 2019. Am J Kidney Dis. 2019;74:682-95.
8. Piscione T, Waters A. Structural and functional development of the kidney. In: Geary DF, Schaefer F (Eds). Comprehensive Pediatric Nephrology. London: Mosby; 2008, pp. 91-130.

Diagnostic Evaluation

Arvind Bagga, RN Srivastava

Common symptoms of renal disorders include edema, hematuria, oligoanuria, dysuria, abnormalities of micturition, flank pain, and ureteric colic. An abdominal mass may be detected by an observant mother or on routine examination. More often, clinical features are mild and subtle, or considered unrelated to a renal problem. Thus, failure to thrive, anemia, rickets, polyuria and polydipsia, skin rash, vague joint pains, low grade fever, and headache are often not suspected to be associated with kidney disease. Awareness of the differences in the pattern of renal diseases at different age groups helps in diagnostic evaluation.

Neonatal period: Congenital anomalies of the kidney and urinary tract are important in this period. These abnormalities are increasingly being detected antenatally on maternal ultrasonographic examination. An abdominal mass in a neonate is most likely to be a multicystic renal dysplasia. Abnormal urinary stream, dribbling of urine, and a persistently enlarged bladder suggest an anomaly of the distal urinary tract. The causes of acute kidney injury in neonates are different from those in older children.

Infancy to 3 years: During infancy, unexplained fever may be the only manifestation of urinary tract infection (UTI). UTI in young infants may also be suggested by nonspecific symptoms such as persistent jaundice, diarrhea, and vomiting. It is important to diagnose UTI since underlying urinary tract anomalies or vesicoureteric reflux may be present. An abdominal mass is likely to be a Wilms tumor or multicystic dysplastic kidney. Hemolytic uremic syndrome (HUS) commonly occurs in this age group. Infants with diarrhea or dysentery who develop oliguria, anemia, and drowsiness should be suspected of having HUS. About 30–40% of patients with minimal change nephrotic syndrome have onset of disease below 3 years, half of whom are between 2 and 3 years. Renal tubular disorders such as renal tubular acidosis (RTA) and Fanconi syndrome may be detected.

3–6 years: Minimal change nephrotic syndrome is common. Acute postinfectious or infection-related glomerulonephritis (GN), rare below the age of 3 years, is usually seen in older children. Patients with refractory rickets should be evaluated in detail.

6–12 years: Acute postinfectious or infection-related GN is usually observed during this period. Previously undetected chronic kidney disease (CKD), symptomatic hypertension, and collagen vascular diseases are common in older children.

Adolescence: Nephrotic syndrome initially starting during adolescence has a greater likelihood of having an underlying non-minimal lesion. The incidence of collagen vascular diseases is higher in this age group. Obesity-related hypertension is recognized more often in adolescents.

CLINICAL FEATURES OF RENAL DISEASE

Hematuria

Gross hematuria is an alarming feature and attracts prompt medical attention. The urine color may vary from frank red to shades of brown, described as tea or cola-colored. Concentrated urine is often mistaken as being abnormal by the parents. Red colored urine may be due to hemoglobinuria (e.g., intravascular hemolysis), methemoglobinuria, and ingestion of food dyes or drugs such as rifampicin and phenothiazines. A brown discoloration of urine is caused by myoglobinuria (following rhabdomyolysis), porphyria, and alkaptonuria (urine turning dark brown on standing), while passage of urate crystals causes pink discoloration of nappies. Urine microscopy is mandatory to confirm the presence of red blood cells (RBCs). Prolonged contact of acidic urine with blood causes oxidation of heme to methemoglobin, which is responsible for the brown color of urine originating from the upper urinary tract.

Gross hematuria in older children is most often due to acute GN. Other causes include renal calculus, hypercalciuria, bleeding/clotting disorders, renal trauma, hemorrhagic cystitis (viral, or due to cyclophosphamide therapy), and urethritis. Surgical causes of gross hematuria (e.g., papilloma of bladder, arteriovenous malformations, tumors, and angiomyolipoma) are uncommon in children and invasive procedures such as cystoscopy are rarely required. In the newborn with hypoxia-ischemia, hematuria may indicate renal venous thrombosis.

Where a cause is not found, subsequent evaluation includes repeated urine microscopy, ultrasound of the urinary tract, estimation of urinary calcium excretion, and serological tests including complement C3 and antinuclear antibody. High resolution computed tomography (CT) may be required if hypercalciuria or family history for renal calculi is present. Significant proteinuria or deranged kidney function with persistent hematuria necessitates percutaneous kidney biopsy. Detection of Munchausen syndrome by proxy requires a high index of suspicion and confirmation by a thorough evaluation. A subset of patients with persistent gross or microscopic hematuria, particularly those with family history of CKD, syndromic features or hypercalciuria, require next-generation sequencing for inherited glomerulopathies or metabolic abnormalities **(Annexure 9.3)**. Evaluation of hematuria is discussed in **Chapter 7**.

Urine with Abnormal Odor

Freshly voided specimen of urine is not unduly offensive. Careful observation may reveal the presence of an underlying metabolic abnormality: maple syrup urine disease, phenylketonuria (musty smell), isovaleric acidemia (sweaty feet smell).

Edema

Facial edema, an important feature of kidney disease, is often mistaken for allergy. Urine should be promptly tested for protein in such patients. Acute GN presents with facial puffiness and gross hematuria. If fluid intake is not restricted edema may rapidly increase and involve the hands, feet, and legs. Edema is turgid and does not readily pit on pressure. Hypertension, and in severe cases, pulmonary edema, may be associated. In nephrotic syndrome, edema develops insidiously starting with puffiness around the eyes that is most noticeable in the morning. Over the next few days, there is swelling over the feet and legs; edema is soft and pits on pressure.

Abnormalities of Micturition

In a boy, a poor urinary stream, especially in the presence of a full bladder, and straining during micturition suggest distal obstruction, most commonly due to posterior urethral valve. Persistent dribbling of urine suggests abnormal ureteric insertion distal to the bladder neck. In all infants with meningomyelocele, a detailed evaluation should be done to detect bladder dysfunction. Retention of urine may be due to neurogenic bladder or obstruction by stone or tumor. Urgent imaging and urological studies should be done.

Enuresis

Nocturnal enuresis without daytime problems is common in young children. There is usually no evidence of renal disease and imaging studies are not required. Daytime voiding abnormalities, such as urgency or frequency may indicate detrusor overactivity or dysfunctional voiding. Secondary enuresis may have an organic basis or be a feature of psychosocial dysfunction. Presence of a poor urinary stream and an enlarged bladder on examination indicate a neuropathic bladder. Clinical examination is required to detect any spinal (sacral dimple, lipoma, tuft of hair) or neurological abnormalities. Ultrasonography, uroflowmetry, micturating cystourethrography, magnetic resonance imaging (MRI) of spine (for spinal dysraphism, tethered cord) may be carried out as required.

Oliguria

Reduced urine output (<0.5 mL/kg/h for >6 hr) is an important feature of renal disease. An underlying cause such as gastroenteritis or other conditions that lead to hypovolemia and decreased renal blood flow can be readily detected. Oliguria is an important feature of moderate or severe acute GN and several other conditions causing serious glomerular injury (e.g., HUS). Oliguria is also present in nephrotic syndrome. An evaluation for intrinsic renal disease or obstructive etiology is required, if volume depletion has been excluded or adequately corrected.

Polyuria

Polyuria (>4 mL/kg/h; >2 L/m^2/day) is an important feature of renal tubular disorders characterized by impaired proximal tubular reabsorption (Fanconi and Bartter syndromes), failure of urine concentrating mechanism (diabetes insipidus), or distal renal tubular disorders. Polyuria, especially when associated with failure to thrive and rickets, needs careful investigation. Other causes of polyuria include excessive fluid intake (psychogenic polydipsia) and osmotic diuresis (diabetes mellitus, mannitol). It is important to distinguish polyuria from frequent passage of small volumes of urine by maintaining a record of voided volumes over at least two 24-hr periods. The water deprivation test is useful in evaluation of some disorders. Polyuria should be distinguished from *pollakiuria* (very frequent voiding of small amounts) in the absence of any kidney disease.

Dysuria, Flank Pain

Burning pain while voiding and suprapubic pain suggest UTI. Flank pain and tenderness in the renal angle are indicative of pyelonephritis especially if fever, chills, and rigors are present.

Ureteric Colic and Passage of Stone or Gravel

These indicate calculus formation in the urinary tract.

Antenatal History

Oligohydramnios during the second trimester or later indicates poor fetal renal function and is associated with intrauterine growth retardation, autosomal recessive polycystic kidney disease, *HNF1B* mutation, renal tubular dysgenesis, renal dysplasia, and obstructive uropathy. Subsequent ultrasonographic evaluation is necessary. Polyhydramnios is associated with antenatal Bartter syndrome, Beckwith-Wiedemann syndrome, and pseudohypoaldosteronism type 1. Antenatal intake of COX-2 inhibitors, angiotensin converting enzyme inhibitors, or angiotensin receptor blockers may be associated with renal tubular dysgenesis and neonatal kidney failure. Renal diseases associated with elevated maternal serum alpha fetoprotein include neural tube defects and congenital nephrotic syndrome.

Birth History

Fetuses with congenital nephrotic syndrome may be noted as having an enlarged placenta. A history of birth asphyxia in a newborn with acute renal failure supports a diagnosis of acute tubular necrosis, and the history of hematuria and enlarged kidneys in a neonate is consistent with renal vein thrombosis. Umbilical artery catheterization is known to predispose to neonatal hypertension as well as to renal artery thrombosis. Presence of a single umbilical artery on neonatal examination should alert to the possibility of multicystic dysplastic kidney, vesicoureteric reflux, and renal dysplasia.

Family History

Consanguinity and positive family history may provide leads to the diagnosis of inherited disorders, including polycystic kidney disease, nephronophthisis, cystinosis, and Bartter and Gitelman syndromes.

Hypertension

Increased blood pressure levels may be detected incidentally, or there may be symptoms such as headache and visual disturbances. The presence of bruits on abdominal auscultation may indicate renal artery stenosis.

Growth Retardation

Physical retardation is an important feature of CKD. Growth retardation is also prominent in renal tubular disorders (e.g., RTA, familial hypophosphatemic rickets, and Fanconi syndrome).

Anemia

Anemia is a striking feature in advanced CKD.

Bony Deformities

Rickets and bony deformities are present in patients with chronic tubulointerstitial diseases and primary renal tubular disorders.

Abdominal Mass

The possibility of multicystic renal dysplasia, polycystic kidney disease, hydronephrosis, and Wilms tumor should be considered. Unilateral hydronephrosis is often secondary to obstruction at the pelviureteric or vesicoureteric junction, while bilateral hydronephrosis indicates posterior urethral valves or vesicoureteric reflux. Bilateral palpable kidneys in the newborn suggest the diagnosis of autosomal recessive polycystic kidney disease.

URINE EXAMINATION

A meticulous examination of urine is important for the diagnosis of renal diseases. The urine specimen should be fresh and relatively concentrated (appearing yellow). Formed elements quickly disintegrate in dilute or alkaline urine. Microscopic examination of uncentrifuged as well as a centrifuged specimen should be done. The presence of red cells and their morphologic characteristics, white cells and casts of various type particularly red cell casts are noted. Various types of crystals can be identified.

Collection of Specimen

The first morning specimen is preferred as it is concentrated. Urine is collected in a clean container and enough quantity sent to the laboratory. For culture, the specimen should be collected in a sterile container and sent to the laboratory immediately, where it should be rapidly plated or stored in a refrigerator at 4°C. Bacteria multiply rapidly at room temperature, which may give false positive results.

Clean-catch urine: A clean-catch specimen is obtained after local cleaning with water. There remains a likelihood of contamination by periurethral and prepucial organisms. In older children, a midstream specimen is obtained. The sample should be collected in a sterile plastic or glass bottle.

Bag collection: In neonates and infants, urine can be collected in sterile bags. The bag is applied after careful cleaning and allowing the skin to dry, and removed immediately once the baby has voided. Urine collection by bag is convenient in infants but gives unacceptably high false positive results on urine culture.

Suprapubic bladder aspiration: The reliable way to obtain a urine specimen in neonates and young infants is by suprapubic aspiration. In children <2 years of age, such a specimen is unlikely to be contaminated and is therefore suitable for diagnosis of UTI. A 5–10 mL syringe with a 22-gauge needle is vertically inserted 1–2 cm above the pubic symphysis to a depth of 2–3 cm. The bladder should be full, which can be confirmed by percussion or on ultrasonography before the procedure.

Bladder catheterization: A urine specimen can also be safely obtained in infants by bladder catheterization, but this requires experience. Careful aseptic precautions are necessary.

Specific Gravity

The specific gravity is measured with a clinical hydrometer or a refractometer. The specific gravity is increased on refrigeration, and in presence of protein, glucose, and radiocontrast media.

pH

Urine pH should be measured on an early morning specimen using a pH meter. The use of pH paper strips is discouraged. Fasting results in low pH values; urine pH is high following meals.

Protein

The boiling test is satisfactory but cumbersome. 10–15 mL urine is taken in a test tube and the upper portion is boiled. If turbidity appears, 3 drops of concentrated acetic acid are added, and the specimen is boiled again. A 0–4+ grading is used to record the concentration of protein. Proteinuria can also be semiquantitatively estimated by precipitation method using 10% sulfosalicylic acid. Five drops of this acid are added to a test tube half filled with urine and turbidity graded from negative to 4+. X-ray contrast media and penicillin may cause false positive reactions. A highly alkaline or dilute urine sample may give false negative reading.

Dipstick methods (e.g., Uristix), widely used to test for proteinuria, are convenient and reliable. The reagent strips are impregnated with tetrabromophenol blue buffered with citrate. Protein binds with the dye and causes color to change from yellow to green. Light chain proteins, globulin, and low molecular weight (LMW) tubular proteins are not detected by this method. Dilute urine may give a false negative result. False positive results occur with very alkaline urine, concentrated specimens, and those contaminated with chlorhexidine or benzalkonium. If the "stick" is left to soak in urine, or there is a delay in reading, false positive reading may occur. Trace reaction on the dipstick corresponds to 5–20 mg/dL urinary protein, 1+ to 30 mg/dL, 2+ to 100 mg/dL, 3+ to 300 mg/dL, and 4+ to >1,000 mg/dL. Composite strips that measure pH, and detect the presence of protein, glucose, ketones, bile pigments, blood, leukocyte esterase, and nitrites are available.

The first morning sample should be assessed since prolonged standing increases protein excretion (orthostatic proteinuria). Normal urine does not contain any albumin, but contains small amounts of tubular protein, chiefly Tamm–Horsfall protein, a glycoprotein from the ascending loop of Henle. Proteinuria in patients with nephrotic syndrome is massive (3–4+) and selective, constituted chiefly by albumin, without loss of higher molecular weight proteins. Selective proteinuria is denoted by a urine immunoglobulin G (IgG) to albumin ratio <0.1. In presence of significant glomerular injury, urine protein contains proteins of higher molecular weight.

In renal parenchymal diseases, proteinuria is often quantified to assess degree of glomerular injury, with persistence of proteinuria or lack of response to therapy indicative of unsatisfactory prognosis. Albuminuria (or microalbuminuria) is the excretion of small amounts of albumin in the urine, about 30–300 mg/g of creatinine, and its presence suggests glomerular injury. LMW proteins, including β_2 microglobulin, α_1 microglobulin, and retinol binding protein, are freely filtered at the glomerulus but totally metabolized or reabsorbed by proximal tubules. Urinary excretion of "tubular" proteins is a marker of impaired proximal tubular function, such as in Fanconi syndrome or Dent disease, and drug-induced tubular injury. Currently used markers of acute tubular necrosis include neutrophil gelatinase associated lipocalin (NGAL), kidney injury molecule 1 (KIM-1), and interleukin 18 (IL-18).

Quantitative Measurement of Urine Protein

Accurate collection of urine over a 24-hr period is required to quantitate protein excretion. A value of >4 mg/m^2/h is considered abnormal and >40 mg/m^2/h indicates heavy proteinuria. Timed collection of urine may be cumbersome and subject to inaccuracy, particularly in young children.

Urine protein/creatinine ratio: An estimate of the severity of proteinuria can be made by the ratio of urinary protein to creatinine (both expressed as mg/dL) on the first morning or timed urine specimen. Random "spot" urine specimens are not ideal, since there is variation over time in protein and creatinine excretion. Values of >2 indicate heavy proteinuria and <0.2 is considered not significant.

Glucose

The older methods (e.g., Benedict test) that detected reducing substances have been replaced by the specific dipstick test, which is based on glucose oxidase reaction.

Blood

Detection of hemoglobin by dipstick is based on an oxidation reaction, with a spotted positive reaction indicating intact RBCs and uniform positivity suggesting presence of free hemoglobin. However, the use of dipstick to detect hematuria is discouraged, because reactions may be false positive (e.g., myoglobin, oxidizing substances, and bacterial colonization) or false negative (e.g., ascorbic acid and other reducing substances).

Microscopic Examination

A fresh, well-mixed specimen should be examined. Presence of cellular elements and casts should be noted. Red cell casts indicate GN **(Fig. 2.1A)**, while clumping of neutrophils (white cell casts) suggests acute pyelonephritis **(Fig. 2.1B)**. Granular casts **(Fig. 2.1C)** result from breakdown of cellular casts or the inclusion of plasma proteins, e.g., albumin or immunoglobulin light chains. The "muddy brown" casts seen in acute tubular necrosis are a type of granular cast. Hyaline or fatty casts are present in proteinuric states or in normal concentrated urine **(Fig. 2.1D)**. Patients with acute tubular necrosis show muddy brown granular or tubular epithelial cell casts **(Fig. 2.1E)**.

Red blood cells and leukocytes can be counted under the high-power field (HPF) and accurately in a counting chamber. With a Fuchs Rosenthal counting chamber, 8,000 RBC/μL and 2,000–8,000 white blood cell (WBC)/μL may normally be seen. Isolated presence of white cells does not confirm UTI. Neutrophils may also be detected in proliferative GN, nephrolithiasis, and interstitial nephritis. More than 10 leukocytes/μL of an uncentrifuged or >5 leukocytes/HPF in a centrifuged specimen is significant. Leukocytes may occasionally be absent despite significant bacteriuria. The presence of any bacteria/HPF in fresh, uncentrifuged urine correlates with a colony count of $>10^5$ organisms/mL indicating significant bacteriuria.

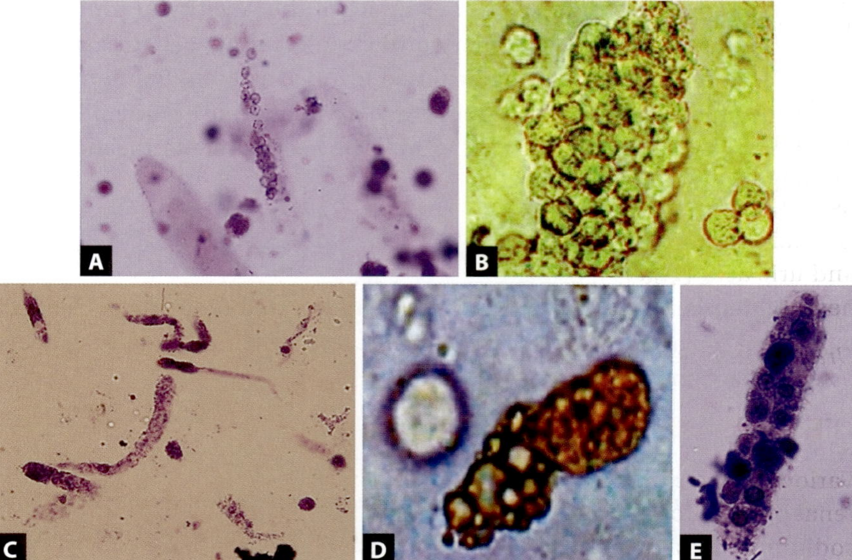

Figs. 2.1A to E: Casts on urine microscopy. (A) Red cell casts and red cells in a patient with acute glomerulonephritis (400×); (B) White cell cast and white cells (500×); (C) Fine and coarse granular casts (500×); (D) Fatty cast in a patient with nephrotic syndrome (400×); and (E) Tubular epithelial cell casts in acute tubular necrosis (500×)

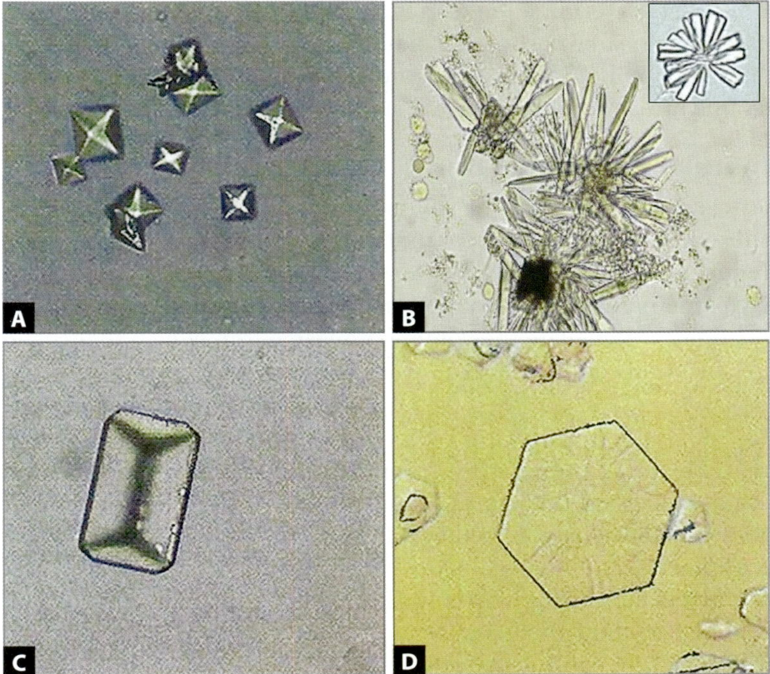

Figs. 2.2A to D: Morphology of urine crystals. (A) Envelope-shaped oxalate dihydrate crystals; (B) Wedge-shaped prisms or (in inset) rosette of calcium phosphate; (C) Coffin lid-shaped triple phosphate; and (D) Hexagonal cystine crystals

Hematuria is defined as the presence of >5 RBC/HPF in a centrifuged specimen. RBC morphology is useful in distinguishing glomerular from nonglomerular causes of hematuria. Dysmorphic RBCs are best detected using phase contrast microscopy but can be identified on light microscopy. Careful examination will identify crystals of cholesterol, oxalate, cystine, and uric acid **(Figs. 2.2A to D)**. Sterile "pyuria" is present in tuberculosis, nephrolithiasis, viral cystitis, and *Chlamydia* infection.

Urine culture: See Chapter 17.

EVALUATION OF KIDNEY FUNCTION

Various aspects of renal function such as glomerular filtration rate (GFR), renal plasma flow (RPF), reabsorption and excretion of substances such as sodium, potassium, calcium, inorganic phosphate, glucose, urea, amino acids, water, and osmoles can be estimated. The mechanisms involved in maximum urinary concentration and urinary acidification can be examined. GFR and renal blood flow can also be determined by radionuclide methods (Chapter 4).

In practice, determination of creatinine clearance as a measure of GFR, water deprivation and vasopressin administration tests to determine urinary concentrating ability, and bicarbonate and fludrocortisone-frusemide tests to examine urinary acidification, are sufficient for diagnostic evaluation.

Glomerular Filtration Rate

Kidney clearance describes the volume of plasma that is completely cleared of a substance by the kidneys per unit of time. Thus, if the urinary excretion rate (equal to the product of the concentration of the substance in urine and urine volume per minute) and the plasma concentration of a substance are known, one can calculate the volume of plasma from which that substance would have been completely removed. The formula for clearance is:

$$C = \frac{U \times V}{P}$$

where, C clearance/minute (mL/min), U urinary concentration (mg/dL), P plasma concentration (mg/dL), and V urine volume/minute (mL/min). Typically, clearance is expressed as mL/min and normalized to 1.73 m^2 body surface area (BSA).

If a given substance is freely filtered and neither reabsorbed nor metabolized by the kidney, its clearance rate would accurately reflect the GFR. Additionally, the substance should be inert, nontoxic to humans, and should not alter renal function. The inert polysaccharide, inulin, which is freely filtered and neither reabsorbed nor secreted by the tubule, has been taken as the reference substance and the measurement of inulin clearance as true GFR. Estimation of inulin clearance requires a continuous intravenous (IV) infusion and bladder catheterization; the chemical assay for inulin is also difficult. Inulin can be substituted by radioisotopes: ^{125}iodine-labeled sodium iothalamate, ^{99m}Technetium-labeled diethylenetriaminepentaacetic acid (DTPA) or ^{51}chromium-labeled ethylenediamine tetra-acetic acid (EDTA), obviating the need for chemical measurements. The radioactive techniques for measuring GFR are accurate and correlate well with inulin studies. However, these methods require availability of nuclear medicine facilities, and are not practical for routine clinical use. Iohexol can be used without being labeled with a radioisotope.

Precise measurement of GFR is not necessary in clinical practice. For practical purposes, plasma creatinine and endogenous creatinine clearance are commonly used as more convenient methods for GFR assessment. Methods of estimating GFR are compared in **Table 2.1**. **Annexures 2.1–2.4** provides links to online calculators for various equations for estimating GFR in children and adults.

Serum Creatinine and Creatinine Clearance

Creatinine is derived from the metabolism of creatine and phosphocreatine, the bulk of which is in muscle. The rate of creatinine production is a function

TABLE 2.1: Methods to estimate glomerular function

Test	*Method*	*Comments*
Plasma creatinine	Random blood sample	Simple; inaccurate with mild renal impairment; reduced with low muscle mass; drugs (cimetidine, trimethoprim) influence renal tubular secretion
Creatinine clearance	24-hr urine collection and blood sample	Urine collections unreliable, difficult in children; overestimates GFR especially with reduced renal function
Estimated GFR	Random blood sample	Avoids urine collection; underestimates GFR in obesity; overestimates GFR in malnutrition; more accurate than plasma creatinine **(Table 2.2)**
Radioisotope based plasma clearance of ^{125}I-iothalamate, ^{51}Cr-EDTA, ^{99m}Tc-DTPA	Single IV injection and minimum of two-timed blood samples	Best approximation to true GFR; needs gamma camera facility; not often needed in clinical practice
Serum cystatin	Random blood sample	Better correlated with GFR than creatinine; levels independent of age, gender, muscle mass
Inulin clearance	Constant IV infusion; collection of timed urine and blood samples	Reference standard; cumbersome in practice
Iohexol	Plasma level 3–4 hr after IV injection	Simple; low osmolality, low risk of toxicity; low (2%) plasma protein binding; no radiation exposure

Cr-EDTA: chromium-labeled ethylenediamine tetra-acetic acid; GFR: glomerular filtration rate; IV: intravenous; Tc-DTPA: Technetium-labeled diethylenetriaminepentaacetic acid

of the muscle mass, which is related to the body size. The production of creatinine and its volume of distribution show very little variation from day-to-day. Since creatinine is chiefly excreted by glomerular filtration, serum creatinine levels reflect changes in GFR. Besides being filtered, a small amount of creatinine is also secreted by the tubules. Creatinine levels are estimated by a number of methods: Jaffe, compensated Jaffe, enzymatic liquid, and dry chemistry methods. Although most assays are traceable to the higher order reference methods (isotope dilution-mass spectrometry, IDMS), there are large interassay variations. Serum creatinine increasingly overestimates GFR at lower GFRs.

The normal levels of serum creatinine range from 0.2–0.5 mg/dL during infancy to 0.4–0.9 mg/dL in older children. Serum creatinine level is not readily affected by prerenal factors. Serum creatinine values are low when the muscle mass is decreased, as in malnutrition. The original Jaffe method is influenced by chromogens such as bilirubin, ketones, some proteins, and cephalosporins.

Creatinine clearance can be calculated by collecting a timed urinary specimen, with a blood sample around the mid-collection period. However, timed urine collections may be inaccurate, difficult to perform and time consuming in children. Noncreatinine chromogens, normally present in plasma (but which do not appear in urine) are measured along with creatinine giving a falsely high value to serum creatinine. This partly compensates for the tubular secretion of creatinine that increases the amount of urinary creatinine. *However, the creatinine clearance overestimates the actual GFR by an inconstant and unpredictable amount.* Plasma creatinine is increased by ingestion of meal high in animal protein, while tubular excretion is impaired by drugs and substances such as cimetidine and trimethoprim.

Formulae for Estimation of GFR

Several formulae have been proposed for estimation of GFR **(*see* Table 2.2 and Annexures 2.1–2.4)**. The modified Schwartz equation is preferred in children, and the most widely used. The improved 2012 Schwartz using the combination of creatinine, cystatin C, and urea performs best in children. The Chronic Kidney Disease Epidemiology Collaboration (CKD-EPI) estimated GFR creatinine equation is preferred in adults with glomerular disease; the 2021 equation, which excludes race from the estimate, is recommended. The Full Age Spectrum (FAS) equation may be used in both adults and children. The multicenter Chronic Kidney Disease in Children (CKiD) study in North America has generated improved GFR estimating formulae, which were validated in children across the GFR range of 15–75 mL/min/1.73 m^2. These include a complex formula and a simple formula that can be used for bedside application **(Table 2.2)**.

Cystatin C

Cystatin C is an LMW (13 kD) nonglycosylated protein produced at a constant rate by all nucleated cells in the body, freely filtered by the glomeruli, not secreted but totally reabsorbed and catabolized by the renal tubules. Little or no cystatin is excreted in the urine. There are no sites of extrarenal metabolism. Serum levels of this product have been proposed as a marker of GFR. Levels in children range from 0.60 to 0.85 mg/L; normal adults have levels between 0.75 and 1.0 mg/L. The superiority of cystatin C over creatinine has been confirmed in a number of studies that have found the former to be better correlated with GFR, independent of age, gender, body composition, and muscle mass. The formula proposed by Filler for estimating GFR using serum cystatin is validated for children **(Table 2.2)**.

Cystatin-based equations are suggested to be better for estimating GFR in early as well as CKD. Cystatin C can be estimated in blood by enzyme immunoassays or immunoturbidimetry.

Radionuclide GFR

Radionuclides are often used to estimate total GFR. An accurate evaluation of GFR is based on the plasma disappearance curve after a single bolus injection of a glomerular tracer, followed by two blood samples around 2–4 hr later. The most commonly used radionuclides for GFR measurements are DTPA, EDTA, and iothalamate. The correlations to inulin clearance are best with DTPA, good with EDTA, and only fair with iothalamate. The estimates do not perform well in neonates **(Table 2.1)**.

Iohexol, a nonionic nonradioactive radiocontrast agent is proposed as an alternative to inulin, since it is eliminated from plasma solely by glomerular filtration and measured easily by high performance liquid chromatography (HPLC). Iohexol is theoretically superior to other exogenous markers because of its low plasma protein binding. Agents with higher plasma protein binding show higher tubular secretion, resulting in overestimation of GFR.

Blood Urea

A normal level of blood urea is often mistakenly regarded to indicate normal kidney function. In a steady state the blood urea may not rise beyond the upper range of normal (40 mg/dL) even when 75% of the renal function is lost. On the other hand, prerenal factors that reduce renal perfusion and decrease GFR, such as dehydration, cause an increase in blood urea levels.

Urea is derived from the metabolism of proteins and is synthesized in the liver. It is distributed throughout the body water, being freely permeable across cell membranes. Urea is readily filtered, reabsorbed as well as secreted by the tubules. 40–60% of filtered urea is reabsorbed by the proximal tubule. The distal tubular reabsorption of urea is high during antidiuresis and low during diuresis. Thus, the state of hydration along with dietary protein intake determines urea excretion and its level in body fluids. Blood urea levels are increased with high protein intake and excessive protein catabolism, trauma, gastrointestinal bleeding, and inhibition of anabolism and increased protein catabolism by corticosteroids or tetracyclines. Reduced dietary protein intake leads to lower levels of urea, as does severe impairment of liver function.

Measurement of Progression of Renal Damage

Patients with chronic renal insufficiency show a linear fall of creatinine clearance with time. Plotting of the reciprocal of serum creatinine against

TABLE 2.2: Equations for estimating glomerular filtration rate (GFR, mL/min/1.73 m^2)

Equation name	*Equation for GFR*
Age <18 years	
Modified Schwartz ("bedside")	$0.413 \times$ height (cm)/Cr
Cystatin C based	$70.69 \times (CysC)^{0.931}$
Chronic kidney disease in children $(CKiD)_{Cr\text{-}CysC}$	$39.8 \times$ [height (cm)/Cr]$^{0.456} \times [1.8/CysC]^{0.418} \times [30/BUN]^{0.079} \times$ [1.076 if male] $\times$ [height (m)/1.4]$^{0.179}$
Pottel equation	107.3/(Cr/Q)
Adults	
Cockroft Gault	[140 – age (year)] $\times$ body weight (kg)/72 $\times$ Cr $\times$ 0.85 (if female)
Modification of Diet in Renal Disease (MDRD)	$175 \times Cr^{-1.154} \times$ age (year)$^{-0.203} \times 0.745$ (if female) $\times$ 1.212 (if African American)
Chronic Kidney Disease Epidemiology Collaboration (CKD-EPI) 2009; 2021	$141 \times \min(Cr/k_1)^{\alpha} \times \max(Cr/k_1)^{-1.209} \times 0.993^{age} \times 1.018$ (if female) $\times$ 1.159 (if African American) $142 \times \min(Cr/k_1)^{\beta} \times \max(Cr/k_1)^{-1.200} \times 0.994^{age} \times 1.012$ (if female)
CKD-EPI $eGFR_{CysC}$ 2012; 2021	$133 \times \min(CysC/k_2)^{-0.499} \times \max(Cr/k_2)^{-1.328} \times 0.996^{age} \times 0.932$ (if female)
CKD-EPI $eGFR_{Cr\text{-}CysC}$ 2012; 2021	$135 \times \min(Cr/k_1)^{\gamma} \times \max(Cr/k_1)^{-0.601} \times \min(CysC/k_2)^{-0.375} \times \max(Cr/k_2)^{-0.711} \times 0.995^{age} \times 0.969$ (if female) $\times$ 1.08 (if African American) $135 \times \min(Cr/k_1)^{\delta} \times \max(Cr/k_1)^{-0.544} \times \min(CysC/k_2)^{-0.323} \times \max(Cr/k_2)^{-0.778} \times 0.996^{age} \times 0.963$ (if female)

Contd...

Contd...

Equation name	***Equation for GFR***
Children and adults	
Full age spectrum (FAS)	107.3/(Cr/Q) for ages 2–40 years 107.3/(Cr/Q) × 0.988^{age-40} for ages >40 years
CKiD $eGFR_{Cr}$ Under 25 years (U25)	$K^{\#1}$ × height (cm)/Cr
CKiD $eGFR_{Cr}$ U25	$K^{\#2}$ × 1/CysC
CKiD and CKD-EPI (For 18–26 years old)	Average of CkiD and CD-EPI

***See* Annexure 2.1** for online calculators for eGFR using various equations

Both low muscle mass and hypoalbuminemia overestimate true GFR. Glucocorticoids may increase CysC, thereby underestimating GFR. The presence of acute kidney injury confounds all estimates.

MDRD equation is not valid for eGFR >60 mL/min/1.73 m^2; CKD-EPI is valid for eGFR >60 mL/min/1.73 m^2; CKD-EPI 2021 equations exclude race in the estimate.

$\alpha = -0.329$ if female and -0.411 if male; $\beta = -0.241$ if female and -0.302 if male; $\gamma = -0.248$ if female and -0.207 if male; $\delta = -0.219$ if female and -0.144, if male

$k_1 = 0.7$ if female and 0.9 if male; $k_2 = 0.8$

$K^{\#1}$ for boys 1–11 years old: $39 \times 1.008^{(age-12)}$; 12–17 years old: $39 \times 1.045^{(age-12)}$; 18–25 years old: 50.8

$K^{\#1}$ for girls 1–11 years old: $36.1 \times 1.008^{(age-12)}$; 12–17 years old: $39 \times 1.023^{(age-12)}$; 18–25 years old: 41.4

$K^{\#2}$ for boys 1–14 years old: $87.2 \times 1.011^{(age-15)}$; 15–17 years old: $87.2 \times 0.960^{(age-15)}$; 18–25 years old: 77.1

$K^{\#2}$ for girls 1–11 years old: $79.9 \times 1.004^{(age-12)}$; 12–17 years old: $79.9 \times 0.974^{(age-12)}$; 18–25 years old: 68.3

max = the maximum of creatinine/(k_1 or k_2) or 1; min = the minimum of creatinine/(k_1 or k_2) or 1

Q values are the mean or median serum creatinine for age-sex-specific healthy population.

BUN: blood urea nitrogen (mg/dL); Cr: creatinine (mg/dL); CysC: cystatin C (mg/L)

time gives a straight line. This method has been suggested to predict the rate of decline of GFR. The CKiD study generated a longitudinal formula helpful in determining current or future changes in GFR based on prior measurements of GFR and changes in certain parameters, given below:

$$eGFR_2 = 40.48\ (iGFR_1)^{0.912} \times [(Ht/SCr_2) \div (Ht/SCr_1)]^{0.514}$$

Where, $eGFR_2$ is the estimated GFR 1 year after baseline, $iGFR_1$ is the iohexol GFR at baseline, Ht/SCr_2 is the height in meters divided by serum creatinine 1 year after baseline, and Ht/SCr_1 is the height in meters divided by serum creatinine at baseline. Limitations of the formula include its applicability to patients with moderate-to-severe CKD and that decline in GFR that actually occurs over 1 year is usually minimal.

Renal Blood Flow

Since >90% para-aminohippurate (PAH) is extracted from the plasma during the first pass through the kidneys, its renal clearance is used as an estimate of RPF. Conventional measurement of PAH clearance requires its continuous infusion followed by timed collection of urine and blood samples. Plasma clearance following single injection of ^{131}I-hippuran is an alternative method. Renal blood flow is calculated by dividing RPF by (1 – hematocrit). Normal values range from 500 to 600 mL/min (about 1200 mL/min/1.73 m^2). Other methods to estimate renal blood flow include color Doppler ultrasound, contrast enhanced ultrasound, and MRI. Measurement of renal blood flow is rarely indicated in clinical practice.

The filtration fraction (FF) is the proportion of plasma entering the renal circulation that is removed from the circulation by glomerular filtration. It is equal to GFR divided by RPF, i.e., ratio of clearance of inulin to clearance of PAH. Normal values of FF range from 17 to 23% (about 20%).

Urinary Concentration

Osmolality depends upon the number of particles in a solution and not on their size or density, which affect the specific gravity. The maximal urine concentration capacity varies with age; while the maximum urine osmolality in neonates is about 700 mOsm/kg, the osmolality in older children and adults can rise up to 1200 mOsm/kg. The first morning urine specimen is usually concentrated with an osmolality of over 600 mOsm/kg. Hyposthenuria (inability to increase urine osmolality more than that of plasma) is characteristic of diabetes insipidus as well as diseases of renal medulla such as nephronophthisis and obstructive uropathy. Polyuria and polydipsia are striking features. In CKD urine osmolality does not rise much above 300–350 mOsm/kg and polyuria and polydipsia are not prominent.

Urinary Concentration Test

Urine concentrating ability needs to be tested in patients with polyuria. If the first morning void after 12 hr of overnight fasting has osmolality exceeding 600 mOsm/kg, no further testing is required. In others, water deprivation testing is indicated.

In the standard water deprivation test, no fluid is allowed after dinner. The bladder is emptied at 8 AM, and all subsequent urine specimens are collected. The child is frequently weighed and carefully observed, particularly if polyuria continues. Water deprivation is stopped if the weight loss exceeds 5% or until three consecutive hourly urine osmolality values are within 10% of each other. Normal children between 2 and 12 years of age can achieve a urine osmolality of over 800 (1000 ± 100) mOsm/kg. Plasma osmolality and sodium levels should be measured at the end of the test to ensure that adequate osmotic stimulus has been provided.

Response to vasopressin: Subsequently, to confirm the lack of renal concentrating ability and distinguish nephrogenic diabetes insipidus (NDI) or arginine vasopressin resistance from central diabetes insipidus (CDI) or arginine vasopressin deficiency, a vasopressin test is performed. Desamino-8-D-arginine vasopressin (dDAVP, desmopressin) is administered nasally (5–10 µg in neonates and infants, 20 µg in children) or by an intramuscular injection (0.4–1.0 µg in infants and young children, 2 µg in older children). Hourly urine collection is done over the next 4 hr. Following administration of dDAVP, patients with NDI fail to show a rise of urine osmolality, which remains below 200–300 mOsm/kg water. Those with CDI and primary polydipsia concentrate urine to varying degrees **(Table 2.3)**.

Persistence of polyuria for years may result in a washout of the medullary countercurrent concentration mechanism. Several days of treatment with dDAVP may be required to elicit an appropriate response in these patients. Where the diagnosis of primary polydipsia is strongly suspected, reduction of fluid intake over several days may restore normal sensitivity of dDAVP.

TABLE 2.3: Water deprivation test

Condition	*Urine osmolality on water deprivation (mOsm/kg)*	*Change in osmolality with dDAVP (mOsm/kg)*
Normal	>800–900	Minimal or no increase
Complete central DI	<300	Substantial increase
Partial central DI	300–800	Increase of >10%
Nephrogenic DI	<200–300	Minimal or no increase
Primary polydipsia	>500	Minimal or no increase

dDAVP: desmopressin; DI: diabetes insipidus

Tests of Urinary Acidification

Acidification mechanisms of the kidney are usually examined in children with suspected RTA.

Urine pH

The pH of a fresh morning specimen is tested with pH meter, which should normally be ≤5.5. UTI with urea splitting organisms makes the urine alkaline. Detection of urine pH below 5.5 virtually excludes distal (type I) RTA.

Urine Anion Gap

Urine anion gap is the difference between concentration of principal urinary cations (sodium plus potassium) and anion (chloride). This difference is expected to estimate the unmeasured anions and cations, which normally include ammonium and bicarbonate. Since the latter is mostly reabsorbed, urine anion gap is chiefly a measure of ammonium excretion. In presence of metabolic acidosis, ammonium excretion is normally stimulated while bicarbonate excretion is minimal. Hence, the urine anion gap should be negative due to obligatory chloride excretion with ammonium. In patients with RTA, due to impaired ammonium synthesis or excretion, the gap remains positive. Given its dependence on diet, the utility of this test is limited in clinical practice.

Sodium Bicarbonate Loading Test

The *bicarbonate threshold* is the plasma bicarbonate level at which bicarbonate appears in the urine. The threshold is determined by increasing the plasma bicarbonate in a stepwise manner to a level of 22–24 mEq/L. 3–5 mL/kg sodium bicarbonate is administered orally or intravenously, which increases the urine pH to >7.4. Levels of bicarbonate and creatinine are measured in blood and random urine specimens. Normally there is no bicarbonaturia unless the plasma bicarbonate level exceeds 20–21 mEq/L.

The urinary bicarbonate threshold is reduced in proximal RTA. The *fractional excretion of bicarbonate* ($FEHCO_3$) is calculated by the formula:

$$FEHCO_3 = \frac{\text{Urine bicarbonate} \times \text{Plasma creatinine} \times 100}{\text{Plasma bicarbonate} \times \text{Urine creatinine}}$$

The normal $FEHCO_3$ is <5%. In proximal RTA, the $FEHCO_3$ usually exceeds 15%. The fractional excretion in patients with distal RTA is usually normal; occasionally it may be increased to 5–10%.

Urine PCO_2

In normal subjects given a bicarbonate infusion to produce high bicarbonate excretion, distal H^+ secretion leads to generation of a high PCO_2 in the urine (measured by collecting the urine under mineral oil). The urine should be concentrated, and fluid intake restricted to obtain maximal response. The magnitude of urine to blood (U–B) PCO_2 gradient is used as an index of distal H^+ secretion. In most patients with distal RTA the U–B PCO_2 gradient is abnormally low (<10 mm Hg compared with >20 mm in normal subjects), reflecting impaired H^+ secretion.

Ammonium Chloride Loading Test

Oral administration of ammonium chloride induces metabolic acidosis to which the kidney responds with maximum urinary acidification. After measuring the baseline urine pH and acid-base status, ammonium chloride 0.1–0.15 g/kg is given orally over 30–45 minutes with fruit juice. A liberal fluid intake is provided. The pH of each urine specimen is measured over the next 6 hr. Blood pH should be measured to determine if acidosis has been induced. If the urine pH falls below 5.3, distal RTA can be ruled out. If urine pH remains >5.5 despite severe acidosis ($TCO_2 < 15$), distal RTA is likely. The furosemide-fludrocortisone test is more convenient to perform and provides similar information as the ammonium chloride test (Chapter 20). Although titrable acid and ammonium can be measured in the urine, their precise estimation is not necessary.

Reabsorption of Phosphate

Inorganic phosphate is freely filtered at the glomerulus and reabsorbed in the proximal tubule. Tubular reabsorption of phosphate is reduced in conditions causing proximal tubular dysfunction, such as Fanconi syndrome and familial hypophosphatemic rickets. Fractional excretion of phosphate ($FEPO_4$) can be determined on a 24-hr urinary specimen with the blood sample obtained around the mid-collection period. Alternatively, a 3–6 hr collection may be done with the blood sample obtained midway.

$$FEPO_4 = \frac{\text{Urine phosphate} \times \text{Plasma creatinine} \times 100}{\text{Plasma phosphate} \times \text{Urine creatinine}}$$

Tubular reabsorption of phosphate is the difference between filtered and excreted phosphate and is expressed as (100 – $FEPO_4$). Its normal range is 85–95% (Chapter 20). Tubular reabsorption of phosphate is influenced by changes in GFR and its dietary intake, and reduced in proximal tubular defects and hyperparathyroidism.

A reliable means for assessing phosphate reabsorption is to measure the tubular maximum for phosphate in relation to the GFR (TmP/GFR, Bijvoet index). This index represents the blood concentration above which most phosphate is excreted and below which most is reabsorbed. TmP/GFR may be derived from the tubular reabsorption of phosphate and plasma phosphorus using a nomogram or calculated directly **(Annexure 6, p 823)**. Normal adults have TmP/GFR between 2.8 and 4.2 mg/dL.

Other Investigations

A few blood tests are often carried out for diagnosis and management of renal disorders. The level of serum albumin is reduced in patients with heavy proteinuria, occasionally to below 1.5 g/dL. Estimation of albumin by bromocresol green colorimetry shows higher levels (by as much as 0.5 g/dL) than that estimated by bromophenol purple. In children with nephrotic syndrome, hypercholesterolemia is typically present. It is related to the severity and the duration of proteinuria.

Antistreptococcal Antibody Titer

Measurement of antibody titer against hemolytic streptococci is important for the diagnosis of poststreptococcal GN. Latex agglutination slide test kits are available, containing polystyrene latex particles coated with stabilized streptolysin O and deoxyribonuclease B (DNAse B) as the antigen that react with antibodies in the patient's serum. A titer of over 200 IU/mL is considered positive. Antistreptolysin O antibody (ASO) titers are elevated in 80% children with preceding *Streptococcal pharyngitis*, but only in 20% with pyoderma. In the latter, antihyaluronidase and anti-DNAse B titers are typically raised. The streptozyme test measures titers against several antibodies.

Serum Complement

Measurement of levels of C3 is important in the diagnosis of infection related GN, C3 glomerulopathy, lupus nephritis, and thrombotic microangiopathy. Levels of C3 may increase in acute inflammatory conditions such as active rheumatoid arthritis. In systemic lupus erythematosus (SLE); reduced levels of complement C3 and C4 reflect disease activity. The normal range of serum C3 is 90–120 mg/dL and C4 20–40 mg/dL.

Serum Immunoglobulins

The levels of serum immunoglobulin A (IgA) are increased in about 30–40% of patients with IgA nephropathy and IgA vasculitis.

Antinuclear Antibodies, Anti-double-stranded Deoxyribonucleic Acid Antibodies

Antinuclear antibodies are directed against chromatin-associated or ribonucleoprotein particles. They are increased in SLE, juvenile rheumatoid arthritis, polyarteritis nodosa, and certain liver diseases. An increase in anti-dsDNA antibodies is diagnostic for SLE. Measurements are made using immunofluorescence as well as enzyme-linked immunosorbent assay (ELISA).

Antineutrophil Cytoplasmic Antibodies

These antibodies, with specificity chiefly against proteinase 3 and myeloperoxidase, are seen in patients with granulomatosis with polyangiitis, microscopic polyarteritis, and in pauci-immune crescentic GN.

RENAL BIOPSY

Expert evaluation of renal histology is important in the diagnosis of various renal parenchymal diseases involving glomeruli, tubulointerstitium, and small blood vessels. The procedure has become much simpler with the use of automatic devices and ultrasonographic visualization of the kidney. The use of automatic, single use needles (e.g., Bard biopsy gun) is easier to manipulate, safer, and provides adequate tissue compared to *Trucut* biopsy.

Indications

Indications for renal biopsy are shown in **Box 2.1**. Obvious indications include rapidly progressive GN, lupus nephritis, systemic vasculitis with renal involvement, and kidney failure of unexplained origin. Kidney biopsy also helps ascertain the diagnosis in unexplained acute and chronic kidney disease, persistent hematuria or proteinuria, with potential implications for management and prognosis. A renal biopsy is not required in uncomplicated cases of postinfectious GN and steroid sensitive nephrotic syndrome. The former condition resolves quickly; in the latter, "minimal lesion" histology can be assumed.

Contraindications and Precautions

While there are no absolute contraindications to performing a biopsy, caution is exercised in presence of any of the following: (*i*) Uncontrolled high blood

BOX 2.1: Indications for renal biopsy

Acute glomerulonephritis: Rapidly progressive glomerulonephritis; delayed resolution; lack of serologic evidence of streptococcal infection; normal C3; systemic features*

Nephrotic syndrome: Steroid resistance; associated persistent hematuria, severe hypertension, elevated creatinine or low complement C3; suspected systemic disorder;* suspected calcineurin inhibitor nephrotoxicity

Hematuria: If persistent and associated with proteinuria, red cell casts, dysmorphic red cells; or azotemia

Proteinuria associated with hematuria; nephrotic proteinuria without other features of nephrotic syndrome

Acute renal failure persisting beyond 2–3 weeks; suspected crescentic glomerulonephritis (GN), acute interstitial nephritis, or unclear etiology

Following renal transplantation for allograft dysfunction

*To monitor course and assess histological activity in systemic diseases

pressure (increased risk of bleeding); (*ii*) Bleeding and clotting disorders (hemophilia, thrombocytopenia, and use of antiplatelet agents); (*iii*) Solitary kidney, except in kidney allograft, when indicated (transplant kidney being close to abdominal wall and easier to biopsy than native solitary kidney); (*iv*) Active pyelonephritis.

Therapy with aspirin, nonsteroidal anti-inflammatory drugs, or warfarin should be stopped 5–7 days before the biopsy and resumed after 2–3 days. Ketamine is avoided in patients with respiratory tract infections, or young infants (<3 months old). If a patient on hemodialysis requires a biopsy, the procedure is performed at least 6 hr after the dialysis, and no anticoagulants should be used for the next 48 hr. For patients on peritoneal dialysis, the dialysis effluent should be drained.

Prebiopsy Work-up

Prior to the procedure, caregivers are counseled regarding the procedure. The history, examination, and investigations are reviewed to rule out significant cardiac or respiratory illness, bleeding diatheses, allergies (especially to povidone, iodine, ketamine, midazolam, and lidocaine), anatomic abnormalities of the spine, chest or abdomen, and subcutaneous infection over biopsy site. Hypertension should be well controlled, and ascites, if any, should not be significant, as the child needs to lie prone for the procedure.

Laboratory Evaluation

The hemoglobin level should be >8 g/dL, platelets should be >75,000/mm^3, and prothrombin, activated partial thromboplastin, bleeding and clotting times should be within normal range, in reports performed within the last 3–4 days. Blood levels of urea and creatinine are estimated. Ultrasonography is done to examine the anatomy, position, and size of both kidneys.

Biopsy Procedure

A renal biopsy is usually performed percutaneously as a daycare procedure under ultrasound guidance. Infants and young children, and patients with solitary kidney and those with CKD should be admitted for biopsy. An open biopsy may be considered in patients with shrunken kidneys, a solitary kidney, or with abnormalities of kidney fusion or position. A written consent is taken from either of the parents or the legal guardian.

The patient should be kept fasting for 4–6 hr prior; clear liquids are allowed until 2 hr before the biopsy. The child lies in a prone position with a folded towel or bed sheet placed under his lower ribs and epigastrium to push the kidneys posteriorly and stabilize their position. Alternatively, the patient may be positioned ipsilateral side down to splint the normal motion of the kidney due to respiration. Biopsy may be done in lateral decubitus or sitting position in patients with marked abdominal distension and ascites. The biopsy site is the angle made by the lower edge of the 12th rib and the lateral border of sacrospinalis. In contrast to native kidneys, allografts are positioned in the right or left lower pelvis and accessed anteriorly.

Most children require conscious sedation with monitoring of vital signs. Allograft biopsies in older cooperative children are performed under ultrasound guidance using local lidocaine. IV midazolam (0.05–0.1 mg/kg; repeated after 10–20 minutes to maximum 0.2 mg/kg) is the preferred sedative. It is often combined with IV ketamine (0.5–1 mg/kg, repeated after 10–20 minutes to maximum 4 mg/kg) and atropine (0.01 mg/kg, maximum 0.5 mg) to reduce excessive secretions. Lidocaine (1%) is carefully infiltrated into the skin, subcutaneous tissue, and the renal capsule.

In absence of ultrasound guidance, the kidney is localized with a "probing" 23-gauge needle. As it enters the capsule a distinct resistance is felt and once in the kidney it moves with respiratory excursions. The length of the needle at that point indicates the depth to which the biopsy needle would need to be inserted. While withdrawing the needle, the tract should be anesthetized. However, most centers prefer to localize and visualize the kidney during biopsy with real time ultrasound. The ultrasound probe may be fitted with an adaptor that enables the biopsy needle to be directed to the lower pole of the kidney.

With either technique, a stab incision is given at the proposed site with an 11-gauge surgical blade. If a Trucut biopsy needle is used, the outer sheath is held steady, and the cutting needle is quickly inserted. The outer sheath is rapidly advanced over the cutting needle and thereafter the entire device is withdrawn. Alternatively, the semiautomatic gun is inserted to the required depth and cores taken by "firing" the gun. Local pressure is applied on the biopsy site for a few minutes, the puncture site is sealed with iodine and pressure dressing applied.

Two-three cores of 8–10 mm length are taken for processing for light microscopy, immunofluorescence and electron microscopy. A pathologist or pathology technician should be present during the procedure to confirm adequacy of samples. The specimen is examined using a hand lens or dissecting microscope for adequacy of glomeruli.

Postbiopsy Monitoring

Heart and respiratory rate, and blood pressure are monitored every 15–30 minutes for one hour, then every 30–60 minutes for the next 2 hr and then every hour for 4–6 hr. At least three urine specimens are inspected for presence of gross hematuria. The patient is kept supine and oral fluids are allowed once conscious.

The patient should stay in the hospital for 6–24 hr after the procedure. Bed rest is advised for 24 hr. At discharge, the vital signs should be normal and there should be no gross hematuria. Patients should not be discharged until resolution of sedation related complications, circulatory compromise, and gross hematuria. Contact sports, cycling, or lifting of heavy objects should be avoided for 1 week. Oral paracetamol is given for pain relief. Treatment with aspirin and warfarin can be restarted after 72 hr, if the procedure was uncomplicated.

Complications

The risk of complications is increased in patients with bleeding diathesis, uncontrolled hypertension, and renal failure. Gross hematuria is the most common complication, which is more common with blind than ultrasound-guided biopsies. In most cases, hematuria disappears over 12–24 hr. In the presence of gross hematuria, ultrasound is done to examine for bleeds, clots or perinephric hematoma. Hematoma may cause pain and transient hypertension. Rarely, hematuria is severe and prolonged.

Oral or IV hydration is useful in preventing hypovolemia and formation of clots. Packed cells are transfused if hemoglobin declines by 10–15% from the baseline. If coagulation is deranged, fresh frozen plasma, cryoprecipitate or desmopressin acetate (DDAVP) should be administered. If hematuria persists, an arteriovenous (AV) fistula should be suspected. The diagnosis is supported by a bruit in the renal area. Such patients require radiographic transcatheter embolization or surgical intervention.

Processing of Kidney Biopsy Specimens

The specimen is removed from the biopsy needle gently, taking care not to stretch or crush the tissue. One core is fixed in buffered 10% formalin or paraformaldehyde for light microscopy, and the other in saline or Michel medium that is snap frozen in the laboratory for immunofluorescence study. For electron microscopy, either a third core is taken or 2 mm tissue is incised from each end of the two cores and fixed in 1–3% glutaraldehyde solution, and rapidly refrigerated. Care must be taken to prevent contamination of fixative fluids while placing the biopsy pieces in their respective vials.

Interpretation of Renal Biopsy

The biopsy tissue should be preserved and processed with utmost care. Thin sections and adequate staining are prerequisites for expert interpretation. A pathologist with adequate experience in renal pathology should examine the specimen and must be provided detailed clinical and laboratory findings.

An adequate biopsy should contain representative portions of the cortex and medulla. A minimum of 10 glomeruli are required to be present for proper evaluation. A focal and segmental lesion may be missed in a biopsy containing fewer than 20 glomeruli. Morphology of glomeruli, tubules, interstitium, and vessels is carefully examined **(Table 2.4)**.

TABLE 2.4: Evaluation of histological features on renal biopsy

Light microscopy	
Glomeruli	Generalized or focal involvement; size, cellularity, crescents Mesangial matrix, cellularity; pattern of sclerosis (global, segmental) Basement membrane; Bowman space
Tubules	Atrophy, degeneration, dilatation, cellularity, basement membrane tubular casts, RBCs, inflammation (tubulitis)
Interstitium	Edema, inflammatory exudates (type of cells), fibrosis
Blood vessels	Afferent, efferent arterioles; interstitial vessels
Immunofluorescence	
Deposits	IgG, IgA, IgM, C3, C4, C1q, fibrin; pattern of deposits (granular and linear) Site: capillary (subepithelial, subendothelial, intramembranous), mesangium
Electron microscopy	
Capillary basement membrane: thickening, thinning, wrinkling; diffuse or focal changes Deposits: site, appearance, abnormal material (fibrin and amyloid) Epithelial cells and foot processes	

Ig: immunoglobulin; RBCs: red blood cells

The histology should be examined by light microscopy using hematoxylin and eosin (H and E), periodic acid-Schiff (PAS), and silver methenamine staining in all cases, and special stains, as necessary. Identification of cortex or medulla, and the number of glomeruli and cells infiltrating the interstitium are best seen on H and E stain. Glomerular structure is best seen on PAS, as it delineates mesangial cells and matrix. PAS and silver-methenamine stain the basement membrane, while Masson trichrome and silver stains identify areas of fibrosis. Vessel wall thickening, medial sclerosis, or fibrinoid necrosis is best seen on PAS stain. Congo red stain for amyloidosis and von Kossa stain for calcification are used occasionally.

The number of glomeruli, their size, presence of any sclerosis, focal or diffuse changes, and presence of crescents or mesangial cell proliferation is reported. Lesions involving <50% of glomeruli are called focal while more than that are called diffuse; if only a part of the glomerulus is involved, it is termed segmental, while involvement of the whole glomerulus is defined as global.

Immunofluorescence examination is done with fluoroscein labeled antisera against immunoglobulins (IgA, IgG, and IgM), light chains (κ and λ), and as required, with components of classic or alternate complement pathway (C1q, C3, C3c, and C4d), albumin and fibrin. The site and pattern of immune deposits is noted. Electron microscopic examination is very useful in several disorders, e.g., thin glomerular basement membrane, irregular thickening with basket weaving (Alport syndrome); dense deposits (dense deposit disease); organized deposits (fibrillary and immunotactoid GN); and zebra bodies with lamellated membrane structures (Fabry disease).

Genetic Testing

Recent advances in techniques for genetic testing leading to the development of efficient approaches to analyse genomic data rapidly, together with the completion of the Human Genome Project, have made a huge impact on the approach to specific diagnosis of various kidney diseases. This allows clinicians and geneticists the option to provide the molecular basis of disease within weeks at affordable prices. The approach to genetic testing differs by underlying disease and setting. While clinical or whole exome sequencing remains the most commonly used technique, copy number variations are confirmed by multiplex ligation-dependent probe amplification. Sanger sequencing is useful if the causative variant has already been determined for an affected family member, e.g., when screening siblings, prenatal testing and in evaluation of potential living related donors. **Annexure 9 (p 845)** provides gene lists for focussed bioinformatics in various clinical contexts.

Annexure 2.1: Online calculator for estimated glomerular filtration rate (eGFR) using the modified Schwartz formula in children https://www.kidney.org/professionals/kdoqi/gfr_calculatorPed *Scan the QR code below or type the following link in browser window:*	
Annexure 2.2: Online calculator for estimated glomerular filtration rate (eGFR) using the CKD-EPI formulae in adults https://www.kidney.org/professionals/gfr_calculator *Scan the QR code below or type the following link in browser window:*	
Annexure 2.3: Online calculator for estimated glomerular filtration rate (eGFR) using the Full Age Spectrum Equation (For age 2-40 years) https://kulak.kuleuven.be/egfr_calculator/ *Scan the QR code below or type the following link in browser window:*	
Annexure 2.4: Online calculator for estimated glomerular filtration rate (eGFR) using the CKiD U25 Equation (For age <25 years) https://qxmd.com/calculate/calculator_822/ckid-u25-egfr-calculator *Scan the QR code below or type the following link in browser window:*	

BIBLIOGRAPHY

1. Chadda V, Garg U, Alon US. Measurement of urinary concentration: a critical appraisal of methodologies. Pediatr Nephrol. 2001;16(4):374-82.
2. Delanaye P, Cavalier E, Pottel H, et al. New and old GFR equations: A European perspective. Clin Kidney J. 2023;16(9):1375-83.
3. Derain Dubourg L, Aurelle M, Chardon L, et al. Tubular phosphate handling: references from child to adulthood in the era of standardized serum creatinine. Nephrol Dial Transplant. 2022;37:2150-6.
4. Evidence reviews for the diagnostic accuracy of eGFR calculations in adults, children, and young people from black, Asian and other minority ethnic groups with CKD: Chronic kidney disease: Evidence review A. London: National Institute for Health and Care Excellence (NICE); 2021.
5. Farrance I, Frenkel R, Choy KW. Uncertainty in measurement and the renal tubular reabsorption of phosphate. Clin Chem Lab Med. 2023;61(12):2178-85.
6. Filler G, Ferris M, Gattineni J. Assessment of kidney function in children, adolescents, and young adults. In: Emma F, Goldstein SL, Bagga A, Bates CM, Shroff R (Eds). Pediatric Nephrology, 8th edition. New York: Springer Nature; 2022, pp. 145-72.
7. Gubbi S, Hannah-Shmouni F, Koch CA, et al. Diagnostic testing for diabetes insipidus. In: Feingold KR, Anawalt B, Blackman MR, Boyce A, Chrousos G, Corpas E, et al., (Eds). Endotext [Internet] 2022. South Dartmouth (MA): MDText. com, Inc.; 2000.
8. Hogan JJ, Mocanu M, Berns JS. The native kidney biopsy: Update and evidence for best practice. Clin J Am Soc Nephrol. 2016;11:354-62.
9. Inker LA, Eneanya ND, Coresh J, et al.; Chronic Kidney Disease Epidemiology Collaboration. New creatinine- and cystatin C-based equations to estimate GFR without race. N Engl J Med. 2021;385(19):1737-49.
10. Inker LA, Titan S. Measurement and estimation of GFR for use in clinical practice: Core curriculum 2021. Am J Kidney Dis. 2021;78(5):736-49.
11. Najafian B, Lusco MA, Alpers CE, et al. Approach to kidney biopsy: Core curriculum 2022. Am J Kidney Dis. 2022;80(1):119-31.
12. Pottel H, Delanaye P, Schaeffner E, et al. Estimating glomerular filtration rate for the full age spectrum from serum creatinine and cystatin C. Nephrol Dial Transplant. 2017;32(3):497-507.
13. Schwartz GJ, Muñoz A, Schneider MF, et al. New equations to estimate GFR in children with CKD. J Am Soc Nephrol. 2009;20(3):629-37.

CHAPTER 3 Imaging of Urinary Tract

Manisha Jana, Arun Kumar Gupta, Amit Gupta

Major advances have taken place in the field of diagnostic imaging. Newer imaging techniques have changed the investigative approach. Expertise, experience, and patience are necessary for the performance of these procedures, especially in infants and young children. Appropriate sedation is used if required.

DIAGNOSTIC PROCEDURES

Plain X-ray Film of the Abdomen

The utility of plain X-ray film of the abdomen has decreased with introduction of ultrasonography and computed tomography (CT). Most disorders can be imaged using these methods, which give much more information than the plain X-ray. The latter still has a role in detecting renal and ureteric calculi, spinal evaluation in neurogenic states, evaluation for metastatic bone disease, and screening for metabolic bone diseases **(Figs. 3.1A and B)**.

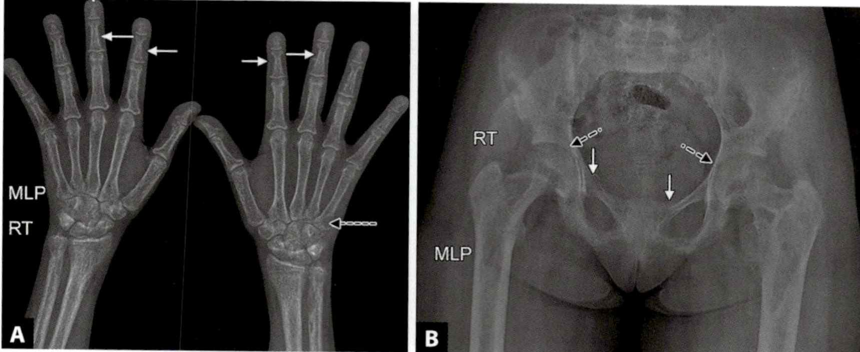

Figs. 3.1A and B: Skeletal radiographs in a case of hyperparathyroidism. (A) Hand radiograph shows areas of subperiosteal resorption, seen most prominently along the middle phalanges (arrows). Well-defined lytic lesion is seen at the base of left 5th metacarpal (dotted arrow); (B) Pelvic radiograph shows Looser zones (arrows) involving bilateral superior pubic rami. Note is made of bilateral coxa profunda (acetabular margin lying medial to ilioischial line; dotted arrows). Diffuse osteopenia is noted in visualized bones in both (A) and (B)

Excretory Urography

Newer techniques, especially ultrasonography, in combination with radionuclide studies have largely replaced excretory urography or intravenous pyelography (IVP). After careful preparation on the previous evening (a liquid diet and laxatives), 2.5–3 mL/kg body weight of a nonionic contrast agent is given intravenously (IV). Ionic contrast materials like meglumine and sodium salts of iodine are not preferred, because the iso-osmolar composition and better safety profile of nonionic compounds decreases contrast reactions. An initial film is taken at 5 minutes after contrast injection, followed by another at 10–15 minutes and a late pelvic film to visualize the urinary bladder. Abdominal compression is avoided in children. Excretory urography should be avoided in neonates because of their poor ability to concentrate the contrast medium. A test dose of the contrast material is not routinely required. The patient should be well hydrated. The IVP has very limited indications, namely complex congenital malformations and genitourinary tuberculosis.

Ultrasonography

Ultrasound examination provides information about the anatomy of the urinary tract. High-resolution images in multiple planes may be obtained, using a high-frequency transducer **(Figs. 3.2A and B)**. The procedure is suited for children since it is painless and requires no sedation or administration of any contrast agent. It can be carried out even at bedside and repeated as often as required. Ultrasound guidance can be used in invasive procedures, e.g., fine-needle aspiration and renal biopsy. The normal kidney has an elliptical shape. All along the margin, there is the low echogenic cortex with evenly

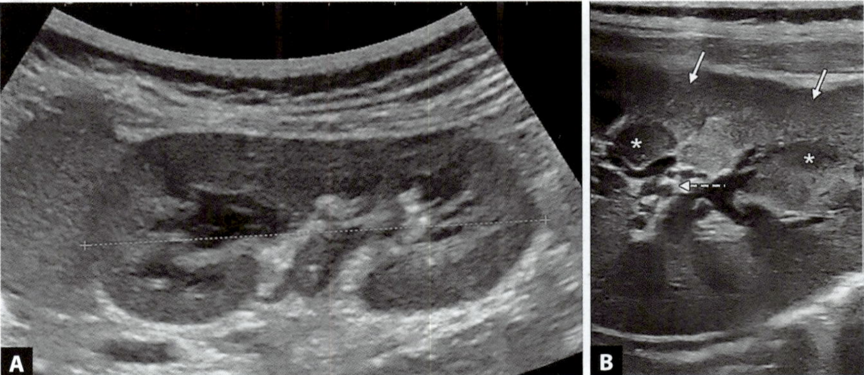

Figs. 3.2A and B: Normal kidney appearance on ultrasound. (A) Low-frequency curvilinear transducer shows the complete longitudinal view of the kidney (between calipers); (B) High-frequency linear frequency transducer shows the corticomedullary differentiation very well with hypoechoic medullary pyramids (asterisks) and comparatively slightly echogenic renal cortex (arrows). Intensely echogenic renal sinus fat is seen in the center of the kidney (dotted arrow)

distributed triangular hypoechoic pyramids. In the center, is the intensely echogenic renal sinus fat. The cortical echotexture in children is hyperechoic compared with liver or spleen. A further increase in echogenicity may be seen in renal parenchymal diseases, but is nonspecific. In neonates, the renal cortex is more echogenic; and corticomedullary differentiation is accentuated **(Figs. 3.3A and B)**. The echogenicity decreases after the first month. Increased medullary tip echogenicity is another normal finding, especially in preterm neonates. Medullary nephrocalcinosis is best detected on high-resolution ultrasound **(Figs. 3.4A and B)**.

Quantitative measurement of renal growth is possible on two-dimensional ultrasonography. Doppler technique when used in conjunction with 2D imaging is informative. Using color Doppler methods, interlobar and even arcuate vessels can be identified. The major drawback of ultrasonography is

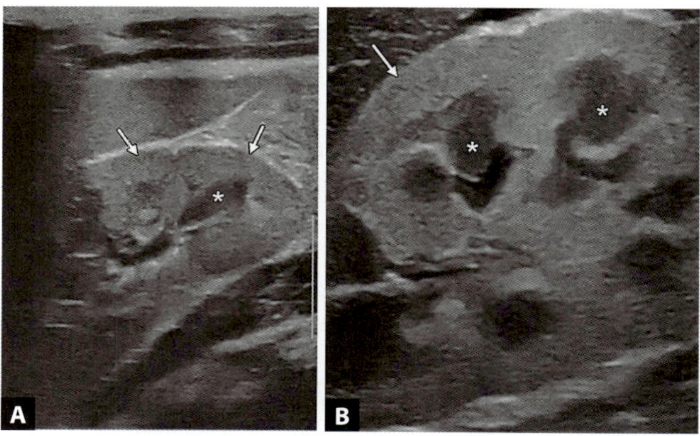

Figs. 3.3A and B: Normal neonatal kidney on ultrasound. (A and B) High-frequency transducer ultrasound images show highly echogenic renal cortex (arrows) as compared to hypoechoic medullary pyramids (asterisks) with accentuated corticomedullary differentiation

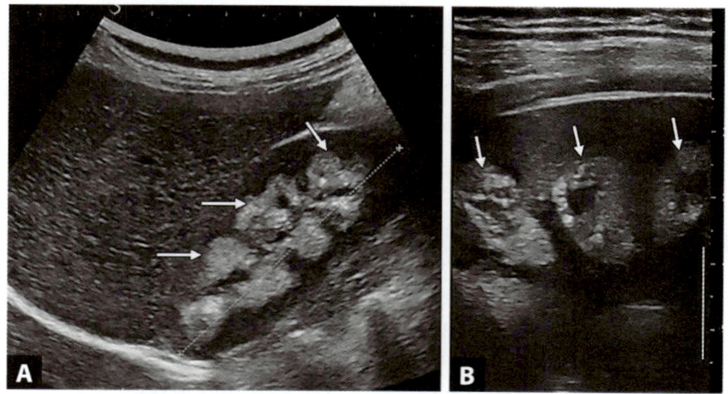

Figs. 3.4A and B: Medullary nephrocalcinosis. (A and B) Ultrasound images show densely echogenic renal medullae (arrows)

TABLE 3.1: Checklist for pediatric urinary tract ultrasound

Kidney	Size, outline; any cysts, nephrocalcinosis or calculi Echogenicity and corticomedullary differentiation Pelvicalyceal dilatation
Renal pelvis	Anteroposterior diameter (in case of hydronephrosis)
Ureter	Dilatation, peristalsis; location of vesicoureteric junction; frequency and volume of ureteric jet
Urinary bladder	Outline, capacity, diverticula; post-void residue

that its performance and interpretation is operator dependent, especially in infants and neonates. A checklist for renal ultrasound can often prove useful **(Table 3.1)**.

Contrast-enhanced ultrasound (CEUS) is an important innovation that has increased the utility of gray scale ultrasound. In India, the approved CEUS agent is composed of sulfur hexafluoride microbubbles. CEUS can assess microvasculature, and hence is also useful in evaluating renal masses **(Figs. 3.5A to C)**.

Antenatal Ultrasonography

Ultrasonography during pregnancy can detect several fetal anomalies. Hydronephrosis, large cystic kidney, and enlarged bladder are common abnormalities in antenatal ultrasonography **(Figs. 3.6A and B)**. Presence of dilatation of urinary system, echotexture of renal parenchyma, appearance of urinary bladder, and the amount of amniotic fluid are carefully examined. Oligohydramnios (<500 mL at 32–36 weeks' gestation) is indicative of poor fetal renal function. Occasionally, delayed maturation of the ureter may cause temporary obstruction that spontaneously resolves. Vesicoureteric reflux (VUR) is the chief cause of dilated urinary tract, and pelviureteric junction obstruction that of isolated hydronephrosis. Increased renal echogenicity, bilateral hydronephrosis, and distended bladder strongly suggest distal urinary tract obstruction. Nonvisualization of bladder may indicate a normally empty bladder or anomalies such as bladder exstrophy or a neuropathic bladder.

Computed Tomography

Computed tomography provides information on anatomy and function of the kidneys. Sedation is required for small children. The main role of CT is for examining mass lesions of the kidney, bladder, or retroperitoneum that secondarily affect the urinary system. The masses may be congenital (teratoma), inflammatory (abscess), traumatic (hematoma), or neoplastic

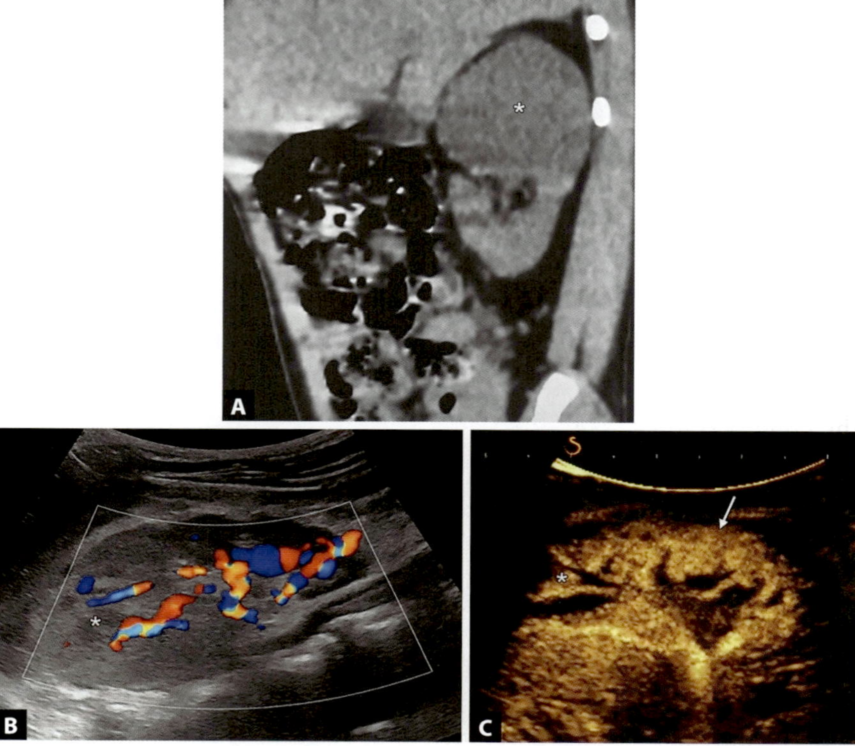

Figs. 3.5A to C: Role of CEUS. (A) Ill-defined hypodensity (asterisk) seen in upper pole of kidney on noncontrast CT suspicious for a mass; (B) Color Doppler shows no significant abnormal vascularity in the upper pole (asterisk) of kidney; (C) CEUS shows similar homogeneous contrast enhancement in the upper pole (asterisk) of kidney similar to the rest of the renal cortex (arrow), confirming it as a "pseudomass". CEUS: contrast-enhanced ultrasound; CT: computed tomography

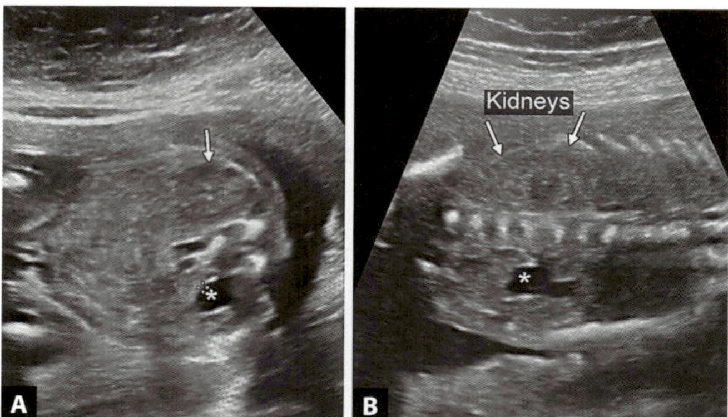

Figs. 3.6A and B: Fetal hydronephrosis. Axial (A) and coronal (B) antenatal ultrasound images show dilated left renal pelvis (asterisk) and mild calyceal dilatation. Contralateral kidney (arrows) is normal

(Wilms tumor, rhabdomyosarcoma). CT can detect a nonfunctioning or a poorly functioning kidney. With the advent of multidetector row CT (MDCT), it is possible to acquire high-resolution images with faster speed and hence, less motion blur in small children. MDCT imaging also enables assessment of renal or retroperitoneal masses (e.g., extent of inferior vena cava thrombus in Wilms tumor). Radiation dose should be kept in mind for the children and unnecessary scanning avoided.

Micturating Cystourethrogram

Micturating cystourethrogram (MCU) is an important procedure for the diagnosis and evaluation of severity of VUR, and detection of the abnormalities of bladder and urethra. The contrast agent is introduced into the bladder through a catheter with strict asepsis. Films are taken when the child is voiding **(Figs. 3.7A and B)**. The procedure is invasive but its indication should be explained to the parents and they should be assured of its safety; adequate time should be spent to allay their anxiety. With advent of superior fluoroscopic equipment, it is possible to perform the investigation with a lesser radiation dose. The catheter should be introduced with strict aseptic precautions. Patients at high risk of sepsis (infants, children with dilated urinary tract, congenital heart disease) should receive prophylactic treatment with oral coamoxiclav or intramuscular (IM) gentamicin 30–60 minutes prior to the procedure.

Magnetic Resonance Imaging

Though there are several advantages of this imaging modality like nonionizing nature, multiplanar imaging capability, and superior soft

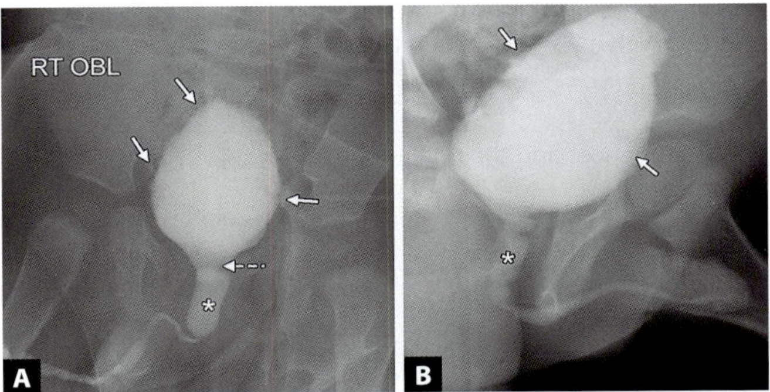

Figs. 3.7A and B: Micturating cystourethrography. (A) Case of posterior urethral valve shows bladder trabeculations (arrows) with dilated posterior urethra (asterisk) with abrupt narrowing of caliber at distal posterior urethra. Note is made of bladder neck hypertrophy (dotted arrow); (B) Case of neurogenic bladder shows an elongated trabeculated urinary bladder (Christmas tree bladder; arrows) with dilated posterior urethra (asterisk)

tissue contrast resolution, its use is limited in children because of motion-related problems and need for sedation and general anesthesia. Normal renal cortex is hyperintense on T1-weighted and relatively hypointense on T2-weighted images whereas normal renal medulla is hyperintense on T2-weighted images **(Fig. 3.8)**. Important uses include MR urography (heavily T2-weighted sequences like HASTE) in cases of hydronephrosis, duplex moiety, and ectopic ureter; and MR angiography in cases of suspected renal artery stenosis. The added advantage of magnetic resonance imaging (MRI) in evaluation of renal masses is that inferior vena cava (IVC) thrombus can be detected without any contrast (thrombi appear hyperintense within hypointense vessel lumen on gradient echo sequence, and isointense on spin echo sequences). Comprehensive list of sequences and their utility is summarized in **Table 3.2**.

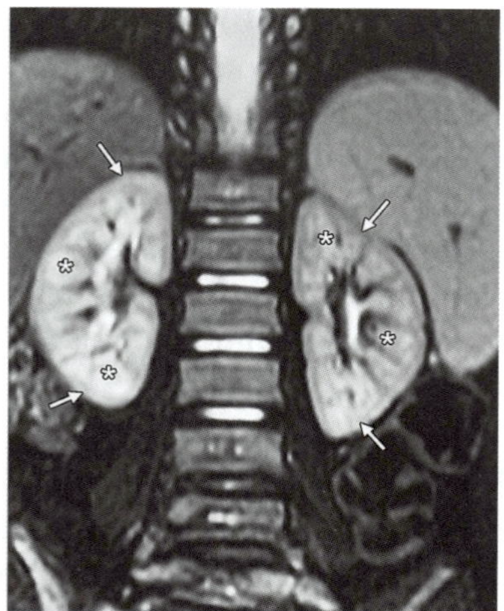

Fig. 3.8: Normal kidneys on T2-weighted MRI show hyperintense medullary pyramids (asterisks) and relatively hypointense renal cortex (arrows). MRI: magnetic resonance imaging

TABLE 3.2: MRI sequences and their utility

Sequence	*Utility*
T1W	Useful for detection of hemorrhage
T2W	Corticomedullary differentiation, cystic kidney diseases, mass lesions
Diffusion-weighted images, ADC map	Characterization of mass lesions
Contrast-enhanced scans	Characterization of mass lesions
Balanced gradient echo (BTFE/TruFISP)	Noncontrast angiography
Time of flight (ToF) sequence	Noncontrast angiography

MRI: magnetic resonance imaging

Digital Subtraction Angiography

Digital subtraction angiography (DSA) is an invasive radiographic procedure performed for diagnosis as well as therapy. The arterial access is usually obtained via femoral route, and after selection of appropriate catheter depending on the artery involved, intra-arterial injection of contrast material is performed. Currently, with the advent of superior quality CT imaging, diagnostic DSA has become a rarity, except for visceral involvement in vasculitis such as polyarteritis nodosa (PAN) **(Figs. 3.9A and B)**. Therapeutic DSA is indicated in the management of renal artery stenosis, in form of angioplasty. In cases of bleeding from a renal tumor such as angiomyolipoma, selective arterial embolization can be life-saving. Embolization is also effective in case of postrenal biopsy arterial injury or pseudoaneurysm.

Special Procedures

Several other imaging procedures are employed to visualize the urinary system, including antegrade pyelogram, retrograde pyelogram, and angiography.

Point-of-care Ultrasound

Point-of-care ultrasound (POCUS) can be defined as the use of advanced ultrasound imaging at the bedside by the treating physician. The pediatrician should have sufficient knowledge and training in order to perform and interpret POCUS. The domain of POCUS in pediatric nephrology is not only limited to nephrologic evaluation, but also to other systemic disorders. In cases of chronic or acute kidney disease, POCUS can be used to evaluate the underlying renal parenchymal disease, assess the suitability for renal biopsy,

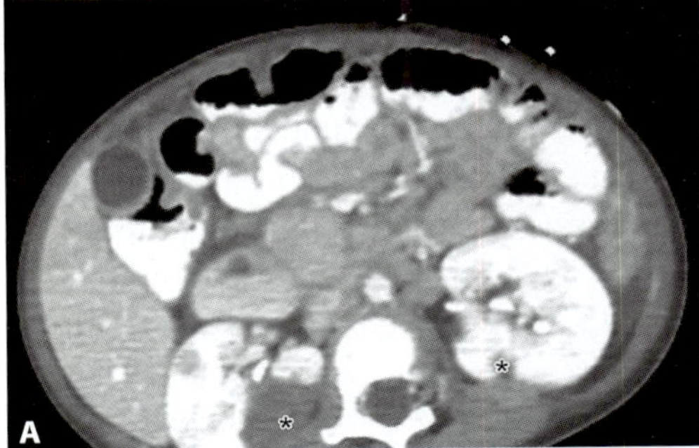

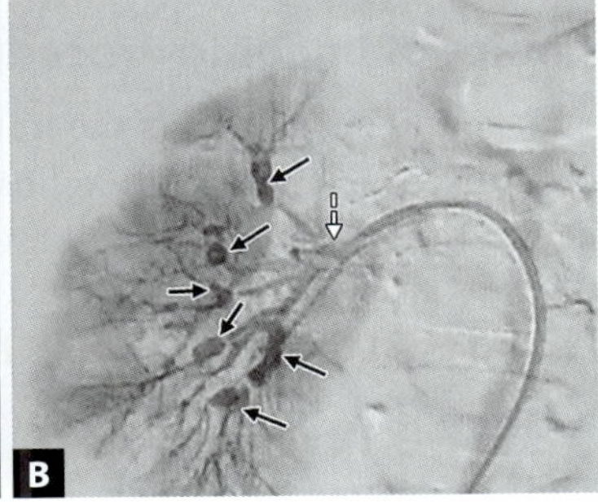

Figs. 3.9A and B: Polyarteritis nodosa. (A) Contrast-enhanced CT shows wedge-shaped nonenhancing areas (asterisks) in bilateral kidneys suggestive of infarcts; (B) Contrast run taken after positioning the catheter tip (dotted arrow) in right renal artery shows multiple contrast outpouchings suggestive of microaneurysms (arrows) arising from interlobar branches of renal artery. CT: computed tomography

TABLE 3.3: Important imaging findings in point-of-care ultrasound

Renal findings	
Chronic renal disease (CKD)	Commonly small kidneys, loss of corticomedullary differentiation, high echogenicity
Acute pyelonephritis	Enlarged hypoechoic kidney, increased corticomedullary differentiation
Hydronephrosis	Splitting of renal sinus fat, fullness of renal pelvis and calyces
Extrarenal findings	
Volume overload	Increased or confluent B lines on lung ultrasound Dilated inferior vena cava (>21 mm), reduced collapsibility (<50%)
Pleural effusion	Anechoic fluid collection in pleural cavity
Pneumothorax	Loss of lung sliding sign on lung ultrasonography Presence of A lines
Cardiogenic shock	Poor cardiac output and contractility Confluent B lines on lung ultrasonography Pleural effusion Distended inferior vena cava
Hypovolemic shock	Decreased cardiac output Increased cardiac contractility Presence of A lines on lung ultrasonography Collapsed inferior vena cava
Cardiac tamponade	Pericardial effusion Collapse of right ventricle in diastole

and offer image guidance during biopsy. POCUS is also used for evaluation of hydration status, monitoring fluid resuscitation, bedside echocardiography, and lung ultrasound **(Table 3.3)**.

Choice of Imaging Procedures

Ultrasound evaluation is the initial procedure in most patients with urinary tract disease. It is often diagnostic (e.g., hydronephrosis, cystic diseases of kidney), or provides information to suggest the next investigation **(Table 3.4)**.

PATHOLOGICAL CONDITIONS

Kidney

The kidney may be absent, hypoplastic, malrotated, or lie ectopic in a low abdominal or pelvic position. Occasionally, the kidneys show crossed ectopia or be ectopically placed and fused (pancake kidney)**(Figs. 3.10A and B)**. Ultrasonography is diagnostic; confirmation may be obtained with excretory urography or radionuclide scan.

TABLE 3.4: Proper selection of imaging procedure depending on clinical indication

Indication	*Suitable radiological investigation*
Antenatal hydronephrosis	Postnatal ultrasound; micturating cystourethrogram (MCU)
Hydronephrosis	Ultrasound
Cystic kidney disease	Ultrasound
Renal vein thrombosis	Ultrasound with Doppler
Renal artery stenosis	Ultrasound with Doppler; CT/MR angiography
Polyarteritis nodosa	Digital subtraction angiography
Renal calculi	Noncontrast CT (dual energy preferable)
Renal mass	Contrast-enhanced CT scan
Urinary obstruction	Ultrasound; retrograde urethrography; MCU

CT: computed tomography; MR: magnetic resonance

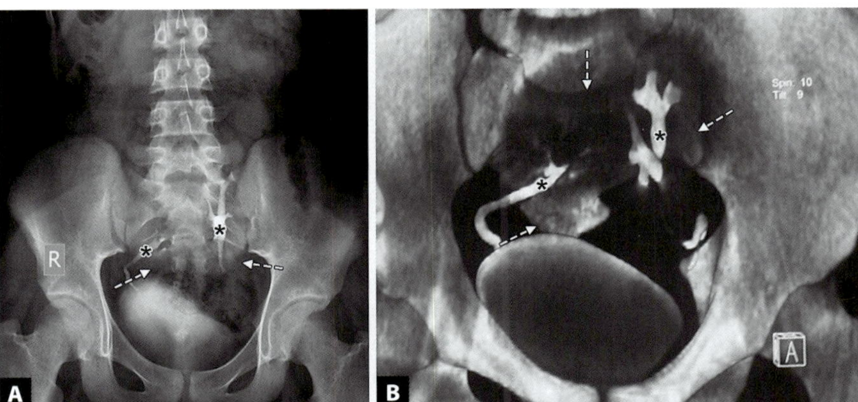

Figs. 3.10A and B: Pancake kidney. (A) Intravenous pyelography image shows opacification of two pelvicalyceal systems (asterisks) ectopically placed in the pelvis with a single nephrogram (dashed arrows); (B) CT urography image similarly shows the two ectopic pelvicalyceal systems (asterisks) opacified in the pelvis with fusion of the parenchyma (dashed arrows) of the two kidneys forming a single pancake kidney. CT: computed tomography

Pelviectasis

Pelviectasis is the most common finding on antenatal ultrasonography. Its detection should be carefully evaluated and the presence of other structural anomalies looked for, as their presence may be associated with other structural and/or chromosomal abnormality. Pelviectasis detected in the second trimester should be followed for increase in the third semester. Mild pelvic dilatation may occasionally be a physiologic variant. MCU and radionuclide studies are carried out in patients with significant postnatal

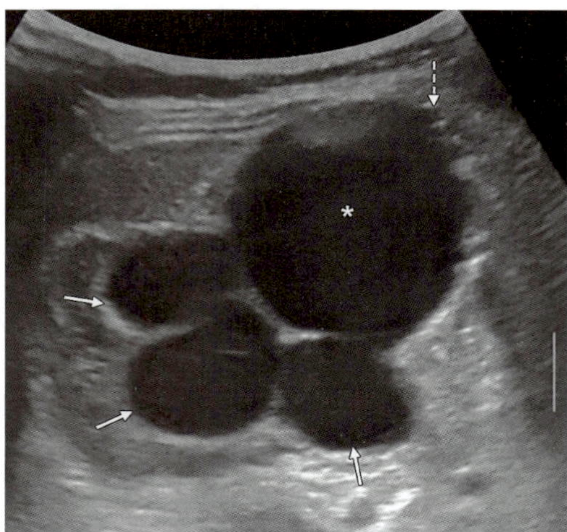

Fig. 3.11: *Pelviureteric junction obstruction (PUJO):* Ultrasonography shows gross dilatation of the renal pelvis (asterisk) out of proportion to the renal calyces (arrows) with abrupt change of caliber at the pelviureteric junction (dashed arrow)

hydronephrosis. Pelviureteric junction obstruction shows hydronephrosis with disproportionate dilation of pelvis, and nonvisualization of distal ureter and ureteric jet **(Fig. 3.11)**.

Cystic Kidney Diseases

Hydronephrosis, commonly due to pelviureteric junction obstruction, is the most common cause of cystic renal mass in older children. Multicystic dysplastic kidney (MCDK) is often diagnosed in neonates. Differentiation between these two conditions can be made on ultrasonography **(Figs. 3.12A and B)**, but further confirmation may be required by radionuclide studies. MCDK shows no uptake on DMSA scan. Other cystic diseases include autosomal recessive polycystic renal disease (ARPKD) **(Fig. 3.13)**, autosomal dominant polycystic kidney disease (ADPKD) **(Figs. 3.14A and B)**, medullary cystic kidney disease, glomerulocystic kidney disease associated with HNF1-beta mutation. Although ultrasonography is adequate for diagnosis, contrast-enhanced CT or MRI may be required in ADPKD to exclude the development of hemorrhage, calculi, or malignancy within a pre-existing cyst. ARPKD can be associated with Caroli disease, congenital hepatic fibrosis, and splenomegaly **(Figs. 3.15A and B)**.

Tumors

The type of tumor depends upon the age at presentation. In neonates and early infancy, congenital mesoblastic nephroma predominates; subsequently Wilms tumor is common. Both have similar morphological appearance

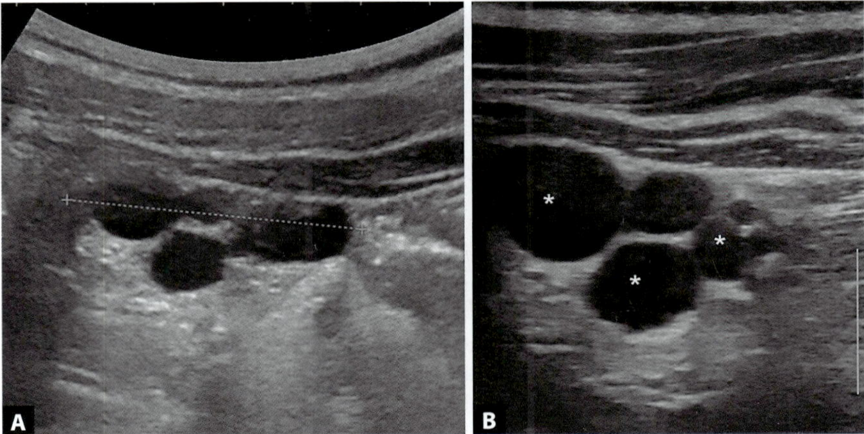

Figs. 3.12A and B: Multicystic dysplastic kidney in a 6-year-old boy. (A) Sagittal ultrasound reveals a small left kidney (between cursors), with no discernible renal parenchyma; (B) High-resolution ultrasound shows variable sized noncommunicating cysts (asterisks)

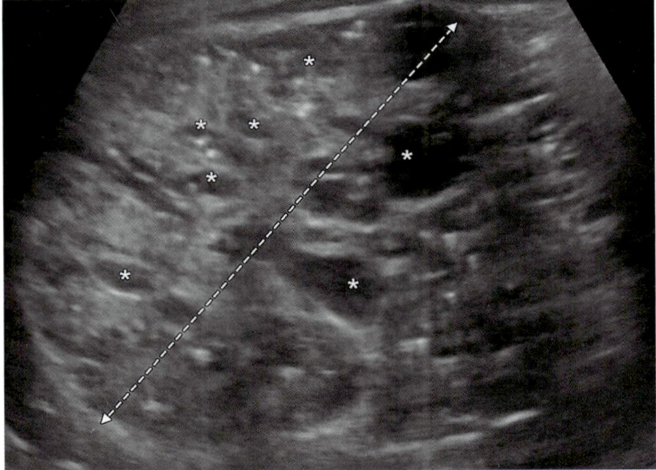

Fig. 3.13: *Autosomal recessive polycystic kidney disease (ARPKD):* Ultrasonography shows an enlarged echogenic kidney (dotted double-headed arrow) with loss of corticomedullary differentiation with innumerable tiny cysts (asterisks) distributed throughout the renal parenchyma

on imaging. Pooling of contrast agent within part of the tumor, either on urography or contrast-enhanced CT, suggests mesoblastic nephroma. Wilms tumor is the most common malignant neoplasm of kidney in children **(Figs. 3.16A and B)**. In most cases, the diagnosis of a solid neoplasm is made on ultrasonography, followed by fine-needle aspiration cytology or a biopsy. Wilms tumor may have an atypical appearance, being predominantly cystic with multiple septa. The tumor is bilateral in 6–10% cases. The renal vein,

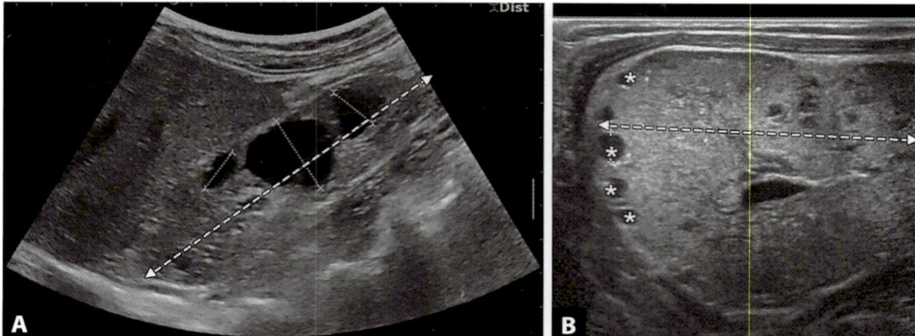

Figs. 3.14A and B: *Autosomal dominant polycystic kidney disease (ADPKD):* (A) Ultrasonography shows multiple large anechoic cysts (between cursors) in the kidney (dotted double-headed arrow) with loss of corticomedullary differentiation; (B) High-resolution image shows an echogenic kidney (dotted double-headed arrow) with loss of corticomedullary differentiation with multiple cysts (asterisks) in the periphery

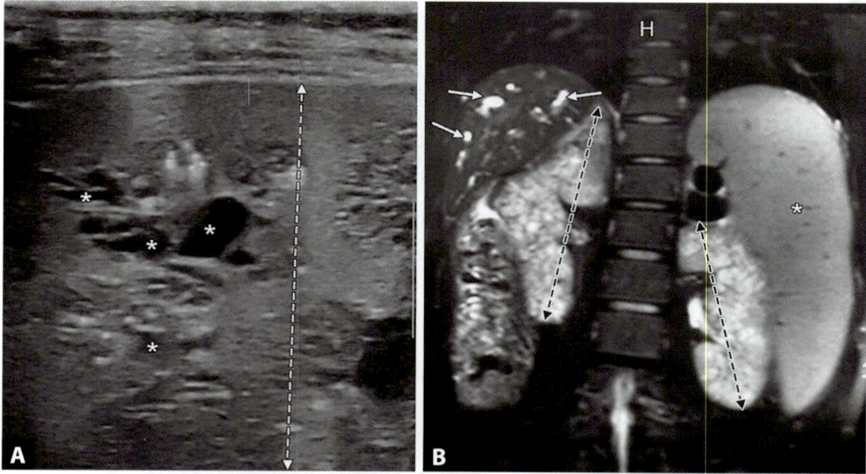

Figs. 3.15A and B: *Autosomal recessive polycystic kidney disease with Caroli disease:* (A) High-resolution ultrasonography shows echogenic kidney (dotted double-headed arrow) with loss of corticomedullary differentiation with innumerable tiny cysts (asterisks); (B) Coronal T2-weighted MRI image shows bilateral enlarged kidneys (dotted double-headed arrows) with innumerable tiny hyperintense cysts. Liver parenchyma also shows multiple dilated intrahepatic biliary ducts (arrows) consistent with Caroli disease. Note is made of enlarged spleen (asterisk). MRI: magnetic resonance imaging

inferior vena cava, and right atrium should be examined to detect a thrombus **(Figs. 3.17A to C)** and chest X-ray and CT scan done for lung metastasis. Patients with Wilms tumor can have intravenous tumor thrombus extension that can migrate to cardiac chambers and cause sudden death. Imaging in the coronal and sagittal plane is required for demonstration of tumor thrombus, which can define the approach of surgical resection.

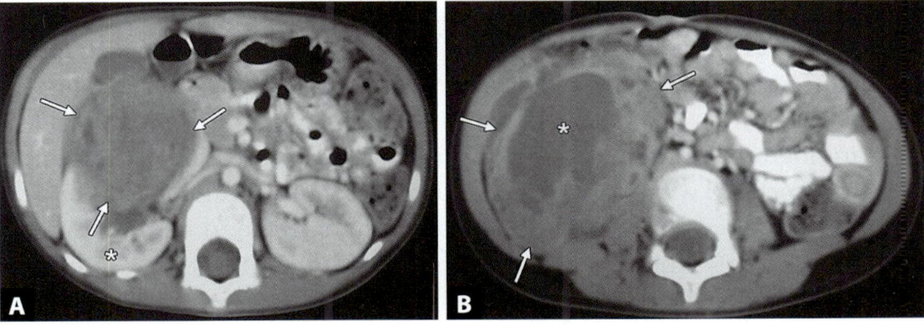

Figs. 3.16A and B: *Wilms tumor:* (A) Contrast-enhanced computed tomography of abdomen shows a heterogeneous mass (arrows) arising from right kidney (asterisk) with an exophytic component; (B) Section caudal to (A) shows the mass (arrows) replacing the entire parenchyma of lower pole of right kidney with large hypodense areas of necrosis (asterisk)

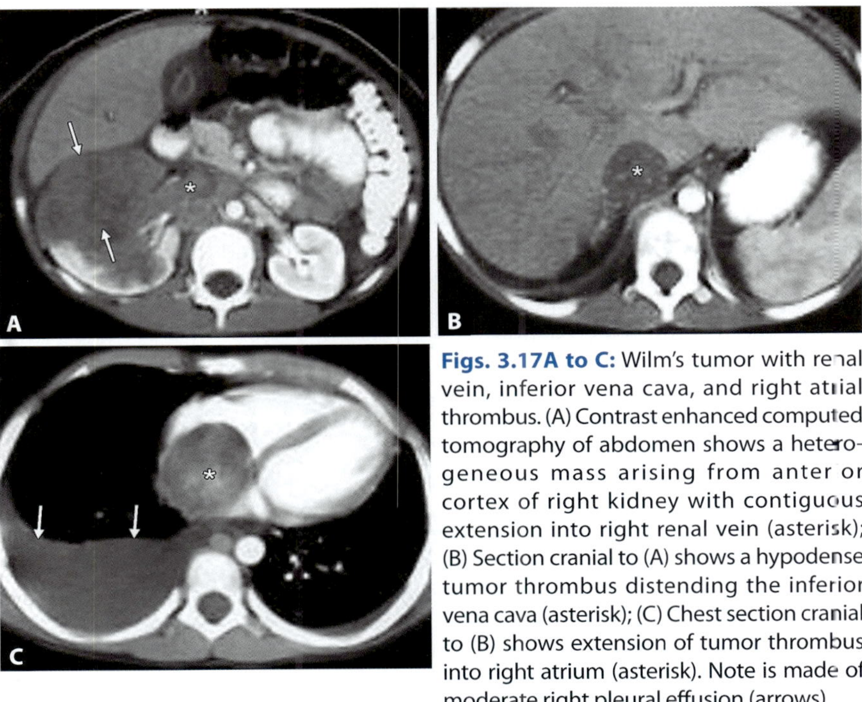

Figs. 3.17A to C: Wilm's tumor with renal vein, inferior vena cava, and right atrial thrombus. (A) Contrast enhanced computed tomography of abdomen shows a heterogeneous mass arising from anterior cortex of right kidney with contiguous extension into right renal vein (asterisk); (B) Section cranial to (A) shows a hypodense tumor thrombus distending the inferior vena cava (asterisk); (C) Chest section cranial to (B) shows extension of tumor thrombus into right atrium (asterisk). Note is made of moderate right pleural effusion (arrows)

Infections of the Kidney

In acute pyelonephritis, ultrasonography may show slightly enlarged kidneys with increased echogenicity and poor corticomedullary demarcation. Renal sinus echoes may be compressed. On Doppler, the resistive index (RI) of the segmental renal arteries is elevated. Although US is helpful in evaluating acute pyelonephritis, CT is a superior modality, but seldom necessary. A renal abscess **(Figs. 3.18A and B)** is usually unilateral; ultrasonography shows a cystic mass with echogenic contents. Perirenal collection, resulting from rupture of a renal abscess, is visualized on ultrasonography and CT imaging. Ultrasonography is also used for guided intervention in these conditions.

Xanthogranulomatous pyelonephritis is a chronic infection of the kidney, usually associated with renal calculi and resulting in nonfunctioning kidney. The disease process can extend to perinephric space and nephrectomy is the treatment of choice. Renal tuberculosis **(Fig. 3.19)** is uncommon in childhood, and is usually associated with pulmonary involvement. Earliest changes are detected on excretory urogram as irregular calyceal margins; advanced cases show focal caliectasis with infundibular stenosis, scarred pelvis and ureteric and vesicoureteric junction (VUJ) strictures.

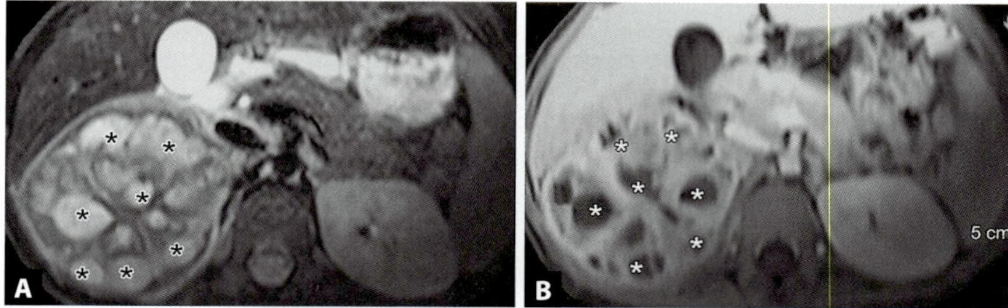

Figs. 3.18A and B: Renal abscesses. (A) Axial T2-weighted MRI shows multiple hyperintense collections (asterisks) in the right renal parenchyma; (B) Axial post-contrast MRI image shows peripheral rim enhancement with central nonenhancing areas in the renal abscesses (asterisks)

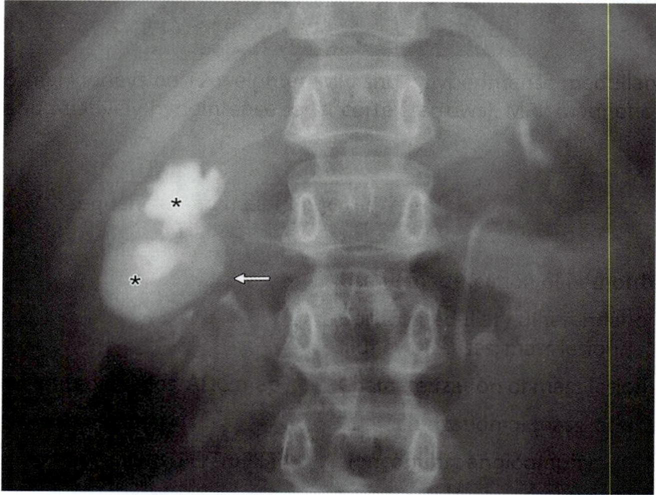

Fig. 3.19: Genitourinary tuberculosis. Intravenous pyelography image showing focal calyceal dilation of upper pole calyces (asterisks) with infundibular stenosis (arrow)

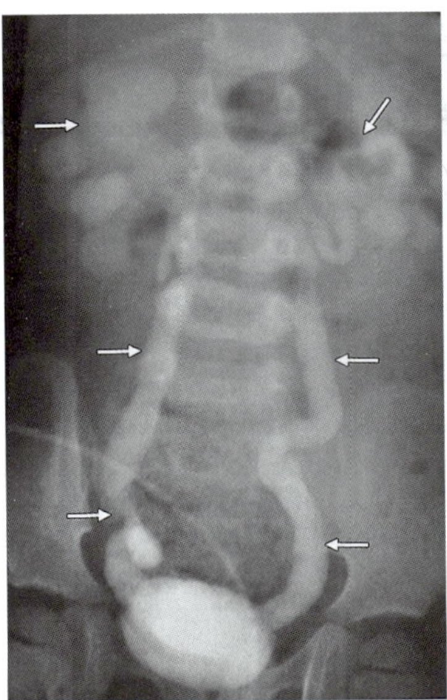

Fig. 3.20: Reflux nephropathy. Micturating cystourethrogram shows bilateral grade 5 vesicoureteric reflux (arrows)

Reflux Nephropathy

The characteristic renal scarring with eventual reduction of kidney size is a sequel of VUR associated with urinary tract infections **(Fig. 3.20)**. The typical lesion is a cortical scar with loss of cortical width and dilatation of the underlying calyx. Lesions are often bilateral, irregular, and asymmetrical, and more frequent at the poles. There is hypertrophy of normal cortical tissue on the same and the contralateral side. Significant lesions are seen on ultrasonography or excretory urography, but DMSA scintigraphy is more sensitive.

Renal Vein Thrombosis

This condition is considered in an infant with a flank mass and hematuria, following an episode of severe dehydration. Ultrasonography shows the affected enlarged kidney, maintaining its shape with diffusely altered echotexture, compressing the renal sinus echoes and poor corticomedullary differentiation **(Figs. 3.21A and B)**. Doppler studies may show normal flow in renal vein since the thrombotic changes start peripherally and propagate centrally. Ultrasonography can distinguish renal vein thrombosis from Wilms tumor, and is useful for follow-up. The kidney may revert to normal or become progressively small, fibrotic, and calcified.

Renovascular Hypertension

Important conditions include Takayasu disease and fibromuscular dysplasia. Ultrasonography with Doppler is useful in diagnosing obstruction in the

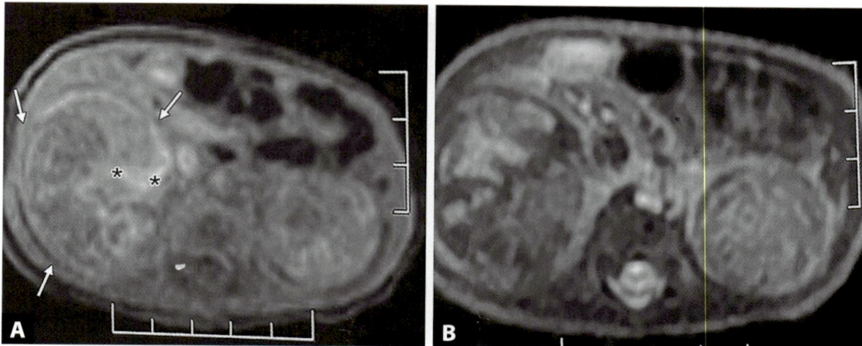

Figs. 3.21A and B: Renal vein thrombosis. (A) Axial T1-weighted MRI shows an enlarged right kidney with areas of T1 hyperintensity suggestive of hemorrhage; (B) Corresponding axial T2-weighted MRI image shows an enlarged right kidney with T2 dark areas within

aorta and renal arteries. Diagnostic angiography is used for evaluation of renal arteries. Selective renal artery catheterization is done if necessary.

Acute and Chronic Kidney Disease

Ultrasonography is a useful investigation for evaluating children with acute kidney injury and chronic kidney disease. It confirms the presence of two kidneys and demonstrates their size, cortical thickness, echogenicity and presence or absence of hydronephrosis, hydroureter, and cystic kidney disease.

Urolithiasis

More than 90% urinary tract stones are radiopaque, only pure uric acid stones being radiolucent. Ultrasonography detects lucent calculi, especially if the collecting system is dilated. Ureteric calculi are difficult to localize on ultrasound unless there is significant dilatation, and the stone is located at either ends of the ureter. High-resolution noncontrast CT is the imaging of choice for renal or ureteric calculi. Bladder calculi are best seen on a plain X-ray film or ultrasound.

Nephrocalcinosis

Calcification is characteristically bilateral and occurs in clusters within the pyramids and corticomedullary areas **(Fig. 3.4)**. CT reveals hyperdensity within the medulla. Ultrasonography is a sensitive modality to detect early nephrocalcinosis. Cortical as well as medullary nephrocalcinosis suggests primary hyperoxaluria **(Figs. 3.22A and B)**.

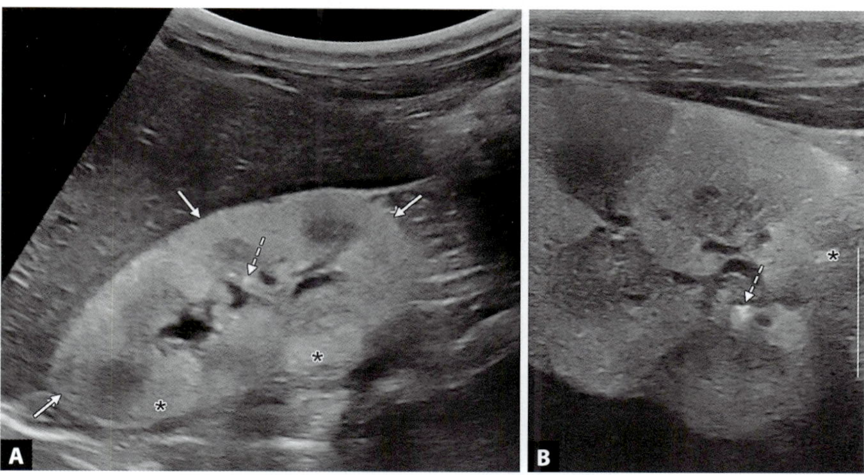

Figs. 3.22A and B: Primary hyperoxaluria. (A) Ultrasonography shows increased echogenicity of renal cortex (arrows) with densely echogenic foci of nephrocalcinosis in both cortices (asterisks) and medulla (dotted arrow); (B) High-resolution ultrasonography shows similar dense echogenic foci in cortex (asterisk) and medulla (dotted arrow)

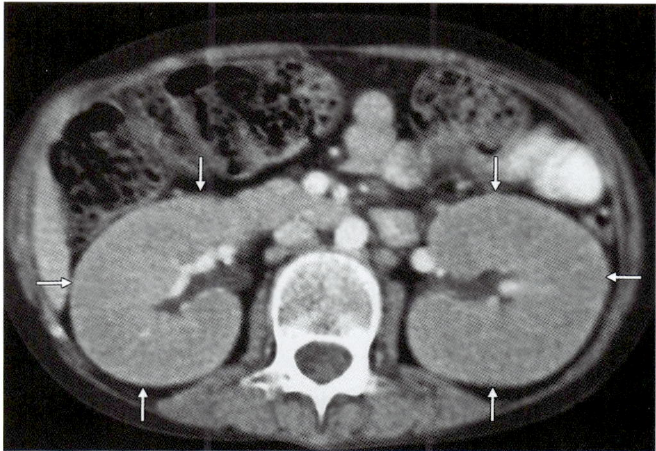

Fig. 3.23: Leukemic involvement of kidneys. Axial contrast-enhanced computed tomography of abdomen reveals bilateral enlarged "faceless" kidneys (arrows) with loss of corticomedullary differentiation

Renal Involvement in Malignancies

Kidney involvement in leukemia can present with diffusely enlarged kidneys with increased echogenicity on ultrasonography. The leukemic deposits appear as focal hypodense lesions on contrast-enhanced CT **(Fig. 3.23)**.

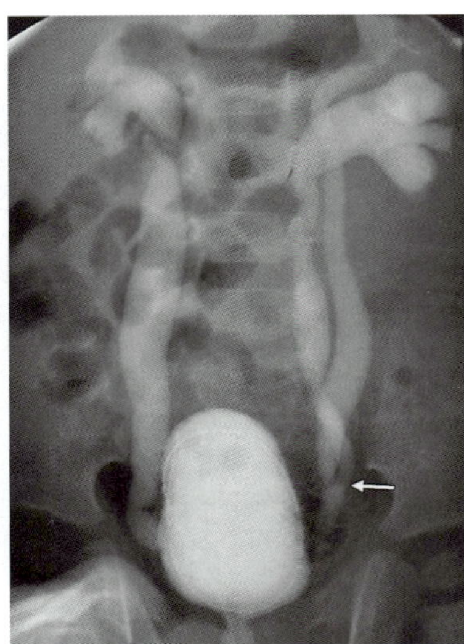

Fig. 3.24: Duplicated ureter. Micturating cystourethrogram image showing bilateral grade 4 vesicoureteric reflux and left-sided partial ureteric duplication joining at the level of distal ureters in hemipelvis (arrow)

Ureters

Ureteric Duplication

These vary from the simple bifid renal pelvis to complete ureteric duplication. The anomaly is of no significance unless associated with ectopic opening of the ureter. Ultrasonography in combination with an appropriate contrast study is necessary for the diagnosis **(Fig. 3.24)**. MR urography is a safe alternative for anatomic delineation of the pelvicalyceal system and ureter, but does not provide functional information.

Ureterocele

A simple ureterocele is usually an incidental finding in an apparently normal child. The characteristic finding on excretory urography is the "cobra head" appearance of the dilated distal ureter **(Figs. 3.25A to C)**. Ectopic ureterocele, on the other hand, is usually seen in symptomatic children. These are commonly associated with ureteral duplication, with the upper moiety opening into the ectopic ureterocele.

Ureteric Obstruction

It may be caused by calculus, stricture, neoplasm, an overlying vessel, or a retroperitoneal or pelvic mass with secondary obstruction of the ureter. A combination of imaging investigations is required to define the exact site and the cause of obstruction.

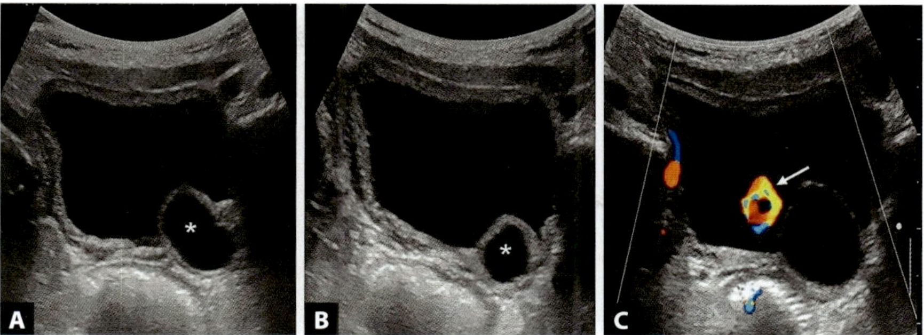

Figs. 3.25A to C: Intravesical ureterocele. (A and B) Dilated ballooned out intravesical part of left ureter (asterisk), showing change in shape with peristalsis. Note the ureteric jet on color Doppler (C) at the tip of the ureterocele, indicating the position of the vesicoureteric junction (arrow)

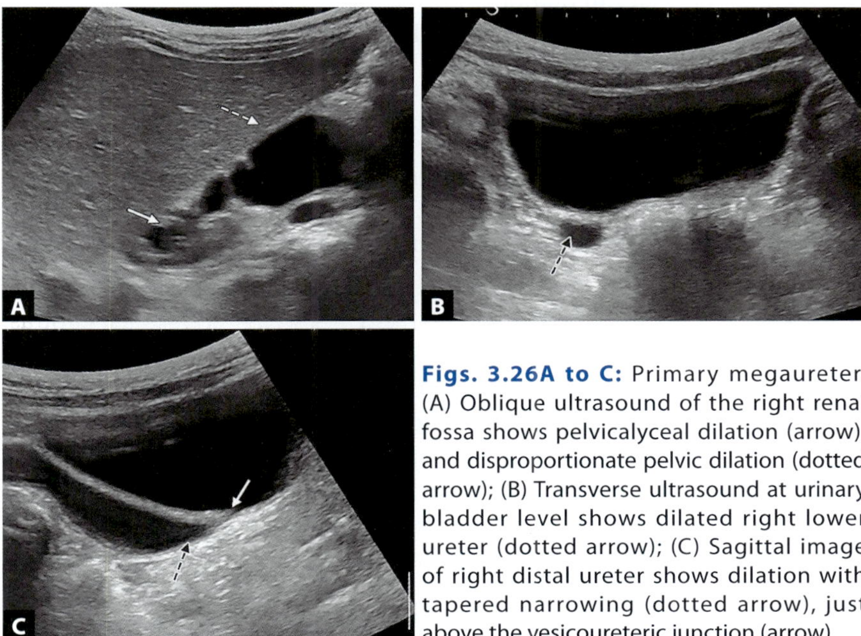

Figs. 3.26A to C: Primary megaureter. (A) Oblique ultrasound of the right renal fossa shows pelvicalyceal dilation (arrow), and disproportionate pelvic dilation (dotted arrow); (B) Transverse ultrasound at urinary bladder level shows dilated right lower ureter (dotted arrow); (C) Sagittal image of right distal ureter shows dilation with tapered narrowing (dotted arrow), just above the vesicoureteric junction (arrow)

Ureterovesical Junction Obstruction

Primary obstruction at this site is usually due to an aperistaltic segment, producing a megaureter **(Figs. 3.26A to C)**. While ultrasonography is useful in detecting this segment on real time scanning, very short segments may be missed and contrast studies are required. Other causes of obstruction at this site include calculus and stricture.

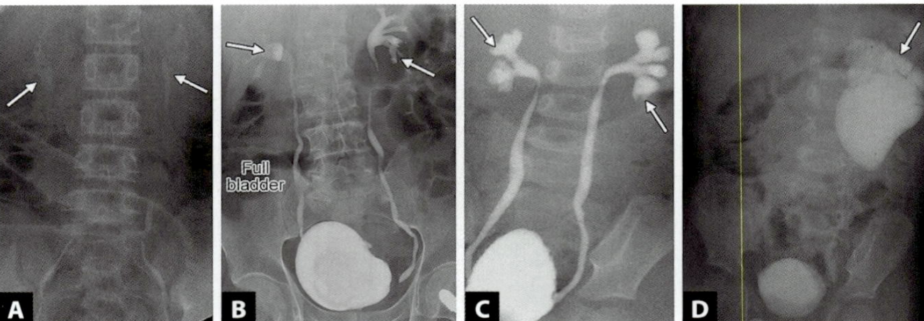

Figs. 3.27A to D: Grading of vesicoureteric reflux (VUR) on micturating cystourethrogram. (A) Bilateral grade 2 VUR (arrows); (B) Bilateral grade 3 VUR (arrows); (C) Bilateral grade 4 VUR (arrows); (D) Left-sided grade 5 VUR (arrow)

Vesicoureteric Reflux

An MCU is necessary to demonstrate VUR and examine the bladder neck and urethra. A standard international system of grading of VUR is used **(Figs. 3.27A to D)**.

Urinary Bladder

Conditions are grouped into congenital (diverticulum), inflammatory (cystitis), neoplastic, traumatic (tear), neurogenic bladder, and calculus. Although ultrasonography is an excellent modality, contrast studies are often required.

Urethra

Posterior urethral valves are an important anomaly, best diagnosed by micturating cystourethrography, which also detects VUR, bladder neck hypertrophy, and severity of outflow obstruction. Spinal dysraphism and prune-belly syndrome **(Figs. 3.28A and B)** may be characterized by detrusor-sphincter dyssynergia that results in functional obstruction. Outflow obstruction may also be due to anterior urethral diverticulum **(Fig. 3.29)**, urethral stricture, and meatal stenosis.

RISKS OF DIAGNOSTIC IMAGING

Radiation Risk

Imaging modalities carry the risk of exposure to ionizing radiation **(Table 3.5)**. While the new generation scanners have means of radiation dose reduction, the basics of radiation protection lies in judicious use of these investigations. Whenever possible, alternative nonionizing radiation modalities such as US or MRI should be substituted. Scan time and irradiated area should be kept to the minimum; use of fluoroscopy is also preferred.

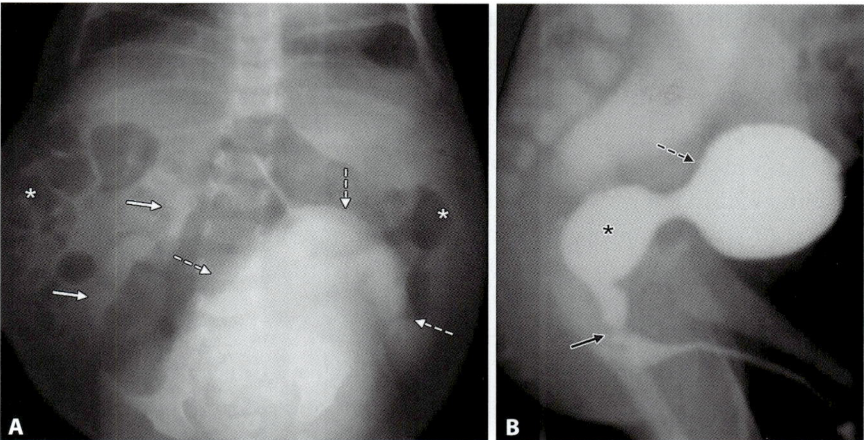

Figs. 3.28A and B: (A) Prune belly syndrome. Micturating cystourethrogram (MCU) shows lateral flank bulges (asterisks), elongated urinary bladder (dotted arrows) and grade 5 reflux into dilated and tortuous right ureter (arrows); (B) MCU shows a "drooping" urinary bladder (dotted arrow), dilated posterior urethra (asterisk), and tapered narrowing at level of membranous urethra (arrow)

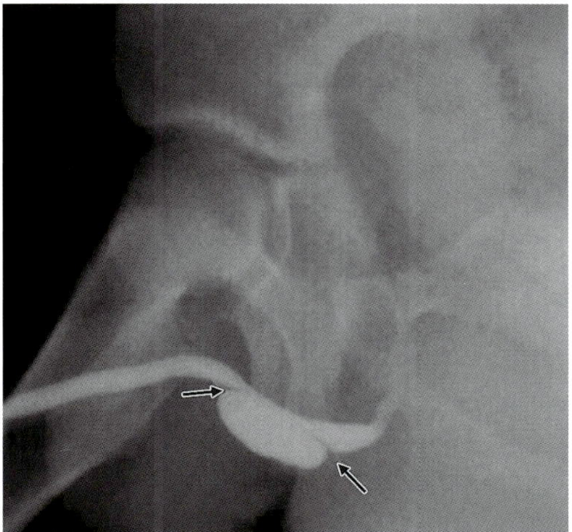

Fig. 3.29: Anterior urethral diverticulum. Retrograde urethrogram showing ventral outpouching with acute angulation with the urethra (arrows)

TABLE 3.5: Radiation risk in different investigations

Imaging modality	*Effective radiation dose*
Chest radiograph	0.02 mSv
Excretory urography	1–2 mSv
Micturating cystourethrography	2–2.5 mSv
CT abdomen (single phase)	3–8 mSv
Digital subtraction angiography	Varies with the scan time

Contrast-induced Kidney Injury

Another risk associated with IVP/CECT is contrast-associated kidney injury/ contrast-induced nephropathy (CA-AKI or CIN). It is defined as a rise in serum creatinine by 0.5 mg/dL or 25%, 2–5 days after contrast injection. KDIGO guidelines have defined CA-AKI as a rise in creatinine by ≥50% from baseline within 7 days after contrast exposure, or ≥0.3 mg/dL from baseline within 48-h after contrast exposure. Measurement of creatinine alone as a marker of kidney function is not as straightforward in children and neonates, as in adults.

The CIN is reported to be associated with a baseline reduced renal function. Its etiology is multifactorial; direct cytotoxicity by iodinated contrast media and sympathetic vasoconstriction are some of the causative factors. High-osmolality contrast media (HOCM) are shown to have a greater association with CIN than low-osmolality contrast media (LOCM) or iso-osmolality contrast media (IOCM). The role of premedication with oral N-acetylcysteine for prevention of CIN is limited. Other than CIN, HOCM can be associated with volume shift and pulmonary edema, especially in neonates and small children. Warming the contrast media may reduce viscosity-associated adverse effects. While injecting iodinated contrast in a very small child, a balanced approach should be followed, so as to optimize image quality and safety.

Nephrogenic Systemic Fibrosis

Nephrogenic systemic fibrosis (NSF) is a multisystem disease affecting primarily the skin and subcutaneous tissue, where there is diffuse fibrosis associated with gadolinium-based contrast media exposure. Considered a potentially fatal disease, it was first described in 2000. Ionic gadolinium is deposited in the tissues, which leads to an inflammatory response and eventual fibrosis. Contractures may develop around the joints, along with skin tightening. Patients with CKD5 (eGFR <15 mL/min/1.73 m^2) and CKD4 (eGFR 15–29 mL/min/1.73 m^2) have a 1–7% chance of developing NSF after one or more exposures to group 1 contrast agents [gadodiamide (Omniscan), gadopentetate dimeglumine (Magnevist), and gadoversetamide (OptiMARK)]. These agents are associated with the highest risk of NSF. Hemodialysis has not shown any benefit in the prevention of NSF. Avoidance of gadolinium-based contrast agents in advanced CKD and substitution with safer alternatives [e.g., gadobenate dimeglumine (Multihance), and gadoteric acid (Dotarem)] are recommended to avoid this adverse effect.

There are myriads of conventional and advanced imaging modalities available at the disposal of pediatricians and radiologists to help diagnose various pathologies of the pediatric urinary tract. The clinicians must be aware of the advantages and drawbacks of these modalities for their efficient utilization, along with their associated risks due to the use of ionizing radiation and contrast agents.

BIBLIOGRAPHY

1. Alejandro MM, Wald R. Contrast-associated acute kidney injury. CJASN. 2020;15(9):1225-27.
2. Berrocal T, Lopez-Pereira P, Arjonilla A, et al. Anomalies of the distal ureter, bladder, and urethra in children: embryologic, radiologic and pathologic features. Radiographics. 2002;22:1139-64.
3. Berry M, Mukhopadhyay S, Chowdhury V, et al. Pediatric Radiology. New Delhi: Jaypee Brothers Medical Publishers; 2004.
4. De Groof J, Dachy A, Breysem L, et al. Cystic kidney diseases in children. Arch Pediatr. 2023;30(4):240-6.
5. Ferro F, Vezzali N, Comploj E, et al. Pediatric cystic diseases of the kidney. J Ultrasound. 2019;22(3):381-93.
6. Grobner T. Gadolinium: a specific trigger for the development of nephrogenic fibrosing dermopathy and nephrogenic systemic fibrosis? Nephrol Dial Transplant. 2006;21(4):1104-8.
7. Hiorns M. Imaging of the urinary tract: the role of CT and MRI. Pediatr Nephrol. 2011;26:59-68.
8. Sethi SK, Raina R, Koratala A, et al. Point-of-care ultrasound in pediatric nephrology. Pediatr Nephrol. 2023;38(6):1733-51.
9. Thomas CC, Jana M, Sinha A, et al. Ultrasound imaging of renal cysts in children. J Ultrasound Med. 2021;40(3):621-35.

Radionuclide Studies

Yogita Khandelwal, Nishikant Avinash Damle

Nuclear medicine plays a crucial role in the management of congenital and acquired conditions of the kidneys and urinary tract in children. The procedures are relatively noninvasive and provide functional assessment in a way that is not possible with structural imaging. Fasting or bowel preparation is not necessary. They have neither systemic toxic effect nor allergic reactions, with minimal absorbed radiation dose [2% of intravenous (IV) urography].

RENAL DYNAMIC IMAGING

Over the last half century, dynamic radionuclide renography has become an indispensable technique in the functional assessment and quantification of renal function and drainage.

Radiopharmaceuticals

Radiopharmaceuticals are cleared from kidneys via glomerular filtration or tubular secretion **(Table 4.1)**. Glomerular agents are used for glomerular filtration rate (GFR) estimation. Tubular agents have greater renal extraction and better kidney-to-background ratio, and are preferred agents for dynamic renal scintigraphy.

- Radiopharmaceuticals that are rapidly eliminated by the kidneys and thus enable evaluation of filtration and drainage function (renal dynamic scintigraphy) namely ^{99m}Technetium-diethylenetriamine pentaacetic acid (^{99m}Tc-DTPA), ^{99m}Technetium-mercaptoacetyltriglycine (^{99m}Tc-MAG3), and ^{99m}Technetium-L, L-ethylenedicysteine (^{99m}Tc-L,L-EC).

TABLE 4.1: Mechanism of renal pharmaceutical agents

Radiopharmaceuticals	*Mechanism*
^{99m}Tc-DTPA	Glomerular filtration (100%)
^{99m}Tc-MAG3	Tubular secretion (100%)
^{99m}Tc-L,L-EC	Tubular secretion (83%)
^{51}Cr-EDTA	Glomerular filtration (100%)

^{51}Cr-EDTA: chromium-51 labeled ethylenediamine tetraacetic acid; ^{99m}Tc-DTPA: ^{99m}Technetium-diethylenetriamine pentaacetic acid; ^{99m}Tc-L,L-EC: ^{99m}Technetium-L, L-ethylenedicysteine; ^{99m}Tc-MAG3: ^{99m}Technetium-mercaptoacetyltriglycine

- Other radiopharmaceuticals are either used exclusively for nonimaging clearance studies namely GFR [chromium-51 labeled ethylenediamine tetraacetic acid (^{51}Cr-EDTA)], or effective renal plasma flow (ERPF) [iodine 131 o-iodohippurate (^{131}I-OIH)] measurements, or for both purposes (^{99m}Tc-DTPA, ^{99m}Tc-MAG3, and ^{99m}Tc-L,L-EC).

Dose of Radiopharmaceuticals

The administered tracer activity to child depends on body weight (0.1 mCi/kg); a minimum dose of 0.5 mCi is given whether ^{99m}Tc-DTPA, MAG3, or LL-EC is used.

Protocol and Procedure

Patient preparation: Ensure good hydration, void bladder before injection, catheterization in patients with increased frequency of micturition, and percutaneous nephrostomy (PCN) clamping.

Protocol: Posterior view (routine) and anterior view (for transplant), and both (ectopic kidneys). Diuretic protocol: Furosemide can be given 15 minutes prior to radiotracer (F-15), with the radiotracer (F0), or 10 minutes after radiotracer injection (F+10). Most common is F0 protocol.

Image acquisition: Blood flow: 1–2 seconds/frame for 60 seconds; dynamic uptake and excretion: 30 seconds/frame for remaining 20 minutes; and static images (prevoid/postvoid and delayed).

Image processing: Draw region of interest (ROI), generate time activity curve (TAC), differential renal function, and GFR/ERPF calculation.

Renogram

A renogram is a TAC that provides a graphical representation of the uptake and elimination of a radiopharmaceutical by the kidneys. The tracer is injected as a bolus and data collection starts immediately and recorded for 20–30 minutes after injection kidneys, background and aorta/iliac vessel. The computer reconstructs the renogram by placing the ROI over the kidneys. Renogram has a characteristic shape and may be considered as having three distinct phases **(Figs. 4.1A to C)**.

1. *Initial blood flow:* The first phase, or the vascular transit phase represents the initial arrival of tracer in kidney. It provides an accurate assessment of renal perfusion. The renal activity during this phase equals or exceeds aorta and should be relatively symmetrical in bilateral kidneys.
2. *Cortical uptake phase:* The second phase or the tubular concentration phase corresponds to the radionuclide taken up by the kidneys and represents the peak of the curve. In a well-hydrated subject, the time to reach the peak lasts approximately 3–5 minutes after the injection.

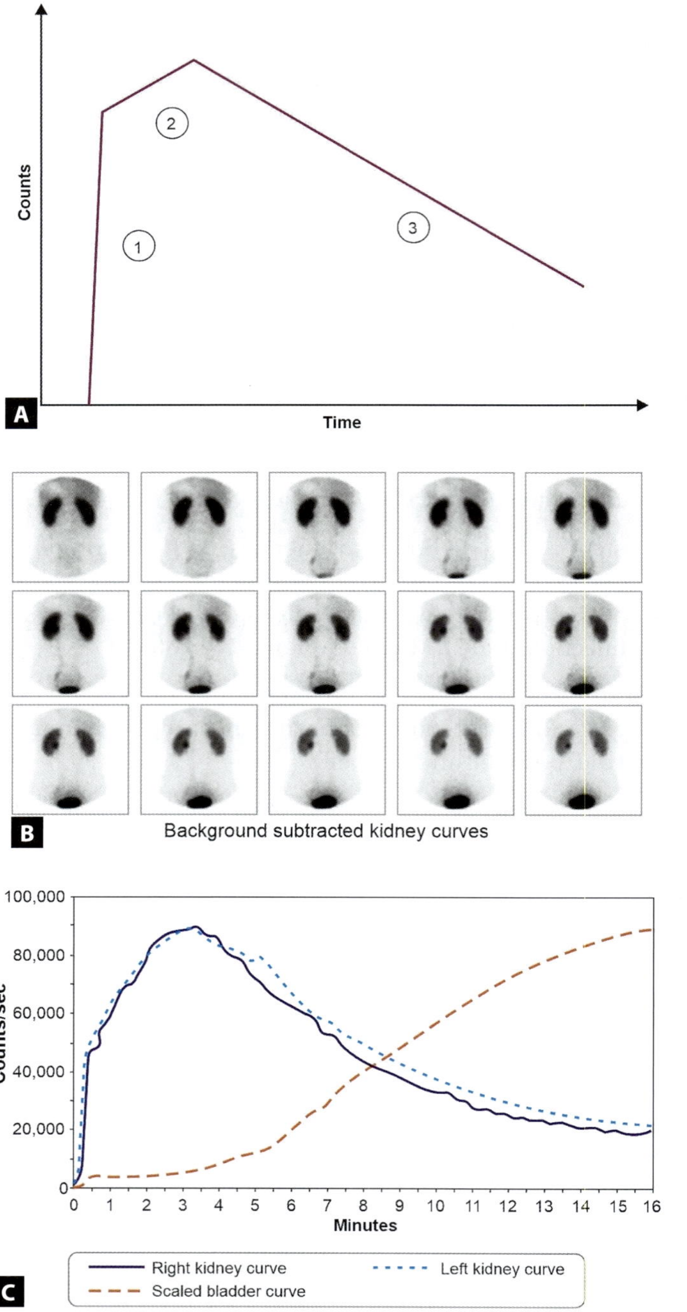

Figs. 4.1A to C: (A) Normal renogram curve divided into three phases; (B) Normal dynamic functional images with prompt symmetrical radiotracer uptake and rapid clearance from the study; (C) Normal ^{99m}Technetium-L, L-ethylenedicysteine (^{99m}Tc-L,L-EC) renogram

3. *Clearance phase:* The third phase or excretion phase is the period of declining amplitude after the peak. The beginning of this phase corresponds to the time at which activity starts moving away from the ROI and shows clearance from the collecting system. The excretory phase normally begins 5 minutes after injection and approaches the baseline about 20 minutes after the injection. It is measured in terms of half-time ($t_{1/2}$), i.e., the time taken for the counts to decline to one-half of the maximum count rate.

Interventions During Renogram

Diuretic renogram: It evaluates both renal function (obstructive uropathy) and urodynamics (hydronephrosis) in single test. By increasing urine flow using a diuretic (such as furosemide), it helps to differentiate obstructive dilatation from nonobstructive dilatation of the upper urinary tract. The increasing pressure in the renal pelvis overcomes the functional obstruction, thus allowing prompt clearing of the radionuclide.

Captopril renogram: Angiotensin-converting enzyme inhibitors (ACEI) renography is useful for diagnosis of reversible renovascular hypertension (RVH). Patients with RVH show a decline in GFR and renal clearance following administrates of ACEI.

Glomerular Filtration Rate

Glomerular filtration rate (GFR) is one the most useful parameter of renal function, and is the sum of filtration rates in each of the functioning nephrons. GFR is measured indirectly through clearance. The clearance of a substance refers to the volume of plasma that is cleared of that substance per unit of time by renal excretion. This is calculated by dividing the excretion rate of a substance by its plasma concentration:

$$\text{Clearance} = (Ux)\, V/(Px)$$

Where, (Ux) = urine concentrations of the substance x

(Px) = plasma concentrations of the substance x

V = urine flow rate (mL/min).

When the substance is freely filtered and not protein-bound, and is not reabsorbed, secreted, or metabolized by the kidney, then its clearance is similar to the GFR. Inulin clearance is the "gold standard" for determination of GFR, but is cumbersome to perform and requires a steady state concentration of inulin. ^{99m}Tc-DTPA is the preferred radionuclide agent because it is inexpensive, easily available, and renal imaging can be simultaneously performed.

The GFR can be estimated either by plasma clearance (plasma sampling method) or upon the tracer uptake by the kidneys (camera method).

Plasma sample radionuclide clearances allow early renal impairment detection and an accurate estimation of hyperfiltration. Among the plasma clearance techniques, single-compartment models require 1–2 blood samples and multi compartment models require multiple blood samples. In adults, external counting procedures that do not require blood samples have become popular because of their simplicity. Camera-based methods are not standardized for children and usually underestimate GFR, thus plasma sample method is recommended. Plasma sampling method has its own limitation including the risk of technical errors.

GFR varies according to age, sex, and body size. Kidneys of newborns and young infants have several functional limitations, including a relatively low GFR. The GFR increases from 13 to 15 mL/min/1.73 m^2 in the premature infant, to 15–60 mL/min/1.73 m^2 in the full-term infant, to 63–80 mL/min/1.73 m^2 at 8 weeks of life. GFR, when corrected for BSA, reaches adult values between 12 and 18 months of age. Tubular functions of the kidney gradually mature with an increase in GFR and reach adult levels by 1–2 years of life.

Pitfalls in Newborn

Renal uptake of dynamic tracers may be lower in newborns than in older children with slower intrarenal transit time and excretion of these tracers. A normal dynamic radionuclide study in newborns during the first or second week of life may demonstrate the tracer's faint, delayed renal uptake with or without appearance in the bladder at the expected times. There may be low plasma clearance of the tracer causing background to be higher throughout the study. Normal newborns may show a relatively low kidney/background ratio in ^{99m}Technetium dimercaptosuccinic acid (^{99m}Tc-DMSA) scan.

Indications for DTPA Renography

- Evaluates hydronephrosis, and for renal obstruction
- Measure differential kidney function
- Estimate GFR and ERPF
- Evaluate for renovascular hypertension

RENAL CORTICAL IMAGING

Renal cortical imaging is a diagnostic scan that assesses the function, size, shape, position, homogeneity, and intensity of tracer uptake in the kidneys. It is considered the gold standard for imaging of the renal parenchyma, especially for renal scarring and acute pyelonephritis. It also offers a method to monitor differential kidney function and evaluate regional kidney function with high sensitivity for detecting cortical defects.

Radiopharmaceutical

^{99m}Tc-Dimercaptosuccinic acid is filtered by the glomerulus and accumulates in the epithelial cells of proximal convoluted tubules *via* megalin/cubulin-mediated endocytosis.

Protocol and Procedure

Dose: ^{99m}Tc-DMSA is administered at a dose of 0.04–0.05 mCi/kg (minimum 0.06 mCi).

Patient preparation: Clinical history with date of most recent infection noted. Patient should void before imaging.

Protocol: After IV injection, delayed static imaging is done after 2–3 hr. Both anterior and posterior view are acquired for differential function. Single photon emission computed tomography (SPECT)/computed tomography (CT) help provide additional information.

Indications

- *Congenital/structural renal abnormalities:* Ectopic kidney, horseshoe kidney, agenesis, dysplastic or multicystic kidney
- Acute pyelonephritis and follow-up; cortical scars in patients with vesicoureteric reflux (VUR), recurrent urinary tract infection (UTI)
- Calculation of differential renal function
- Characterization of renal masses

Image Interpretation

The ^{99m}Tc-DMSA scintigraphy is useful to identify the degree of renal damage and to assess recovery and/or residual renal damage. The high sensitivity of DMSA scintigraphy for early diagnosis and localization of pyelonephritis (sensitivity 90–96% and specificity 95–98%) is well established. Similarly, this imaging is the most sensitive technique for detecting renal scars **(Fig. 4.2)**.

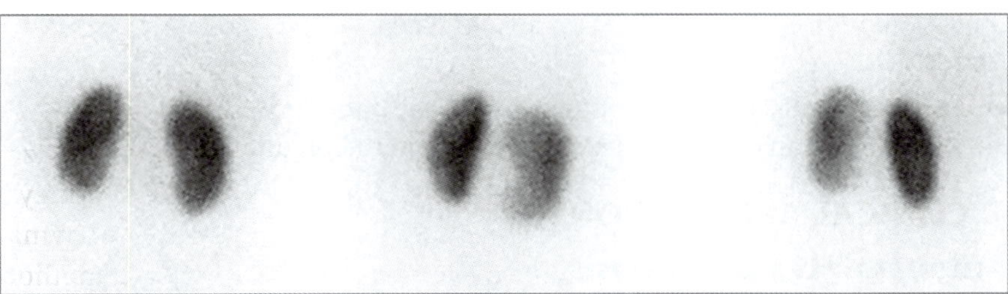

Fig. 4.2: Normal dimercaptosuccinic acid (DMSA) scintigraphy in a 12-year-old boy with posterior urethral valves (PUV), following fulguration

Classification of renal scars according to DMSA scan (Snellen classification):

- No more than two scarred areas
- More than two scars with some areas of normal parenchyma in between
- Generalized damage to whole kidney
- End-stage shrunken kidney; little or no uptake on DMSA scintigraphy (<10% overall function)

RADIONUCLIDE CYSTOGRAPHY

Radionuclide cystography (RCG) is a satisfactory investigation for the diagnosis and follow-up of patients with VUR. Advantages of RCG include low gonadal radiation exposure [100–200 times less than with micturating cystourethrogram], high temporal resolution, and high sensitivity for detection of patients with VUR. However, RCG cannot delineate anatomy of the bladder and urethra. Two types of RCG are described, direct and indirect. Direct radionuclide cystography (DRCG) is done commonly. Indirect radionuclide cystography (IRCG) does not require bladder catheterization or suprapubic puncture and is done following IV injection of the radiopharmaceutical (such as ^{99m}Tc-DTPA/MAG3/LL-EC), followed by voiding films.

Radiopharmaceutical

DRCG requires filling of the radionuclide (mostly ^{99m}Tc-sulfur colloid) into the urinary bladder either by catheterization or directly by suprapubic puncture till maximum distension of the bladder.

Protocol and Procedure

Dose: ^{99m}Tc-sulfur colloid dose is 0.25–0.5 mCi in infants, and 0.5–1.0 mCi in children.

Protocol: Patient lies supine under the gamma camera and bladder is filled till maximum capacity; static prevoid image is taken. Patient is asked to void and dynamic scan is taken 2 seconds/frame for 120 seconds, followed by a static postvoid image.

Indications

- Initial diagnosis of VUR; follow-up of these patients
- Quantification of postvoid residual urine in the bladder

CLINICAL APPLICATIONS

Antenatal Hydronephrosis

It is most frequently diagnosed abnormality in prenatal ultrasound. Spontaneous resolution occurs in 50% of cases with mild hydronephrosis.

Hydronephrosis is one of the chief indications for radionuclide evaluation of the kidneys in children. It enables serial monitoring of function of individual kidneys. It is safer to follow neonatal hydronephrosis nonoperatively till there is clear evidence of obstruction. The first renal scintigraphy should be done between 4–6 weeks of age.

Decreased split function at the initial assessment or functional loss in serial studies is often used as an indication for surgery. However, none of the available diagnostic parameters including the degree of hydronephrosis, level of initial functional impairment, and the washout pattern are accurate enough to predict which child will benefit from surgical intervention. Impaired cortical transit of tracer with the absence of activity in subcortical structures of the kidney within 3 minutes of tracer injection predicts risk of deterioration. The combination of ultrasound and diuretic renography provides, the necessary anatomic and functional information needed for management **(Fig. 4.3)**.

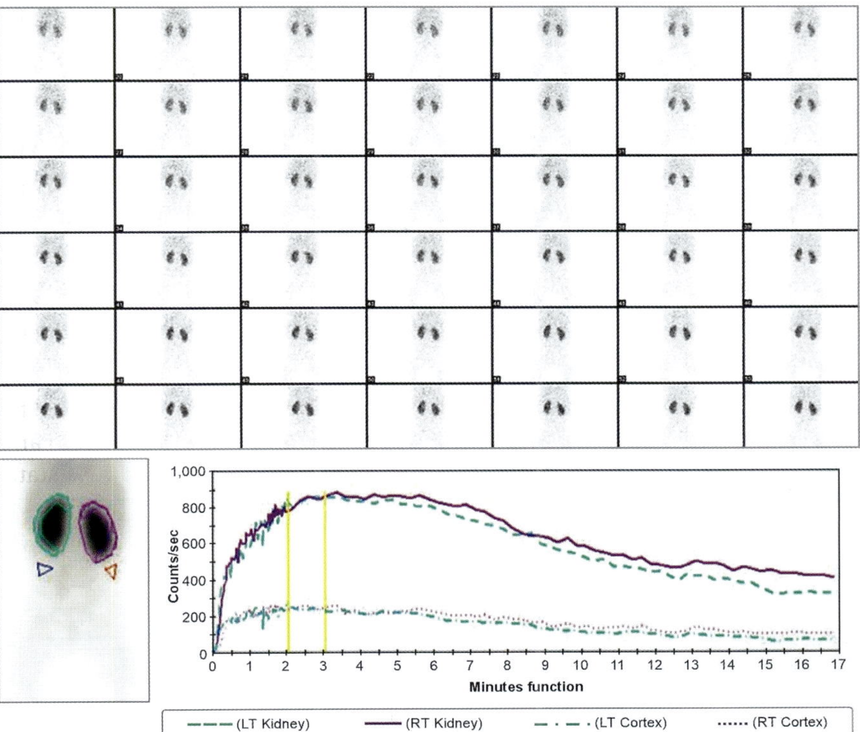

Fig. 4.3: A 1-year-old boy with bilateral antenatal hydronephrosis. On follow-up, renal dynamic scintigraphy, planar and renogram curve shows bilateral kidneys with normal function and drainage. LT: left; RT: right

Obstructive Uropathy

Obstruction of the urinary tract can lead to recurrent infection, progressive loss of nephrons, diminished function, and parenchymal atrophy. Diuretic renography is indicated, especially to differentiate it from nonobstructed dilatation.

In dynamic studies, the hydronephrotic kidney initially appears as a rim of tracer concentration in the renal parenchyma surrounding an area devoid of tracer, corresponding to the renal pelvis and collecting system. The size of the photon-deficient area depends on the degree of dilatation and the position of the pelvis in relation to the cortex (intrarenal vs. extrarenal). As the study progresses, the pelvicalyceal system begins to fill with radiotracer as it leaves the renal parenchyma. The rate of appearance of the tracer in the pelvicalyceal system depends on the function of the hydronephrotic kidney. Depending on the severity and duration of the obstruction, tracer may begin to accumulate in the renal pelvis within 3–6 minutes despite severe dilatation; however, this may be slower with prolonged severe obstruction **(Fig. 4.4)**.

It has been suggested that in preoperative patients in whom the cortical time-activity curves appear more nearly normal than the total kidney curve, there is a strong likelihood of improvement after the obstruction is relieved. Conversely, abnormal cortical curves may be associated with a poor prognosis for functional improvement. In some cases, it is possible to identify the site of obstruction at the ureterovesical junction or pelviureteric junction.

Differentiating obstructed from dilated nonobstructed systems is done by imaging after IV injection of furosemide (diuretic renography). The loop diuretic furosemide inhibits sodium and chloride resorption, markedly

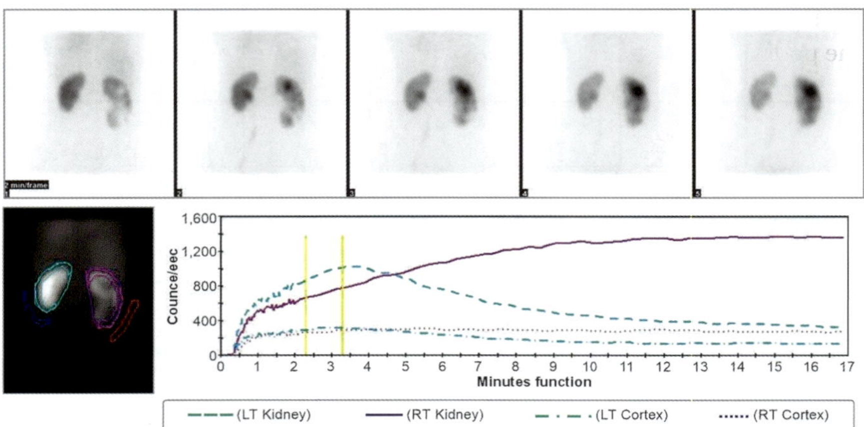

Fig. 4.4: A 14-year-old boy with right grade III hydronephrosis showing normal functioning left kidney with normal drainage and right hydronephrotic kidney with obstructive drainage on ^{99m}Technetium-L, L-ethylenedicysteine (^{99m}Tc-LL-EC) renogram. LT: left; RT: right

increasing dilute urine flow, and renal washout. If mechanical obstruction is present, prolonged retention of the tracer is seen. While a nonobstructive washout pattern ($t_{1/2}$ <10 minutes) rules out obstruction, an obstructive washout pattern is sometimes false positive. In such cases, even a split function of >40% on the hydronephrotic side may be inadequate to rule out obstruction and therefore serial monitoring of the affected kidney function is necessary **(Fig. 4.4)**. Therefore, single study might not have prognostic value, and serial studies provide a better indication of the natural progression of hydronephrosis and screen for presence of obstruction.

Congenital Urinary Tract Anomalies

Early diagnosis of congenital urinary tract anomalies is of considerable significance in order to preserve kidney function and to prevent complications such as infection, obstructive uropathy, and calculus formation. In the evaluation of neonatal abdominal masses, ultrasound is the initial study recommended. It can differentiate renal from extrarenal masses. Once the mass is identified to be arising from kidney, radionuclide studies are used for assessing the functional status. The possible causes for neonatal renal masses are congenital hydronephrosis, multicystic kidney disease, infantile polycystic kidneys, renal vein thrombosis, or mesoblastic nephroma. Whenever serial monitoring of renal function is required, e.g., following surgery, evaluation in posterior urethral valves, exstrophy bladder, and other congenital anomalies, radionuclide studies are useful because they show both absolute and split renal function. Symptomatic mobile kidney, ectopic kidneys **(Figs. 4.5 and 4.6)** and horseshoe-shaped kidneys can be diagnosed by radionuclide studies.

Dysplastic kidneys are more prone to infection and scarring. Ultrasound is the preferred method for assessing morphological abnormalities, but DMSA

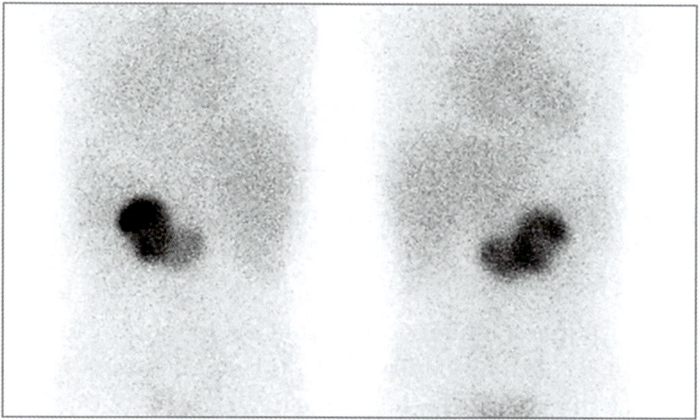

Fig. 4.5: ^{99m}Technetium dimercaptosuccinic acid (^{99m}Tc-DMSA) scan showing crossed fused renal ectopia

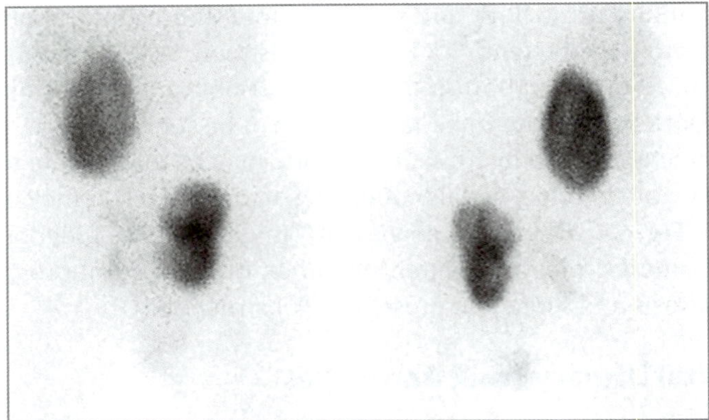

Fig. 4.6: A 14-year-old girl showing left ectopic kidney ^{99m}Technetium dimercaptosuccinic acid (^{99m}Tc-DMSA) renal scan (anterior and posterior views) with normal functioning right kidney

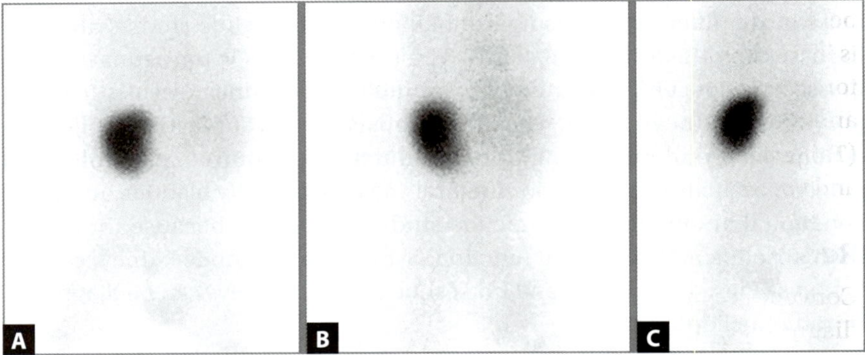

Figs. 4.7A to C: ^{99m}Technetium dimercaptosuccinic acid (^{99m}Tc-DMSA) left renal scan (posterior, right posterior oblique, and left posterior oblique) showing right multicystic dysplastic kidney with no function in a 1-month-old boy. Left kidney shows normal morphology and function

scintigraphy is required to assess their function. A dysplastic kidney is typically asymmetrically smaller and has substantially decreased, inhomogeneous, or absent uptake. Radiotracer uptake is completely absent in congenital multicystic dysplastic kidney **(Figs. 4.7A to C)**.

Urinary Tract Infection

Various expert groups have recommended evaluation of urinary tract in all children with UTI. An abdominal USG is recommended to evaluate the structure of the kidneys and bladder once the diagnosis of UTI is confirmed. A MCUG is done to look for VUR. Imaging (ultrasonography and DMSA scans) aids differentiation between upper or lower UTI, evaluates renal involvement, enables detection of associated urinary tract malformation, and allows recognition of atypical disease. If the infection is diagnosed early and treated effectively, the abnormalities in renal cortical function found in acute pyelonephritis may resolve without scarring. ^{99m}Tc-DMSA is helpful in the diagnosis of acute pyelonephritis, especially in newborns and young children, because clinical signs and symptoms can be nonspecific and is associated with lower radiation dose and contrast injection risks.

^{99m}Tc-DMSA scintigraphy is the method of choice in monitoring for complications of acute pyelonephritis. The cortical abnormalities persist as renal scarring, roughly 6 months following acute infection. Approximately 50–90% of children with febrile UTI have a cortical defect on the DMSA scan **(Figs. 4.8A to C)**.

Vesicoureteric Reflux

Micturating cystourethrography provides excellent anatomic details of the bladder and the urethra and in patients with reflux outlines the anatomy of the pelvicalyceal systems, the ureters, and their insertion into the bladder. DRCG is in most cases a stress test of the ureterovesical junction. DRCG is indicated for evaluation of VUR following medical and/or surgical management and serial evaluation of bladder dysfunction (e.g., neurogenic bladder) **(Table 4.2)**. VUR may be present intermittently or during most of the filling and voiding phases of the radionuclide cystogram **(Figs. 4.9A to C)**.

Renovascular Hypertension

Conventional radionuclide studies are not reliable screening tests for the diagnosis of renovascular hypertension, particularly in the presence of

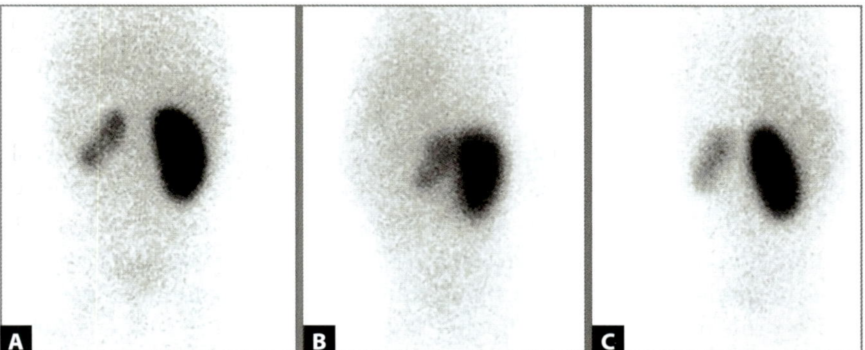

Figs. 4.8A to C: ^{99m}Technetium dimercaptosuccinic acid (^{99m}Tc-DMSA) renal scan (posterior, left posterior oblique, and right posterior oblique) of a 1-year-old girl with history of recurrent urinary tract infection (UTI) showing small right kidney with irregular cortical margins suggestive of scarring. Left kidney with normal morphology and function

TABLE 4.2: Interpretation of direct radionuclide cystography (DRCG)

DRCG reflux grade	*Radiological grade*	*Reflux level*
A	I	Ureter
B	II–III	Pelvis
C	IV–V	Pelvis with dilatation

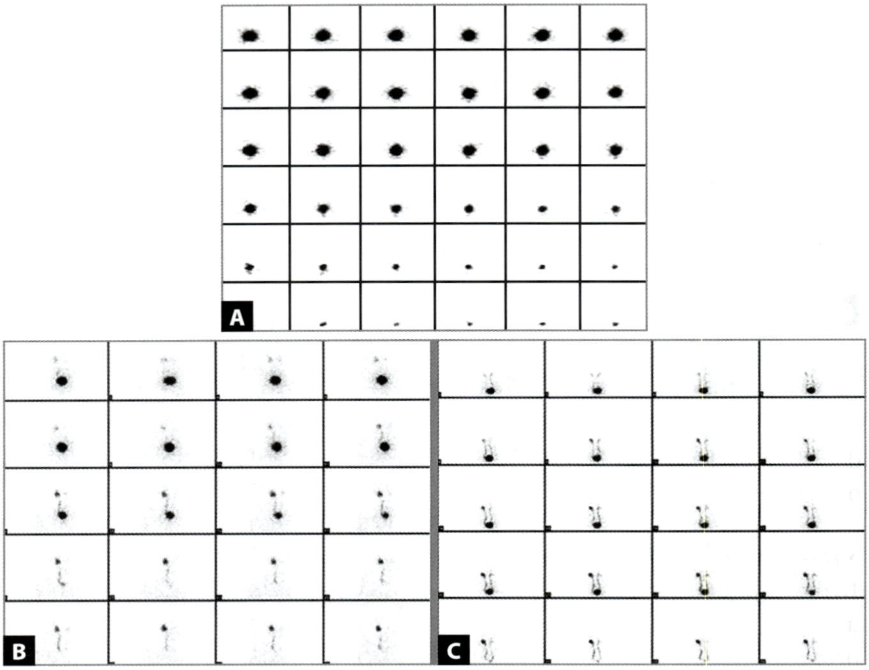

Figs. 4.9A to C: Direct radionuclide cystography (DRCG). (A) Normal DRCG study showing no vesicoureteric reflux during voiding; (B) A 7-year-old boy with grade C right vesicoureteric reflux (VUR); (C) A 6-year-old boy with grade C right VUR and grade B left VUR

bilateral or segmental renal artery stenosis. The efficacy of renal scan for the diagnosis of renovascular hypertension is improved by the use of ACEI.

The ACEI such as captopril, block the formation of angiotensin II, resulting in dilatation of the efferent arterioles and a decrease in the transcapillary pressure gradient. This led to a significant decrease in net filtration pressure and a drop in GFR of the affected kidney, proving the hemodynamic significance of renal artery stenosis. The effect of an ACEI on renal study manifests at varying degrees of decreased extraction of the tracer and delayed visualization of the collecting system **(Figs. 4.10A and B)**, whereas with the use of tubular agents, prolonged retention of the tracer is seen. Because it is easier to detect cortical retention of tracer than it is to appreciate its focal

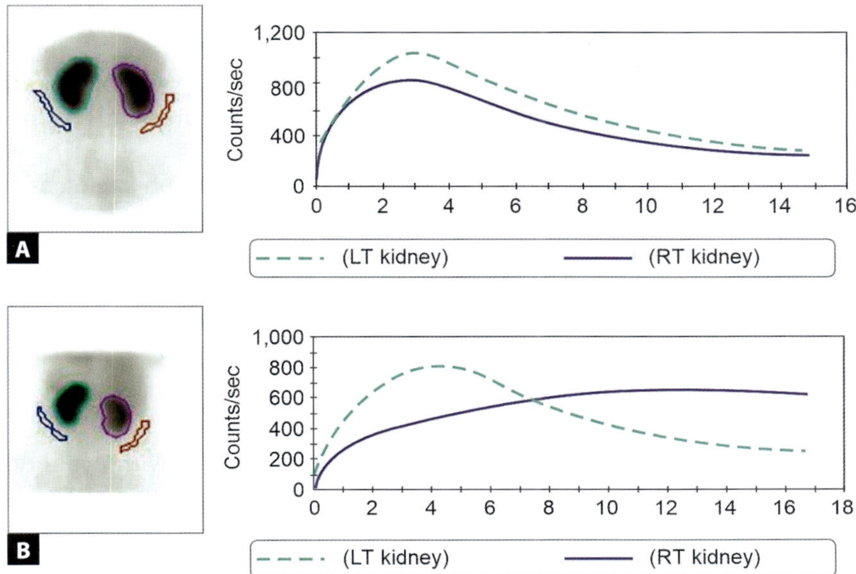

Figs. 4.10A and B: (A) Baseline renogram and (B) Captopril renogram. Captopril renogram shows worsening of renal function in RT kidney. LT: left; RT: right

decreased extraction, MAG3 may be more useful than DTPA for the detection of segmental renal artery stenosis.

Ideally, a baseline study is obtained followed by a repeat examination either 1 hr after oral administration of captopril (1 mg/kg, up to 50 mg) or 10 minutes after an IV injection of enalapril (0.03 mg/kg). Findings include an increase in the differential renal uptake, an increase in cortical transit time, a prolongation of time to peak, and retention of tracer in the renal parenchyma.

With tubular agents, in comparison to the baseline study, unilateral prolonged parenchymal retention after ACEI in the absence of outflow tract obstruction is a high probability for RVH (>90%). In this group of patients, the degree of narrowing of the renal artery is between 70 and 95%. However, a rising renogram is seen even on baseline in patients with >95% renal artery stenosis with sufficient collaterals. Upon captopril administration, function may or may not change. With glomerular agents such as Tc-DTPA, a reduction of relative uptake or absolute individual kidney GFR of >10% indicates a high probability of RVH. However, ACEI-induced changes of relative renal uptake of 5–9% are considered as intermediate probability. Scintigraphic abnormalities in unilateral renal artery stenosis can be appreciated visually by inspecting the images and the renal time-activity curves. In the presence of bilateral renal artery stenosis, narrowing is usually asymmetrical, as is the effect of captopril on each kidney.

It is necessary to distinguish between renal artery stenosis demonstrated by angiography and renovascular hypertension demonstrated by captopril renography. Captopril renography is useful for predicting the patients who are likely to derive benefit from revascularization. In patients with renal artery stenosis, hypertension mediated by renin angiotensin system is cured by revascularization whereas hypertension due to other mechanisms are unaffected by surgery.

Recent studies of new radiopharmaceuticals have focused on angiotensin receptors. The angiotensin II subtype 1 receptor (AT1R) has been linked to the development and progression of renovascular hypertension. AT1R positron emission tomography (PET) measurements have been reported with the radioligand ATR1 C11-KR 31173, renin receptors, and vascular endothelial growth factor receptors.

Renal Infarction

Renal infarction is a rare event that can occur in patients with cyanotic congenital heart disease, polycythemia, atrial fibrillation, dehydration, or trauma. Aortic thrombus formation and renal infarction are also complications of prolonged umbilical artery catheterization. DMSA scintigraphy shows decreased or no tracer uptake, or at times focal perfusion defect(s) in the affected kidney(s).

Acute Kidney Injury

Although not used routinely, radionuclide studies might predict functional recovery in patients with acute kidney injury. Improvements in scintigraphic function precede biochemical changes by 1–2 days.

Kidney Transplantation

Multiple imaging modalities are used to evaluate the transplanted kidney. Radionuclide studies are useful after renal transplantation to assess surgical results and can detect and discriminate complications such as urinoma or lymphocele. They are carried out to assess graft perfusion and function and can detect rejection or recovery of function 24–48 hr before changes in the clinical course. The initial uptake in renal allografts with short cold and warm ischemic times is normal and occasionally more intense than in a normally functioning kidney. If diuresis is brisk, the intrarenal transit time is normal or faster. In the absence of complications, the tracers by the transplant become identical to those of normal kidneys.

There are three clinical settings in which imaging of the newly transplanted kidneys plays a role. First, if no significant function is noted immediately after transplantation, the possibilities are vascular occlusion (arterial or venous thrombosis), hyperacute rejection, and unusually severe prolonged acute tubular necrosis. In the former two conditions, there will be no visualization of the transplanted kidney in a renogram, but in the last condition, there is intense uptake in the kidney **(Fig. 4.11)**. Acute tubular necrosis is unusual in live-related renal transplants, but common with kidneys from deceased donors. If tracer activity within the transplant is similar to the background on the renal scan, it indicates severe depression of renal function, unlikely to recover from the injury. The second situation to consider in allograft imaging is when the allograft that was functioning well ceases to function suddenly. In addition to the above possibilities, cyclosporine toxicity and acute rejection **(Fig. 4.12)** have to be considered. The distinction is difficult unless serial studies are performed. Thirdly, an allograft with good function might develop a local complication.

A baseline evaluation of the transplant is obtained during the immediate postoperative period. These studies are performed to determine the adequacy

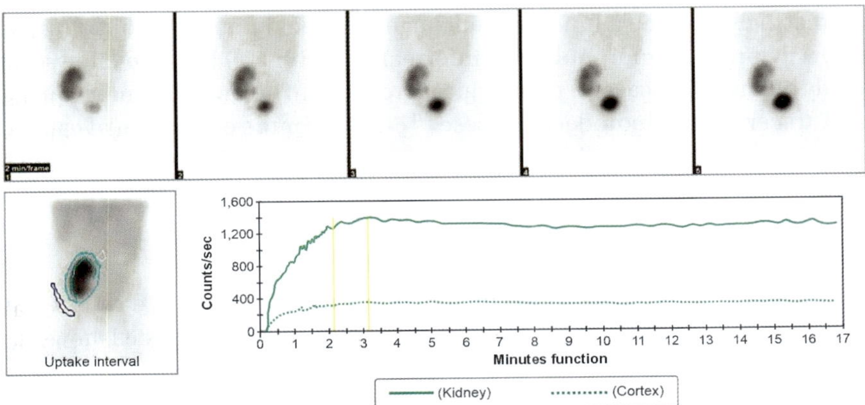

Fig. 4.11: Renal scintigraphy in patient with acute tubular necrosis after renal transplant

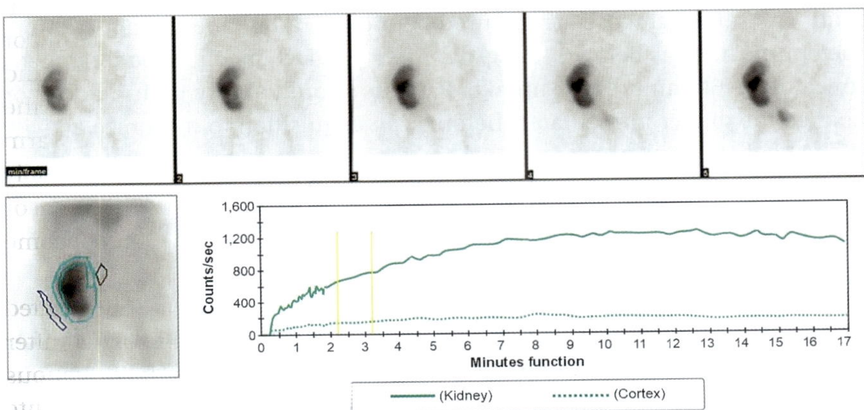

Fig. 4.12: Renal scintigraphy showing transplant kidney in right iliac fossa with early acute graft rejection

of perfusion of the graft and assess the graft function. Subsequent studies are performed depending on clinical progress. Time-to-peak activity, $t_{1/2}$ of the excretory phase of the renogram, bladder appearance time, aorta-to-kidney ratio, and kidney-to-background ratio are used in the evaluation of renal function. Several perfusion indices are obtained which differentiate between normal and impaired perfusion. The changes in ERPF and excretion index as a measure of urinary excretion help to differentiate between acute rejection, chronic rejection, acute tubular necrosis, and obstruction.

POSITRON EMISSION TOMOGRAPHY

Positron emission tomography imaging with specific tracers provides valuable insights into metabolic activity, inflammation, and neoplastic disorders within the kidneys. Since its introduction in clinical practice, PET/CT has increasingly become a fundamental diagnostic tool in pediatric oncology. It not only provides morphological information (with CT) but also allows the study of physiological and pathological processes. The most commonly used PET tracer is F-18 fluorodeoxyglucose (^{18}F-FDG) for the evaluation of cancer. ^{18}F-FDG permits metabolic assessment with quantitative and semiquantitative analysis helping to better characterize lesions and predict therapy outcome.

Patient Preparation and Precaution

Brief history should be taken at scheduling, and a minimum of 15 days interval between chemotherapy and 2–3 months of radiotherapy is suggested, however depending on clinical indication, an early PET/CT can be done. The patient should be able to lie still for approximately 30 minutes, hence at the time of scheduling appropriate measures need to be taken for sedation. Fasting is required for 4–6 hr before ^{18}F-FDG injection. Glucose-containing IV fluids and parenteral nutrition should be discontinued and replaced by saline IV fluid. The serum glucose is measured before the radiotracer administration, the optimal level is below 140 mg/dL. After ^{18}F-FDG injection, patient needs to wait for ~60 minutes for uptake. Patients should empty their bladder or change the diaper immediately before scan acquisition to minimize activity in the bladder.

The administered activity should be lowest possible dose. The recommended dose is 0.1 mCi/kg with minimum dose of 0.7 mCi.

Normal Physiological Uptake on ^{18}F-FDG PET/CT

Brain shows intense FDG uptake as it is an obligate glucose user. FDG is excreted via urine, therefore increased uptake is noted in kidneys, ureter, and bladder. Moderate activity is noted in liver, and spleen should be less intense than liver. Variable activity is noted in bowel, myocardium, thymus, salivary glands, tonsils, testes, and uterus. The major challenge in young patient is brown fat uptake noted in neck, supraclavicular, costovertebral junction, upper mediastinum, and suprarenal regions. A favorable approach to reduce brown fat uptake is to provide warm ambient temperature of the room or provide cold blanket during uptake phase. Premedication to reduce brown fat includes oral propranolol, IV fentanyl, or oral diazepam.

Clinical Applications

Wilms Tumor

Wilms tumor is the most frequent pediatric renal tumor occurring mostly in children <5 years old. The role of FDG-PET in Wilms tumor has not been well established. Various studies have explored its role in treatment response, identify recurrence, and evaluation of sites of extrarenal Wilms tumor.

Renal Cell Carcinoma

The peak incidence of renal cell carcinoma is between 9 and 15 years. Although the usefulness of FDG PET/CT in primary RCC remains unclear, it can be used for postoperative surveillance and restaging as an adjunct when conventional imaging is not conclusive.

Rhabdomyosarcoma

Rhabdomyosarcoma is the most common soft tissue sarcoma in children. They can occur anywhere in the body, the genitourinary tract is the second most common primary location. FDG PET/CT can be useful in staging, treatment response and restaging/relapse for patients affected by RMS **(Fig. 4.13)**. It is more sensitive for identifying nodal metastases.

Post-transplant Lymphoproliferative Disorder

The risk of post-transplant lymphoproliferative disorder (PTLD) is the highest in recipients of bowel grafts and lowest in recipients of kidney grafts. Diagnostic modalities such as X-ray, ultrasonography, CT, magnetic resonance imaging, and PET are essential for diagnosis, assessment of response, and monitoring of this disease. A constellation of imaging findings and certain clinical features may be helpful in the diagnosis of PTLD. Both nodal and extranodal involvement is common **(Fig. 4.14)**. Adenotonsillar activity can be a marker for PTLD. FDG-PET after a few cycles of therapy is an excellent predictor for sustained remission.

Neuroblastoma

Neuroblastoma is the most common extracranial solid malignancy and usually occurs in patients under 5 years old. Unfortunately, up to 50% of cases are present as metastatic disease at the diagnosis. Several imaging

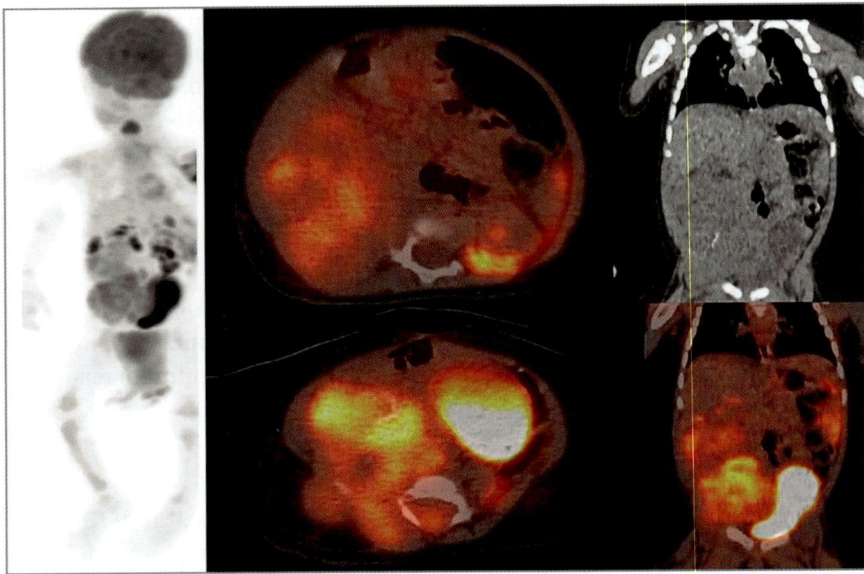

Fig. 4.13: A 6-month-old boy with rhabdomyosarcoma showing fluorodeoxyglucose (FDG) avid large soft tissue mass in abdominal and pelvic region closely abutting right kidney

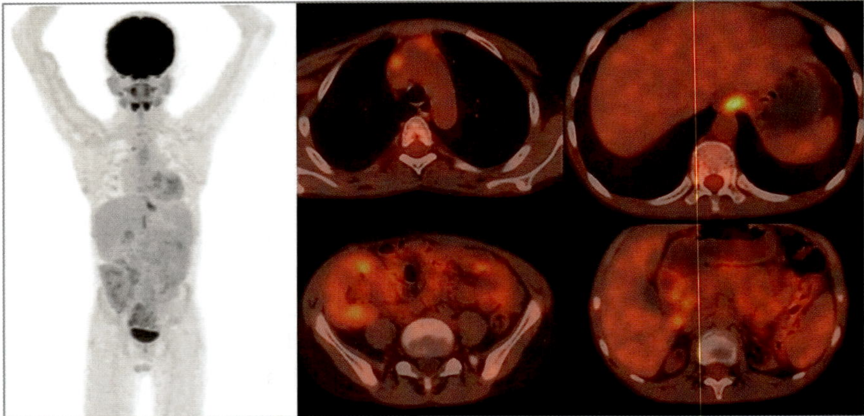

Fig. 4.14: A 12-year-old boy with post-transplant kidney in renal fossa shows thickening in pylorus and first part of duodenum with prevascular and paraesophageal lymph node suggestive of lymphproliferative disorder

modalities have been used for staging and therapy of neuroblastoma. Metaiodobenzylguanidine (MIBG) conjugated with iodine-123(^{123}I) and iodine-131(^{131}I) can be used for the detection of metastatic disease and treatment of relapsed and refractory neuroblastoma, respectively.

As for PET/CT two types of tracers are currently used in neuroblastoma: The first one is ^{18}F-FDG and the second one is the group of gallium-68 (^{68}Ga) conjugated somatostatin analogues DOTATOC (DOTA-d-Phe1-Tyr3-octreotide), DOTANOC (DOTA-1-Nal3-octreotide), and DOTATATE.

IODINE-131 METAIODOBENZYLGUANIDINE (^{131}I-MIBG) SCINTIGRAPHY

Radiopharmaceutical

Metaiodobenzylguanidine is an analogue of noradrenaline and guanethidine. MIBG is labeled with ^{131}I or ^{123}I. ^{123}I is not available in India. Tracer localization is dependent upon the adrenergic innervation and the level of catecholamine secretion in tumors **(Fig. 4.15)**.

Medications interfering with the adrenergic system should be discontinued. These include selected antihypertensives, antipsychotics, tricyclic antidepressants, opioids, tramadol, and sympathomimetic drugs. SPECT/CT can be done for anatomical localization.

Indications

- For detection and staging of neuroblastoma.
- For planning and assessing response to ^{131}I-MIBG radionuclide therapy.

Normal physiological uptake is seen in the liver, salivary glands, myocardium, and excretion into urinary bladder. Abnormal lesions are seen as focal areas of increased tracer uptake.

Advancements in nuclear medicine technology continue to drive innovations in pediatric renal imaging and therapy. Additionally, the

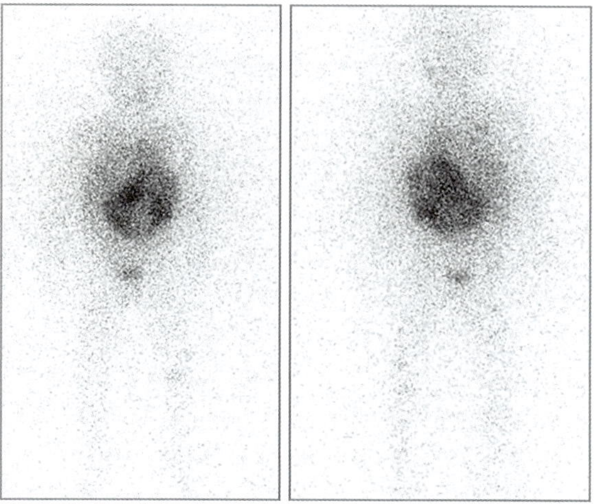

Fig. 4.15: A 1-year-old boy with large left suprarenal mass with increased uptake on iodine-131 metaiodobenzylguanidine (^{131}I-MIBG) scan suggesting neuroblastoma

integration of hybrid imaging modalities such as single-photon emission computed tomography (SPECT/CT), PET/CT and PET/MRI holds promise for the comprehensive evaluation of pediatric renal disorders with improved anatomical and functional information. Thus, with continued advancements and innovations, nuclear medicine remains an important aspect in the comprehensive management of pediatric renal conditions.

BIBLIOGRAPHY

1. Bar-Sever Z, Shammas A, Gheisari F, et al. Pediatric nephro-urology: Overview and updates in diuretic renal scans and renal cortical scintigraphy. Semin Nucl Med. 2022;52(4):419-31.
2. Durand E, Chaumet-Riffaud P, Grenier N. Functional renal imaging: new trends in radiology and nuclear medicine. Semin Nucl Med 2011;41(1):61-72.
3. Faust WC, Diaz M, Pohl HG. Incidence of post-pyelonephritic renal scarring: A meta-analysis of the dimercapto-succinic acid literature. J Urol. 2009;181(1):290-7.
4. Riccabona M, Avni FE, Blickman JG, et al. Imaging recommendations in pediatric uroradiology: Minutes of the ESPR workgroup session on urinary tract infection, fetal hydronephrosis, urinary tract ultrasonography and voiding cystourethrography. Pediatr Radiol. 2008;38(2):138-45.
5. Skoog SJ, Peters CA, Arant BS, et al. Pediatric Vesicoureteral Reflux Guidelines Panel Summary Report: Clinical practice guidelines for screening siblings of children with vesicoureteral reflux and neonates/infants with prenatal hydronephrosis. J Urol. 2010;184(3):1145-51.
6. Taylor AT. Radionuclides in nephrourology: Pitfalls and diagnostic applications, Part 2. J Nucl Med. 2014;55(5):786-98.

Congenital Anomalies of the Kidney and Urinary Tract

Ranjeet Wishram Thergaonkar

Congenital anomalies of the kidney and urinary tract (CAKUT) have an estimated incidence of 3–6 per 1,000 live births and account for 30–40% of kidney failure in Indian children. The term "CAKUT" refers to a spectrum of disorders encompassing developmental abnormalities of kidney and urinary tract involving the kidneys (glomeruli and tubules derived from the mesenchyme), and the lower tract (collecting ducts, renal pelvis, and ureter, derived from the ureteric bud).

NORMAL DEVELOPMENT

The renal parenchyma originates from the metanephros, the most caudal of the three blocks of the nephric cord, while the renal collecting ducts, calyces, and ureters are derived from the ureteric bud, an outpouching of the nephric (Wolffian) duct. The nephric cord and the nephric duct are both derivatives of the intermediate mesoderm **(Fig. 5.1)**. For ease of understanding, renal development is divided into the following stages—ureteric budding, branching morphogenesis, nephrogenesis, and renal patterning.

Ureteric budding begins in the 5th week of gestation as glial-derived neurotrophic factor (GDNF), secreted by the metanephric mesenchyme, stimulates the GFRA1-RET coreceptors in the nephric duct. Stimulation of the GFRA1-RET coreceptors activates the downstream PI3K-AKT-ETV4/ETV5, ERK, and PLCγ pathways to effect ureteric budding. Many molecules stimulate and inhibit GDNF as well as RET secretion so that ureteric budding and induction of nephrogenesis is limited to a single area. A GDNF-independent pathway, relying on fibroblast growth factor 7 (FGF-7), FGF-10 and FGF-20, and their receptors FGFR1 and FGFR2 is also described. The relation between GDNF dependent and independent pathways is unclear; it is postulated that the latter fine-tunes the former **(Fig. 5.2)**.

Branching morphogenesis occurs as the ureteric bud undergoes repeated organized branching (usually a T-shaped bifurcation and sometimes trifurcation, followed by elongation) up to 15 generations by the 22nd week of gestation to form a network of 65,000 collecting ducts **(Fig. 5.3)**. This process occurs under continued stimulation of the GDNF-GFRA1/RET signaling that receives positive feedback from WNT11, which is secreted by the ureteric tips.

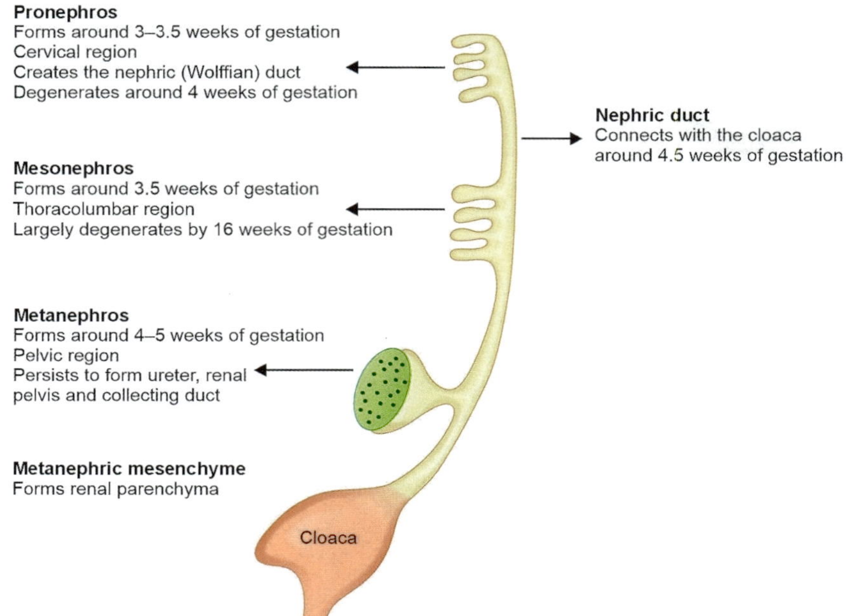

Fig. 5.1: Early events in the development of the kidney and urinary tract

The number of nephrons in the developed kidney exceeds the expected number of 2^{15} (32,768) because 4–7 nephrons are induced in each of the terminal collecting ducts that have completed their branching. Such nephrons are organized in "arcades", where the connecting tubules of multiple nephrons open into the ampulla of a terminal collecting duct. Even after the arcades are formed, the terminal branch of the last generation of branching elongates past the arcade and develops more ampullae that induce nephrons. These steps are crucial for adequate nephron endowment of the developing kidney.

Nephrogenesis, the process of nephron development, begins as the metanephric mesenchyme organizes itself around the branches of the ureteric bud. Cap mesenchyme organizes itself into pretubular aggregates followed by renal vesicles under the influence of *WNT9B* signaling by the ureteric bud tips **(Fig. 5.3)**. At the cellular level, mesenchyme differentiates into epithelium (mesenchymal-epithelial transformation) under the influence of *WNT4*. At the same time, *SIX2* and *SALL1* signaling ensure that there is a constant replenishment of a population of progenitor cells. Renal vesicles elongate and curl to form to form "comma"-shaped bodies and further to form "S"-shaped bodies. Vascular cells migrate into the distal cleft of the "S"-shaped body to begin to form glomeruli under the influence of vascular endothelial growth factor (VEGF) secreted by podocyte precursors. Vascular cells express platelet-derived growth factor (PDGF)—essential for the formation of the mesenchyme. The first glomeruli are formed

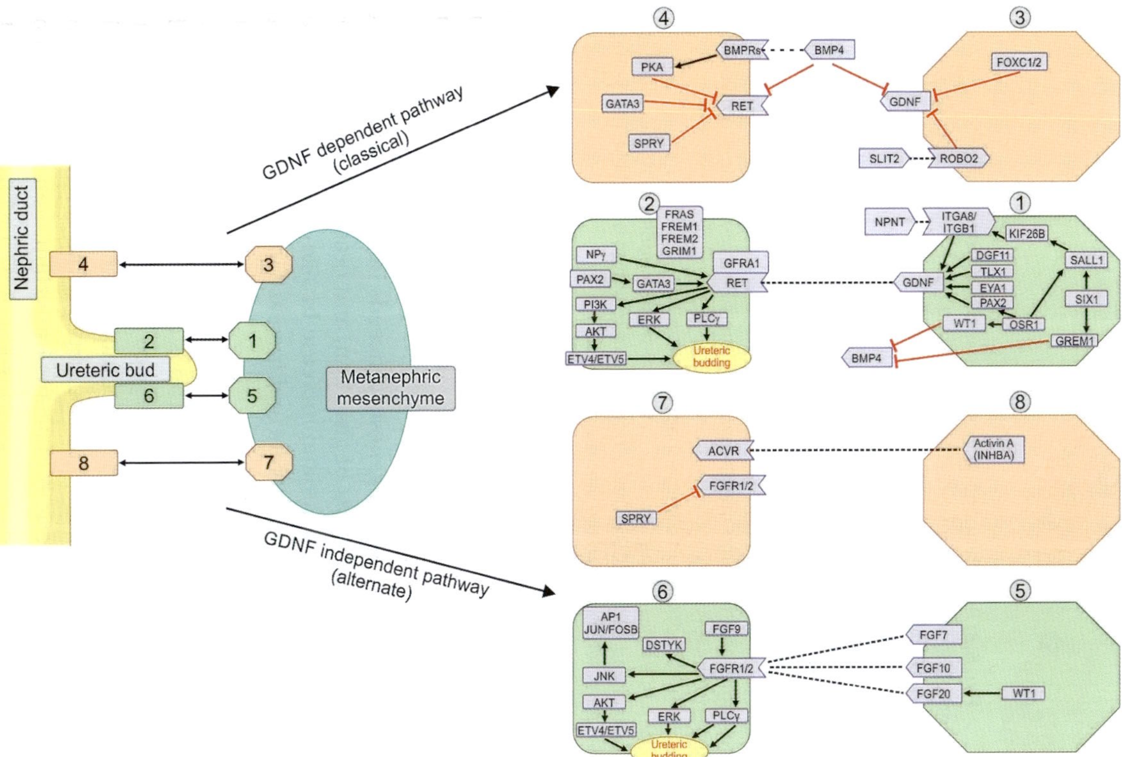

Fig. 5.2: Molecular signaling during ureteric budding. Black arrows with heads indicate stimulatory pathways, red arrows with flat heads indicate inhibitory pathways and dotted lines indicate receptor-ligand interaction. Pathways for events 1–8 indicated on the left pane are detailed in graphics on the right. GDNF: glial-derived neurotrophic factor

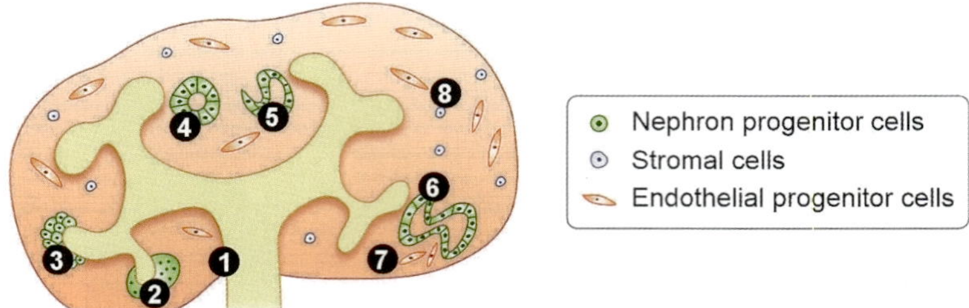

Fig. 5.3: Branching morphogenesis and nephrogenesis

1. Branching morphogenesis begins with the ureteric bud (Ret+, Wnt11+) penetrating the metanephric mesenchyme and continues with serial branching for approximately 15 generations while inducing nephrogenesis. The first 6–10 generations give rise to the renal pelvis and calyces and subsequent generations give rise to collecting ducts.
2. Nephrogenesis starts with the ureteric bud and its branches inducing some metanephric mesenchymal cells to condense on their tips to form cap mesenchyme (Six2+, Cited 1+, and Gdnf+).
3. The cap mesenchyme organizes into pretubular aggregates containing 4–30 cells.
4. Pretubular aggregates undergo mesenchymal-epithelial transformation to give rise to renal vesicles (Wnt4+, Pax8+).
5. Renal vesicles "unwind" to form comma-shaped bodies.
6. Comma-shaped bodies further unwind to form S-shaped bodies with vascularization at the proximal end (Notch-ICD+) (away from the ureteric bud branches). The S-shaped bodies will ultimately fuse with the ureteric stalk.
7. Endothelial progenitor cells (Flk1+, Tie2+) – differentiate into the glomerulus, afferent and efferent arterioles as well as venules (angiogenesis).
8. Stromal cells (Foxd1+, RAR+) provide a supporting milieu, form the kidney capsule and delineate zones within the kidney, and also give rise to non-epithelial cells such as mesangial cells and pericytes.

at ~8 weeks of gestation. Nephrogenesis proceeds in a centripetal fashion, is most active after the 20th week of gestation, and ceases between the 36th and 38th week of gestation. Postnatal increase in size of kidneys is due to enlargement of glomerular diameters and increase in tubular volume and length.

During renal patterning (occurring simultaneously with nephrogenesis), the proximal-distal polarity of the nephron is determined as renal vesicles organize into comma-shaped bodies followed by S-shaped bodies on their journey to becoming nephrons. The exact molecular signaling responsible for patterning of the renal vesicle is unclear, but the role of WNT9B released by the branches of the ureteric bud seems important. Renin-angiotensin signaling is important for renal angiogenesis, as well as maintenance of the mesenchymal-epithelial transformation, especially in the proximal tubule. Blood vessels develop through branching of existing vessels as well as angiogenesis (differentiation of endothelial cell precursors within metanephric mesenchyme) **(Fig. 5.4)**. At the macroscopic level, the cortex-medullary patterning of the kidney occurs between 22 and 34 weeks.

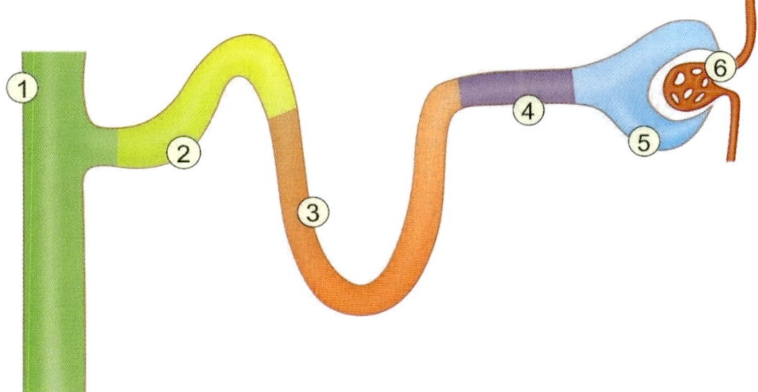

Fig. 5.4: Nephron patterning. The S-shaped bodies differentiate to form the definitive nephron with collecting duct (1), distal convoluted tubule expressing DLL1 and BRN1 (2), loop of Henle (expressing BRN1) (3), proximal tubule (expressing NOTCH proteins and JAGGED1) (4), Bowman's capsule (expressing WT1 and VEGF) (5), and glomerulus (expressing PDGF) (6). Notch2 signaling is essential for the designation of proximal nephron fate and Lhx1 for the distal nephron

The kidneys are initially positioned opposite S1 but reach their normal position in the renal fossae opposite L1 by 9 weeks. Renal ascent occurs due to the "pull" caused by growth of the heart, lungs, and the liver along the transverse axis. Concurrent rotation of the kidneys through 90° due to increase in growth of the lateral lip of the hilum ensures that the pelves are oriented medially. There is concomitant migration of the blood supply till the renal arteries in the anatomical position become the final source **(Figs. 5.5A to D)**. The sonic hedgehog (SHH) pathway has a role in preventing renal fusion during ascent.

As the kidneys develop, there is simultaneous development of the urinary tract. The development of the urinary bladder begins with the "division" of the cloaca at 4–6 weeks into the urogenital sinus (bladder) and the rectum. The superior most part of the urogenital sinus forms the urinary bladder, which is initially continuous with the allantois. The next (pelvic) part of the urogenital sinus gives rise to the entire urethra in females, and prostatic and membranous urethra in males. The penile urethra in males develops from the urethral grooves as it folds whilst being incorporated into the developing phallus. The distal most (glandular) part of the male urethra develops after inward movement of the ectodermal cells of the glans. The remnants of the allantois form the fibrous cord called the urachus that connects the bladder to the umbilicus. The proximal part of the ureteric bud not in contact with the metanephric mesenchyme elongates and finds insertion inside the developing urinary bladder as the proximal nephric duct involutes **(Figs. 5.6A and B)**.

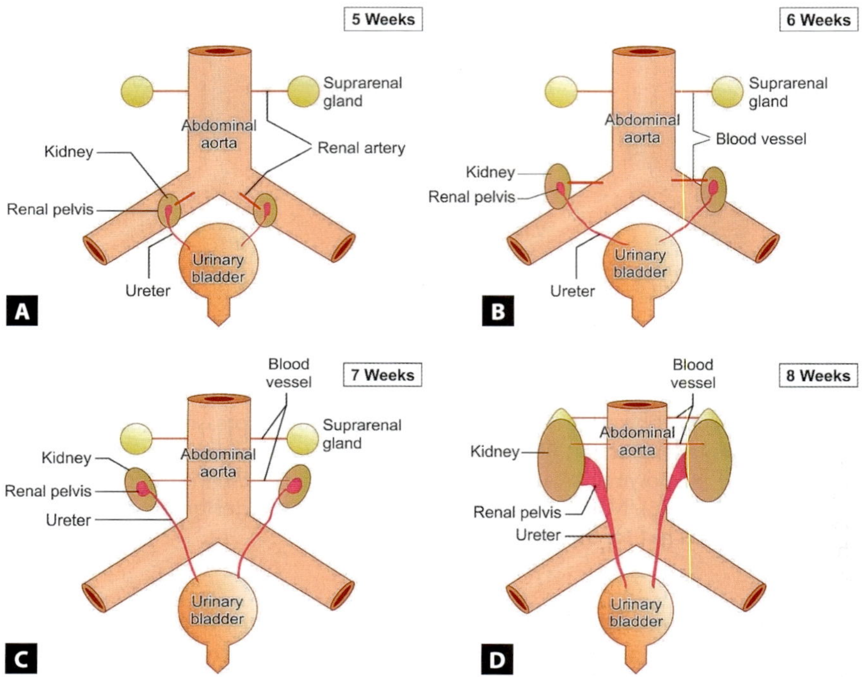

Figs. 5.5A to D: "Ascent" of the kidneys during renal development

ETIOLOGY OF CONGENITAL ANOMALIES OF THE KIDNEY AND URINARY TRACT

Interference with ureteric budding negatively leads to renal agenesis, and positively leads to multiple ureters, typically duplex kidneys. Interference with branching morphogenesis and nephrogenesis leads to renal hypoplasia and dysplasia. Interference with renal ascent leads to disorders of ectopia and fusion.

The etiology of CAKUT is complex. Pathogenic variants in genes translating into signaling molecules are associated with renal agenesis, renal hypoplasia, and dysplasia **(Annexure 9.1, p 845)**. Since these signaling molecules may be involved in the development of other organ systems, there may be syndromic association of CAKUT **(Table 5.1)**. CAKUT may also be oligosyndromic (CAKUT being the first or leading clinical feature) **(Table 5.2)**. Environmental factors also play a role. Maternal malnutrition is associated with reduced nephron endowment. Maternal exposure during pregnancy to angiotensin-converting enzyme (ACE)-inhibitors, aminoglycosides, nonsteroidal anti-inflammatory drugs (NSAIDs), corticosteroids, retinoids, alcohol, and cocaine are associated with CAKUT.

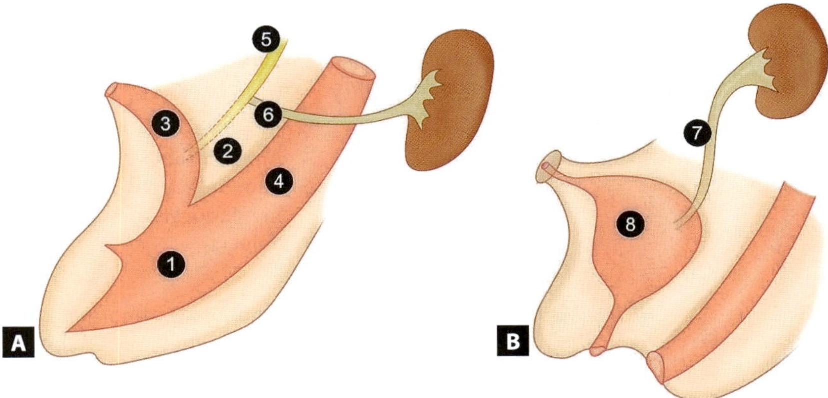

Figs. 5.6A and B: The cloaca (1) is divided by the urorectal septum (2) into primitive urogenital sinus (3) and the anorectal canal (4). The nephric duct (5) initially opens into the primitive urogenital sinus and itself gives rise to the ureteric bud (6). The superior part of the primitive urogenital sinus later gives rise to the urinary bladder. However, the nephric duct (5) proximal to the ureteric bud involutes and the ureteric bud (6) elongates, so that the ureter (7) later opens directly into the urinary bladder (8)

TABLE 5.1: Important syndromes associated with CAKUT

Syndrome; inheritance	*Gene/ cytoband/ chromosome*	*Renal manifestations*	*Extrarenal manifestations*
Alagille; AD	*JAG1* (notch signalling)	Agenesis, hypoplasia, cystic dysplasia, ureteropelvic junction obstruction, vesicoureteral reflux	Broad forehead, triangular face, deep set eyes posterior embryotoxon, congenital heart disease, infantile cholestasis, vertebral anomalies, intellectual disability
Beckwith Wiedemann; AD	11p15.5	Renal dysplasia, cortical cysts, medullary cysts, large kidneys, nephrocalcinosis, nephrolithiasis	Macrosomia, hemihypertrophy, hyperinsulinism, omphalocele, cryptorchidism
Branchio-oto-renal, AD	*EYA1, SIX1, SIX5**	Hypoplasia, vesicoureteral reflux, ectopic kidney	Hearing loss, abnormal pinna, preauricular pit, high-arched palate
Cat eye syndrome, AD	22q11	Agenesis	Colobomas, down slanting palpebral fissures, preauricular pit or skin tag

Contd...

Contd...

Syndrome; inheritance	*Gene/ cytoband/ chromosome*	*Renal manifestations*	*Extrarenal manifestations*
Caudal regression; AD, AR	*VANGL1*	Agenesis, ectopic kidney, hypoplasia, hydronephrosis, fused ureters	Anterior sacral hemidefect, anterior sacral meningocele, neural tube defects
CHARGE association; AD	*CHD7, SEMA3E*	Horseshoe kidney, hydronephrosis	Colobomas, abnormal pinna, tetralogy of Fallot, septal defects, growth retardation, genital anomalies
Down syndrome	Trisomy 21	Dysplasia, duplex system	Short stature, flat occiput, upslanting palpebral fissures, clinodactyly, intellectual delay
Fraser syndrome; AR	*FRAS1, FREM2, GRIP1**	Agenesis, hypoplasia	Unusual hairline, cryptophthalmos, syndacytyly, genital anomalies
Craniofacial microsomia 1 (Goldenhar); AD	*SF3B2*	Agenesis, ectopy, multicystic dysplasia	Hemifacial microsomia, mandibular hypoplasia, maxillary hypoplasia, epibulbar dermoid, microtia, preauricular skin tags, hearing loss, macrostomia
Hypoparathy-roidism, sensori-neural deafness and renal dysplasia (HDR) syndrome; AD	*GATA3**	Agenesis, dysplasia, vesicoureteral reflux	Hyperparathyroidism, sensorineural hearing loss, Müllerian anomalies (girls)
Kallman; XL, AR, AD	*ANOS1, KAL1, FGFR1, FGF8, PROKR2, PROK2*	Agenesis, vesicoureteral reflux	Anosmia, hypogonadotropic hypogonadism
Mayer-Rokitansky-Küster-Hauser	Unknown	Agenesis, ectopia	Aplasia/hypoplasia of uterus and upper two-thirds vagina, aplastic Fallopian tubes
Ochoa syndrome; AR	*HPSE2, LRIG2*	Lower urinary tract dysfunction	Peculiar facies, constipation

Contd...

Contd...

Syndrome; inheritance	*Gene/ cytoband/ chromosome*	*Renal manifestations*	*Extrarenal manifestations*
Pallister–Hall; AD	*GLI3* (sonic hedgehog pathway)	Agenesis, hydronephrosis, hydroureter, renal ectopia, horseshoe kidney	Polydactyly, asymptomatic bifid epiglottis, hypothalamic hamartoma, laryngotracheal cleft
Renal coloboma; AD	*PAX2**	Hypoplasia, dysplasia, multicystic dysplasia	Optic nerve coloboma
Renal-hepatic-pancreatic dysplasia; AR	*EVC, EVC2*	Cystic dysplasia	Pancreatic fibrosis, hepatic dysgenesis skeletal abnormalities
Rubinstein Taybi; AD	*CREBBP*	Agenesis, ectopia, ureteric duplication	Intellectual disability, broad thumbs and halluces, peculiar facies
Simpson Golabi Behmel; XL	*GPC-3*	Medullary cystic dysplasia	Overgrowth syndrome; heart defects, coarse facies intestinal malrotation, hypotonia, hydrocephalus
Smith Lemli Opitz; AR	*DHCR7*	UPJ obstruction, hydronephrosis, vesicoureteral reflux, cystic dysplasia	Growth retardation intellectual deficit, microcephaly, anteverted nares
Syndromic microphthalmia; AD	*BMP4*	Hypoplasia	Anophthalmia, microphthalmia, craniofacial anomalies, disorders of sexual development, intellectual disability
Townes Brocks; AD	*SALL1*	Hypoplasia, dysplasia, multicystic dysplasia	Intellectual disability, large ears, broad thumb, triphalangeal thumb
Turner syndrome	Monosomy X	Horseshoe kidney	Short stature, lymphedema, hypergonadotropic hypogonadism, coarctation
Zellweger syndrome; AR	*PEX*	Cystic dysplasia, hydronephrosis	Neurological abnormalities, hearing, visual loss, hepatomegaly hypotonia

AD: autosomal dominant; AR: autosomal recessive; XL: X-linked
See **Annexure 9.1** for list of genes associated with CAKUT
* Indicates that the gene may be associated with oligosyndromic or non-syndromic CAKUT

TABLE 5.2: Nonsyndromic and oligosyndromic causes of CAKUT

Disease; inheritance	*Gene/cytoband/ chromosome*	*Renal manifestations*	*Extrarenal manifestation*
Renal cysts and diabetes syndrome; AD	*HNF1B*	Agenesis, cystic dysplasia, oligophrenia	Müllerian anomalies, hypospadias, and impaired glucose tolerance
Renal tubular dysgenesis; AR, AD	*AGT, AGTR1, REN*	Reduced number and shorter proximal tubules, atrophic loops of Henle, tightly packed glomeruli	Large ears, low-set ears, limb positioning defects, arthrogryposis, lung hypoplasia (Potter sequence), and skull ossification defect
	BMP4	Hypoplasia	Cleft lip, microphthalmia
Vesicoureteral reflux; AD?	1p13; 3p12 *(ROBO2)*; 8q11 *(SOX17)*; 4p15 *(SLIT2)*; 6p21 *(TNXB)*	Vesicoureteral reflux, hydroureter, hypoplasia, dysplasia, and duplex kidneys	Joint laxity (*TNXB*)

AD: autosomal dominant; AR: autosomal recessive
See **Annexure 9.1 (p 845)** for list of genes associated with CAKUT

INDIVIDUAL DISORDERS

Congenital Solitary Kidney (Single Functioning Kidney)

Congenital solitary kidney (CSK), seen in 1:1,000–1:2,000 live births, may be the result of any of the following conditions **(Figs. 5.7A to C)**.

Unilateral Renal Agenesis

Renal agenesis refers to the complete absence of one or both kidneys without identifiable rudimentary tissue **(Fig. 5.7A)**. Unilateral renal agenesis (URA) is diagnosed if antenatal ultrasonography at 18–22 weeks' gestation fails to detect a kidney in the renal fossa. The incidence of unilateral agenesis is ~0.3 per 1,000 live births. There is a male (1.2–3.1:1) and slight left-sided preponderance. URA may be associated with urogenital tract anomalies on the same side (e.g., seminal vesicle hypoplasia and absence of the vas deferens), cardiac anomalies (atrial or ventricular septal defects), and/or gastrointestinal anomalies (anal atresia).

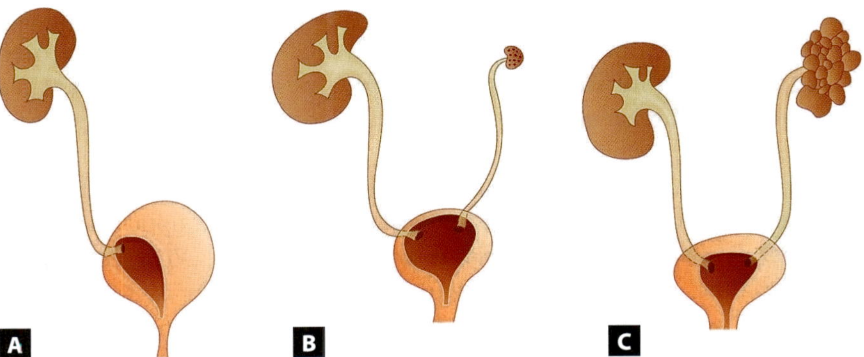

Figs. 5.7A to C: Causes of congenital solitary kidney. (A) Unilateral renal agenesis. The trigone is absent on the affected side; (B) Renal aplasia; (C) Multicystic dysplastic kidney

Unilateral agenesis occurs due to a developmental failure of the ureteric bud and the metanephric mesenchyme. Unilateral agenesis may occur due to mutations in many genes, such as *RET* (10q11.2), *BMP4* (14q22-q23), *FRAS1* (4q21.21), *FREM1* (9p22.3), or *UPK3A* (22q13.31). Maternal diabetes mellitus or use of specific drugs during pregnancy may also cause renal agenesis. URA may be associated with anomalies of the paramesonephric duct. An embryological classification is proposed for Müllerian anomalies associated with renal agenesis: type 1 occurring before 4th week gestation, and associated with unicornuate uterus; type II occurring in the early part of the 4th week of gestation and associated with didelphys uterus and obstruction of the ipsilateral horn and vagina; and type III occurring later without association with Müllerian anomalies.

Syndromic associations of renal agenesis include:

- Neurofacioskeletal syndrome with or without renal agenesis; *HS2ST1*; recessive inheritance (OMIM 619194)
- Microcephaly, facial dysmorphism, renal agenesis, and ambiguous genitalia syndrome; *CTU2*; recessive inheritance (OMIM 618142)
- Müllerian duct aplasia, URA, and cervicothoracic somite anomalies; MURCS (OMIM 277000) (OMIM 601076) I/II
  - Mayer–Rokitansky–Kuster–Hauser syndrome, types I–II
  - Klippel–Feil deformity, conductive deafness, and absent vagina
- Hirschsprung disease with polydactyly, renal agenesis, and deafness (OMIM 235740)
- Uterus bicornis bicollis with partial vaginal septum and unilateral hematocolpos with ipsilateral renal agenesis (OMIM 192050)
- Aniridia, partial, and psychomotor retardation (OMIM 206750)
- Microcephaly, congenital heart disease, hyposegmented lungs (OMIM 601355)

- Hypoparathyroidism, sensorineural deafness, and renal disease; HDR; *GATA3*; dominant transmission (OMIM 146255): Also termed hypoparathyroidism, sensorineural deafness, and renal dysplasia syndrome; Barakat syndrome; nephrosis, nerve deafness, and hypoparathyroidism
- Papillorenal syndrome (PAPRS): Also known as renal coloboma syndrome—optic nerve coloboma with renal disease; coloboma of optic nerve with renal disease; optic coloboma, vesicoureteral reflux (VUR), and renal anomalies; renal-coloboma syndrome with macular abnormalities; CAKUT with or without ocular abnormalities; dominant inheritance, *PAX2* (OMIM 120330)
- Bifid nose with or without anorectal and renal anomalies; *FREM1* (OMIM 608980)
- Diaphragmatic hernia, congenital (OMIM 142340)
- Vertebral, cardiac, tracheoesophageal, renal, and limb defects; VCTERL; *WBP11*; dominant inheritance (OMIM 619227)
- RET protooncogene; *RET*; dominant inheritance (OMIM 164761)
- Multinucleated neurons, anhydramnios, renal dysplasia, cerebellar hypoplasia; *CEP55*; recessive inheritance (OMIM 236500)
- Fraser syndrome 1; *FRAS1*; recessive inheritance (OMIM 219000)
- Renal cysts and diabetes syndrome; *HNF1B;* dominant inheritance (137920)
- Thymic-renal-anal-lung dysplasia (OMIM 274265)
- Neurofacioskeletal syndrome with or without renal agenesis; *HS2ST1*; recessive inheritance (OMIM 604844)
- Hypogonadotropic hypogonadism 1 with or without anosmia (Kallmann syndrome 1); *ANOS1*; X-linked (OMIM 308700)
- Renal-hepatic-pancreatic dysplasia; *NEK8*; recessive (OMIM 615415)
- DiGeorge syndrome; *TBX1;* dominant inheritance (OMIM 188400)
- Pallister–Hall syndrome (PHS; OMIM 146510)
- Hypothalamic hamartoblastoma, hypopituitarism, imperforate anus, and postaxial polydactyly; *GLI3;* dominant inheritance (OMIM 146510)
- Meckel syndrome; *KIF14;* recessive inheritance (OMIM 616258)
- Branchiootorenal syndrome; *EYA1*; dominant inheritance (OMIM 601653)
- Fanconi anemia; *FANCB*; X-linked recessive (OMIM 300514)
- Scalp-ear-nipple syndrome; *KCTD;* dominant inheritance (OMIM 181270)
- Bifid nose with or without anorectal and renal anomalies; *FREM1*; and recessive inheritance (OMIM 608944)
- Gonadal dysgenesis, dysmorphic facies, retinal dystrophy, myopathy; *PPP2R3C*; recessive inheritance (OMIM 618419)
- Chromosome 16p11.2 deletion syndrome (OMIM 611913)

Renal Aplasia

This is said to occur if antenatal ultrasonography at 18–22 weeks' gestation shows a rudimentary kidney on one side that shows <5% function on ^{99m}Tc-dimercaptosuccinic acid (DMSA) scan after birth **(Fig. 5.7B)**. Renal aplasia is the most severe form of a combination of renal hypoplasia and renal dysplasia (see below).

Multicystic Dysplastic Kidney

The condition **(Fig. 5.7C)** is described below.

Undefined Congenital Solitary Kidney

The above term includes conditions when no antenatal ultrasonography is performed at 18–22 weeks of gestation, but when performed during or after the third trimester shows an empty renal fossa.

Clinical Features

Congenital solitary kidney is usually detected on antenatal ultrasonography, but may be detected later for unrelated causes or during evaluation of urinary tract infection (UTI) and chronic kidney disease. On antenatal ultrasonography, CSK may be missed because of confusion with a suprarenal gland, or wrongly diagnosed because of ectopic location. CSK is likely to have a favorable outcome in the presence of compensatory enlargement (length >2–2.5 SD for age, or ≥95th percentile for height). It is unclear whether compensatory enlargement occurs due to increase in nephron number or nephron size. Compensatory enlargement may occur anytime from the antenatal period to 2 years of age.

The CSK is at greater risk of other anomalies such as VUR (20%), megaureter (7%), pelviureteric junction obstruction (5%), duplex kidney (3%), renal cysts **(Fig. 5.8)**, ureterocele, and posterior urethral valves (1% each). UTIs occur in ~30% patients. Associated extrarenal anomalies include those of the gastrointestinal tract (16%), cardiovascular and nervous systems (15% each), and musculoskeletal system (13%); hypospadias, undescended testes, and Müllerian malformations are not uncommon.

The prevalence of hypertension in childhood is not increased compared to general population, but is slightly higher in adults. Proteinuria is present in 3–20% children, and 40–45% adults with CSK (compared to <0.3% of the general population). Most patients with CSK have low normal estimated glomerular filtration rate (eGFR) (usually 80–90 mL/min/1.73 m^2). Risk factors for decline in renal function include absence of compensatory enlargement, prematurity, low birthweight, UTI, hypertension, and proteinuria.

The Dutch longitudinal study, Kidney of MONofunctional Origin (KIMONO), on over 400 children with congenital and early-acquired single

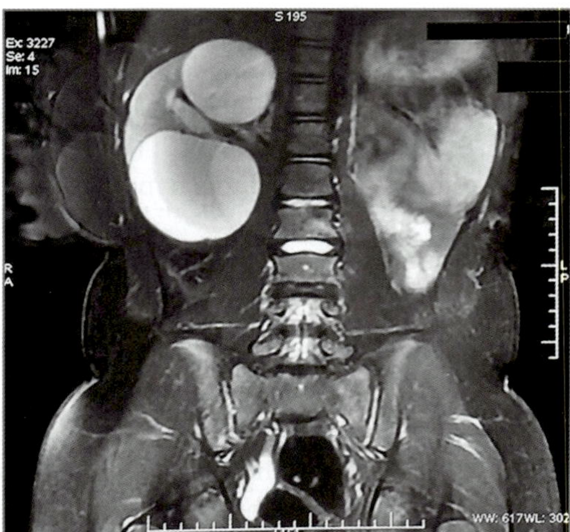

Fig. 5.8: Congenital solitary kidney in a 12-year-old boy with ballotable mass in right hypochondrium and lumbar region. MR urography revealed an empty left renal fossa; the right kidney showed large cysts in each pole. Renal function tests were normal

functional kidney showed that approximately one in three children with single kidney had signs of kidney injury [hypertension, proteinuria, reduced eGFR, and/or use of ACE inhibitor and angiotensin receptor blocker (ARB)] at a mean age of 6.4 years. Approximately 25% had hypertension by 5 years, and 19% had proteinuria by 10 years. The median age to kidney injury in children with single kidney was ~15 years. Patients with ipsilateral CAKUT had higher incidence of kidney injury, compared to those without ipsilateral CAKUT. The cohort also showed that individuals with early-acquired single kidney had higher incidence of kidney injury compared with those with its congenital absence.

Management

The initial evaluation of a patient includes: (*i*) head-to-toe examination for extrarenal anomalies; (*ii*) measurement of blood pressure; (*iii*) renal imaging; (*iv*) assessing kidney function (estimating serum creatinine); and (*v*) evaluation for proteinuria.

While office blood pressure is sufficient to look for hypertension in most cases; ambulatory blood pressure monitoring is recommended periodically to detect masked hypertension, especially if office measurements indicate elevated blood pressure. In addition to ascertaining the diagnosis of CSK, postnatal ultrasonography is important to assess for compensatory enlargement. Further imaging is therefore indicated only after febrile UTI or if obstructive uropathy is suspected. Nuclear scintigraphy (^{99m}Tc DMSA or MAG3 scans) to confirm CSK, or imaging for VUR (micturating cystourethrography) is not routinely advised. Genetic testing may be considered in patients with additional anomalies or a positive family history **(*see* Annexure 9.1, p 845)**.

Ultrasonography report should include kidney length, cortical thickness, echogenicity, corticomedullary differentiation and the presence of cysts, pelvic anteroposterior diameter, presence of calyceal, and/or ureteral dilatation, and bladder parameters (wall thickness, ureteroceles). Nomograms for renal length for age or height are fallacious in the presence of conditions that alter the anatomy such as hydronephrosis, ectopic location, and duplex collecting systems. Evaluation in girls should include examination for Müllerian malformations by a detailed pelvic ultrasonography at 9–12 years of age.

Dietary protein, weight control: High dietary protein intake is associated with higher risk for chronic kidney disease (CKD) or faster CKD progression, because it leads to afferent arteriolar vasodilatation that in turn increases intraglomerular pressure. A high-protein diet leads to an initial increase in GFR; in the long-term, increased intraglomerular pressure may lead to glomerular hyperfiltration and loss of kidney function. Children should consume the recommended dietary intake for protein; higher intakes are avoided. The diet should include adequate fiber from plant-based sources; high in complex carbohydrates including fruits, vegetables, whole grains and legumes, and low in animal-based protein such as meat, saturated fat, refined grains, sweets, and processed food. These dietary strategies also help with weight maintenance.

Dietary sodium: A high-sodium diet leads to increased intraglomerular pressure, causing glomerular hyperfiltration and renal injury. Diet with >3–4 g/day of sodium should be avoided in individuals at risk of developing future CKD, including those with a solitary kidney.

Adequate hydration: Adequate to generous fluid intake (>2.5 L/day) is advised in patients with solitary functioning kidney and eGFR >60 mL/min per 1.73 m^2, as long as there is no hyponatremia.

Smoking cessation: Smoking is a risk factor for CKD and may worsen its progression. Persons with single kidney are advised to avoid smoking.

Contact sports: Most experts advise against participation in contact sports for children with single functioning kidney. There is limited consensus on which sports activities lead to the highest rate of renal trauma. Sports such as skiing, snowboarding, sledding, off-road biking, horse racing, and horseback riding are more often associated with high-grade injury and renal loss than football. Certain sports, especially biking in difficult terrain, bike-racing, snow sports, and equestrian activities might predispose to a higher risk of renal trauma and should be avoided. While flank pads and belts, intended to protect against urologic injuries exist, these devices have not been formally tested with regards to their degree of protection, especially in patients with ectopic kidneys and following transplantation.

Blood pressure control: Blood pressure should be measured at each clinic visit. Ambulatory blood pressure monitoring helps define the severity of hypertension, and detects white coat and masked hypertension. Blood pressure targets are between the 75–90th percentile, and are best achieved by healthy lifestyle, interventions in diet, and careful use of ACE inhibitor or ARB.

Follow-up: For follow-up, children are divided into three risk groups: (*i*) low (renal length > 50th percentile in the first 2 years of life and ≥95th percentile thereafter, with absence of ipsilateral CAKUT); (*ii*) medium (absence of compensatory enlargement and/or presence of ipsilateral CAKUT); and (*iii*) high (presence of decreased eGFR, hypertension, or proteinuria). In low-risk patients, follow-up ultrasound examination and assessment of proteinuria are advised annually until 3 years of age, and every 5 years thereafter. Office blood pressure is measured annually. In those with medium risk, ultrasonography is performed as above, but assessment of proteinuria, blood pressure, and serum creatinine is advised yearly. In high-risk cases, monitoring is more frequent and individualized. All children should be followed up till adolescence and transitioned to adult care thereafter, since puberty is a time when deterioration in kidney function may occur. Girls should undergo abdominopelvic ultrasound between thelarche and menarche.

Bilateral Renal Agenesis

Bilateral renal agenesis is less common with an estimated incidence of 0.13 per 1,000 live births. A few cases of bilateral renal agenesis are due to mutations in *RET*, *FGF20* (8p22), *ITGA8* (10p13), *GREB1L* (18q11), and *GFRA1* (10q26) genes. Antenatal diagnosis is achieved with ultrasonography showing reduced amniotic fluid and high-resolution ultrasonography showing empty renal fossae and absence of renal arteries. Postnatal presentation is usually in the form of the usually fatal oligohydramnios (Potter) sequence consisting of flattened nose, receding chin, low set ears, epicanthus, and severe pulmonary hypoplasia.

Renal Hypoplasia

Renal hypoplasia refers to arrested development of an otherwise normal kidney with reduced size, due to multiple causes including reduced nephron endowment, and defects in ureteric branching, morphogenesis, and nephron induction. Pathogenic variants in genes responsible for these processes, and epigenetic and environmental influences may also have a role **(*see* Annexure 9.1)**. Histology of the kidney shows normal tissue morphology. From a clinical perspective, renal hypoplasia is defined as a reduction in kidney size to less than two standard deviation scores (SDS) below mean with normal corticomedullary differentiation.

Segmental Hypoplasia (Ask–Upmark Kidneys)

In this form of hypoplasia, there is reduction in the number of renal lobes. The kidney has one or more transverse grooves that overlie a dilated calyx **(Fig. 5.9)**. Histologically, it contains few glomeruli or tubules and has loose interstitial tissue with dilated veins and thick-walled arteries. Renin secretion from these hypoplastic lobules results in hypertension. The underlying medulla is rudimentary with collecting ducts often set inside mesenchymal tissue. The presentation is usually during infancy or childhood, with recurrent UTI and hypertension; VUR is commonly associated.

Oligomeganephronia

Congenital oligomeganephronia is a form of renal hypoplasia characterized by reduced renal size (sum of both kidney lengths <80% that of a one kidney of a child of same age), absent corticomedullary boundaries, 5–6 renal pyramids, and reduced number of nephrons that are substantially increased in size. Histology shows reduced number of glomeruli; existing glomeruli and tubules are enlarged **(Figs. 5.10A and B)**. As the disease progresses, segmental sclerosis, tubular atrophy, and interstitial fibrosis are seen. Children with this disorder, more often boys than girls, are born preterm or with low birthweight. Patients present during infancy with anorexia, vomiting, polyuria, proteinuria, and failure to thrive. The disorder is progressive and leads to kidney failure in early childhood.

Simple Hypoplasia

This refers to a kidney that is reduced in size (weight of one kidney <50% expected, or weight of both kidneys <33% expected). The number of lobes is reduced; the nephrons show normal histology. If unilateral, the contralateral kidney may show compensatory enlargement. Diagnosis is made on ultrasonography.

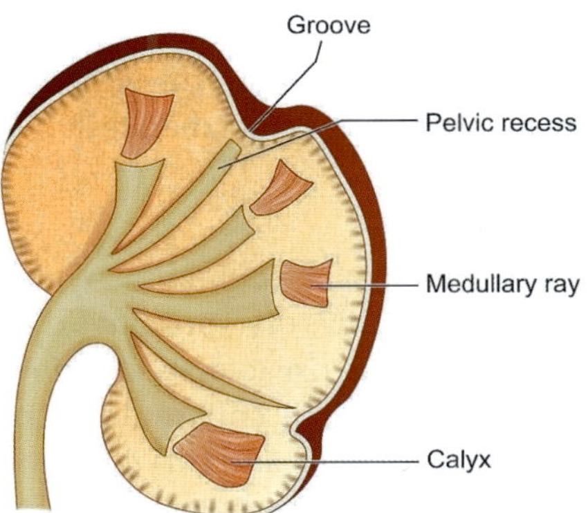

Fig. 5.9: Segmental hypoplasia

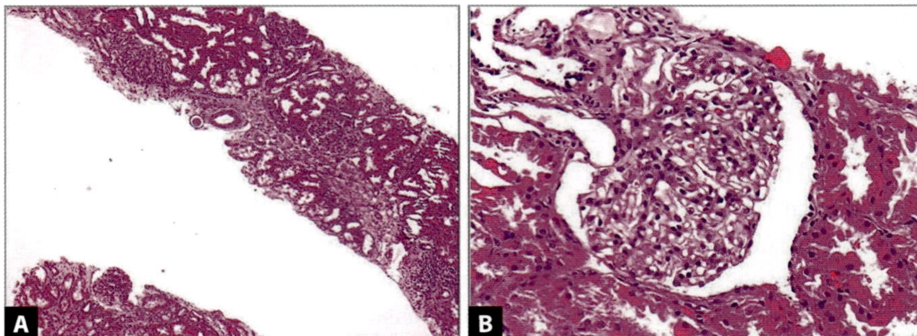

Figs. 5.10A and B: Oligomeganephronia. An 18-month-old boy presented with recurrent episodes of vomiting. Blood urea and serum creatinine were elevated; ultrasound showed normal-shaped kidneys with slightly reduced size but within 2 standard deviations of length for age. Kidney biopsy shows paucity of glomeruli in the renal cortex **(Fig. A, HE, 4x)**. However, each glomerulus was markedly hypertrophied with patent capillary loops **(Fig. B, HE, 20x)**. *Courtesy:* Prof. Geetika Singh, Department of Pathology, AIIMS

Cortical Hypoplasia

The number of generations of nephrons are reduced, along with reduced size of cortical pyramids and medullary rays. The diagnosis is histological, using radial glomerular counts. While the normal count is 12–14, cortical hypoplasia is said to occur when the number is reduced below 10. The number of lobes is not reduced. Cortical hypoplasia may be an isolated finding or occur in association with segmental hypoplasia, oligomeganephronia, or simple hypoplasia.

Oligonephronia

The term refers to reduced nephron endowment (not to be confused with oligomeganephronia) caused by early cessation of nephrogenesis. However, nephron number counting is difficult in clinical practice. Antenatal causes include maternal malnutrition, gestational hyperglycemia, chronic illnesses and infections, and exposure to medications. Association with variants in *PAX2, RET1,* and *EAY1* is described. Low birthweight, prematurity, and small for gestational age are associated; the chief manifestation is hypertension.

Renal Dysplasia

Renal dysplasia refers to the histological finding of abnormal metanephric differentiation. This includes findings of (*i*) primitive ducts lined by cuboid or squamous epithelium that may give rise to cysts of various sizes, and therefore divergent macroscopic features; (*ii*) collarettes of mesenchymal tissue (spindle-shaped fibromuscular cells); and (*iii*) lobar disorganization. Renal dysplasia is rarely proven histologically since biopsy is not indicated. Therefore, the ERKNET 2022 statement on nonobstructive kidney dysplasia proposes sonographic criteria as the chief surrogate parameters. *The finding of reduced corticomedullary differentiation is accepted as a sonological hallmark of renal dysplasia.* Diffuse cortical thinning and the presence of cysts are supportive, but not mandatory. Poor prognostic factors include bilateral dysplasia, dysplasia of a solitary kidney, lack of compensatory enlargement of the contralateral kidney, VUR, and postobstructive state.

Clinical assessment includes examination for syndromic associations. Renal functions (creatinine, pH, and bicarbonate; and urine biochemistry) are tested in newborns after 48–72 hr. Detailed ultrasonography, with assessment of kidney length and volume, corticomedullary differentiation, cortical thinning, description of cysts, pelvic anteroposterior diameter, ureteric and calyceal dilatation, and bladder anomalies, is performed and recorded. *Nuclear scintigraphy or micturating cystourethrography is not routinely recommended.*

A genetic cause underlies approximately 10–15% patients with nonobstructive, nonsyndromic, or oligosyndromic disease **(*see* Annexure 9.1, p 845)**. Genetic testing has limited utility for reproductive counseling, but helps by (*i*) providing clear cause to the families; (*ii*) giving hope of nonrecurrence in the next pregnancy in the case of *de novo* pathogenic variant; (*iii*) planning personalized medical support such as screening for systemic findings; and (*iv*) furthering medical knowledge. Genetic testing should be considered in patients with bilateral, syndromic, or familial kidney dysplasia. Sonographic screening of first-degree relatives is useful to detect hypertension or diabetes mellitus (e.g., *HNF1B* variants). Other than antenatal ultrasonography, prenatal testing is not recommended in pregnancies following a previous child with renal dysplasia.

Children with unilateral renal dysplasia should be followed up annually till 18 years, with physical examination, blood pressure, proteinuria, and ultrasonography of the contralateral kidney. Children with bilateral dysplasia require twice-a-year follow-up into adulthood with blood pressure and proteinuria. GFR is estimated twice a year during infancy, and then tailored to regular ultrasound and biochemical findings. Hypertension and proteinuria are managed using ACE inhibitors or angiotensin receptor blockers.

Multicystic Dysplastic Kidney

Multicystic dysplastic kidney (MCDK) is a form of renal dysplasia with incidence of 1:3,600–1:4,300 live births, with higher frequency on the left side and in boys. The kidney is replaced by multiple noncommunicating cysts of various sizes arranged in reniform shape and absence of any identifiable renal parenchyma. The condition is usually asymptomatic and identified on ultrasonography. The risk of hypertension is ~3%, and that of malignancy is <0.1%. Compensatory enlargement of the contralateral kidney is seen in approximately 85% of patients. Urological abnormalities are seen in approximately 30%, including VUR in 14%. Genital anomalies such as seminal cyst, Gartner cyst, and blind hemivagina may be associated. Spontaneous involution is seen in ~50% of patients. The management is on the lines of congenital solitary kidney, as described above.

Renal Ectopy and Fusion

Renal ectopy and fusion anomalies arise from a disruption of the normal migration of the kidneys. Renal ectopy occurs in approximately 1:1,000 population. The ectopy may be simple (on the same side) or crossed (on the opposite side). Renal ectopy may occur in association with other anomalies such as VUR and renal dysplasia, genitourinary anomalies such as cryptorchidism and hypospadias, and Müllerian anomalies (Mayer-Rokitansky-Küster-Hauser syndrome) or with extrarenal anomalies (CHARGE, VACTERL association).

Horseshoe Kidney

Horseshoe kidney is the most common renal fusion anomaly characterized by ectopic location, malrotation, and aberrant blood vessels. Population prevalence is 1:400–1:600 with male preponderance (approximately 2:1). The embryological origin of the horseshoe kidney is unclear. Fluctuations in the growth of the embryo resulting in ventral flexion of the caudal portion and ectopic mesenchymal tissue are proposed. Ascent of the horseshoe kidney might also be "held back" by the inferior mesenteric artery.

The fusion is usually at the lower poles (~90%), and occasionally at the upper pole resulting in an inverted U shape (5–10%)—both varieties have an "isthmus" between the two kidneys. Very rarely, both poles are fused resulting in a *disc kidney*. The fusion may be in the midline (~42%) causing a U shape or lateral (~58%) resulting in an L shape. The isthmus is narrow and with predominance of fibrous tissue in approximately 20%. Horseshoe kidney is commonly associated with non- or incomplete rotation, hyperrotation, or even reverse rotation. The renal calyces are located in the upper pole in the upper one-third of the renal masses. The ureters often have kinks; duplex ureters with ectopic opening are known. The isthmus may have independent ureteric drainage.

The arterial supply of the horseshoe kidney is from a single renal artery on each side in 5% cases. Chief sources of arterial supply include the common iliac artery (40%) and the contralateral renal artery (25%); rarer sources include the sacral artery, internal and external iliac arteries, iliolumbar artery, and phrenic artery. The isthmus may receive blood supply from the aorta, a renal artery, or a common iliac artery.

Horseshoe kidney is usually asymptomatic and diagnosed on ultrasonography; symptoms may be present due to urolithiasis or UTI.

Urolithiasis occurs in 16–60% adults and 3% children. Urinary stasis due to ureteric abnormalities is the chief cause; metabolic causes (hypercalciuria, hyperoxaluria, hyperuricosuria, and hypocitraturia) and coexistence of medullary sponge kidney are reported. UTI associated with obstructive uropathy (pelviureteric junction obstruction) and urolithiasis is common. Horseshoe kidneys are at higher risk of malignancy, including renal cell carcinoma (50%), transitional cell carcinoma (20%), and Wilms tumor (20%). These kidneys are also at risk of injury because of their inferior location. Extrarenal associations include chromosomal anomalies (horseshoe kidneys are seen in 67%, 14–20% and 1% of patients with Edward, Turner and Down syndrome, respectively), vertebral anomalies and abnormalities of central nervous system **(Figs. 5.11A and B)**.

Pelvic Kidney

This is a condition in which the kidney does not cross the pelvic brim and is associated with an anteriorly oriented renal pelvis as well as aberrant blood supply. The incidence is ~1:2,200–3,000. The arterial supply may be single, double, or triple, and the origin may be from the bifurcation of the aorta, iliac artery, or hypogastric artery. Patients are usually asymptomatic; symptoms may be present due to urolithiasis, UTI, or pelviureteric junction obstruction. The ectopic kidney may have reduced function as assessed by dynamic scintigraphy. Malignancies are very rarely reported, renal cell carcinoma being the most common. Surgical approach to management of urolithiasis or pelviureteric junction obstruction might pose anatomical challenges.

Crossed Renal Ectopia

Crossed renal ectopia is a condition in which a ureter in the normal bladder crosses the midline to an ectopic kidney on the opposite side of the body. The condition is estimated to occur in 1:1,000 live births, with predominance in boys (3:2). Left-to-right ectopia is more common than right to left. There are four types of crossed ectopia; the first, crossed fused ectopia has six subtypes **(Figs. 5.12 and 5.13)**.

The origin of renal ectopia is unclear, but occurs between 4- and 8-week gestation. As per the mechanical theory, abnormal position of the umbilical artery obstructs the ascent of the kidney which takes the path of least resistance to the other side. As per an alternate theory, the ureteral bud crosses to the other side of the body and induces the metanephric mesenchyme of the other side. Crossed ectopia can be associated with VUR, hydronephrosis, and renal hypoplasia and/or dysplasia. Crossed ectopia is usually asymptomatic and may be associated with nonspecific abdominal pain; diagnosis during evaluation of hematuria, hypertension, nephrolithiasis, and CKD is also reported.

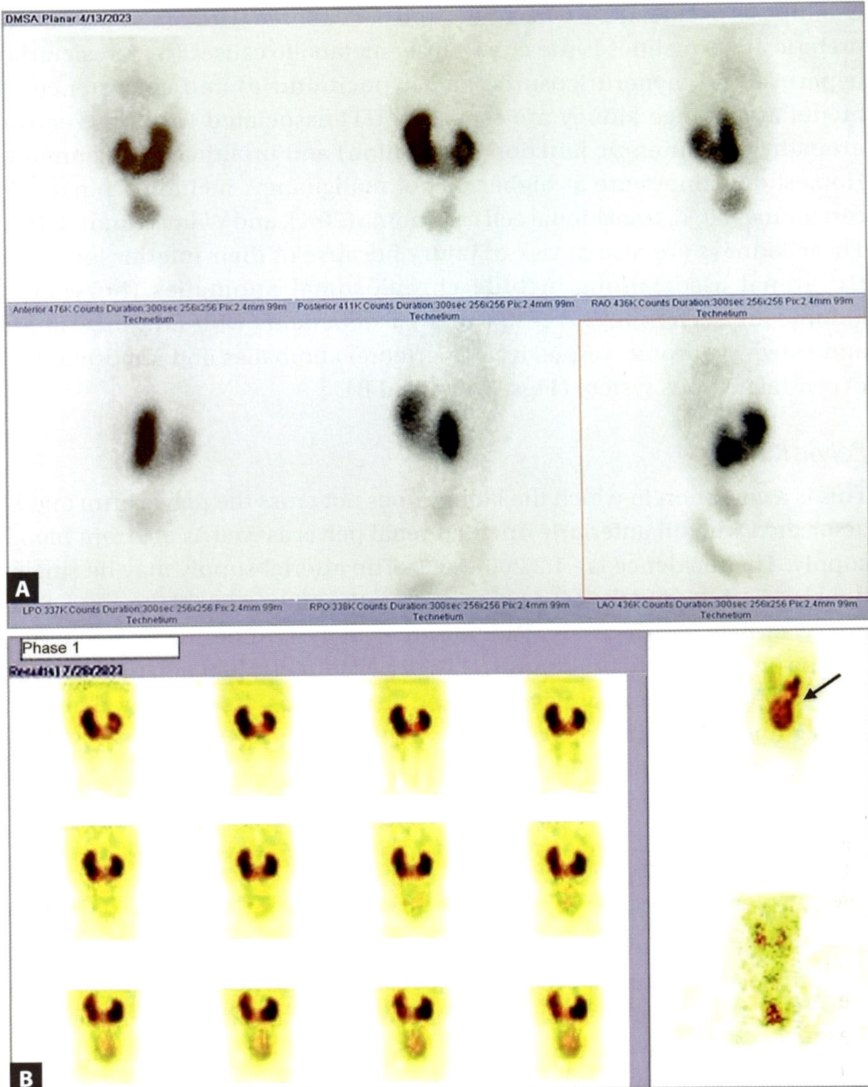

Figs. 5.11A and B: Horseshoe kidney in a 2-year-old boy with recurrent urinary tract infection. Ultrasonography showed horseshoe kidney and ureteric dilatation on the right. Micturating cystourethrography was negative for vesicoureteral reflux. (A) ^{99m}Tc dimercaptosuccinic acid (DMSA) scan shows U-shaped horseshoe kidney with a photopenic isthmus; (B) L,L, ethylenedicysteine (LLEC) scintigraphy shows slow nonobstructive drainage on the right side (black arrow)

Duplex Kidneys

Duplex kidney refers to a kidney with two pelvicalyceal systems; the estimated population prevalence is 0.2–2%. Based on ureteric drainage, it may be classified into four varieties **(Figs. 5.14A to D)**; another classification is based on features of the upper moiety **(Figs. 5.15A to E)**.

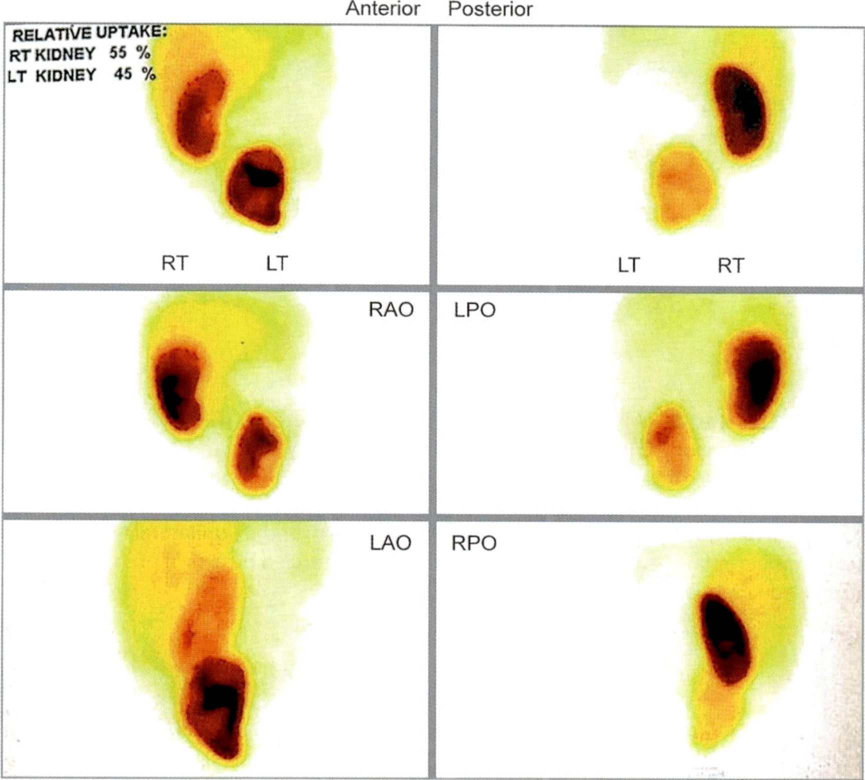

Fig. 5.12: ^{99m}Tc dimercaptosuccinic acid (DMSA) scan in a 10-year-old boy with left-sided pelvic kidney with irregular outline on ultrasonography. DMSA scan confirms left pelvic kidney with adequate tracer uptake, irregular outline, and slightly reduced differential function. LT: left; RT: right

The developmental origin of duplex systems is understood to be either the branching of the ureteric bud before contact with the metanephric mesenchyme (bifid pelvis/ureter), emergence of an additional ureteric bud rostral to the original ureteric bud; both buds either interacting with metanephric mesenchyme independently (double ureters) or rarely merge before approaching the metanephric mesenchyme (inverted Y-ureteral duplication).

Two principles dictate the opening site of the ureters—(*i*) Weigert–Meyer law states that the upper moiety drains into the bladder at a point inferior to the point at which the lower moiety drains; (*ii*) Mackie Stevens relationship states that the moiety with hypodysplasia drains aberrantly while the moiety with normal tissue drains normally.

Patients with duplex kidneys are often asymptomatic; however, UTI due to VUR, urinary dribbling from an ectopic ureter, or obstructive uropathy due to ureterocele may cause symptoms. The evaluation of renal

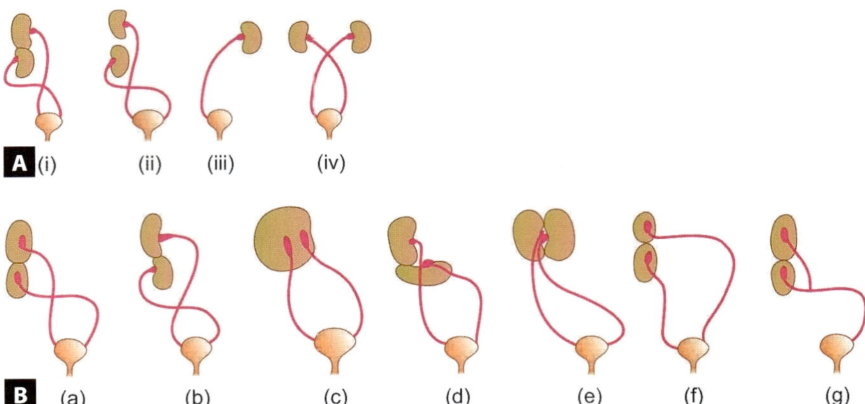

Figs. 5.13A and B: (A) Four types of crossed renal ectopia (CRE) are described—(i) CRE with fusion; (ii) CRE without fusion; (iii) Solitary CRE; and (iv) Bilateral CRE; (B) The first type of CRE (CRE with fusion) has 6 subtypes: (a) unilateral fused kidney (inferior ectopia); (b) S-shaped kidney; (c) lump kidney; (d) L-shaped kidney; (e) disc kidney (also described as subtype of horseshoe kidney); and (f) unilateral fused kidney (superior ectopia). A seventh type, the "Y-type" characterized by fusion of the ureters of the fused kidneys (g) has also been described

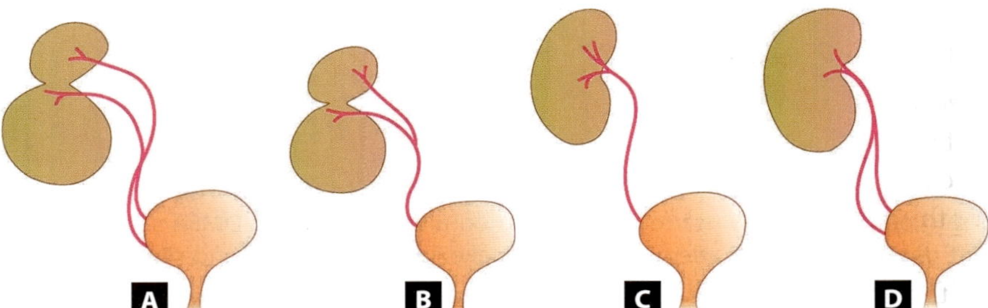

Figs. 5.14A to D: Types of duplex system based on ureteric drainage—(A) double ureters; (B) bifid ureters, (C) bifid renal pelvis, and (D) Inverted Y-ureteral duplication where two ureteral orifices drain from a single normal kidney (rare)

duplication includes evaluation of morphology, ureter status, and function of individual moieties. Management options include renal preservation (antibiotic prophylaxis for VUR, reimplantation of ectopic ureter), or renal resection (heminephrectomy, nephrectomy) based on function of the renal moieties.

Vascular Anomalies

Aberrant renal arteries, often considered an anatomical variant, may be a source of hypertension and need consideration prior to renal donor nephrectomy. The nutcracker phenomenon, or compression of the left renal vein in the fork formed by the abdominal aorta and superior mesenteric

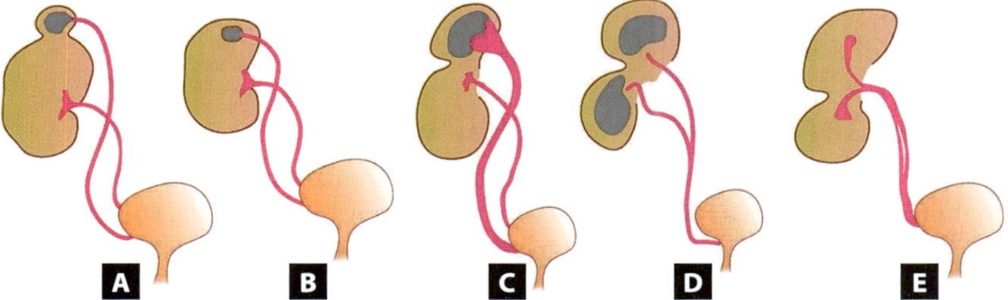

Figs. 5.15A to E: Classification of duplex kidneys based on features of the upper moiety. (A) Appendant: mini upper pole moiety located above the lower one; (B) Embedded: tiny upper moiety located within the interior top of the lower one and with same capsule; (C) Hydronephrotic—ureter is dilated and hydronephrotic and, as a consequence, the upper moiety may be as large as the lower; (D) Dual poor: both moieties small with "Y"-shaped ureters with ectopic orifices; and (E) Dual well—upper moiety nearly as big as the lower one without apparent dilatation of the "Y" or double ureters

artery, may be associated with exercise induced or postural hematuria, proteinuria, flank pain, and left varicocele. Conservative management is the norm. However, surgical correction (left renal vein transposition) or endovascular repair may occasionally be required.

Anomalies of Ureters

Retrocaval ureter is a rare anomaly in which the ureter passes posterior to the inferior vena cava. It occurs almost invariably on the right. Clinical features include abdominal pain, hematuria, infection, and urolithiasis in the second or third decade of life.

Ectopic ureters have their orifices caudal to the usual site on the trigone of the urinary bladder. Ectopic ureter is a frequent accompaniment of duplex kidneys. In males, the most common site is the posterior urethra (50%), followed by the seminal vesicle (33%), vas deferens, prostate, and epididymis. In females, the common sites are the bladder neck and upper urethra (33%), vaginal vestibule (33%), vagina (25%), cervix, and uterus.

CONCLUSION

Development of the kidney and urinary tract involves ureteric budding, branching morphogenesis, nephrogenesis and patterning. These processes are regulated by a complex genetic network but are also affected by environmental factors such as nutrition and teratogens. Interference in these processes can lead to renal agenesis, renal hypoplasia, renal dysplasia, duplex kidneys and vesicoureteral reflux. While developing, the kidneys also undergo relative ascent from the pelvis to the lumbar region. Interference with this process can lead to renal ectopia and fusion. CAKUT may be diagnosed incidentally or on evaluation after UTI. Management is aimed at prevention of UTI and mechanical injury whilst preserving renal function by screening for and treating hypertension and proteinuria.

BIBLIOGRAPHY

1. Balawender K, Cisek A, Cisek E, et al. Anatomical and clinical aspects of horseshoe kidney: a review of the current literature. Int J Morphol. 2019;37:12-6.
2. Bonsib SM. Renal hypoplasia, from grossly insufficient to not quite enough. Adv Anat Pathol. 2020;27:311-30.
3. Dressler GR. Advances in early kidney specification, development and patterning. Development. 2009;136:3863-74.
4. Hutchinson KA, Halili L, Guerra A, et al. Renal function in children with a congenital solitary functioning kidney: A systematic review. J Pediatr Urol. 2021;17:556-65.
5. Jain S. Kidney development and related anomalies. In: McManus LM, Mitchell RN (Eds). Pathobiology of Human Disease—A Dynamic Encyclopedia of Disease Mechanisms. Philadelphia: Elsevier; 2014, pp. 2701-15.
6. Kohl S, Avni FE, Boor P, et al. Definition, diagnosis and clinical management of non-obstructive kidney dysplasia: a consensus statement by the ERKNet Working Group on Kidney Malformations. Nephrol Dial Transplant. 2022;37:2351-62.
7. Kozlov VM, Schedl A. Duplex kidney formation: developmental mechanisms and genetic predisposition. F1000Res. 2020;9:F1000.
8. La Scola C, Ammenti A, Bertulli C, et al. Management of congenital solitary kidney: Recommendations of Italian Society of Pediatric Nephrology. Pediatr Nephrol. 2022;37:2185-207.
9. Loganathan AK, Bal HS. Crossed fused renal ectopia in children: a review of clinical profile, surgical challenges and outcome. J Pediatr Urol. 2019;15:315-21.
10. Papagiannopoulos D, Gong E. Revisiting sports precautions in children with solitary kidneys and congenital anomalies of the kidney and urinary tract. Urology. 2017;101:9-14.
11. Psooy K. Sports and the solitary kidney: What parents of a young child with a solitary kidney should know. Can Urol Assoc J. 2014;3:67-8.
12. Taghavi K, Kirkpatrick J, Mirjalili SA. The horseshoe kidney: anatomy and embryology. J Pediatr Urol. 2016;12:275-80.

Fluid, Electrolyte, and Acid-base Disorders

Georgie Mathew

Perturbations of fluid, electrolyte, and acid-base homeostasis are commonly encountered in practice. Some of these are life-threatening emergencies that require rapid evaluation and prompt management. A clear understanding of the physiological mechanisms is necessary for the diagnosis of the underlying etiology of various disorders and their treatment.

SODIUM AND WATER HOMEOSTASIS

Disorders of sodium and water, though familiar to all practising clinicians, are often misunderstood. The level of plasma Na^+ is chiefly a function of water intake and excretion and not that of sodium balance. Hyponatremia indicates the primary problems affecting water intake that cannot be excreted conversely, hypernatremia indicates the loss of water that has not been replaced. Hypovolemia principally represents loss of Na^+ and water.

Total body water (TBW) constitutes 90% of body weight in early fetal life, declining to 60% by 1–2 years, which remains constant thereafter. Though adult females can have a smaller proportion of TBW (~50–60%), a significant difference can be seen in individuals with high fat content. TBW is distributed in two major compartments: (*i*) 55–75% is intracellular fluid (ICF) and (*ii*) 25–45% is extracellular fluid (ECF). The ECF is distributed between intravascular (plasma) and extravascular (interstitial) spaces in a ratio of 1:3 **(Figs. 6.1A to E)**. The solute concentration of fluid, measured as osmolality, is expressed as milliosmoles per kilogram of water (mOsm/kg). The major solutes contributing to ECF osmolality are Na^+ and its accompanying anions Cl^- and HCO_3^- (usually poor membrane permeability), whereas K^+ and organic phosphate esters [adenosine triphosphate (ATP), creatinine phosphate, and phospholipids] are the major solutes in ICF.

This discordant solute content of ECF and ICF is maintained across membranes by the presence of Na^+/K^+-ATPase pump which pumps sodium actively out of cells. The operation of most of the other pumps/channels depends on the voltage distribution across the membrane created by the Na^+/K^+-ATPase pump. It is also helped by the presence of albumin in the ECF and the resultant Gibbs–Donnan effect. Water distributes between ECF and ICF compartments to achieve osmotic equilibrium. Capillary hydrostatic pressure and colloid osmotic pressure determine water movement within the

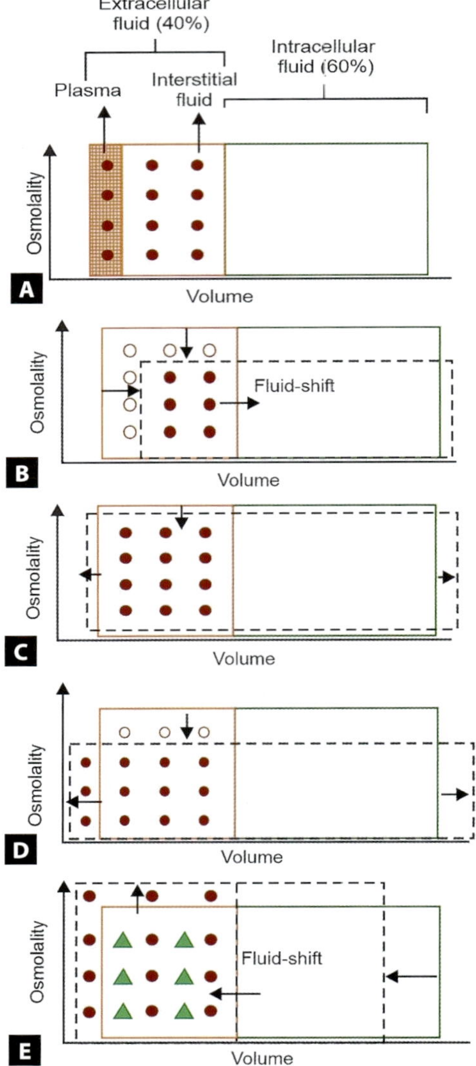

Figs. 6.1A to E: Abnormalities of sodium and water homeostasis. (A) *Normal body composition*. Nearly 60% of the body weight is water. Of this two-thirds is intracellular fluid (ICF), while the rest is extracellular fluid (ECF), which is distributed between the interstitial and intravascular compartments in a 3:1 ratio. (B) *Hypotonic hyponatremia*. Sodium and water are lost; water is conserved by vasopressin to defend against volume depletion. Hypotonic replacement fluids aggravate hyponatremia. While total body water is decreased, water shifts from ECF to ICF along the gradient of osmolality, leading to ECF volume depletion with pronounced signs of dehydration and relatively mild ICF expansion. (C) *Euvolemic hyponatremia*. These patients typically have an excess of total body water and slightly decreased serum sodium. Nevertheless, patients appear normal or have subtle signs of fluid overload. (D) *Hypervolemic hyponatremia*. Effective circulatory volume is depleted causing sodium and water retention in the kidneys. Increase in water is more than increase in sodium causing hyponatremia, edema, and hypotonicity. (E) *Hypertonic hyponatremia*. Glucose acts as an effective osmole at high concentration in diabetic ketoacidosis (DKA). Accumulation of effective osmoles in the ECF results in water shift from ICF to ECF, causing hyponatremia. Symptoms of hyponatremia are absent because osmolality is increased. During correction of DKA, glucose moves back into cells, fluid shifts from ECF to ICF, and serum sodium rises. If hyponatremia persists it may lead to excessive fluid shift into ICF causing cerebral edema

ECF compartment, i.e., between intravascular and interstitial spaces. While sodium balance is critical for the size of ECF space, water balance decides the fate of individual cell size.

Changes in the effective arterial blood volume are mediated by sensors in the afferent glomerular arterioles (for renin secretion), carotid sinus (sympathetic activity), and by the atria and ventricles (secreting natriuretic peptides). Usually, loss of ECF volume leads to reduction in tissue perfusion, except in heart failure and cirrhosis due to reduction in cardiac output and vasodilation. In both conditions, reduced tissue perfusion stimulates sodium retention with attempts to normalize ECF but tissue perfusion remains compromised due to the underlying condition.

It is important to differentiate between concepts of total and effective osmolality. Solutes, such as sodium and potassium with their anions that are restricted to ECF or ICF compartments, contribute to water movement and thus determine the effective osmolality of that compartment. In contrast, solutes such as urea and glucose do not contribute to water shifts as they diffuse freely across cell membranes and are therefore known as ineffective osmoles. Glucose, however, acts as an effective osmole in high concentrations, such as in diabetic ketoacidosis. Plasma osmolality is estimated directly using osmometers, or calculated as follows:

$$\text{Plasma osmolality (mOsm/kg)} = 2\,(\text{Na}^+) + (\text{glucose})/18 + (\text{blood urea nitrogen})/2.8$$

Normal plasma osmolality is maintained strictly within 1–2% of the normal range (285–295 mOsm/kg). The normal sodium concentration in the ECF is 135–145 mEq/L. Changes in sodium concentration in the ECF are linked to changes in ECF volume, and are associated with dysregulated water balance. Water balance is maintained by volume regulation (baroreceptors in the great vessels) and osmoregulation (central osmoreceptors in anterolateral hypothalamus). Since sodium is the principal determinant of effective ECF osmolality, increased serum osmolality (interpreted as decreased body water) leads to increased arginine vasopressin (AVP) secretion causing renal conservation of water and *vice versa*. Volume depletion also leads to nonosmotic AVP release, sympathetic system activation, and renal conservation of water by activating the renin-angiotensin-aldosterone system (RAS). However, as hypovolemia worsens, volume regulation takes precedence over osmoregulation, so volume depletion stimulates AVP despite hyponatremia. Angiotensin II amplifies osmosensory pathways and explains the potentiation of AVP release during states with low effective circulatory volume. This mechanism is responsible for the occurrence of hyponatremia in edema-forming states.

Plasma tonicity, or effective plasma osmolality, is an important concept. Osmoreceptors in the hypothalamus sense tonicity and determine the water's transcellular distribution, which moves from an area of low tonicity (higher water content) to that of high tonicity (lower water content). The principal difference between plasma tonicity and osmolality is that tonicity reflects the solute concentration that does not cross the cell membrane easily (sodium salts). Urea concentration does not affect tonicity as it freely equilibrates across the cell membrane (as is ethanol), while it determines plasma osmolality. Plasma tonicity is calculated by reducing the urea component from plasma osmolality calculation. Both hypo- and hypernatremia affect plasma tonicity, resulting in water transport across the cells and particularly leading to the neurologic symptoms of dysnatremia.

Changes in plasma tonicity, sensed by the hypothalamic osmoreceptors, affect water intake and its excretion by influencing thirst and antidiuretic hormone (ADH) release. These cells respond to changes as small as 1% in plasma osmolality, which is tightly regulated between 285 and 295 mOsm/kg of H_2O. In situations characterized by hypertonicity/hypernatremia, thirst is the chief defence mechanism and occurs prior to ADH secretion. Even though thirst is centrally regulated, it is sensed peripherally as oropharyngeal mechanoreceptors mediate a sensation of dry mouth and its cessation. Hypernatremia is rare in a patient with normal thirst mechanism and access to water, and is seen in critically ill children or infants without access to free water. ADH signaling by vasopressin 2 (V2) receptors leads to insertion of aquaporin 2 channels in the luminal membrane of the collecting duct, leading to water reabsorption. Suppression of ADH is the primary protective mechanism against development of hyponatremia. Below the lower limit of normal serum osmolality, ADH secretion is miniscule with maximal urinary dilution, below 100 mOsm/kg of H_2O. Clinical scenario in which this mechanism does not function well is seen in reduced effective circulating blood volume, or in the syndrome of inappropriate antidiuresis (SIAD). Above the osmotic threshold, a relatively linear rise in ADH secretion is observed.

Clinicians must understand that there are no normal values of Na^+ and H_2O excretion by the kidneys. As these disorders are intertwined, often occur concurrently, and with varying severity, the clinician must assess if the Na^+ and H_2O handling is appropriate for the given clinical scenario.

In conditions of Na^+ and H_2O imbalance, the first step is to assess life-threatening changes in ECF volume and manage that appropriately (volume resuscitation or removal). The next step is to grade the severity of defect in Na^+ balance and clinically determine the ECF volume (serial body weight being the most sensitive indicator). Laboratory estimations of plasma and urine osmolality provide clues regarding defects of water balance. Following establishment of defects in Na^+ and H_2O balance, appropriate diagnostic and therapeutic steps help navigate through the clinical problem.

Hyponatremia

Hyponatremia is defined as serum sodium concentration <135 mEq/L. A majority of hyponatremia (~70%) seen in patients are mild (130–134 mEq/L) and usually does not pose any clinical problems. Another important distinction is to be made between acute hyponatremia, when the condition develops or is presumed to have developed within the past 48 hr, and chronic hyponatremia that is otherwise. Acute and severe hyponatremia is often symptomatic.

Serum Na^+ reflects water content relative to body cations. Pseudohyponatremia (factitious hyponatremia) is a laboratory artifact caused by displacement of serum water by hyperlipidemia and hyperproteinemia, if sodium is measured by flame photometry. Indirect ion-selective electrode (IISE) potentiometry is the currently used Na^+ assay worldwide and direct IISE, used in blood gas analysis, do not report this problem. The spuriously low levels of Na^+ are usually minor; 1 mEq/L decrease in serum Na^+ requires 500 mg/dL increase in serum triglycerides or 4 g/dL increase in serum proteins. Corrected serum Na^+ can be calculated **(Flowchart 6.1)**.

Etiology

Hyponatremia is explained if an obvious cause is present, e.g., vomiting or diarrhea **(Box 6.1)**. Hyponatremia commonly results from disorders impairing electrolyte-free water excretion (aquaresis) by the kidneys, mediated chiefly by the ADH, and can occur in some cases of aquaresis independent of ADH, and rarely from excess water intake that overwhelms aquaresis. While low, normal, or high levels of total body Na^+ may be present in hyponatremia, the classification is based on the patient volume status so that the ratio of body Na^+ to water is always low. Serum osmolality is always low, although hyperosmolality occurs in conditions where effective osmoles accumulate in the ECF followed by dilutional hyponatremia **(Fig. 6.1E)**. The latter is seen in DKA and following mannitol administration. Corrected serum Na^+ may be calculated **(Flowchart 6.1)**.

Hypotonic (Hypovolemic) Hyponatremia (Fig. 6.1B)

Hypotonic hyponatremia typically occurs due to Na^+ loss coupled with free water loss (or excess free water retention). The electrolyte-mixed water loss may occur from kidneys or other sources such as the skin, gut, and third spaces. Diarrhea is the most common extrarenal cause in children **(Box 6.1)**. Homeostatic response to maintain intravascular volume results in low urine sodium (<30 mEq/L), due to avid reabsorption at the tubular level to maintain volume status and significant elevation in ADH production.

In diarrheal loss, as most of the fluid that is lost is hypotonic or isotonic to plasma, appropriate ADH secretion leads to concentrated urine with reduced urine volume and maintenance of serum Na^+. Replacement of these losses with hypotonic solutions (free water orally or IV) can lead to free water retention and consequent hyponatremia. Urinary salt wasting due to tubulointerstitial damage or skin losses (e.g., high sweat Na^+ in cystic fibrosis) can lead to excess Na^+ loss without water retention and hypotonic hyponatremia. Patients receiving thiazide diuretics are at higher risk of

Flowchart 6.1: Approach to hyponatremia. Urinary sodium ≤30 mEq/L suggests low effective circulatory volume even in patients receiving diuretics. RAS: renin-angiotensin-aldosterone system

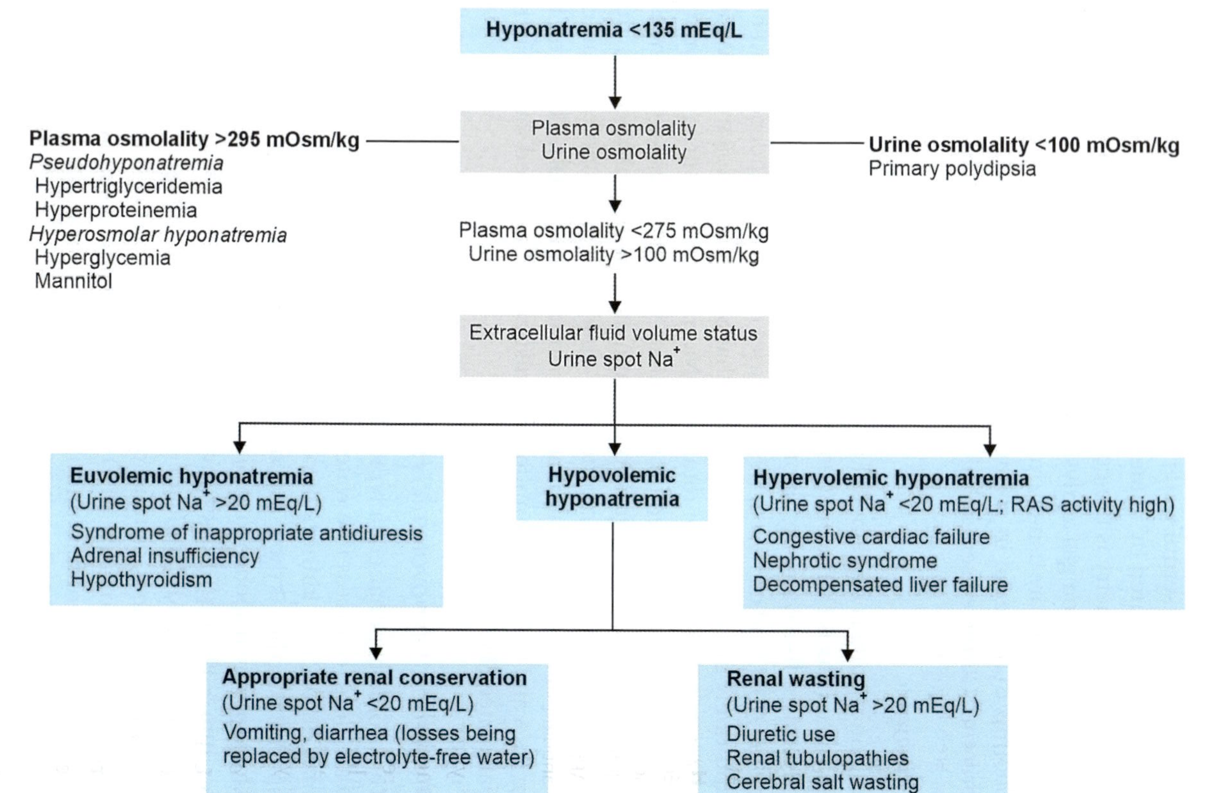

BOX 6.1: Etiology of hyponatremia

Hypotonic (hypovolemic)

Extrarenal

Gastrointestinal loss: Diarrhea, vomiting, fistulas
Cutaneous loss: Excessive sweating, cystic fibrosis
Third-space loss: Burns, pancreatitis, peritonitis
Postoperative (hypotonic fluids, third space loss, vomiting)

Renal

Diuretics (thiazides and loop diuretics), osmotic diuresis
Tubulopathies: Bartter, Gitelman, and Fanconi syndromes
Medullary or tubular damage: Nephronophthisis, tubulointerstitial nephritis, ARPKD
Mineralocorticoid deficiency, pseudohypoaldosteronism
Cerebral salt wasting

Euvolemic

SIAD: Classic, nephrogenic (activating mutation in AVPR2)
Water intoxication: Near drowning in fresh water, tap water enema, hypotonic IV fluids
Hypothyroidism
Glucocorticoid deficiency
Malnutrition

Hypervolemic

Edema forming states: Nephrotic syndrome, cirrhosis, congestive cardiac failure, sepsis
Renal insufficiency: Acute kidney injury, chronic kidney disease

ARPKD: autosomal recessive polycystic kidney disease; SIAD: syndrome of inappropriate antidiuresis

hyponatremia than those receiving loop diuretics. Loop diuretics dissipate the medullary concentration gradient, blunt urinary concentration that prevents free water retention, and protects against aggravation of hyponatremia. Aldosterone deficiency (congenital adrenal hyperplasia) or aldosterone resistance [pseudohypoaldosteronism (PHA)] results in hyponatremia, hyperkalemia, and metabolic acidosis.

Corrections for pseudohyponatremia: Na^+ decreases by 1.6 mEq/L for 100 mg/dL increase in glucose; Na^+ decreases by 2 mEq/L for 1000 mg/dL increase in triglycerides; Na^+ decreases by 0.25 mEq/L for 1 g/dL increase in protein.

Urine and serum osmolality should be measured in the first morning urine and fasting serum samples respectively. Urine spot Na^+ should be performed prior to initiation of IV fluids containing sodium.

Hypervolemic Hyponatremia (Fig. 6.1D)

In edema forming states (nephrotic syndrome, cirrhosis, and cardiac failure), the effective circulating volume is decreased, due to third space fluid loss or poor cardiac output. Decreased effective renal perfusion leads to renal sensing of a state of hypovolemia, causing retention of salt and water. Urine Na^+ concentration is low (<30 mEq/L). In acute kidney injury, oliguria results in an expanded intravascular volume, hyponatremia, and variable high urine Na^+ concentration.

Euvolemic Hyponatremia (Fig. 6.1C)

Hyponatremia occurs with normal or slightly expanded ECF volume chiefly in the SIAD **(Box 6.2)**. In homeostatic conditions, AVP levels are very low when plasma osmolality <280 mOsm/kg; ADH progressively increases above this cutoff, with thirst being stimulated at 5–10 mOsm/kg levels higher.

Reliable and reproducible assays for copeptin, a 39-aminoacid glycopeptide from the C-terminal part of pre-proAVP, have resulted in better delineation of five different patterns of AVP secretion in SIAD. Type A is characterized by very high levels that are unresponsive to osmotic changes, typically seen in nonregulated/ectopic AVP secretion (e.g., bronchogenic carcinoma). An abnormally low osmotic threshold characterizes type B with linear increase in AVP with rising osmolality (reset osmostat). In type C, an abnormal AVP response is observed only at low osmolality, potentially due to dysfunction of inhibitory neurons in the hypothalamus; type D shows undetectable AVP levels, either because of secretion of an unidentified antidiuretic substance from tumor cells, or alternatively, a gain-of-function mutation in the V2 receptor (i.e., nephrogenic SIAD). Type E shows linear decrease in AVP secretions with increasing serum osmolality (reset barostat).

BOX 6.2: Diagnostic criteria for syndrome of inappropriate antidiuresis (SIAD)

Essential criteria
Hyponatremia serum Na^+ <135 mEq/L
Effective serum osmolality <275 mOsm/kg
Inappropriate urinary concentration (urine osmolality >100 mOsm/kg)
Clinical euvolemia
Urine sodium >20–30 mEq/L, with normal dietary salt and water intake
Absence of adrenal, thyroid, pituitary, renal insufficiency, or diuretic use

Supplemental criteria
Fractional sodium excretion >0.5%#
Low serum uric acid <4 mg/dL#
Low serum urea <21.6 mg/dL#
Fractional urea excretion >55%#
Fractional uric acid excretion >12%#
Failure to correct hyponatremia with 0.9% saline infusion
Correction of hyponatremia through fluid restriction

#Signifies extracellular volume expansion

Consumption of considerably large amounts of water exceeding renal free water excretion and malnutrition similarly causes hyponatremia. Sodium and urea (breakdown product of proteins) are the principal urinary solutes. In chronic malnutrition, the quantum of solutes required to generate a minimal urine osmolality becomes a limiting factor to produce a certain volume of urine. A positive water balance thereby ensues, and chronic hyponatremia occurs in malnourished children not consuming enough sodium and protein to produce solutes for adequate water excretion.

In hospitalized patients, hyponatremia is frequently seen, chiefly due to administration of hypotonic intravenous (IV) fluids and inappropriate production of AVP. Potent stimuli of AVP secretion include pain, stress, nausea, positive pressure ventilation, and medications; AVP secretion thus occurs despite normovolemia **(Box 6.3)**.

Cerebral Salt Wasting

Some patients with neurological diseases may present with features that resemble SIAD, but in fact are secondary to cerebral salt wasting. The distinction is important because the management differs. In cerebral salt wasting, natriuretic peptides such as B-type natriuretic peptide or adrenomedullin leads to secondary activation of AVP due to volume loss. Urinary urate and urea excretion are normal or high despite volume contraction. Consequently, hypouricemia, hypouremia, and a normal or

BOX 6.3: Etiology of the syndrome of inappropriate antidiuresis (SIAD)

Central nervous system
Infections: Meningoencephalitis, brain abscess
Demyelination, Guillain–Barré syndrome
Malignancies
Pituitary surgery, head trauma, intracranial hemorrhage
Cerebral hypoxia

Pulmonary
Infections: Pneumonia, tuberculosis
Positive pressure ventilation, bronchial asthma, pneumothorax

Medications
Vasopressin analogs: Desmopressin, oxytocin
Increased vasopressin release: Carbamazepine, chlorpropamide, vincristine, cyclophosphamide
Decreased prostaglandins synthesis: Nonsteroidal anti-inflammatory drugs, paracetamol
Others: Haloperidol, amitriptyline, serotonin-reuptake inhibitors, morphine

Malignancy
Leukemia, lymphoma, Hodgkin disease
Other stimuli for vasopressin release: Pain, nausea, surgery
Nephrogenic SIAD, due to gain of function mutation in *AVPR2*

TABLE 6.1: Comparison of syndrome of inappropriate antidiuresis (SIAD) and cerebral salt wasting

	SIAD	*Cerebral salt wasting*
Serum sodium	Low	Low
Body fluid status	Increased	Decreased
Central venous pressure	Normal to high	Decreased
Serum uric acid Fractional excretion (FE) uric acid FE uric acid after hyponatremia correction	Decreased High (>11%) <11%	Decreased High (>11%) >11%
Serum osmolality	<280 mOsm/kg	Decreased
Urine osmolality	>100 mOsm/kg	Increased
Urine: serum osmolality ratio	<1	>1
Urine output	Normal	Increased
Urea/creatinine ratio	Normal to low	Normal to low
Serum aldosterone	Decreased	Normal to low
Serum renin	Decreased	Normal to low
Natriuretic peptide type B	Increased	Increased
Fractional excretion of phosphate	Normal (<10%)	High (>20%)

even low urea-to-creatinine ratio are characteristic **(Table 6.1)**. ECF volume depletion is the only feature which differentiates cerebral salt wasting from SIAD. Since clinical assessment of volume status may be inaccurate, measurement of central venous pressure might be necessary.

Classification and Clinical Features

Serum sodium concentration between 130 and 135 mEq/L is classified as mild, 125 and 129 mEq/L as moderate, and <125 mEq/L as severe hyponatremia. Symptoms of hyponatremia are more common when serum sodium concentration is below 125 mEq/L. Hyponatremia, which develops or is presumed to have developed in ≥48 hr is termed "chronic". Children are at higher risk than adults for developing hyponatremic encephalopathy.

Hyponatremic encephalopathy is a medical emergency that presents subtle and nonspecific symptoms such as nausea, vomiting, irritability, restlessness, apathy, change in personality, and disturbance in gait. Severe manifestations include altered sensorium, seizures, and coma. The severity of symptoms reflects the degree of cerebral edema due to intracellular shift of water from the hypotonic plasma. The brain adapts to low plasma osmolality by extruding out potassium and idiogenic osmoles (organic solutes—inositol, taurine, and glutamine) in an attempt to lower intracellular osmolality and restore cell volume. This osmotic adaptation takes about 48 hr.

Cerebral edema is precipitated if fluid shifts occur rapidly before the brain has time to adapt. This threshold is used to define acute (<48-hr) or chronic (>48-hr) hyponatremia. During treatment of hyponatremia, these adaptive responses make neurons vulnerable to sustain damage by intracellular dehydration if plasma sodium returns to normal rapidly. A consequence of this damage is osmotic demyelination syndrome, which is diagnosed on MRI by hyperintense pontine and extrapontine lesions. In clinical practice, the distinction between acute and chronic hyponatremia is often unclear at initial evaluation.

Hyponatremia should therefore be assumed as chronic, and corrected gradually (~10–12 mEq/L/day). Patients who develop the demyelination syndrome show a biphasic course, with neurological improvement followed by deterioration with mutism, dysarthria, lethargy, spastic quadriparesis, and pseudobulbar palsy.

Approach to Hyponatremia

A stepwise approach to hyponatremia is outlined in **Flowchart 6.1**. Estimation of ECF volume status is the first step in algorithmic approach to differential diagnosis of hypotonic hyponatremia. Since clinical assessment of ECF volume status is imprecise, this is assessed by urinary osmolality and spot urine sodium levels. Clinical features suggest the differential diagnosis and guide management.

Treatment of Hyponatremia

Symptomatic hyponatremia requires early recognition and prompt management. In hypovolemic hyponatremia with hypotension, volume resuscitation with normal saline takes precedence over treatment of hyponatremia even at the risk of sudden increase in serum sodium. The brain serves as a reasonable barometer in rapidly developing (<12 hr) hyponatremia and emergent central nervous system (CNS) dysfunction can usually be managed by hypertonic saline boluses (4–5 mL/kg given over 20–60 minutes). After CNS symptoms have stabilized, further corrections can be performed. In patients with asymptomatic/chronic hyponatremia, especially absence of CNS dysfunction, slow correction is prudent.

Isotonic saline should be primarily used for management of hypovolemic hyponatremia, with a prompt response. Recent studies have supported oral urea therapy in chronic SIAD. Vaptans produce significant and prompt aquaresis; however, effects are variable and often serious overcorrection of Na^+ is reported; should be used only with caution and supervision, after all other measures have been exhausted.

Flowchart 6.2 outlines the management of hyponatremia. Close biochemical and clinical monitoring is provided during management.

Flowchart 6.2: Management of hyponatremia. Rise of serum Na^+ should not exceed 0.5 mEq/hr or 10 mEq/L in the first 24-hr, and additional 8 mEq/L during every next 24-hr, until Na^+ level of 130 mEq/L. CSW: cerebral salt wasting; RRT: renal replacement therapy; SIAD: syndrome of inappropriate diuresis

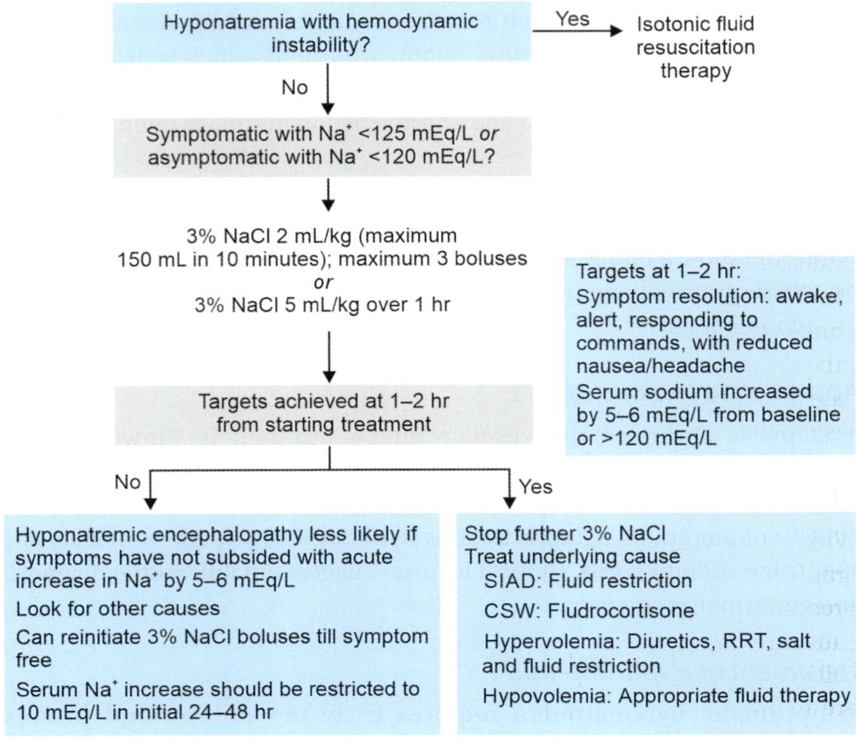

Chronic hyponatremia should be slowly corrected over 48–72 hr to avoid the risk of osmotic demyelination. Hyponatremic encephalopathy is unlikely if no clinical improvement occurs despite an acute rise in serum Na^+ of 5–6 mEq/L. In such cases, infusion of 3% hypertonic saline is continued aiming for an additional 1 mEq/L/h increase in serum Na^+ concentration while appropriate diagnosis is established. SIAD can be managed with water restriction to match for the insensible water loss and urine output. If required, cautious coadministration of furosemide (1–2 mg/kg) and NaCl (1–2 g/day) might help in promoting hypotonic fluid loss. Refractory SIAD may be managed, by experts, using lithium/demeclocycline or tolvaptan.

Hypernatremia

Hypernatremia is defined as serum Na^+ level >145 mEq/L. Hypernatremia is always a state of plasma hyperosmolality, although ECF volume may be variable. Protective mechanisms against developing hypernatremia are the ability to increase AVP secretion to concentrate urine and a powerful thirst mechanism. The degree of hypernatremia is mild unless the thirst mechanism is abnormal or access to water is limited. The latter occurs in infants, physically handicapped, patients with impaired mental status, postoperative state, and in critically ill children requiring assisted ventilation.

Etiology

Hypernatremia occurs due to relative water deficiency in proportion to total body sodium **(Box 6.4)**. The source of water deficit is either renal or extrarenal. A frequent cause of hypernatremia is the inability to establish adequate breast feeding in otherwise healthy term or near-term (≥35 weeks of gestation) exclusively breastfed newborns of primiparous mothers. The underlying cause of hypernatremic dehydration is inadequate water intake. Most children with diarrhea do not have hypernatremia because they consume enough hypotonic fluids to compensate for losses. Improperly mixed oral rehydration solutions are a common cause of pure Na^+ gain causing hypernatremia during episodes of diarrhea. Renal water loss is responsible for hypernatremia in diabetes insipidus and osmotic diuresis.

Clinical Features

With hypernatremia and hypertonicity, water moves down its osmotic gradient, leading to a contracted ICF volume. The ECF volume is relatively preserved, and thus clinical signs of dehydration may be masked, potentially causing profound dehydration before medical attention is sought. Brain cell volume decreases, and hence, the important features of hypernatremia are neurological consisting of altered mental status, lethargy alternating

BOX 6.4: Etiology of hypernatremia

Hypotonic fluid loss

Gastrointestinal loss: Diarrhea, vomiting, and lactulose

Renal

- Osmotic diuresis: Incorrect mixing of infant formula, diabetes mellitus
- Polyuric phase of acute tubular necrosis
- Postobstructive polyuria

Pure water deficit

Respiratory, skin: Fever, preterm newborns on radiant warmer/phototherapy

Inadequate intake: Poor access to water, inadequate breastfeeding, altered thirst perception

Renal

- Central diabetes insipidus: Partial or complete
- Nephrogenic diabetes insipidus: Hereditary, acquired (hypokalemia, tubulointerstitial disease, obstructive uropathy, therapy with amphotericin)

Pure increased sodium load

Sodium chloride intoxication (oral, IV, enema); sodium bicarbonate therapy

Improperly mixed oral rehydration solutions

with irritability, high pitched cry in infants, neuromuscular irritability, focal neurologic deficits, and occasionally coma or seizures. As the brain moves away from the meninges, due to intracellular dehydration, tension on bridging veins causes increased risk of subarachnoid, subdural, and intracerebral hemorrhage. Thrombotic complications due to severe dehydration and possibly hypercoagulability include stroke, dural sinus thrombosis, peripheral thrombosis, and renal vein thrombosis. Hypernatremia may be associated with hyperglycemia and mild hypocalcemia.

Diagnostic Approach

Flowchart 6.3 indicates the approach to evaluating a patient with hypernatremia. History of polyuria and gastrointestinal fluid loss is obtained in all cases of hypernatremia. The normal renal response to hypernatremia is excretion of a minimal amount of maximally concentrated urine. If urine osmolality is >600 mOsm/kg in a child with hypernatremia, extrarenal hypotonic fluid losses are suspected. Central diabetes insipidus and the genetic forms of nephrogenic diabetes insipidus result in massive urinary water losses and very dilute urine. Water losses are less profound, and urine may have almost same osmolality as plasma in conditions causing secondary nephrogenic diabetes insipidus, like obstructive uropathy and medullary damage.

Management

In chronic hypernatremia, brain cells accumulate idiogenic osmoles to increase intracellular osmolality to defend against intracellular dehydration. These dissipate slowly during correction of hypernatremia. With rapid correction of hypernatremia, osmotic gradient may drive water intracellularly, producing cerebral edema manifesting as seizure, brain herniation, and death. Therefore, cautious correction of serum sodium level, not exceeding 12 mEq/L/24-hr is important **(Box 6.5)**. Hyperglycemia may be seen, but insulin is not recommended since it might increase idiogenic osmoles in the brain. Hypocalcemia is common and the addition of calcium gluconate to rehydration fluid is often indicated.

Renal replacement therapy is indicated for hypernatremia with concurrent renal failure and volume overload, with high Na^+ dialysate baths to prevent rapid fall of Na^+.

Patients with diabetes insipidus should have unrestricted access to free water. Management aims at decreasing urine volume through use of vasopressin analogs (central diabetes insipidus), low osmolar load (dietary restriction of sodium), and hydrochlorothiazide (2–4 mg/kg/day) with or without amiloride (0.3 mg/kg/day). Volume resuscitation in children with

Flowchart 6.3: Approach to hypernatremia. Assessment of volume status and urine osmolality allows determination of the underlying etiology
*Copeptin cut-off values are different for arginine and hypertonic saline stimulated tests
Δ: change, AVP: arginine vasopressin; DI: diabetes insipidus; ECF: extracellular fluid; sOsm: serum osmolality; uOsm: urine osmolality; uNa: urine sodium

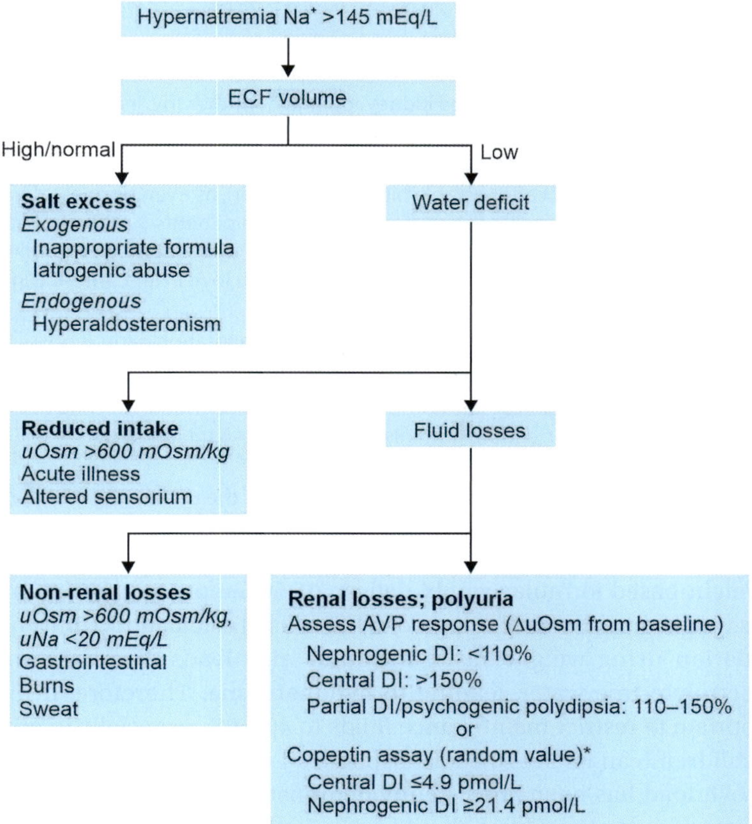

diabetes insipidus should preferably be with 5% dextrose water to prevent solute load and worsening hypernatremia. Therapy for salt overload is targeted at removal of excess salt by loop diuretics or renal replacement therapy if associated with renal failure.

FLUID MANAGEMENT IN HOSPITALIZED CHILDREN

There have been significant improvements in the quantity and level of evidence on the use of maintenance IV fluids in hospitalized children. The Holliday-Segar formula is still used globally to determine the fluid volume in ill (and critically ill) children, despite significant paucity of data to support its use.

BOX 6.5: Correction of hypernatremic dehydration

Restore intravascular volume with 1–2 boluses of 20 mL/kg normal saline over 20 minutes (till restoration of intravascular volume)

Determine time for correction, based on initial Na^+ concentration:

- Serum Na^+ level: Time to achieve ~145 mEq/L target
- 145–157 mEq/L: 24-hr
- 158–170 mEq/L: 48-hr
- 171–183 mEq/L: 72-hr
- 184–196 mEq/L: 84-hr (may need kidney replacement therapy, if oliguric)

In moderate-to-severe chronic hypernatremia (>157 mEq/L), after establishing intravascular repletion, initial fluid for correction should contain 77–154 mEq/L of Na^+ (with 20 mEq/L KCl after establishing urine output), as even normal saline (osmolarity 308 mOsm/L) will provide free water in such patients (~200 mL/L free water when serum Na^+ >190 mEq/L). Initially, higher Na^+ content may be obtained in severe hypernatremia by adding 3% saline; fluids with lower Na^+ content can be used in the maintenance phase

Fluid rate: 1.25–1.5 times maintenance; institute oral rehydration early, if possible

Monitor serum Na^+ q 4-hr; should not fall by >0.5 mEq/L/hr or >8–12 mEq/day

Adjust fluid on basis of clinical status and serum Na^+ concentration; if child develops seizures (due to rapid correction) administer 3% NaCl (4–6 mL/kg over 30 minutes)

Replace ongoing losses as they occur; identify and treat the underlying cause

Weight-based formulae would deliver 20–50% more volume in children of this weight group when compared to BSA-based calculation. Conventional calculation using weight-based formulae also leads to overestimation of electrolyte-free water, leading to hyponatremia. Therefore, it may be appropriate to restrict maintenance fluids to 40–60%, especially in critically sick children (can be 50–70% for hospitalized noncritically ill children), as fluid overload has been consistently demonstrated to be an independent predictor of mortality. Fluids should be limited to around 400 mL/m^2 (with replacement of urine output/other losses) in acute kidney injury/chronic kidney disease (AKI/CKD) with oliguria.

Hypotonic fluids have been extensively used in all children <18 years of age, irrespective of age, etiology, severity of illness, and underlying diagnosis. The American Academy of Pediatrics, European Society of Pediatrics, and other expert groups now recommend that isotonic fluids be used for maintenance fluid therapy in all children, irrespective of the reason for admission, excluding neonates <28 days of age, and certain disease states. Multiple meta-analysis emphasizes a significant reduction in the risk of hyponatremia with use of isotonic fluids.

Balanced salt solutions (Plasma-Lyte, Ringer's lactate) are being increasingly used in critically ill children. These solutions, when compared to normal saline, reduce the chloride load to the patient and help in preservation of acid-base balance. Though recent evidence does not point to any mortality benefits in critically ill children with balanced salt solution when compared to normal saline, reduction in time in hospital and hypokalemia incidence was noted. No difference in the incidence of hyponatremia was observed between the two solutions.

There is no single IV maintenance fluid (volume or composition) for children; individualized therapy is required, with close monitoring for the incident adverse events. Parenteral fluid therapy must be replaced as soon as feasible in children by enteral route of fluid/nutrition administration.

DISORDERS OF POTASSIUM HOMEOSTASIS

Normal potassium (K^+) homeostasis maintains plasma K^+ concentration within a specific, narrow range to maintain ionic balance across excitable tissues. The amount of potassium in the ECF constitutes <2% of the total body potassium content and 98% of exchangeable K^+ resides in the intracellular compartment. This distribution between ECF and ICF compartments is maintained by the Na^+/K^+-ATPase pump which actively transports potassium in and sodium out of the cell in a 2:3 ratio, maintaining cellular resting membrane potential that is crucial for neuromuscular function and cardiac conduction. Normal plasma K^+ concentration is strictly regulated between 3.5–5 mEq/L. Higher levels are observed in newborns, ranging from 4 to 6 mEq/L in term and 5.5 to 7 mEq/L in preterm infants.

The kidney is primarily responsible for maintaining body K^+ content; which involves about 60–80 mEq in the ECF compartment **(Fig. 6.2)**. To reduce the effects of transient and potentially harmful increases in plasma K^+, there are a few physiological mechanisms for transcellular shifts, which occur immediately before renal excretory mechanisms can set in. The third but minor element, in K^+ homeostasis, is the gastrointestinal tract.

Multiple factors influence the distribution of potassium between the ICF and ECF. Insulin release after a meal plays a vital role in the transcellular shift of dietary K^+ before renal excretion. In insulin-responsive tissues, insulin causes glucose transporter type 4 (GLUT-4) channels to be inserted, which stimulate K^+ uptake by increasing the activity of Na^+/K^+-ATPase pump. Differential regulation of insulin-mediated glucose and K^+ uptake is seen in metabolic syndrome and CKD. Catecholamines, acting through β_2 receptors, increase the Na^+/K^+-ATPase pump activity, leading to shift of K^+ transcellularly in the muscle, to prevent abnormal increase in K^+ during exercise. Medications that stimulate β_2 receptors, also produce similar effects, and is clinically applied in the emergent management of hyperkalemia.

The skeletal muscle plays a vital role in the K^+ balance. In hyperchloremic acidosis, reduced extracellular pH will reduce both the Na^+/H^+ exchange pump (NHE) and the electrogenic sodium bicarbonate cotransporter (NBCe) **(Figs. 6.3A and B)**. Reduced inward Na^+ leads to reduced Na^+/K^+-ATPase

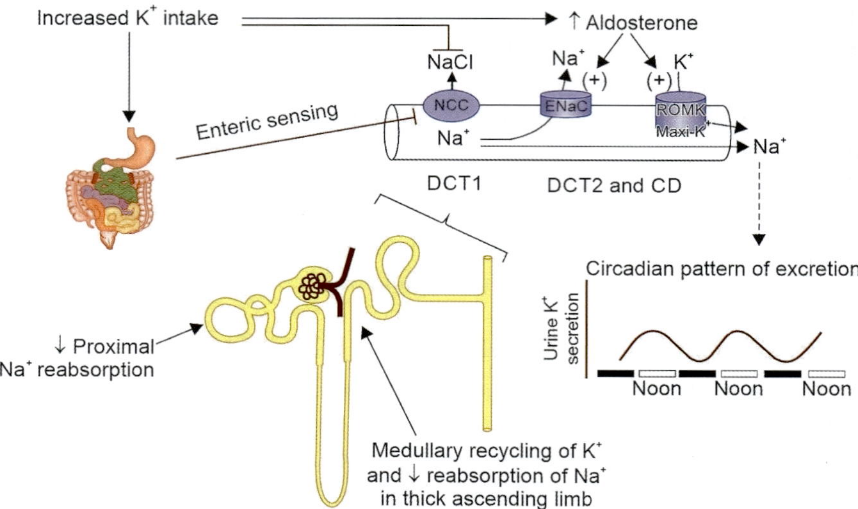

Fig. 6.2: Handling of potassium (K^+) load, from dietary sources and tissue breakdown, by the kidneys. Urinary K^+ secretion and expression of K^+ transporters exhibit a circadian pattern. Gene expression of ROMK is higher in the day and during periods of activity (renal K^+ excretion is greater), while H^+/K^+ ATPase expression follows the inverse pattern. Lines ending with arrowheads and straight lines signify stimulation and inhibition, respectively. CD: collecting duct; DCT: distal convoluted tubule; ENaC: epithelial sodium channel; NCC: sodium chloride cotransporter; ROMK: renal outer medullary potassium channel

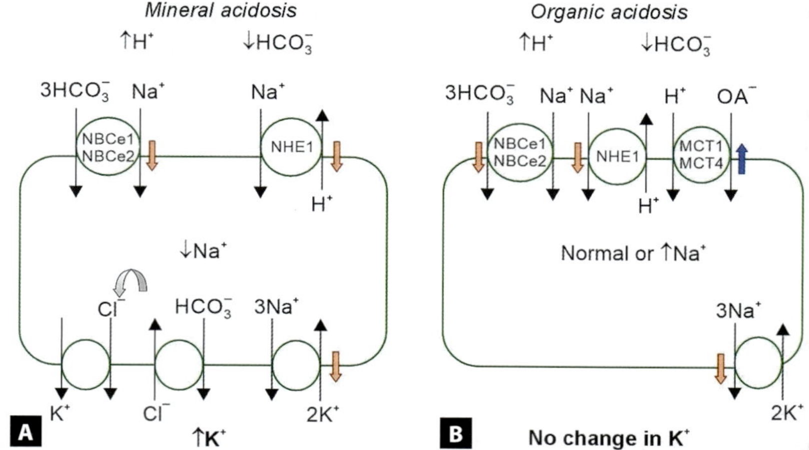

Figs. 6.3A and B: The skeletal muscle plays an essential role in the K^+ balance during mineral and organic acidosis. During mineral (hyperchloremic normal anion gap) metabolic acidosis, the extracellular acidosis slows the rate of the sodium hydrogen exchanger (NHE1; *SLC9A1*) and electrogenic sodium bicarbonate cotransporter 1 (NBCe1; *SLC4A4*), reducing intracellular Na^+ and Na^+/K^+-ATPase activity, resulting in hyperkalemia. The influx of Na^+ *via* monocarboxylate transporters (MCT) during organic acidosis maintains intracellular Na^+ and does not result in significant hyperkalemia

activity, resulting in reduced transcellular shift and hyperkalemia. Low extracellular bicarbonate concentrations lead to efflux of K^+ and bicarbonate, by the combined action of the Cl^-/HCO_3^- exchanger and K^+/Cl^- cotransport. Organic acidosis (H^+ anion other than Cl^-) is typified by inward movement of the organic anion and H^+ through the monocarboxylate transporter (MCT1, 4) that causes a reduction in intracellular pH, activating both NHE and NBCe. Due to increased intracellular Na^+, the activity of the Na^+/K^+-ATPase pump remains intact, facilitating transcellular K^+ shifts and maintaining normokalemia.

The internal K^+ balance alters with changes in plasma tonicity as well. Effective osmoles (glucose, mannitol, sucrose, etc.) accumulating in the extracellular space create an osmotic efflux of water from the ICF. The resultant increased intracellular K^+ concentration also favors K^+ efflux through permeable channels.

The principal driver of the K^+ balance is the nephron, which freely filters plasma K^+. Reabsorption in the proximal tubule (60–70%) occurs in the paracellular pathway (proportionate to Na^+ and water) and the ascending limb of Henle (15–20%) via the $Na^+/K^+/2Cl^-$ pump. Reabsorption is largely independent of K^+ intake. The late distal convoluted tubule and cortical collecting duct, collectively known as the aldosterone sensitive distal nephron, is the main site of renal K^+ excretion and regulation. Tubular K^+ secretion is predominantly driven by the apical membrane depolarisation and negative transepithelial potential difference (lumen-negative orientation) generated by the amiloride-sensitive epithelial sodium channels (ENaC). Aldosterone (stimulated by volume depletion) increases insertion of ENaC into the apical membrane of the principal cells of the cortical collecting duct, which stimulates potassium excretion. Aldosterone increases both the number and duration of the open state of the ENaC. Inward rectifying K^+ channels (ROMK; also called Kir1.1) in the principal cells and big K^+ (BK; also called Maxi-K, slo1 or $K_{Ca}1.1$) channels in the principal and intercalated cells have an important role in K^+ secretion. K^+ secretion via the ROMK channels are intrinsically limited by intracellular Mg^{2+} and release of this inhibition in hypomagnesemia might result in refractory hypokalemia. The luminal fluid flow rate principally activates the BK channels.

The effect of dietary K^+ on renal excretion is summarized as follows. High oral K^+ (palaeolithic and fruit-based diets) and higher K^+ plasma levels are sensed by the Kir4.1/5.1 channels located in the basolateral membranes of the distal convoluted tubule (DCT), leading to depolarization of the membrane. Subsequent inhibition of the regulatory WNK kinase-SPAK (with no lysine kinases; Ste20-related protein/alanine-rich kinase) pathway leads to decreased sodium chloride cotransporter (NCC) activity. An increase in the distal Na^+ delivery due to NCC inhibition leads to increased K^+ secretion as outlined above. The feed-forward mechanism, triggered by splanchnic sensing of K^+, can trigger renal excretory mechanisms (dephosphorylation and decreased NCC activity in the DCT) independent of renal regulation. This mechanism also has a diurnal variation, peaking in the afternoon to coincide with dietary intake and activity, and reaching a nadir at night. High K^+ diets (in the long term) can potentially lead to natriuresis and explain their blood pressure lowering effect. On the other hand, a diet deficient in K^+ (and having high Na^+, as in high/ultrahigh processed foods) leads to increased NCC activity, and sodium retention and results in salt sensitive hypertension.

The role of aldosterone in renal K^+ excretion is vital. Aldosterone (triggered by low blood pressure, low Na^+/Cl^- sensing by the macula densa → renin secretion) acts on the mineralocorticoid receptor (MR) in the aldosterone sensitive distal nephron. Aldosterone will activate these channels in the nephron—ENaC in the principal cells, apical H^+/ATPase and H^+/K^+-ATPase in α-intercalated cells, apical bicarbonate/chloride exchanger (pendrin) in β-intercalated cells, and the basolateral Na^+/K^+-ATPase in all these cells. Depending on the physiology, aldosterone can increase the following—Na^+ absorption, K^+ excretion, acid excretion, bicarbonate excretion, or chloride reabsorption.

A peculiar "aldosterone paradox" pattern results in salt retention without K^+ secretion in hypovolemic conditions, and *vice versa* in hyperkalemia. The aldosterone paradox in hypovolemia occurs due to angiotensin II, which stimulates proximal Na^+ reabsorption by stimulating the NCC and inhibits the ROMK channel in the distal nephron. Angiotensin II also activates (by dephosphorylation of MR) apical H^+/ATPase, H^+/K^+-ATPase and Cl^-/HCO_3^- exchanger, leading to electroneutral NaCl absorption while preventing excess K^+ secretion. Vasopressin release, in hypovolemia, results in water reabsorption.

Thus, the key determinants of K^+ secretion along the aldosterone sensitive distal nephron include distal Na^+ delivery (and lumen negative potential difference), luminal fluid flow, plasma K^+, aldosterone concentration, and acid-base status.

Hypokalemia

Hypokalemia is defined as serum potassium <3.5 mEq/L. Hypokalemia is usually mild, with levels in the 3.0–3.5 mEq/L range but can be moderate to severe (<3.0 mEq/L).

Etiology

The etiology of hypokalemia can be broadly classified into these categories—spurious hypokalemia (resulting from uptake of K^+ into cells after sampling; occurs predominantly in warm environments), transcellular shifts with normal total body stores, and true depletion of body stores due to chronic reduction in intake or losses (*via* urine, skin, or gut) **(Boxes 6.6 and 6.7)**.

BOX 6.6: Causes of hypokalemia

Spurious hypokalemia Cellular K^+ uptake after blood sampling; hot weather

Shift of potassium from ECF to ICF Normal total body K^+

Activation of β_2 adrenergic receptors
- Endogenous: Catecholamine excess
- Exogenous: β-adrenergic agonists

Insulin action
- Endogenous: Refeeding syndrome, insulinoma
- Exogenous: Treatment of diabetic ketoacidosis

Metabolic alkalosis
Hypokalemic periodic paralysis
Expanded effective circulatory volume
Enhanced mineralocorticoid activity

True potassium depletion

Extrarenal losses
- Poor intake: Malnutrition
- Gastrointestinal loss: Vomiting, diarrhea, laxative abuse, congenital chloride diarrhea
- Skin loss: Excessive sweating, burns, cystic fibrosis

Renal losses **(Box 6.7)**

BOX 6.7: Causes of hypokalemia due to renal losses

With metabolic acidosis
Renal tubular acidosis (proximal and distal; ***see* Table 20.1**)
Medications: Acetazolamide, amphotericin B, outdated tetracycline **(*see* Table 20.2)**

With metabolic alkalosis
Bartter and Gitelman syndromes **(*see* Tables 20.4 and 20.7)**
Loop, thiazide diuretics
Posthypercapnia
Mineralocorticoid excess states: Renovascular stenosis, glucocorticoid remediable hypertension, apparent mineralocorticoid excess, Liddle syndrome **(*see* Table 25.9)**

Without specific acid base disturbances
Recovery from acute kidney injury
Amphotericin, cisplatin, aminoglycosides
Hypomagnesemia
Interstitial nephritis

Spurious hypokalemia occurs when cells take up potassium after blood sample has been drawn and left at room temperature, e.g., in patients with high leukocyte counts. This has been noted in patients with conditions such as acute leukemia (from the significant increase in the metabolically active cells) and in high environmental temperature. This is avoided if plasma (or serum) is rapidly separated from the cells and stored at 4°C. Since potassium is ubiquitous in the diet, hypokalemia secondary to inadequate intake is unusual. More often, a relatively low intake is complicated by excessive loss in vomit or diarrhea. The potassium content in gastric secretions is 20 mEq/L and in diarrheal fluid 10–80 mEq/L. ECF depletion, in such cases, leads to activation of the renin-angiotensin-aldosterone axis, worsening the potassium deficiency. Renal loss of potassium occurs in tubulopathies, tubular damage, and use of diuretics. Excessive mineralocorticoid activity is the main cause of hypokalemia associated with metabolic alkalosis and hypertension. Evaluation of these disorders is discussed in **Chapter 20**.

Shift of K^+ into the cells is an important cause of hypokalemia with normal total body stores of K^+. Metabolic alkalosis and increased endogenous or exogenous insulin/β_2 adrenergic receptor activation are important causes. Hypokalemic periodic paralysis is an uncommon condition, characterized by recurrent episodes of hypokalemia (often with hypophosphatemia and hypomagnesemia) with muscular weakness or paralysis. These episodes are often triggered after exercise, a carbohydrate rich meal or administration of insulin/β_2 adrenergic receptor agonist agents in susceptible individuals. The disease is caused by mutations in *CACNA1S, SCN4A, KCNJ2,* and *KCNJ18* and may be seen in thyrotoxicosis.

Clinical Features

Mild hypokalemia (3–3.5 mEq/L) is often asymptomatic; symptoms manifest when K^+ level is below 2.5–3.0 mEq/L. It is important to understand that there is no definite cutoff level for development of symptoms. Initial electrocardiographic changes include ST depression, which progress to wide P waves, flat T waves, and development of U waves at lower serum levels. Severe degrees of hypokalemia can produce apparent QT prolongation with giant U waves (differentiated from large T waves in having a broad base; the apparent QT prolongation being a QU interval). Lower levels are associated with weakness, rhabdomyolysis and cardiac conduction abnormalities **(Fig. 6.4)**. Hypokalemia increases the potential for digitalis-induced

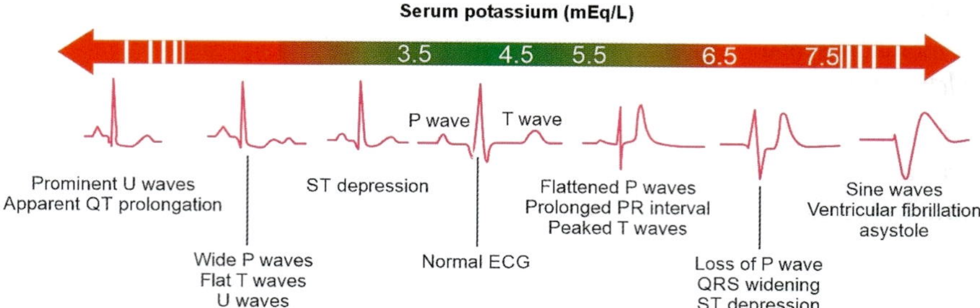

Fig. 6.4: Electrocardiographic manifestations of hyper- and hypokalemia. Characteristic changes are depicted in order of severity. The changes in hyperkalemia correspond to serum potassium levels, while those of hypokalemia do not always relate to serum potassium concentration

arrhythmias, such as supraventricular tachycardia, ventricular tachycardia, and heart block. Paralysis usually occurs below levels <2.5 mEq/L and involves skeletal muscles (beginning with lower extremities, progressing to trunk and upper extremities, may affect respiratory muscles) and smooth muscles (paralytic ileus, urinary retention). Chronic hypokalemia may cause impaired renal concentrating ability, polyuria, renal cysts, and poor somatic growth.

Evaluation

Spurious hypokalemia is excluded by absence of characteristic electrocardiogram (ECG) changes. The clinical setting usually provides clues to etiology. As most patients with true body K^+ depletion have either a gastrointestinal or renal cause of K^+ wasting, etiology is often apparent. The combination of clinical features, blood pressure, along with investigations that include blood pH, electrolytes, urea and creatinine, and urine K^+ and chloride enable a diagnosis in most cases **(Flowchart 6.4)**. The estimation of spot urinary K^+, fractional excretion of K^+, and potassium to creatinine (K^+/Cr) ratio are useful. Spot urine K^+ level alone might be misleading, because hypokalemia can cause polyuria and a relatively low value could represent a large urinary loss. The urine spot K^+/Cr ratio should be assessed keeping in view the potassium retaining state of the growing child and the increase in plasma creatinine with muscle mass. In presence of hypokalemia, fractional excretion of potassium <6% is consistent with an appropriate renal response. While these indices enable differentiation of transient transcellular shifts from losses of potassium, they do not always differentiate extrarenal from renal wasting of potassium because volume loss in extrarenal conditions triggers secondary activation of renin-angiotensin-aldosterone axis causing renal excretion of potassium. In hypovolemic states, high urine potassium index (urine K^+/sum of K^+ and Na^+) >0.6 indicates appropriate aldosterone response to hypovolemia. Urinary chloride levels help evaluate patients with metabolic alkalosis and hypokalemia **(Chapter 20)**.

Management

Oral and IV K^+ preparations are available for managing hypokalemia. The oral route is safe and absorption is fast and effective. IV supplementation is usually indicated by the following:

- Likelihood of cardiac arrhythmias
- Possibility of intracellular shift (e.g., during management or recovery of diabetic ketoacidosis, refeeding syndrome)
- Severe muscle weakness with respiratory muscle involvement
- Large ongoing losses
- Severe hypokalemia (<2.5 mEq/L)

Flowchart 6.4: Approach to hypokalemia based on urine potassium concentration (UK^+), fractional excretion of potassium (FEK), urine potassium/creatinine ratio (K^+/Cr), blood pressure, and presence of acidosis or alkalosis

*Levels 2.5–3.5 mEq/L require only oral correction if asymptomatic; levels <2.5 mEq/L (even asymptomatic) require IV correction

#Fractional excretion of K^+ >6% and spot urine K^+ >20 mEq/L suggest urinary wasting

AME: apparent mineralocorticoid excess; CAH: congenital adrenal hyperplasia; DKA: diabetic ketoacidosis; GRA: glucocorticoid remediable aldosteronism; RTA: renal tubular acidosis

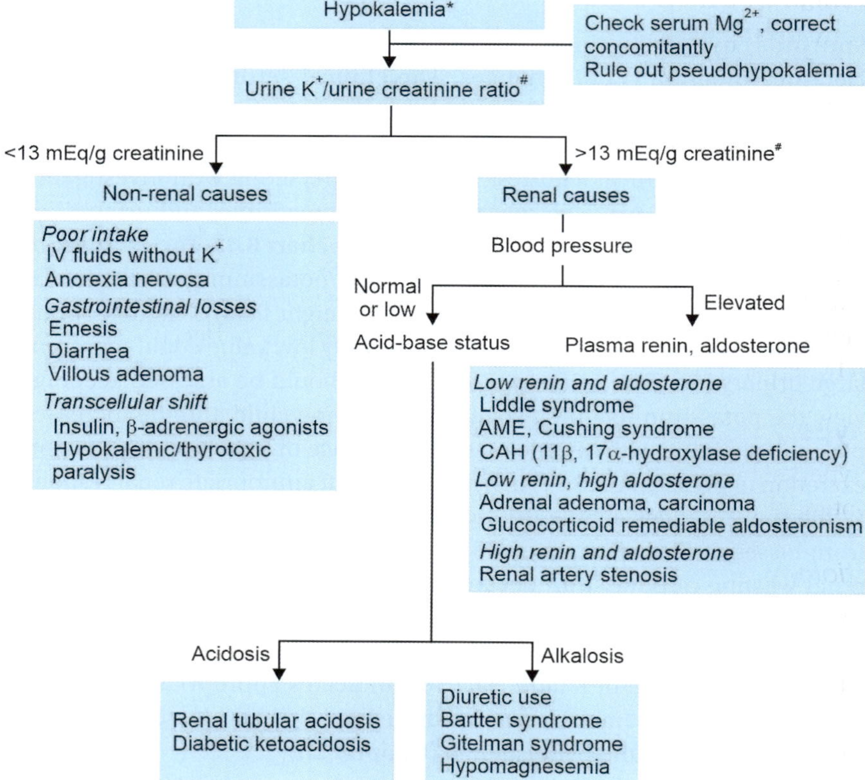

The aim of therapy is to raise serum potassium to a safe range (>3 mEq/L). Intracellular stores need to be corrected initially before changes in serum K^+ are noted (correction of serum K^+ from 2–3 mEq/L requires 400–600 mEq and correction from 3 to 4 mEq/L is achieved after 100–200 mEq K^+, for an adult). Hence, correction from very low levels of plasma K^+ would take place slowly and must be performed under expert guidance and close monitoring.

Potassium chloride (15%) is the preferred agent (2 mEq/mL; 0.5–1 mEq/kg per dose) given as IV infusion over 1–2 hr. Dose of K^+ required (mEq) is calculated as follows: (3.0 – measured K^+) × body weight × 0.04. This formula is based on the rationale that plasma volume is nearly 4% of body weight

(60% of blood volume of 70–80 mL/kg) and is needed to rapidly increase plasma K^+ to 3 mEq/L from the current levels. Infusion rate should not exceed 1 mEq/kg/h and concentration of K^+ should not exceed 60 mEq/L (peripheral line) and 80 mEq/L (central line), to avoid thrombophlebitis and venous spasm. The use of IV potassium phosphate (94 mg phosphate and 4.4 mEq potassium/mL; infused at 0.06 mEq/kg/h over 4–6 hr) is useful in situations requiring concomitant phosphate supplements.

While children with chronic hypokalemia tolerate low plasma K^+ levels without significant symptoms, it is prudent to correct all clinical situations of hypokalemia with utmost urgency and care. Associated magnesium deficiency may render the treatment ineffective and hypomagnesemia should be managed appropriately.

Mild hypokalemia is managed with oral potassium supplements (1–4 mEq/kg/day in divided doses). Oral formulations of potassium chloride (10%; 20 mEq/15 mL) are used in situations with alkalosis, and potassium citrate (usually available as potassium citrate with citric acid; 2 mEq/mL) in patients with renal tubular acidosis. Potassium sparing diuretics such as spironolactone, triamterene, or amiloride are useful in specific situations, but should be used cautiously with supplemental potassium because of the risk of hyperkalemia.

Hyperkalemia

Hyperkalemia, defined as serum potassium level above 5.5 mEq/L, is a potentially life-threatening condition.

Etiology

Spurious hyperkalemia occurs as a result of K^+ moving out of the cells during or after the blood draw. The chief cause of the problem is mechanical trauma during venipuncture (excessive suction, inappropriately small needle bores, and use of tourniquets); a reddish tint to the plasma (or serum) provides a clue. Hemolysis of the specimen might occur during transport, due to significant delay in processing, high temperatures, and in hemolytic states. Autosomal dominant familial pseudohyperkalemia, caused by mutations in *ABCB6* (2q36) is due to a thermosensitive (<37°C) passive efflux of K^+ from the ICF. Significant leukocytosis and thrombocytosis can also elevate plasma (or serum) K^+ due to efflux after clotting.

As cellular and renal adaptations prevent substantial K^+ accumulation in the ECF, true hyperkalemia occurs in the following situations:

- Increased K^+ load, especially acute loading or associated with impaired urinary excretion: Transfusion of stored blood, massive transfusions, or abnormally large doses (erroneous charting) can result in hyperkalemia, especially in infants.

- Net release of intracellular K^+ can occur in extracellular hypertonicity, tumor lysis, rhabdomyolysis, and hyperkalemic periodic paralysis.
- Impaired urinary K^+ secretion in AKI or CKD with low glomerular filtration rate (GFR) (<15 mL/min/1.73 m^2), drugs impairing renal excretion of K^+, deficiency of aldosterone, or from intrinsic inability of the distal nephron to secrete potassium into the tubular lumen **(Box 6.8)**. Hypoaldosteronism may be primary (Addison disease) or secondary resulting in hyperkalemia with urinary salt wasting, volume depletion, and hypotension. Similar features may be seen in patients with obstructive uropathy and renal tubular acidosis type IV. Drugs affecting the RAS,

BOX 6.8: Causes of hyperkalemia

Spurious
Hemolysis, leukocytosis, thrombocytosis
Familial pseudohyperkalemia (*ABCB6* mutation)

Shift of potassium from intracellular to extracellular compartment
Metabolic acidosis
Hyperkalemic paralysis (thyrotoxicosis; *CACNA1S, SCN4A, KCNJ2, KCNJ18* mutations)
Cellular breakdown (e.g., tumor lysis syndrome)

Increased intake; release from damaged cells
Potassium supplements
Transfusion of old blood
Massive intravascular hemolysis
Rhabdomyolysis, tumor lysis, malignant hyperthermia

Decreased excretion
Acute kidney injury and chronic kidney disease
Renal tubular acidosis (RTA) type IV **(*see* Tables 20.1, 20.2 and 20.8)**
Medications: Potassium sparing diuretics, trimethoprim, pentamidine, nonsteroidal anti-inflammatory drugs, angiotensin-converting enzyme inhibitors, angiotensin receptor blockers, calcineurin inhibitors

Mineralocorticoid deficiency, resistance
Normal plasma aldosterone
Sickle cell disease, systemic lupus erythematosus
Obstructive uropathy
Type I RTA (voltage defect; ***see* Chapter 20**)
Angiotensin-converting enzyme inhibitors, potassium sparing diuretics, trimethoprim

Low plasma aldosterone
Congenital adrenal hyperplasia, Addison disease
Chronic tubulointerstitial nephritis

High plasma aldosterone
Pseudohypoaldosteronism type 1 and type 2 (Gordon syndrome; ***see* Chapter 20**)
Obstructive uropathy

including those that inhibit renin release from juxtaglomerular cells, inhibit aldosterone release from adrenals and cause MR/ENaC blockade, can cause hyperkalemia.

Pseudohypoaldosteronism is a heterogeneous group of disorders characterized by hyperkalemia, metabolic acidosis, and normal renal function. PHA type I is caused by either autosomal dominant mutations in the mineralocorticoid receptor (MR) gene (*NR3C2*; type 1A) or autosomal recessive loss of function mutations of amiloride sensitive sodium channel (ENaC α, β, and γ subunits; *SCNN1A, SCNN1B,* and *SCNN1G,* respectively; type 1B). PHA type II (Gordon syndrome), caused by loss of function mutations in lysine-deficient protein kinase 1 and 4 (*WNK1, WNK4, KLHL3, CUL3*), presents with volume expansion, suppressed renin and reduced mineralocorticoid induced K^+ excretion, leading to hypertension, hyperkalemia, and hyperchloremic acidosis.

Clinical Features

Akin to hypokalemia, hyperkalemia also affects the excitable tissues of the body. Patients rarely present with symptoms, hyperkalemia being detected on laboratory tests. In patients with serum potassium level >6.5 mEq/L, ECG changes are apparent and correlate with the degree of hyperkalemia **(Figs. 6.3A and B)**. Peaking of T-wave, ST-segment depression, widening of the PR interval, and widening of the QRS interval are sequential and predictable changes of progressive hyperkalemia. Cardiac toxicity is more evident if there is rapid rise in serum potassium level, or there is an underlying cardiac problem and in patients receiving digitalis. Neuromuscular manifestations include paresthesias and fasciculations; some patients have ascending paralysis (usually sparing trunk, head, and respiratory muscles). Hyperkalemia also impairs acidification by reducing ammoniagenesis and limits net acid excretion.

Evaluation

The etiology of hyperkalemia is suggested by clinical evaluation. Estimation of blood levels of creatinine, renin, aldosterone, and urinary K^+ excretion is required for definitive diagnosis. Transtubular potassium gradient (TTKG) reflects K^+ secretion in the cortical collecting duct under the action of aldosterone, and helps in assessing the renal response to hyperkalemia.

$$\text{Transtubular gradient of potassium} = \frac{\text{Urine potassium} \times \text{Serum osmolality}}{\text{Serum potassium} \times \text{Urine osmolality}}$$

Urinary K^+, adjusted for urine and serum osmolality, is an estimate of luminal K^+ in the cortical collecting duct that is only influenced by water removal in the medullary collecting duct. Since serum potassium is an estimate of peritubular K^+ concentration, the TTKG provides an estimate of the gradient at level of the cortical collecting duct. While estimating TTKG, the urinary Na^+ should be >25 mEq/L (to ensure that K^+ secretion is not limited by insufficient Na^+ delivery) and urine osmolality should exceed serum osmolality. Normally in the presence of hyperkalemia, TTKG exceeds 7 due to increased secretion of K^+ in the collecting duct under the influence of aldosterone. A value <5 signifies inappropriate aldosterone effect. An increase in TTKG to >7 within 2–4 hr of administering 0.05–2 mg of fludrocortisone distinguishes patients who have mineralocorticoid deficiency versus resistance, where TTKG remains <7. While TTKG assumes negligible absorption of osmoles distal to the collecting duct, this has been questioned in recent research.

Management

Spurious hyperkalemia should be excluded. Therapeutic measures are instituted immediately if serum K^+ level >6.5 mEq/L, or if there are ECG changes. The goals of emergency management are to counteract the cardiac toxicity and to shift K^+ into the intracellular space. While IV calcium gluconate rapidly stabilizes the myocardial cell membrane to prevent cardiac arrhythmia, β_2-adrenergic agonist, insulin-dextrose, and sodium bicarbonate enable cellular uptake of K^+ and reduce its blood levels **(Table 6.2)**. IV dextrose/insulin or β_2-adrenergic agonist is the best supported recommendations. Their combination is more effective than either alone. There is no difference of efficacy between IV versus nebulized β_2-adrenergic agonist. Potassium-containing fluids and medications that lead to hyperkalemia must be discontinued. Measures to reduce total body K^+, such as resins and diuretics need to be simultaneously initiated. The underlying cause should be identified and treated.

Sodium zirconium cyclosilicate, a selective K^+ binder ion exchange resin, selectively binds monovalent cations (K^+ and NH_4^+) due to its specific binding site geometry and is being used for acute and chronic hyperkalemia in children. It is also useful in improving metabolic acidosis due to its NH_4^+ binding action from the gut.

Hemodialysis is the modality of choice in refractory hyperkalemia, renal failure, or tumor lysis where accelerated tissue breakdown releases large amounts of K^+, and rapid correction is desired. The largest amount of potassium removal occurs during the first hour of hemodialysis; serum K^+ reaches its nadir at ~3 hr and a total of 50–80 mEq/L of K^+ may be removed in 4 hr. Peritoneal dialysis is 15–20% as effective as hemodialysis, and is not as useful in brisk lowering of K^+ levels. Continuous renal replacement therapy has a role in critically sick, hemodynamically unstable patients who cannot undergo hemodialysis.

TABLE 6.2: Management of hyperkalemia

Medication	*Dose*	*Onset of action; duration of effect*	*Adverse events*
Calcium gluconate, 10%	0.5–1 mL/kg over 5–10 minutes, under ECG monitoring; repeat 5–10 minutes (maximum total dose 30 mL)	1–3 minutes; 30–45 minutes	Hypercalcemia, tissue necrosis, contraindicated in digoxin intoxication
Dextrose/ insulin	Regular insulin 0.1 U/ kg with 2 mL/kg of 25% dextrose over 30 minutes; repeat q 30–60 minutes or infusion of 25% dextrose at 1–2 mL/ kg/hr with insulin 0.1 U/ kg/hr	Decrease of 0.5–1.5 mEq/L in 15–30 minutes; 2–4 hr	Hypoglycemia, hyperosmolality, volume overload
Nebulized, IV salbutamol	Inhaled: 0.2 mg/kg (maximum 5 mg) IV: 4–5 µg/kg over 15 minutes	Decline 0.5–1.5 mEq/L in 20–30 minutes (IV) and 90 minutes (nebulized); 2–4 hr	Tachycardia
Sodium bicarbonate, 7.5%	1–2 mEq/kg over 30–60 minutes	5–20 minutes; 2 hr	Unpredictable; not effective without acidosis; risk of sodium, volume overload
Furosemide	1–2 mg/kg	Intermediate action	Ototoxicity, nephrotoxicity
Ion exchange resins	Sodium polystyrene sulfonate 1 g/kg q 8 h per oral (PO) or per rectal (PR)	Removes 0.5–1.0 mEq/L in exchange for 2–3 mEq/L of Na^+ in 1–2 hr; 4–6 hr	PO: Nausea, constipation, paralytic ileus; diarrhea if preparations are premixed with sorbitol PR: Cecal perforation
Sodium zirconium cyclosilicate	<3 years: 0.5–2.5 g (max 5 g) 3–12 years: 2.5–5 g (max 5 g) >12 years: 5–10 g (max 10 g) Dosed once to thrice daily	Acute reduction of 1–2 mEq/L can be seen in 6–8 hr	Mild edema/fluid retention, nausea, constipation
Patiromer	Exchanges Ca^{2+} for K^+; also binds Mg^{2+}	6–8 hr	Constipation, flatulence, hypomagnesemia

DISORDERS OF CALCIUM HOMEOSTASIS

Serum concentration of calcium is a poor reflection of total body stores, since 99% Ca^{2+} is stored in the bones in combination with phosphorus and magnesium. Calcium exists as three forms in the plasma—ionic (48%) that is the physiologically active, albumin bound (40%), and complexed with anions such as phosphate, sulfate, lactate, citrate, and bicarbonate (12%). Consequently, low serum albumin levels lower total Ca^{2+} without altering the ionized component whereas, alkalosis and infusion of anions (citrate, in massive blood transfusions) decrease the ionized component by increasing the complexed component. Calcium stores depend on its dietary intake, absorption from gastrointestinal tract, and renal excretion. Renal resorption of Ca^{2+} occurs passively in the proximal tubule (70%), by paracellular pathway in thick ascending limb of Henle (20%), and actively in distal convoluted tubule (5–10%), and collecting duct (5%) **(Figs. 6.5A to C)**.

Response to hypocalcemia (reduction in ionized Ca^{2+}), sensed by the calcium sensing receptor (CaSR) in the parathyroid gland, leads to immediate parathyroid hormone (PTH) secretion. PTH affects the following change: (*i*) Enhanced bone resorption, via increased NF-κB ligand receptor activator (in osteoblasts) and subsequent RANK-RANKL-mediated Ca^{2+} resorption (by osteoclasts), (*ii*) Stimulate urine Ca^{2+} reabsorption in the distal nephron (increased TRPV5 channel activity), (*iii*) Upregulates circulating 1,25$(OH)_2$ vitamin D levels, by stimulating 1-α hydroxylase and downregulating 24-hydroxylase enzymes, and (*iv*) Stimulating phosphaturia by downregulating NaPi-2a and NaPi-2c channels in the proximal tubule (increasing excretion of phosphate).

The response to hypercalcemia is inverse of the steps mentioned above and is partly mediated by the release of calcitonin from parafollicular cells of the thyroid gland. In addition to the parathyroid gland, CaSR receptor is also present on the renal tubular epithelium, basolateral surface in thick ascending limb of Henle, and apical surface in collecting ducts. In the loop of Henle, hypercalcemia sensed by CaSR, inhibits the ROMK channel and subsequently reduces the function of the sodium-potassium-chloride channel (NKCC2); leading to the loss of transepithelial voltage required for paracellular calcium uptake. This results also in the urinary loss of Na^+, K^+, Ca^{2+}, and Mg^{2+} in the urine, along with polyuria. This might result in depletion of the intravascular volume and predisposes to AKI. Hence, the first step of hypercalcemia management is infusion of normal saline; use of loop diuretics might worsen AKI. At the renal collecting duct, hypercalciuria sensed by the CaSR, downregulates the water channel aquaporin 2, causing a concentrating defect that prevents formation of kidney stones.

Genetic defects of CaSR receptor can involve either loss or gain of function, the former results in hypercalcemia and the latter in hypocalcemia.

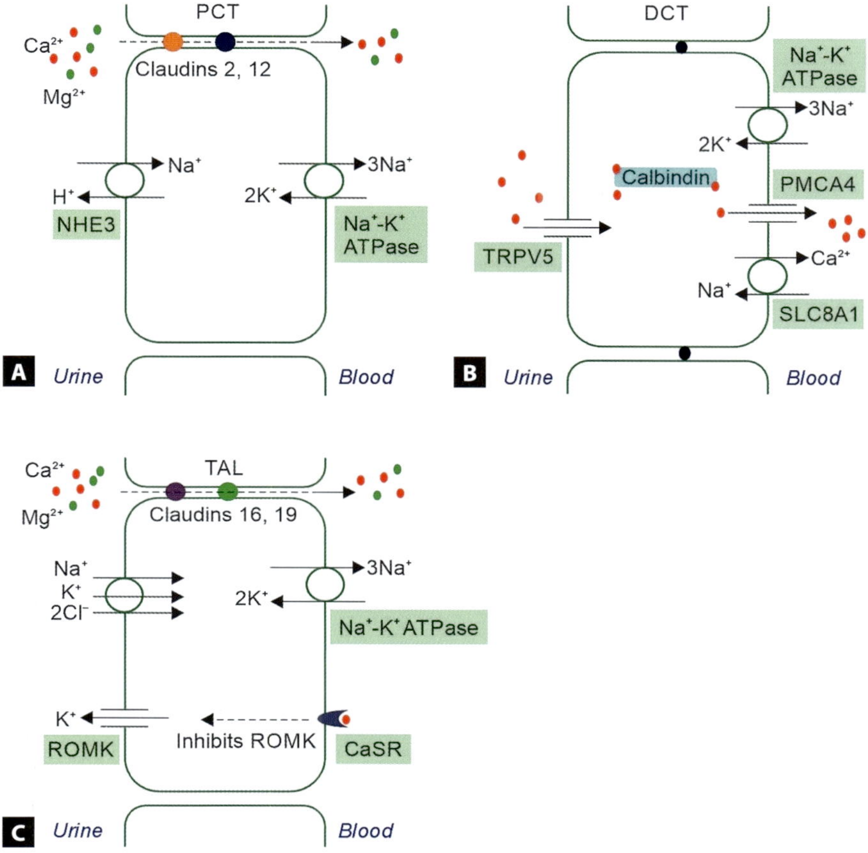

Figs. 6.5A to C: Renal calcium absorption at the proximal convoluted tubule (PCT), thick ascending limb (TAL) of loop of Henle, and the distal convoluted tubule (DCT). CaSR: calcium sensing receptor; NHE3: sodium hydrogen exchanger; PMCA4: plasma membrane Ca^{2+} transporting ATPase-4; ROMK: renal outer medullary potassium channel; SLC8A1: sodium calcium exchanger; TRPV5: transient receptor potential vanilloid channel 5

Calcimimetic agents, that are allosteric activators of CaSR, are used in the management of secondary hyperparathyroidism with CKD.

Hypocalcemia

Hypocalcemia is defined as total serum calcium >9 mg/dL. A common cause of pseudohypocalcemia is hypoalbuminemia in which total serum calcium is low, but the ionized fraction is not affected. Serum calcium can be corrected for alterations in serum albumin, although in ill patients or in those with changes in albumin, pH, or one of the complexing anions, ionized Ca^{2+} should be measured directly.

BOX 6.9: Causes of hypocalcemia

Low/ineffective PTH
Postparathyroidectomy
Chronic kidney disease
Pseudohypoparathyroidism

Decreased PTH level
Dysgenesis of parathyroid gland
DiGeorge syndrome (22q11 deletion)
Kenny–Caffey syndrome (associated with osteosclerosis)
Hypoparathyroidism, sensorineural deafness, and renal disease (HDR) syndrome (with deafness and renal dysplasia)
Autoimmune destruction of parathyroid gland: Type 1 polyendocrinopathy
Inadvertent damage during surgery, neck radiation
Infiltration: Hemosiderosis, Wilson disease
Hypomagnesemia

Vitamin D deficiency/resistance (*see* Chapter 22)

Activating mutations of calcium sensing receptor (autosomal dominant)
Tissue sequestration
Hyperphosphatemia
Tumor lysis syndrome
Acute pancreatitis
Osteoblastic bone metastasis
Chelators: Citrate, foscarnet, ethylenediaminetetraacetic acid (EDTA)
Medications: Bisphosphonates, cinacalcet, etelcalcetide, phenytoin, calcitonin, fluoride

PTH: parathyroid hormone

Etiology

Hypocalcemia is caused either by perturbation in vitamin D metabolism **(Chapter 22)**, deficiency of PTH, end-organ resistance to PTH or excess tissue consumption of calcium **(Box 6.9)**. Hypoparathyroidism may be genetic (e.g., DiGeorge syndrome), autoimmune, or due to infiltration, infection, or surgery of the gland. In pseudohypoparathyroidism, there is either secretion of ineffective PTH or end-organ resistance to its action. Severe hypomagnesemia inhibits secretion of PTH and therefore causes secondary hypocalcemia. Excessive removal of (ionized) calcium from the circulation occurs due to binding with phosphate in rhabdomyolysis and tumor lysis, with fat in pancreatitis, and in "hungry bone syndrome" following parathyroidectomy in patients with CKD.

Clinical Features

Hypocalcemia may often be asymptomatic. The signs and symptoms are related to the severity and duration of hypocalcemia **(Box 6.10)**. Acute symptoms are related to neuromuscular irritability or cardiac conduction defects.

BOX 6.11: Causes of hypercalcemia

Increased parathyroid hormone (PTH) levels
Parathyroid adenoma: Isolated, or multiple endocrine neoplasia syndrome
Inactivating mutations of calcium sensing receptor
Chronic kidney disease

Excessive vitamin D effect
Vitamin D overdose
Sarcoidosis, tuberculosis, Hodgkin lymphoma: Ectopic 1α-hydroxylase activity
Idiopathic hypercalcemia of infancy: 24-hydroxylase deficiency
William syndrome: Augmented recruitment of vitamin D receptor
Hypophosphatasia: Increased synthesis of calcitriol

Increased bone resorption/reduced calcium incorporation
Humoral hypercalcemia of malignancy: PTH-related peptide excess
Jansen metaphyseal dysplasia: Activating mutation of PTH/PTHrp receptor
Vitamin A overdose
Prolonged immobilization
Adynamic bone disease (with calcium and calcitriol supplementation)

Medications
Thiazides; calcium, vitamin D and A supplements, lithium, antacids
Milk-alkali syndrome

Clinical Features

The severity of symptoms relates to the blood level of Ca^{2+}, with patients having severe hypercalcemia (>14 mg/dL) more likely to be symptomatic. Gastrointestinal and neurological symptoms are common, but nonspecific and include lethargy, drowsiness, irritability, hypotonia, nausea, vomiting, and constipation. Severe hypercalcemia may lead to peptic ulcers, pancreatitis, stupor, and coma. Cardiac manifestations are hypertension and short QT interval, but arrhythmias are rare. Hypercalcemia causes polyuria and volume depletion, which enhances Ca^{2+} reabsorption potentiating the hypercalcemia. This may lead to renal dysfunction and acute kidney injury. Prolonged severe hypercalcemia may cause nephrocalcinosis, metastatic calcifications, and band keratopathy. Clinical features are nonspecific in infants and present as failure to thrive, weakness, lethargy, hypotonia, and rarely seizures.

Diagnostic Approach

An approach to evaluation of a patient with hypercalcemia is shown in **Flowchart 6.6**.

Management

Hypercalcemia is often accompanied by dehydration. For mild hypercalcemia (<12 mg/dL) in asymptomatic children, avoiding dehydration and reducing dietary calcium are sufficient. In children with moderate hypercalcemia

Flowchart 6.6: Evaluation of hypercalcemia
*Rare etiologies of hypoparathyroid hypercalcemia include hypophosphatasia, congenital lactase deficiency, and Jansen metaphyseal chondrodysplasia

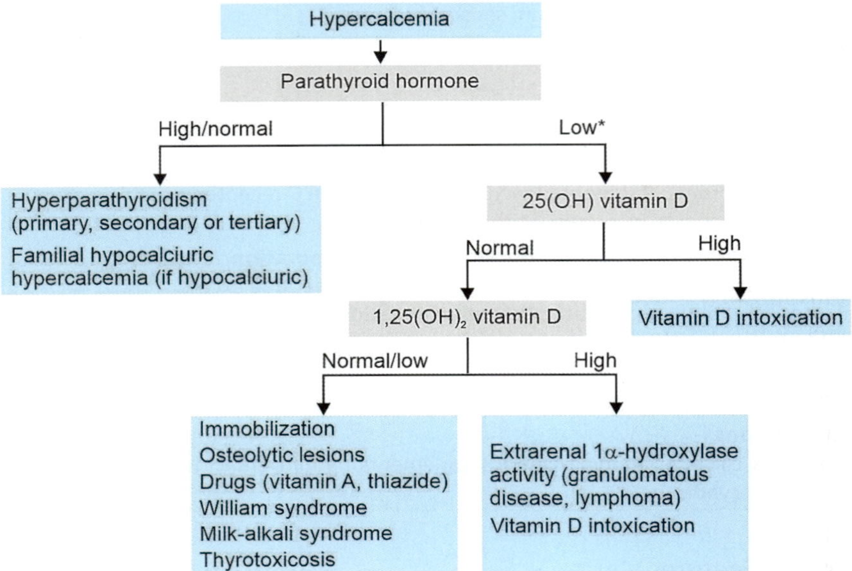

(12–14 mg/dL), aggressive rehydration with IV saline is instituted at 1.5–2 times maintenance rate, which decreases the renal sodium-dependent calcium reabsorption. Reabsorption is further decreased by addition of loop diuretics (furosemide 1 mg/kg/dose q6 h). Hypokalemia and hypomagnesemia should be monitored. These maneuvers reduce serum calcium by approximately 1–3 mg/dL. Bisphosphonates should be used with caution in those with moderate hypercalcemia to avoid symptomatic hypocalcemia.

Rapid correction of hypercalcemia is necessary in symptomatic patients or those with severe hypercalcemia (>14 mg/dL). In addition to IV hydration followed by furosemide, administration of bisphosphonates and calcitonin can be considered. Bisphosphonates (pamidronate) block osteoclastic activity within 2–4 days following IV administration. Pamidronate (0.25–1 mg/kg/dose) or zoledronic acid (0.25–0.5 mg/kg) can be administered as infusion over 4 hr, for 1–3 days as necessary days. Adverse events include high-grade fever, myalgia, and hypocalcemia.

IM or SC calcitonin (4–8 IU/kg, every 12 hr) has a rapid, and short-lasting effect due to development of tachyphylaxis over 24–48 hr. Rarely, patients with severe hypercalcemia with renal failure require peritoneal or hemodialysis using low-calcium dialysate. Hydrocortisone (1 mg/kg/dose every 6 hr IV) is beneficial in vitamin D intoxication, granulomatous disease, or paraneoplastic syndrome. Primary hyperparathyroidism requires surgical intervention.

Children with CKD and secondary hyperparathyroidism require interventions to decrease PTH secretion with calcimimetics (cinacalcet hydrochloride), low calcemic vitamin D analogs, and parathyroidectomy **(Chapter 22)**. Cinacalcet allosterically activates the CaSR decreasing PTH secretion. Vitamin D analogs including 22-oxacalcitriol, 19-nor-1,25-dihydroxyvitamin D2 (paricalcitol), and 1α-hydroxyvitamin D2 (doxercalciferol) directly inhibit PTH secretion without affecting intestinal calcium and phosphorus absorption. Subtotal or total parathyroidectomy with autotransplantation is indicated when serum PTH is persistently >800 pg/mL.

DISORDERS OF PHOSPHORUS METABOLISM

Phosphorous is critical for most biological activities, including biochemical energy transfer via ATP, maintenance of genetic information with nucleotides, intracellular signaling via cyclic adenosine monophosphate, membrane structure integrity via phospholipids, and muscle contraction. Along with this, it exists as hydroxyapatite in the mineralized bone as a major constituent (~80–90% of the entire phosphorous body pool). The remaining 10–15% exists in a readily exchangeable form in the soft tissues and extracellular fluid. One-third of plasma phosphorous exists as the inorganic form (Pi), and nearly 80% is protein bound. Phosphate in bone and body fluids also provides a high-capacity buffer.

Although ubiquitous across food groups, dairy products, meat, nuts, beans, and legumes are rich sources of phosphorus. Normal age defined ranges of serum phosphorus are 1–3 years: 3.8–6.5 mg/dL, 4–11 years: 3.7–5.6 mg/dL, 12–15 years: 2.9 to 5.4 mg/dL, and 16 to 18 years: 2.7 to 4.7 mg/dL. Plasma phosphate levels show significant diurnal variation and association with food intake. Circulating phosphorous levels exchange in equilibrium with the intestinal uptake and renal reabsorption. Intestinal phosphorous absorption (along the entire intestine; small intestine more than the colon) occurs predominantly by passive paracellular pathway through the luminal concentration. A small, saturable and energy-dependent pathway occurs through the sodium phosphate cotransporter 2b (NaPi2b; SLC34A2) across the apical brush-border membrane. The expression of NaPi2b channels is inducible by 1,25-dihydroxyvitamin D, during hypophosphatemia. Nicotinamide or nicotinic acid inhibits this transport, and is sometimes used in management of hyperphosphatemia of CKD.

The kidney is the primary organ regulating Pi concentration in the circulation. Reduction in the GFR proportionally reduces Pi delivery to the PCT and increases Pi in the circulation. As dietary phosphate is usually more than the daily requirement, the gut is unable to compensate for a chronic decrease in GFR. Tubular maximum of Pi reabsorption, corrected for GFR (TmP/GFR), serves as a measure of renal reabsorption threshold as this factors the net inflow of Pi (from gut, bone, and soft tissues), the tubular reabsorption and GFR. TmP/GFR progressively reduces with age, reflecting the phosphate balance. Renal phosphate reabsorption via the NaPi2a (SLC34A1), located in the proximal tubule is regulated chiefly by PTH and fibroblast growth factor 23 (FGF23). Another channel, NaPi2c (SLC34A3), is present in the PCT of deep nephrons and handles ~10% of the renal phosphate load. Normally, 80–90% of the filtered load is reabsorbed. Vitamin D enhances and PTH opposes reabsorption. Renal CaSRs in the proximal tubule enhance phosphate reabsorption to counteract the effect of PTH.

The FGF23, a hormone secreted by osteocytes and osteoblasts, is the key regulator of phosphate homeostasis with potent phosphaturic action, by reducing NaPi2a and NaPi2c channels in the PCT. The activity of FGF23 is controlled by PHEX (phosphate-regulating neutral endopeptidase homolog; Xp22.11) and DMP1 (dentin matrix acidic phosphoprotein; 4q22.1). FGF23 requires its cofactor klotho (KL; 13q13) to act on the FGF receptor 1 (FGFR1). FGF23 inhibits 1-α hydroxylase in the kidney, while stimulating the enzyme 24-hydroxylase that catabolizes calcitriol. Calcitriol inhibits PTH production and stimulates FGF23 production. Mutations involving regulators of the homeostatic pathway cause hereditary disorders of phosphate wasting.

In homeostasis, adults usually have a neutral phosphorous balance and children are in a negative balance till completion of growth, with respect to intake. Hypo- or hyperphosphatemia almost always reflect an underlying disease. Acute changes in either direction are common in critically ill children, and can contribute to morbidity and mortality.

Hypophosphatemia

Hypophosphatemia is defined as serum phosphorus concentration less than the age defined cut-offs. Serum levels of phosphorus depict <1% of total body stores, as it is chiefly an intracellular ion. Important causes of hypophosphatemia are listed in **Box 6.12**. Processes that stimulate cellular uptake and usage of phosphorus (glycolysis and respiratory alkalosis) and anabolic hormones (insulin during therapy of diabetic ketoacidosis, refeeding syndrome and steroids) cause transcellular shift of phosphorus into cells. A transient decrease in plasma phosphorus, in the presence of depleted total body stores of phosphorus may cause severe symptomatic hypophosphatemia. Increased renal excretion (FGF or PTH mediated) is usually the cause of chronic hypophosphatemia than decreased dietary consumption or absorption. Rapid skeletal consumption of calcium and phosphate occurs following parathyroidectomy (hungry bone syndrome).

Hypophosphatemia, secondary to excessive renal loss of phosphorus, is seen in X-linked and autosomal dominant forms of hypophosphatemic rickets, Fanconi syndrome, hyperparathyroidism, vitamin D deficiency,

BOX 6.12: Causes of hypophosphatemia

Decreased intestinal absorption
Prolonged vomiting
Fat malabsorption
Premature infants
Phosphate binders, intake of phosphate binding antacids

Transcellular shift into the intracellular compartment
Insulin
Refeeding syndrome in malnutrition
Respiratory alkalosis
Hungry bone syndrome (following parathyroidectomy)

Renal losses
Hyperparathyroidism
X-linked hypophosphatemic rickets
Autosomal recessive and dominant hypophosphatemic rickets
Hereditary hypophosphatemia with hypercalciuria
Tumor-induced osteomalacia
McCune–Albright syndrome (fibrous dysplasia)
Fanconi syndrome
Vitamin D deficiency
Vitamin D-dependent rickets types 1 and 2
Dent disease
Following renal transplantation
Diuretics, glucocorticoids

vitamin D dependence, and Dent disease **(*see* Chapter 22)**. Renal excretion, as mentioned before, depends primarily on the phosphate load presented to the proximal tubule by glomerular filtration. Maximal tubular reabsorption can be calculated from plasma phosphate and creatinine with corresponding urinary values. As plasma values show significant diurnal and dietary variation, it is necessary to collect blood after overnight fasting. The blood sample should be collected at the midpoint of the timed (3–6 hr) or along with the spot urine sample. From these, TmP/GFR can be derived using available nomograms or mathematical formulae.

Chronic hypophosphatemia is the common denominator in calcipenic and phosphopenic rickets; low phosphate levels lead to impaired apoptosis of chondrocytes in the growth plate cartilage. The bony changes are attributable to hypophosphatemia, and the hypocalcemic complications are limited to neuromuscular irritability, seizures, tetany, and dilated cardiomyopathy.

Clinical Features

Mild hypophosphatemia is asymptomatic. Severe acute hypophosphatemia is associated with depletion of ATP, which leads to neuromuscular features including proximal myopathy, impaired cardiac contractility, paresthesia, tremors, and peripheral neuropathy. Hemolysis and rhabdomyolysis may rarely occur in acute hypophosphatemia. Chronic hypophosphatemia is associated with rickets.

Management

Severe hypophosphatemia (<1 mg/dL) in critically ill, intubated patients, or those with clinical sequelae of hypophosphatemia are managed with IV replacement therapy. Sick patients with moderate hypophosphatemia (1.0–2.5 mg/dL) who require assisted ventilation also need IV replacement. Those with mild to moderate hypophosphatemia should be managed with oral supplements. IV sodium or potassium phosphate (94 mg or 3 mmol phosphate/mL) is infused at a dose of 2.5–5 mg/kg over 4–6 hr (0.3–1 mL/h). Close monitoring for hyperphosphatemia, hyperkalemia, hypocalcemia, hypotension, and arrhythmias is required. Most oral phosphate formulations provide 250 mg of phosphate, with either 7 mEq each of sodium and potassium, or 14 mEq of potassium; dose of oral phosphate supplement is 50–75 mg/kg/day.

Chronic hypophosphatemia (usually due to monogenic renal wasting) is managed with supplementation with 20–60 mg/kg per day of elemental phosphorous (four to six divided dose better), calcitriol 20–30 ng/kg per day and monitoring closely for hypercalciuria. Calcimimetics may be required for persistent secondary hyperparathyroidism. Chronic FGF-mediated hypophosphatemia can be managed with burosumab, a monoclonal antagonist of FGF23. Burosumab is given as subcutaneous injections, every 2–4 weekly, with starting doses at 0.4–0.8 mg/kg (maximum 2 mg/kg and 90 mg/dose). Significant improvements in fasting phosphate levels, bone strength, radiological features, and height have been reported.

Hyperphosphatemia

Hyperphosphatemia is defined as serum phosphorus concentration exceeding the normal age defined range. Renal insufficiency is the chief etiology. Derangement of serum Ca^{2+} levels is almost always associated. While hypoparathyroidism and pseudohypoparathyroidism are associated with hypocalcemia, vitamin D excess, and osteolytic malignancies cause hypercalcemia. Phosphate-containing enemas raise serum phosphorus concentration in young children and in patients with extracellular volume depletion. Rhabdomyolysis and tumor lysis syndrome in presence of reduced kidney function are also associated with hyperphosphatemia.

Clinical Features

Moderate and even severe acute hyperphosphatemia is asymptomatic. The decline in total and ionized Ca^{2+} concentration can result in tetany.

Chronic hyperphosphatemia is associated with metastatic calcification, especially in CKD. While previous publications suggest that the serum calcium-phosphate product (≥55–70 mg^2/dL^2) is a risk factor for vascular disease, this is not substantiated by current literature. The formation of metastatic calcifications is multifactorial and complex process, with multiple promotional and inhibitory factors.

Management

The phosphorus intake is curtailed and phosphate binders used to reduce intestinal absorption **(Chapter 22, 26)**. However, a low phosphate diet is difficult to implement, and can affect bone growth. Severe, acute hyperphosphatemia in individuals with reduced kidney function requires dialysis (peritoneal, hemodialysis, or continuous renal replacement therapy). Chronic hyperphosphatemia with metastatic calcifications, often seen due to low FGF23 or end-organ resistance, is difficult to manage. Therapies used for hyperphosphatemia with tumoral calcinosis include many agents including acetazolamide, probenecid, and renal replacement therapy in severe cases.

DISORDERS OF MAGNESIUM HOMEOSTASIS

An adult has approximately 1 mol (~20–24 g) of Mg^{2+} in the body; half is present in the bone and the rest is distributed in other tissues, with only 1–2% in the ECF, akin to K^+. Intracellular Mg^{2+} is a cofactor for many enzymes that are involved in ATP metabolism, along with an important role in nerve and muscle conduction. Magnesium also acts as second messenger in T cells; mutations in *MAGT1* are linked to human immunodeficiency. The normal serum Mg^{2+} concentration is 1.7–2.2 mg/dL. Approximately 30–40% of Mg^{2+} in the diet is absorbed in the intestine; this can vary from 10 to 65% depending on the body stores and dietary intake. The relation between dietary intake and absorption is curvilinear, indicating a paracellular passive transport (distal jejunum and ileum) and a saturable transcellular pathway (through TRPM6 and TRPM7 channels; cecum and colon). The saturable transport functions predominantly with low or normal Mg^{2+} intake, and the passive transport predominates when intake is elevated. The paracellular pathway also increases absorption when the transcellular pathway is deficient. CNNM4 (cyclin and CBS domain divalent metal cation transport mediator 4; a Na^+/Mg^{2+} antiporter) and SLC41A1 are transporters that mediate the efflux of Mg^{2+} from the intestine to the bloodstream. The kidney excretes about 1–4% of the magnesium filtered at the glomerulus. In childhood, Mg^{2+} balance remains negative due to bone growth and after attaining bone maturation, the body maintains a neutral Mg^{2+} balance. Absorbed Mg^{2+} circulates in the ionized form (~50–60%), protein-bound (~30–40%), and the remaining is present as soluble complexes with anions (phosphates and citrate).

Renal reabsorption occurs in the proximal tubule (15%), thick ascending limb (70%), and distal convoluted tubule (10%)**(Figs. 6.5A to C)**. Mg^{2+} is predominantly absorbed through the paracellular pathway, stimulated by the transepithelial potential difference (lumen negative) created by the NKCC and Na^{+}/K^{+}-ATPase channels. Claudin 2 and claudin 12 channels are thought to mediate the reabsorption of Mg^{2+} in the PCT. While the reabsorption in the PCT and loop of Henle takes place predominantly via the paracellular pathways (claudin 16 and claudin 19), the transcellular pathway via the TRPM6 channel operates primarily in the DCT. Along with these, cyclin M2 (CNNM2) and SLC41A3 are also directly involved in Mg^{2+} transport. Claudin 10/14, epidermal growth factor (EGF) and CNNM2 channels are also involved in the regulation of Mg^{2+} transport proteins. EGF regulates TRPM6 activity, and its plasma membrane availability.

Fractional excretion of magnesium is calculated by the following formula:

$$\text{FeMg (percent)} = \frac{(\text{Urine Mg}^{2+} \times \text{serum creatinine})}{(0.7 \times \text{serum Mg}^{2+} \times \text{urine creatinine})} \times 100$$

The fractional excretion of Mg^{2+} is 3–5% with normal diet; renal conservation mechanisms can reduce it <0.5% in states of negative balance. With negative Mg^{2+} balance, equilibrium with bone stores occur after several weeks. If there is reduced intake with increased kidney excretion, symptomatic hypomagnesemia can occur rapidly. As kidney is the major organ regulating Mg^{2+} excretion, loss of renal function leads to significant extracellular Mg^{2+} retention. Conversely, the kidney can increase Mg^{2+} excretion 10-fold when serum Mg^{2+} concentration doubles.

Hypomagnesemia

Hypomagnesemia is defined as serum concentration <1.7 mg/dL. However, serum magnesium levels at times are an inaccurate marker for total body stores. Other methods, which have been proposed to predict total body stores include ionized Mg^{2+} levels, total red blood cell Mg^{2+} levels, and the Mg^{2+} loading test. Total RBC Mg^{2+} levels may better predict magnesium status, since the cation may be pulled out from red cells during hypomagnesemia. The etiology of hypomagnesemia is shown in **Box 6.13**.

Clinical features of hypomagnesemia are difficult to distinguish from hypokalemia, hypocalcemia, and metabolic alkalosis, which are usually also present. Neuromuscular excitability is often the first clinical feature. Tremors, tetany, positive Chvostek and Trousseau signs, cramps, choreoathetosis, vertical nystagmus, delirium, coma, and even depression is reported as CNS manifestations. ECG changes include flat T wave, wide QRS complexes, U waves and prolonged QT interval, and arrhythmias (including torsades de pointes). Digoxin toxicity is heightened as intracellular K^{+} is often depleted and Na^{+}/K^{+}-ATPase is inhibited. High fractional excretion of Mg^{2+} (exceeding 5%) in presence of hypomagnesemia suggests renal magnesium wasting.

BOX 6.13: Causes of hypomagnesemia

Decreased intake
Parenteral nutrition
Proton pump inhibitors
Malnutrition
Anorexia nervosa

Redistribution
Hungry bone syndrome
Refeeding syndrome
Acute pancreatitis
Insulin therapy during diabetic ketoacidosis therapy

Increased losses
Extrarenal losses
Acute and chronic diarrhea, malabsorption, intestinal fistula
Prolonged nasogastric suction
Excessive sweating and burns
Renal losses
Thiazide or loop diuretics
Renal transplantation
Hypercalcemia
Drugs: Calcineurin inhibitors, amphotericin B, cisplatin, cetuximab, aminoglycoside
Diuretic phase of acute tubular necrosis
Postobstructive diuresis
Diabetes mellitus (due to polyuria)
Genetic disorders: Variants in *CLDN16/19, TRPM6, FXYD2, KCNA1, EGF, CNNM2, RRAGD,* and *ATP1A1*

Chronic hypomagnesemia is observed in many metabolic diseases. Magnesium deficiency is known to affect glycemic control. Magnesium, along with citrate and pyrophosphate, is antilithogenic factors, and nephrocalcinosis/urolithiasis is seen in many monogenic disorders of Mg^{2+} metabolism. Hypokalemia associated with hypomagnesemia is due to lack of inhibition of ROMK channels. Refractory hypocalcemia in the setting of hypomagnesemia is contributed by impaired secretion of, and end-organ resistance to PTH.

Management

In a patient with hypomagnesemia, it is recommended to check Ca^{2+}, K^{+}, phosphate, creatinine, and ECG to manage concomitant abnormalities. In asymptomatic patients, oral supplementation (magnesium gluconate, oxide, or hydroxide) is sufficient at a dose of 100–200 mg/kg/dose q 4–6 hr. The maintenance dose is 30–60 mg/kg/day. The formulation, magnesium oxide (400 mg tablet) contains 240 mg of elemental magnesium. The dose is increased gradually; diarrhea is seen at higher dosages.

Alternatively, 0.2 mL/kg of 50% magnesium sulfate (500 mg/mL) may be given IM. Parenteral administration is necessary for symptomatic patients or those with level < 1.0 mg/dL. This is given as magnesium sulfate 25–50 mg/dose (maximum 2 g) by IM injection or slow IV infusion over 20–30 min q 6-h for three to four doses. Special caution is required during renal insufficiency; IV calcium gluconate should be available as antidote. Close monitoring for magnesium levels, hypotension, heart block, and respiratory depression is necessary. Associated hypokalemia and hypocalcemia should be appropriately treated.

The underlying cause should be appropriately treated. Amiloride, a K^+ and Mg^{2+} sparing diuretic, may benefit symptomatic patients with chronic renal losses refractory to supplementation.

Hypermagnesemia

Hypermagnesemia (serum Mg^{2+} >2.2 mg/dL) may occur in patients with renal failure given magnesium containing laxatives, and in infants born to mothers who have received magnesium for preeclampsia. Clinical features include respiratory depression, hypotension, hypotonia, hyporeflexia, paralysis, and coma. IV calcium gluconate 100 mg/kg rapidly, but transiently, reverses the toxic effects of magnesium (doses can be repeated). IV saline with loop diuretics may be employed to increase urine magnesium excretion in patients with preserved kidney function. Hemodialysis may be required in patients with renal failure (~50% reduction in magnesium levels with three to four dialysis is seen).

METABOLIC ACIDOSIS AND ALKALOSIS

Maintenance of acid-base balance is crucial for normal physiological processes. Homeostatic mechanisms maintain arterial pH (7.35–7.45), pCO_2 (35–45 mm Hg), and bicarbonate (20–28 mEq/L) within a narrow range. The pH of body fluids is calculated using the Henderson-Hasselbalch equation: where, pK is the dissociation constant of the acid.

$$pH = pKa + \log [HCO_3^-/pCO_2]$$

Alterations in either the serum bicarbonate concentration or in the partial pressure of carbon dioxide can lead to altered pH. Changes in pH are resisted by intracellular buffers (hemoglobin, protein, and phosphate) and extracellular buffers (bicarbonate and ammonia).

$$H_2O + CO_2 \rightleftharpoons H_2CO_3 \rightleftharpoons H^+ + HCO_3^-$$

During metabolic acidosis more carbon dioxide is generated leading to hyperventilation and subsequent respiratory compensation which tends to bring the pH back to normal **(Fig. 6.6)**. Respiratory compensation occurs within minutes and is completed by 12–24 hr. In contrast, renal compensation is slowly achieved in 2–5 days **(Table 6.3)**. Kidneys regulate bicarbonate resorption of HCO_3^-, mostly in proximal convoluted tubules, and through excretion of H^+ in the distal tubules **(Fig. 6.6)**. Hydrogen ions are excreted as free H^+ ions, as titratable acid (dihydrogen phosphate) or as ammonium.

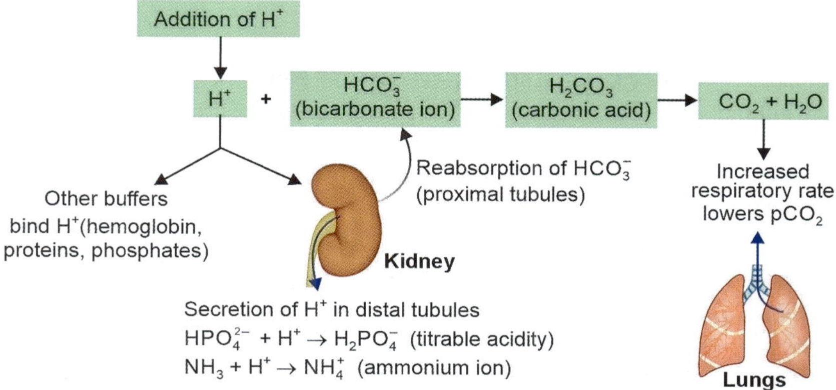

Fig. 6.6: Principles of acid-base homeostasis

TABLE 6.3: Compensation for primary acid-base disorders

Disorder	*Primary event*	*Compensation*	*Expected compensation*
Metabolic acidosis	↓ $[HCO_3^-]$	↓ pCO_2	pCO_2 ↓ by 1–1.5 mm Hg for 1 mEq/L ↓ $[HCO_3^-]$
Metabolic alkalosis	↑ $[HCO_3^-]$	↑ pCO_2	pCO_2 ↑ by 0.5–1 mm Hg for 1 mEq/L↑ $[HCO_3^-]$
Respiratory acidosis: Acute (<24-hr) Chronic (3–5 days)	↑ pCO_2	↑ $[HCO_3^-]$	$[HCO_3^-]$ ↑ by 1 mEq/L for 10 mm Hg ↑ pCO_2 $HCO_3^-]$ ↑ by 4 mEq/L for 10 mm Hg ↑ pCO_2
Respiratory alkalosis: Acute (<24-hr) Chronic (3–5 days)	↓ pCO_2	↓ $[HCO_3^-]$	$[HCO_3^-]$ ↓ by 1–3 mEq/L for 10 mm Hg ↓ pCO_2 $[HCO_3^-]$ ↓ by 2–5 mEq/L for 10 mm Hg ↓ pCO_2

The appropriate respiratory or renal compensation can be calculated and a mixed acid-base disorder is suspected when the compensation in a given patient differs from the predicted values **(Table 6.3)**.

Metabolic Acidosis

Primary metabolic acidosis is characterized by arterial pH <7.35 due to a low plasma bicarbonate concentration (<24 mEq/L; <20–22 mEq/L in neonates) and low to normal pCO_2 (<40 mm Hg).

Etiology

Metabolic acidosis may be caused by renal or extrarenal loss of bicarbonate, production of organic acids (diabetic ketoacidosis and lactic acidosis),

BOX 6.14: Causes of metabolic acidosis[1]

High anion gap metabolic acidosis (normochloremic)
Kidney dysfunction: Glomerular filtration rate <15 mL/1.73 m^2/min]
Extrarenal origin
Diabetic ketoacidosis
Lactic acidosis
Fasting ketoacidosis
Inborn errors of metabolism
Poisoning: Methanol, ethylene glycol, paraldehyde, salicylates

Normal anion gap metabolic acidosis
Gastrointestinal bicarbonate loss (urinary anion gap negative)
Diarrhea
Ureterosigmoidostomy
Pancreatic or biliary losses
Cholestyramine
Renal: Proximal bicarbonate loss/distal acidification defect (urinary anion gap positive)
Renal tubular acidosis
Interstitial nephritis
Uremic acidosis (GFR 15–30 mL/1.73 m^2/min)
Acetazolamide
Potassium sparing diuretics
Diminished mineralocorticoid activity

[1]*See* Chapter 20

inadequate excretion of daily acid load in kidney dysfunction, and ingestion of toxins **(Box 6.14)**. Intestinal secretions have high concentration of bicarbonate, and removal of bile, pancreatic, or intestinal secretions leads to metabolic acidosis. Ureterosigmoidostomy leads to metabolic acidosis by two mechanisms—firstly ammonium ions absorbed by colonic mucosa are metabolized in liver to release H^+; secondly, colonic Cl^--HCO_3^- exchanger absorbs urinary chloride and excretes HCO_3^-. The diagnosis and evaluation of renal tubular acidosis are discussed in **Chapter 20**.

Clinical Features

Rapid, deep breathing (Kussmaul respiration) is the chief clinical feature. Other features are nausea, vomiting, abdominal pain, stupor, and coma. Consequences of metabolic acidosis include reduced cardiac contractility, arterial vasodilatation, hypotension, and resistance to catecholamines (if pH <7.2). Chronic metabolic acidosis leads to demineralization of bones and growth retardation.

Evaluation

Clinical evaluation provides clues for the underlying cause of metabolic acidosis. Blood creatinine should be measured to rule out kidney failure.

Blood pH, pCO_2, bicarbonate, and base excess should be estimated. Base excess, defined as the amount of H^+ ions required to return the pH of blood to 7.35 if the pCO_2 was held constant at 40 mm Hg, estimates the metabolic component of the abnormality. More negative base excess suggests severe metabolic acidosis. Expected respiratory compensation for metabolic acidosis is then calculated as:

$$\text{Compensated } pCO_2 = [1.5 \times \text{serum } HCO_3^- + 8] \pm 2$$

Inadequate or excessive changes in pCO_2 suggest a mixed disorder.

Anion Gap

Plasma anion gap (AG) is used to divide metabolic acidosis into disorders which present with a high or normal AG **(Box 6.14; Figs. 6.7A to D)**. This gap is a measure of unmeasured anions in the plasma, primarily phosphates, sulfates, acidic protein moieties, and nonvolatile acids.

$$\text{Anion gap} = \text{Unmeasured anions} - \text{Unmeasured cations}$$
$$= \text{Serum sodium} - [\text{chloride} + \text{bicarbonate}]$$

The normal plasma AG is 8–12 mEq/L. Metabolic acidosis resulting from bicarbonate loss (normal AG) can be differentiated from acidosis due to accumulation of nonvolatile acids (high AG). Bicarbonate loss stimulates

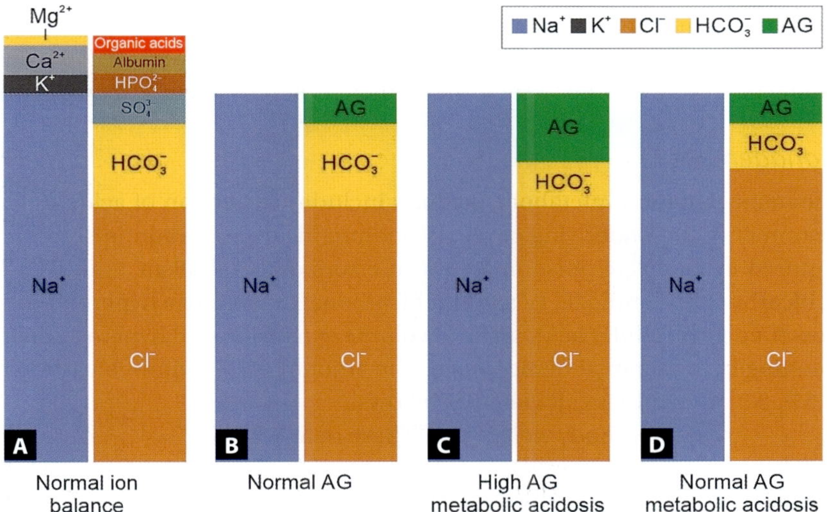

Figs. 6.7A to D: Gamblegram depicting the concept of anion gap (AG) in metabolic acidosis. The total anion and total cation concentrations (measured in mEq/L) must be equal. (A) If only Na^+, Cl^-, and HCO_3^- are considered, an anion gap (AG) normally exists. (B) High AG metabolic acidosis reduces the HCO_3^- without changing Cl^- and thereby increases the AG in a reciprocal fashion. (C) Normal AG, or hyperchloremic metabolic acidosis, reduces the HCO_3^- and increases the Cl^- in a reciprocal fashion. These relationships assume that the other anions and cations in serum are initially in their normal ranges and stable

equivalent chloride reabsorption by the proximal tubule, and the AG remains normal. Serum albumin has a net negative charge of about 2.5 mEq/g; this is the largest component of the normal AG. Hence, hypoalbuminemia warrants correction as per the formula:

$$\text{Corrected AG} = \text{Observed AG} + 2.5^{*}\,(4.5 - \text{albumin in g/dL})$$

Adequacy of renal response to acidosis, in case of normal AG metabolic acidosis, is given by the urine AG that is calculated as follows:

$$\text{Urinary anion gap} = (\text{urine Na}^{+} + \text{urine K}^{+}) - \text{urine Cl}^{-}$$

The urine AG is an indirect estimate of renal ammonium excretion. Appropriate response to systemic metabolic acidosis is an increase in urine ammonium and chloride excretion (since ammonium is excreted as ammonium chloride). The increase in urine chloride concentration results in negative urine AG if metabolic acidosis is secondary to extrarenal loss of bicarbonate. A positive urine AG in presence of systemic acidosis indicates impaired ammonium excretion and a renal etiology **(Box 6.14; *see* also Chapter 20)**.

D-lactic acidosis is a rare form of metabolic acidosis that affects patients with short bowel syndrome or other intestinal malabsorption, due to fermentation of unabsorbed glucose into D-lactate and other organic acids. Quantitation of D-lactate requires special techniques; the condition should be suspected in patients with unexplained high anion gap metabolic acidosis in appropriate clinical settings. Neurological involvement such as confusion, cerebellar ataxia, slurred speech, incontinence, and nystagmus may be seen.

Management

The management of metabolic acidosis includes correction of acidosis and treatment of the underlying cause. IV sodium bicarbonate administration is required in salicylate poisoning, inborn errors of metabolism, and pH ≤7.0 or bicarbonate <5 mEq/L. IV sodium bicarbonate may cause hypernatremia, worsened intracellular acidosis, ECF volume expansion and hyperosmolality resulting in intracranial hemorrhage. The amount of IV sodium bicarbonate (7.5%, 0.9 mEq/mL) is calculated as follows:

$$\text{Body weight (kg)} \times \text{base deficit} \times 0.3$$

The medication is given as 1:1 dilution, infused over 2 hr. Correction of acidosis might precipitate hypokalemia and hypocalcemia, which should be monitored.

Sodium bicarbonate is not indicated in patients with lactic acidosis, where therapy should be directed toward improving oxygen supply to tissues. Oral bicarbonate therapy with sodium bicarbonate, sodium citrate, or potassium citrate (1–2 mEq/kg/day) is initiated in chronic acidosis. Refractory metabolic acidosis may require hemodialysis or peritoneal dialysis. In refractory lactic acidosis, bicarbonate-based dialysate (rather than lactate-based solutions) is preferred. Intoxications, such as ethylene glycol poisoning are managed with hemodialysis.

Veverimer, a polyamine polymer that selectively binds to H^+ and Cl^- from the gut and removes them in feces, is an emerging treatment option for metabolic acidosis in CKD.

Metabolic Alkalosis

Metabolic alkalosis is defined as high blood pH (>7.45) and increased serum bicarbonate (>26 mEq/L). Plasma pH differentiates primary metabolic alkalosis from metabolic compensation during respiratory acidosis. The pH is generally <7.35 in compensated respiratory acidosis since the metabolic compensation does not overcorrect the pH into the alkalotic range. Expected respiratory compensation for alkalosis is given by:

$$\text{Compensated } paCO_2 = 0.7 \times [\text{serum } HCO_3^- - 22] \text{ or serum } HCO_3^- + 15$$

If actual compensation is less than expected, a mixed respiratory and metabolic disorder is suspected.

Etiology

Causes of metabolic alkalosis are listed in **Box 6.15**. When H^+ and Cl^- are lost from any extrarenal site, chloride is avidly retained by the kidneys and bicarbonate forms the primary anion in distal tubules. Bicarbonate is

BOX 6.15: Causes of metabolic alkalosis[1]

Chloride responsive
Loop or thiazide diuretics
Persistent vomiting, nasogastric suction, congenital hypertrophic pyloric stenosis
Villous adenoma; congenital chloride-losing diarrhea
Cystic fibrosis
Posthypercapnia

Chloride unresponsive
Normal blood pressure
Bartter syndrome
Gitelman syndrome
Elevated blood pressure
Renovascular stenosis
Renin secreting tumor
Adrenal hyperplasia, adenoma, and carcinoma; Cushing syndrome
Congenital adrenal hyperplasia: Deficiency of 11β hydroxylase or 17α-hydroxylase
Glucocorticoid remediable aldosteronism
Liddle syndrome
Apparent mineralocorticoid excess
Licorice ingestion; exogenous steroids
Milk-alkali syndrome; bicarbonate use; blood transfusion

[1]*See* Chapter 20

reabsorbed with simultaneous H^+ secretion. To maintain electroneutrality, tubular Na^+ and K^+ are lost with accompanying water loss. Volume depletion activates the renin-angiotensin-aldosterone axis, further compounding hypokalemia. This state of ECF volume depletion, hypochloremic metabolic alkalosis, and hypokalemia is termed contraction alkalosis. Hypokalemia maintains metabolic alkalosis by increasing renal ammoniagenesis and renal H^+ secretion. Since alkalosis is driven by hypochloremia, it is responsive to administration of chloride (IV, orally).

Metabolic alkalosis might also be the result of retention of bicarbonate. This usually results from altered mineralocorticoid activity resulting in increased distal Na^+ reabsorption, increased K^+ secretion and increased intravascular volume. The resulting alkalosis is driven and compounded by hypokalemia. Rarely, in the presence of reduced GFR, excessive ingestion of alkali (milk, calcium carbonate) may lead to alkalosis. Alkalosis in these patients does not respond to chloride administration.

Clinical Features and Diagnosis

Mild metabolic alkalosis is asymptomatic. Symptoms occur in severe alkalosis due to decrease in Ca^{2+} and K^+. Neuromuscular irritability, paresthesia, fatigue, muscle cramps, tetany, seizures, confusion, stupor, and cardiac arrhythmias may occur. Alkalosis shifts the oxygen hemoglobin dissociation curve to the left causing tissue hypoxemia. The compensatory hypoventilation may cause difficulty in weaning from mechanical ventilation.

A history of diuretic use, vomiting, nasogastric suction, administration of licorice or steroids, and history suggestive of significant respiratory illness is important **(Flowchart 6.7)**. Subtle, chronic volume contraction is detected by measuring urine chloride concentration, which will be <20 mEq/L. Urinary chloride wasting with volume depletion is seen in Bartter and Gitelman syndromes where hyperaldosteronism secondary to volume contraction causes hypokalemia, which maintains metabolic alkalosis **(Chapter 20)**.

Management

Mild or moderate metabolic alkalosis or alkalemia rarely requires correction. Treatment of chloride responsive states includes management of the underlying state, volume repletion, and correction of chloride and potassium deficits. Normal saline with added potassium chloride is the fluid of choice. Proton pump inhibitors minimize gastric acid loss in patients with continuous gastric drainage. Patients with metabolic alkalosis associated with use of loop diuretics may need supplemental potassium chloride or therapy with a potassium sparing diuretic. In primary hyperaldosteronism, treatment with spironolactone or amiloride is useful. Management of potassium losing tubulopathies includes fluid replacement, potassium

Flowchart 6.7: Approach to a patient with metabolic alkalosis and hypokalemia. AME: apparent mineralocorticoid excess; CAH: congenital adrenal hyperplasia; GRA: glucocorticoid remediable aldosteronism; NG: nasogastric

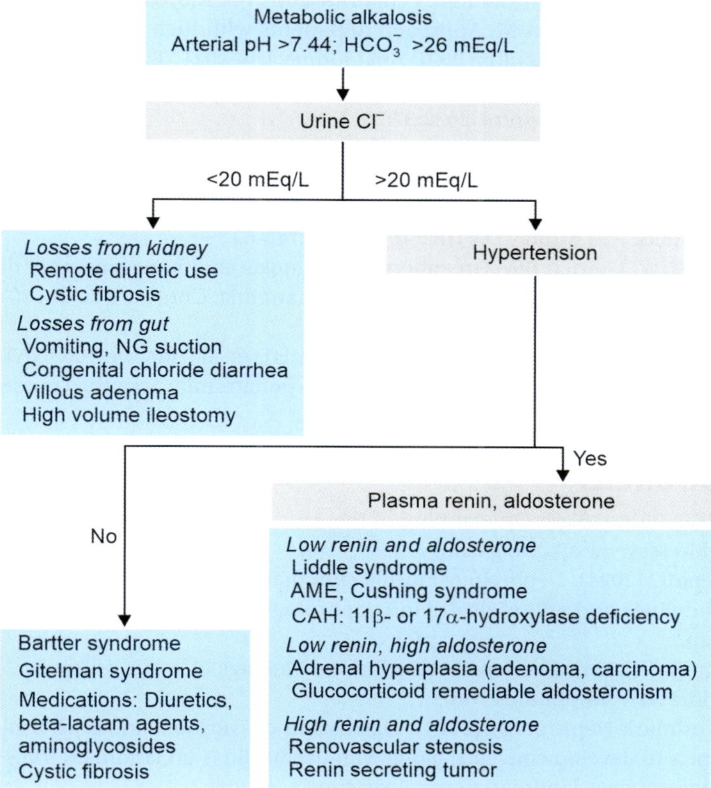

chloride supplementation, and therapy with indomethacin or ibuprofen. Acetazolamide is sometimes used in patients with chloride-resistant metabolic alkalosis with normal kidney function.

BIBLIOGRAPHY

1. Adrogué HJ, Madias NE. The syndrome of inappropriate antidiuresis. N Engl J Med. 2023;389:1499-509.
2. Amer BE, Abdelwahab OA, Abdelaziz A, et al. Efficacy and safety of isotonic versus hypotonic intravenous maintenance fluids in hospitalized children: an updated systematic review and meta-analysis of randomized controlled trials. Pediatr Nephrol. 2024;39:57-84.
3. Bagga A, Sinha A. Renal tubular acidosis. Indian J Pediatr. 2020;87:733-44.
4. Brossier DW, Tume LN, Briant AR, et al.; Metabolism Endocrinology and Nutrition section of the European Society of Pediatric and Neonatal Intensive Care. ESPNIC clinical practice guidelines: intravenous maintenance fluid therapy in acute and critically ill children: A systematic review and meta-analysis. Intensive Care Med. 2022;48:1691-708.

5. Emmett M. Metabolic alkalosis: A brief pathophysiologic review. Clin J Am Soc Nephrol. 2020;15:1848-56.
6. Feld LG, Neuspiel DR, Foster BR, et al. Clinical practice guideline: Maintenance intravenous fluids in children. Pediatrics. 2018;142:e20183083.
7. Fenves AZ, Emmett M. Approach to patients with high anion gap metabolic acidosis: Core curriculum 2021. Am J Kidney Dis. 2021;78:590-600.
8. Haffner D, Leifheit-Nestler M, Grund A, et al. Rickets guidance: Part I-diagnostic workup. Pediatr Nephrol. 2022;37:2013-36.
9. Palmer BF, Clegg DJ. Physiology and pathophysiology of potassium homeostasis: Core curriculum 2019. Am J Kidney Dis. 2019;74:682-95.
10. Ray E, Mohan K, Ahmad S, et al. Physiology of a forgotten electrolyte-magnesium disorders. Adv Kidney Dis Health. 2023;30:148-63.
11. Seay NW, Lehrich RW, Greenberg A. Diagnosis and management of disorders of body tonicity-hyponatremia and hypernatremia: Core curriculum 2020. Am J Kidney Dis. 2020;75:272-86.
12. Sterns RH, Rondon-Berrios H, Adrogue HJ, et al.; for the PRONATREOUS Investigators. Treatment guidelines for hyponatremia: Stay the course. Clin J Am Soc Nephrol. 2024;19:129-135.

RESOURCES

1. AJKD Blog (2024). Official blog of the American Journal of Kidney Diseases. Address: www.ajkdblog.com.
2. NephJC (2024). Nephrology journal club that uses Twitter to discuss research, guidelines and editorials driving nephrology forward. Address: www.nephjc.com.
3. Topf JM (2024). Precious bodily fluids—Musings of a salt whisperer. [online] Address: www.pbfluids.com.
4. Landmark Nephrology (2024). Discussion on various landmark trials, basic topics to develop concepts, along with useful slides on landmark trials as well. Address: www.landmarknephrology.com.
5. Life in the fast lane (2024). ECG Library Content. Address: https://litfl.com/ecg-library.

Hematuria and Proteinuria

Arvind Bagga, Geetika Singh, Aditi Sinha

Asymptomatic, isolated hematuria, and proteinuria are commonly observed in apparently healthy children. A careful clinical and laboratory evaluation is required. The presence of both hematuria and proteinuria indicates significant glomerular disease and requires detailed investigation.

HEMATURIA

Epidemiology and Definition

Urine dipsticks are very sensitive and detect even small numbers of red blood cells (RBCs), especially if the specimen is concentrated. The urine dipstick relies on peroxidation of a reagent (tetramethylbenzidine) incorporated into the dipstick, by hemoglobin peroxidase. Since small numbers of RBCs (<5 RBCs/high-power field on microscopic examination) in the urine are physiologic and do not signify hematuria, the urine dipstick cannot be used to diagnose "true" hematuria. Occasionally, the presence of substances other than RBCs, such as hemoglobin and myoglobin, can cause discoloration of the urine dipstick. Thus, for the diagnosis of hematuria, a microscopic examination of the urine sediment is essential. Other false positives on the dipstick include the presence of nonheme oxidizing agents and contaminants in urine, such as bleach. Microbial peroxidases, such as in urinary tract infection, may also be responsible for a false positive test. False negatives may be seen, if the urine is very dilute or if reducing substances such as ascorbic acid are present.

Microscopic hematuria is defined as the presence of >5 RBCs/high-power field on a centrifuged urine specimen (or >5 RBCs/mm^3 on unspun specimen) and is found in 4–5% of all urine specimens in American school children (8–12 years of age), more so in girls and increases with age. It is generally benign when present in isolation, without concomitant proteinuria. Persistent microscopic hematuria, defined as microscopic hematuria on two to three occasions, occurs in <1% of children. Large school-screening programs, chiefly from Japan, China, and South Korea, report isolated microscopic hematuria in 0.4–0.5% cases, while 0.03–0.7% have both hematuria and proteinuria. Gross hematuria (visible discoloration of the urine due to the presence of RBCs) occurs is <0.1% cases. There is increasing evidence that persistent hematuria, especially if associated with proteinuria, is a risk factor for chronic kidney disease.

Microscopic Hematuria

Since isolated microscopic hematuria most often resolves spontaneously, it is prudent to repeat urinalysis on multiple occasions on fresh urine specimens. The urine specimen is examined for RBC morphology **(Figs. 7.1A to D)** and for other formed elements. If the child is otherwise healthy and hematuria resolves, no further evaluation is needed. Detailed evaluation may be warranted if microscopic hematuria persists.

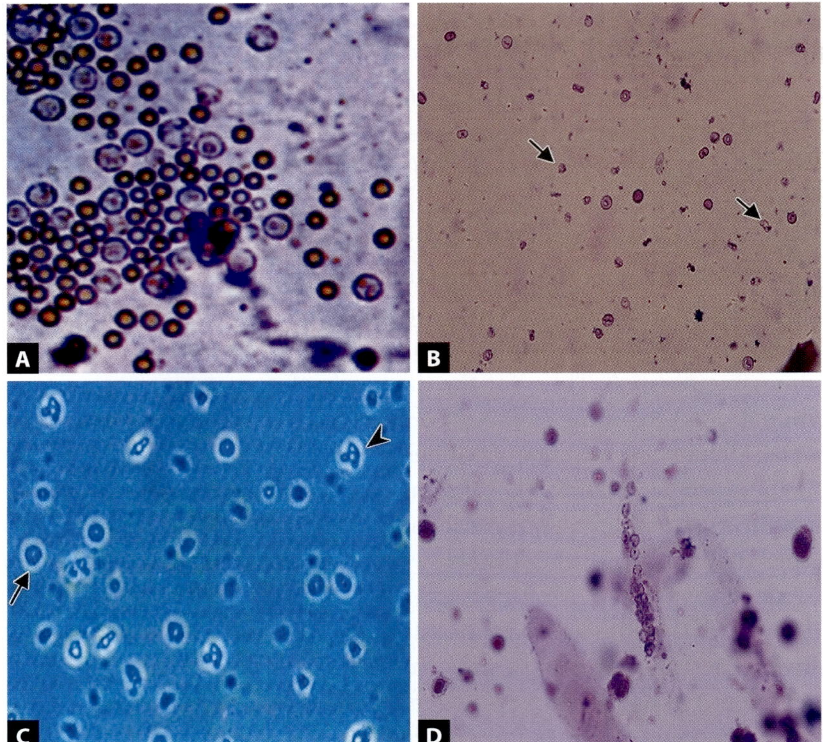

Figs. 7.1A to D: Urinalysis for hematuria. (A) Red cells in a patient with idiopathic hypercalciuria. Note the normal morphology (400 x); (B) Glomerular hematuria. The variation in morphology of red cells is obvious even under bright light; arrows indicate dysmorphic red cells. (C) Phase contrast microscopy showing dysmorphic red cells (arrowhead) as well as normal red cells (arrow). There is marked variation in the size and shape of cells. (D) Red cell casts confirm glomerular origin of hematuria.

Epidemiologic studies suggest that in 60–80% of children with persistent microscopic hematuria, no identifiable cause can be found using noninvasive means. Common identified causes include idiopathic hypercalciuria, poststreptococcal glomerulonephritis (GN), immunoglobulin A (IgA) nephropathy, and thin basement membrane disease. A limited work up in this setting is appropriate, including a random urine calcium-to-creatinine ratio for hypercalciuria, and screening of family members for microscopic hematuria to evaluate for familial GN. However, if the patient has microscopic hematuria along with proteinuria or other associated signs or symptoms, it is necessary to rule out significant renal diseases, using a complete work-up as for gross hematuria. Idiopathic persistent microscopic hematuria resolves in the majority of children. At 1-year follow-up, only one-third of children have persistent urinary abnormalities, and by 5 years, the proportion is even lower.

Gross Hematuria

The likelihood of identifying an underlying cause is much greater in patients with gross hematuria, chief causes being hypercalciuria, renal calculi, infection-related GN, and IgA nephropathy. A complete work-up is therefore needed in patients with gross hematuria. History, physical examination, and urinalysis can identify if the source of the bleeding is the renal parenchyma (glomerular hematuria) or the collecting system (nonglomerular hematuria) **(Table 7.1 and Flowchart 7.1)**. If the source can be identified, the patient should be evaluated further for various etiologies **(Box 7.1)**. If the source of hematuria is not identified, examining the child and the urine again at time of an episode of gross hematuria may be of value. **Flowcharts 7.1 and 7.2**

TABLE 7.1: Approach to a patient with hematuria

	Parenchymal, intrarenal (glomerular hematuria)	*Collecting system, extrarenal (nonglomerular hematuria)*
Appearance of urine	Tea colored	Bright red, blood clots
Pattern of hematuria	Hematuria throughout urinary stream	Initial, terminal hematuria
Urinary symptoms	Painless	Dysuria, urgency, frequency
Associated features	Sore throat, hypertension, edema	Fever, colicky pain
Family history	Deafness, renal failure	Renal stones, urinary infection
Proteinuria	≥2+ on dipstick; PCR >1 mg/mg	Trace to 1+; PCR <1 mg/mg
Urinary findings	Red cell casts; dysmorphic red cells	Crystals, eumorphic red cells

PCR (first morning spot) urine protein to creatinine ratio

Flowchart 7.1: Approach to evaluation of gross hematuria. Also see Table 7.1. C3: complement C3; GN: glomerulonephritis; RBC: red blood cell

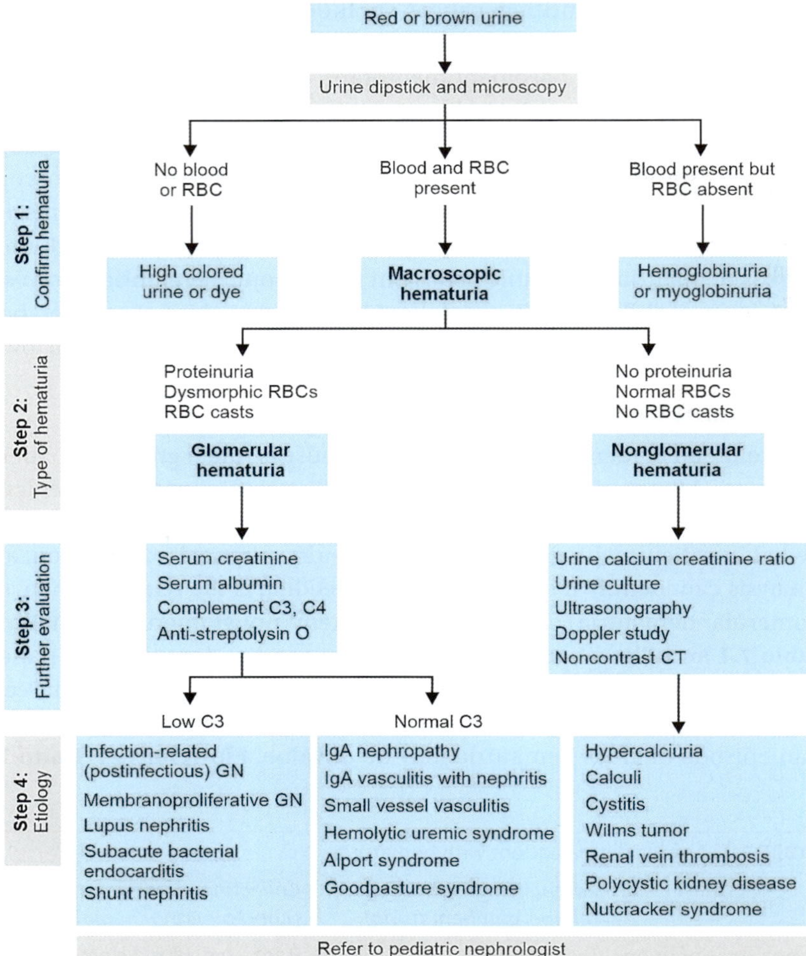

outline the plan for evaluation in patients with gross hematuria and persistent microscopic hematuria, respectively.

Evaluation for Glomerular Hematuria

Urine culture is important to detect a urinary infection, although most children with pyelonephritis have other features (fever, flank pain, and pyuria), and occasionally gross hematuria. Since GN is an important cause of renal hematuria, detailed investigations are required. These include estimation of blood levels of creatinine, urea, protein, albumin, and cholesterol, appropriate serologies (antistreptolysin O and streptozyme

BOX 7.1: Causes of hematuria

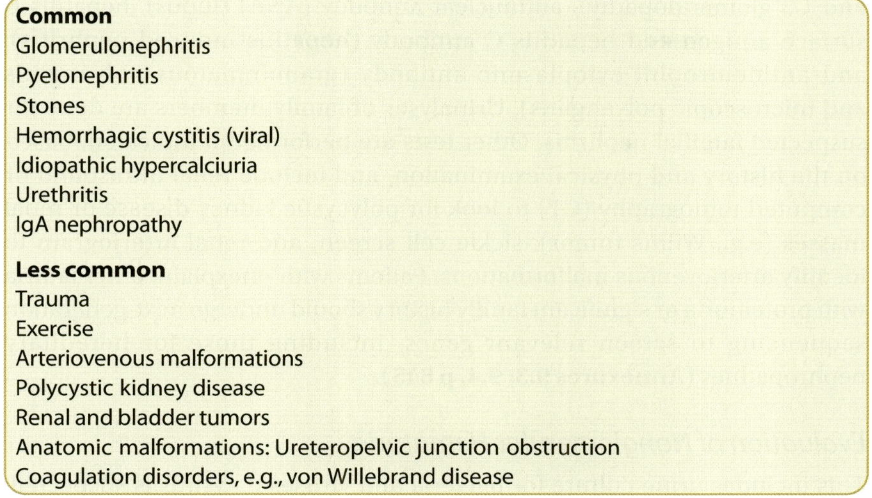

Common
Glomerulonephritis
Pyelonephritis
Stones
Hemorrhagic cystitis (viral)
Idiopathic hypercalciuria
Urethritis
IgA nephropathy

Less common
Trauma
Exercise
Arteriovenous malformations
Polycystic kidney disease
Renal and bladder tumors
Anatomic malformations: Ureteropelvic junction obstruction
Coagulation disorders, e.g., von Willebrand disease

Flowchart 7.2: Approach to evaluation of persistent microscopic hematuria

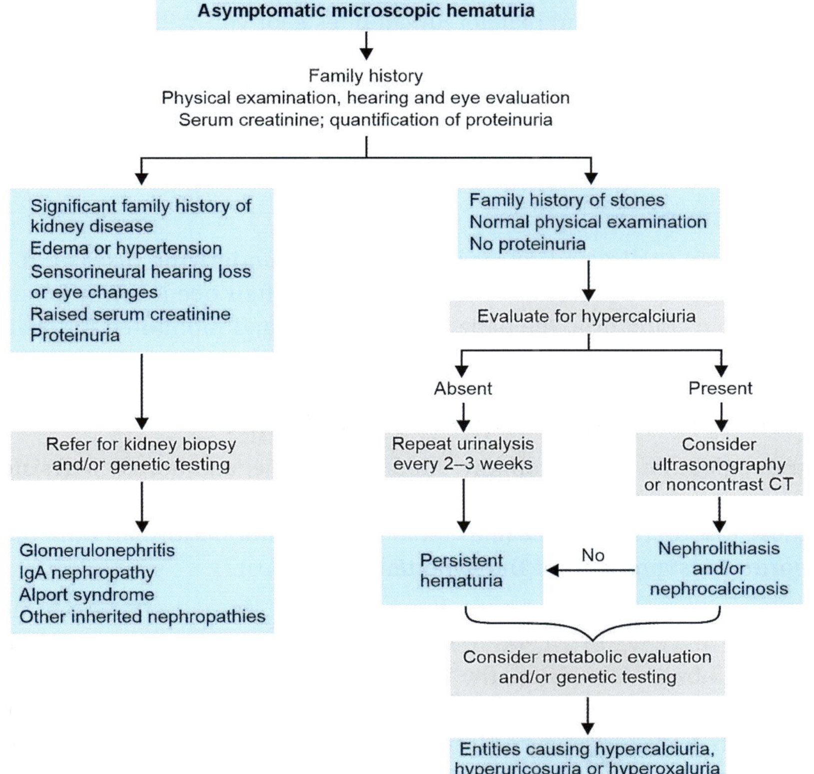

for postinfectious GN), complement C3 and C4 (postinfectious GN, lupus, and C3 glomerulopathy), antinuclear antibody (ANA) (lupus), hepatitis B surface antigen and hepatitis C antibody (hepatitis-induced nephritis), and antineutrophil cytoplasmic antibody (granulomatous polyangiitis and microscopic polyangiitis). Urinalyses of family members are done for suspected familial nephritis. Other tests are performed if indicated, based on the history and physical examination, and include renal ultrasound or computed tomography (CT) to look for polycystic kidney disease or renal masses (e.g., Wilms tumor), sickle cell screen, and renal arteriogram to identify arteriovenous malformations. Patients with unexplained hematuria with proteinuria or significant family history should undergo next-generation sequencing to screen relevant genes, including those for hereditary nephropathies **(Annexures 9.3; 9.4, p 845)**.

Evaluation of Nonglomerular Hematuria

This includes urine culture for bacteria and viruses if cystitis is suspected, early morning urine for spot calcium-to-creatinine ratio to screen for hypercalciuria (followed by 24-hr calcium excretion), X-ray abdomen, and ultrasonography. Where indicated, a noncontrast helical CT scan is done to look for renal stones and platelet function tests for von Willebrand disease. Invasive tests including cystourethroscopy or retrograde pyelography (for AV malformations, hemangiomas, or polyps) are seldom required. Next-generation sequencing is useful in patients with metabolic abnormalities, including hypercalciuria and hyperuricosuria **(Annexures 9.3; 9.7, p 845)**.

Management

Management is directed toward the identified underlying disease. If the evaluation does not yield a diagnosis, which often occurs with isolated microscopic hematuria, the patient is counseled and monitored for change in clinical features and for appearance of hypertension or proteinuria.

PERSISTENT MICROSCOPIC HEMATURIA

Immunoglobulin A nephropathy, Alport syndrome, and occasionally other diseases may initially manifest with microscopic hematuria. The incidence of these disorders is not clear, as renal biopsy is not performed until other abnormalities (proteinuria and hypertension) appear.

Immunoglobulin A Nephropathy

Immunoglobulin A nephropathy is the most common form of primary GN worldwide, although there are differences in its prevalence in different regions. Its prevalence varies from 5 to 140 per million children per year and represents 5–30% of kidney biopsies performed across the globe.

The condition is common in Japan, Korea, Taiwan and Australia, and less frequent in Europe and USA. The condition is not uncommon in children in India.

IgA nephropathy is characterized by the presence of predominant or codominant IgA deposits in the glomeruli. Other conditions that could result in similar immunofluorescence findings include IgA vasculitis, systemic lupus erythematosus, chronic liver disease, psoriasis, dermatitis herpetiformis, celiac disease, and non-Hodgkin lymphoma.

Pathogenesis

The pathogenesis of IgA nephropathy is now better understood. Multiple pathophysiological "hits", in a genetically predisposed individual, may result in the disease **(Flowchart 7.3)**. Galactose deficient IgA (GD-IgA) is produced in the mucosa after stimulation by various antigens, including microbes. Individuals prone to IgA nephropathy maintain high-systemic levels of GD-IgA, against which IgG- or IgA-directed autoantibodies can be stimulated. This leads to circulating immune complexes containing the autoantibody and the GD-IgA. Through specific and nonspecific interactions, these complexes accumulate in the mesangium, and generate molecular and cellular immune responses. Over time, this process can lead to the characteristic findings of hematuria and proteinuria, and also drives glomerular and tubulointerstitial sclerosis. Some patients show activation of the alternate complement pathway with C3 and properdin deposition. Plasma levels of IgA are increased in a proportion of patients, but do not correlate with severity of histologic lesions.

Clinical Features

Recurrent gross hematuria is the typical presentation. Flank pain may be associated. Episodes of gross hematuria immediately follow upper respiratory infections (synpharyngitic hematuria), but microscopic hematuria may persist. Microscopic or gross hematuria is more common in children than in adults; children also have higher estimated glomerular filtration rate (eGFR) and lower urine protein excretion. Occasionally, the disorder manifests with acute nephritic features or with heavy proteinuria and nephrotic syndrome, and rarely, with rapidly progressive GN.

Diagnosis

Urinalysis shows presence of RBC and RBC casts with variable degree of proteinuria. The severity of proteinuria should be quantified, since it useful for the management and prognosis of these patients. Serum IgA levels are elevated in 10–15% patients; serum C3 is normal in most cases.

The diagnosis of IgA nephropathy is made on biopsy that shows focal or diffuse proliferation of mesangial cells with increase in mesangial matrix **(Fig. 7.2A)**. Severe cases show segmental fibrinoid necrosis, capsular adhesions,

Flowchart 7.3: Pathogenesis of IgA nephropathy. A four hit hypothesis is proposed. Ig: immunoglobulin; Gal-def: galactose-deficient

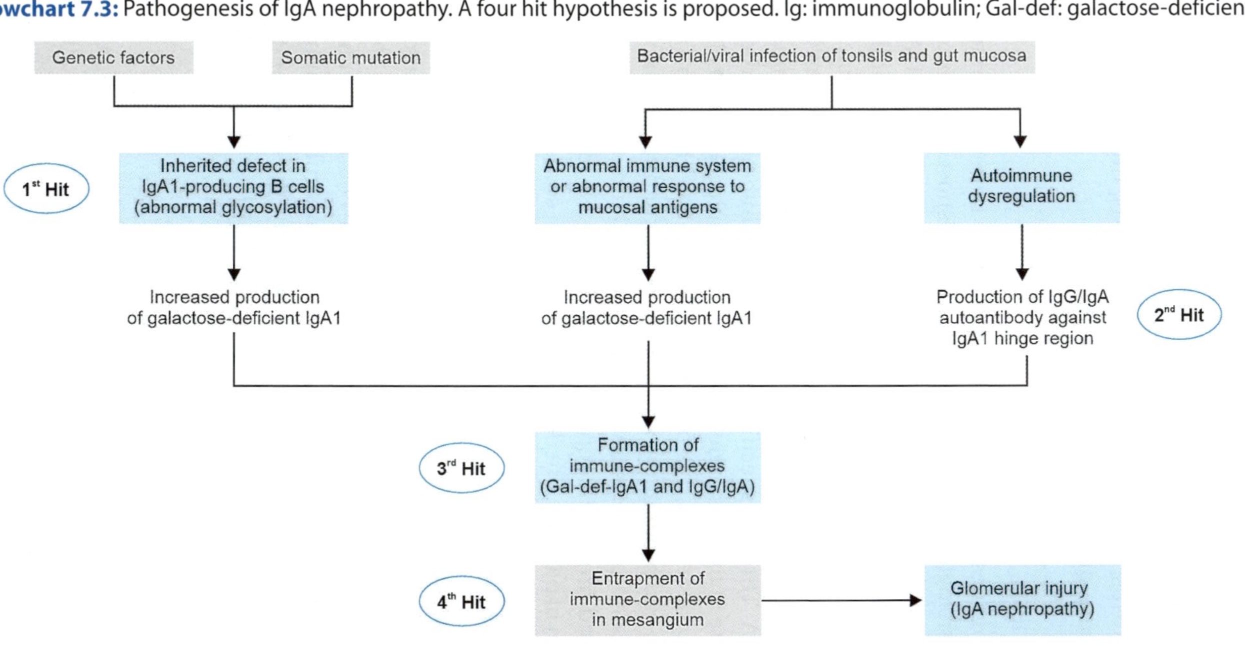

and crescents. Proliferative lesions are observed early in the course and gradually decrease after a few months, when focal segmental sclerosis or hyalinosis may persist. The mesangial deposits are predominantly composed of polymeric IgA1 **(Figs. 7.2B and C)**. Electron microscopy reveals deposits in mesangium, subendothelial, and subepithelial spaces **(Fig. 7.2D)**.

The revised MEST-C Oxford classification incorporates scores for mesangial hypercellularity (M), endocapillary proliferation (E), segmental glomerulosclerosis (S), tubular atrophy/interstitial fibrosis (T), and crescents (C) **(Table 7.2 and Figs. 7.3A to E)**. The classification has been validated as a predictor for renal outcome both in adults and children. Staining for KM-55, an antibody directed against galactose-deficient IgA, allows discrimination between mucosal-derived and systemically derived IgA **(Figs. 7.4A to D)**.

Treatment

Treatment of IgA nephropathy is determined based on findings on kidney biopsy, degree of proteinuria, and kidney function **(Table 7.3)**. The primary

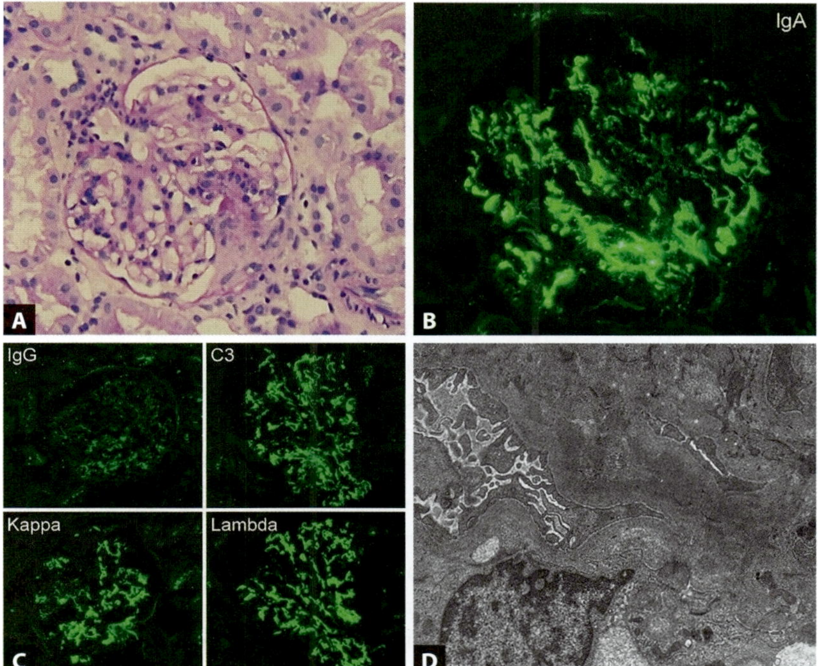

Figs. 7.2A to D: Histology of IgA nephropathy. (A) Light microscopy showing moderate mesangial proliferation and segmental sclerosis (H&E); (B) Immunofluorescence showing positive staining for IgA in mesangial areas; (C) Immunofluorescence showing focal mesangial staining for C3 and kappa and lambda light chains; (D) Electron microscopy shows subendothelial and mesangial deposits

TABLE 7.2: MEST-C criteria in the updated Oxford Classification of IgA nephropathy

Histological variable	*Definition*	*Score*
Mesangial hypercellularity	More than four mesangial cells in any mesangial area	*M0:* <50% of glomeruli showing mesangial hypercellularity *M1:* >50% of glomeruli showing mesangial hypercellularity
Endocapillary hypercellularity	Hypercellularity due to increased number of cells within glomerular capillary lumina	*E0:* No endocapillary hypercellularity *E1:* Any glomeruli showing endocapillary hypercellularity
Segmental glomerulosclerosis	Adhesion or sclerosis (obliteration of capillary lumina by matrix) in part; not the whole glomerular tuft	*S0:* Absent *S1:* Present in any glomeruli
Tubular atrophy, interstitial fibrosis	Estimated percentage of cortex showing tubular atrophy or interstitial fibrosis, whichever is more	*T0:* 0–25% of cortical area *T1:* 26–50% of cortical area *T2:* >50% of cortical area
Cellular, fibrocellular crescents	Percentage of glomeruli with cellular or fibrocellular crescents	*C0:* Absent *C1:* 0–25% of glomeruli *C2:* >25% of glomeruli

M: mesangial hypercellularity; E: endocapillary hypercellularity; S: segmental glomerulosclerosis; T: tubular atrophy/interstitial fibrosis; C: crescents

target of therapy is to achieve reduction of proteinuria (Up/Uc <0.2 mg/mg), normalization of kidney functions and reduction of blood pressure to <90th percentile. Recent KDIGO guidelines emphasize that all patients with IgA nephropathy with significant proteinuria should be managed with angiotensin-converting enzyme (ACE) inhibitors or angiotensin II receptor blocker (ARB), salt restriction, and optimal blood pressure control. Patients with crescentic GN should be managed with three to six doses of IV methylprednisolone and IV cyclophosphamide, followed by tapering doses of oral steroids and mycophenolate mofetil or azathioprine for at least 12–18 months. In patients with heavy proteinuria and/or severe histological changes, treatment with oral prednisolone has been proposed. Other medications, including cyclophosphamide, mycophenolate and azathioprine have been used with variable results. Calcineurin inhibitors are considered in patients presenting with nephrotic syndrome and kidney biopsy showing focal segmental glomerulosclerosis (FSGS) with predominant

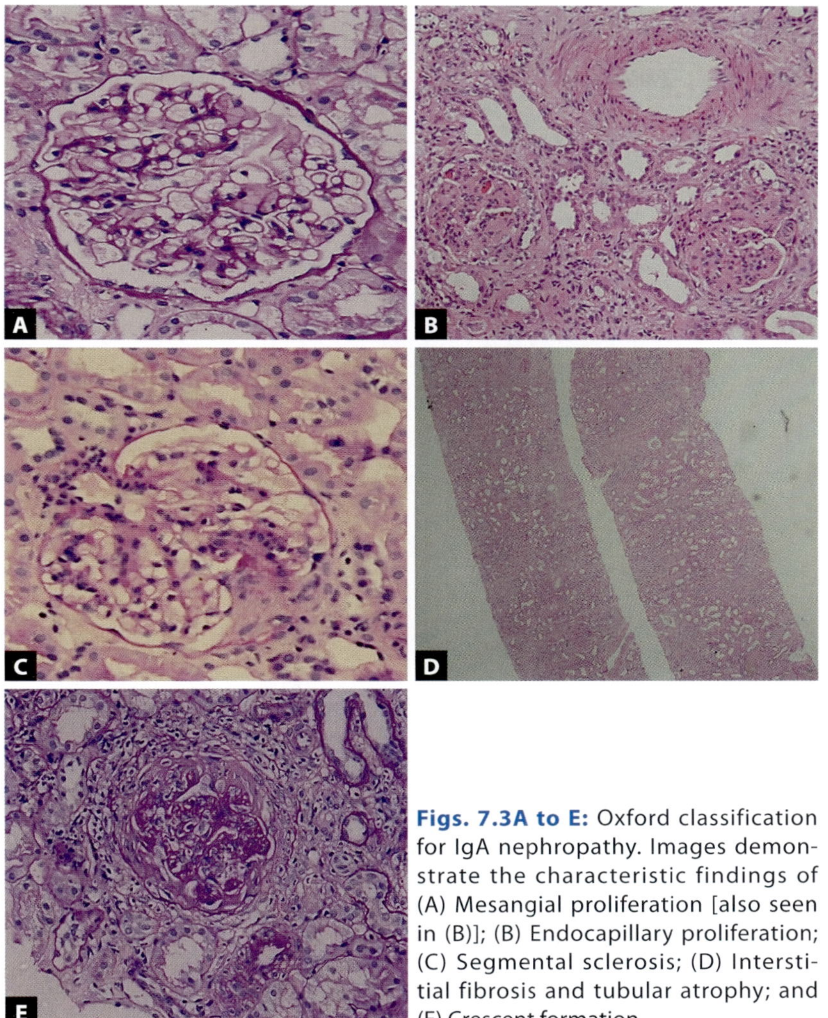

Figs. 7.3A to E: Oxford classification for IgA nephropathy. Images demonstrate the characteristic findings of (A) Mesangial proliferation [also seen in (B)]; (B) Endocapillary proliferation; (C) Segmental sclerosis; (D) Interstitial fibrosis and tubular atrophy; and (E) Crescent formation

IgA deposits. Patients with advanced disease eGFR <30 mL/min/1.73 m^2 and chronicity on kidney biopsy are best managed with supportive therapy, as immunosuppressive medications are unlikely to be effective.

Enteric-coated slow-release formulation of budesonide has been tested in clinical trials with some success, and the medication was recently approved by the United States Food and Drug Administration (US FDA) for adults with IgA nephropathy and proteinuria. Studies using sparsentan, a dual endothelin and angiotensin receptor antagonist, are also promising. There is limited and unproven evidence on oral therapy with omega-3 fatty acids (6–12 g/day; as fish oil), which is therefore not currently recommended. The role of B-cell inhibition and complement blockers is being examined.

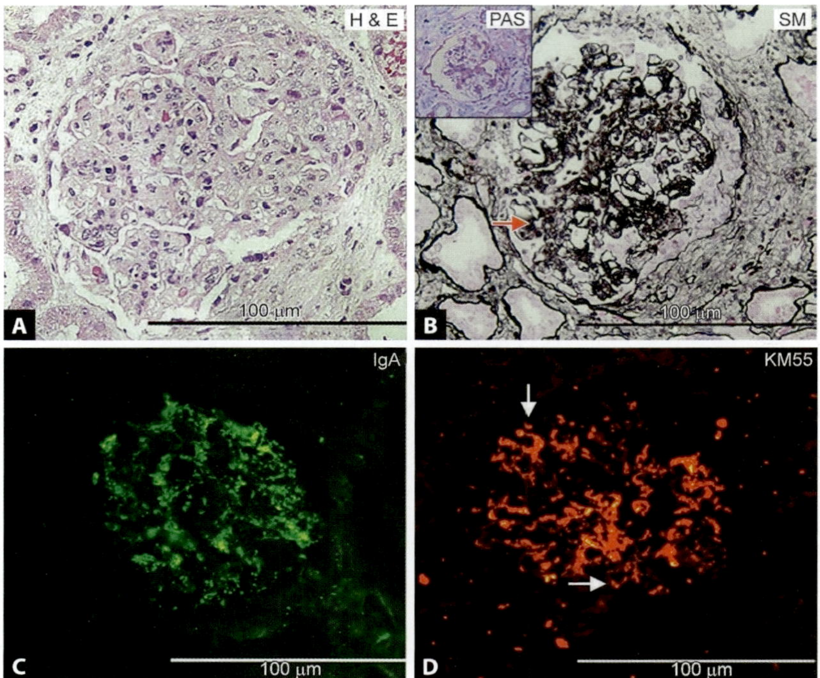

Fig. 7.4A to D: IgA nephropathy secondary to chronic liver disease. (A) Light microscopy indicates endocapillary hypercellularity including neutrophils and a cellular crescent (hematoxylin-eosin, ×40); (B) Segmental reduplication of the glomerular basement membrane (red arrow) (Jones methenamine silver, ×40), while other glomeruli show mesangial hypercellularity (inset, Periodic acid Schiff, ×20); (C) Immunofluorescence for IgA shows 2+ mesangial granular staining (IgA-FITC, ×20); (D) Staining for KM55, an antibody directed against galactose-deficient IgA, shows 3+ mesangial granular staining with capillary-wall extension (white arrows), suggesting mucosal-derived IgA (KM55-phycoerythrin, ×20)

Prognosis and Natural History

The prognosis in children is better than in adults. Approximately 10% children with IgA nephropathy progress to advanced CKD by 10 years from diagnosis, and an additional 20–30% will progress within 20 years. Monitoring of blood pressure, blood creatinine, urinalysis, and protein excretion is recommended. Factors indicating poor outcome include heavy proteinuria, impaired kidney function, and severe kidney histology. A risk prediction tool, developed by the International IgA Network that employs ethnicity, clinical and MEST-C score, has been shown to satisfactorily predict kidney-specific endpoints of 50% decline in kidney function or end-stage kidney disease (ESKD) **(*see* Annexure 7.1)**. A similar tool for children predicts the risk of 30% decline in eGFR or ESKD **(*see* Annexure 7.2, p 203)**.

TABLE 7.3: Treatment of IgA nephropathy based on clinical features and histology

Clinical presentation	*Kidney histology*	*Therapy*
Isolated microscopic/gross hematuria; normal eGFR >90 mL/min/1.73 m^2; no proteinuria (Up/Uc <0.2 mg/mg)	MEST score 0	No specific treatment; monitor urine protein 3–6 monthly
Proteinuria (Up/Uc 0.2–0.6 mg/mg); eGFR >90 mL/min/1.73 m^2	MEST score 0	ACEi or ARB for 3-months to decrease proteinuria, Up/Uc <0.2 mg/mg If reduction not achieved: Prednisolone 1 mg/kg/day for 4 weeks; AD for 6-months Follow up 3–6 monthly for proteinuria; blood pressure; eGFR
Proteinuria (Up/Uc 0.6–2 mg/mg); eGFR >90 ml/min/1.73 m^2	Mesangial proliferation (M1) lesion	Prednisolone 1 mg/kg/day for 3–6 months; 0.5 mg/kg AD for 3–6 months; reduce by 0.2 mg/kg AD every month for 3 months Concomitant therapy with ACEi or ARB
Any of the following: (*i*) nephrotic proteinuria (Up/Uc >2 mg/mg); (*ii*) nephrotic syndrome; (*iii*) eGFR <60 mL/min/1.73 m^2	Mesangial (M1) or endocapillary (E1) proliferation; tubular atrophy (T1, T2)	Prednisolone 2 mg/kg/day for 4 weeks; 1.5 mg/kg AD for 4 weeks; 1 mg/kg AD for 6 months; 0.5 mg/kg AD for 6 months Cyclophosphamide 2 mg/kg/day for 12 weeks; follow by MMF (800–1000 mg/m^2/day) or azathioprine (1–2 mg/kg/day) for ~2-yr Prefer cyclosporine or tacrolimus if nephrotic syndrome with biopsy showing FSGS Concomitant therapy with ACEi or ARB
Nephrotic syndrome	Mesangial IgA deposits; minimal change disease	Treat as minimal change disease (prednisolone); ACEi or ARB
Acute nephritic syndrome	Mesangial or endocapillary proliferation; no crescents	Prednisolone 1 mg/kg/day for 1–2 months; then AD; taper ~1-yr MMF (800–1000 mg/m^2/day) or azathioprine (1–2 mg/kg/day) for ~2-yr
Rapidly progressive glomerulonephritis*	Crescents (C1, C2)	IV methylprednisolone (10–20 mg/kg; three doses); prednisolone (1 mg/kg/day for 4 weeks, 1 mg/kg AD for 3–6 months, 0.5 mg/kg AD for 6–12 months) IV cyclophosphamide 500 mg/m^2 monthly for 6 months; follow by MMF (800–1000 mg/m^2/day; preferred) or azathioprine (1–2 mg/kg/day) for ~2-yr
Advanced disease; eGFR <30 mL/min/1.73 m^2	High chronicity index (T2, global glomerulosclerosis)	Cautious use of ACEi if eGFR < 25; limited role for immunosuppression; therapy for advanced CKD

*Plasma exchange may be considered in patients with dialysis dependence

ACEi: angiotensin converting enzyme inhibitor; AD: alternate days; ARB: angiotensin receptor blocker; eGFR: estimated glomerular filtration rate; FSGS: focal segmental glomerulosclerosis; MMF mycophenolate mofetil; Up/Uc: spot urine protein to creatinine ratio

Patients with ESKD require dialysis or transplantation. Living-related transplant is not contraindicated. Recurrent IgA deposition in allograft is reported in up to 20–30% of patients, but graft loss is rare. The risk of recurrence is higher in younger patients, and in those whose disease has progressed rapidly. Recurrent IgA nephropathy is managed as disease in native kidneys.

Alport Syndrome

Alport syndrome occurs in three genetic forms—(*i*) X-linked (80% of all patients), (*ii*) autosomal recessive (15%), and (*iii*) dominant illness (5%) **(Table 7.4)**. The X-linked form is more severe, and results from mutations in *COL4A5* localized to the X chromosome (Xq22). The type of mutation in this gene has a significant impact on the course of disease in affected males, with the age at ESKD being strongly correlated with the *COL4A5* genotype. The risk of ESKD by age 30-year is 90% for deletions and nonsense mutations, 70% for splicing mutations, and 50% for missense mutations. In most families with X-linked illness, the age at ESKD is fairly similar among affected males.

Homozygous or heterozygous mutations in *COL4A3* or *COL4A4* (located on chromosome 2q) result in the autosomal recessive and dominant forms respectively. Individuals with the autosomal recessive form of the disease carry a high risk of ESKD by 30 years of age. Individuals with heterozygous *COL4A3* or *COL4A4* mutations who exhibit isolated microscopic hematuria, previously known as thin basement membrane nephropathy or disease, are now included as autosomal dominant Alport syndrome. Patients with autosomal dominant disease show slower progression of kidney disease and lower rates of ESKD; hearing and ocular findings are also less common. Sex and genotype chiefly determine the severity of kidney, auditory, and ocular disease **(*see* Table 7.2)**.

The onset of X-linked Alport syndrome in boys is usually below 10 years of age, with persistent microscopic hematuria or recurrent episodes of gross hematuria that may follow upper respiratory tract infections. Proteinuria appears later and initially may be mild and intermittent. Steroid resistant nephrotic syndrome is also described. Males with X-linked disease show progressive kidney disease and 80% require renal replacement therapy by 40 years of age. Females with X-linked Alport syndrome have milder disease and 10–15% reaches ESKD by 45 years.

High-frequency sensorineural hearing impairment is common in male patients with X-linked Alport syndrome (50–80%). A variety of associated ocular defects including anterior lenticonus, macular and perimacular retinopathy (characterized by multiple white and yellow dots and macular flecks, which do not affect vision), recurrent corneal erosions, and cataract are observed in 30–50% cases. Other abnormalities include elliptocytosis, midface hypoplasia, mental retardation, esophageal leiomyomatosis,

TABLE 7.4: Distinguishing features between genetic forms of Alport syndrome

	X-linked		*Autosomal recessive*	*Autosomal dominant*
	Males	***Females***		
Gene	*COL4A5*	*COL4A5*	*COL4A3* or *COL4A4*	*COL4A3* or *COL4A4*
Hematuria; proteinuria	100%; 100%	100%; 75%	100%; 100%	Variable
Sensorineural deafness	50% by 15-yr 90% by 40-yr	10% by 40-yr 20% by 60-yr	>60%	Rare
Eye findings	~40%	~10%	~40%	Rare
End-stage kidney disease	50% by 25-yr 80% by 40-yr 100% by 60-yr	~30% by 60-yr	100%	Uncommon
Electron microscopy: GBM width	Early: Thin Late: Thick and thin	Early: Thin Late: Thin; or thick and thin	Early: Thin Late: Thick and thin	Early: Thin Late: Thin; or thick and thin
α5(IV) in GBM	Absent	Mosaic in 60%	Absent	Present
α5(IV) in Bowman capsule and distal TBM	Absent	Mosaic in 60%	Present	Present

GBM: glomerular basement membrane; TBM: tubular basement membrane
Hearing loss occurs earlier in X-linked disease due to deletions, nonsense, or splice site variants, compared to missense mutations
Eye findings are usually seen in adolescents or young adults; especially among males with X-linked disease, and autosomal recessive forms
Large deletions, truncating, and nonsense variants in *COL4A5* are associated with rapid decline of kidney function, compared to splice site and missense variants

hyperprolinuria, and aortic abnormalities, especially in individuals with contiguous microdeletions involving *COL4A5* and either *AMMECR1* or *COL4A6*.

Histology

In the initial stages, light microscopic changes on kidney biopsy may be insignificant or nonspecific. Subsequently, increase in mesangial matrix with segmental proliferation **(Fig. 7.5A)**, presence of lipid laden foam cells, and irregular thickening of capillary walls may be seen **(Fig. 7.5B)**. Some patients show changes of FSGS on biopsy.

Electron microscopy shows thickening of glomerular basement membrane (GBM), splitting and splintering of lamina densa (basket weave pattern), and presence of electron dense granulations within its layers (**Figs. 7.5C and D**). In early stages, marked thinning of the lamina densa may be seen. Thick, normal, and thin segments of the GBM may be present on ultrastructure in the same capillary loop. Such widespread abnormalities of the GBM are strongly indicative of Alport syndrome. These changes are seen to a lesser degree in the basement membrane of Bowman capsule and tubules.

Immunostaining for α chains of type IV collagen might distinguish the X-linked from the autosomal forms of the disease. Patients with X-linked Alport syndrome have altered expression of α3α4α5 and α5α5α6 collagen trimers in renal basement membranes. Therefore, immunostaining of the GBM, Bowman capsule and tubular basement membrane for α3(IV), α4(IV) and α5(IV) chains is negative. While patients with autosomal recessive disease have negative staining for these chains on the GBM, positive staining is found for α5(IV) in Bowman capsule, tubular basement membrane, and collecting duct basement membrane, because of unimpaired expression of α5α5α6 trimers. Heterozygous carriers of single *COL4A3* or *COL4A4* mutation show normal immunostaining for these chains on the GBM. The α5α5α6 trimer is a normal component of the epidermal basement membrane. Therefore, male patients with X-linked disease can be diagnosed by lack of immunostaining for α5(IV) on skin biopsy.

Diagnosis

The diagnosis is based on the findings of hematuria with or without proteinuria, hypertension, and renal failure in association with—(*i*) familial hematuria, (*ii*) sensorineural deafness in the patient or an affected relative, and (*iii*) progression to renal failure. Thick and split GBM and abnormal GBM distribution of α3 to α5 type IV collagen chains are specific markers of the disease. Identification of the mode of inheritance is necessary for genetic counseling.

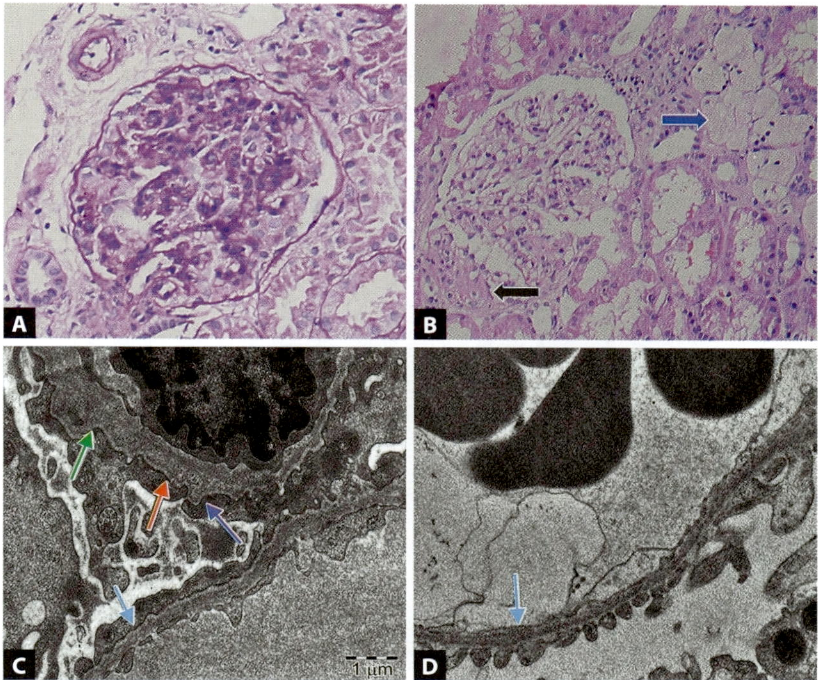

Figs. 7.5A to D: Alport syndrome. Light microscopy can show non-specific glomerular histology, including (A) Mesangial proliferation (Periodic acid Schiff; 20x); (B) Focal segmental glomerulosclerosis (black arrow) with interstitial foam cells (blue arrow) (Periodic acid-Schiff, 20x); (C and D) Transmission electron microscopy shows characteristic thick (red arrow) and thin (blue arrow) segments of glomerular basement membrane, lamellation (green arrows) and rarefaction, resulting in a "basket weaving" appearance, along with tenting (purple arrow) of the external surface (uranyl acetate-lead citrate; 2550x)

Next-generation sequencing allows for rapid simultaneous analysis of variants in *COL4A3*, *COL4A4,* and *COL4A5*. If the suspicion of the diagnosis is not high, a broad panel including other *FSGS* genes and familial nephropathies may be tested. Important differential diagnoses are listed in **Table 7.5**. If clinical suspicion is high and the next-generation sequencing is negative, multiplex ligation-dependent probe amplification may be considered to detect intragenic deletions or duplications, which account for 10–15% of cases of X-linked Alport syndrome. Asymptomatic family members may be screened by urinalysis, followed by Sanger sequencing to confirm the variant found in the index patient.

Course

The course of Alport syndrome is variable. Hearing impairment, ocular changes, persistent proteinuria, and severe histologic changes indicate

TABLE 7.5: Monogenic disorders associated with glomerular hematuria in children[1,2]

Disorder	*Gene defect*	*Inheritance pattern*	*Clinical features*	
			Renal	*Extra-renal*
Alport syndrome[3]	*COL4A3* *COL4A4* *COL4A5*	AD, AR AD, AR X linked	Microscopic hematuria; progressive CKD based on genotype	Lenticonus, central fleck retinopathy, sensorineural hearing loss
Alport syndrome with diffuse leiomyomatosis (ATS-DL)	*COL4A5-6* deletion; breakpoint in intron 2 of *COL4A6*	X linked	Same as Alport syndrome	Benign smooth muscle tumors of esophagus, tracheobronchial tree and female genital tract; congenital cataract
AMME complex, AMME syndrome, ATS-MR	Contiguous gene deletion of *COL4A5*, *FACL4* & *AMMECR1*	X linked	Same as Alport syndrome	Midface hypoplasia, intellectual disability, and elliptocytosis
HANAC syndrome	*COL4A1*	AD	Microscopic hematuria, renal cysts	Tortuous retinal arteries, intracranial aneurysms, leukoencephalopathy, and muscle cramps
CFHR5 (Cypriot) nephropathy	*CFHR5*	AD	Microscopic hematuria since first decade; ESKD in 80% men beyond 50-year-old; MPGN pattern	None described
MYH9-related disease[4]	*MYH9*	AD	Proteinuria and microscopic hematuria in one-fourth by second–third decade	Thrombocytopenia, giant platelets, Dohle body-like inclusions in leukocytes, sensorineural hearing loss, and cataract

Contd...

Contd...

Disorder	Gene defect	Inheritance pattern	Clinical features	
			Renal	Extra-renal
Glomerulopathy with fibronectin deposits (fibronectin glomerulopathy)	*FN1*	AD	Hematuria, proteinuria and hypertension; ESKD by second–fifth decade in 50%	None described

[1]Consider testing for genes associated with steroid resistant nephrotic syndrome in children presenting with hematuria and proteinuria

[2]Familial clustering and association with 6q22-q23 loci have been described in IgA nephropathy; no single gene with Mendelian inheritance has been identified

[3]Thin basement membrane nephropathy is now termed autosomal dominant Alport syndrome

[4]Previously termed Fechtner syndrome (thrombocytopenia, giant platelets, and Dohle body-like inclusions in leukocytes, Alport syndrome-like nephritis, hearing loss, and cataracts), May–Hegglin anomaly (thrombocytopenia, giant platelets, and Dohle body-like inclusions in leukocytes), Epstein syndrome (thrombocytopenia, deafness, and nephritis; no leukocyte inclusion bodies), or Sebastian syndrome (May–Hegglin anomaly, with different ultrastructural appearance of the leukocyte inclusions)

AD: autosomal dominant; AMME: Alport syndrome, midfacial hypoplasia, mental retardation and elliptocytosis; AR: autosomal recessive; ATS -MR: Alport syndrome with mental retardation; CFHR: complement factor H related; ESKD: end-stage kidney disease; HANAC: hereditary angiopathy with nephropathy, aneurysms, and muscle cramps; MYH9: heavy chain of non-muscle myosin of class II, isoform A

unsatisfactory outcome. *COL4A5* genotype has an important effect on the rate of progression in males with X-linked disease. Patients with autosomal recessive disease show natural history similar to boys with X-linked disease.

Management

Therapy with ACE inhibitors is recommended in patients with proteinuria (urine protein to creatinine ratio > 0.2 mg/mg, or protein excretion exceeding 4 mg/m^2/h), and may be considered at diagnosis in asymptomatic boys with X-linked disease. The preferred agents include ramipril (starting dose 1–2 mg/m^2/day, increase by 1–2 mg/m^2 every 2–3 months to 6 mg/m^2/day) or enalapril (0.3–0.6 mg/kg/day). ARB (losartan, valsartan, and irbesartan) may be used in patients showing poor tolerance to ACE inhibitors. Losartan is given at a dose of 12.5 mg/m^2/day and can be increased to 50 mg/m^2. Bardoxolone methyl, an Nrf2 activator that reduces oxidative stress and inflammation, was not shown to be useful in retarding disease progression in Alport syndrome. The combination of sodium glucose like transporter 2 (SGLT2) inhibitors and ACE inhibitors is being investigated in a clinical trial (DOUBLE PROTECT). Preclinical gene therapies targeting specific mutations, e.g., nonsense read-through and exon skipping with antisense oligonucleotides, appear promising.

Results following renal transplantation are good, except for two issues. First-degree relatives at risk for ESKD should not be accepted as donors. Secondly, crescentic anti-GBM GN may occur in 3–5% allografts, usually in the first post-transplant year. The circulating antibody is directed against the missing collagen constituent of the GBM, typically the α5(IV) or the α3(IV) chains.

Autosomal Dominant Alport Syndrome

Patients with this entity, formally termed benign familial hematuria or thin basement membrane disease, show isolated, usually nonprogressive microscopic hematuria, thin GBM on electron microscopy, and a heterozygous *COL4A3* or *COL4A4* variant. Recent genetic studies suggest that AD Alport syndrome may be much more common than presumed in earliest studies. Usually, there is no proteinuria, hypertension, hearing or ocular defects, nor progression to ESKD. On ultrastructure, diffuse attenuation of the GBM (<200–250 nm) is characteristic; lamellation is not seen **(Fig. 7.5D)**. Immunostaining for type IV collagen α3 and α4 chains on histology is normal. The prognosis is favorable, but patients should be monitored annually for proteinuria or hypertension.

MYH9 Nephropathy or MYH9-related Disorder (MYH9-RD)

MYH9 encodes nonmuscle myosin heavy chain IIA (NMMHC-IIA) that is expressed in podocytes. Pathogenic heterozygous variants in this gene result in features similar to Alport syndrome. The clinical features of this autosomal dominant disorder include proteinuria with or without hematuria, seen in 30% of patients. Most patients with nephropathy shown progressive kidney disease in adulthood. Many patients also show thrombocytopenia with giant platelets. Döhle-like bodies are basophilic aggregates within leukocytes that represent the mutated NMMHC-IIA. Sensorineural hearing loss may present after the first decade; early-onset cataract is seen in approximately 20% patients. The condition has been called May–Hegglin anomaly or Sebastian, Fechtner or Epstein syndrome based on the constellation of clinical features. Examination of peripheral smear and genetic testing aid in confirming the diagnosis **(Table 7.5)**.

Fibrillary Nephropathy or Fibrillary Glomerulonephritis

This is a rare proliferative glomerular disease characterized by distinctive, randomly oriented, and nonbranching fibrillary deposits with a mean diameter of 12–25 nm. The condition typically presents in third to fifth decades of life, and is often associated with hepatitis C infection, paraproteinemia, autoimmune disease, diabetes mellitus, or malignancy. Light microscopy reveals mesangial proliferation and variable endocapillary proliferation. On immunofluorescence, the fibrils stain for polyclonal IgG, C3, and κ and λ light chains as "smudged" deposits, chiefly in the mesangium. Electron microscopy reveals randomly arranged fibrils of 12–25 nm in the mesangium and GBM. The fibrils do not stain for Congo red. Immunofluorescence or immunohistochemical staining of the fibrils for DNAJ heat shock protein family member B9 (DNAJB9) confirms the diagnosis, even in the absence of electron microscopy. The prognosis for fibrillary GN is poor, therapeutic options are limited, and the disease might recur after transplantation.

PROTEINURIA

Proteinuria is associated with progressive renal disease, but may be a transient finding during stress, including exercise, fever, and dehydration. Excess urinary protein loss can result from: (*i*) increased permeability of the glomeruli to the passage of serum proteins (glomerular proteinuria); (*ii*) decreased reabsorption of proteins by the renal tubules (tubular proteinuria); (*iii*) increased secretion of tissue protein into the urine (secretory proteinuria). Proteinuria may be present in up to 10% of routine urine testing in children, although this decreases to 0.1% with repeated testing. The prevalence increases with age, peaks during adolescence, and is higher in girls.

Detection of Proteinuria

Normal protein excretion in urine is <4 mg/m^2 per hour or <150 mg/1.73 m^2 per day **(Table 7.6)**. Albumin constitutes ~15% of daily urine protein excretion in healthy children; other plasma proteins (e.g., beta-2 microglobulin) and Tamm–Horsfall protein constitute the remaining 85%.

TABLE 7.6: Definitions of proteinuria

	Dipstick	*24-hr urine protein excretion, mg/m²/h (g/m²/day)*	*First morning spot urine protein to creatinine ratio, mg/mg*	*24-hr urine albumin to creatinine ratio, mg/g (albuminuria category)*[1]
Physiologic	Nil, trace	<4 (0.1)	<2 years: <0.5 ≥2 years: <0.2	<30 (A1)
Pathologic				
Non-nephrotic proteinuria	1+, 2+	4–40 (0.1–1)	0.2–2	30–300 (A2)
Nephrotic range proteinuria	3+, 4+	>40 (>1)	>2	>300 (A3)

[1]Based on the Kidney Disease Improving Global Outcomes (KDIGO) criteria for classification of chronic kidney disease in adults

Urine Dipstick

The urine dipstick (impregnated with tetrabromophenol blue) is a screening test for the presence of proteinuria. Based on the intensity of the color change (proportionate to the amount of protein present), the dipstick can be read as negative or trace; 1+ (30 mg/dL protein), 2+ (100 mg/dL), 3+ (300 mg/dL), and 4+ (1000 mg/dL or more). The test primarily detects albuminuria and is less sensitive for other proteins.

False positive tests can occur if the dipstick is kept in the urine too long and the buffer leaches out. It may also occur in the presence of hematuria, pyuria, and bacteriuria, in presence of pyridium and chlorhexidine in urine, and after administration of radiographic contrast, penicillin, or cephalosporins. Concentrated urine (specific gravity >1.025) and alkaline urine (pH >8.0) can also show false positive results. *False negative tests* may be seen if the urine is dilute (specific gravity <1.010) or acidic (pH <4.5). This may also occur in nonalbumin proteinuria, because albumin binds better to the dye than do other proteins.

Sulfosalicylic Acid Test

An alternative method for measuring urine protein is the sulfosalicylic acid precipitation of protein in urine. This technique estimates all the proteins present, including albumin and low molecular weight proteins. The test is performed by mixing one-part urine with three parts 3% sulfosalicylic acid. The resultant turbidity is graded as no turbidity (0); slight turbidity (0.01–0.15 g/L); turbidity through which print can be read (0.15–0.3 g/L); white cloud without precipitate through which heavy black lines on a white background are seen (0.4–1 g/L); white cloud with precipitate through which heavy black lines cannot be seen (1–3 g/L); and flocculent precipitate (>5 g/L).

Quantitation of Proteinuria

Quantitative methods detect all proteins including low-molecular-weight proteins. *A 24-hr urine collection* is cumbersome in children because of difficulties of collection and the need to correct the protein excretion rate for body surface area. Urine dipstick testing correlates with 24-hr urinary protein estimation. Abnormal proteinuria is defined as protein excretion >4 mg/m^2/hr. Proteinuria >40 mg/m^2/hr is considered nephrotic range **(Table 7.6)**.

Another method is to measure the concentration of protein and creatinine in *single voided sample* and express as a ratio (Up/Uc). The first morning sample is recommended as it eliminates any effect of posture (orthostatic proteinuria). This is a reasonably reliable surrogate for a 24-hr urine collection in young children. A first morning spot urine protein to creatinine ratio of >0.2 mg/mg indicates proteinuria, which is considered nephrotic range if it exceeds 2 mg/mg **(Table 7.6)**.

Etiology

When proteinuria is detected, it is important to determine whether it is intermittent or persistent. The former is benign in the majority and can be transient and postural. **Box 7.2** lists important conditions presenting with proteinuria.

BOX 7.2: Conditions presenting with proteinuria

Glomerular proteinuria
Nephrotic syndrome: Minimal change disease, focal segmental glomerulosclerosis, congenital nephrotic syndrome, and membranous nephropathy
Hepatitis B and C nephropathy, HIV nephropathy
Reflux nephropathy
Amyloidosis
Associated hematuria: C3 glomerulopathy, postinfectious GN, IgA nephropathy, IgA vasculitis, lupus nephritis, Alport syndrome, and MYH9-related disease

Tubular proteinuria
Tubular damage: Aminoglycosides, amphotericin B, cisplatin, non-steroidal anti-inflammatory agents, radiocontrast media
Heavy metal nephropathy (e.g., gold, lead, cadmium, and copper) (*see* **Table 7.7**)
Proximal renal tubular acidosis (Fanconi syndrome), e.g., Dent disease
Interstitial nephritis: Infections and medications
Pyelonephritis

Intermittent or transient proteinuria
Postural (orthostatic)
Fever, cold exposure
Stress, exercise

Intermittent Proteinuria

In intermittent proteinuria, protein is detected in only some urine samples. Intermittent proteinuria can also occur after exercise or in association with stress, dehydration, cold exposure, or fever. *Orthostatic (postural) proteinuria* is defined as an elevated protein excretion when the child is upright but normal protein excretion during recumbency. It is related to alterations in renal or glomerular hemodynamics and is benign. The diagnosis is made by demonstrating that the protein to creatinine ratio in the first morning urine is <0.2 mg/mg, and higher in a sample taken at least 4–6 hour after the patient has been upright. No treatment is required for children with orthostatic proteinuria.

Persistent Proteinuria

Persistent proteinuria is defined as proteinuria of ≥1+, on multiple occasions over 4 weeks or more. The presence of persistent proteinuria requires evaluation. Persistent nonorthostatic proteinuria occurs in two main situations. *Glomerular proteinuria* occurs in disorders that cause increased permeability of glomerular capillaries allowing filtration of large molecular-weight proteins such as albumin. Conditions that lead to glomerular proteinuria include nephrotic syndrome, various glomerulopathies, and reflux nephropathy. *Tubular proteinuria* results from defective tubular resorption of low-molecular-weight proteins such as β2 microglobulin (as in Fanconi syndrome), tubulointerstitial nephritis, acute tubular necrosis, and some hereditary tubulopathies.

The amount of protein is larger in patients with glomerular disease compared to a tubular disease (tubular proteinuria is typically <1 g/day). Since glomerular diseases are more common than tubular disorders, the former should be excluded in patients with asymptomatic isolated proteinuria or proteinuria accompanied by hematuria. It is important to exclude acute nephritic or nephrotic syndrome as these are distinct clinical entities which require specific management.

Evaluation

A step-by-step approach is recommended to evaluate isolated proteinuria in an asymptomatic child. However, if the child has signs and symptoms that suggest renal disease, detailed investigations are initiated.

History and Examination

History is taken for clues that suggest an underlying etiology. These include history of (*i*) edema, hematuria, polyuria, or nocturia; symptoms of GN or renal failure; (*ii*) rashes and joint pain; history of connective tissue disorders;

(*iii*) recurrent urinary tract infections; and (*iv*) family history of polycystic kidney disease, renal failure, or deafness. Important physical signs include (*i*) growth failure, anemia, hypertension, and bone disease; (*ii*) features of acute nephritic or nephrotic syndrome; (*iii*) palpable purpuric rash, photosensitivity, and arthritis; and (*iv*) palpable flank masses: hydronephrosis or polycystic kidneys.

Investigations

In an asymptomatic child, the first step is to determine whether the proteinuria is persistent. Patients with persistent proteinuria (≥1+ on multiple occasions over 4 weeks or more) need further investigations. If proteinuria is absent on subsequent testing, the initial proteinuria may be *transient* and related to fever or severe exercise, and no further investigations are required. The patient should be reassured and a urine dipstick test for protein repeated at 3–6 months.

For orthostatic proteinuria, the urine is examined two times a day for 1 week, with the first sample voided in the morning as soon as the child wakes up and the last voided in mid-afternoon or evening. The diagnosis is suggested with normal protein excretion (negative urine dipstick test, or UP/C ratio ≤0.2 mg/mg) in the spot, first-morning urine sample after the patient has been supine for the entire night, and increased excretion (positive urine dipstick, or UP/C ratio >0.2), 4–6 hr after the patient is upright. No further investigations are required, and the urine should be rechecked for proteinuria in 1 year.

Approach to Proteinuria

If proteinuria on dipstick *recurs* or is *persistent*, the next step is to quantify its amount and type. Quantification of proteinuria may be done either as early morning spot urine protein to creatinine ratio or a 24-hr protein excretion. A spot urine protein to creatinine ratio that exceeds 0.2 mg/mg or 24-hr urinary protein >150 mg/1.73 m^2 confirms significant proteinuria that requires evaluation for the presence of kidney disease.

Urinalysis

Patients with the combination of hematuria with proteinuria require evaluation for an underlying glomerular disorder. Microscopic examination of a fresh specimen is necessary. Urine culture is done in patients with suspected urinary tract infection. Measurement of excretion of low-molecular proteins such as β_2-microglobulin and retinol-binding protein indicates tubular proteinuria.

Blood Examination

These include, wherever necessary, one or more of the following investigations: (*i*) renal function tests, electrolytes, total protein and albumin, and lipid profile; (*ii*) serum complement C3 and C4; (*iii*) antistreptolysin O, anti-DNAse B titers; (*iv*) serology for hepatitis B, hepatitis C, and HIV; and (*v*) ANA; antidouble stranded DNA antibodies; antineutrophil cytoplasmic antibodies (ANCA).

Renal Imaging

Ultrasonography is useful in identifying congenital or acquired anatomic abnormalities of the kidneys or urinary tract. A dimercaptosuccinic acid (DMSA) scan is a sensitive test for detecting reflux nephropathy that might be due to an underlying vesicoureteric reflux. Doppler sonography may be useful for detecting the nutcracker syndrome, a rare cause of proteinuria in children.

Indications for Renal Biopsy

A kidney biopsy is required in patients with: (*i*) persistent significant proteinuria >1 g/1.73 m^2 per day, except in steroid sensitive nephrotic syndrome; (*ii*) persistent proteinuria associated with urinary sediment abnormalities (microscopic hematuria); (*iii*) elevated serum creatinine or decreased glomerular filtration rate, except in patients with resolving GN; (*iv*) persistent low C3 levels for >3 months; (*v*) clinical or serological evidence of collagen vascular disease or vasculitis (systemic lupus, IgA vasculitis, and ANCA-associated vasculitis).

Additional Evaluation

Audiometry is recommended in patients with family history of nephritis, renal failure, or sensorineural deafness. Eye examination may show lenticonus, keratoconus, and macular degeneration in patients with Alport syndrome.

Next-generation sequencing for genetic causes of FSGS and hereditary nephropathies (e.g., Alport syndrome, MYH9 nephropathy, and Fabry disease) should be considered in patients with extrarenal syndromic features, family history of proteinuric kidney disease, isolated nephrotic range proteinuria without nephrotic syndrome and an identifiable cause, or features of Fanconi syndrome or hypercalciuria (e.g., Dent disease)**(Annexure 9.4)**. Genetic testing is also useful in patients in whom kidney histology indicates diffuse mesangial sclerosis (*WT1*, *PLCE1*, and *LAMB2*) or electron microscopy shows basket-weaving of the GBM (Alport syndrome), or intracellular zebra bodies (Fabry disease).

Management

The family is reassured if the proteinuria is transient or orthostatic, and the child is asymptomatic, has no associated hematuria, and has normal blood pressure, and eGFR. However, 6–12 months' follow-up is important as long as significant proteinuria persists. Patients with persistent proteinuria should initially receive a physical examination, including measurement of blood pressure, urinalysis, and blood tests for creatinine, urea, and albumin, every 6–12 months. There is no dietary restriction, and patients can participate in normal physical activities.

The therapy of persistent proteinuria is directed at the diagnosis and management of the underlying cause. In patients with glomerular disorders, nonspecific reduction of proteinuria may be achieved following treatment with an ACE inhibitor or ARB. Therapy with either of these agents results in reduction of glomerular proteinuria by 25–40%, in a dose- and time-dependent manner. Combined therapy of ACE inhibitors with ARB, aliskiren, or aldosterone is not recommended for additional reduction of proteinuria.

Studies in adult patients show that therapy with SGLT2 inhibitors (dapagliflozin and empagliflozin) or finerenone, a highly selective, nonsteroidal mineralocorticoid antagonist, reduces glomerular proteinuria by 30–40%. A few longer-term studies also suggest that this translates into stabilization of the slope of GFR decline in patients with proteinuric chronic kidney disease. The role of these medications in children with proteinuria is being investigated.

Patients with proteinuria and either of the following—active urinary sediment, hematuria, nephrotic range proteinuria, sustained stage II hypertension, low levels of C3, impaired kidney function, or signs and symptoms of a vasculitic disorder require prompt referral. Similarly, children with a suspected tubular or interstitial disease also require expert opinion for precise diagnosis and potential therapies.

Nail-Patella Syndrome

This condition, inherited in an autosomal dominant manner, is caused by mutations in the gene *LMX1B,* which maps to 9q34, and encodes the LIM-homeodomain protein LMX1B. Clinical features include nail abnormalities (usually symmetric; thumb nails maximally affected; nails absent, hypoplastic, or dystrophic with ridges, pits, and/or triangular lunulae), absent or hypoplastic patella **(Fig. 7.6A)**, iliac horns (rarely palpable; usually seen on X-ray film **(Fig. 7.6B)**, deformed elbow joints (decreased extension, pronation, supination, and/or pterygia), and impaired urinary concentration and acidification. Edema, proteinuria, microscopic hematuria, and hypertension are seen in 30–50% of patients. Open angle glaucoma and sensorineural hearing loss are uncommon.

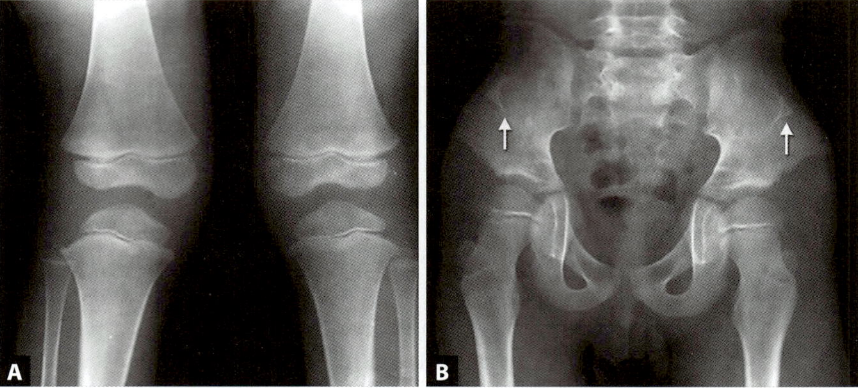

Figs. 7.6A and B: Radiographs from a child with nail-patella syndrome; (A) Absent patellae on knee X-ray; (B) X-ray pelvis shows prominent iliac horns (arrows)

Light microscopic changes are nonspecific showing FSGS and hypercellularity. Electron microscopic findings are characteristic, showing mottled and moth-eaten appearance of GBM. Intramembranous fibrils are seen, with the 65 nm periodicity of collagen. *LMX1B* sequencing is diagnostic in the majority of patients; 80–85% show mutations in exons 2–6. Once a mutation is found, other family members can have targeted testing. Chronic renal failure may occur in 5–10% cases. Pathogenic or likely pathogenic heterozygous variants in *LMX1B* are also described in patients with autosomal dominant FSGS without extrarenal features. Therapy with ACE inhibitor and/or ARB is beneficial in reducing the severity of proteinuria.

Fabry Disease

This is a rare, X-linked recessive disorder of sphingolipid metabolism, due to mutations in *GLA*, located on Xq 22.1. Deficiency of the lysosomal enzyme, α-galactosidase A, leads to accumulation of globotriaosylceramide (Gb3). There are characteristic skin lesions (angiokeratomas), autonomic neuropathy, premature coronary and cerebral vascular disease (arrhythmias, chest pain, heart failure, and stroke), corneal opacities (cornea verticillata, seen on slit-lamp examination), anemia, hepatosplenomegaly, and lymphadenopathy. Children often show acroparesthesias and abdominal cramps. Sensorineural and conductive hearing loss may be present in childhood.

Kidney disease manifests as proteinuria in male hemizygotes and rarely in female heterozygotes. ESKD occurs in the fourth or fifth decade. Histology shows enlarged epithelial cells with abundant cytoplasm and numerous vacuoles giving a foamy appearance. Electron microscopic findings are distinctive **(Figs. 7.7A and B)**. The diagnosis is confirmed by demonstrating

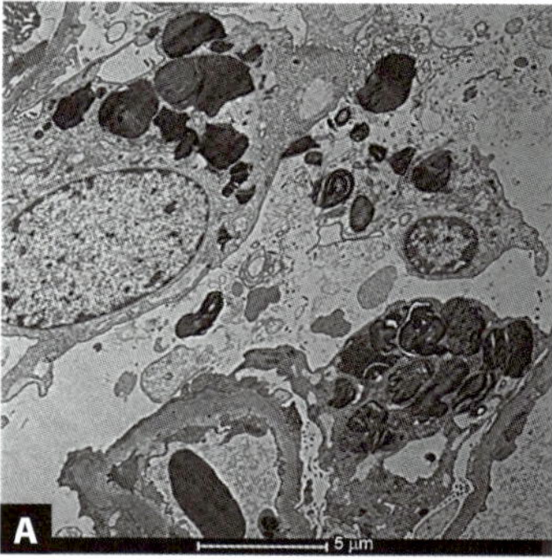

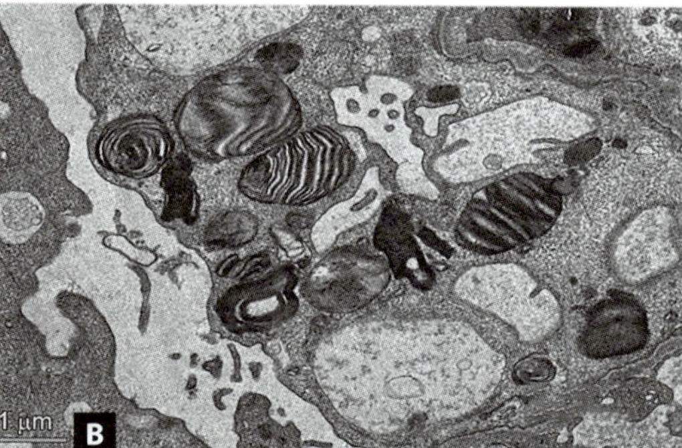

Figs. 7.7A and B: Electron microscopy in Fabry disease reveals (A) Diffuse globotriaosylceramide deposits or inclusions in all kidney cells and (B) Characteristic globotriaosylceramide concentric lamellar bodies (myelin figures or "zebra" bodies) within podocytes

decreased enzyme activity in plasma leukocytes or cultured skin fibroblasts. Sequencing of *GLA* may be necessary to detect female heterozygotes.

Recombinant enzyme replacement with fortnightly infusions of agalsidase alpha or agalsidase beta is safe and well tolerated, and results in reduced neuropathic pain, gastrointestinal symptoms, improved exercise tolerance, as well as delayed progression of heart and kidney dysfunction. Therapy may be initiated for neuropathic pain, gastrointestinal disturbances, decline in kidney function, proteinuria, and cardiac manifestations. Some missense variants do not affect the catalytic site of the enzyme but impair their folding and function within liposomes. Migalastat, an amino sugar, is a chemical chaperone that corrects the conformation of the enzyme and increases its catalytic activity. This medication is approved for use in adults with *GLA* variants that affect enzyme folding.

Amyloidosis

Amyloidosis is a group of systemic and local diseases characterized by extracellular deposition of insoluble fibrillar protein aggregates in various organs. Amyloid fibrils originate from ~20 different proteins. Amorphous eosinophilic deposits on hematoxylin and eosin staining bind to Congo red and have a characteristic apple green birefringence under polarized light **(Figs. 7.8A to D)**. Electron microscopy reveals randomly oriented, 8–12 nm nonbranching fibrils; X-ray diffraction indicates a beta-pleated sheet structure.

Kidney involvement (renal amyloidosis) is observed in three forms: (*i*) immunoglobulin light-chain (AL) or primary amyloidosis; (*ii*) amyloid A (AA) or secondary amyloidosis; and (*iii*) hereditary amyloidosis, the most common among which is leukocyte cell-derived chemotaxin-2 (LECT2) amyloidosis. In AL amyloidosis, fibrils are composed of N-terminal amino acid

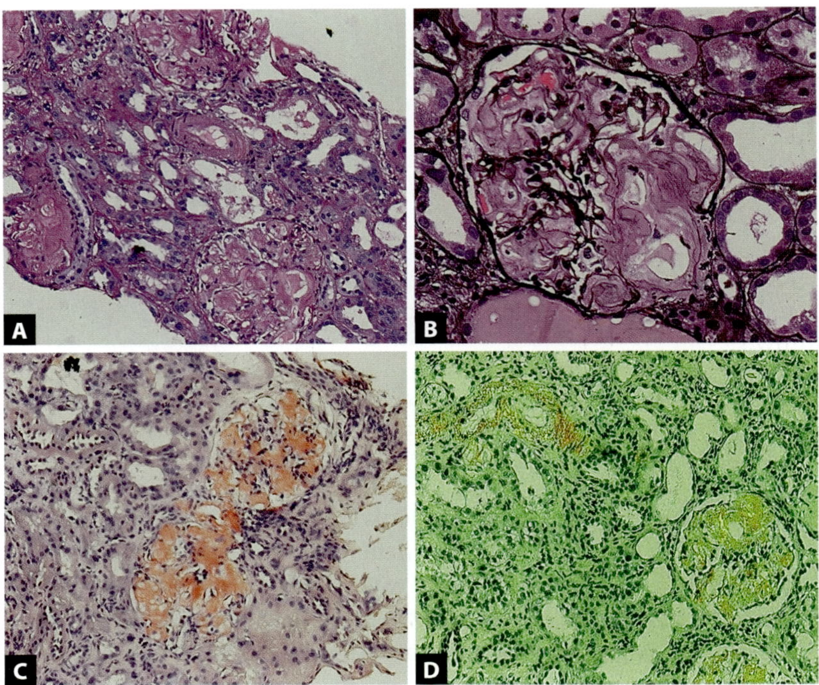

Figs. 7.8A to D: Renal amyloidosis secondary to systemic-onset juvenile idiopathic arthritis in a 12-year-old boy. (A) Periodic acid Schiff images on light microscopy showing fluffy deposits within glomeruli; (B) Jones silver methenamine stain showing mesangial expansion with deposits; (C) Glomerular deposits stain with Congo red; (D) These deposits show apple red birefringence under polarized light in slides stained with Congo red

residues of the variable region of an immunoglobulin light chain produced by clonal expansion of plasma cells or plasmacytic B cells. The light chain is more often λ than κ; the most common λ subtype is VI. AA amyloidosis results from the deposition of the N-terminal end of the acute phase reactant serum amyloid A (SAA) protein in certain chronic inflammatory states. SAA is produced in the liver and circulates with high-density lipoprotein. Rare hereditary forms of amyloidosis result from tissue deposition of aberrant proteins due to mutations in genes encoding transthyretin (ATTR), fibrinogen A α-chain (AFib), apolipoprotein A-I (apo A-I) or A-II (apo A-II), lysozyme (ALys), gelsolin (AGel), and LECT2 peptide.

Patients with AL amyloidosis are typically older than 50 years (men: women 2:1). Up to 20% cases have multiple myeloma. Patients present with weight loss, fatigue, light-headedness, dyspnea, pedal edema, peripheral neuropathy (often carpal tunnel syndrome), and orthostatic hypotension. Examination may reveal cardiomyopathy, hepatosplenomegaly, and macroglossia. Multiple organs are affected, including kidneys (50%), heart

(40%), and peripheral nerves (~25%). AA amyloidosis occurs in chronic inflammatory diseases, such as rheumatoid arthritis, other inflammatory arthritides, inflammatory bowel disease, or familial Mediterranean fever (FMF); in patients with chronic urinary infections, decubitus ulcers, untreated osteomyelitis, or bronchiectasis; and in chronic heroin addicts with history of subcutaneous drug injections. Patients with hereditary amyloidosis present like AL amyloidosis; however, most present in adulthood, with higher serum creatinine and lower proteinuria than either AL or AA amyloidosis. LECT2 defects, a recently described inherited form of amyloid, is more common than AL amyloidosis in certain populations, e.g., Punjabis, Latinos from the southwest United States, Native Americans, and Egyptians. The condition chiefly affects kidneys and liver and often progresses to ESKD. Hereditary amyloidosis due to LECT2 fibrils affects all kidney compartments, AFib causes massive glomerular obliteration, and apolipoproteins A-I, A-II, A-IV, affect tubulointerstitial and medullary compartments.

Amyloidosis is diagnosed on tissue biopsy, typically liver and kidney; other sites, according to symptoms, include fat pad or bone marrow aspirate, and rectal, gingival, or skin biopsy. Whole-body scintigraphy following injection of radiolabeled serum amyloid P component enables noninvasive diagnosis, especially in AA amyloidosis, as well as semiquantification of disease load and monitoring of therapeutic response. AL amyloidosis is suggested by the presence of serum or urine monoclonal M protein on electrophoresis, serum or urine paraproteins ("spike" on immunofixation), and serum-free light chains with an abnormal κ- to λ-light chain ratio, suggesting plasma cell dyscrasia. Light chain assay is the most sensitive and helps monitor response to therapy. Mass spectrometry and laser dissection of glomeruli are recently used modalities that accurately diagnose all types of glomerular amyloid.

Regardless of etiology, patients with nephrotic syndrome require judicious use of diuretics and salt restriction; orthostatic hypotension is managed with compression stockings, fludrocortisone, and midodrine. Specific management differs by etiology. Young healthy patients with AL amyloid are offered autologous stem cell transplant (ASCT), whereas older patients with comorbidities receive chemotherapy. If required, kidney transplantation in AL amyloid may be performed before or after ASCT. The treatment of AA amyloid focuses on controlling the underlying inflammation, e.g., anti-inflammatory or immunosuppressive agents, including biologics, in rheumatoid arthritis and inflammatory bowel disease; chronic colchicine therapy in FMF; surgical débridement of infected tissue; and antibiotics for chronic infection. Patients with AA amyloid who require kidney transplant, typically those with FMF, show satisfactory outcomes. Certain forms of hereditary amyloidosis are amenable to liver transplantation. Isolated kidney transplantation in hereditary amyloidosis, e.g., for fibrinogen A α-chain disease, is associated with high rates of recurrence, hence, combined liver and kidney transplantation is preferred.

DRUG-INDUCED PROTEINURIA

Occasionally, therapy with certain drugs is associated with glomerular injury that leads to proteinuria or hematuria. Mechanistically, these may be caused by direct cellular toxicity to podocytes, endothelium or mesangial cells, or immune-mediated injury. Cessation of therapy with the offending agent is usually associated with reversal of the lesions and clinical and biochemical improvement. **Table 7.7** lists drugs that cause glomerular injury by these mechanisms. Drug-induced podocytopathies present with either nephrotic

TABLE 7.7: Medication induced proteinuria or hematuria

Histology	*Examples*
Podocytopathy (minimal change disease; focal segmental glomerulosclerosis, collapsing glomerulopathy)	Nonsteroidal anti-inflammatory drugs (NSAIDs): indomethacin and celecoxib Lithium Bisphosphonates: Pamidronate and zoledronate mTOR inhibitors: Everolimus and sirolimus Interferon Androgenic anabolic steroids VEGF targeting therapies: Bevacizumab; ramucirumab; aflibercept
IgA nephropathy	Vancomycin, ceftriaxone, metronidazole Carbamazepine Cyclosporine Acetaminophen Amiodarone Furosemide ICI: Ipilimumab, pembrolizumab, nivolumab
Lupus-like lesions	TNF-α inhibitors Procainamide Hydralazine Quinidine Low risk: Carbamazepine, methyldopa, captopril, acebutolol, chlorpromazine, isoniazid, minocycline, and ICI
Membranous nephropathy	Gold therapy, penicillamine, bucillamine Lithium Captopril NSAIDs and celecoxib Gefitinib, nivolumab, and adalimumab Mercaptopropionyl, chlorpropamide, and aprotinin
Miscellaneous lesions	Allopurinol, atorvastatin, cocaine/levamisole, denosumab, hydralazine, isotretinoin, phenytoin, febuxostat, foscarnet, methamphetamine, sofosbuvir in kidney transplant recipient, and protease inhibitors

ICI: immune-checkpoint inhibitors; TNF: tumor necrosis factor; VEGF: vascular endothelial growth factor

syndrome or nephrotic range proteinuria, with or without acute kidney injury. Kidney biopsy might show minimal change disease (MCD), FSGS, or collapsing glomerulopathy. Mesangial injury leading to IgA nephropathy has been described following use of some medications. Drug-induced autoimmunity has been reported most commonly in the form of membranous nephropathy, encountered with penicillamine, gold salts, captopril, lithium, and nonsteroidal anti-inflammatory drugs (NSAIDs) (celecoxib), and recently with adalimumab, chemotherapeutic agents like epidermal growth factor receptor tyrosine kinase inhibitors and immune-checkpoint inhibitors (nivolumab), and organic mercurials (in skin-lightening creams).

Annexure 7.1: Online calculator for risk of 50% decline in kidney function or end-stage kidney disease (ESKD) in adult patients with IgA nephropathy https://qxmd.com/calculate/calculator_499/international-iganpredictiontool-adults#	
Annexure 7.2: Online calculator for risk of 30% decline in kidney function or end-stage kidney disease (ESKD) in pediatric patients with IgA nephropathy https://qxmd.com/calculate/calculator_713/international-igan-prediction-tool-at-biopsy-pediatrics	

BIBLIOGRAPHY

Hematuria

1. Bergstein J, Leiser J, Andreoli S. The clinical significance of asymptomatic gross and microscopic hematuria in children. Arch Pediatr Adol Med. 2005;159:353-5.
2. Kashtan CE, Ding J, Gregory M, et al. Clinical practice recommendations for the treatment of Alport syndrome. Pediatr Nephrol. 2013;28:5-11.
3. Pade KH, Liu DR. An evidence-based approach to the management of hematuria in children in the emergency department. Pediatr Emerge Med Pract. 2014;11:1-13.
4. Phadke KD, Vijayakumar M, Sharma J, Iyengar A; Indian Pediatric Nephrology Group. Consensus statement on evaluation of hematuria. Indian Pediatr. 2006;43:965-73.
5. Rosenstock JL, Markowitz GS. Fibrillary glomerulonephritis: An update. Kidney Int Rep. 2019;4:917-22.
6. Savige J, Gregory M, Gross O, Kashtan C, Ding J, Flinter F. Expert guidelines for the management of Alport syndrome and thin basement membrane disease. J Am Soc Nephrol 2013;24:364-75.
7. Taylor J, Flinter F. Familial hematuria: When to consider genetic testing. Arch Dis Child. 2014;99:857-61.

IgA Nephropathy

1. Barbour SJ, Coppo R, Er L, et al; International IgA Nephropathy Network. Updating the International IgA nephropathy prediction tool for use in children. Kidney Int. 2021;99:1439-50.
2. Cambier A, Gleeson PJ, Flament H, Le Stang MB, Monteiro RC. New therapeutic perspectives for IgA nephropathy in children. Pediatr Nephrol. 2021;36:497-506.
3. Caster DJ, Lafayette RA. The treatment of primary IgA nephropathy: Change, change, change. Am J Kidney Dis. 2024;83:229-40.
4. Coppo R, D'Arrigo G, Tripepi G, et al. ERA-EDTA Immunonephrology Working Group. Is there long-term value of pathology scoring in immunoglobulin A nephropathy? A validation study of the Oxford Classification for IgA Nephropathy (VALIGA) update. Nephrol Dial Transplant. 2020;35:1002-09.
5. Coppo R. Treatment of IgA nephropathy in children: A land without guidance. Pediatr Nephrol. 2021;36:491-6.
6. Dixon A, Blanchette E, Kendrick J. A lack of KDIGO guidelines for adolescents and young adults with IgA nephropathy. Pediatr Nephrol. 2024;39:297-304.

Proteinuria

1. Bokenkamp A. Proteinuria–Take a closer look. Pediatr Nephrol. 2020;35:533-41.
2. Feitosa VA, Neves PDMM, Jorge LB, Noronha IL, Onuchic LF. Renal amyloidosis: A new time for a complete diagnosis. Braz J Med Biol Res. 2022;55:e12284.
3. Hogan JJ, Markowitz GS, Radhakrishnan J. Drug-induced glomerular disease: Immune-mediated injury. Clin J Am Soc Nephrol. 2015;10:1300-10.
4. Larkins NG, Teixeira-Pinto A, Craig JC. A narrative review of proteinuria and albuminuria as clinical biomarkers in children. J Pediatr Child Health. 2019;55:136-42.
5. Lenders M, Nordbeck P, Kurschat C, et al. Treatment of Fabry disease with migalastat-outcome from a prospective 24 months observational multicenter study (FAMOUS). Eur Heart J Cardiovasc Pharmacother. 2022;8:272-81.
6. Markowitz GS, Bomback AS, Perazella MA. Drug-induced glomerular disease: direct cellular injury. Clin J Am Soc Nephrol. 2015;10:1291-9.
7. Nader R, Angel-Korman A, Havasi A. Amyloidosis and the kidney: An update. Semin Nephrol 2022;42:151343.
8. Spada M, Baron R, Elliott PM. The effect of enzyme replacement therapy on clinical outcomes in pediatric patients with Fabry disease-A systematic literature review by a European panel of experts. Mol Genet Metab. 2019;126:212-23.
9. Viteri B, Reid-Adam J. Hematuria and proteinuria in children. Pediatr Rev. 2018;39:573-87.

Acute Glomerulonephritis and Rapidly Progressive Glomerulonephritis

Jitendra Meena, Geetika Singh, Arvind Bagga

Acute glomerulonephritis (AGN; acute nephritic syndrome) is a group of disorders of variable severity and combination of hematuria, edema, hypertension, oliguria and diminished glomerular filtration rate (GFR), and fluid and salt retention. AGN can be caused by infections, systemic vasculitis, and primary glomerulopathies such as immunoglobulin A (IgA) nephropathy **(Box 8.1)**. Infections are considered one of the most common triggers for AGN. While various microorganisms can cause AGN, the term infection-related glomerulonephritis (IRGN) is typically reserved for bacterial infection triggering the GN. Among the IRGN, AGN occurring after a latency period of β-hemolytic streptococcal infection [poststreptococcal glomerulonephritis (PSGN)] is the prototype and most common cause of AGN in childhood, accounting for approximately 80% of cases. In the other instances of IRGN, a bacterial infection such as *Staphylococcus* is usually ongoing during episodes of AGN.

The past decades have witnessed a shift in epidemiology and outcome of AGN. The burden of PSGN is declining globally, but remains an important

BOX 8.1: Etiology of acute glomerulonephritis

Infection-related glomerulonephritis

Postinfectious: Streptococci, staphylococci, pneumococci, meningococci, *T. pallidum*, *S. typhi*, and *Leptospira*

Glomerulonephritis with active infection: Infection of shunts, prostheses, and bacterial endocarditis (*S. aureus*, *S. viridans*, *S. mutans*, and HACEK group of fastidious gram negative bacilli)

P. malariae, *P. falciparum*, toxoplasma, and filaria

Hepatitis B and C, cytomegalovirus, parvovirus, echovirus, Ebstein-Barr virus, coxsackie virus, and varicella

Systemic vasculitis

IgA vasculitis

Microscopic polyangiitis, granulomatous polyangiitis, and eosinophilic granulomatosis with polyangiitis

Other disorders

C3 glomerulopathy

IgA nephropathy

Hereditary nephropathy

Systemic lupus erythematosus

problem in Asia, especially among children. In developed countries, a significant proportion of cases afflicts the elderly or the immunocompromised. In adults, staphylococcal infections are now as common as streptococcal infections. The sites of infection include skin, upper respiratory tract, lung, heart, oral mucosa, teeth, and deep-seated abscess in the abdomen. The underlying etiology and severity of the disease determine the outcome of the condition. In contrast to childhood and epidemic PSGN, which resolve, other causes of IRGN have a less satisfactory prognosis, with a proportion developing chronic kidney disease.

POSTSTREPTOCOCCAL ACUTE GLOMERULONEPHRITIS

PSGN is an important cause of AGN in developing countries. PSGN occurs 1–6 weeks following pharyngitis, impetigo, or rarely a middle ear infection, and is caused by group A β-hemolytic streptococci. Commonly implicated nephritogenic strains are M-protein strains 1, 4, 12, and 25 (pharyngitis) and 2, 42, 49, 57, and 60 (skin infection). Less than 2% of children infected with nephritogenic strains of streptococci develop clinical features of AGN. While the precise nephritogenic antigen is not known, potential antigens include M protein, endostreptosin, preabsorbing antigen, nephritis strain associated protein, streptococcal pyrogenic exotoxin B, or nephritis-associated plasmin receptor (NaPlr). Host factors, which might be determined genetically, are important in forming antibodies to streptococcal antigens. The risk of developing AGN in epidemics varies from 5% following pharyngitis to ~25% following skin infections caused by β-hemolytic streptococcus type 49. Subclinical episodes occur 4–10 times more frequently than overt clinical disease. Asymptomatic contacts of patients with PSGN may have abnormal urinary findings, commonly microscopic hematuria.

Glomerular injury in PSGN results from the deposition of immune complexes in the glomerular capillaries, which may occur from the deposition of circulating immune complexes containing nephritogenic antigen, or in situ formation of immune complexes from nephritogenic antigen implanted within subepithelial glomerular sites **(Flowchart 8.1)**. These immune complexes result in activation of complement, infiltration of neutrophils, proliferation of glomerular cells, and expansion of mesangial matrix. Molecular mimicry between streptococcal antigens and normal glomerular antigens that react with antibodies against streptococcal antigens, and direct activation of the complement cascade by implanted streptococcal antigens are other pathogenic mechanisms.

Pathology

Glomerular abnormalities are characterized by proliferative and exudative changes. Glomeruli are diffusely enlarged, and the lobular pattern is

Flowchart 8.1: Pathogenesis of postinfectious glomerulonephritis. Poststreptococcal glomerulonephritis is the prototype
*Typical examples of nephritogenic antigen are nephritis-associated plasmin receptor (NAPlr) and streptococcal cationic proteinase exotoxin B (SPeB)
GBM: glomerular basement membrane

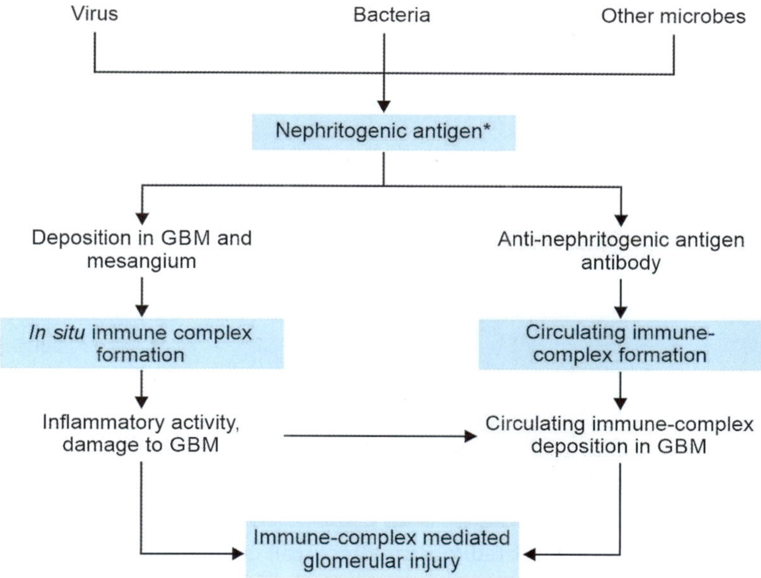

accentuated. Hypercellularity due to the proliferation of both endothelial and mesangial cells and early neutrophilic infiltration is striking, with obliteration of the capillary lumen resulting in glomeruli that appear bloodless **(Figs. 8.1A and B)**. Capillary basement membrane and the arterioles do not show significant abnormality. Epithelial cell proliferation and crescents are uncommon. In a small proportion of cases, extensive crescentic changes are present that are associated with a rapidly progressive course and unsatisfactory outcome.

Immunofluorescence examination shows granular deposits of IgG and C3 along the capillary walls and in the mesangium. C1q and C4 deposits may also be seen. Deposits of C3 and IgG, along the capillary walls (starry sky appearance) are noted in the early phase of the disease **(Fig. 8.1C)**. Mesangial deposits are noted typically if the biopsy is performed during 4–6 weeks of illness. A "garland pattern" with dense, confluent deposits along the capillary loops sparing the subendothelial and mesangial locations **(Fig. 8.3C)**, correlates with heavy proteinuria. Electron microscopy shows electron-dense subepithelial deposits or "humps" **(Fig. 8.1D)**, which tend to disappear after 6 weeks. These subepithelial humps are most characteristic of PSGN; although they can be observed in other forms of AGN. The histological

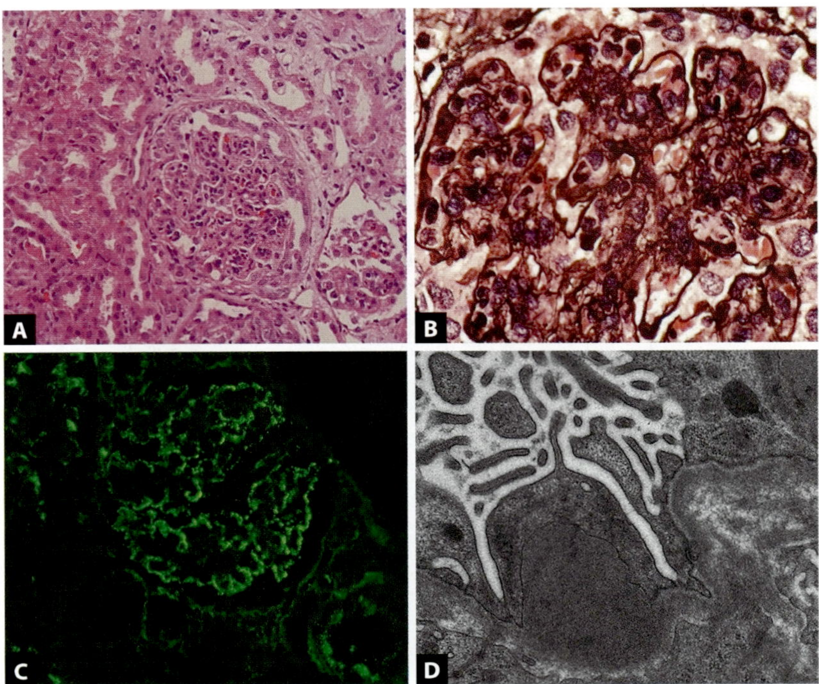

Figs. 8.1A to D: Infection-related (poststreptococcal) glomerulonephritis. (A) Hematoxylin and eosin-stained image shows enlarged, relatively bloodless glomerulus with increased cellularity, neutrophilic infiltration, and few open capillary lumina; (B) Jones methenamine silver confirms moderately severe proliferation and neutrophilic infiltration; (C) Immunofluorescence shows coarse, "lumpy bumpy" granular deposits of IgG with 3+ intensity; similar deposits were noted for C3, IgM, kappa, and lambda; (D) Electron microscopy shows classical subepithelial "hump"

abnormalities resolve rapidly, and within 6–8 weeks there is considerable decrease in exudative changes. Mild mesangial hypercellularity may persist for 1–2 years.

Clinical Features

In most cases, there is a history of preceding upper respiratory tract or skin infection. The latent period is 1–2 weeks in the former and 2–4 weeks in the latter. Pharyngitis may be occasionally mild and clinically not noticed. Active or healed lesions of impetigo may be present when AGN develops. During an epidemic of streptococcal throat infection, many subclinical cases occur that have only microscopic hematuria, and hypocomplementemia, normal, or high blood pressure.

PSGN affects children between the ages of 5–14 years and is rare below the age of 3 years. A male preponderance (male to female ratio of 2) is reported. The severity of PSGN is variable; mild cases may have microscopic hematuria

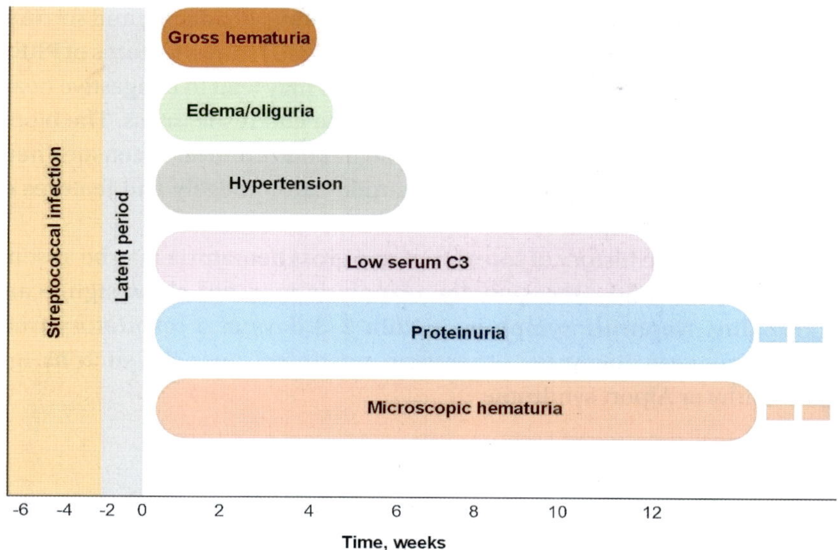

Fig. 8.2: Chronology of clinical events and biochemical abnormalities during and following poststreptococcal infection-related glomerulonephritis

with slight proteinuria; those with the severe illness have oliguria and hypertension. Hematuria (80–95%) is the chief manifestation, followed by edema and hypertension. Urine is red to brown, smoky, or cola-colored. Gross hematuria may only last a few hours and resolve by 2 weeks **(Fig. 8.2)**. Rarely, the symptoms may relapse following exercise or viral illness. Some degree of oliguria is usually associated, but persistent anuria is infrequent and suggests rapidly progressive GN. Edema is noted in 70–90% of children with PSGN. If fluid intake is unrestricted, edema extends to the hands and legs. Edema is turgid and not flaccid, as in nephrotic syndrome. Hypertension, noted in 60–80% of patients hospitalized with PSGN, is an important finding. Severe hypertension with retinal changes should lead to suspicion of underlying renal disease.

Atypical Presentations

In a small proportion of patients, PSGN may have an atypical presentation. A mixed picture of AGN and nephrotic syndrome may be present. The child has gross hematuria, hypertension, generalized edema, and heavy proteinuria. In such cases, the glomerular lesions are invariably severe, and extensive crescent formation may be present. In some patients, oliguria and azotemia are the chief features, and gross hematuria and edema are absent.

Children may present with altered sensorium caused by posterior reversible leukoencephalopathy syndrome (PRES). Drowsiness is observed in 0.5–10% of hospitalized patients; nausea, vomiting, headache, and seizures might be present. Magnetic resonance imaging (MRI) shows features of PRES. Occasionally, expansion of extracellular volume may lead to congestive heart failure and pulmonary edema. There is dyspnea and restlessness. The blood pressure is high, but in later stages, when heart failure and shock ensue, there may be hypotension. Chest X-ray shows mild cardiomegaly and features of pulmonary edema.

Sometimes, the history of sore throat and gross hematuria may be absent, and the edema mild. Occasionally, urinalysis may not show significant abnormality. Nephritic symptoms within 2–3 days of a respiratory tract infection suggest diagnoses other than postinfectious GN, such as IgA nephropathy or Alport syndrome.

Laboratory Investigations

Gross hematuria is present in a majority of moderate to severe cases. Proteinuria is seen in 60–95% cases but is usually mild; it may be in the nephrotic range in 10–25% patients. Microscopic examination shows dysmorphic red cells, red cell casts, and neutrophils. The urine may contain a large number of neutrophils, which is mistakenly regarded as urinary tract infection. Casts are examined on a fresh, uncentrifuged specimen since they disintegrate on standing and centrifugation. Hyaline and granular casts may also be seen.

Levels of blood urea and creatinine are elevated. Patients with severe acute kidney injury (AKI) may have hyponatremia, hyperkalemia, and acidosis. Increased distal tubular reabsorption of sodium and water leads to hypervolemia and expansion of extracellular volume. Plasma levels of renin and aldosterone are decreased. Chest X-ray may show cardiomegaly and pulmonary congestion. Mild dilutional anemia is noted; thrombocytopenia may suggest other etiology of AGN, such as systemic lupus erythematosus (SLE) or hemolytic uremic syndrome (HUS).

Documenting evidence of preceding streptococcal infection is crucial for confirming the diagnosis of PSGN. High antistreptolysin O (ASO) titer is observed in 60–80% of cases. In pyoderma, ASO titer is less commonly elevated, but anti-DNAse B is often raised. Combining these tests provides better sensitivity (96%) and specificity (89%), than either test alone. The rise in ASO titer begins 1–3 weeks after the streptococcal infection, peaks at 3–5 weeks, and falls to insignificant levels in 6–8 months. The titers are not related to the disease severity or prognosis. Titers of both ASO and anti-DNAse B are influenced by age, seasonal, and geographical variations; hence there is no universally accepted upper normal value. Early antibiotic treatment may also attenuate antibody response. Hence, demonstrating rising titers (fourfold) in a paired serum sample is preferable. Streptozyme test detects several streptococcal antibodies but has low diagnostic accuracy and is not used routinely. Titers of antizymogen antibodies are highly sensitive and specific for streptococcal infection but are not available routinely. Streptococci can rarely be cultured from the throat or skin infection.

Approximately 70–95% of patients have low serum C3 levels that return to normal in 8–10 weeks. Serum C5 levels are mildly reduced; C4 levels are normal. Persistent hypocomplementemia (>12-weeks) is rare in PSGN and suggests an alternative condition such as C3 glomerulopathy, lupus nephritis or GN related to endocarditis or occult abscesses. Levels of C3 do not correlate with severity of the disease. Patients with anti-C1q antibodies have severe clinical presentation with hypertension, proteinuria, and unfavorable outcomes.

Kidney biopsy is not required in typical cases of PSGN, except in patients with initial presentation of rapidly progressive GN and if serum C3 levels remains depressed. **Box 8.2** summarizes the indications for biopsy, which is chiefly done to assess prognosis, or for the diagnosis of other conditions such as systemic vasculitis, lupus erythematosus, C3 glomerulopathy, or HUS.

Management

The treatment is chiefly supportive; mild cases are managed at home, those with moderate or severe edema, hypertension, and oliguria require hospital care. Daily weight, urine output, and blood levels of urea, creatinine, and electrolytes are monitored. With careful management, the child should lose weight depending on the degree of edema. Circulatory congestion and edema can be treated with salt and water restriction and judicious use of diuretics. Moderate-to-severe hypertension responds to treatment with furosemide (1–4 mg/kg/day) and calcium channel blockers (nifedipine and amlodipine). Rarely do cases with PSGN require therapy with IV labetalol, sodium

BOX 8.2: Indications for biopsy in acute glomerulonephritis

At presentation
Rapidly progressive glomerulonephritis
Systemic features: Fever, rash, joint pain, and heart disease
Nephrotic state (heavy proteinuria and hypoalbuminemia)
Normal complement C3 level

During follow-up
Oliguria, severe acute kidney injury (AKI) persisting beyond 7–10 days
Gross hematuria persisting beyond 2–3 weeks
Nephrotic range proteinuria beyond 2–3 weeks
Hypocomplementemia (low C3) persisting beyond 12 weeks
Persistent proteinuria (Up/Uc >0.5 mg/mg) beyond 6 months
Persistent microscopic hematuria beyond 12–18 months

Severe AKI is defined as stage 2–3

nitroprusside, and nicardipine for hypertensive emergencies. Angiotensin-converting enzyme inhibitors such as enalapril are useful in lowering blood pressure, but should be avoided in the acute phase as they may be associated with AKI and hyperkalemia.

Patients with severe AKI require management of fluid and electrolyte abnormalities, with dialysis support as when indicated. Indications for starting dialysis are similar to that of any patients with AKI, such as refractory hyperkalemia, metabolic acidosis, fluid overload (>10–15%), and symptomatic uremia. Appropriate supportive measures are instituted in patients with acute pulmonary edema and shock. Furosemide is given at a dose of 1–3 mg/kg; multiple doses are not necessary and might be associated with ototoxicity.

Most patients with PSGN have self-limiting disease and do not require immunosuppressive therapy. Patients with rapidly progressive GN with crescentic GN on biopsy are managed with immunosuppressive therapy, i.e., combination of IV methylprednisolone (10–15 mg/kg/dose, for three to six doses) and IV cyclophosphamide (500–750 mg/m^2/dose every 4 weeks, for six doses). Immunosuppressive therapy is also considered in cases with severe AKI and diffuse proliferative GN on kidney biopsy **(Flowchart 8.2)**.

Penicillin or erythromycin is given for 7 days in cases with active pyoderma or throat infection. Antibiotic therapy does not influence the course of the disease but prevents the spread of streptococcal infection from patients with positive cultures. During epidemics, antimicrobial prophylaxis may be considered for close contact of patients with streptococcal infection to prevent the development of PSGN.

Course and Prognosis

The symptoms resolve in the first week with the loss of edema and a decline in levels of blood pressure. Gross hematuria rapidly clears, but microscopic hematuria may be detected for 6–12 months or longer. Occasionally, mild-to-moderate hypertension may persist for a few weeks. The long-term prognosis of PSGN in children is excellent; even patients with severe disease show recovery. The development of chronic kidney disease following PSGN is rare but has been reported in recent studies. Risk factors for unfavorable outcome include severe kidney dysfunction at presentation, crescents on kidney biopsy, and persistent proteinuria. Since kidney function impairment may ensue many years after disease onset, children with crescentic GN need follow-up with monitoring of blood pressure, proteinuria, and serum creatinine.

Immunity to streptococcal M-protein is type-specific and long-lasting, and nephritogenic serotypes are limited in number. Recurrent episodes of PSGN are rare, and penicillin prophylaxis is not recommended.

Flowchart 8.2: Management of poststreptococcal glomerulonephritis (GN). The choice and duration of immunosuppressive therapy is empirical and based on severity of presentation and/or kidney histological findings. RPGN: rapidly progressive glomerulonephritis
*See Box 8.2 for indications of kidney biopsy

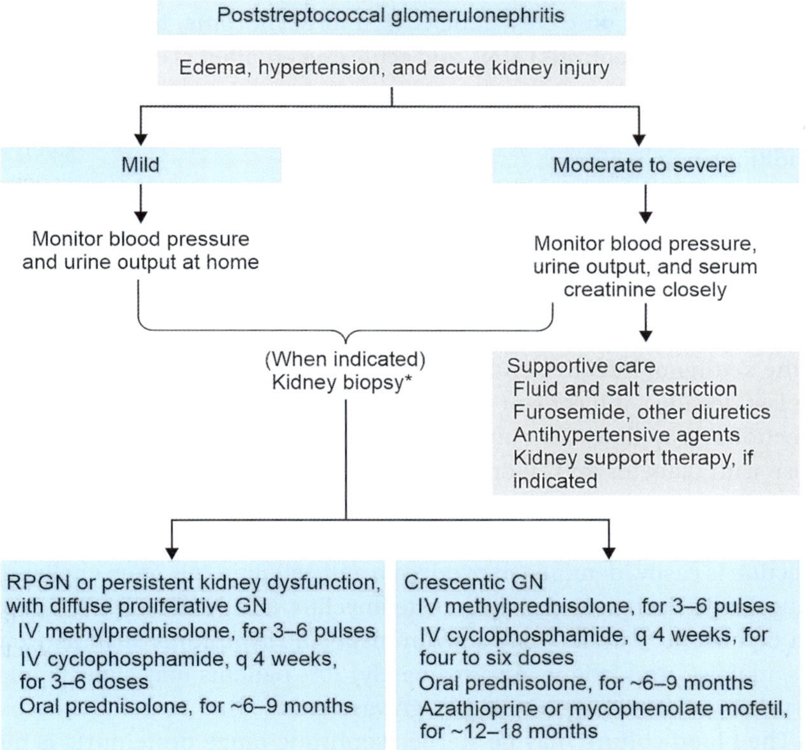

Children with AGN without evidence of preceding streptococcal infection should be followed for several years, with regular urinalysis and estimation of blood pressure. Renal biopsy is considered if mild-to-moderate proteinuria persists, or if there is decline in renal function.

ACUTE NEPHRITIC SYNDROME

Widespread use of antibiotics and improved living conditions have markedly reduced the incidence of streptococcal infections and PSGN in developed countries. Infections with methicillin-resistant *Staphylococcus aureus* are increasingly reported to result in proliferative GN. Other bacterial, viral, and parasitic agents have also been implicated **(Box 8.1)**. In patients with AGN associated with infections other than group A *Streptococcus*, the onset is often insidious, course protracted, and may lead to chronic kidney disease.

It is important to distinguish these patients from PSGN because appropriate antibiotic therapy would lead to the resolution of the disease.

Other conditions that may cause the acute nephritic syndrome include IgA vasculitis (Henoch–Schönlein purpura), C3 glomerulopathy, SLE, bacterial endocarditis, infected hydrocephalus shunt, microscopic polyangiitis, idiopathic crescentic GN, Alport syndrome, IgA nephropathy, acute interstitial nephritis (AIN), and acute exacerbation of chronic GN. Since patients with PSGN usually recover between 1 and 2 weeks, the persistence of abnormalities or a rapid deterioration should alert the physician to other conditions.

Staphylococcus Infection-associated Glomerulonephritis

Staphylococcus infection-associated glomerulonephritis (SAGN) is characterized by AGN in the setting of acute ongoing infection with *Staphylococcus*. Traditionally, staphylococci are implicated in triggering AGN in the setting of infective endocarditis and shunt nephritis. However, over the last decades, it has been reported to cause proliferative GN with acute infections as well. SAGN chiefly affects the elderly population, especially those with diabetes and IV drug abusers. Infection with both *S. aureus* and *S. epidermidis* can lead to SAGN. The chief features are microscopic hematuria, nephrotic range proteinuria, and severe AKI. While the source of infection is easily identified in pyoderma and cellulitis, it is often challenging to localize in deep-seated abscess, osteomyelitis, and dental infections. Fever can be absent; patients may show nonspecific symptoms such as weight loss, malaise, and fatigue. Approximately, 20% patients may show palpable purpura similar to that observed in IgA vasculitis.

The blood culture may be sterile. Nephrotic range proteinuria is more frequently seen in SAGN than in PSGN. Hypocomplementemia is seen in 30–50%; a few show positive antineutrophilic cytoplasmic antibody (ANCA) serology. Histological findings include mesangial proliferation, diffuse proliferative GN, and crescentic GN. Immunofluorescence shows mesangial and occasionally capillary wall deposition of IgA and C3. SAGN is considered IgA-dominant GN, but IgA predominance is not seen in all patients.

Therapy aims to eliminate the source of infection. Patients with deep-seated abscesses require 4–6 weeks antibiotic therapy to control the underlying infection. Long-term outcome is worse in cases with SAGN than PSGN.

Nephritis in Subacute Bacterial Endocarditis

Acute glomerulonephritis in patients with subacute bacterial endocarditis or infected prosthetic valves is indicated by moderate proteinuria and microscopic hematuria. Gross hematuria and hypertension are uncommon. Blood urea levels are elevated; C3 and C4 levels are low and rheumatoid factor may be positive. Circulating immune complexes may be detected. The common causative organisms are *S. aureus*, *S. epidermidis*, *S. viridans*, and gram-negative bacteria. With decline in rheumatic fever, more cases are due to native valve endocarditis, associated with hemodialysis and caused by staphylococci. Renal histological abnormalities are similar to those observed in PSGN; crescentic GN is seen in ~50% cases. Focal and segmental lesions showing infarcts, vasculitic GN without demonstrable immune complex deposits, and interstitial nephritis may be present.

Presentation with Osler nodules, Janeway lesions, and splinter hemorrhages is rare, and fever, with or without arthralgias, purpura, leukocytosis, and raised erythrocyte sedimentation rate, is noted. While the cardiac lesion is demonstrated by echocardiography, the renal disease manifests as microscopic hematuria and proteinuria, with deranged renal functions noted in up to one-third of patients. Treatment consists of eradication of the causative pathogens with appropriate antibiotics. Removal of the prosthesis may be necessary. Normalization of serum C3 indicates the resolution of nephritis; urinary abnormalities may persist for weeks to months. With early and adequate treatment, the prognosis is satisfactory.

Shunt Nephritis

Infection of the ventriculoatrial or ventriculoperitoneal shunt, and long-term indwelling catheters may lead to immune complex-mediated GN. Renal involvement is indicated by mild proteinuria and microscopic hematuria, and acute nephritic syndrome. Systemic features such as fever, joint pain, pallor, purpuric rash, and weight loss are associated. Serum C3 levels are low; blood culture or culture from shunt or catheter shows causative organisms, usually coagulase-negative staphylococci.

Renal histology shows features of postinfectious GN; abnormalities may resemble membranoproliferative GN (MPGN). Immunofluorescence shows C3 and IgM deposits, and occasionally IgG. Treatment consists of the removal of the shunt or indwelling catheter and the eradication of infection with the use of appropriate antibiotics. On long-term, some patients may have residual kidney dysfunction.

Viral Glomerulopathy

Association between viral infection and involvement of kidney has been described in various clinical scenarios over the last few decades. Glomerular injury is chiefly associated with systemic viral infection. **Table 8.1** describes the most common viral infections resulting in various patterns of glomerular injury. Often it is challenging to establish the causative link between infective agents and glomerular disease.

TABLE 8.1: Common viral infections and glomerular injury

Virus	*Patterns of glomerular injury*
Hepatitis B	Membranous nephropathy, focal segmental glomerulosclerosis, and IgA nephropathy
Hepatitis C	Immune complex glomerulonephritis and membranous nephropathy
HIV	HIVAN (collapsing glomerulopathy) and immune complex glomerular disease
SARS-CoV-2	Collapsing glomerulopathy and thrombotic microangiopathy

HIV: human immunodeficiency virus; HIVAN: HIV-associated nephropathy; IgA: immunoglobulin A; SARS-CoV-2: severe acute respiratory syndrome coronavirus 2

Glomerulonephritis Associated with Hepatitis B

Kidney involvement in hepatitis B is common in certain parts of the world. The chief glomerular pattern of injury associated with hepatitis B infection is membranous nephropathy; MPGN, mesangial proliferative GN, and polyarteritis nodosa (PAN) may occasionally occur. Most likely implicated antigens in immune deposition are hepatitis B surface antigen (HBsAg), hepatitis core antigen (HBcAg), and hepatitis B e antigen (HBeAg); of these HBeAg is the smallest and likely to traverse the basement membranes. Almost ~90% of patients with hepatitis B virus-associated membranous nephropathy show circulating HBeAg in serum. Most patients with hepatitis B-associated membranous nephropathy resolve spontaneously and hence do not require specific therapy. Spontaneous resolution is also associated with systemic clearance of HBeAg in children with chronic hepatitis B viral infection. KDIGO guidelines recommend that immunosuppression (rituximab or cyclophosphamide) be deferred till virological remission is achieved in patients with hepatitis B viral infection and anti-PLA2R antibody-mediated membranous nephropathy.

Membranoproliferative GN is the second most common glomerular pattern of injury in hepatitis B infected patients. HBsAg with IgG is most commonly found on kidney biopsy in subendothelial space in these patients. Some reports also describe mixed cryoglobulinemia in the setting of prolonged hepatitis B virus infection. Patients with cryoglobulinemia may show AKI, nephrotic syndrome, and systemic vasculitis.

When indicated therapy with interferon, and nucleos(t)ide analogs such as entecavir and tenofovir are recommended. Recent guidelines do not recommend the use of pegylated interferon-based regimens due to adverse effects. Medications such as entecavir (0.015 mg/kg/day; 0.5 mg maximum) and tenofovir disoproxil fumarate (8 mg/kg/day, 300 mg maximum), or tenofovir alafenamide (25 mg/day) are administered orally and have good safety profile, but require prolonged therapy.

Glomerulonephritis Associated with Hepatitis C

Glomerular injury in hepatitis C virus infection is mediated by immune complex formation in the glomerular basement membrane (GBM). Hepatitis C virus infection most commonly results in MPGN; some also show cryoglobulinemia. The patients present with nephrotic syndrome but may also have features of AGN. Similar to hepatitis B viral infection, PAN is also reported in patients with hepatitis C infection. Presentation with AKI is rare in patients with hepatitis C and glomerular disease. Kidney dysfunction in setting of hepatitis C infection is likely due to acute tubular necrosis or hepatorenal syndrome in patients with chronic liver disease.

KDIGO guidelines on management of hepatitis C virus infection in patients with glomerular diseases suggest that kidney biopsy is not mandatory since precise renal histology might not dictate therapy with direct acting antiviral (DAA) drugs. Immunosuppressive therapy is not recommended in treatment of the GN associated with hepatitis C infection, However, recent guidelines suggest that immunosuppressive medications along with DAA therapy be considered in patients with rapidly progressive glomerulonephritis (RPGN), systemic flare of cryoglobulinemic vasculitis, and nephrotic syndrome with complications.

DAA therapy is the cornerstone of management for hepatitis C virus infection. Latest WHO guidelines recommend combination regimen comprising of sofosbuvir/daclatasvir (400 mg/60 mg for >25 kg body weight; 200 mg/30 mg for 14–25 kg body weight) for 12 weeks as first-line therapy for hepatitis C virus infection in children and adolescents. Sustained virological response should be documented prior to discontinuation of DAA. In patients with decompensated cirrhosis, the duration of sofosbuvir/daclatasvir regimen is 24 weeks. Other DAA combination regimen approved for children include sofosbuvir/velpatasvir for 12 weeks and glecaprevir/pibrentasvir for 8 weeks.

Coronavirus and Glomerular Disease

Acute kidney injury was an important clinical feature observed during COVID-19 pandemic in children. AKI was chiefly caused by hemodynamic instability apart from cytokine storm leading to kidney injury. While acute tubular necrosis was common biopsy findings, other pathological findings observed on kidney biopsy include collapsing glomerulopathy, pauci-immune crescentic GN, membranous nephropathy, thrombotic microangiopathy, and podocytopathy. Severe acute respiratory syndrome coronavirus 2 (SARS-CoV-2) can cause direct injury by activation of complement and coagulation pathway and immune dysregulation.

Collapsing glomerulopathy is the most common glomerular disease observed in COVID-19, manifesting with severe AKI and heavy proteinuria, typically affecting the patients with high-risk variant allele of *APOL1* gene. No specific therapy is reported for collapsing glomerulopathy but about ~25% received treatment with corticosteroids and/or cyclosporine. The overall prognosis is unsatisfactory. Noncollapsing podocytopathy has also been reported in COVID-19 which mimics the clinical features of collapsing glomerulopathy but usually have better prognosis. Similar to other viral infections [influenza, human immunodeficiency virus (HIV), cytomegalovirus, and Epstein-Barr virus] SARS-CoV-2 can also lead to thrombotic microangiopathy due to direct endothelial injury mediated by hyperinflammatory state and uncontrolled complement activation. Patients with thrombotic microangiopathy manifest with severe AKI, hypertension, hematuria, and subnephrotic range proteinuria.

Other Virus-associated Diseases

Human immunodeficiency virus is associated with a number of renal syndromes, including HIV nephropathy, HIV-associated immune-complex GN, thrombotic microangiopathy, vasculitis, and electrolyte disorders. Medications used in the management of HIV infection can cause renal dysfunction (pentamidine and sulfonamides) or nephrolithiasis (indinavir). HIV-associated nephropathy (HIVAN) is characterized by nephrotic range proteinuria, azotemia, normal to large kidneys on ultrasonography, and collapsing glomerulopathy.

Dose adjustment should be made for patients treated with nucleoside or nonnucleoside reverse transcriptase inhibitors when the GFR is <50 mL/min; no dose adjustment is required for those receiving protease inhibitors. The combination of renin-angiotensin-aldosterone system (RAAS) inhibitors and antiretroviral therapy can slow the progression of HIV nephropathy. Patients with collapsing glomerulopathy may show rapid loss of kidney function.

Other viruses that might result in an immune complex GN (rarely, nephrotic syndrome) include parvovirus B19, mumps, measles, varicella, and dengue virus.

Acute Interstitial Nephritis

Acute interstitial nephritis is an immune-mediated injury to tubulointerstitial compartment of kidneys with relative sparing of glomeruli. The condition might account for ~10% children with AKI. Medications, infections, and systemic disorders (SLE and Sjögren syndrome) are the common etiologies in children. Medications incriminated includes antibiotics (ampicillin, ciprofloxacin, methicillin, and rifampicin), proton-pump inhibitors, and NSAIDs. Nonspecificity of symptoms often delays the diagnosis. Some patients may present with the triad of fever, rash, and arthralgia. Clinical features vary from asymptomatic urinary abnormalities to nonoliguric AKI.

Urinalysis shows leukocyturia and leukocyte casts; eosinophiluria (>1% of leukocytes) and hematuria are uncommon.

Tubulointerstitial nephritis with uveitis (TINU) accounts for 2–5% of all the cases of AIN. It is syndrome characterized by occurrence of tubulointerstitial nephritis and uveitis in absence of a systemic disorder, although kidney and ocular symptoms often have asynchronous presentation. TINU should be suspected in any child manifesting with nephritis or uveitis due to unknown etiology. Uveitis is typically bilateral anterior and usually diagnosed after onset of AIN. Experts suggest ophthalmological screening at 3-monthly intervals for at least 1 year following onset of AIN. On the other hand, patients with uveitis should be screened for TINU by urinalysis, and screening for beta-2 microglobulin. TINU is proposed to be caused by autoimmune disease triggered by viral infections, medications, or environmental factors. Studies have revealed an association with HLA-DRB1*0102. Therapy is not standardized, but includes treatment with steroids and mycophenolate mofetil.

Kidney biopsy is the gold standard for diagnosis. Histology shows interstitial inflammatory abnormalities with damage to tubular cells. Inflammation with T cells, monocytes, macrophages, plasma cells, and eosinophils is patchy, mostly in the deep cortex and outer medulla. Immunofluorescence is unremarkable, except for some C3 deposition in anti-GBM disease and IgG deposition in tubular basement membranes in IgG-4 related kidney diseases.

Course and Treatment

Removal of the offending agent leads to rapid recovery. Patients who develop AKI, especially if prolonged, show residual impairment of renal function. Therapy with prednisolone, initially 1–2 mg/kg/day and tapered over 3–4 weeks, may hasten recovery. In patients with severe AKI, 4–6 pulses of IV methylprednisolone (15–20 mg/kg/day) improve renal function. The long-term prognosis of AIN is excellent in most patients, except those presenting very late.

RAPIDLY PROGRESSIVE GLOMERULONEPHRITIS

Rapidly progressive glomerulonephritis is a rare condition in children, characterized by clinical features of GN and rapid loss of kidney function. Histology shows crescentic extracapillary proliferation in Bowman space affecting majority of glomeruli. RPGN is a medical emergency, which if untreated rapidly progresses to irreversible loss of kidney function. Prompt evaluation and specific therapy are necessary to ensure satisfactory outcome.

Definition

The RPGN is a clinical syndrome characterized by an acute nephritic illness accompanied by rapid loss of kidney function over days to weeks.

The histological correlation is the presence of crescents (crescentic GN), usually involving 50% or more glomeruli. The presence of crescents is a histologic marker of severe glomerular injury, which may occur in a number of conditions including postinfectious GN, IgA nephropathy (Chapter 7), SLE (Chapter 10), renal vasculitis (Chapter 9), and C3 glomerulopathy (Chapter 13). The severity of clinical features correlates with the proportion of glomeruli that show crescents. While patients with circumferential crescents involving >80% of glomeruli present with more severe acute kidney injury, those with noncircumferential crescents in <50% of glomeruli have a relatively milder course.

Although the terms RPGN and crescentic GN are used interchangeably, similar presentation might occur in conditions without crescents, including HUS, diffuse proliferative GN, and rarely with AIN. **Box 8.3** lists common conditions that present with RPGN in childhood.

Pathophysiology

Crescent formation is usually a nonspecific inflammatory response to severe injury to the glomerular capillary wall. While the underlying inciting reason may differ, the final pathway is often similar. In immune complex crescentic GN, the underlying trigger is deposition of immune complexes in the

BOX 8.3: Causes of rapidly progressive glomerulonephritis (RPGN)

Immune complex GN
Postinfectious GN: Poststreptococcal nephritis, infective endocarditis, shunt nephritis, *Staphylococcus aureus* sepsis, and other infections
Systemic disease: Systemic lupus erythematosus, IgA vasculitis, cryoglobulinemia, mixed connective tissue disorder, and juvenile rheumatoid arthritis
Primary GN: IgA nephropathy, C3 glomerulopathy, membranous nephropathy, and C1q nephropathy

Pauci-immune crescentic GN
Microscopic polyangiitis, granulomatosis with polyangiitis, renal limited vasculitis, eosinophilic granulomatosis with polyangiitis
Idiopathic crescentic GN
Medications: Penicillamine, hydralazine, hydrocarbons, propylthiouracil

Antiglomerular basement membrane GN
Anti-GBM nephritis, Goodpasture syndrome, postrenal transplantation in Alport syndrome

Postrenal transplantation
Recurrence of IgA nephropathy, IgA vasculitis, C3 glomerulopathy, systemic lupus erythematosus

RPGN without crescents
Hemolytic uremic syndrome
Acute interstitial nephritis
Diffuse proliferative GN

GBM: glomerular basement membrane; GN: glomerulonephritis; IgA: immunoglobulin A

glomerular capillary tufts. These immune complexes may be formed in the circulation or within the glomerular capillary wall itself.

Pauci-immune crescentic GN is associated with ANCA, directed against either myeloperoxidase (MPO), or proteinase 3 (PR3), or both. ANCAs are proposed to activate neutrophils and set off an inflammatory cascade, which subsequently causes endothelial and microvascular injury, and damage to the glomerular capillary wall. Activated neutrophils results in extrusion of neutrophil extracellular traps (NETs) extruded from the cell containing entrapped MPO, PR3, and complement components. Following this, they undergo a form of cell death, NETosis. NETs also mediate direct injury to endothelium, transfer MPO/PR3 to vascular endothelium for antigen presentation, and activate the alternate complement pathway. Involvement of the alternate complement pathway, specifically anaphylatoxin C5a and C5a receptor (CD88) has been shown in recent studies. It is proposed that there may be an amplification loop wherein activated neutrophils release properdin, activate the alternate pathway and generate C5a, resulting in additional neutrophil priming and their activation.

Finally, in anti-GBM GN, there are circulating IgG antibodies directed against the noncollagenous domain of α chain of type IV collagen present in the GBM and/or alveolar basement membrane.

Crescent Formation

Crescents are defined by the presence of two or more layers of cells in Bowman space, and composed chiefly of coagulation proteins, macrophages, T cells, fibroblasts, and parietal and visceral epithelial cells. The initial event in formation of crescents is the occurrence of a physical gap in the glomerular capillary wall and the GBM, mediated by macrophages and T lymphocytes. Breaks in the integrity of the capillary wall lead to passage of inflammatory mediators and plasma proteins into the Bowman space with fibrin formation, influx of macrophages and T cells, and release of inflammatory cytokines, e.g., interleukin-1 (IL-1) and tumor necrosis factor-α. Activated neutrophils and mononuclear cells also release matrix metalloproteinases, procoagulant tissue factor, and serine proteinases.

Similar breaks in the Bowman capsule allow cells and mediators from the interstitium to enter Bowman space and for contents of the latter to result in interstitial inflammation. Proliferating parietal and visceral epithelial cells comprise a key component of the crescents. The stage of inflammation is followed by development of fibrocellular and fibrous crescents. The expression of fibroblast growth factors and transforming growth factor-β is important for fibroblast proliferation and production of type I collagen, responsible for transition from cellular to fibrocellular and fibrous crescents. The plasminogen-plasmin system is responsible for fibrinolysis and resolution of crescents.

Epidemiology and Classification

Based on pathology and immunofluorescence staining patterns, crescentic GN is classified as discussed below.

Immune Complex Crescentic GN

These patients form a heterogeneous group in which multiple stimuli lead to proliferative GN with crescents. Immunohistology shows granular deposits of immunoglobulin and complement along capillary walls and in the mesangium. The causes include infections, systemic diseases, and primary GN.

- *Systemic infections:* Poststreptococcal GN can rarely present with crescentic histology. While most patients recover, the presence of nephrotic range proteinuria, sustained hypertension, and crescents is associated with unsatisfactory outcome. Other infectious illnesses associated with crescentic GN include infective endocarditis, infected atrioventricular shunts, and visceral abscesses. Crescentic GN might be associated with infection with resistant *S. aureus,* hepatitis B and C virus, leprosy, and syphilis.
- *Systemic immune complex disease:* RPGN with glomerular crescents might be seen in patients with IgA vasculitis (Henoch-Schönlein purpura), and class IV/less commonly class III lupus nephritis.
- *Primary GN:* Patients with IgA nephropathy, C3 glomerulopathy, and membranous nephropathy may occasionally present with rapid loss of renal function and crescents on biopsy.

Pauci-immune Crescentic GN

This form of GN is characterized by few or no immune deposits on immunofluorescence microscopy. This includes renal-limited vasculitis, and renal manifestations of microscopic polyangiitis, granulomatosis with polyangiitis (formerly Wegener's granulomatosis), or eosinophilic granulomatosis with polyangiitis (formerly Churg-Strauss syndrome). Most (80%) show ANCA in blood and are collectively classified as ANCA-associated vasculitides. Some cases of ANCA positive disease might be induced by drugs, including penicillamine, propylthiouracil, minocycline, and hydralazine (see Chapter 9).

Approximately 10–20% of patients with pauci-immune crescentic GN are ANCA negative. These patients are younger, and have fewer constitutional and extrarenal symptoms, but more proteinuria than those who are ANCA-positive.

Anti-GBM Crescentic GN

This condition is uncommon in childhood, accounting for <10% cases in children. The nephritogenic autoantibody is directed against a 28 kDa monomer located on the α3 chain of type IV collagen (Goodpasture antigen). In addition, approximately 5% of patients with Alport syndrome who receive a renal allograft show anti-GBM autoantibodies and anti-GBM nephritis within the first year of the transplant. Unlike de novo anti-GBM nephritis, pulmonary hemorrhage is not observed because the patient's lung tissue does not contain the putative antigen. The risk of post-transplantation anti-GBM nephritis is low in subjects with normal hearing, late progression to end-stage kidney disease, or females with X-linked Alport syndrome.

Idiopathic RPGN

This group includes patients with immune complex crescentic GN who do not fit into any identifiable category, and those with ANCA-negative pauci-immune disease. The proportion of cases varies across different regions.

The decline in the incidence of postinfectious GN has resulted in a change in the profile of crescentic GN. However, immune complex GN is still the most common pattern of crescentic GN in children accounting for 60–70% cases. Pauci-immune crescentic GN, while common in adults, is less frequent in children, accounting for ~20–25% cases.

Clinical Features

The spectrum of presenting features in RPGN is variable, and includes macroscopic hematuria (60–90% patients), oliguria (60–100%), hypertension (60–80%), and edema (60–90%). The illness is often complicated by occurrence of hypertensive emergencies, pulmonary edema, and cardiac failure. Occasionally, RPGN may have an insidious onset with initial symptoms of fatigue or edema. Nephrotic syndrome is rare and seen in patients with less severe renal insufficiency. Systemic complaints, involving the upper respiratory tract (cough and sinusitis), skin (vasculitic rash), musculoskeletal (joint pain and swelling) and nervous system (seizures and altered sensorium) are common in patients with pauci-immune RPGN, with or without ANCA positivity. Patients with anti-GBM antibody disease present with hemoptysis and, less often, pulmonary hemorrhage. Similar complications are found in granulomatosis with polyangiitis, systemic lupus, IgA vasculitis, and severe GN with pulmonary edema. The severity of clinical, laboratory, and histological features is maximum with anti-GBM disease, followed by pauci-immune GN and finally immune complex crescentic GN.

Investigations

Hematuria, characterized by dysmorphic red cells and red cell casts, is seen in all patients; most also have gross hematuria. A variable degree of nonselective proteinuria (2+ to 4+) is present in >65% patients. Urinalysis shows leukocyte, granular, and tubular epithelial cell casts. Severe AKI is often present at diagnosis. Anemia, if present is mild; peripheral smear shows normocytic normochromic red cells.

Serology

Serological investigations assist in evaluation of the cause and monitoring disease activity **(Box 8.4 and Flowchart 8.3)**. Low levels of total hemolytic complement (CH50) and C3 are seen in PSGN and SLE. Patients with lupus may additionally show reduced levels of C4, and antinuclear antibodies. Dense deposit disease is associated with low C3. Positive ASO titers and antideoxyribonuclease B suggest streptococcal infection in the past 3 months.

Elevated levels of ANCA suggest an underlying vasculitis, and are present in most patients with pauci-immune crescentic GN. Most ANCA have specificity for MPO or PR3. They should be screened by indirect immunofluorescence and positive tests confirmed by both PR3-enzyme-linked immunosorbent assay (ELISA) and MPO-ELISA (see also Chapter 9). Some patients may show antibodies to human lysosome-associated membrane protein-2 (hLAMP-2). Approximately 10–20% patients with granulomatosis with polyangiitis or microscopic polyangiitis have negative assays for ANCA. P-ANCA autoantibodies may occasionally be present in 20–30% patients with anti-GBM GN, and occasionally in idiopathic immune complex RPGN, inflammatory bowel disease, rheumatoid arthritis, and systemic lupus.

High titers of anti-GBM IgG antibodies, demonstrated by immunofluorescence or ELISA, are seen in anti-GBM nephritis or Goodpasture syndrome and correlate with disease activity. About 5% of ANCA positive samples are also anti-GBM positive and ~20–30% of anti-GBM positive samples are ANCA

BOX 8.4: Diagnostic evaluation of patients with rapidly progressive glomerulonephritis

Blood counts; peripheral smear; reticulocyte count; ESR, coagulation profile
Blood levels of urea, creatinine, and electrolytes
Urinalysis: Proteinuria; microscopy for erythrocytes and leukocytes, casts
Complement levels (C3, C4, CH50); additional evaluation based on biopsy findings
Antistreptolysin O, antinuclear antibody, antidouble stranded DNA antibodies
Anti-neutrophil cytoplasmic antibodies (ANCA): Indirect immunofluorescence and ELISA
Kidney biopsy (light microscopy, immunofluorescence, electron microscopy)

Required in specific instances
Anti-GBM IgG antibodies
Blood levels of cryoglobulin, hepatitis B and C serology
Chest: Radiograph, CT (patients with Goodpasture syndrome and vasculitides)
Sinuses: Radiograph, CT (patients with granulomatosis with polyangiitis)

ELISA: enzyme-linked immunosorbent assay; GBM: glomerular basement membrane; IgG: immunoglobulin G

Flowchart 8.3: Evaluation of crescentic glomerulonephritis. Etiological diagnosis is suggested by pattern of immunofluorescence, levels of complement C3, and presence of antineutrophil cytoplasmic antibodies (ANCA). ANA: Antinuclear antibodies; GBM: glomerular basement membrane; GN: glomerulonephritis; IgA: immunoglobulin A

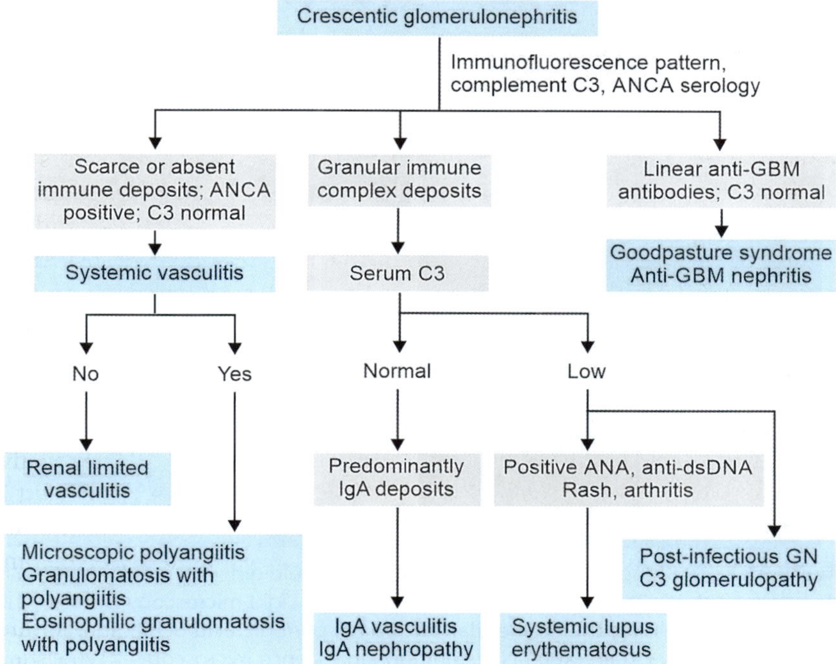

positive. Serology for ANCA is therefore recommended in all patients with either anti-GBM antibodies in blood or linear IgG deposition along the GBM. The initial clinical outcome for these patients is similar to that of anti-GBM disease, though relapses may occur.

Renal Histology

Light microscopy: Renal histological findings in various forms of crescentic GN are similar. A glomerular crescent is an accumulation of two or more layers of cells that partially or completely fill the Bowman space **(Figs. 8.3A to D)**. The crescent size varies from circumferential to segmental depending on the plane of the tissue section and the underlying disease. Crescents in anti-GBM nephritis or ANCA-associated disease are usually circumferential, while they are often segmental in immune complex GN. Interstitial changes range from acute inflammatory infiltrate to chronic interstitial scarring and tubular atrophy. Once the glomerular capillary loop is compressed by the crescent, tubules that derive their blood flow from that efferent arteriole show ischemic changes.

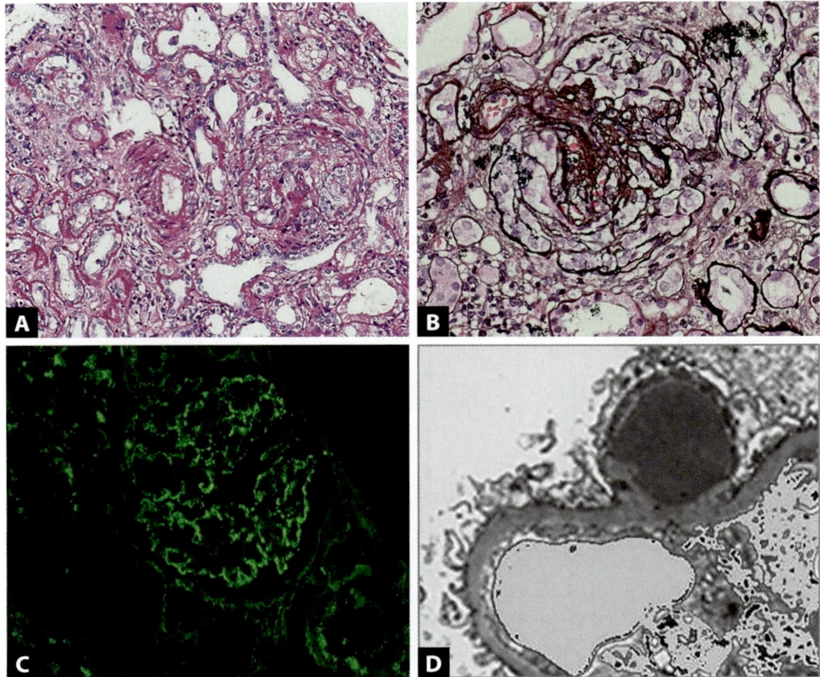

Figs. 8.3A to D: Kidney histology findings in a 9-year-old girl with rapidly progressive glomerulonephritis 2 weeks after sore throat and fever. Light microscopy shows cellular crescents compressing the glomerular tuft on (A) periodic acid Schiff and (B) Jones methenamine silver stain (X800); (C) Immunofluorescence microscopy (X1200) shows IgG deposits in typical "garland" pattern; (D) Electron microscopy shows a subepithelial "hump", indicating a diagnosis of poststreptococcal glomerulonephritis

Crescents may be completely cellular or show variable scarring and fibrosis. Cellular crescents are characterized by proliferation of macrophages, epithelial cells, and neutrophils **(Fig. 8.4A)**. Fibrocellular crescents show admixture of collagen fibers and membrane proteins amongst the cells **(Fig. 8.4B)**. In fibrous crescents, the cells are replaced by collagen **(Fig. 8.4C)**. Renal biopsies from patients with vasculitis show crescents in various stages of progression indicating episodic inflammation. Early lesions have segmental fibrinoid necrosis with or without an adjacent small crescent. Severe acute lesions show focal or diffuse necrosis in association with circumferential crescents. Features of small vessel vasculitis, affecting interlobular arteries **(Fig. 8.4D)** and rarely angiitis involving the vasa recta might be seen.

Immunohistology and electron microscopy: The presence, location, and nature of immune deposits on immunofluorescence and electron microscopy help determine the underlying cause of crescentic GN. Crescents stain strongly for fibrin on immunofluorescence. Mesangial deposits of IgA are found

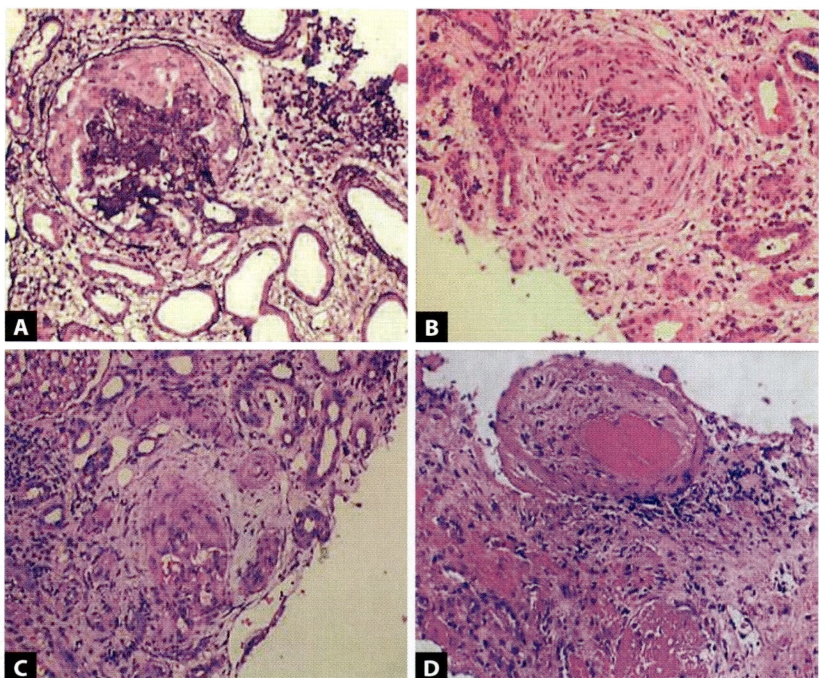

Figs. 8.4A to D: Histopathological spectrum of crescents. (A) Cellular crescent compressing the glomerular tuft. Silver methenamine stain (×800); (B) Fibrocellular crescent with compression of glomerular tuft and partial sclerosis. There is chronic interstitial inflammation, tubular atrophy, and interstitial fibrosis (H&E ×800); (C) Fibrous crescent compressing glomerular tuft (H&E ×800); (D) Pauci-immune crescentic glomerulonephritis, with a small artery showing features of active vasculitis with neutrophil infiltration of vessel wall, fibrin deposition, and luminal occlusion by a thrombus. Perivascular area shows interstitial hemorrhage and inflammation (H&E ×600)

in IgA nephropathy and IgA vasculitis. Postinfectious GN is characterized by granular, subepithelial deposits of IgG and C3 **(Fig. 8.3C)**. "Full house" capillary wall and mesangial deposits of granular IgG, IgA, IgM, C3, C4, and C1q are seen in SLE. Immune complex-mediated MPGN is characterized by immunoglobulin and complement deposits, while C3 glomerulopathy is characterized by complement deposits in the absence of significant immunoglobulins. Electron microscopy usually shows subendothelial and mesangial deposits. Anti-GBM disease is characterized by linear staining of the GBM with IgG (rarely IgM and IgA) and C3 **(Figs. 8.5A to C)**.

The third group of crescentic GN may have few or no immune deposits by immunofluorescence or electron microscopy. The majority of these patients are ANCA positive, though some may have ANCA-negative, pauci-immune crescentic GN.

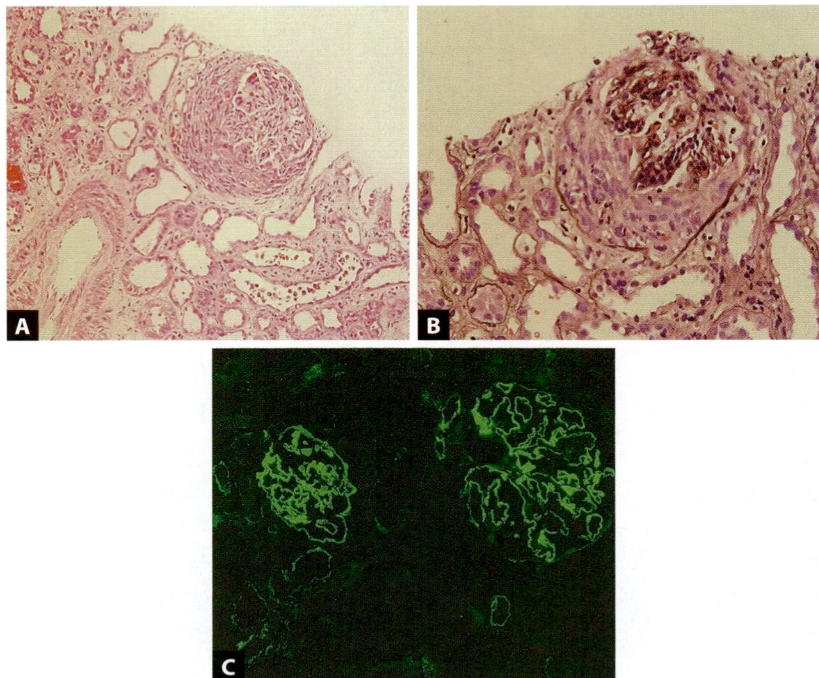

Figs. 8.5A to C: Antiglomerular basement membrane (GBM) nephritis in a 12-year-old boy presenting with rapidly progressive glomerulonephritis. Light microscopy shows fibrous to fibrocellular crescents with compression of glomerular tuft on (A) hematoxylin and eosin (×800) and (B) Jones methenamine silver (×1200). There is chronic interstitial inflammation, tubular atrophy, and interstitial fibrosis (A); (C) Immunofluorescence microscopy (×1200) shows linear deposition of IgG on the capillary wall

Evaluation and Diagnosis

It is necessary to make an accurate and rapid diagnosis in RPGN as treatment strategies vary and delay in instituting treatment results in risk of irreversible disease. All patients should undergo a kidney biopsy promptly. While the majority shows the presence of crescentic GN, the detection of thrombotic microangiopathy (affecting interlobular arteries and arterioles), or diffuse proliferative GN is not unusual. The diagnosis of the etiology of crescentic GN depends on integration of clinical data and findings on serology and renal histology **(Box 8.4 and Flowchart 8.3)**. In this way, anti-GBM disease or ANCA-associated RPGN is distinguished from other conditions.

Treatment

Empiric therapy with IV pulses of methylprednisolone (15–20 mg/kg, maximum 1 g/day) for 3–6 days should be initiated in patients with severe disease. This empiric initial therapy does not alter the histologic abnormalities on a kidney biopsy that is performed soon after. Plasmapheresis can be considered in the initial phase, especially if the patient presents with hemoptysis.

More specific therapy is started once the diagnosis is established. Treatment of RPGN typically comprises two phases—(*i*) *induction* of remission and (*ii*) *maintenance*. The first phase aims at control of inflammation and the associated immune response. Once remission is induced, the maintenance phase attempts to prevent further renal damage and relapses. All patients with RPGN, irrespective of the underlying diagnosis will benefit from supportive management including maintenance of fluid and electrolyte balance, provision of adequate nutrition, and control of infections and hypertension.

Steroids: After the initial IV pulses, steroids are typically given as high-dose oral prednisone (1 mg/kg daily) for 4 weeks, with tapering to 0.5 mg/kg daily by 3 months and alternate day prednisone for 6–12 months. Based on recent studies, a reduced-dose, oral glucocorticoid-tapering regimen could be considered for a patient with new onset or relapsing ANCA-associated vasculitis.

Cyclophosphamide: It is administered IV at frequency of 3–4 weeks, for a total of six doses. While the medication can also be given orally for 12 weeks, the cumulative dose and risk of side effects is higher. Pulse cyclophosphamide dosing may, however, be associated with a greater risk of relapses, exposing patients to further immunosuppression. The dose of oral and IV cyclophosphamide is 2 mg/kg/day and 500–750 mg/m^2, respectively. The IV dose should be adjusted to maintain a nadir leukocyte count, 2 weeks' posttreatment, of 3000–4000/cu mm.

Rituximab: B-cell depletion with rituximab has been shown to have similar efficacy than cyclophosphamide in many studies with fever side effects. It has been used successfully in patients with refractory lupus nephritis and in granulomatosis with polyangiitis, at a dose of 375 mg/m^2/week for four doses.

Azathioprine: Most patients with ANCA-associated disease need long-term maintenance immunosuppression with azathioprine due to the risk of relapses. The duration of maintenance treatment is debatable, with most patients of pauci-immune crescentic GN treated for 2–4 years.

Mycophenolate mofetil: MMF has been used chiefly during the maintenance phase of therapy. The KDIGO recommends azathioprine as the first choice for maintenance therapy in ANCA vasculitis, and considering MMF as an alternative in patients who are allergic to or intolerant of azathioprine.

Newer Agents

A number of agents including intravenous immunoglobulin (IVIG), monoclonal anti-CD52 antibody (alemtuzumab or CAMPATH 1-H) and belimumab (a monoclonal antibody that prevents the survival of B lymphocytes by blocking the binding of soluble human B lymphocyte stimulator protein, BLyS to receptors on B lymphocytes) have been used with variable success in patients with granulomatosis with polyangiitis and other vasculitides. Additionally, complement-targeted therapy may reduce steroid exposure in these patients. Trials using C5a receptor inhibitor, avacopan shows that the medication is well tolerated and safe and has a steroid sparing effect.

Plasmapheresis

Plasmapheresis or plasma exchange has been used for the treatment of crescentic GN with variable success. The mechanism of action is not clear, but is believed to involve removal of pathogenic autoantibodies, complement and coagulation factors and cytokines. Plasma exchange has been shown to have therapeutic benefit in anti-GBM disease with clearance of antibodies, lower serum creatinine, and improved patient and renal survival. However, adults who were anuric with severe azotemia, dialysis dependent or those who had >85% crescents on renal biopsy showed minimal benefit. The role of intensive plasma exchange has been examined in patients with ANCA-associated vasculitis with variable success. Some, but not all studies, have shown benefits in terms of ability to withhold dialytic support and lower risk of progression to end-stage kidney disease.

Anecdotal reports suggest the efficacy of plasmapheresis in patients with RPGN due to lupus, IgA vasculitis and severe proliferative GN, and in life-threatening pulmonary hemorrhage. However, a recent meta-analysis (nine randomized trials; 387 adult patients) on renal vasculitis or idiopathic RPGN, did not show evidence that adjunctive plasma exchange improved renal and patient survival.

According to recent KDIGO Clinical Practice Guidelines, the routine use of plasma exchange is not recommended for patients presenting with eGFR <50 mL/min/1.73 m^2, but can be considered in those with more severe AKI or in those with alveolar hemorrhage and hypoxemia. The dose recommended is 60 mL/kg volume replacement. For ANCA associated vasculitis, seven treatments over 14 days are prescribed and for vasculitis with anti-GBM antibodies, daily exchanges are done for 14 days or until anti-GBM antibodies are undetectable.

Immune Complex Crescentic GN

Therapy for these patients depends on the underlying disease. The treatment of IgA nephropathy and lupus nephritis presenting with RPGN is discussed in their respective chapters. Patients with idiopathic immune complex crescentic GN should be treated similarly to those with pauci-immune crescentic GN. An approach to the management of PSGN with crescents is shown in **Flowchart 8.2**.

Pauci-Immune Crescentic GN (See Small Vessel Vasculitis, Chapter 9)

Anti-GBM Crescentic GN

Prompt institution of plasma exchange is necessary in these patients. Double volume exchange is done daily, and subsequently on alternate days until anti-GBM antibodies are no longer detectable (usually 2–3 weeks). The patients are also treated with IV methylprednisolone (20 mg/kg on alternate days) followed by high-dose oral prednisolone. Coadministration of cyclophosphamide (2 mg/kg daily for 3 months) is effective in suppressing further antibody production. Pulmonary hemorrhage responds to plasma exchange and IV steroids. As anti-GBM disease does not usually have a relapsing course, long-term maintenance therapy is not required and steroids can be tapered over the next 6–9 months. Patients treated early in the course of their illness do satisfactorily.

A proportion of patients with anti-GBM nephritis also show positive ANCA, most often P-ANCA. While the precise significance of the dual positivity is unclear, their outcome is similar to classical anti-GBM disease. In view of a risk of relapses, these patients require a longer course of maintenance immunosuppressive therapy (as for ANCA associated GN).

Outcome

The outcome for patients has improved in the last decades, such that almost 60–70% patients show normal kidney function on the long term. Patients with poststreptococcal crescentic GN have a better prognosis, with most showing spontaneous improvement. The prognosis is better in patients with poststreptococcal crescentic GN with subepithelial, rather than subendothelial or intramembranous deposits. Outcomes in patients with pauci-immune crescentic GN, C3 glomerulopathy, and idiopathic RPGN are less favorable than IgA vasculitis or systemic lupus. ESKD may occur on the long-term in up to 25% patients with ANCA-associated vasculitis.

The outcome is determined by the severity of renal failure at presentation and promptness of intervention, renal histology, and underlying diagnosis. Studies have shown that the use of plasma exchange, high percentage of normal glomeruli, and absence of glomerulosclerosis, tubular atrophy and arteriosclerosis, were associated with better renal recovery. The potential for recovery corresponds with the relative proportion of cellular or fibrous components in the crescents, and the extent of tubulointerstitial scarring and fibrosis.

Post-transplant Recurrence

It is suggested that patients with ANCA positive vasculitis should have sustained remission for 1 year before considering a transplant. A positive ANCA titer at the time of transplantation does not increase the risk of allograft recurrence. While the use of immunosuppression following transplantation and different antigenic characteristics of the allograft prevent severe recurrences, better graft survival might increase this risk. Conditions associated with higher risk of histological recurrence include C3 glomerulopathy, IgA nephropathy, IgA vasculitis, and lupus. Graft losses are uncommon and occur in <5% cases. In patients with anti-GBM disease who develop end-stage renal disease, transplantation should be deferred until anti-GBM antibodies are undetectable for 12 months, at which point disease recurrence is unlikely.

BIBLIOGRAPHY

Acute Glomerulonephritis

1. Amaro D, Carreño E, Steeples LR, Oliveira-Ramos F, Marques-Neves C, Leal I. Tubulointerstitial nephritis and uveitis (TINU) syndrome. Br J Ophthalmol. 2020;104:742-7.
2. Balasubramanian R, Marks SD. Postinfectious glomerulonephritis. Pediatr Int Child Health. 2017;37:240-7.
3. Deoliveira M, Sikri H, Yu SM, He JC. Viral glomerulopathy. Glomerular Dis. 2023;3:148-54.
4. Khandelwal P, Krishnasamy S, Govindarajan S, et al. Anti-factor H antibody associated HUS following SARS-CoV-2 infection. Pediatr Nephrol. 2022;37:2151-6.
5. Kidney Disease: Improving Global Outcomes (KDIGO) Glomerular Diseases Work Group. KDIGO 2021 Clinical Practice Guideline for the Management of Glomerular Diseases. Kidney Int. 2021;100:S1-S276.
6. Kidney Disease: Improving Global Outcomes (KDIGO) Hepatitis C Work Group. KDIGO 2022 Clinical Practice Guideline for the Prevention, Diagnosis, Evaluation, and Treatment of Hepatitis C in Chronic Kidney Disease. Kidney Int. 2022;102:S129-S205.
7. Klomjit N, Zand L, Cornell LD, Alexander MP. COVID-19 and glomerular Diseases. Kidney Int Rep. 2023;8:1137-50.
8. Ong LT. Management and outcomes of acute post-streptococcal glomerulonephritis in children. World J Nephrol. 2022;11:139-45.
9. Ruebner RL, Fadrowski JJ. Tubulointerstitial nephritis. Pediatr Clin North Am. 2019;66:111-9.
10. Sethi S, De Vriese AS, Fervenza FC. Acute glomerulonephritis. Lancet. 2022;399:1646-63.

Rapidly Progressive Glomerulonephritis

1. Berden AE, Ferrario F, Hagen EC, et al. Histopathologic classification of ANCA-associated glomerulonephritis. J Am Soc Nephrol. 2010;21:1628-36.

2. Hiemstra TF, Walsh M, Mahr A, et al. Mycophenolate mofetil vs azathioprine for remission maintenance in antineutrophil cytoplasmic antibody-associated vasculitis: a randomized controlled trial. JAMA. 2010;304:2381-8.
3. Hoschek JC, Dreyer P, Dahal S, Walker PD. Rapidly progressive renal failure in childhood. Am J Kidney Dis. 2002;40:1342-7.
4. Kuang H, Jiang N, Jia XY, Cui Z, Zhao MH. Epidemiology, clinical features, risk factors and outcomes in anti-glomerular basement membrane disease: A systematic review and meta-analysis. Autoimmun Rev. 2024;23:103531.
5. Morgan MD, Harper L, Williams J, Savage C. Anti-neutrophil cytoplasm-associated glomerulonephritis. J Am Soc Nephrol. 2006;17:1224-34.
6. Raff A, Hebert T, Pullman J, Coco M. Crescentic post-streptococcal glomerulonephritis with nephrotic syndrome: Is aggressive therapy warranted? Clin Nephrol. 2005;63:375-80.
7. Rovin BH, Adler SG, Barratt J, et al. Executive summary of the KDIGO 2021 guideline for the management of glomerular diseases. Kidney Int. 2021;100:753-79.
8. Sinha A, Puri K, Dinda AK, Bagga A. Etiology and outcome of crescentic glomerulonephritis. Indian Pediatr. 2013;50:283-8.
9. Walsh M, Catapano F, Szpirt W, et al. Plasma exchange for renal vasculitis and idiopathic rapidly progressive glomerulonephritis: A meta-analysis. Am J Kidney Dis. 2011;57:566-74.
10. Kidney disease improving global outcomes (KDIGO) ANCA vasculitis work group. KDIGO 2024 clinical practice guideline for the management of antineutrophil cytoplasmic antibody (ANCA). Associated vasculitis. Kidney Int. 2024;105:571-5116.
11. Meena J, Nangla P, Ojha, et al. Etiology, clinical profile, and outcomes of crescentic glomerulonephritis in children: a systematic review. Pediatr Nephrol. 2024 Sep 16. doi: 10.1007/s00467-024-06521-3.

Systemic Vasculitis

Arvind Bagga

Systemic vasculitis comprises a heterogeneous group of disorders with multiorgan involvement and myriad clinical presentations. These conditions may involve small (arterioles, capillaries, and venules), medium (e.g., renal, hepatic, mesenteric, and coronary arteries), or large (aorta, large branches) sized vessels and are classified by the *smallest* vessel affected. Kidneys are frequently affected and their involvement is a chief cause of morbidity and mortality. Prompt recognition and initiation of therapy, and judicious follow-up are necessary for optimal management.

EPIDEMIOLOGY AND ETIOPATHOGENESIS

The annual incidence of primary vasculitis in children and adolescents is approximately 20 per 100,000. Ethnicity has an influence on the incidence, prevalence, disease manifestations, and outcome. Kawasaki disease and Takayasu arteritis are more common in the Asian population. Various genetic, environmental, and immune factors have an important role in disease susceptibility and pathogenesis. Antineutrophil cytoplasmic antibodies (ANCA) have an important role in certain vasculitides. Antecedent infections, especially streptococcal, have been implicated in some forms including immunoglobulin A (IgA) vasculitis, granulomatosis with polyangiitis (GPA), and polyarteritis nodosa (PAN).

PATHOLOGY

Takayasu arteritis is a large vessel vasculitis characterized by focal granulomatous inflammation with multinucleated giant cells that progress to fibrosis and vascular narrowing. PAN and Kawasaki disease have predilection for medium-sized arteries, renal, and coronary arteries respectively, and are characterized by focal necrotizing vasculitis and inflammatory aneurysms. The presence of arteritis and glomerulonephritis (GN) indicates small vessel vasculitis. Leukocytoclastic vasculitis, typically observed in IgA vasculitis and hypersensitivity vasculitis, is characterized by neutrophilic inflammation, scattered nuclear debris (leukocytoclasia), and necrosis of small-sized vessels. Renal histology, in most conditions, shows focal and segmental proliferative glomerulonephritis. The severity of the lesions can vary from mild proliferative changes to formation of extensive crescents.

DIAGNOSIS

The clinical features of systemic vasculitides are varied and depend on the size, site, and extent of the affected vessels. Recognition of these conditions can be challenging as presenting symptoms may be nonspecific with fever, malaise, and generalized aches and pain. With evolving vascular damage more obvious and specific features such as purpura, and organ involvement such as GN may appear. A detailed history should include recent illnesses, drug exposure, and a family history. Blood pressure is measured in all four extremities, peripheral pulses palpated, and major vessels auscultated for bruit. Skin is examined for petechiae and purpura. Evidence of peripheral neuropathy is sought and fundoscopy done to examine retinal vasculature.

Hemogram and C-reactive protein are examined to detect acute phase reactants as markers of systemic inflammation. Urinalysis is done for evidence of glomerular involvement. Kidney and liver functions tests and serology for antibodies [antinuclear antibody (ANA) and ANCA] and complement (C3 and C4) are done, as required. Imaging studies [computed tomography and magnetic resonance (CT, MR)] or conventional angiography help detect abnormalities of blood vessels, especially medium and large vessels. Renal biopsy is performed if there is evidence of glomerular involvement.

CLASSIFICATION

A classification of major childhood vasculitis, based on the size of the affected vessel, was jointly proposed by the Pediatric Rheumatology European Society (PRES) and European League against Rheumatism (EULAR) in 2005 (**Box 9.1**). Criteria for classification of major childhood vasculitic disorders are detailed in **Box 9.1**.

SMALL VESSEL VASCULITIS

IgA Vasculitis

With an estimated incidence of 6–20 cases per 100,000 children annually, IgA vasculitis (previously termed Henoch-Schönlein purpura or anaphylactoid purpura) is the chief childhood systemic vasculitis, accounting for almost one-half of all cases. The condition affects children between the ages of 3 and 10 years. Tissue biopsy shows leukocytoclastic vasculitis predominantly affecting the small blood vessels, with IgA deposits. Seasonal trends with predilection for winter and spring and antecedent upper respiratory infections suggest an infectious trigger with bacterial or viral infections such as group A β hemolytic streptococcus, *Staphylococcus aureus*, influenza, parainfluenza, and Epstein-Barr viruses. IgA-dominant immune deposits are found in small vessels.

BOX 9.1: Classification of childhood vasculitis

Predominantly large vessel vasculitis
Takayasu arteritis
Predominantly medium-sized vessel vasculitis
Childhood polyarteritis nodosa
Kawasaki disease
Predominantly small vessel vasculitis
Granulomatous
Granulomatosis with polyangiitis
Eosinophilic granulomatosis with polyangiitis
Nongranulomatous
IgA vasculitis
Microscopic polyangiitis
Hypocomplementemic urticarial vasculitis
Isolated cutaneous leukocytoclastic vasculitis
Other vasculitides
Behçet disease
Vasculitis associated with connective tissue diseases (lupus, rheumatoid arthritis, and sarcoidosis)
Isolated vasculitis of central nervous system
Secondary to infection (hepatitis B), malignancy, and drugs, including hypersensitivity vasculitis
Cogan syndrome
Unclassified

Clinical Features

The illness is characterized by nonthrombocytopenic purpura, arthritis or arthralgia, abdominal pain, and kidney involvement. Purpuric rash usually appears on the extensor aspects of legs and glutei, and often also affects arms and face **(Figs. 9.1A to C)**. The rash may initially be maculopapular or urticarial but soon becomes purpuric and disappears over the next 2 weeks. Arthralgia or arthritis affects large joints in 60–65% patients and is usually oligoarticular and self-limited. Gastrointestinal manifestations, observed in 70–85% patients, include abdominal pain, melena, and occasionally intussusception. The rash may occasionally be absent or follow abdominal or joint involvement. Rarely pulmonary hemorrhage and neurological features (seizures, stroke, and changes in mental status) are present.

Immunoglobulin A vasculitis might uncommonly present during infancy (Seidlmayer syndrome). Distinctive clinical features include acute onset of purpura with ecchymoses, inflammatory edema of limbs and face, and medallion-like distribution of skin lesions on the face, auricles, and extremities. Kidney involvement occurs in about one-third, usually within the first 4–6 weeks, and almost always within 6 months. Urinalysis is necessary for >6 months, and optionally for 12 months from initial presentation of systemic

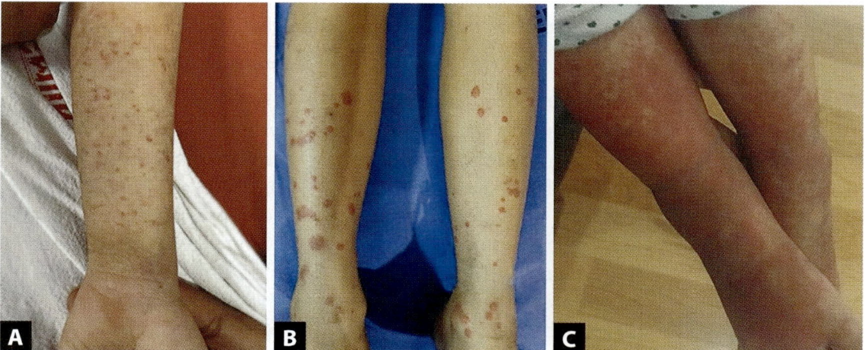

Figs. 9.1A to C: Skin rash in IgA vasculitis. Lesions range from (A) pin-head size or larger palpable nonblanching erythematous petechiae and papules, to (B) palpable purpuric macules and papules, and (C) extensive confluent purpuric lesions, observed chiefly on the limbs. Older individuals may show hemorrhagic bullae and vesicles (not shown)

disease. Isolated microscopic hematuria with or without mild proteinuria is most common. Occasionally, features of nephritic or nephrotic syndrome may be present. In two-thirds of cases, the disease runs its entire course within 4 weeks of onset. Risk factors for renal involvement include older age at onset, persistent rash, severe abdominal symptoms, and low factor XIII activity. Approximately 15–40% of patients have at least one recurrence of IgA vasculitis with rash and abdominal pain. Each such episode is usually similar but shorter and milder than the preceding one.

Diagnosis

The classification criteria are outlined in **Table 9.1**. In cases of purpura with atypical distribution, demonstration of leukocytoclastic vasculitis with IgA deposition is required on skin biopsy performed at the edge of a fresh cutaneous lesion. Indications for kidney biopsy include the presence of significant or persistent proteinuria, nephrotic or nephritic syndrome, acute kidney injury (AKI), and isolated microscopic hematuria that persists beyond a month. Renal histology shows focal and segmental proliferative GN. Mesangial proliferation is predominant but infiltration with neutrophils may be present. The severity of lesions varies from mild proliferative changes to severe proliferation with crescents **(Figs. 9.2A to E)**. Immunofluorescence shows predominant mesangial IgA deposits. Renal histological features are often indistinguishable from idiopathic IgA nephropathy.

Treatment

Symptomatic treatment is provided with rest and analgesia for joint pains. Corticosteroids are not recommended for prevention of nephritis

TABLE 9.1: Classification criteria for common vasculitides

	Criteria	*Comments*
IgA vasculitis	*Mandatory:* Purpura or petechiae (not related to thrombocytopenia) with lower limb predominance, and at least one of the following: (*i*) acute abdominal pain: may include intussusception, gastrointestinal bleeding; (*ii*) leukocytoclastic vasculitis or proliferative glomerulonephritis with predominant IgA deposits; (*iii*) acute-onset arthritis or arthralgia; (iv) renal involvement*	• Finding of IgA predominance in biopsy specimens is useful in doubtful or atypical cases • Joint involvement is common in children; renal involvement underlines the importance of prospective monitoring for hematuria/proteinuria
Polyarteritis nodosa	*Mandatory criterion:* Angiographic abnormalities such as aneurysm, stenosis or occlusion, *or* histopathology showing necrotizing vasculitis, of medium or small sized artery, plus one of the following: (*i*) skin involvement: livedo reticularis, nodules, and ischemic changes; (*ii*) myalgia, muscle tenderness; (*iii*) hypertension; (*iv*) peripheral neuropathy; and (*v*) renal involvement*	• Emphasis on mandatory criteria of angiographic or histopathological findings • While conventional angiogram is the current standard, future studies may establish a place for other techniques • Hepatitis B associated illness is classified separately
Granulomatosis with polyangiitis	Presence of at least three of the following: (*i*) histology: granulomatous inflammation within vessel wall, perivascular, or extravascular area; (*ii*) upper airway involvement: chronic purulent or bloody nasal discharge, nasal septal perforation, or chronic sinusitis; (*iii*) laryngotracheobronchial stenosis; (*iv*) pulmonary involvement on chest X-ray or CT (nodules, cavities, and infiltrates); (*v*) ANCA positive (ELISA and immunofluorescence); (*vi*) renal involvement*	• Emphasis on CT findings and specific upper and lower respiratory tract involvement • Recognition of frequent subglottic stenosis in children • Isolated disease with orbital or upper airway involvement to be separated from the widespread form

Contd...

Contd...

	Criteria	*Comments*
Takayasu arteritis	*Mandatory criterion:* Angiography showing aneurysm/dilatation of aorta or its main branches plus one of the following: (*i*) decreased peripheral artery pulse and/or claudication of extremities; (*ii*) bruit over the aorta and/or its major branches; (*iii*) blood pressure difference >10 mm between the extremities; (*iv*) systemic hypertension; and (*v*) elevated acute phase reactants (ESR and C-reactive protein)	• Important to differentiate noninflammatory conditions such as fibromuscular dysplasia or mid-aortic syndrome • Combination of pulse deficit and claudication, and inclusion of hypertension makes classification more specific • Raised acute phase reactants associated with angiographic changes allow early classification

ANCA: antineutrophil cytoplasmic antibodies; CT: computed tomography; ELISA: enzyme-linked immunosorbent assay; ESR: erythrocyte sedimentation rate; GFR: glomerular filtration rate

*Proteinuria (>0.3 g/24 h, >30 mmol/mg of urine albumin/creatinine ratio, ≥2+ on dipstick on spot morning sample); hematuria (>5 red cells/hpf, active urinary sediment); impaired renal function (measured or estimated GFR <50% normal)

Source: Ozen S, et al. 2010

in IgA vasculitis. Indications for using corticosteroids include severe gastrointestinal manifestations, orchitis, and severe kidney involvement **(Table 9.2)**. Prednisolone is administered at a dose of 1–2 mg/kg/day for a week, followed by gradual reduction of the dose over 2–3 weeks. Therapy with pulse corticosteroids may be considered in patients with severe extrarenal features, including bullous and necrotic skin lesions, neurologic involvement (vasculitis, nonhypertensive nonmetabolic encephalopathy), diffuse alveolar hemorrhage, and severe orchitis or myocarditis.

Renal disease is mild in the majority and does not require specific therapy. The Kidney Disease: Improving Global Outcomes (KDIGO) recommendations suggest that children with IgA vasculitis and persistent proteinuria be initially treated with angiotensin converting enzyme inhibitors (ACEI) or angiotensin receptor blockers (ARB). Children with persistent proteinuria after a trial of ACEI or ARBs may be offered a 6-month course of corticosteroids. Patients with severe nephritis or nephrotic syndrome should be treated with corticosteroids and cytotoxic drugs. Treatment of crescentic GN comprises of intravenous (IV) methylprednisolone and IV cyclophosphamide. Plasma exchanges may be considered in refractory disease.

The European consensus (SHARE, Single Hub, and Access point for pediatric Rheumatology in Europe initiative) on the diagnosis and treatment of IgA vasculitis, based on expert opinion of pediatric rheumatologists,

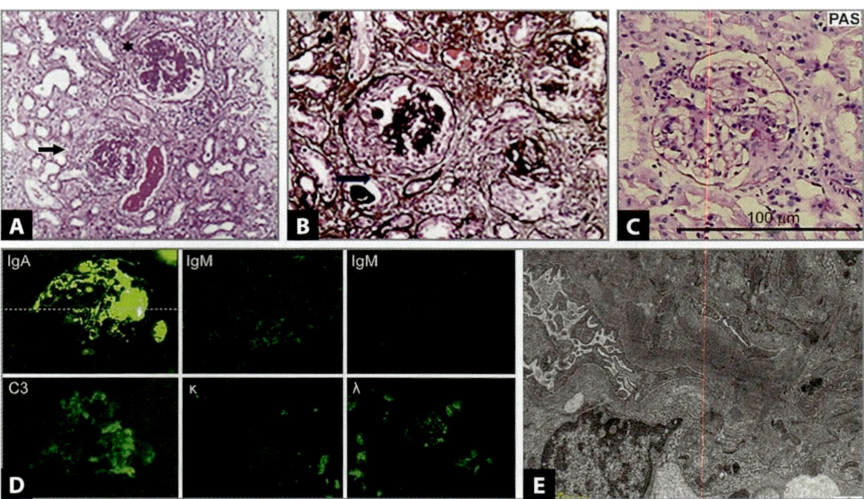

Figs. 9.2A to E: Kidney biopsy in a 5-year-old girl with gross hematuria and palpable purpura due to IgA vasculitis. Light microscopy shows (A) glomeruli with mesangial hypercellularity, mesangial sclerosis (*) and overlying crescent (arrow) (Periodic acid-Schiff; 10x); (B) variable glomerulosclerosis with a cellular crescent with Bowman capsule disruption (arrow) (Jones' silver methenamine; 40x); and (C) mesangial hypercellularity and segmental sclerosis (hematoxylin and eosin; 40x). (D) Immunofluorescence shows mesangial deposits of IgA (2–3+) with capillary wall extension, 1+ mesangial deposits of C3 and lambda accentuation. (E) Electron microscopy reveals electron dense deposits in the mesangium. *Courtesy:* Prof Geetika Singh, Department of Pathology, AIIMS, New Delhi

TABLE 9.2: Options for management of IgA vasculitis

Illness	*Supportive*	*Oral steroids*	*IV steroids*	*Plasmapheresis*
Rash, edema, and arthritis	Yes, NSAIDs			
Severe rash, edema	Yes	Yes		
Severe abdominal colic	Yes	Yes		
Orchitis	Yes	Yes		
Nephrotic proteinuria*	Yes	Yes	Occasionally	
Rapidly progressive GN*	Yes	Yes	Yes	Occasionally
Pulmonary hemorrhage*	Yes	Yes	Yes	Yes

GN: glomerulonephritis; NSAID: nonsteroidal anti-inflammatory drug

*Simultaneous use of corticosteroid and immunosuppressive agents (cyclophosphamide, azathioprine) is recommended

differs from the KDIGO recommendations in advocating prompt initiation of corticosteroid therapy in patients with IgA vasculitis and evidence of nephritis, without awaiting response to a 6-month trial with ACEI/ARB. This opinion, which is overall consistent with pediatric nephrology practice, is based on the consideration that the disease in children has an acute onset, rapid development, and high possibility of regression with immunosuppression. While recognizing the lack of evidence from controlled pediatric studies, the SHARE guidelines suggest that mild cases of IgA vasculitis with normal kidney function and mild-to-moderate proteinuria be treated with oral prednisolone as first-line treatment, with pulse steroids and/or additional immunosuppression reserved as second-line therapies. Patients with moderate IgA vasculitis [defined by estimated glomerular filtration rate (eGFR) reduction or persistent proteinuria along with <50% crescents] require a more aggressive approach, with treatment with steroid pulses considered first-line **(Table 9.3)**. Adjunctive therapy with ACEI/ARB is recommended to prevent long-term damage. Guidelines from the International Pediatric Nephrology Association are awaited.

Outcome

Renal involvement although usually self-limited, can be severe with extensive glomerular crescentic changes and can lead to end stage kidney disease in <1%. Persistent heavy proteinuria, hypertension and severe AKI, and histology showing crescentic GN indicate an unsatisfactory outcome.

Patients requiring renal transplantation do well, and the disease rarely recurs in the allograft, although insignificant mesangial IgA deposits may be present.

Antineutrophil Cytoplasmic Antibodies-associated Small Vessel Vasculitis

Systemic small vessel vasculitis include microscopic polyangiitis, GPA (Wegener granulomatosis), eosinophilic granulomatosis with polyangiitis (EGP, Churg-Strauss syndrome), and renal limited vasculitis (idiopathic crescentic GN). Patients with renal limited vasculitis present with pauci-immune necrotizing crescentic GN without extrarenal manifestations of systemic vasculitis. These conditions have characteristic clinical manifestations and test positive for antineutrophil cytoplasmic antibodies (ANCA).

Microscopic Polyangiitis

Microscopic polyangiitis is a necrotizing vasculitis of small vessels with few or no immune deposits and is distinguished from classic PAN by the presence of extensive glomerular involvement. It usually presents with renal

TABLE 9.3: Management of IgA vasculitis with nephritis

Kidney involvement	***Immunosuppression****
Subnephrotic range proteinuria (Up/Uc 0.2–2 mg/mg) with normal renal function (eGFR >60 mL/min/1.73 m^2), no proliferation on histology (M0, E0, C0)	Prednisolone 1 mg/kg/day (maximum 60 mg/day) for 4 weeks; taper over 3–6 months
As above, but with histology indicating proliferative activity without crescents (M1 and/or E1, C0)	• Prednisolone 1 mg/kg/day for 4 weeks; taper over 6 months • Cyclophosphamide 2–2.5 mg/kg/day for 12 weeks
Moderate nephritis, as indicated by any of the following: Nephrotic range proteinuria (Up/Uc ≥2 mg/mg), reduced renal function (eGFR <60 mL/min/1.73 m^2), and histology indicating proliferative activity without sclerosis or crescents (M1 and/or E1, S0, C0)	• Prednisolone 1 mg/kg/day for 4 weeks; taper over 6 months • Cyclophosphamide 2–2.5 mg/kg/day for 12 weeks • Maintenance with MMF 900–1,200 mg/m^2/day; *or* azathioprine 2–2.5 mg/kg/day for 24 months
Any proteinuria (Up/Uc >0.2 mg/mg) with normal renal function, and histology indicating segmental sclerosis without crescents (M0-1 and/or E0-1, S1, C0)	• Prednisolone in tapering doses over 2 years • Calcineurin inhibitors for 1–2 years
Severe nephritis, as indicated by rapidly progressive glomerulonephritis or histology indicating crescents in >10% glomeruli (C1)	• IV Methylprednisolone 20–30 mg/kg/day; maximum 1 g/day for 3–6 days • IV Cyclophosphamide 500 mg/m^2/dose q monthly for 6 doses; followed by • MMF 900–1,200 mg/m^2/day; *or* azathioprine 2–2.5 mg/kg/day for 2–3 years
Severe, refractory IgA vasculitis	Rituximab 375 mg/m^2 IV, 2 doses 1 week apart; subsequent doses based on the severity of renal disease at initiation of therapy

eGFR: estimated glomerular filtration rate; IgA: immunoglobulin A; MMF: mycophenolate mofetil

*Additional therapy with ACE-I/ARB is administered in all categories, except in patients with eGFR <30 mL/min/1.73 m^2

impairment associated with proteinuria, hematuria, and hypertension. Malaise, fever, anorexia, and weight loss are common. Rashes, arthralgia, myalgia, and pulmonary hemorrhage may be present. Renal biopsy shows focal, segmental necrotizing GN with fibrinoid necrosis, and thrombosis of glomerular tuft segments surrounded by neutrophils. There may be extensive crescent formation. Glomerular immune deposits are scarce or absent, hence the term *pauci-immune crescentic GN.*

Granulomatosis with Polyangiitis

The GPA (formerly termed Wegener granulomatosis) is characterized by granulomatous inflammation of the respiratory tract with necrotizing vasculitis affecting small- to medium-sized vessels and a necrotizing GN. The classification criteria for GPA are outlined in **Table 9.1**.

Diagnosis

Serology: Antibodies directed against neutrophil cytoplasmic antigens (ANCA) may be found in patients with microscopic polyarteritis. These antibodies may also be associated with other small vessel vasculitis. An indirect immunofluorescence assay detects two patterns of staining **(Figs. 9.3A to D)**. The first, strongly associated with GPA, is a diffuse granular staining throughout the neutrophil cytoplasm and termed cytoplasmic ANCA (cANCA). It usually corresponds to specificity for the enzyme proteinase 3 (PR3). The second pattern is a concentration of fluorescence

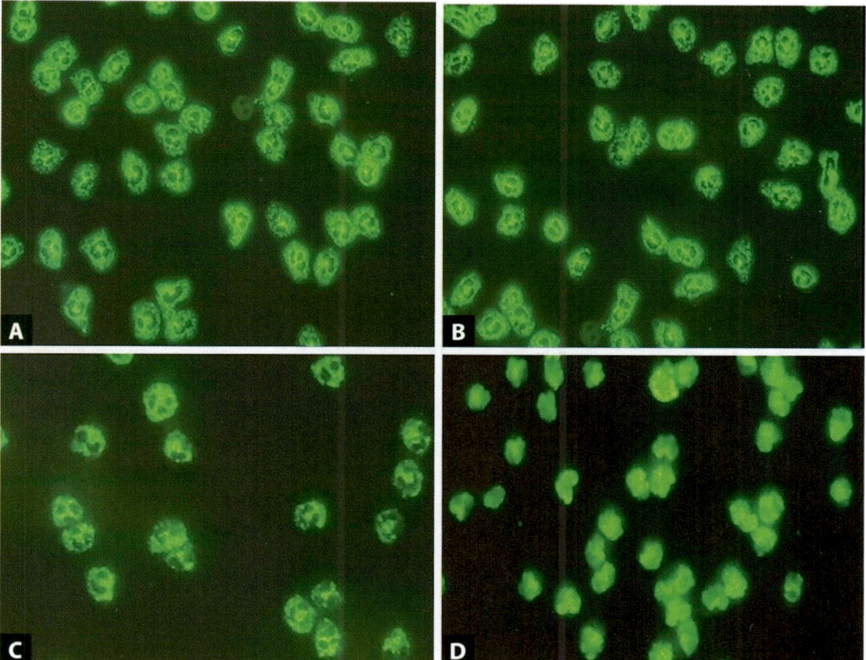

Figs. 9.3A to D: Antineutrophil cytoplasmic antibodies (ANCA) stained by indirect immunofluorescence. (A) Formalin-fixed and (B) ethanol-fixed images show diffuse cytoplasmic staining with coarse granular and central interlobular accentuation of neutrophils, consistent with cytoplasmic or c-ANCA. (C) Formalin-fixed and (D) ethanol-fixed images show coarse granular perinuclear immunofluorescence outlining the nuclear lobes of neutrophils, consistent with perinuclear or p-ANCA. *Courtesy:* Dr Danveer Bhadu, Department of Rheumatology, AIIMS, New Delhi

around the nucleus, called perinuclear ANCA (pANCA), and usually associated with antibodies directed against the enzyme myeloperoxidase (MPO). For diagnostic accuracy, screening for ANCA should include a high-quality immunochemical analysis for antigen specificity (PR3 or MPO), such as by enzyme-linked immunosorbent assay (ELISA). About 80–85% patients with microscopic polyangiitis have either pANCA or cANCA, the majority having the former.

Some patients with classic features of pauci-immune crescentic GN are ANCA negative. A negative ANCA result does not rule out these diseases. These patients have the same prognosis and should receive the same treatment as those who are ANCA positive. Some patients who are ANCA negative might show autoantibodies to human lysosome-associated membrane protein-2 (hLAMP-2) that binds native glomerular but not neutrophil hLAMP-2. Persistence of ANCA positivity, an increase in titers, or change in ANCA from negative to positive does not precisely predict the course of the disease or occurrence of a relapse, and should not be used to guide therapy.

Histology: Kidney biopsy should be done promptly in a patient with clinical features of small-vessel vasculitis with positive MPO- or PR3-ANCA serology. If biopsy is not feasible immediately, especially in a setting of rapidly progressive GN, appropriate therapy is commenced, and biopsy done as soon as feasible. The typical histopathological finding is that of pauci-immune crescentic GN **(Figs. 9.4A to D)**.

Treatment

Therapy of microscopic polyangiitis, GPA, and other ANCA-associated vasculitides is similar, and consists of induction and maintenance phases **(Flowchart 9.1)**.

Induction therapy: Induction therapy for new-onset ANCA-associated vasculitis is best given by the combination of glucocorticoids in combination with cyclophosphamide or rituximab **(Table 9.4)**. *IV cyclophosphamide and IV glucocorticoids are preferred for induction therapy in patients with markedly reduced or rapidly declining kidney function (serum creatinine > 4 mg/dL).* The combination of two IV doses of cyclophosphamide with rituximab can also be considered in this setting. Rituximab is preferred in children and adolescents where steroid sparing will be beneficial, relapsing disease and PR3-ANCA positive disease. While once-daily oral therapy with cyclophosphamide is as effective as once-monthly IV therapy, the latter is preferred in view of relatively lower toxicity, and ability to ensure compliance. Therapy with prednisone is tapered, to a dose of ~5–7.5 mg/day by 4 months. Therapy with avacopan, a C5a receptor antagonist, might be used for induction in patients at risk of glucocorticoid toxicity.

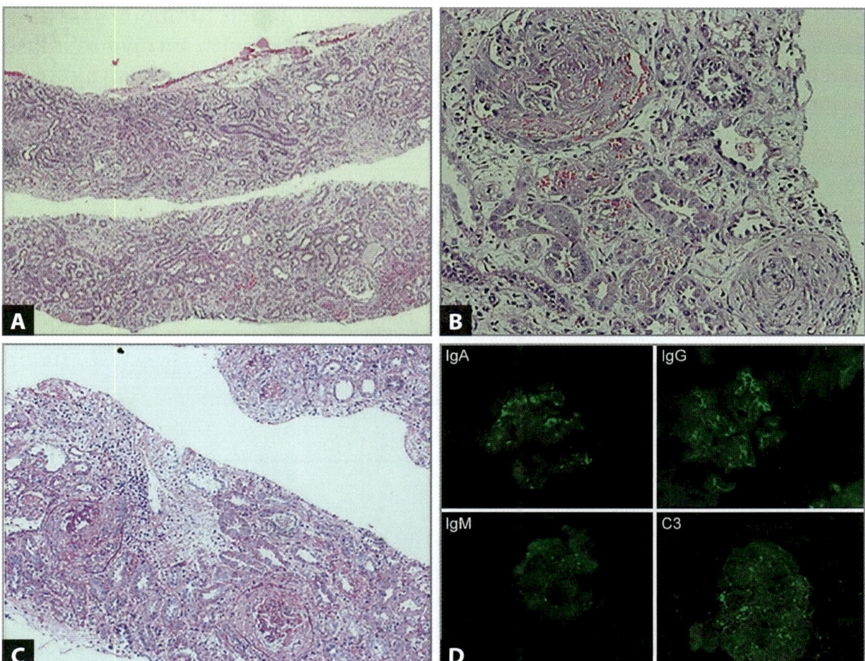

Figs. 9.4A to D: Kidney histology in a 11-year-old boy presenting with rapidly progressive glomerulonephritis and high titers of myeloperoxidase antineutrophil cytoplasmic antibodies (MPO-ANCA). (A) Low power view on light microscopy shows sclerosed and viable glomeruli along with mild tubulointerstitial atrophy (hematoxylin and eosin; 10x). High power view shows cellular and fibrocellular crescents with necrotizing lesions: (B) Hematoxylin and eosin; 40x and (C) Periodic acid Schiff; 40x. (D) Immunofluorescence was negative for immunoglobulin A (IgA), IgG, IgM, and C3.
Courtesy: Dr Adarsh Barwad, Department of Pathology, AIIMS, New Delhi

The role of plasma exchange in ANCA-associated vasculitis is debatable. Indications for plasma exchange include (*i*) serum creatinine >3.4 mg/dL requiring dialysis, or rapidly increasing serum creatinine; (*ii*) patients with diffuse alveolar hemorrhage with hypoxemia; (*iii*) overlap syndrome of ANCA vasculitis with antiglomerular basement membrane (GBM) antibodies; and (*iv*) illness that is refractory to standard therapy. The dosing and duration of plasma exchanges vary, with aggressive therapy for patients with pulmonary hemorrhage or anti-GBM antibodies. The usual dosing is with 60 mL/kg volume replacement, preferably with fresh frozen plasma.

A treatment algorithm for patients with ANCA-associated vasculitis with kidney involvement is given in **Flowchart 9.1**. Induction immunosuppressive therapy may be discontinued if patients are dialysis dependent after 3 months, and do not have extrarenal features of vasculitis.

Maintenance therapy: It follows induction treatment and is an important strategy that prevents the occurrence of relapses. Maintenance therapy is

Flowchart 9.1: Management of antineutrophil cytoplasmic antibodies (ANCA)-associated vasculitis. Induction immunosuppression with intravenous (IV) glucocorticoids and IV cyclophosphamide is preferred in patients with rapidly progressive glomerulonephritis and other manifestations of severe organ-threatening injury. Glucocorticoids should then be tapered over 3–4 months. MMF: mycophenolate mofetil

*Rituximab is preferred in patients with relapsing disease, PR3 ANCA positivity, and where significant steroid-sparing is desirable. Therapy in repeated courses may be used as maintenance immunosuppression, as detailed in text

**Indications for plasmapheresis are listed in text

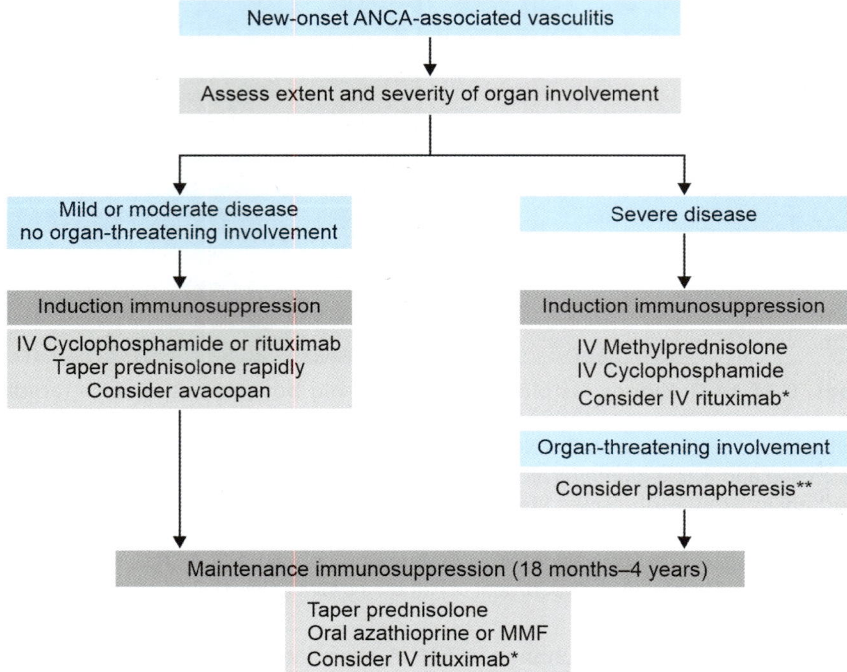

provided with either mycophenolate mofetil (MMF) or azathioprine, and low-dose prednisone. Rituximab is preferred as maintenance therapy in patients with relapses, PR3-ANCA disease, elderly patients, instances where corticosteroid sparing is important, allergy to azathioprine, or intolerance to MMF. Azathioprine or MMF may be preferred in children with low baseline IgG (<300 mg/dL), hepatitis B exposure, and/or limited availability of rituximab.

The optimal duration of maintenance therapy is 18 months–4 years. Recommendations for dosing and duration of maintenance therapy are given in **Table 9.4**. When considering stoppage of maintenance therapy, the risk of relapse should be considered and patients informed of the need for attention if symptoms recur. Factors that increase the risk of relapse are: (*i*) Baseline: Diagnosis of GPA, PR3-ANCA positive disease, extensive disease,

TABLE 9.4: ANCA-associated vasculitis: Dosing and duration of induction and maintenance therapy

Induction therapy	
Glucocorticoids	IV: Methylprednisolone 20–30 mg/kg/day (maximum 1 g/day) for 3–6 days[1] Oral: Prednisolone 1–2 mg/kg/day for 1 month, then tapered over 3-4 months
Cyclophosphamide	PO: 2 mg/kg/day for 3 months IV cyclophosphamide[#] 0.5–1.0 g/m^2 monthly for six doses; or 500 mg 2 weekly for 6 doses
Rituximab	375 mg/m^2/week for 4 weeks, or 750 mg/m^2 at weeks 0, 2
Cyclophosphamide with rituximab	Rituximab 375 mg/m^2/week for 4 weeks, with IV cyclophosphamide 15 mg/kg at weeks 0 and 2
Maintenance therapy	
Prednisolone	Continued at 5–7.5 mg/m^2/day for 2 years; then reduced by 1 mg every 2 months
Azathioprine	Start at 1.5–2 mg/kg/day at complete remission for 18–24 months, decrease to 1 mg/kg/day until 4 years after diagnosis; then taper by 25 mg every 3 months
Mycophenolate mofetil	2,000 mg/1.73 m^2 at complete remission for 2-years; reduce to 1,000–1,500 mg/1.73 m^2 until 4 years after diagnosis
Rituximab[†]	Continue for 18 months–4 years, after induction of remission. Rituximab may be dosed on a fixed schedule, or upon reappearance of CD19+ B cells and/or ANCA

ANCA: antineutrophil cytoplasmic antibodies; GFR: glomerular filtration rate

[1]Recent KDIGO guidelines advise that use of reduced-dose prednisolone and rituximab is as effective and associated with lower risk of infections

[#]Recent KDIGO guideline recommend IV Cyclophosphamide dose of 15 mg/kg at weeks 0, 2, 4, 7, 10, and 13 (if required, additionally at weeks 16, 19, 21, and 24). Reduce oral dose by 0.5 mg/kg/day and IV dose by 2.5 mg/kg for GFR <30 mL/min/1.73 m^2

[†]MAINRITSAN MAINtenance of Remission Using RITuximab in Systemic ANCA-associated Vasculitis; RITAZAREM Rituximab versus azathioprine as therapy for maintenance of remission for antineutrophil cytoplasm antibody associated vasculitis; MAINRITSAN: 500 mg for 2 doses at complete remission; repeat 500 mg at 6, 12, and 18 months; RITAZAREM: 1,000 mg infusion after induction of remission; repeat 1000 mg at 4, 8, 12, and 16 months

and ear-nose-throat disease; (*ii*) After diagnosis: History of relapse, ANCA positivity at end of induction, rise in ANCA titers; and (*iii*) Therapy related: Lower cyclophosphamide dose, and withdrawal of immunosuppressive medications.

Methotrexate is avoided either for induction or maintenance in patients with kidney disease, especially if eGFR is <60 mL/min per 1.73 m^2. Patients with relapsing disease (life- or organ-threatening) should again receive induction therapy, preferably with rituximab. Refractory kidney disease or lung hemorrhage can be treated by increase in dose of IV or oral glucocorticoids, or with use of rituximab if cyclophosphamide induction was used previously, or vice versa. Plasma exchanges may be considered for refractory disease, and in patients with lung hemorrhage with hypoxemia.

Patients with ANCA-associated vasculitis should be transplanted once they are in complete clinical remission for ≥6 months. Persistence of ANCA titers should not delay transplantation.

MEDIUM VESSEL VASCULITIS

Polyarteritis Nodosa

Childhood PAN is a necrotizing vasculitis associated with aneurysmal nodules along the walls of medium-sized muscular arteries in skin, joints, peripheral nerves, gastrointestinal tract, and other organs. It is the third most common childhood vasculitis after IgA vasculitis and Kawasaki disease. The onset is between 9 and 11 years and overall disease course is associated with fewer relapses and improved survival compared to adult-onset disease. Clinical features relate to vascular insufficiency mostly in the skin, muscles, kidneys, and gastrointestinal tract. Involvement of the heart, peripheral, and central nervous systems is less common and lungs are spared. Presenting features include malaise, fever, weight loss, abdominal pain, myalgia, and arthralgia. Renal involvement occurs in 50–60% of cases manifesting with hematuria and hypertension. In addition, testicular pain, neurological features such as focal deficits, hemiplegia, visual loss, mononeuritis multiplex, and ischemic heart disease may develop. Ruptured arterial aneurysms may result in massive intraabdominal hemorrhage. Painful subcutaneous nodules when present along affected vessels are characteristic.

Laboratory investigations show anemia, raised ESR, and thrombocytosis. Hepatitis B surface antigen may be detected in a few patients. The presence of vasculitis is confirmed on biopsy of involved muscle. The most valuable investigation is renal and hepatic angiography, which shows irregularity, stenosis, or occlusion of involved vessels **(Figs. 9.5A to D)**. Aneurysms in medium-sized artery observed on angiography (e.g., in renal, mesenteric, or coronary arteries) are suggestive, but are not specific as they can be seen in other forms of vasculitis. Childhood PAN differs from microscopic polyangiitis through the absence of necrotizing GN and the absence of ANCA.

The initial treatment is with corticosteroids alone or in conjunction with cyclophosphamide, followed by maintenance agents such as MMF or azathioprine for 2–3 years. In patients with severe organ damage, plasmapheresis is used. The role of biologic agents and rituximab in the management is being examined. Addition of antiplatelet drugs is recommended, especially in patients showing evidence of ischemia. Once controlled, the disease is self-limiting but early withdrawal of therapy may lead to relapses. The prognosis is variable with mortality ranging from 10 to 20% despite aggressive therapy.

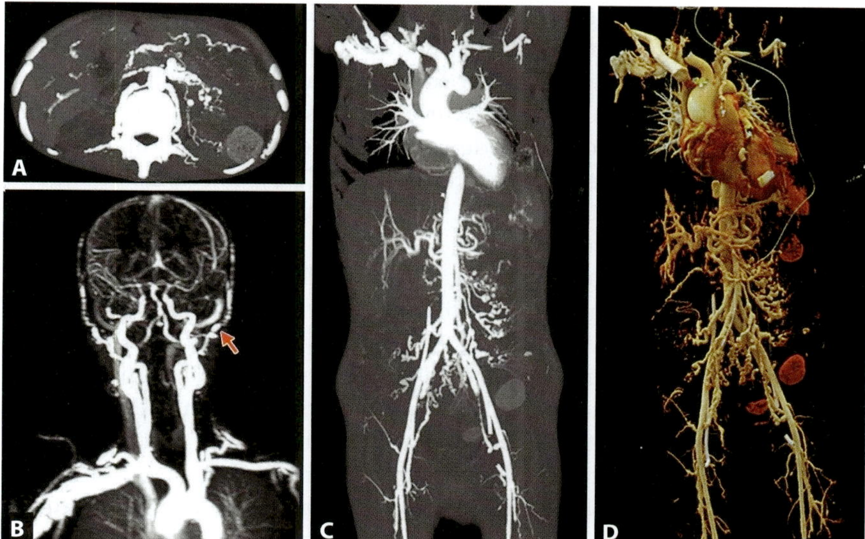

Figs. 9.5A to D: Polyarteritis nodosa (PAN) in a 12-year-old boy presenting with fever and weight loss for one month, followed by seizures and altered sensorium. Computed tomography and angiography show beaded arteries with alternating stenosis and dilatation characteristic of PAN: (A) Along the celiac axis and mesenteric and hepatic arteries in axial image of the abdomen; (B) External carotid, superficial temporal artery, and vertebral arteries in coronal images of the brain, and (C and D) Multiple visceral vessels in CT coronal reconstructed images. *Courtesy:* Prof Manisha Jana, Department of Radiodiagnosis, AIIMS, New Delhi

Deficiency of Adenosine Deaminase 2

Deficiency of adenosine deaminase 2 (ADA2) is a monogenic form of vasculitis, due to mutations in *ADA2* (previously termed *CECR1*). The disease closely mimics PAN. Features that suggest the diagnosis include early age at onset, family history of similar disease, presentation with ischemic or hemorrhagic stroke and livedo reticularis, presence of cytopenias, and absence of thrombocytosis. Low activity of ADA2 supports the diagnosis. Patients do not respond satisfactorily to conventional immunosuppressive therapy, but respond well to monoclonal medications inhibiting tumor necrosis factor (anti-TNF antibodies). Hematopoietic stem cell transplantation is curative for hematological abnormalities.

Kawasaki Disease

Kawasaki disease is an acute vasculitis occurring in young children. The diagnostic criteria include fever for 5 or more days, with 4 of the following 5 criteria: (*i*) bilateral nonpurulent conjunctival injection; (*ii*) changes in oral/mucosal cavity; (3) a polymorphic rash which is chiefly truncal;

(*iv*) swelling of extremities or periungual desquamation; and (*v*) cervical lymphadenopathy. Other features include irritability, abdominal pain, vomiting, diarrhea, arthralgia, and arthritis. Increase in hepatic transaminase enzymes and intermittent sterile pyuria is common. Renal involvement is uncommon. Investigations include complete blood counts, inflammatory markers, liver function tests, electrocardiogram (EKG), and echocardiogram. Complications include coronary artery aneurysms, coronary artery thrombosis, and myocarditis.

Treatment is aimed at decreasing systemic inflammation and preventing development of coronary aneurysm and thrombosis. Therapy is started with IV immunoglobulin (2 g/kg IV over 10–12 hr, while monitoring carefully for infusion reactions and fluid overload). Therapy may be repeated if fever persists beyond 36 hr of the first infusion. Other options for refractory disease, tested anecdotally, include pulse corticosteroids and biologicals agents, including anti-interleukin-1 (anakinra and canakinumab), and TNF inhibitors (infliximab, etanercept). High-dose aspirin is started at 30–80 mg/kg/day until the patient is afebrile for 48 hr and continued at 3–5 mg/kg/day for 6–8 weeks. The use of corticosteroids is controversial and limited to patients not responding to therapy with intravenous immunoglobulin (IVIG) and/or those at risk of developing coronary aneurysms.

LARGE VESSEL VASCULITIS

Takayasu Arteritis (Nonspecific Aortoarteritis)

Takayasu arteritis is a granulomatous vasculitis that predominantly affects the aorta and its major branches, most commonly the renal, subclavian, and carotid arteries. It is a common cause of renovascular hypertension in children in India and East Asian countries. Majority of cases are diagnosed during adolescence with a female preponderance. Demonstration of angiographic abnormalities on conventional imaging, CT, or MR **(Figs. 9.6A and B)** of the aorta or its main branches is necessary for diagnosis, which should include at least one of the features listed in **Table 9.1**.

An early phase of the disease is characterized by systemic features such as fever, anorexia, weight loss, cough, joint pains, and anemia, which often go unrecognized. Subsequently, hypertensive complications and features of renovascular hypertension and heart failure may develop. Patients may have claudicating pain in the extremities, absent pulses, and bruits. Occasional patients show glomerular lesions, chiefly mesangioproliferative glomerulonephritis. Although conventional angiography shows stenosis or occlusion of involved vessels, the procedure is invasive and cannot detect thickened vessel walls, an early sign of inflammation. Cross-sectional images on CT and MR angiograms and positron emission tomography (PET) may show vessel wall thickening in acute stages.

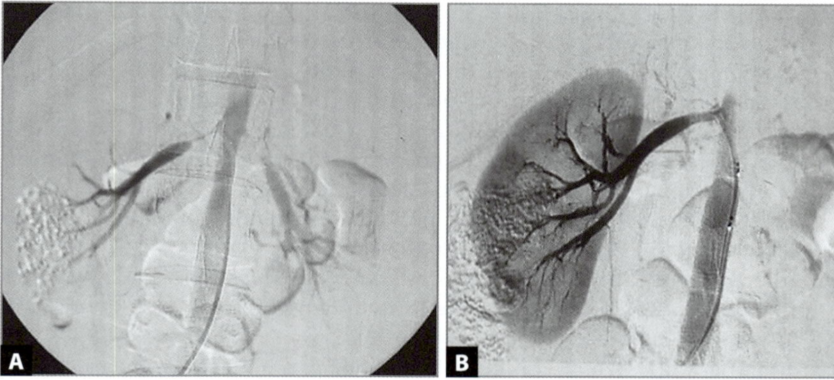

Figs. 9.6A and B: Takayasu aortoarteritis in a 10-year-old girl with severe hypertension. Digital subtraction angiogram showing (A) bilateral renal artery stenosis, and (b) dilated right renal artery after angioplasty in the same patient. *Courtesy:* Prof Sanjeev K Sharma, Department of Cardiac Radiology, AIIMS, New Delhi

The acute stage is best treated with corticosteroids, often in combination with cyclophosphamide and/or MMF. Therapy with anti-TNF agents and tocilizumab has been used in patients with refractory disease. Recent guidelines indicate a preference for TNF-inhibitors over tocilizumab in patients with refractory disease. Hypertension is controlled with appropriate medications. After the inflammatory phase is over and stenosis has developed, reconstructive vascular surgery or balloon angioplasty is employed. Patients with critical cranial or vertebrobasilar involvement may benefit from therapy with aspirin or another antiplatelet agent.

BIBLIOGRAPHY

1. Butters C, Curtis N, Burgner DP. Kawasaki disease fact check: Myths, misconceptions and mysteries. J Paediatr Child Health. 2020;56:1343-45.
2. Di Santo M, Stelmaszewski EV, Villa A. Takayasu arteritis in pediatrics. Cardiol Young. 2018;28:354-61.
3. Maz M, Chung SA, Abril A, et al. 2021 American College of Rheumatology/ Vasculitis Foundation guideline for the management of giant cell arteritis and Takayasu arteritis. Arthritis Rheumatol. 2021;73:1349-65.
4. McCrindle BW, Rowley AH, Newburger JW, et al; American Heart Association Rheumatic Fever, Endocarditis, and Kawasaki Disease Committee of the Council on Cardiovascular Disease in the Young; Council on Cardiovascular and Stroke Nursing; Council on Cardiovascular Surgery and Anesthesia; and Council on Epidemiology and Prevention. Diagnosis, Treatment, and Long-Term Management of Kawasaki Disease. Circulation. 2017;135:e927-99.
5. Ozen S, Marks SD, Brogan P, et al. European consensus-based recommendations for diagnosis and treatment of immunoglobulin A vasculitis - The SHARE initiative. Rheumatology (Oxford). 2019;58:1607-16.

6. Ozen S, Pistorio A, Iusan SM, et al. EULAR/PRINTO/PRES criteria or Henoch-Schönlein purpura, childhood polyarteritis nodosa, childhood Wegener granulomatosis and childhood Takayasu arteritis: Ankara 2008. Part II: Final classification criteria. Ann Rheum Dis. 2010;69:798-806.
7. Padmanabhan A, Smith CL, Aqui N, et al. Guidelines on use of therapeutic apheresis in clinical practice: Evidence based approach from the American Society for Apheresis. J Clin Apheresis. 2019;34:171-354.
8. Peruzzi L, Coppo R. IgA vasculitis nephritis in children and adults: One or different entities? Pediatr Nephrol. 2021;36:2615-25.
9. Pinto B, Deo P, Sharma S, et al. Expanding spectrum of DADA2: A review of phenotypes, genetics, pathogenesis and treatment. Clin Rheumatol. 2021;40:3883-96.
10. Sag E, Batu ED, Ozen S. Childhood systemic vasculitis. Best Pract Res Clin Rheumatol. 2017;31:558-75.
11. Schnabel A, Hedrich CM. Childhood vasculitis. Front Pediatr. 2019;6:421.
12. Watts RA, Hatemi G, Burns JC, et al. Global epidemiology of vasculitis. Nat Rev Rheumatol. 2022;18:22-34.
13. Welzel T, Winskill C, Zhang N, et al. Biologic disease modifying antirheumatic drugs and Janus kinase inhibitors in pediatric rheumatology-What we know and what we do not know from randomized controlled trials. Pediatr Rheumatol Online J. 2021;19:46.

CHAPTER 10

Lupus Nephritis

Arvind Bagga

Systemic lupus erythematosus (SLE) is a chronic, multisystem, and autoimmune disorder characterized by widespread inflammation of connective tissues affecting the skin, joints, kidneys, heart, lungs, and nervous system. SLE is most often diagnosed in women during the second to fourth decades of life, but ~20% of cases are diagnosed before the age of 18 years. Compared to adulthood-onset disease, childhood SLE is associated with more severe clinical features, higher prevalence of multiorgan system involvement, including nephritis and neuropsychiatric, hematological and cutaneous features, higher rates of macrophage activation syndrome and vasculitis, more frequent disease flares, and higher mortality. Nephritis is seen in 60–80% cases of SLE in children and constitutes an important determinant of prognosis.

CLINICAL FEATURES

Common clinical features include fever, a characteristic malar rash, mucocutaneous involvement, arthralgia, or arthritis. Proteinuria, urinary casts, thrombocytopenia, hemolytic anemia, hypertension, seizures, lymphadenopathy, Raynaud phenomena, and pleuritis may be present. Renal involvement is seen in almost half of the children with features ranging from minor abnormalities on urinalysis to severe renal insufficiency. Deranged renal function at onset is seen in 50% patients with about 2% presenting with acute renal failure requiring renal replacement therapy. A small proportion present with a rapidly progressive renal failure with crescentic glomerulonephritis. Patients are prone to arterial and venous thrombosis.

DIAGNOSIS

Criteria developed by the European League against Rheumatology and American College of Rheumatology (EULAR/ACR) in 2019 are used to classify childhood SLE **(Table 10.1)**. The diagnosis of SLE is made if the entry criterion of a positive antinuclear antibody is met, at least one additive clinical criterion is present, and the additive criteria add to a score of 10 or higher. In patients with positive antinuclear antibody (ANA), presence of class III or IV lupus nephritis **(Table 10.2)** on kidney biopsy is sufficient to diagnose SLE.

TABLE 10.1: European League Against Rheumatism/American College of Rheumatology 2019 classification criteria for systemic lupus erythematosus

*Entry criterion**	*Threshold*		
Antinuclear antibody	≥1:80 on Hep-2 cells, or an equivalent positive test		
*Additive criteria***	Diagnosis of SLE requires ≥1 clinical criterion/a and ≥10 points		
Clinical domains and criteria	*Weight*	*Clinical domains and criteria*	*Weight*
Constitutional Fever	 2	*Musculoskeletal* Joint involvement	 6
Mucocutaneous Nonscarring alopecia Oral ulcers Subacute cutaneous or discoid lupus Acute cutaneous lupus	 2 2 4 6	*Hematological* Leukopenia Thrombocytopenia Autoimmune hemolysis	 3 4 4
Renal involvement Proteinuria >0.5 g/day Kidney biopsy class II or V nephritis Kidney biopsy class III or IV nephritis	 4 8 10	*Neuropsychiatric* Delirium Psychosis Seizure	 2 3 5
Serosal Pleural or pericardial effusion Acute pericarditis	 5 6		
Immunological domains and criteria	*Weight*	*Immunological domains and criteria*	*Weight*
Antiphospholipid antibodies Anticardiolipin antibodies, anti-β2 glycoprotein 1 antibodies, or lupus anticoagulant	 2	*Complement proteins* Low C3 or low C4 Low C3 and low C4	 3 4
SLE-specific antibodies Anti-Smith or anti-dsDNA antibodies	 6		

* Entry criterion must be met to classify as SLE; can apply additive criteria only if it is met
**A criterion should not be counted if an alternative explanation is more likely than SLE; a criterion should be present on ≥1 occasion; the criteria need not be met simultaneously; and within each domain, only the highest weighed criterion is counted

Serological tests include antinuclear antibody [positive in 95% cases by enzyme-linked immunosorbent assay (ELISA)]; usually shows a homogeneous diffuse pattern on immunofluorescence and a peripheral pattern with active disease, antidouble stranded DNA (anti-dsDNA) (specific to SLE; high titers correlate with lupus nephritis) and complement C3, C4. Investigations that help in diagnosis and determination of severity include

TABLE 10.2: Histological classifications of lupus nephritis

WHO	*ISN/RPS nomenclature*	*Description*	*Changes from WHO classification*
Class I	Minimal mesangial lupus nephritis	Normal appearing glomeruli by LM with immune deposits confined to the mesangium by IF or by IF and EM	Elimination of "normal biopsy" category; lack of renal abnormalities by LM, IF, and EM does not qualify as class I
Class II	Mesangial proliferative lupus nephritis	Mesangial proliferation by LM and mesangial deposits by IF; isolated small immune deposits by IF or EM involving the peripheral capillary walls may be present. Any subendothelial deposits by EM qualify as classes III or IV	Class II includes mesangial proliferation of any degree as studies fail to show a difference in prognosis with mild, moderate, or severe mesangial proliferation
Class III **(Figs. 10.1A to D)**	Focal lupus nephritis[1] (<50% of glomeruli) (A) active; (A/C) active and chronic; (C) chronic lesions	Focal lupus nephritis involving <50% of glomeruli; affected glomeruli display segmental endocapillary proliferative lesions, with or without capillary wall necrosis and crescents, with subendothelial deposits	"Focal" replaces "focal proliferative" and "diffuse" replaces "diffuse proliferative". *A/C/AC:* Used to indicate activity and/ or chronicity
Class IV **(Figs. 10.2A and B)**	Diffuse lupus nephritis[2] (≥50% of glomeruli) (A), (A/C), (C)	Involvement of 50% or more glomeruli in the biopsy; lesions may be segmental (S) or global (G)	Subcategories for predominantly segmental (IV-S) and global (IV-G) lesions. For assessing glomerular lesions, both active and sclerotic lesions are counted
Class V **(Figs. 10.3A to C)**[3]	Membranous lupus nephritis	Membranous lesion with subepithelial immune deposits and mesangial hypercellularity. Any subendothelial deposits (on IF or EM) warrant a combined diagnosis of class III and V or class IV and V **(Figs. 10.4A to C)**	Biopsy with features of both diffuse and membranous lupus nephritis is accorded separate diagnosis of class IV and V, emphasizing the importance of the proliferative lesion
Class VI **(Fig. 10.5C)**	Advanced sclerosing lupus nephritis	Biopsies with >90% global glomerulosclerosis and clinical or pathologic evidence of sclerosis attributed to lupus nephritis	Absence of ongoing active glomerular disease

[1]Indicate proportion of glomeruli with active or sclerotic lesions

[2]Indicate proportion of glomeruli with fibrinoid necrosis and with cellular crescents

[3]Diagnosis of combined class III/IV and V requires membranous involvement of ≥50% of glomerular capillary surface area of ≥50% of glomeruli by LM or IF **(Figs. 10.4A to C)**

complete blood counts, erythrocyte sedimentation rate, C-reactive protein, and renal and liver function tests. Urinalysis and 24-hr protein excretion (or urine protein/creatinine ratio) are performed to evaluate renal involvement.

Other than ANA, various autoantibodies are present in patients with lupus. Screening for these antibodies, collectively termed "extractable nuclear antigens" is useful, although the prevalence varies, from 54 to 93% for anti-dsDNA, 17–52% for anti-Smith, 22–50% for antiribonucleoprotein (RNP), 33–54% for anti-Ro/SS-A, and 14–32% for anti-La/SS-B. Anti-Smith antibodies are highly specific to SLE and associated with central nervous system and kidney disease. Antiphospholipid antibodies (anticardiolipin antibodies and lupus anticoagulant) should be examined in patients with recurrent thrombosis, livedo reticularis, chorea, cerebrovascular accidents, and hypertension.

Rarely, lupus may be monogenic, secondary to one of various defects in genes encoding immune pathogenetic pathways, such as the complement system, phagocyte oxidase system, apoptosis, nucleic acid repair, DNA degradation, DNA sensing, type I IFN, and B-cell development. The condition should be suspected in patients presenting with early-onset severe disease, especially with kidney and central nervous system involvement. Screening for complement deficiencies, using CH50, AP50, C3, and C4 (or other validated classic and alternative complement pathway assays) may provide a clue to the diagnosis; genetic studies are confirmatory.

EVALUATION

All patients diagnosed with SLE should undergo comprehensive evaluation, at baseline and periodically, to define the disease extent and severity **(Box 10.1)**. European evidence-based recommendations for management of childhood SLE recommend that all patients be evaluated at regular intervals for parameters of disease activity using one of the two standardized validated disease activity instruments, namely Systemic Lupus Erythematosus Disease Activity Index (SLEDAI 2000 or SLEDAI-2K) or pediatric British Isles Lupus Assessment Group index 2004 (pBILAG-2004).

Renal Histology

Renal biopsy is carried out to plan the treatment and determine prognosis. The World Health Organization (WHO) classification of lupus nephritis is shown in **Table 10.2**. **Figures 10.1 to 10.7** show representative histological images. A revised classification proposed by the International Society of Nephrology and Renal Pathologic Society emphasizes the utility of activity and chronicity indices while reporting biopsies and standardizes definitions. The most severe type, diffuse proliferative lupus nephritis (class IV, **Figs. 10.2A and B**) is seen in 40–50% children, and focal lesions (class III, **Figs. 10.1A to D**) in 30%. Interstitial infiltration with T cells and macrophages, and tubulitis are

BOX 10.1: Evaluation at onset in patients with childhood-onset systemic lupus erythematosus

Blood investigations
Hemoglobin, total and differential leukocyte count, platelet count, erythrocyte sediment rate
Peripheral smear with reticulocyte count
C-reactive protein
Direct Coombs test
Urea, creatinine, sodium, potassium, calcium, phosphorus, alkaline phosphatase, alanine and aspartate aminotransferases, total protein, albumin, cholesterol
Free T3 and T4, thyroid-stimulating hormone
Complete lipid profile
Anti-HBs antibody
Antiphospholipid antibodies, lupus anticoagulant, anticardiolipin antibodies

Urinalysis
Urine microscopy
Urine protein to creatinine ratio (PCR) or 24-hr urine protein and creatinine

Imaging, additional evaluation
Ultrasound of kidneys
Chest X-ray
Electrocardiography, echocardiography
Retinal examination **(Figs. 10.8A and B)**

Additional evaluation (indications)
Kidney biopsy (if proteinuria, gross or microscopic hematuria, or acute kidney injury)
Pulmonary function test (if respiratory signs and symptoms)
Bone densitometry (symptoms of osteoporosis)
Bleeding and clotting time, prothrombin time, activated partial thromboplastin time (before biopsy)
Antibodies against extracted nuclear antigens

seen in 70%. The presence of immune deposits in mesangial, subepithelial, and subendothelial sites is striking. Immunoglobulin G (IgG) is the dominant immunoglobulin; IgM, IgA, C3, C4, and C1q are frequently present **(Figs. 10.6A to C)**. The simultaneous presence of all immunoglobulins, C3, C4, and C1q is suggestive of SLE, even if serological tests are negative. Patients with class I or II histology, absent or few immunoglobulin deposits that are confined to the mesangium, but with nephrotic range proteinuria are considered to have *lupus podocytopathy*. Electron microscopy in these cases shows diffuse and severe podocyte effacement and minimal mesangial deposits **(Fig. 10.7A)**.

TREATMENT

Multidisciplinary care is necessary for children and adolescents with SLE. General management includes administration of a steroid sparing agent, hydroxychloroquine sulfate (HCQS, 4–6 mg/kg/day) and application of a

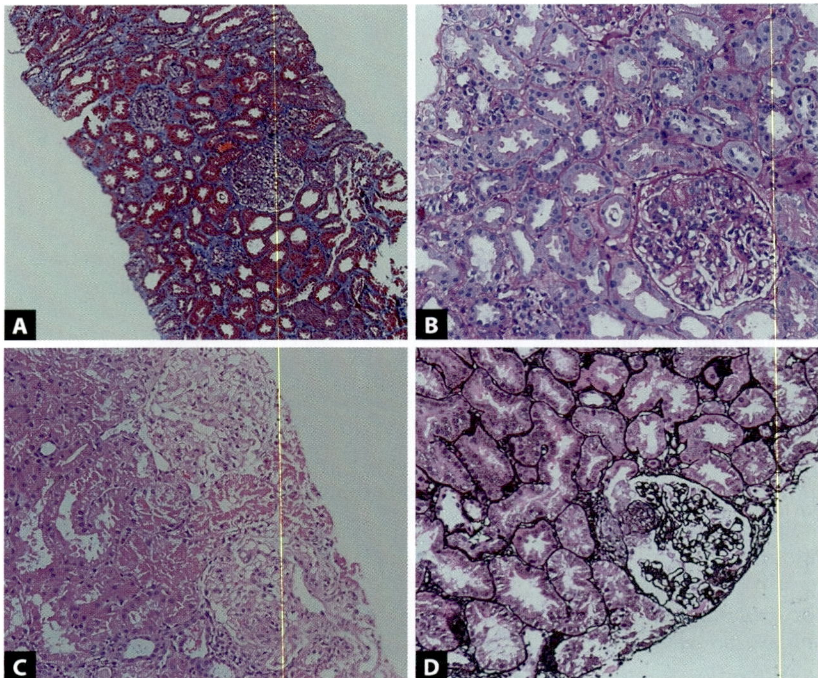

Figs. 10.1A to D: Class III lupus nephritis. (A) Representative photomicrograph showing segmental endocapillary hypercellularity in one of the three glomeruli (Masson's trichome, 100X); (B) High power image of the same glomerulus displaying segmental endocapillary hypercellularity with mononuclear cells obliterating capillary lumina (Periodic acid Schiff, 200X); (C) Representative photomicrograph of another case showing segmental necrotizing lesion in one of the two glomeruli (Hematoxylin & eosin, 100X); (D) High power image of the same glomerulus displaying segmental tuft necrosis with fibrin and overlying small cellular crescent (Jones methenamine silver, 200X). *Courtesy:* Dr Adarsh Barwad, Department of Pathology, AIIMS, New Delhi

sunscreen in children with skin disease and arthritis. Therapy with HCQS is associated with lower rates of kidney flare, higher rates of response to therapy, improved lipid profile, and higher bone mass. Naproxen (15–20 mg/kg/day) or ibuprofen (40 mg/kg/day) is recommended for patients with systemic and musculoskeletal features. Angiotensin-converting enzyme inhibitors are used for management of hypertension and/or proteinuria, and hydroxymethylglutaryl-coenzyme A (HMG-CoA) reductase inhibitors for dyslipidemia. Patients with SLE show high prevalence of vitamin D deficiency, chiefly due to photosensitivity and sun avoidance. Association of exacerbation of disease activity with vitamin D deficiency has prompted recommendations for correcting deficiency with 60,000 IU vitamin D_3 weekly for 4–6 weeks, followed by 1,000 IU vitamin D_3 daily.

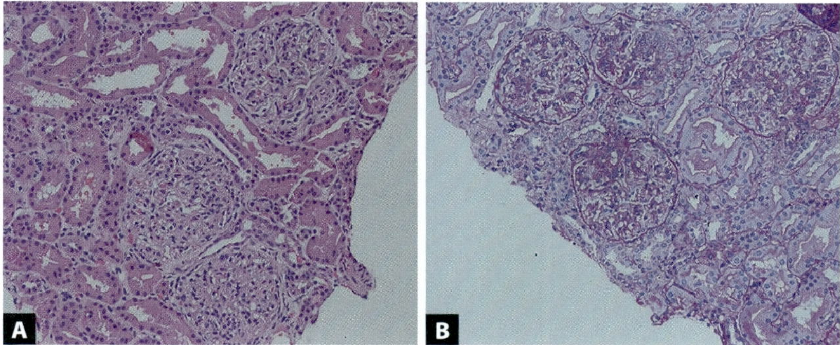

Figs. 10.2A and B: Class IV lupus nephritis. (A) Representative photomicrograph showing segmental to diffuse endocapillary hypercellularity in all the glomeruli (Hematoxylin & eosin, 200X); (B) Another image of the same case displaying diffuse mesangial and endocapillary hypercellularity with mononuclear cells obliterating capillary lumina. In addition, one cellular crescent is also identified (Periodic acid Schiff, 200X). *Courtesy:* Dr Adarsh Barwad, Department of Pathology, AIIMS, New Delhi

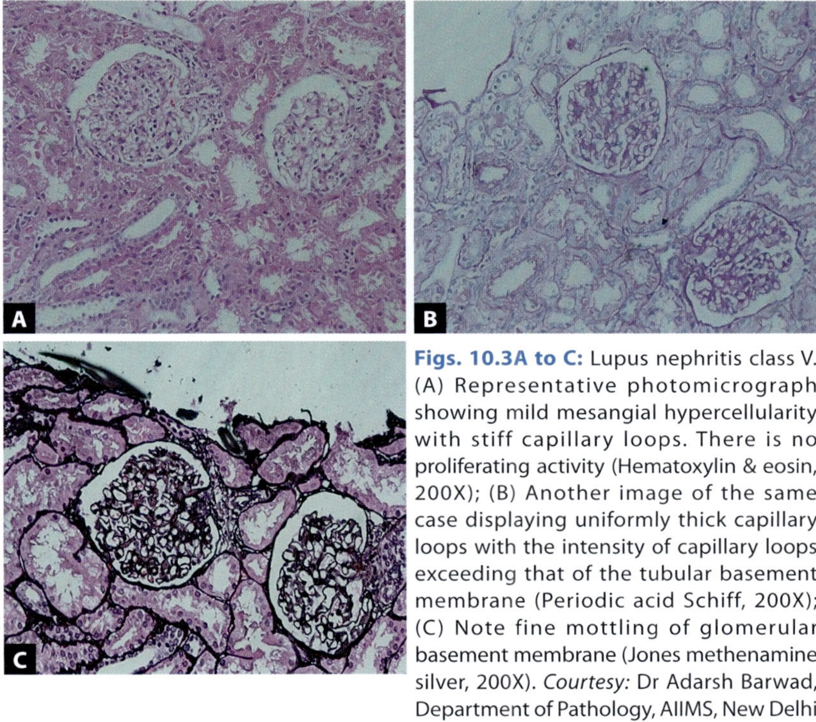

Figs. 10.3A to C: Lupus nephritis class V. (A) Representative photomicrograph showing mild mesangial hypercellularity with stiff capillary loops. There is no proliferating activity (Hematoxylin & eosin, 200X); (B) Another image of the same case displaying uniformly thick capillary loops with the intensity of capillary loops exceeding that of the tubular basement membrane (Periodic acid Schiff, 200X); (C) Note fine mottling of glomerular basement membrane (Jones methenamine silver, 200X). *Courtesy:* Dr Adarsh Barwad, Department of Pathology, AIIMS, New Delhi

Induction Immunosuppression

The treatment of lupus nephritis depends on its severity **(Table 10.3)**. No specific medications are required for mild lupus nephritis (classes I–II). In moderate-to-severe nephritis (classes III and IV), remission is induced

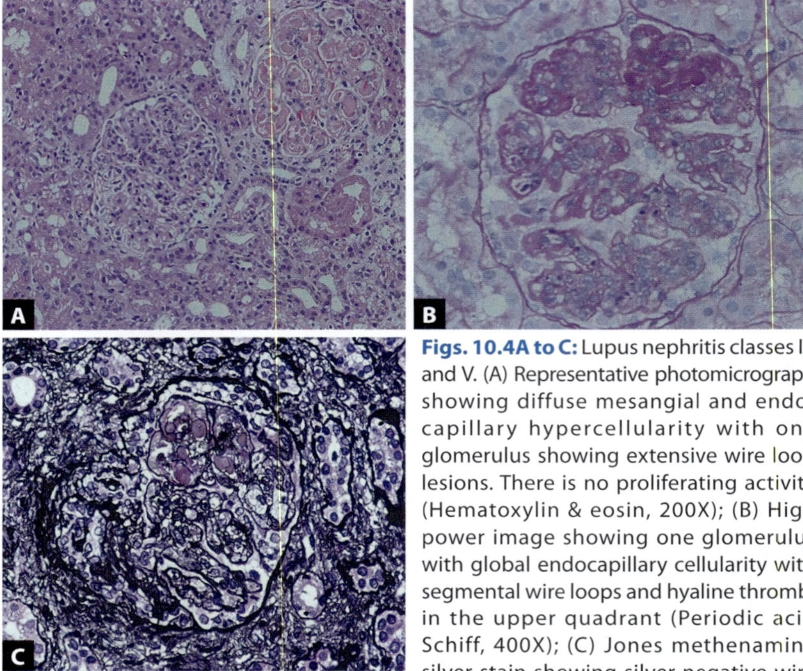

Figs. 10.4A to C: Lupus nephritis classes IV and V. (A) Representative photomicrograph showing diffuse mesangial and endocapillary hypercellularity with one glomerulus showing extensive wire loop lesions. There is no proliferating activity (Hematoxylin & eosin, 200X); (B) High power image showing one glomerulus with global endocapillary cellularity with segmental wire loops and hyaline thrombi in the upper quadrant (Periodic acid Schiff, 400X); (C) Jones methenamine silver stain showing silver negative wire loops, diffuse spikes and crater formation, hyaline thrombi in the upper quadrant of the glomerulus, a fibrocellular crescent on the left side (Jones methenamine silver, 400X).
Courtesy: Dr Adarsh Barwad, Department of Pathology, AIIMS, New Delhi

with IV followed by oral steroids, along with IV cyclophosphamide pulses. Prednisolone is initially given at a dose of 0.8–1.0 mg/kg/day for 2–4 weeks and then gradually tapered to a maintenance dose of 0.1–0.15 mg/kg/day by 6 months. Cyclophosphamide is given intravenously every 4 weeks for 6 pulses; oral therapy (2 mg/kg daily for 3-4 months) may be considered in patients with class II nephritis. While an important component of most induction protocols for classes II–IV lupus nephritis, therapy with cyclophosphamide carries the risk of infections; long-term toxicity is unlikely in the doses indicated above. Therapy with mycophenolate mofetil (MMF) is as effective as IV cyclophosphamide for induction of remission, with a better safety profile.

Triple drug therapy with a calcineurin inhibitor may be considered in patients with estimated glomerular filtration rate (eGFR) $\geq$ 45 mL/min/1.73 m^2 who also have heavy proteinuria due to podocyte injury. Alternatively, triple drug therapy with belimumab may be preferred in patients with high risk of nephritic flares or advanced CKD (eGFR < 30 mL/min/1.73 m^2).

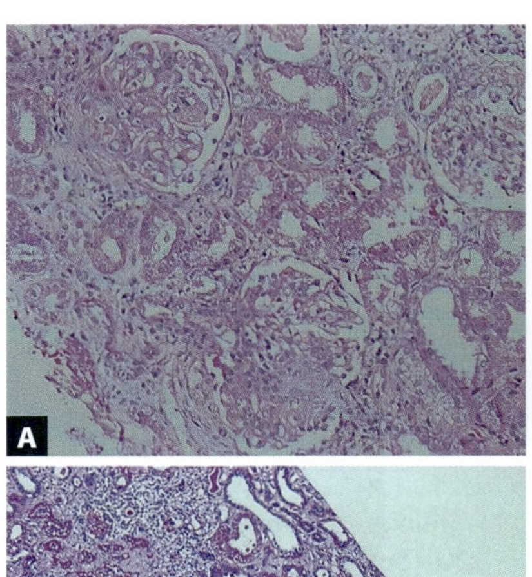

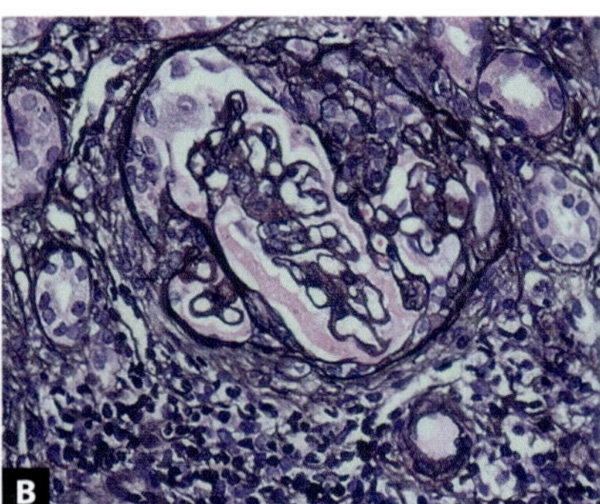

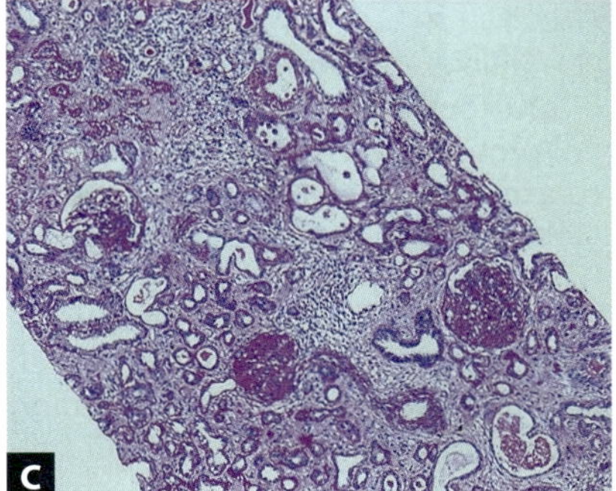

Figs. 10.5A to C: Chronic lesions in lupus nephritis. (A) Histological photomicrograph of follow-up biopsy in a patient with lupus nephritis class IV, showing chronic changes in the form of segmental sclerosis in two of the three glomeruli. One glomerulus also showed segmental wire loop like lesion (Hematoxylin & eosin, 200X); (B) High power image shows one glomerulus with segmental sclerosis and overlying fibrocellular crescent. The glomerular basement membrane displays reduplication with silver negative material representing immune complexes (wire loops) (Jones methenamine silver, 400X); (C) Histological photomicrograph of a case of lupus nephritis class VI showing all glomeruli in advanced stage of sclerosis, along with high chronicity in the background tubulointerstitial compartment in the form of tubular atrophy, interstitial fibrosis, and moderate chronic inflammation (Hematoxylin & eosin, 100X). *Courtesy:* Dr Adarsh Barwad, Department of Pathology, AIIMS, New Delhi

In patients with rapidly progressive renal failure or those showing sudden deterioration of renal function, 3–6 daily or alternate day doses of IV pulse methylprednisolone (15–20 mg/kg/dose) are used before administering oral corticosteroids. Plasma exchange and IV immunoglobulin may be helpful in some patients.

Maintenance Therapy

Following induction, cyclophosphamide is replaced with MMF (first choice) or azathioprine. A calcineurin inhibitor may be used if MMF or azathioprine is not tolerated. Patients who have received triple therapy during induction may remain on belimumab or calcineurin inhibitors for an extended duration of ~2 years. Low-dose therapy with prednisolone is continued, except when escalation is required for features of extrarenal lupus. Most patients require 3 or more years of maintenance therapy.

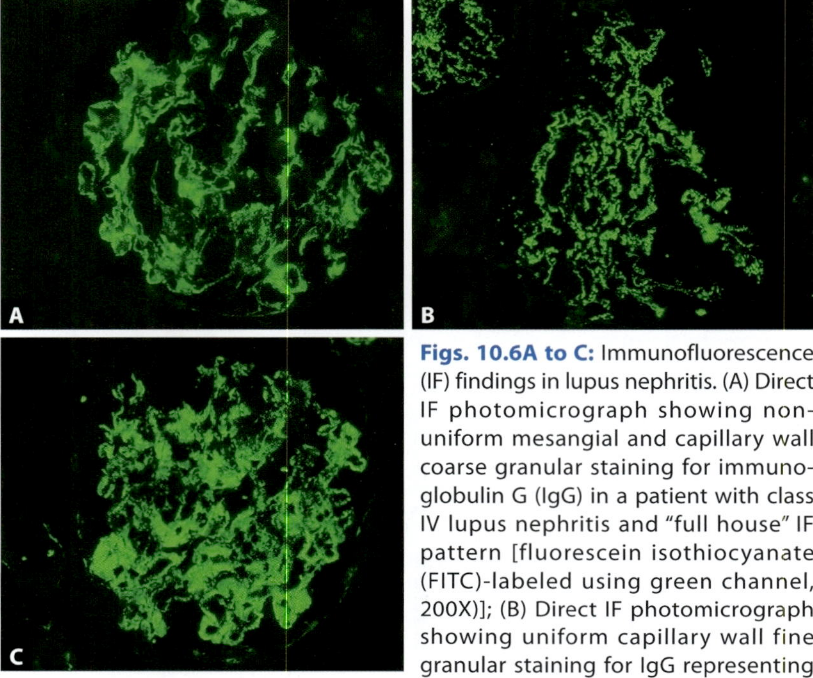

Figs. 10.6A to C: Immunofluorescence (IF) findings in lupus nephritis. (A) Direct IF photomicrograph showing non-uniform mesangial and capillary wall coarse granular staining for immunoglobulin G (IgG) in a patient with class IV lupus nephritis and "full house" IF pattern [fluorescein isothiocyanate (FITC)-labeled using green channel, 200X)]; (B) Direct IF photomicrograph showing uniform capillary wall fine granular staining for IgG representing full-house IF pattern of class V lupus nephritis (FITC-labeled using green channel, 200X); (C) Direct IF photomicrograph showing mesangial and capillary wall fine granular staining for IgG. In addition, there is segmental coarse granular capillary wall staining, representing subendothelial deposits of wire loops, in a case of lupus nephritis class IV+V (FITC-labeled using green channel, 200X). *Courtesy:* Dr Adarsh Barwad, Department of Pathology, AIIMS, New Delhi

Patients with class V nephritis **(Figs. 10.3A to C)** are treated with a combination of prednisolone and MMF, with satisfactory response in the majority. Alternate therapies include cyclophosphamide, calcineurin inhibitors, or rituximab.

PROGNOSIS

Screening for new features (rash, arthritis, serositis, seizures, and psychosis), laboratory analyses (blood count, creatinine, and urinalysis), and serologic tests (blood C3, anti-dsDNA, anti-Ro/SSA, anti-La/SSB, antiphospholipid, and anti-RNP) are used for monitoring the course of the disease. Patients should be evaluated for comorbidities, including acute and chronic infections, hypertension, dyslipidemia, and autoimmune disorders **(Box 10.1)**. Patients receiving HCQS should have a baseline retinal examination, followed by annual retinal testing, especially after 5 years of use **(Figs. 10.8A and B)**.

TABLE 10.3: Treatment of lupus nephritis

WHO Class	*Treatment*
I. Minimal mesangial lupus nephritis	No specific therapy Treat as dictated by extrarenal manifestations
II. Mesangial proliferative lupus nephritis • With no or minimal proteinuria • With moderate to heavy proteinuria	• Treat as dictated by extrarenal manifestations; hydroxychloroquine sulfate (HCQS) • Consider lupus podocytopathy • Prednisone (1–1.5 mg/kg/day for 4–6 weeks, then tapered[1]); azathioprine (AZA) (1–2 mg/kg/day) or mycophenolate mofetil (MMF)
III and IV. Focal, diffuse lupus nephritis	• *Induction:* IV methylprednisolone 10–30 mg/kg/day for 1–3 days depending on disease severity; prednisone 0.8–1.0 mg/kg/day for 2–4 weeks, and taper to 0.1–0.15 mg/kg by 6-month, and one of the following: – IV cyclophosphamide 0.5–1.0 g/m^2 monthly for six doses; or 500 mg 2 weekly for 6 doses; or 2.0 mg/kg/day orally for 3 months – Mycophenolate mofetil (MMF) 1,000–1,200 mg/m^2/day for 6 months – MMF as above, and tacrolimus (trough 4–6 ng/mL), or voclosporin (23.7 mg twice daily), or cyclosporine. The duration of therapy with any of the calcineurin inhibitors is 2–3 years – Belimumab with MMF, or low-dose cyclophosphamide. Duration of therapy with belimumab ~2.5 years • *Maintenance:* Low-dose prednisolone (0.1–0.2 mg/kg/day) and MMF (1,000–1,200 mg/m^2/day in two divided doses), or azathioprine (1.5–2 mg/kg/day). Therapy with MMF is preferred, except in pregnancy • *Alternative agents for maintenance therapy:* Belimumab and calcineurin inhibitors
V. Membranous lupus nephritis • Normal function, non-nephrotic proteinuria • Persistent nephrotic proteinuria	• ACE-I/ARBs; other therapy dictated by extrarenal features; HCQS • Corticosteroids with oral MMF • *Alternate agents:* Cyclophosphamide, calcineurin inhibitors, rituximab, or azathioprine
VI. Advanced sclerosis lupus nephritis	Treat as dictated by extrarenal manifestations; HCQS
Relapse	Consider original induction and maintenance regimen; consider other therapies; repeat biopsy if suspected change in histology, high creatinine, or worsening proteinuria
Resistant disease	Consider alternative initial treatment regimen; consider treatment with rituximab, IV immunoglobulin, or calcineurin inhibitors

[1]Prednisolone is tapered by 2.5–5 mg/week when prednisolone dose is 20–40 mg/day; 2.5 mg/week for dose of 10–20 mg/day; and 1 mg every 2–4 weeks for doses below 10 mg/day

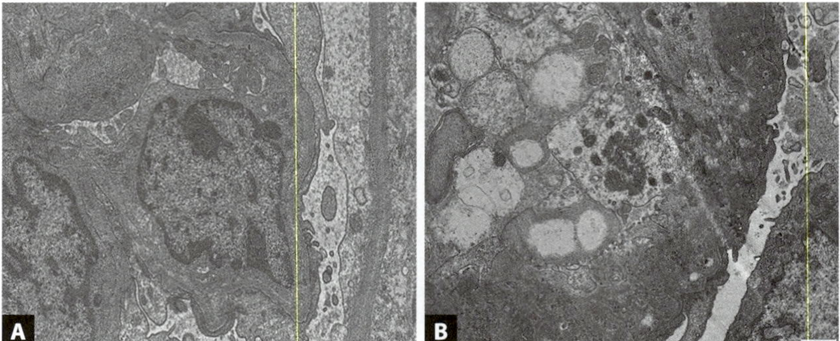

Figs. 10.7A and B: Electron microscopy findings in lupus nephritis. (A) Ultrastructural photomicrograph of a case of lupus podocytopathy showing diffuse effacement of foot processes. The morphology of the glomerular basement membrane was unaltered. There were no immune complexes in the form of unorganized electron dense deposits in mesangial, subendothelial, or subepithelial location (uranyl acetate, 4000X); (B) Ultrastructural photomicrograph of a case of lupus nephritis class V showing abundant subepithelial electron dense deposits of varying sizes, representing subepithelial immune complexes. A few tubuloreticular inclusions were also identified as electron-dense, irregular structures within the cytoplasm of endothelial cells (uranyl acetate, 4000X). *Courtesy:* Dr Adarsh Barwad, Department of Pathology, AIIMS, New Delhi

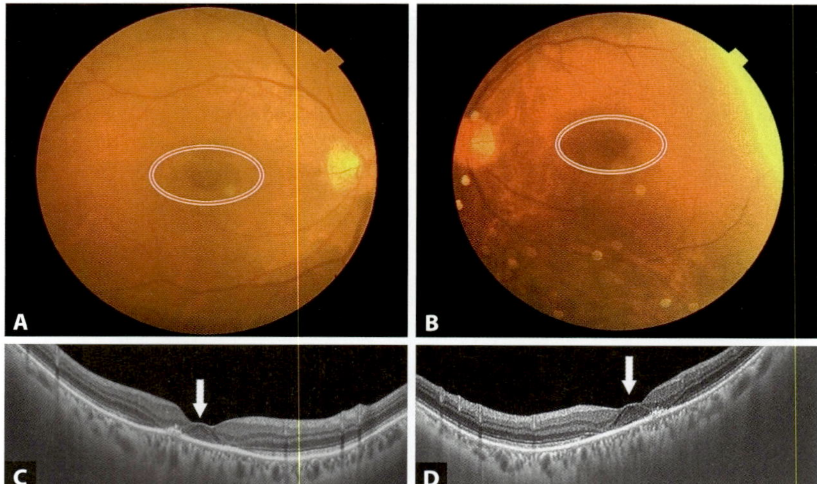

Figs. 10.8A to D: Bulls eye appearance of macula following chronic use of hydroxychloroquine sulfate (HCQS). HCQS destroys the macular rod and cone photoreceptors while sparing the foveal cones. The typical appearance is caused by migration of retinal pigmentary epithelium into these destroyed areas, causing pigment laden cells to be detected in the outer nuclear and outer plexiform layers. Color fundus photography of right (A) and left (B) eyes shows pigmentary mottling around the perifoveal region with blunting of foveal reflex (red circles). (C and D) Optical coherence tomography (OCT) of the corresponding area shows "flying saucer" sign with outer retinal atrophy in the perifoveal region. *Courtesy:* Dr. N Shaikh, Dr. R Chawla, Dr Rajendra Prasad Centre for Ophthalmic Sciences, AIIMS, New Delhi

Childhood-onset lupus nephritis carries a worse prognosis than the disease in adults. Patients with SLE show increased mortality when compared to the general population. Early mortality is related to infections or lupus activity, while kidney failure and malignancies account for late mortality. Relapses of lupus nephritis occur in approximately one-third of treated patients and are associated with adverse kidney outcomes, such as deterioration of renal function and higher risk for end-stage kidney failure. However, mortality from renal failure has declined with the use of effective therapies. Transplantation in patients with lupus nephritis has similar long-term graft survival when matched to controls, with <10% likelihood of recurrence in the graft.

BIBLIOGRAPHY

1. Alperin JM, Ortiz-Fernández L, Sawalha AH. Monogenic lupus: A developing paradigm of disease. Front Immunol. 2018;9:2496.
2. Charras A, Smith E, Hedrich CM. Systemic lupus erythematosus in children and young people. Curr Rheumatol Rep. 2021;23:20.
3. Groot N, de Graeff N, Avcin T, et al. European evidence-based recommendations for diagnosis and treatment of childhood-onset systemic lupus erythematosus: the SHARE initiative. Ann Rheum Dis. 2017;76:1788-96.
4. Khandelwal P, Govindarajan S, Bagga A. Management and outcomes in children with lupus nephritis in the developing countries. Pediatr Nephrol. 2023;38:987-1000.
5. Oni L, Wright RD, Marks S, et al. Kidney outcomes for children with lupus nephritis. Pediatr Nephrol. 2021;36:1377-85.
6. Rovin BH, Ayoub IM, Chan TM, et al. Executive Summary of the KDIGO 2024 Clinical Practice Guideline for the Management of Lupus Nephritis. Kidney Int. 2024;105:31-34.
7. Trindade VC, Carneiro-Sampaio M, Bonfa E, et al. An update on the management of childhood-onset systemic lupus erythematosus. Pediatr Drugs. 2021;23:331-47.

Steroid Sensitive Nephrotic Syndrome

Arvind Bagga, Aditi Sinha

Nephrotic syndrome, characterized by edema, heavy proteinuria (>1 g/m^2 per day; >40 mg/m^2/h), and hypoalbuminemia (serum albumin <3 g/dL), is a rare disease affecting approximately 1.2–16.9 (mean 2.9) per 100,000 children annually. A higher incidence of the illness is seen in Southeast and East Asia, compared to Europe, North America, and Oceania.

Most cases in childhood are idiopathic, and an underlying systemic illness (e.g., amyloidosis, lupus, and IgA vasculitis) is found in <10% patients. More than 85% of patients with idiopathic nephrotic syndrome show remission following therapy with oral corticosteroids. Almost 70–75% of patients show more than one episode of the disease. While patients with steroid-sensitive nephrotic syndrome experience disease relapses at varying frequency throughout childhood, the long-term outcome is usually favorable. About 10–15% of patients do not respond to corticosteroids, either at onset (initial steroid resistance) or following a subsequent relapse (late steroid resistance). Management of patients with steroid-resistant nephrotic syndrome is challenging, particularly if the disease does not respond to next line therapy with calcineurin inhibitors (CNIs). This chapter summarizes the current understanding on the etiopathogenesis of nephrotic syndrome and principles of management of steroid-sensitive disease. Steroid-resistant nephrotic syndrome is discussed in Chapter 12.

PATHOLOGY

Almost 80% patients with nephrotic syndrome do not show significant glomerular changes on light microscopy, no deposits on immunofluorescence examination, and effacement of podocytes with disruption and disorganization of actin filaments on electron microscopy, termed minimal change disease. About 40–70% patients with steroid-resistant nephrotic syndrome and 5–8% with steroid-sensitive disease have focal segmental glomerulosclerosis (FSGS), characterized by sclerosis involving a segment of the glomerular tuft. A proportion of patients with FSGS show variable degrees of mesangial proliferation. A small proportion of patients with steroid resistance, particularly older (>12 years old) children, show membranous nephropathy, C3 glomerulopathy (membranoproliferative glomerulonephritis), or IgA nephropathy.

PATHOGENESIS

The glomerular filtration barrier consists of capillary endothelial fenestrations, glomerular basement membrane (GBM), and interdigitating podocyte foot processes. Proteinuria in nephrotic syndrome results from dysfunction of podocytes, leading to loss of the selective filtering function. **Figure 11.1** summarizes the prevailing hypotheses on pathogenesis of nephrotic syndrome.

In about 15–20% of cases of initial steroid resistance, the disease is caused by mutations in genes encoding structural elements of the podocyte slit diaphragm or cytoskeleton (*NPHS1, NPHS2, CD2AP, TRCP6*, and *ACTN4*), GBM proteins (*LAMB2, COL4A5*), mitochondrial genes (*COQ2*), or transcription factors (*WT1, LMX1B*). While loci on MHC class II, *HLA-DQ* and *HLA-DR*, and few non-HLA loci (*CALHM6/DSE, TNFSF15, BTNL2*, and *KIRREL2*) are reported as risk alleles for steroid-sensitive nephrotic syndrome, they appear insufficient to cause disease alone. A multiple hit hypothesis is proposed in steroid-sensitive disease, wherein risk alleles interact with environmental factors, leading to immune disturbances, podocyte dysfunction, and proteinuria. Environmental triggers for relapses of nephrotic syndrome include respiratory viruses, Epstein–Barr virus (EBV), other infections, aero- and food allergens, and insect bites.

The majority of cases of nephrotic syndrome, particularly steroid-sensitive disease, are considered to be associated with immune dysfunction. Experimental evidence suggests that alterations in cell-mediated immunity may lead to T helper type 2 (Th2) polarization and the release of an uncharacterized circulating factor that increases glomerular permeability. Studies also suggest an imbalance between Th17 and regulatory T cells that potentially causes persistent activation of Th2 cells; alternatively, deficient action by regulatory T cells might be responsible for inadequate censoring of podocyte CD80 (B7-1) expression that is upregulated in models of minimal change disease. Nephrotic syndrome is associated with immunodeficiency, polyendocrinopathy, and enteropathy (IPEX) syndrome, an X-linked disease due to variants in *FOXP3* that inactivate T regulatory cells.

The rapidity with which relapses follow minor infections suggests the involvement of innate immunity, likely involving activation of toll-like receptors and nuclear factor kappa signaling in antigen-presenting cells, which might influence humoral immune responses. Recent reports also suggest the pathogenic role of B cell abnormalities, given the response to therapy with anti-CD20 medications (rituximab and ofatumumab), and the presence of autoantibodies to nephrin, slit diaphragm, CD40, and ubiquitin carboxyl-terminal hydrolase L1 (UCHL1) in plasma of patients with nephrotic syndrome (**Fig. 11.1**). Reconstitution of switched memory B cells (isotype switching from IgM to IgG production) is an important predictor of post-rituximab relapses, supporting the importance of B-cells in the pathogenesis.

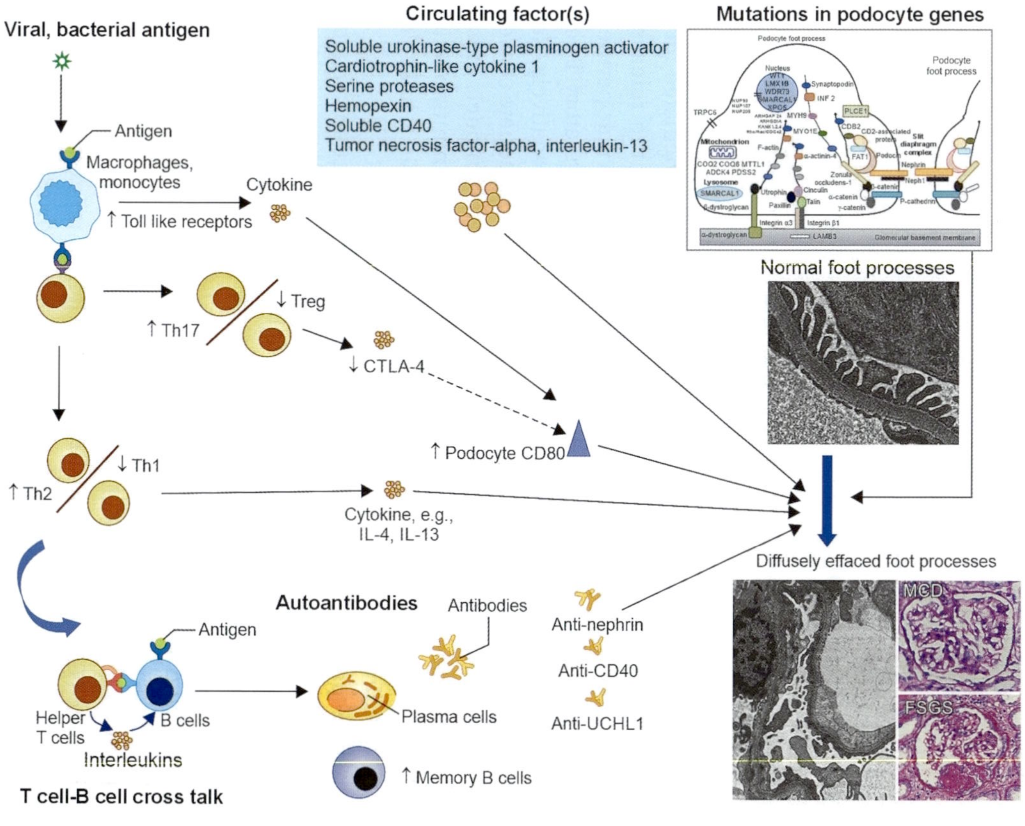

Fig. 11.1: Pathogenesis of nephrotic syndrome in childhood. In most patients with steroid sensitive disease, minor infections trigger relapses, likely through stimulation of naïve immune responses. Signaling through toll like receptors triggers cytokine secretion; some cytokines may act directly or indirectly on the podocytes. Alternatively, antigen presentation to helper T cells might alter the balance of Th2/Th1 and Th17/T-regulatory cells or influence T-B cells cross-talk, resulting in the production of pathogenic cytokine(s) that alter podocyte permeability, or result in podocyte CD80uria. Both reduced T-regulatory cells and increased memory B cells are linked to relapses. Recent studies suggest the presence of circulating autoantibodies such as anti-nephrin, anti-UCHL1, anti-CD40 and anti-slit diaphragm antibodies. Risk alleles involving MHC class II loci as well as non HLA-loci has also been proposed in the pathogenesis of steroid sensitive disease. Steroid-resistant nephrotic syndrome is postulated to result from either circulating factors or pathogenic variants in genes encoding podocyte proteins (see text)

Steroid-resistant nephrotic syndrome is considered to be mediated by a "soluble mediator", a hypothesis that is supported by recurrence of nephrotic range proteinuria immediately post-transplant in 30–50% of patients with idiopathic FSGS who develop kidney failure. It is supported by experimental evidence in which nephrotic plasma induces changes in distribution of podocyte cytoskeletal and slit diaphragm proteins, foot process effacement, and increase in vascular permeability. The proposed circulating factors include interleukin-13, tumor necrosis factor-α, heparanase, hemopexin, cardiotrophin-like cytokine-1, C-maf-inducing protein, soluble urokinase-type plasminogen activator receptor, vascular endothelial growth factor, anti-CD40, anti-nephrin or anti-slit diaphragm antibody, and soluble CD40 ligand. However, none of these factors have been shown to be implicated unequivocally.

The precise immune perturbations underlying nephrotic syndrome and the identity of the circulating factor remain elusive. Given lack of understanding of the pathogenesis of proteinuria, the rationale for using immunosuppressive therapies remains empiric and is guided chiefly by clinical studies. Almost all medications used for nephrotic syndrome have been shown to inhibit or modify humoral or cellular immune responses. Podocytes are also potential targets for these interventions, including for corticosteroids, levamisole, and CNIs.

CLINICAL FEATURES

The onset of minimal change disease is usually between the ages of 2 and 6 years. The condition is more common in boys (60–70%) and occurrence in siblings is rare. When nephrotic syndrome starts after the age of 12–16 years, the chances of a significant underlying lesion are higher. The onset is insidious with swelling around the eyes and facial puffiness, noticeable in the morning but resolving when the child is ambulatory. In some cases, an upper respiratory tract infection may be present, but the child looks well. The facial puffiness may be mistakenly ascribed to allergy, conjunctivitis, mumps, or dental infection. The swelling increases to result in edema and anasarca. Mild diarrhea is not uncommon, probably due to intestinal edema. Occasionally, anasarca is associated with gross hematuria and oliguria. Such cases present a picture of nephrotic and nephritic syndrome, and require detailed evaluation including a kidney biopsy.

DEFINITIONS

Nephrotic syndrome is defined by the occurrence of edema in the presence of hypoalbuminemia and nephrotic range proteinuria. **Table 11.1** provides key definitions of disease course of nephrotic syndrome. "Frequent relapsers" include patients with "steroid dependence", a term that identifies a subgroup of patients who fail to sustain remission once steroids are discontinued

TABLE 11.1: Definitions of disease course in steroid-sensitive nephrotic syndrome

Nephrotic syndrome	Edema, heavy proteinuria (>1 g/m^2 per day; >40 mg/m^2/h), and hypoalbuminemia (serum albumin <3 g/dL)
Remission	Urine protein nil or trace (Up/Uc <0.2 mg/mg) for 3 consecutive early morning specimens
Relapse	Urine protein >3+ (Up/Uc >2 mg/mg) for 3 consecutive early morning specimens, having been in remission previously
Frequent relapses	2 or more relapses in the 6 months following therapy of the initial episode; ≥3 relapses in any 12 months
Steroid dependence	Two consecutive relapses when on alternate day steroids, or within 14 days of its discontinuation
Steroid resistance	Lack of complete remission despite therapy with daily prednisolone at a dose of 2 mg/kg (60 mg/m^2) daily for 6 weeks[1,2] *Initial resistance:* Steroid resistance at onset of disease *Late resistance:* Steroid resistance during therapy of a relapse
Complicated relapse	Relapse associated with life-threatening complications: (*i*) hypovolemia requiring inpatient care, (*ii*) severe infection (peritonitis, cellulitis, and meningitis), or (*iii*) thrombosis
Significant steroid toxicity	Patients with hyperglycemia (fasting glucose >100 mg/dL, postprandial glucose >140 mg/dL, or HbA1c >5.7%), obesity (body mass index more than the equivalent of 27 kg/m^2 in adults), short stature (height <–2 SDS for age) with height velocity (<–3 SDS for age), raised intraocular pressure, cataract, myopathy, osteonecrosis, or psychosis
Difficult-to-treat sensitive nephrotic syndrome	Both of the following: (*i*) frequent relapses, or significant steroid toxicity with infrequent relapses; and (*ii*) failure of ≥2 steroid sparing agents (including levamisole, cyclophosphamide, and mycophenolate mofetil)
Stable remission	Sustained remission or infrequent relapses during immunosuppressive therapy

SDS: standard deviation score; Up/Uc: spot urine protein to creatinine ratio
[1]Therapy in the last 2 weeks may be given on alternate days in patients with steroid toxicity
[2]In guidelines of International Society of Pediatric Nephrology (IPNA) and KDIGO, patients with partial remission at 4 weeks and complete remission at 6 weeks are defined as "late responders"

or given on alternate days. Patients with two or more relapses in the first 6 months or three relapses in any 12 months are classified as frequent relapses. Complicated relapses are that which are associated with a life-threatening complication, such as hypovolemia requiring inpatient care, severe bacterial infection (peritonitis, cellulitis, and meningitis), or thrombosis. Significant steroid toxicity identifies patients with complications of steroid therapy that requires near-total avoidance of corticosteroid therapy, and the use of potent medications to prevent disease relapses.

Given the natural history of disease, relapses may continue to occur even while on immunosuppressive therapy; hence, both sustained remission and infrequent relapses are considered acceptable and imply "stable remission". The subgroup of patients that continues to manifest frequent relapses (or infrequent relapses in the presence of significant steroid toxicity) despite the use of two or more steroid-sparing agents (such as levamisole, cyclophosphamide, or mycophenolate mofetil) is termed "difficult-to-treat", and merits use of potent but potentially toxic agents.

The diagnosis of steroid resistance is based on demonstration of nonresponse (3–4+ proteinuria, edema, or hypoalbuminemia) despite therapy with prednisone in adequate doses for 6 weeks. Therapy with pulse corticosteroids is not required to confirm steroid resistance. The evaluation and management of steroid-resistant nephrotic syndrome is discussed in Chapter 12. Patients with frequent relapses and steroid resistance are at high risk of complications due to the morbidities associated with the illness and toxicity of medications. These patients, and those below the age of 1 year, should be managed by pediatric nephrologists.

EVALUATION

Investigations at the onset of illness include urinalysis, and blood levels of urea, creatinine, albumin, cholesterol, electrolytes, and blood counts **(Box 11.1)**. Quantitative estimation of urine protein, by repeated early morning spot urine protein to creatinine ratios or a timed (12- or 24-hr) collection is required if nephrotic range proteinuria is uncertain. Urine microscopy is normal, except for occasional hyaline or granular casts and/or

BOX 11.1: Investigations at the first episode of nephrotic syndrome

Urinalysis; quantitative estimation of protein by first morning spot urine protein to creatinine ratio (Up/Uc)[1]
Complete blood counts
Blood urea, creatinine, electrolytes, total protein, albumin, and cholesterol
Tuberculin test

Additional evaluation (if indicated):
Complement C3, C4, antinuclear antibody, antistreptolysin O (gross or persistent microscopic hematuria; sustained hypertension; acute kidney injury without hypovolemia; suspected secondary cause[2])
Serum transaminases; hepatitis B surface antigen; antibody against hepatitis C virus (history of jaundice or liver disease)
Chest radiography (positive tuberculin test or history of contact; suspected lower respiratory tract infection)
Kidney biopsy (*see* **Box 11.2**)

[1]24-hour protein excretion is seldom necessary
[2]Systemic lupus, IgA vasculitis, C3 glomerulopathy

microscopic hematuria. A tuberculin test is considered in view of the risk of activation of latent infection in young children.

Additional investigations are rarely necessary. Patients with positive tuberculin test or history of contact should undergo chest radiography. Serologies to rule out lupus (antinuclear antibody), antistreptolysin O, and/or complement C3 and C4 are only need in patients with atypical presentation suggesting glomerulonephritis, such as gross or persistent microscopic hematuria, sustained hypertension, or extrarenal features (rash and arthralgia). An ultrasonography is not necessary unless the child is planned for kidney biopsy or has gross hematuria or acute kidney injury (AKI). Routine screening for chronic viral infections is not recommended.

Most patients with steroid-sensitive nephrotic syndrome do not require a kidney biopsy. A biopsy is required at onset if a cause other than minimal change disease is suspected, such as clinical features suggesting a secondary cause, or presence of gross or persistent microscopic hematuria or AKI not attributable to hypovolemia **(Box 11.2)**. Age thresholds are perhaps not relevant in mandating the need for kidney biopsy at disease onset. Young infants with nephrotic syndrome and older infants with steroid resistance are considered for next-generation sequencing to determine a genetic cause, avoiding the need for a kidney biopsy. Adolescents presenting with nephrotic syndrome should receive a trial of corticosteroids before considering biopsy, unless there are atypical features (hematuria, hypertension, extrarenal features, or low C3). A kidney biopsy is necessary in patients with steroid-resistant nephrotic syndrome, except in patients with syndromic or familial disease, where genetic screening has higher diagnostic and prognostic role. Kidney biopsy is also suggested before initiating therapy with calcineurin inhibitors (CNI), and following their prolonged use, to rule out histological nephrotoxicity.

Since relapses might occur through childhood and timely intervention prevents morbidities, parents are taught to maintain a record of proteinuria (by dipstick or boiling), infections, and medications received. During relapses, blood investigations are done if complications are suspected. Complete blood counts help to rule out systemic infection and hypovolemia. Blood urea, creatinine, albumin, and electrolytes are recommended in children presenting with severe edema, hypovolemia, dehydration or oligoanuria,

BOX 11.2: Indications for kidney biopsy in nephrotic syndrome

- Persistent microscopic hematuria or gross hematuria
- Acute kidney injury despite correction of hypovolemia
- *Systemic features:* Fever, rash, arthralgia; suspected secondary cause
- Low complement C3 level
- Initial or late corticosteroid resistance
- Prior to therapy with calcineurin inhibitors; prolonged (>30–36 months) therapy with these agents; reduced kidney function during their use

and following prolonged use of diuretics. Annual re-evaluation is recommended even in patients with infrequent relapses in order to monitor growth and detect hypertension. Blood levels of creatinine, albumin, and electrolytes are assessed every 1–2 years in patients with relapsing illness, and more frequently if on immunosuppressive medications, as discussed later.

MANAGEMENT

Initial Episode

Collaborative efforts by the International Study of Kidney Diseases in Children (ISKDC) and Arbeitsgemeinschaft für Pädiatrische Nephrologie (APN) defined the therapy of nephrotic syndrome in the 1970s to 1990s. Subsequent randomized controlled trials (RCTs) using varying doses and duration of predniso(lo)ne therapy have formed the bases for multiple guidelines and recommendations by the Kidney Disease: Improving Global Outcomes (KDIGO), Indian Society of Pediatric Nephrology, and International Pediatric Nephrology Association. Meta-analysis of these studies suggests that the initial duration of predniso(lo)ne therapy should be for 8–12 weeks. Prolonging initial therapy is not associated with benefits in terms of lower risk of relapses and lower proportion of patients with frequent relapses, and may be at the cost of steroid toxicity **(Table 11.2)**.

TABLE 11.2: Management of serious infections

Infections	*Diagnosis*	*Treatment*
Peritonitis	Ascitic fluid: >100 white cells/mm^3, >50% neutrophils Ascitic fluid: Culture, latex agglutination, PCR	Ceftriaxone or cefotaxime for 7–10 days Ampicillin and gentamicin/amikacin for 7–10 days[a]
Pneumonia	Chest X ray; blood culture; sputum for Gram stain, culture	*Oral:* Amoxicillin, co-amoxiclav, cefuroxime for 10–14 days[a] *Parenteral*: Ceftriaxone; or ampicillin and amikacin for 7–10 days
	Throat swab for H1N1 by PCR	Oseltamivir for 5 days
	Tuberculin test; pleural tap, gastric aspirate, sputum: acid fast bacilli, CBNAAT	Therapy as per National Tuberculosis Elimination Program
Cellulitis	Pus for culture, sensitivity Blood culture	*Parenteral:* Co-amoxiclav; cloxacillin with ceftriaxone for 7–10 days[a]
Sepsis	Complete blood counts; C-reactive protein, procalcitonin; blood culture	Ceftriaxone and amikacin for 10–14 days[a]
Varicella	Characteristic skin lesions	IV acyclovir (1,500 mg/m^2/day in three doses) or oral acyclovir (80 mg/kg/day in four doses) for 7–10 days

CBNAAT: cartridge-based nucleic acid amplification test; PCR: polymerase chain reaction
[a]*Penicillin allergy*: Clarithromycin, azithromycin, clindamycin, or vancomycin

Flowchart 11.1: Evaluation and management at presentation of nephrotic syndrome. Genetic studies may be considered, at onset of disease, before therapy with prednisolone, in patients with onset below 9 months, family history of steroid resistance, features of inherited syndromes, and specific histology (e.g., diffuse mesangial sclerosis). Syndromic features include impaired statural growth, skeletal, neurodevelopmental and ocular abnormalities, deafness, genital ambiguity, and facial dysmorphism

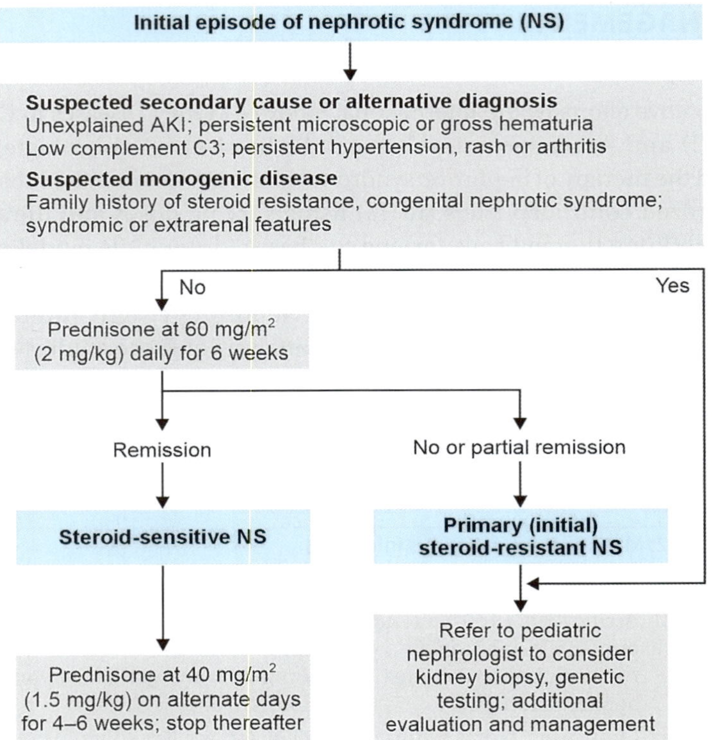

Flowchart 11.1 shows the approach to managing patients with the first episode of nephrotic syndrome. Only prednisolone or prednisone is recommended and is administered in single or divided doses; there is no evidence to support the use of deflazacort of other corticosteroids. Prednisolone may be dosed by body surface area (BSA) or weight. Weight-based dosing is more convenient since estimating surface area is cumbersome and often inaccurate. BSA-based dosing is preferred in young children to avoid relative underdosing, which may potentially be associated with increased risk of relapses.

Therapy for Relapse

Almost 70–75% of patients with steroid-sensitive disease exhibit disease relapses, often within a year since onset. Almost half the relapses are precipitated by minor, usually upper respiratory tract infections. Proteinuria during infections may be transient; hence, it is advisable to await resolution of infection, thus avoiding the need for corticosteroid therapy. However, 3+/4+ proteinuria that lasts for 3 days or longer is unlikely to resolve spontaneously, and has conventionally, albeit empirically, been treated with prednisolone at 60 mg/m^2/day (2 mg/kg/day; maximum 60 mg) in single or divided doses until remission (protein trace/nil for 3 consecutive days), followed by 40 mg/m^2 (1.5 mg/kg, maximum 40 mg) on alternate days for 4 weeks **(Flowchart 11.1)**. Dosing based on BSA and weight is associated with similar outcomes.

Daily therapy is usually required for <2 weeks. If proteinuria persists, daily therapy with prednisolone may be extended to maximum 6-weeks; lack of remission despite such treatment indicates late steroid resistance that is managed similar to initial resistance (Chapter 12). While recent studies suggest that reduced dose or briefer duration of therapy with prednisolone is effective in inducing and maintaining remission, the optimal dose and duration of therapy requires further examination. The management of the subsequent course of nephrotic syndrome is summarized in **Flowchart 11.2**.

Management of Frequent Relapses

Frequent relapses and steroid dependence are more common in patients with age at onset <3 years, delayed time to initial remission, brief corticosteroid therapy at onset, and short duration of initial remission. Prolonged therapy with high-dose prednisolone is associated with significant steroid toxicity, as well as behavior problems, cataract, glaucoma, hypertension, avascular hip necrosis, and diabetes **(Figs. 11.2A to C)**. Relapses are associated with significant complications, including infections, thrombosis, and dyslipidemia. Hence, patients with frequent relapses or steroid dependence are treated with long-term alternate day steroids, or alternative steroid sparing agents to maintain remission while limiting exposure to steroids. Most guidelines do not specify the order or choice of therapy. However, they do advise that therapy be based on steroid threshold and severity of relapses, presence of adverse effects of steroid therapy, patient age, cost of therapy, adherence, and patient preferences.

Table 11.3 summarizes recommendations on dose, duration and adverse effects and precautions during therapy, while **Flowchart 11.2** outlines an approach to the choice and order of therapies. This categorization relies on the definitions discussed earlier, including the presence of significant steroid toxicity, complicated relapses, stable remission, and difficult-to-treat steroid-sensitive disease. The approach suffices in most patients, but might be modulated in individual cases. For example, long-term therapy with prednisolone on alternate days is advocated as the first-line therapy; however, patients diagnosed with steroid dependence soon after initial

Flowchart 11.2: Approach to the management of disease relapses in nephrotic syndrome. Patients with frequent relapses, steroid dependence, and steroid resistance should be referred for management by specialists. Decisions on choice of noncorticosteroid immunosuppressive agents for frequent relapses and steroid dependence are based on efficacy, safety, and costs and their availability (see text). Management of patients with steroid resistance is discussed in Chapter 12

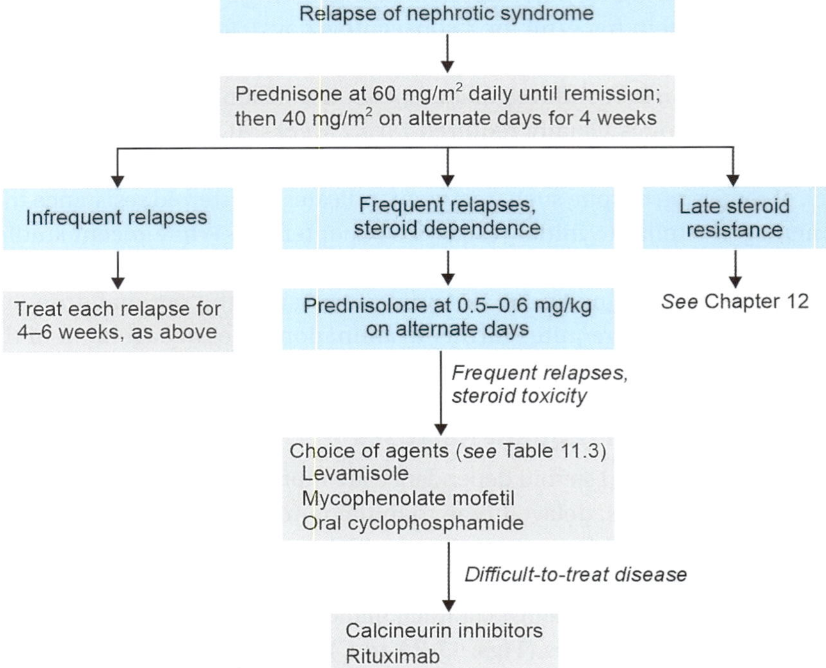

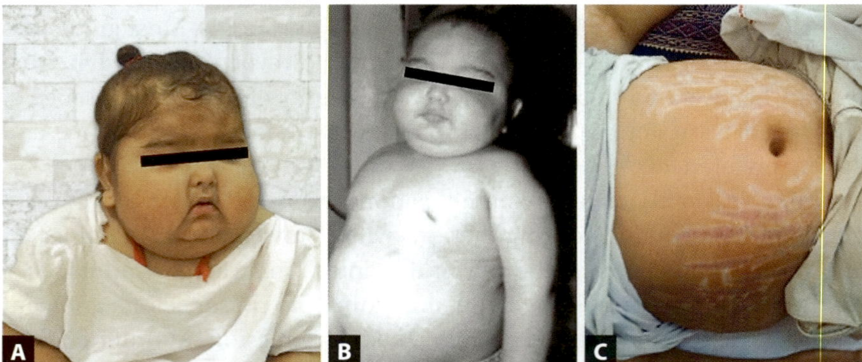

Figs. 11.2A to C: Steroid toxicity in patients with nephrotic syndrome. (A) 2-year-old with frequent relapses. Note the cushingoid facies and increased growth of hair. (B) 4-year-old showing similar facies and truncal obesity. (C) Abdominal striae in an 8-year-old with steroid resistance

TABLE 11.3: Immunosuppressive agents for frequently relapsing and steroid-dependent nephrotic syndrome

Drug	*Dose and duration*	*Adverse effects; precautions*
Prednisolone	0.5–0.6 mg/kg on alternate days for 6–12 months;[a] the same dose is given daily during infections to prevent relapses	Weight gain, Cushingoid features; reduced height velocity; hypertension; raised intraocular pressure; cataract; impaired glycemic tolerance Monitor anthropometry, blood pressure and blood glucose q 3–6 months; eye evaluation q 6–12 months
Levamisole	2–2.5 mg/kg on alternate days for 1–3 years	Neutropenia, vasculitic rash; raised transaminases, seizures Monitor blood counts q 2–3 months; transaminases q 3–6 months; ANCA q 6 months Discontinue therapy if ANCA positive, skin rash, neutropenia
Cyclophosphamide	2–2.5 mg/kg/day orally for 8–12 weeks	Leukopenia, alopecia, blue nails; risk of gonadal toxicity and malignancies Initiate therapy during remission; maintain hydration; monitor blood counts q 2 weeks; withhold drug during serious infection or if total leukocyte count <4,000/mm^3 Second course of therapy should not be given
Mycophenolate mofetil	800–1,200 mg/m^2/day in divided doses for 1–3 years; AUC >45 mg*h/L	Abdominal pain, diarrhea, nausea; viral warts; leukopenia; elevated transaminases Monitor blood counts q 2–3 months; transaminases q 3–6 months
Calcineurin inhibitors	Given for 1–3 years	*Both:* Nephrotoxicity, hyperkalemia, hepatotoxicity
Cyclosporine	4–5 mg/kg/day in two divided doses; target 12-hr trough 80–120 ng/mL	Monitor creatinine, potassium at 2 weeks, and then q 3–6 months along with liver function tests, glucose, uric acid, magnesium, and lipids
Tacrolimus	0.1–0.2 mg/kg/day in two divided doses; target 12-hr trough 4–8 ng/mL	*Specific to cyclosporine:* Gum hyperplasia, hirsutism; hypertension; dyslipidemia *Specific to tacrolimus:* Tremors, seizures, headache; diarrhea; glucose intolerance; hypomagnesemia
Rituximab	375 mg/m^2 as slow IV infusion, 2 doses 1 week apart (consider 1–2 additional doses if B cells not depleted, i.e., >5/μL, or >1% of CD45+ cells)	Chills, fever; serum sickness; bronchospasm; neutropenia; *P. jirovecii* pneumonia; acute lung injury; hypogammaglobulinemia; reactivation of hepatitis B or JC virus Rule out acute and chronic infections before therapy Monitor CD19 counts; blood counts; IgG levels; consider cotrimoxazole prophylaxis

AUC: area under the curve (therapeutic drug monitoring); ANCA: antineutrophil cytoplasmic antibody

[a]May reduce dose further if remission is sustained

therapy or with significant steroid toxicity at diagnosis of frequent relapses are considered directly for steroid-sparing therapies. Therapy with cyclophosphamide is avoided in young patients and in pubertal or postpubertal boys, and therapy with CNI might be preferred to mycophenolate mofetil (MMF) in very young patients with significant steroid toxicity.

Long-term, Alternate-day Steroids

Prednisolone is tapered to a dose of 0.5–0.6 mg/kg on alternate days to keep the disease in remission without significant adverse effects and maintained for 6–12 months. The dose may be lowered further and given for 12–18 months, if effective in reducing relapses or maintaining remission without causing steroid toxicity. Patients on long-term therapy with prednisolone require monitoring for toxicity through frequent assessment of weight, height and blood pressure, ocular toxicity, and hyperglycemia **(Box 11.1)**.

Almost one-half of the relapses follow minor infections, usually of the upper respiratory tract. Controlled studies have shown that administering a small daily dose of prednisolone for 5–7 days during infections effectively prevents infection-associated relapses. Therefore, expert guidelines advise a short course of low-dose (10–15 mg/m^2) daily prednisolone, at the onset of upper respiratory tract infection(s), in children with frequently relapsing nephrotic syndrome who are already taking low-dose alternate-day prednisolone, especially in those with history of repeated infection-associated relapses. There is no consensus on initiating therapy with low-dose prednisone in patients who are not already receiving alternate-day therapy.

Corticosteroid-sparing Agents

The additional use of an alternative agent should be considered in patients with prednisolone threshold for maintaining remission >0.5–0.6 mg/kg on alternate days, or with features of corticosteroid toxicity (**Box 11.1**). Patients should ideally be in steroid-induced remission prior to initiation of steroid-sparing agents, such as cyclophosphamide, levamisole, MMF, CNIs, or rituximab. Therapy with mizoribine, azathioprine, and chlorambucil is not currently recommended.

Levamisole

This is an effective steroid-sparing agent, especially in patients with frequent relapses or mild steroid dependence. Results from multiple controlled trials suggest 35–40% reduction in risk of relapses following 6–12 months therapy with levamisole. The risk of relapses appears to be comparable for levamisole, MMF, or cyclophosphamide. Levamisole is given at a dose of 2–2.5 mg/kg on alternate days, while monitoring for therapy-related adverse effects

(Table 11.3). Since levamisole does not reduce steroid requirement substantially, patients with high threshold or marked steroid toxicity do not do well on this therapy. Chief adverse effects include leukopenia, flu-like syndrome, raised transaminases, occurrence of positive antineutrophil cytoplasmic antibody (ANCA), and vasculitis.

Mycophenolate Mofetil

Mycophenolate mofetil (MMF) inhibits inosine monophosphate dehydrogenase, thus inhibiting lymphocyte proliferation. Several uncontrolled retrospective and prospective studies report that MMF (dose 600–1,200 mg/m^2/day or 20–33 mg/kg/day) has steroid-sparing effects and reduces relapse rates without causing significant toxicity in patients with frequent relapses or steroid dependence. MMF was comparable to levamisole, but inferior to cyclosporine in maintaining satisfactory remission or reducing the frequency of relapses in prospective studies. MMF is perhaps more effective in young children, and more effective than levamisole in patients with steroid dependence.

Side effects of MMF therapy include leukopenia, abdominal pain, and diarrhea. Therapy with MMF should be monitored by drug levels, targeting area under the curve >45–60 mg*h/L or trough levels >2–3 μg/mL. In absence of facilities for therapeutic drug monitoring, therapy may be initiated at the lower end of dose range and escalated as tolerated, to 1,000–1,200 mg/m^2, if patients continue to relapse.

Alkylating Agents

Therapy with cyclophosphamide results in ~40–50% reduction in the risk of relapses and high proportions of patients in sustained remission at 1–2 years follow-up. Therapy with cyclophosphamide is more effective in patients with frequent relapses than in steroid dependence, and in patients older than 5–7 years. Adverse effects include leukopenia, hemorrhagic cystitis, alopecia, nausea and vomiting, and with prolonged use, gonadal toxicity and malignancies. Therapy with chlorambucil is avoided due to its toxicity, including the risk of seizures. Given concerns of toxicity, therapy with cyclophosphamide usually follows failure of levamisole or MMF and should be limited to one 12-weeks' course (cumulative dose ~168 mg/kg).

Therapy with cyclophosphamide should be initiated during remission. Prednisolone is co-administered at a dose of ~1 mg/kg on alternate days during therapy with cyclophosphamide; the medication may be stopped after 1–2 months. The efficacy of IV and oral cyclophosphamide is perhaps similar; the former might be preferred if there are concerns about compliance with oral therapy.

Calcineurin Inhibitors

Cyclosporine A (CsA) and tacrolimus maintain remission and enable steroid sparing in 60–90% patients with steroid-dependent nephrotic syndrome who fail treatment with alkylating agents. There are limited prospective studies on the efficacy of these agents in patients with steroid-sensitive nephrotic syndrome. Few controlled trials found that cyclosporine was associated with reduced risk of relapse as compared to prednisolone, alkylating agents, or MMF. Tacrolimus is often preferred due to lack of cosmetic adverse effects (hirsutism and gum hyperplasia) **(Table 11.3)**.

Chief adverse effects include acute and chronic nephrotoxicity (both agents), hypertension and hyperlipidemia (chiefly CsA), and diarrhea, hypomagnesemia and hyperglycemia (chiefly tacrolimus). Given their superior efficacy but high risk of toxicity, therapy with CNI, either CsA or tacrolimus, is reserved for patients with difficult-to-treat steroid-sensitive nephrotic syndrome. These agents are also preferred in patients with high threshold relapses or significant steroid toxicity if other agents cannot be used. With either agent, therapy should be given for at least 12 months with monitoring of drug levels (target trough 4–7 ng/mL for tacrolimus; 80–150 ng/mL for CsA).

Rituximab

Multiple case series have reported benefits of B cell depletion with rituximab in patients with difficult-to-treat steroid-dependent nephrotic syndrome. Treatment with one or more doses of rituximab results in remission lasting 6–18 months, with 25–83% patients showing sustained remission. In a large series from this center, therapy with rituximab was associated with ~80% reduction in relapse rates. Studies suggest that rituximab has similar or superior efficacy as compared to CNIs.

Adverse effects are common after therapy with rituximab. Therapy with rituximab is associated with high risk of infusion reactions, delayed adverse events, serious infections, and high risk of reactivation of hepatitis B virus infection. Hypogammaglobulinemia is common, and significant and persistent reduction in blood IgG levels may be seen in ~10% patients given the drug. Risk factors for rituximab-associated hypogammaglobulinemia include its administration in young children (below 7–8 years of age), repeated doses of rituximab, pre-existing low levels of IgG, and concomitant use of MMF.

Based on considerations of safety as well as efficacy, most current guidelines recommend that therapy with rituximab be limited to patients with difficult-to-treat nephrotic syndrome. Therapy is administered while in steroid-induced remission, after ensuring that acute infections, tuberculosis, and chronic viremia have been ruled out. Therapy should be avoided in young children (<5–7 years old). The medication is given as a slow IV infusion at a dose of 375 mg/m^2 IV once a week for two doses, under specialist supervision.

If B cell depletion (CD19+ cells <1% of CD45+ cells, or <5 cells/μL) is not achieved, a maximum of four infusions may been given. Patients should be monitored for infections, leukopenia, and hypogammaglobulinemia during follow-up. B cell recovery usually occurs by 6–9 months and is associated with risk of relapses. Options to sustain remission include redosing after recurrence of frequent relapses, redosing when B cell repopulation is expected or detected, or use of additional immunosuppression (e.g., with MMF). Prophylactic antibiotics (cotrimoxazole: 150 mg/m^2 or 5 mg/kg of trimethoprim on alternate days) should be considered in patients receiving intense immunosuppression.

Supportive Care

Patients with steroid-sensitive nephrotic syndrome are at significant risk of complications associated with disease relapses as well as adverse effects due to medications. The principles of supportive care are outlined in **Table 11.4**. Parents should be explained the natural history of disease and

TABLE 11.4: Principles of supportive care to reduce symptoms and/or complications

Diet and lifestyle	Ensure adequate caloric and protein intake; avoid restricting physical activity During moderate-to-severe edema: Increase protein intake and restrict salt intake
Growth	Monitor anthropometry q 6–12 months
Hypertension	Monitor blood pressure q 6–12 months; prefer ACEi/ARB to treat hypertension
Infections	Vaccinate against common pathogens as in national program; avoid live vaccines while on immunosuppression Ensure vaccination against pneumococcus, varicella, influenza, and hepatitis B infections Consider IV varicella zoster immunoglobulin, or oral acyclovir in susceptible patients exposed to varicella or to zoster Consider cotrimoxazole prophylaxis in patients receiving immuno-suppression with more than one non-steroidal medication
Hypovolemia	Rule out in all patients with edema, particularly in a setting of vomiting, diarrhea, low intake or fever **(*see* Flowchart 11.3)** Avoid diuretics and ACEi/ARB; administer oral or IV fluids, consider IV albumin (20–25%; 0.5–1 g/kg over 4-hr)
Edema	Rule out hypovolemia; manage as outlined in **Flowchart 11.3**
Thrombosis	Rule out in setting of hypovolemia with specific clinical features; administer low-molecular weight heparin
Acute kidney injury (AKI)	Monitor for AKI during relapse with edema or hypovolemia, particularly if receiving ACEi/ARB, diuretics, NSAIDs, radiocontrast or nephrotoxic drugs; manage as per standard guidelines

ACEi: angiotensin-converting enzyme inhibitor; ARB: angiotensin receptor blocker; NSAIDs: nonsteroidal anti-inflammatory drugs

the need for long-term monitoring, while emphasizing on ensuring normal diet and physical activity as for healthy children. Patients with frequently relapsing illness, requiring repeated use of high-dose corticosteroids, should be monitored for hypertension, growth retardation, obesity, and ocular complications. Given the risk of hypothalamo pituitary suppression, patients who have been treated with oral corticosteroids for >2 weeks within the past 1 year should receive prednisolone at 15 mg/m^2 (or equivalent doses of hydrocortisone) during conditions associated with physiological stress (fever ≥38°C, systemic infections, inadequate oral intake, lethargy, dehydration, invasive surgery, dental surgery, trauma, and large burns). "Stress" dosing is not required during uncomplicated viral or bacterial infections.

Disease relapses are associated with risk of hypovolemia, edema, severe infections, and AKI. These conditions should be managed appropriately. **Flowchart 11.3** outlines the management of patients presenting with edema, the most common complication associated with relapses. Hypovolemia

Flowchart 11.3: Management of edema and hypovolemia. Text provides details on assessment of hypovolemia and severity of edema and management

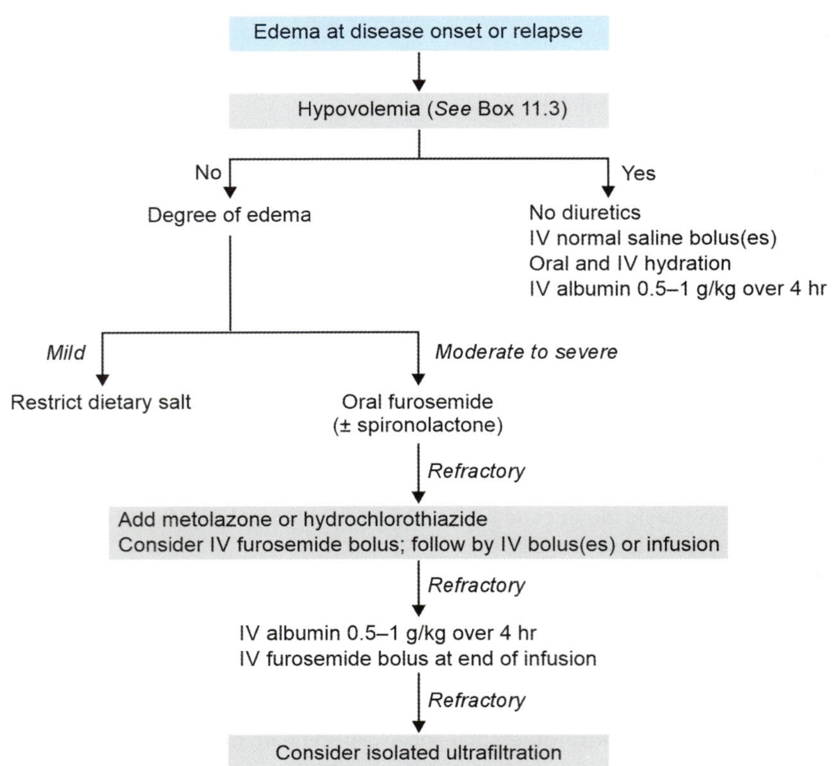

needs to be excluded in all children presenting in relapse with or without edema, particularly in a setting of vomiting, diarrhea, reduced oral intake, or unsupervised diuretic use. Clinical features of hypovolemia include abdominal pain, vomiting or postural pulses or hypotension **(Box 11.3)**. Biochemical parameters that indicate hypovolemia include an elevated hematocrit and an increased blood urea (mg/dL) to creatinine (mg/dL) ratio >100, low fractional excretion of sodium (<0.5%), and high urinary potassium index (>0.6). Patients with hypovolemia need to receive intravenous fluids and/or albumin, in order to restore circulating volume and also reduce the risk of thrombosis.

The severity of edema may be graded empirically as: mild if ≤7% increase in body weight, moderate if 7–15% increase in body weight, and severe if >15% increase in body weight. Patients with mild edema usually do not require diuretics; edema resolves with reduction in salt intake and therapy of relapse **(Flowchart 11.3)**. Oral furosemide is usually sufficient in managing moderate edema associated with steroid-sensitive disease. Spironolactone should be added to prevent hypokalemia if furosemide use is prolonged (>48 hr). More severe cases benefit with additional use of a thiazide diuretic, or switch to IV furosemide; IV albumin is required in a subgroup of patients, particularly those with concomitant hypovolemia and nonresponse to hydration. Doses of commonly used diuretics are given in **Table 11.5**.

Patients with nephrotic syndrome are at risk of infections due to encapsulated organisms, as well as due to concomitant immunosuppression. Live vaccines should not be administered to children on immunosuppressive medications **(Table 11.6)**. Specific vaccines for children with nephrotic syndrome are listed in **Table 11.7**.

BOX 11.3: Features of hypovolemia during relapse

Clinical features:
Abdominal pain, vomiting, lethargy
Prolonged capillary refill time; cold extremities
Tachycardia, low-volume pulses
Low blood pressure; postural hypotension

Biochemical indices:
Elevated hematocrit
Blood urea (mg/dL) to creatinine (mg/dL) ratio >100
Fractional excretion of sodium <0.5%
Urinary potassium index [urine K^+/(urine Na^++ K^+)] >0.6

Ultrasonography: Decreased inferior vena cava diameter, increased collapsibility index

$$\text{Fractional excretion of sodium} = \frac{\text{Urine Na}^+ \times \text{serum creatinine}}{\text{Serum Na}^+ \times \text{urine creatinine}} \times 100$$

TABLE 11.5: Diuretics used in the management of edema of nephrotic syndrome

Medication	*Site of action*	*Route; dose mg/kg/day*	*Half-life, hr*	*Duration of effect, hr*	*% oral bioavailability*	*% eliminated by kidneys*	*Adverse effects*
Furosemide	NKCC2; thick ascending limb of Henle	Oral: 1–6 IV: 1–4 Infusion: 0.1–1 mg/kg/h	1.5–2	6–8	20–80	65	Hypovolemia; hypokalemia, metabolic alkalosis; hypercalciuria, hypomagnesemia
Torsemide	NKCC2; thick ascending limb of Henle	Oral: 5–10 mg/d	3–4	12	80	20	Not approved for use children with nephrotic syndrome.
Hydrochlo-rothiazide	NCCT2; distal convoluted tubule	Oral: 1–2	~2.5	~24	70	95	Hyponatremia, hyperuricemia, hypomagnesemia, hyperlipidemia, hyperglycemia
Metolazone	NCCT2; distal convoluted tubule	Oral: 0.2–0.4		~24	65	95	
Spironolactone	Mineralocorticoid receptor; collecting duct	Oral: 1–4	~1.6	~3	65	0	Hyperkalemia, gynecomastia, muscle cramps (spironolactone); abdominal pain, anorexia (amiloride)
Amiloride	Epithelial sodium channel; collecting duct	Oral: 0.1–0.6	6–9	~24	15–25	100	
Acetazolamide	Sodium hydrogen exchanger 3; proximal tubule	Oral: 5–30	6–9	16	100	100	Metabolic acidosis, hypersensitivity; paresthesias, dysgeusia, polyuria, fatigue
Mannitol	All along the tubule	Oral: 0.25–1 g/kg/dose	0.5–1.7	~2	Negligible	80	Pulmonary edema, hypernatremia

TABLE 11.6: Principles of immunization with live vaccines in patients with nephrotic syndrome

Immunosuppression	*Advice*
Receiving high-dose prednisolone (≥2 mg/kg/d; ≥20 mg/day if >10 kg) for <14 days	Vaccinate immediately after discontinuing treatment
Receiving high-dose prednisolone (≥2 mg/kg/d; ≥20 mg/day if >10 kg) for >14 days	Vaccinate 1 month after discontinuing corticosteroids
Receiving low–moderate dose prednisolone (<2 mg/kg/d or equivalent; <20 mg/d)	No live vaccines, until discontinuation of steroid therapy
Low-dose alternate day prednisolone and pressing need for vaccine	Live vaccine may be administered
Patients receiving cyclophosphamide	Avoid live vaccines until off therapy for 3 months
Patients receiving calcineurin inhibitors, levamisole, or mycophenolate mofetil	Avoid live vaccines until off therapy for 1 month
Therapy with rituximab	Avoid live vaccines until after B-cell recovery (~6–9 months)
Immunocompetent siblings and household contacts	Do not administer oral polio vaccine; may receive measles-mumps-rubella, rotavirus and varicella vaccines
Household contacts older than 1 year	Administer influenza vaccine annually

TABLE 11.7: Specific vaccines for patients with nephrotic syndrome[a]

Vaccine	*Age*	*Previously received*	*Vaccine*	*Schedule*
Pneumococcal: *Conjugate* (PCV, 13-valent) *Polysaccharide*, (23-valent, PPSV23)	6–72 months	Completely immunized (3 doses at 6, 10, 14 weeks; booster 12–15 months)	PCV13/10	One dose ≥2-year-old
			PPSV23	One dose when ≥2-year-old (given ≥8 week after PCV13/10 dose[b])
		No, or incompletely immunized	PCV13/10	Two doses, ≥8 week apart[c]
			PPSV23	One dose when ≥2-year-old (given ≥8 week after PCV13/10 dose[b])
	≥72 months	Completely immunized	PPSV23	1 dose[b]
		No, or incompletely immunized	PCV13/10	1 dose
			PPSV23	1 dose (given ≥8 week after last PCV13/10 dose[b])
Varicella[d]	>15 months	No evidence of immunity[e]	Live attenuated	Two doses 4–8 week apart
Influenza	>6 months		Inactivated	Annually
Hepatitis B	Any	No, or anti-HBs <10 mIU/mL	Subunit (10 µg/0.5 mL)[f]	3 doses at 0, 1, and 6 months; *or* accelerated with ≥4 week gap between doses 1 and 2, ≥8 week between doses 2 and 3, and ≥16 week between doses 1 and 3[f]

[a]Efficacy of vaccines might be attenuated while on high-dose corticosteroids or other immunosuppression
[b]Repeat after 5 year if still experiencing disease relapses
[c]If the two doses are administered at <1-year-old, give one additional dose during 2nd year of life
[d]Avoid in patients <15 months; administer while off immunosuppression **(Table 11.6)**
[e]Immunity refers to past diagnosis of varicella or herpes zoster, verified by a physician; documented receipt of 2 doses of vaccine 4–8 weeks apart; or serological evidence of immunity
[f]Consider postvaccination testing for adequacy (anti-HBs antibody ≥10 mIU/mL) and administering higher (20 µg) or additional doses

OUTCOMES

Most patients with steroid-sensitive nephrotic syndrome show satisfactory outcomes, and the disease tends to resolve by late adolescence. The frequency of relapses declines with age. However, 15–25% patients may continue to have active disease in adulthood, maintaining the features of childhood onset disease with rapid response to glucocorticoids. Factors associated with risk of relapse in adulthood include age at onset before 3–4 years, and frequently relapsing disease course. Fewer than 1% children develop kidney failure. Morbidity due to severe infections, associated with disease relapses and immunosuppression, has declined with prompt diagnosis and immunization practices; however, they remain the chief cause of hospitalization and mortality. Steroid toxicity remains a major concern, particularly in patients with frequent relapses or steroid dependence, including short stature, obesity, hypertension, metabolic bone disease, diabetes mellitus, and ocular complications. Patients who continue to relapse in adolescence or have features of steroid toxicity should be transitioned into care by nephrologists.

BIBLIOGRAPHY

1. Banh THM, Hussain-Shamsy N, Patel V, et al. Ethnic differences in incidence and outcomes of childhood nephrotic syndrome. Clin J Am Soc Nephrol. 2016;11:1760-8.
2. Campbell RE, Thurman JM. The immune system and idiopathic nephrotic syndrome. Clin J Am Soc Nephrol. 2022;17:1823-34.
3. Chan EY, Yap DY, Colucci M, et al. Use of rituximab in childhood idiopathic nephrotic syndrome. Clin J Am Soc Nephrol. 2023;18:533-48.
4. Chanchlani R, Parekh RS. Ethnic differences in childhood nephrotic syndrome. Front Pediatr. 2016;4:39.
5. Emma F, Montini G, Gargiulo A. Equations to estimate prednisone dose using body weight. Pediatr Nephrol. 2019;34:685-8.
6. Hahn D, Samuel S, Willis NS, et al. Corticosteroid therapy for nephrotic syndrome in children. Cochrane Database Syst Rev. 2020;2020:CD001533.
7. Hjorten R, Anwar Z, Reidy KJ. Long-term outcomes of childhood onset nephrotic syndrome. Front Pediatr. 2016;4:53.
8. International Study of Kidney Disease in Children. The primary nephrotic syndrome in children. Identification of patients with minimal change nephrotic syndrome from initial response to prednisolone. A report of the International Study of Kidney Disease in Children. J Pediatr. 1981;98:556-64.
9. Kaku Y, Ohtsuka Y, Komatsu Y, et al.; Japanese Society for Pediatric Nephrology. Clinical practice guidelines for pediatric idiopathic nephrotic syndrome. Clin Exp Nephrol. 2015;19:34-53.
10. KDIGO. (2024). Clinical practice guideline for management of nephrotic syndrome in children. [online] Available from https://kdigo.org/wp-content/

uploads/2024/04/KDIGO-2024-Nephrotic-Syndrome-in-Children-Guideline-Public-Review-Draft.pdf. [Last accessed June, 2024]

11. Kidney Disease: Improving Global Outcomes Glomerular Diseases Work Group. KDIGO 2021 Clinical Practice Guideline for Management of Glomerular Diseases. Kidney Int. 2021;100:S1-S276.
12. Kopp JB, Anders HJ, Susztak K, et al. Podocytopathies. Nat Rev Dis Primers. 2020;6:68.
13. Lane BM, Cason R, Esezobor CI, et al. Genetics of childhood steroid sensitive nephrotic syndrome: An update. Front Pediat. 2019;7:8.
14. Larkins NG, Liu ID, Willis NS, et al. Non-corticosteroid immunosuppressive medications for steroid-sensitive nephrotic syndrome in children. Cochrane Database Syst Rev. 2020:CD002290.
15. Marchel DM, Gipson DS. Adult survivors of idiopathic childhood onset nephrotic syndrome. Pediatr Nephrol. 2021;36:1731-37.
16. Meena J, Bagga A. Current perspectives in management of edema in nephrotic syndrome. Indian J Pediatr. 2020;87:633-40.
17. Mühlig AK, Lee JY, Kemper MJ, et al. Levamisole in children with idiopathic nephrotic syndrome: Clinical efficacy and pathophysiological aspects. J Clin Med. 2019;8:860.
18. Querfeld U, Weber LT. Mycophenolate mofetil for sustained remission in nephrotic syndrome. Pediatr Nephrol. 2018;33:2253-65.
19. Salfi G, Casiraghi F, Remuzzi G. Current understanding of the molecular mechanisms of circulating permeability factor in focal segmental glomerulosclerosis. Front Immunol. 2023;14:1247606.
20. Sinha A, Bagga A, Banerjee S, et al.; Expert Group of Indian Society of Pediatric Nephrology. Steroid Sensitive Nephrotic Syndrome: Revised Guidelines. Indian Pediatr. 2021;58:461-81.
21. Sinha A, Bagga A. Rituximab therapy in nephrotic syndrome: Implications for patients' management. Nat Rev Nephrol. 2013;9:154-69.
22. Sinha A, Hari P, Sharma PK, et al. Disease course in steroid sensitive nephrotic syndrome. Indian Pediatr. 2012;49:881-7.
23. Tarshish P, Tobin JN, Bernstein J, et al. Prognostic significance of the early course of minimal change nephrotic syndrome: report of the International Study of Kidney Disease in Children. J Am Soc Nephrol. 1997;8:769-76.
24. Trautmann A, Boyer O, Hodson E, et al.; International Pediatric Nephrology Association. IPNA clinical practice recommendations for the diagnosis and management of children with steroid-sensitive nephrotic syndrome. Pediatr Nephrol. 2023;38:877-919.
25. Trautmann A, Vivarelli M, Samuel S, et al.; International Pediatric Nephrology Association. IPNA clinical practice recommendations for the diagnosis and management of children with steroid-resistant nephrotic syndrome. Pediatr Nephrol. 2020;35:1529-61.
26. Vasudevan A, Thergaonkar R, Mantan M, et al.; Expert Group of Indian Society of Pediatric Nephrology. Consensus Guidelines on Management of Steroid-Resistant Nephrotic Syndrome. Indian Pediatr. 2021;58:650-66.

27. Veltkamp F, Rensma LR, Bouts AHM; LEARNS consortium. Incidence and relapse of idiopathic nephrotic syndrome: Meta-analysis. Pediatrics. 2021;148:e2020029249.
28. Vivarelli M, Gibson K, Sinha A, et al. Childhood nephrotic syndrome. Lancet. 2023;402:809-24.
29. Wang L, Li Q, Wang L, et al. The role of Th17/IL-17 in the pathogenesis of primary nephrotic syndrome in children. Kidney Blood Press Res. 2013;37:332-45.
30. Watanabe A, Feltran LS, Sampson MG. Genetics of nephrotic syndrome presenting in childhood: Core curriculum 2019. Am J Kidney Dis. 2019;74:549-57.
31. Watts AJB, Keller KH, Lerner G, et al. Discovery of autoantibodies targeting nephrin in minimal change disease supports a novel autoimmune etiology. J Am Soc Nephrol. 2022;33:238-52.

Steroid Resistant Nephrotic Syndrome

Aditi Sinha, Geetika Singh, Arvind Bagga

Idiopathic nephrotic syndrome, characterized by proteinuria, hypoalbuminemia, and edema, is a rare condition that affects 12–16 per 100,000 children. The majority of patients achieve complete remission of proteinuria following therapy with prednisolone. Patients who fail to do so are termed as steroid-resistant nephrotic syndrome (SRNS). This condition, affecting 5–10% of cases presenting in childhood, has a difficult course with frequent complications, adverse effects of therapy, and high risk of progression to kidney failure.

DEFINITIONS

A diagnosis of SRNS is considered in patients who do not show resolution of proteinuria despite treatment with daily prednisone. The dose and duration of steroid therapy for defining SRNS have varied. While the International Study of Kidney Disease in Children (ISKDC) defined nonresponse following 8-weeks' prednisone therapy (4 weeks each of daily and intermittent treatment), other guidelines had defined steroid resistance at the end of 4 weeks. Since a small proportion of patients enter remission between 4 and 6 weeks, current guidelines by the Indian Society of Pediatric Nephrology (ISPN) define steroid resistance following 6-weeks' daily therapy with prednisolone at 2 mg/kg (60 mg/m^2). The International Pediatric Nephrology Association (IPNA) and Kidney Disease Improving Global Outcomes (KDIGO) define steroid resistance in patients showing nonresponse at 4 weeks or partial remission at 6 weeks.

Table 12.1 lists common definitions of disease and its course. Children who do not achieve complete remission during the first episode are referred to as initial SRNS; patients who develop steroid resistance later in the course are termed late (secondary) SRNS. This distinction has relevance, since the two categories of patients have differences in pathophysiology, histology, response to second-line immunosuppression, disease progression, and risk of post-transplant recurrence.

EPIDEMIOLOGY

Data from retrospective and prospective series suggests that SRNS is observed in 12% [95% confidence interval (CI): 2–27] children with idiopathic nephrotic syndrome. The prevalence of SRNS is 0.5–2 per 100,000 children, with higher

TABLE 12.1: Definitions of disease course in steroid-resistant nephrotic syndrome (SRNS)

Nephrotic-range proteinuria	Up/Uc >2 mg/mg, or dipstick 3+/4+, on ≥3 consecutive occasions
Steroid resistance (SRNS)	Lack of complete remission following 6 weeks of daily therapy with prednisolone at a dose of 2 mg/kg (60 mg/m^2)*,†
Initial (primary)	Steroid resistance documented after initial therapy of nephrotic syndrome
Late (secondary)	Steroid resistance following therapy of a relapse, having been in remission previously (initial steroid-sensitivity)
Secondary FSGS	Maladaptive injury in systemic conditions (e.g., obesity, hypertension) or podocyte injury by viruses, toxins, or drugs
Complete remission	Up/Uc ≤0.2 mg/mg or negative or trace dipstick, on ≥3 consecutive occasions; serum albumin ≥3 g/dL; and no edema
Partial remission	Up/Uc >0.2 and ≤2 mg/mg or dipstick 1+/2+, on ≥3 consecutive occasions; serum albumin ≥3 g/dL; and no edema
Nonresponse	Up/Uc >2 mg/mg or dipstick 3+/4+; serum albumin <3 g/dL; or edema
Relapse	Recurrence of nephrotic-range proteinuria with or without edema in a child who was previously in remission
Monogenic SRNS	Pathogenic or likely pathogenic variant, defined by American College of Medical Genetics and Genomics, in a gene known to be associated with nephrotic syndrome **(Annexure 9.4, p 845)**
CNI-refractory/ resistant SRNS	Nonresponse to cyclosporine A or tacrolimus, given in adequate doses and titrated to blood levels, for 6 months
Multidrug-resistant SRNS	Nonresponse to ≥6 months of therapy with each of two mechanistically distinct nonsteroidal agents in standard doses
Recurrence of nephrotic syndrome in allograft	Persistent proteinuria (Up/Uc >1 mg/mg) if previously anuric; or increase of Up/Uc by >1 mg/mg if proteinuric at time of transplant (in absence of other apparent causes)
Congenital NS	Onset of nephrotic syndrome within 3 months of birth

CNI: calcineurin inhibitor; FSGS: focal segmental glomerulosclerosis; NS: nephrotic syndrome; Up/Uc urine protein to creatinine ratio in spot (first morning void) or 24-hr sample

*Therapy during the last 2 weeks may be given on alternate days in patients with features of steroid toxicity

†International Pediatric Nephrology Association 2020 guidelines define steroid resistance as nonresponse at 4 weeks, or persistent partial response at 6 weeks (including 2 weeks confirmation period), with or without 3 pulses of intravenous methylprednisolone at 500 mg/m^2 (15 mg/kg)

proportions reported from Asia and Africa. Data from registries suggests that almost one-third (32%; 95% CI: 26–37%) patients with initial SRNS have a monogenic basis (see below).

PATHOGENESIS

Podocytes have a key role in the pathogenesis of idiopathic SRNS, as suggested by diffuse effacement of podocyte foot processes observed on electron microscopy. In the early phase of focal segmental glomerulosclerosis (FSGS), podocyte injury leads to attenuation of its cell body, foot process effacement, pseudocyst formation, and microvillus transformation; interstitial fibrosis with tubular atrophy follows later.

A proportion of SRNS is mediated by alterations in the structural components of the foot process due to mutation(s) in corresponding genes **(Fig. 12.1)(Annexure 9.4, p 845)**. Alternatively, podocytes may be the target

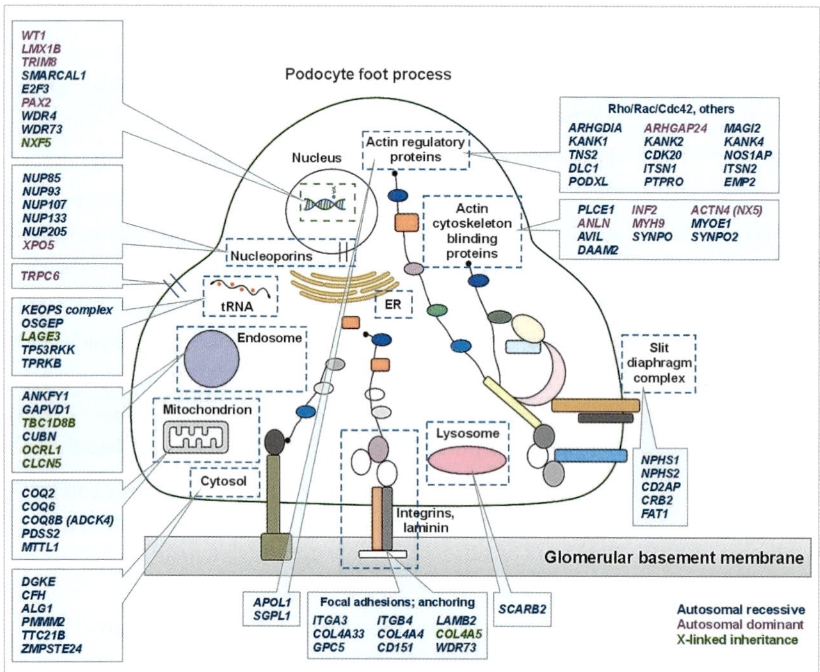

Fig. 12.1: Sites of expression of the genes implicated in monogenic steroid-resistant nephrotic syndrome. The cartoon represents the foot processes of podocytes, which interdigitate to form the glomerular slit membrane, considered critical for the integrity of the glomerular filtration barrier. Genes implicated in causing monogenic steroid resistance are depicted according to the location of the proteins encoded by them. **Annexure 9.4 (p 845)** lists all relevant genes. ER: endoplasmic reticulum; tRNA: transfer ribonucleic acid

of yet unidentified circulating factor(s) that cause dysfunction of the filtration barrier **(Fig. 12.1 and Table 12.2)**. While some patients with initial SRNS have monogenic disease, all patients with late SRNS and most with initial SRNS are perhaps mediated by circulating factor(s). Distinction between the two mechanisms impacts management and outcomes.

TABLE 12.2: Postulated circulating factors in nephrotic syndrome, their proposed mechanisms of action, and supportive evidence

Postulated factors	*Proposed mechanisms; experimental and/or clinical evidence*
Soluble urokinase-type plasminogen activator receptor (suPAR)	Activates podocyte αvβ3-integrin, causing cytoskeletal rearrangement, reduced nephrin and podocin expression, increased *TRPC6* expression, and albuminuria in mice; serum levels elevated in FSGS *versus* MCD, and recurrent *versus* nonrecurrent FSGS Not confirmed in later studies; levels correlate inversely with eGFR and directly with inflammation; predicts progression of CKD
Tumor necrosis factor-alpha (TNFα)	Induces proteinuria in rats; present in supernatant of cultured lymphocytes from patients with FSGS; inhibition of TNFα ameliorates the effects of recurrent FSGS plasma on podocytes; urinary levels high in relapse TNFα did not increase glomerular permeability *in vitro*; TNFα inhibitor (adalimumab) does not induce remission in FSGS
Serum serine proteases; podocyte VASP	Vasodilator stimulated phosphoprotein (VASP) phosphorylated in relapse by serum proteases; podocyte motility depends on VASP phosphorylation
Vascular endothelial growth factor (VEGF)	VEGF knockout rats lack endothelial fenestrations and show renal injury However, serum levels are not increased in relapse; VEGF infusion in rats does not cause proteinuria
Factor inhibited by galactose	Oral administration of galactose inhibits activity of unknown factor; reduces glomerular permeability Benefits of oral administration not confirmed in a controlled trial
Anti-CD40 antibody; soluble CD40 ligand (sCD40L)	sCD40L binds to podocyte CD40 to redistribute nephrin and increase permeability of rat glomeruli; effect inhibited by CD40-sCD40L inhibitors Anti-CD40 and sCD40L elevated in plasma of patients with recurrent FSGS; sCD40L present in PEX effluent in recurrent FSGS However, levels of sCD40L are also elevated in inflammatory conditions not associated with proteinuria; levels predict change in renal function

Contd...

Contd...

Postulated factors	*Proposed mechanisms; experimental and/or clinical evidence*
Podocyte CD80 (B7-1)	Podocyte CD80 expression, induced by ligands of toll-like receptors (lipopolysaccharide), is associated with foot process effacement in cultured podocytes and proteinuria; CD80 shown to be of podocyte origin; podocyte CD80 expression is increased in biopsies with FSGS Inhibition of CD80 signaling by abatacept induced remission in refractory FSGS (but this was not confirmed in later studies)
Hemopexin	Reversible proteinuria in rats and cytoskeletal rearrangement in podocytes; serum levels are lower and protease activity higher in relapse
Interleukin (IL) 13	Overexpression of IL-13 induces proteinuria in rats; increased T-cell IL-13 expression and serum IL-13 levels in relapse *versus* remission
Interleukin 8	Increases heparan sulfate catabolism to alter GBM charge; induces proteinuria in animal models that is abolished by anti-IL-8; serum and urinary IL-8 elevated in relapse *versus* remission; IL-8 infusion does not increase permeability *in vitro*
Cardiotropin-like cytokine 1 (CLC-1)	Increases glomerular permeability and decreases nephrin expression in glomeruli and cultured podocytes; effects inhibited by JAK2 or STAT3 inhibition; plasma level elevated in active FSGS or recurrent FSGS; JAK/STAT pathway upregulated in FSGS
Antinephrin antibodies	Elevated levels in minimal change disease, primary FSGS and recurrent FSGS compared to secondary FSGS, membranous nephropathy and controls; associated with fine granular staining for IgG on kidney biopsy

CKD: chronic kidney disease; eGFR: estimated glomerular filtration rate; FSGS: focal segmental glomerulosclerosis; JAK2: janus kinase 2; MCD: minimal change disease; PEX: plasma exchange; STAT3: signal transducer and activator of transcription 3; *TRPC6*: Transient receptor potential cation channel 6

Pathology

Histopathologically, SRNS is characterized by a primary podocytopathy, represented by either minimal change disease (MCD) **(Figs. 12.2A to C)** or FSGS **(Figs. 12.3A to C)**, each accounting for about 40% cases. A small proportion of patients show mesangial proliferative glomerulonephritis. Uncommon pathologies, such as diffuse mesangial sclerosis **(Figs. 12.4A to D)** and collapsing glomerulopathy **(Figs. 12.5A and B)** are associated with monogenic cause or viral infections, respectively. In older children and adolescents, biopsy may show C3 glomerulopathy, membranous nephropathy, immunoglobulin A (IgA) nephropathy, or secondary forms of FSGS. Patients with secondary forms of FSGS typically have focal (<50%) foot process effacement.

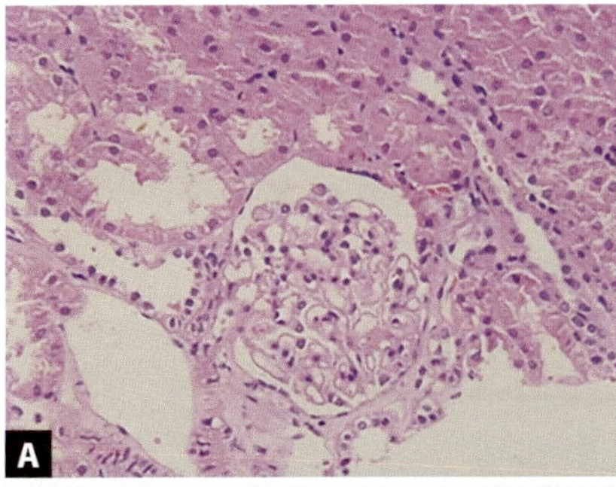

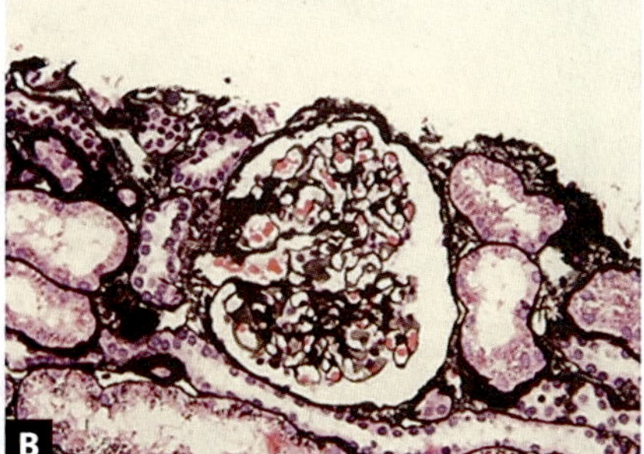

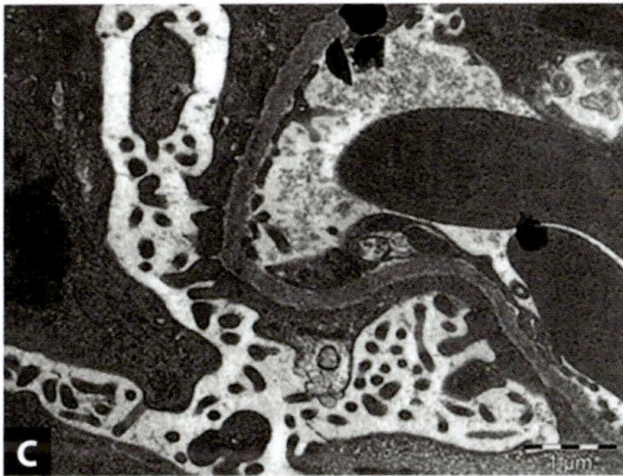

Figs. 12.2A to C: Minimal change disease. Panels show a morphologically unremarkable glomerulus on (A) Periodic acid-Schiff staining (20×); (B) Jones silver methenamine staining (20×); and (C) Transmission electron microscopy reveals diffuse foot process effacement, actin condensation, and microvillous transformation, the ultrastructural hallmarks of podocyte injury in primary podocytopathy (Uranyl acetate-lead citrate; 2550×)

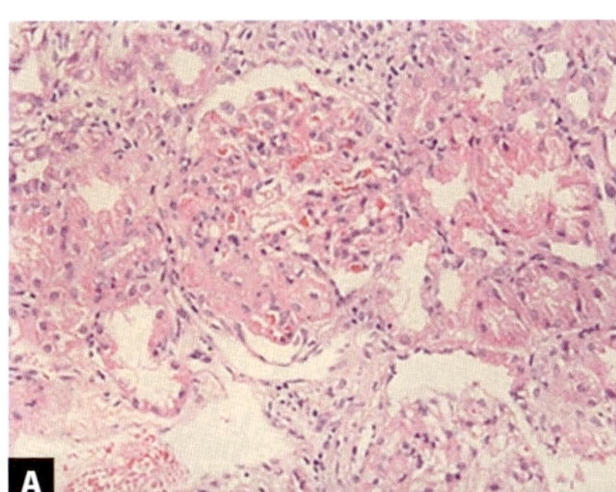

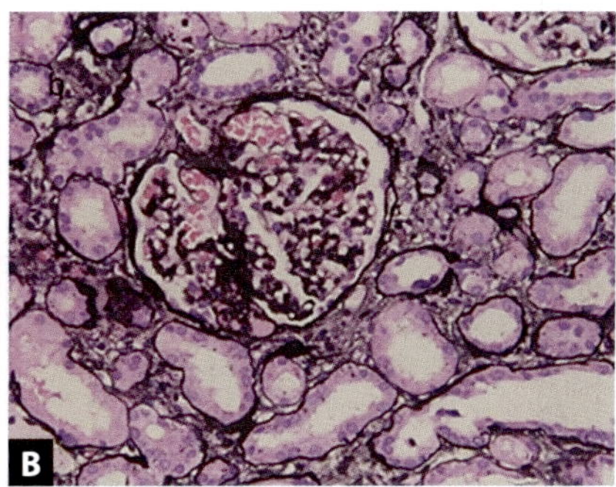

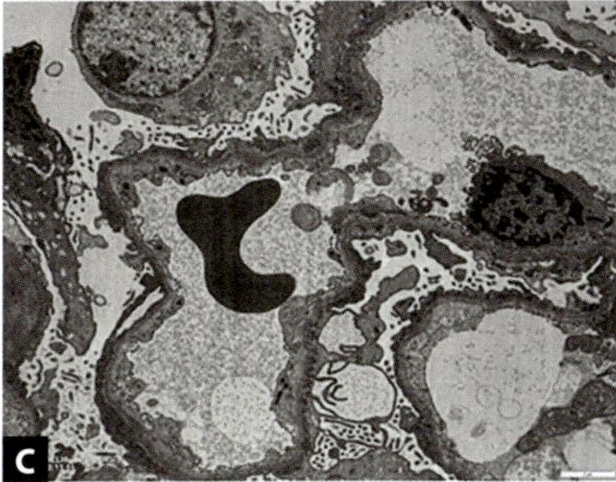

Figs. 12.3A to C: Focal segmental glomerulosclerosis not otherwise specified (FSGS-NOS). (A) The sclerotic segment at 6 o'clock is "crowned" by epithelial cells. Note the irregularly thickened Bowman capsule (Periodic acid-Schiff; 20×); (B) The collagenized sclerotic segment at 8 o'clock stains blue, while peripheral hyalinosis noted at 11 o'clock position stains pink (Masson trichrome; 20×); and (C) Transmission electron microscopy, as in all primary podocytopathies, is characterized by diffuse foot process effacement (Uranyl acetate-lead citrate; 2550×)

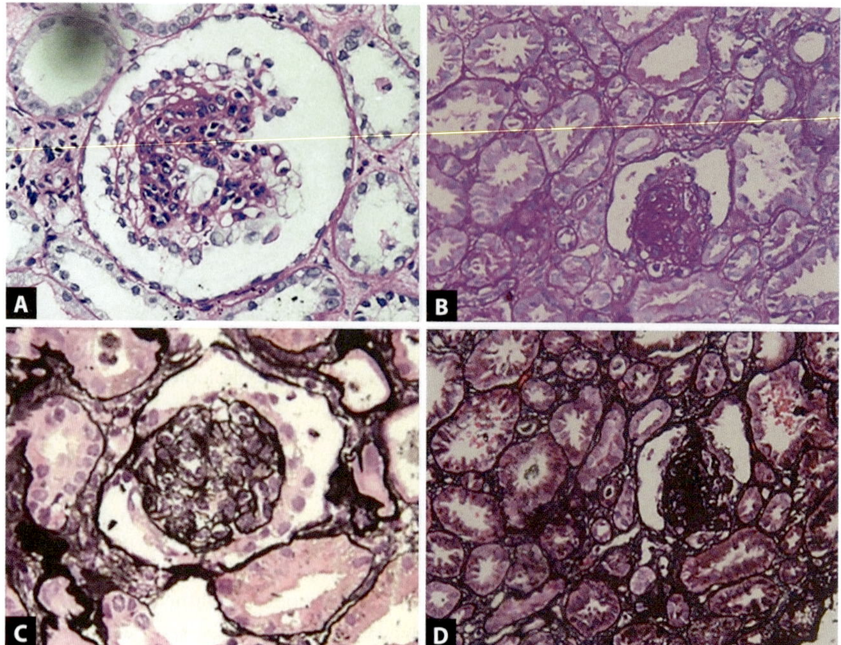

Figs. 12.4A to D: Diffuse mesangial sclerosis. (A and B) There is global mesangial sclerosis with a "crown" of visceral epithelial cells. The mesangium appears sclerotic and hypercellular without open capillary loops (Periodic acid-Schiff; 40× and 20×); (C and D) Note the classic mesangial knotting or "yarn ball" appearance and crowning with a single layer of visceral epithelial cells (Jones methenamine silver; 40× and 20×)

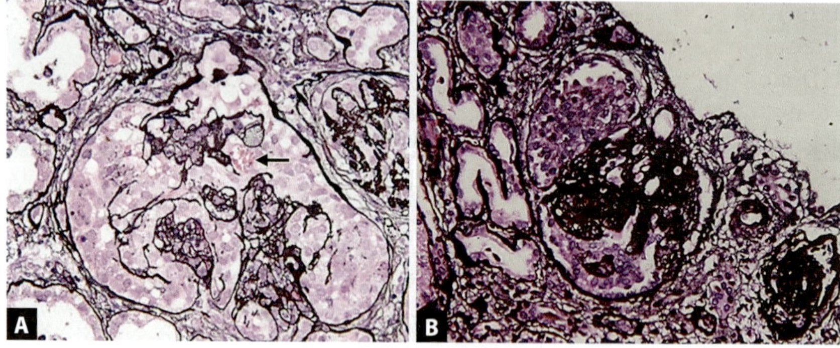

Figs. 12.5A and B: Collapsing glomerulopathy: The glomerular tuft is globally collapsed or imploded by markedly hypertrophic and hyperplastic visceral epithelial cells, displaying conspicuous nucleoli and protein resorption droplets (arrow) (Jones methenamine silver; 30×, 20×)

Monogenic Disease

SRNS may be caused by mutations in genes encoding components of the slit diaphragm, podocyte actin cytoskeleton, mitochondrial proteins, lysosomal proteins, nuclear transcription factors, and the glomerular basement membrane (GBM) **(Fig. 12.1)**. Next-generation sequencing (NGS) has facilitated the identification of almost 90 causative genes **(Annexure 9.4)**. The genetic mutations may be inherited in autosomal recessive (*NPHS1, NPHS2,* and *PLCE1*) or dominant fashion (*INF2, TRPC6,* and *ACTN4*) or both (*WT1*). SRNS caused by mutations in the recessive genes presents early in childhood, while that due to dominant genes shows variable penetrance and severity, and often presents in late childhood or young adulthood.

Data from registries suggests that ~30% children with SRNS may have an underlying genetic cause, with the proportions varying from 80% in patients with congenital nephrotic syndrome, to 50–70% with syndromic or familial SRNS. The genes implicated include *NPHS1, NPHS2, WT1, PLCE1,* and *LAMB2,* genes coding coenzyme Q10 pathway, *INF2, TRPC6,* and *CD2AP*. Recent reports emphasize the frequency of mutations in genes encoding type IV collagen (*COL4A3, COL4A4,* and *COL4A5*) and laminin alpha 5 (*LAMA5*), presenting with SRNS. **Tables 12.3** and **12.4** list findings on clinical examination or histology, mediated by specific genes. While most patients with monogenic SRNS do not respond to immunosuppression, partial or complete remission of proteinuria is reported following therapy with steroids or cyclosporine for specific genetic defects (*WT1, EMP2, TNS2, DLC1, CDK20, ITSN1, ITSN2*). Partial remission might follow CoQ10 supplementation in patients with defects in CoQ pathway (*COQ2, COQ6, ADCK4, PDSS2*). Certain syndromic forms of monogenic SRNS require follow up for significant extrarenal manifestations. Normally, alternative splicing at intron 9 of *WT1* is responsible for two *WT1* isoforms, with (+) or without (–) three amino acids lysine-threonine-serine (KTS), between zinc fingers 3 and 4. Donor splice site heterozygous mutations at this location affect the KTS +/– ratio that leads to gonadal dysgenesis, pseudohermaphroditism, and the risk of gonadoblastoma.

Circulating Factors

The majority of cases of SRNS are proposed to result from a putative soluble "circulating factor" that results from the immune dysregulation in SRNS. The strongest clinical evidence of a circulating permeability factor is the recurrence of proteinuria, within hours following renal transplantation, from the healthy allograft in a recipient with end stage kidney disease (ESKD) due to FSGS. Studies on podocyte cells in culture and in animal experiments show disruption of podocyte focal complexes, changes in podocyte motility, and

TABLE 12.3: Genes associated with syndromic forms of steroid resistance and key phenotypic features[1]

Syndrome	*Gene*	*Protein*	*Function*	*Inheritance*	*Associated features; histology*
Denys-Drash syndrome	*WT1*	Wilms tumor protein	Podocyte development	AD	Male pseudohermaphroditism, Wilms tumor; DMS
Frasier syndrome				AD	Male pseudohermaphroditism, gonadoblastoma; FSGS
Pierson syndrome	*LAMB2*	Laminin beta-2	Links GBM to cytoskeleton	AR	Microcoria, abnormal lens; DMS
Schimke immune-osseous dysplasia	*SMARCAL1*	SWI/SNF related, matrix associated, actin dependent regulator of chromatin, subfamily A-like protein	Chromatin bundling; gene transcription	AR	Bone dysplasia, immunodeficiency, ischemic cerebral lesions; FSGS
Nail-patella syndrome	*LMX1B*	LIM homeodomain transcription factor 1, beta	Podocyte, GBM development	AD	Hypoplastic nails and patellae, iliac horns; FSGS
Charcot-Marie-Tooth disease, intermediate E	*INF2*	Inverted formin 2	Actin regulation	AD	Neuropathy, deafness; FSGS
Galloway-Mowat syndrome	11 genes **(Table 12.4)**	Proteins with WD40 repeat-domains; KEOPS complex, nucleoporins	Unknown	AR; XL	Microcephaly, intellectual disability, hiatal hernia, optic atrophy; FSGS

Contd...

Contd...

Syndrome	*Gene*	*Protein*	*Function*	*Inheritance*	*Associated features; histology*
Mitochondrial respiratory-chain disease	*MTTL1*	Mitochondrial tRNA leucine 1	Mitochondrial tRNA	Maternal	MELAS, diabetes mellitus, deafness; FSGS
	COQ2	Polyprenyltransferase	Coenzyme (Co) Q10 biosynthesis	AR	Encephalomyopathy, hypotonia, seizures, lactic acidosis; FSGS
	COQ6	Ubiquinone biosynthesis monooxygenase *COQ6*	CoQ10 biosynthesis	AR	Sensorineural deafness; FSGS
	PDSS2	Decaprenyl diphosphate synthase, subunit 2	CoQ10 biosynthesis	AR	Encephalomyopathy, hypotonia, seizures, lactic acidosis; FSGS
Sphingosine phosphate lyase insufficiency syndrome (SPLIS)	*SGPL1*	Sphingosine-1-phosphate lyase-1	Sphingolipid catabolism	AR	Adrenal, other endocrine abnormalities; cranial nerve deficits, peripheral neuropathy, sensorineural hearing loss; developmental delay; immunodeficiency; ichthyosis
Action myoclonus renal failure	*SCARB2*	Scavenger receptor class B member 2	Lysosomal protein synthesis	AR	Progressive myoclonus epilepsy; collapsing FSGS

AD: autosomal dominant; AR: autosomal recessive; DMS: diffuse mesangial sclerosis; FSGS: focal segmental glomerulosclerosis; GBM: glomerular basement membrane; KEOPS: kinase, endopeptidase and other proteins of small size; MELAS: mitochondrial encephalomyopathy, lactic acidosis, and stroke-like symptoms; tRNA: transfer ribonucleic acid; XL: X-linked

[1]**Annexure 9.4** provides list of all genes to be screened through next-generation sequencing

TABLE 12.4: Specific phenotypes that indicate the etiology of monogenic steroid-resistant nephrotic syndrome*

Systemic feature(s)	*Genes implicated*
Intellectual disability, developmental delay, microcephaly	*WDR4, WDR73; OSGEP, TP53RK, TPRKB, LAGE3, GON7, YRDC; NUP107, NUP133; PRDM15* (Galloway–Mowat syndrome); *NUP85, NUP93, NUP160, NUP205; TRIM8*
Seizure, ataxia, encephalopathy	*COQ8B, COQ2, COQ6, PDSS2, MTTL1*
Failure to thrive, intellectual disability, developmental delay, hypotonia, and epilepsy	*ALG1* (congenital disorder of glycosylation)
Microcoria, cataract, myopia, nystagmus	*LAMB2*
Coloboma, microphthalmia, ptosis, syndactyly	*FAT1*
Myoclonic seizures; hearing loss	*SCARB2* [action myoclonus renal failure syndrome (AMRF)]
Epidermolysis bullosa	*ITGB4, ITGA3*
Heart block, arrhythmias	*NXF5*
Skeletal abnormalities	*SMARCAL1* (Schimke immuno-osseous dysplasia), *LMX1B* (nail patella syndrome)
Immunodeficiency	*SMARCAL1* (Schimke immuno-osseous dysplasia), *FOXP3* (IPEX syndrome); *SGPL1* (SPLIS)
Thrombocytopenia, giant platelets; neutrophil Dohle bodies	*MYH9*
Microangiopathic hemolytic anemia; thrombocytopenia	*DGKE*
Peripheral neuropathy	*INF2* (Charcot-Marie-Tooth disease)
Polyuria, rickets, glucosuria, aminoaciduria	*CLCN5, OCRL1, CUBN*
Microscopic hematuria; sensorineural hearing loss	*COL4A3, COL4A4, COL4A5, MYH9, INF2, SGPL1, MTTL1, COQ6*
Kidney cysts	*TTC21B, CRB2*
Congenital anomalies of the kidney and urinary tract	*PAX2, CRB2*
Diffuse mesangial sclerosis	*WT1, LAMB2, PLCE1, NPHS1, ARHGDIA*

IPEX: immune dysregulation, polyendocrinopathy, enteropathy, X-linked syndrome; SPLIS: sphingosine phosphate lyase insufficiency syndrome

*Specific syndromes are detailed in **Table 12.3**

foot process effacement following exposure to sera from patients with FSGS or relapse of nephrotic syndrome. Sera from patients with FSGS induces proteinuria or increased permeability of glomeruli to albumin.

However, identifying the putative factor remains elusive. Numerous factors have been identified including heparanase, hemopexin, angiopoietin-like 4 (ANGPTL4), cardiotrophin-like cytokine-1 (CLCF-1), and soluble urokinase plasminogen activator receptor (suPAR) **(Table 12.2)**. Apart from circulating factors, dysfunction or dysregulation of T lymphocytes have also shown to be involved in the pathogenesis of SRNS. Increase in podocyte B7-1 expression has been shown to cause podocyte dysfunction due to actin reorganization in a variety of animal models of proteinuria as well as in post-transplant FSGS recurrence.

Maladaptive Response to Injury

Secondary forms of FSGS result from maladaptive response of podocytes to conditions: (*i*) promoting hyperfiltration (obesity, acquired solitary functional kidney, and uncontrolled hypertension); (*ii*) leading to podocyte injury (viral infections: hepatitis B and C, parvovirus, and human immunodeficiency virus (HIV); exposure to toxins or medications: heavy metals, anti-vascular endothelial growth factor (anti-VEGF) monoclonals, pamidronate, lithium, and interferon); (*iii*) causing metabolic disturbances (mitochondrial disorders and diabetes mellitus); (*iv*) malignancy (e.g., lymphoma); and (*v*) deposition of abnormal protein (amyloid). Many of these conditions, associated with increased single nephron glomerular filtration rate (GFR), lead to intraglomerular hypertension, glomerular hypertrophy, and podocyte activation, stress and denudation with deposition of extracellular matrix and glomerular sclerosis.

CLINICAL FEATURES

Clinical features are discussed in Chapter 11. SRNS is diagnosed following nonresponse to steroids in either the initial episode (initial SRNS), or following nonresponse during therapy of a subsequent relapse (late SRNS). A detailed history and physical examination are done to rule out alternative diagnoses, syndromic association, and familial disease, and to detect complications. History of jaundice and systemic features (rash, joint pains, and palpable purpura) suggest a secondary cause. Skeletal, neurological, eye, ear, and urogenital abnormalities, developmental delay, dystrophic nails, and small or absent patella indicate syndromic cause **(Tables 12.3 and 12.4)**. Hypertension and gross hematuria may be observed in a proportion of cases.

It is important to distinguish SRNS from nephrotic range proteinuria without edema, seen in various primary or secondary glomerulonephritides (systemic lupus, C3 glomerulopathy, and IgA vasculitis), systemic disease (obesity and hypertension), reflux nephropathy, and other chronic kidney disease (CKD), chronic viral infections (hepatitis B or C and HIV), and certain tubulopathies (Dent disease and cystinosis). FSGS secondary to maladaptive repair, such as with low nephron endowment and obesity-related glomerulopathy, typically presents in adolescence or adulthood without edema, and with subnephrotic range proteinuria and normal serum albumin levels.

At onset of the disease, it is difficult to distinguish patients with steroid resistance from those with steroid sensitive nephrotic syndrome. However, some features might indicate that the child does not have MCD. For example, patients with onset during infancy have a higher likelihood of monogenic SRNS. Patients presenting with nephrotic syndrome in adolescence are likely to have nonminimal change histology, particularly if accompanied by microscopic hematuria, low complement C3, or hypertension. Patients with initial and late SRNS do not show phenotypic differences at onset. Patients with late SRNS are diagnosed within 2 years of disease onset, and often respond satisfactorily to noncorticosteroid immunosuppressive agents. While progression to kidney failure is rare, the risk of recurrence of disease in the allograft is several-fold higher than for patients with initial SRNS.

Monogenic SRNS is suspected in patients with onset in infancy (particularly if <9 months old), extrarenal features **(Table 12.3)**, consanguinity, and family history of nephrotic syndrome, proteinuria, CKD or ESKD in siblings, parents, or cousins. Details of disease in affected family members are collected, including age at onset, histological findings, results of genetic testing, response to immunosuppression, age at ESKD, and the pattern of inheritance. Almost half of the cases with familial SRNS have a monogenic basis of disease. The likelihood of finding a monogenic cause decreases with age: While 50–70% cases of SRNS in infancy have a genetic basis, the proportion with monogenic SRNS falls to 25% at 1–6 years, 18% at 7–12 years, and 11% in adolescence. Phenocopies of monogenic disorders, such as Alport syndrome, Dent disease, cystinosis, fibrillary nephropathy, and Fabry disease, might erroneously be managed as idiopathic SRNS, underscoring the role of genetic testing and detailed phenotyping **(Annexure 9.4)**.

EVALUATION

Evaluation at diagnosis of SRNS intends to: (*i*) confirm the diagnosis; (*ii*) rule out syndromic diagnosis, systemic disease, infections, and secondary etiologies; (*iii*) establish histological diagnosis; (*iv*) examine for monogenic etiology, where appropriate; and (*v*) determine baseline kidney function and proteinuria **(Table 12.5)**.

Urinalysis and specific serologies help in ruling out most glomerulonephritis. Serologic testing for hepatitis B and C, and HIV is useful before initiating immunosuppression. These chronic infections are asymptomatic, may not be detected by histology unless associated with

TABLE 12.5: Evaluation and monitoring in patients with steroid-resistant nephrotic syndrome

Investigations	*Frequency of reevaluation: Specific indication*
Urinalysis, including microscopy	q 6–12 months
Urine protein to creatinine ratio in spot (first morning void) or 24-hr urine	q 3–6 months (more frequently until remission)
Complete blood counts	q 6–12 months (more frequently until remission)
Blood creatinine, estimated GFR, electrolytes, calcium, total protein, albumin	q 3–6 months (more frequently until remission, or if CKD 4–5)
Fasting glucose, glycosylated hemoglobin (HbA1c)	q 6–12 months
Alkaline phosphatase, parathyroid hormone, 25-hydroxyvitamin D	q annually (more frequently if CKD 4–5)
Total, low density and high-density cholesterol; triglycerides	q annually
Thyroid functions (T3, T4, and TSH)	q annually if persistent proteinuria
Ultrasonography of kidneys	If indicated
Kidney biopsy; All, except if monogenic cause suspected*	After >2–3 years CNI therapy; drop in eGFR; increased proteinuria
Physical examination, including anthropometry; blood pressure	q 3–6 months
Family history, neurological examination, pubertal assessment, vaccination review	q annually, or when indicated
Toxicities related to specific medications	See **Table 12.6**
Evaluation: Specific indication	
Next generation or whole exome sequencing	Initial resistance*
Hepatitis B surface antigen; hepatitis C, HIV antibodies	Before therapy with CNI or monoclonal antibodies
Complement C3, C4; antinuclear antibody	Suspected lupus; persistent hematuria
For extrarenal disease	Features of systemic disease;^1 monogenic cause or phenocopy^2

CKD: chronic kidney disease; CNI: calcineurin inhibitors; FSGS: focal segmental glomerulosclerosis; GFR: glomerular filtration rate; HIV: human immunodeficiency virus; TSH: thyroid stimulating hormone; T3: triiodothyronine; T4: thyroxine

^Examples: [1]joint pain or swelling, weight loss, alopecia, jaundice, malar rash; palpable purpura, arthralgia; [2]see **Tables 12.3 and 12.4**

*Genetic testing is prioritized in those with infantile onset, familial disease; syndromic or extrarenal features; nonresponse to CNI therapy; and before transplantation. **Annexure 9.4** provides list of genes in which variants are prioritized

atypical lesions (e.g., collapsing or membranous nephropathy), often require antiviral therapy, and if left untreated, might lead to symptomatic disease following immunosuppression. Ultrasonography is useful in ruling out reflux nephropathy and congenital anomalies of kidneys.

Following a diagnosis of idiopathic SRNS, it is essential to quantify proteinuria and estimate GFR [estimated GFR (eGFR)] to establish a baseline for subsequent assessment of response to management. Since 24-hr urine collection is often cumbersome and/or inaccurate in young children, first morning urine protein to creatinine ratio (Up/Uc) is preferred. Trends in proteinuria, quantified by either method, help assess the response to therapy **(Table 12.5)**. Parents are explained the need for dipstick monitoring for proteinuria on the first morning void.

Schwartz eGFR is usually normal at baseline, but requires monitoring particularly in patients with hypovolemia, those receiving therapy with calcineurin inhibitors (CNI), angiotensin converting enzyme inhibitors (ACEi), or angiotensin receptor blockers (ARBs), and those with persistent nonresponse. Low eGFR at baseline or follow-up indicates either acute kidney injury (AKI) associated with hypovolemia, fluid loss, infections, and medication toxicity, or progression of CKD in patients with persistent nonresponse, recurrent AKI, unfavorable histology (e.g., diffuse mesangial sclerosis) or monogenic cause, or chronic tubulointerstitial disease.

Patients with persistent proteinuria are at risk of malnutrition, dyslipidemia, thrombosis, and subclinical hypothyroidism or hypovitaminosis D **(Table 12.5)**. Children with advanced CKD should be monitored for its complications, including growth failure, mineral bone disease, and anemia.

Kidney Histology

Kidney biopsy is an important diagnostic and prognostic tool in children with SRNS. Kidney biopsy is recommended in all patients with SRNS before instituting specific treatment. However, biopsy is not mandatory in familial, congenital nephrotic syndrome, infantile-onset SRNS, and/or syndromic SRNS, in whom next generation sequencing (NGS) carries higher likelihood of providing clinically useful and prognostic information. A biopsy helps (*i*) distinguish MCD from FSGS, membranous nephropathy, and mesangioproliferative glomerulonephritis that might differ in their response to immunosuppression and prognosis; (*ii*) identify proliferative lesions (e.g., IgA nephropathy, C3 glomerulopathy, and lupus nephritis) that require to be managed differently; (*iii*) detect glomerular injury secondary to other conditions (e.g., arteriosclerosis and intimal changes in hypertension; mesangial expansion in diabetes; tubulointerstitial changes and periglomerular fibrosis in reflux nephropathy; foam cells and tubulointerstitial chronicity in Alport syndrome); (*iv*) identify unusual histologies associated with adverse outcomes (collapsing glomerulopathy and diffuse mesangial sclerosis); and (*v*) inform on prognostic factors (e.g., degree of glomerulosclerosis, interstitial fibrosis, and tubular atrophy). The initial kidney biopsy forms a baseline for comparison with a repeat biopsy that may be performed to detect CNI-induced nephrotoxicity, and in patients in whom disease progression or change in histology is suspected.

Biopsies are examined by light, immunofluorescence, and electron microscopy. A core of tissue containing at least 20 glomeruli is considered necessary to confidently exclude FSGS. While light microscopy is the most informative, immunofluorescence helps exclude membranous nephropathy, IgA nephropathy, or C3 glomerulopathy, and electron microscopy evaluates the ultrastructure to confirm a primary podocytopathy (idiopathic FSGS or MCD), indicated by diffuse effacement of foot processes and lack of electron dense deposits. Electron microscopy is also useful in diagnosing secondary FSGS (focal or <40% foot process effacement), glomerulonephritis (electron dense immune deposits), and inherited GBM disorders such as Alport syndrome and myosin heavy chain 9 (MYH9)-related disease (variably thick and thin segments of GBM, basket-weaving pattern).

Minimal change histology **(Figs. 12.2A to C)** has better response to therapy and higher rates of kidney survival compared to FSGS. FSGS may have distinctive patterns, as outlined in the Columbia classification, which is, however, not validated in children. The FSGS not otherwise specified [FSGS-not otherwise specified (NOS)] is the most common variant **(Figs. 12.3A to C)**, while the collapsing, tip, perihilar, and cellular variants are less common. Collapsing FSGS **(Figs. 12.5A and B)**, observed in patients with HIV nephropathy, parvovirus B19 infection, or intravenous (IV) drug abuse, has the worst prognosis, while the NOS and tip variants have favorable outcomes. A perihilar pattern is observed in FSGS secondary to obesity or low nephron endowment and is accompanied by glomerular enlargement. Diffuse mesangial sclerosis **(Figs. 12.4A to D)** is an uncommon histology, often seen in infants with significant variants in *WT1*, *PLCE1*, *NPHS1* or *LAMB2*, and rapid progression to ESKD.

Genetic Testing

The IPNA and KDIGO advise genetic testing for all patients with initial SRNS using NGS for a comprehensive panel of genes **(Annexure 9.4)**. Guidelines from the ISPN limit the use of genetic testing to patients with initial SRNS who have high likelihood of a monogenic cause. These include patients with: (*i*) congenital nephrotic syndrome; (*ii*) patients with onset in infancy; (*iii*) family history of SRNS; (*iv*) nonresponse to 6-months therapy with CNI; (*v*) patients with extrarenal or syndromic features suggesting monogenic disease; and (*vi*) prior to kidney transplantation. This approach to testing is more feasible where facilities for NGS are not widely available or cannot be afforded by all patients, and test results are often interpreted and acted upon by clinicians rather than by trained medical geneticists.

Clinical or whole exome sequencing is recommended, with bioinformatics focused on variants in ~90 genes relevant to SRNS, including phenocopies. NGS should be performed by certified laboratories that report the pathogenicity of prioritized variants based on criteria proposed by the American College of Medical Genetics and Genomics. Sanger sequencing is the preferred method for patients in whom a specific disease-causing mutation has been found in another affected family member, or if the phenotype is specific for a particular gene, as in syndromic SRNS **(Table 12.3)**. Sanger sequencing is also used to confirm allele segregation for compound heterozygous variants, and to validate findings of NGS. Where screening is required, Sanger sequencing is preferred for testing siblings or parents, and potential living-related donors of an index patient with monogenic SRNS.

MANAGEMENT

The management of patients with SRNS is challenging because of variable response to therapy, adverse effects related to disease or therapies, presence of comorbidities, risk of progression to ESKD, and likelihood of post-transplant recurrence. The goal of therapy is to achieve complete or partial remission of proteinuria that is associated with lower rates of disease complications and progression to ESKD. Definitions of response are provided in **Table 12.1**. Various noncorticosteroid immunosuppressive strategies used to induce and sustain remission of proteinuria are summarized in **Table 12.6** and discussed below. Each of these requires careful monitoring for adverse effects.

Calcineurin Inhibitors

Therapy with CNI, either cyclosporine or tacrolimus, is recommended as initial therapy for patients with SRNS. Registries, such as the PodoNet (Europe), RaDAR (United Kingdom), and NEPTUNE (United States), report favorable response to therapy with CNI in 41–76% patients of nongenetic etiology. Systematic reviews indicate that therapy with CNI for 6–12 months results in remission of complete or partial remission of proteinuria in 70% (95% CI: 64–75) patients. Remission is 2–3 times more likely following therapy with CNI as compared to no treatment or therapy with IV cyclophosphamide. The rates of remission are similar for therapy with cyclosporine and tacrolimus, with no difference in rates of AKI, histological nephrotoxicity, or hypertension.

Guidelines by the ISPN, the IPNA, and the KDIGO recommend CNI as first-line therapy for patients with SRNS. Tacrolimus is preferred since it is not associated with cosmetic adverse effects, including hypertrichosis and gingival hyperplasia that are frequent with cyclosporine. Cyclosporine is preferred in young children since it is available as a suspension, while

TABLE 12.6: Agents used to induce and/or maintain remission of steroid-resistant nephrotic syndrome

Medication	*Dose*	*Medication target*	*Adverse effects*	*Monitoring*
Tacrolimus	0.1–0.2 mg/kg/day in two divided doses	Trough level 4–8 ng/mL[1]	*Both:* Acute and chronic nephrotoxicity, hyperkalemia, and hepatotoxicity *Tacrolimus*: Seizures, tremors, and headache; diarrhea; glucose intolerance, diabetes; hypomagnesemia *Cyclosporine:* Gingival hyperplasia, hypertrichosis; hypertension; dyslipidemia	*Both:* Screen for adverse effects Monitor creatinine, potassium at 2 weeks, then q 3 months; liver function tests, uric acid, magnesium, lipids, glucose q 6 months Avoid if eGFR <30 mL/min/1.73 m^2 Consider drug interactions
Cyclosporine	3–5 mg/kg/day in two divided doses	Trough level 80–120 ng/mL[1]		
Mycophenolate mofetil	1,000–1,200 mg/m^2/day in two divided doses	Mycophenolic acid AUC >50 mg*h/L[2]	Leukopenia; abdominal pain and diarrhea; liver dysfunction; paresthesia; weight loss; viral warts; teratogenic	Hemogram, liver functions q 3–6 months Avoid if planning pregnancy
Cyclophosphamide	500–750 mg/m^2 IV, q monthly for 6 months	Not applicable	Leukopenia, hemorrhagic cystitis, vomiting, and infections; gonadal toxicity and malignancies	Withhold if total leukocyte count <4,000/mm^3 Ondansetron, mesna prevent adverse effects
Rituximab	375 mg/m^2 q weekly for 2–4 doses	CD19% <1% or <5 cells/µL	Infusion reactions; serum sickness; acute lung injury; neutropenia; *P. jirovecii* pneumonia; reactivation of hepatitis B and JC virus; hypogammaglobulinemia	Blood counts; hepatitis, HIV serology; IgG level Monitor CD19, blood counts, IgG Trimethoprim 150 mg/m^2 on alternate day for 3–6 months
ACEi, ARB	As per medication used	Not applicable	Hyperkalemia; AKI; teratogenic	Do not combine ACEi and ARB *Avoid if:* hypovolemia; eGFR <30 mL/min/1.73 m^2 (AKI; CKD 4–5)

[1]12-hr after last dose; measured 2-weekly until target reached; then q 3 months or if suspecting toxicity, noncompliance, lack of response or drug interactions

[2]Abbreviated AUC at three points (C_0: 12-hr trough, $C_{0.5}$: 30 minutes after dose, C_2: 2 hr after dose) MPA-AUC = 7.75 + (6.49*C_0) + (0.76*$C_{0.5}$) + (2.43*C_2)

ACEi: angiotensin converting enzyme inhibitor; AKI: acute kidney injury; ARB: angiotensin receptor blocker; AUC: area under the curve; CKD: chronic kidney disease; IgG: immunoglobulin G; GFR: glomerular filtration rate; HIV: human immunodeficiency virus; P: *Pneumocystis*

tacrolimus is only available as capsules that young children are unable to swallow. Cyclosporine is also preferred in patients at risk of diabetes and those with seizures. The dose, adverse effects, and monitoring while on CNI therapy is summarized in **Table 12.6**. Both medications are given in two divided doses, along with tapering prednisolone; once daily formulation of tacrolimus is also effective. Prednisolone is tapered over 6–9 months. The dose of CNI is titrated to maintain trough levels within a target range of 80–150 ng/mL for cyclosporine and 4–8 ng/mL for tacrolimus. Interaction with other medications might affect drug trough levels. Low levels are associated with nonresponse and relapses, while high levels increase risk of nephrotoxicity. *CNI therapy is contraindicated in children with reduced kidney function.*

Response to therapy with CNI is usually achieved at median of 8–12 weeks. Patients who do not respond to CNI despite 6 months of adequate dose and drug trough levels are labeled as CNI resistant. These patients are considered for genetic testing followed by alternative immunosuppressive strategies or discontinuation of CNI therapy.

Following CNI-induced remission, ~60% patients experience disease relapses that are often steroid responsive. Therapy compliance and adequacy of dosing with drug trough levels must be ensured in patients experiencing frequent relapses. The optimal duration of treatment with CNI for patients with partial or complete remission is not clear. While guidelines recommend at least 12-months' therapy, most experts would continue CNI for 24–36 months with careful monitoring for adverse effects. Nephrotoxicity is observed in 10–25% patients receiving prolonged CNI treatment. Risk factors for nephrotoxicity include high doses, elevated trough levels and prolonged duration of CNI therapy, heavy proteinuria, initial steroid resistance, and hypertension during therapy.

The disease may relapse following discontinuation of CNI therapy; these relapses may be steroid sensitive or resistant. Multiple case series indicate satisfactory efficacy of switching therapy from CNI to either mycophenolate mofetil (MMF) or rituximab. Therefore, following 24–36 months CNI therapy, subsequent treatment options include: (*i*) discontinue CNI therapy if patient has been in sustained remission or has infrequent relapses; consider steroid-sparing therapies if frequent relapses occur following therapy discontinuation; (*ii*) continue CNI therapy, especially if relapses are frequent; perform kidney biopsy if treatment is prolonged beyond 36 months; and (*iii*) electively switch to IV rituximab or oral MMF in patients with multiple steroid-sensitive relapses or evidence of CNI or steroid toxicity.

Intravenous Cyclophosphamide

Intravenous cyclophosphamide, administered every month for 6 months, has been the chief alternative to CNI, typically in situations where CNI therapy is not accessible or feasible, or is contraindicated due to adverse effects. Complete or partial remission is reported in 15–50% of patients; a significant proportion develop serious adverse effects. Oral cyclophosphamide is not recommended as therapy for SRNS, since it is associated with unsatisfactory remission, similar to prednisolone alone.

Mycophenolate Mofetil

The MMF is the ester prodrug of mycophenolic acid (MPA), which inhibits inosine monophosphate dehydrogenase, a key enzyme in de novo purine biosynthesis in proliferating B and T lymphocytes. MPA blunts cell-mediated immune responses, inhibits lymphocyte recruitment, and reduces mesangial cell proliferation and activation. While its lack of renal, hemodynamic, and metabolic adverse effects makes MMF an attractive alternative to CNI, it has unsatisfactory efficacy in inducing remission. Long-term remission while on MMF was reported in one-sixth of patients in the PodoNet registry and in one-third of patients in a National Institute of Health (NIH)-funded clinical trial where patients with FSGS received therapy with a combination of MMF and oral pulse dexamethasone.

However, therapy with MMF appears to be useful in maintaining remission in patients with CNI-dependent SRNS and/or features of CNI toxicity. Attention to therapeutic drug monitoring is necessary to maintain an area under the curve of >45–60 µg*h/mL, which appears to be an important determinant of response to MMF. Close monitoring for adverse effects, including gastrointestinal disturbances and myelosuppression, is necessary, particularly at high doses **(Table 12.6)**.

Rituximab

Rituximab is an important second-line therapy in children with CNI-resistant SRNS. This monoclonal antibody binds to CD20 on the surface of B lymphocytes, inducing their apoptosis, affecting T-B cell cross-talk and T-cell function, including T-regulatory and T-helper cell 17 (Th17) balance. Although previously proposed, there is no evidence that rituximab has a direct effect on the podocyte actin cytoskeleton.

Despite the initial promise, rituximab has limited efficacy in inducing remission in patients with steroid- and CNI-resistant nephrotic syndrome. While systematic reviews indicate complete or partial remission in 30–40% patients with CNI-refractory SRNS who receive rituximab, this is an overestimate due to inclusion of patients with CNI-dependent SRNS, concomitant therapies, and short follow-up. The response to rituximab is reportedly better in patients with late *versus* initial SRNS and MCD *versus* FSGS.

On the other hand, just like MMF, therapy with rituximab appears to be a useful strategy to maintain remission of CNI-dependent SRNS, especially in patients with prolonged CNI use or toxicity. Studies reporting switch of therapy from CNI to rituximab indicate satisfactory rate of complete or partial remission, reduced immunosuppressive drug requirement, and improved eGFR. However, relapses often recur once B cells repopulate, with need for additional strategies to sustain remission.

Therapy with rituximab is associated with a high risk of infusion reactions. Chills, fever, and urticaria are common; serious reactions, including bronchospasm, hypotension, and anaphylaxis, and serum sickness may occur. B cell depletion is associated with high risk of serious infections (5.3/100 patient-years in one registry data) and reactivation of hepatitis B infection. An important delayed complication is hypogammaglobulinemia that might be severe and persistent in ~10% patients. The risk of hypogammaglobulinemia is higher in young children, those receiving concomitant therapy with MMF, and following multiple courses of therapy. Other adverse events include neutropenia, *P. jirovecii* pneumonia, severe lung injury, and progressive multifocal leukoencephalopathy.

Rituximab is conventionally administered at a dose of 375 mg/m^2 IV at weekly intervals, targeting CD19 cell count <5/µL or <1% of lymphocyte count. While two doses usually suffice, up to four doses might be required to achieve B cell depletion. The clearance of rituximab is accelerated in proteinuria, due to which frequent redosing might be necessary to sustain B cell depletion. Given the concerns of serious adverse events, the optimal dosing strategy remains uncertain. Individual centers vary in their practice of repeating doses of rituximab following relapses or repopulation of B cells, or switch to MMF to maintain rituximab-induced remission.

Pulse Corticosteroids

Initial studies had examined IV methylprednisolone (20–30 mg/kg for 6 alternate days; once a week for 8 doses, fortnightly for 4 doses, monthly for 8 doses, and bimonthly for 4 doses) or IV dexamethasone (4–5 mg/kg per dose), usually in combination with oral cyclophosphamide. While complete or partial remission was reported in 30–50% patients, there was high risk of steroid toxicity (hypertension, high glucose, and steroid psychosis) and systemic infections. This strategy is currently not recommended.

Combination of Immunosuppressive Agents

Anecdotal reports suggest that the combination of CNI and MMF might enable remission in patients with CNI-refractory disease. Polytherapy with rituximab, IV methylprednisolone, and MMF, led to remission in one series of patients with CNI-refractory SRNS; hypogammaglobulinemia and infections were common complications. Combinations of immunosuppression must be reserved for cautious use at experienced centers, following counseling, close vigilance for infections, and under cover of antibiotic prophylaxis.

Newer Agents

Low-density Lipoprotein Apheresis or Immunoadsorption

Lower lipid levels improve macrophage function, reduce endothelial dysfunction, prevent lipid-induced toxicity, improve renal blood flow, and reduce inflammation. Immunoadsorption (IA) using Liposorber® LA-15 or LA-40 filters (Kaneka Pharma America LLC), based on dextran sulfate cellulose adsorption, for 12–15 sessions over 10–12 weeks, with or without concomitant steroids, cyclosporine and statins, was associated with complete and partial remission in ~70% patients. Other reports have shown satisfactory data with either IA or low density lipoprotein (LDL) apheresis, but more studies are clearly required.

Monoclonal Agents

Ofatumumab is a fully human anti-CD20 antibody that has been reported to induce remission in anecdotal cases of CNI- and rituximab-refractory SRNS and rituximab- and plasmapheresis-refractory post-transplant recurrent FSGS. However, the therapy was deemed futile in a placebo-controlled randomized controlled trial (RCT). *Abatacept*, a fusion protein of cytotoxic T-lymphocyte-associated protein 4 (CTLA-4) and immunoglobulin, blocks the CD28:CD80/CD86 interaction that blunts the costimulatory signal for T-cell activation. Although encouraging results were reported in a series of patients with primary CNI-refractory SRNS or post-transplant recurrent FSGS treated with abatacept (10 mg/kg IV once, repeated every 15–30 days), subsequent studies have not shown similar results. *Adalimumab* blocks tumor necrosis factor (TNF)-α. Two small RCTs [FONT-I and FONT-II (The Novel Therapies for Resistant Focal Segmental Glomerulosclerosis phase I and II)] found low rates of remission in patients with FSGS treated with this agent (24 mg/m^2 subcutaneously biweekly for 16 weeks). *Fresolimumab* targets transforming growth factor-β (TGF-β), which is implicated in the pathogenesis of fibrosis in FSGS. Following initial promise in a phase I trial in adults with FSGS, no response was documented in a subsequent phase II study.

Other Medications

Following anecdotal reports suggesting that oral *galactose* (0.2 g/kg twice daily, maximum 30 g/day) binds to a "serum circulating factor", inhibiting its activity and reducing proteinuria in refractory FSGS, unsatisfactory results were reported in subsequent trials that evaluated its efficacy. Similarly, studies using *adrenocorticotropic hormone (ACTH) gel* (80 U/1.73 m^2 twice weekly, or tetracosactide 1 mg weekly) did not show satisfactory results in children with steroid-resistant or steroid-dependent disease.

Supportive Care

Steroid resistance is associated with risks of hypertension, dyslipidemia, hypoalbuminemia, hypercoagulable state, and steroid-induced obesity. Besides immunosuppression, therapy is directed at decreasing proteinuria using pharmacologic agents and management of related symptoms and complications.

Antiproteinuric Therapy

The most important strategy to minimize residual proteinuria and manage hypertension is the blockade of the renin-angiotensin-aldosterone (RAS) system with either ACEi or ARBs to decrease proteinuria and slow the progression of CKD. The agents most often used include enalapril, lisinopril, ramipril, losartan, valsartan, irbesartan, and telmisartan. Therapy with any of these agents reduces proteinuria in a time- and dose-dependent manner, to the tune of ~30%, especially when consuming a low salt diet. Adverse effects include reduction in eGFR, and risk of hyperkalemia and anemia; persistent cough may follow therapy with ACEi.

Combinations of ACEi and ARB are not advocated in view of the high risk of adverse effects, including hyperkalemia and AKI. The efficacy and safety of sodium-glucose cotransporter-2 inhibitors (SGLT2i; dapagliflozin and empagliflozin), and nonselective mineralocorticoid antagonists (finerenone) in reducing proteinuria in children with SRNS is being examined.

Sparsentan is a dual-acting ARB and highly selective endothelin type A receptor antagonist which has shown promise in reducing proteinuria in two RCTs (DUET and DUPLEX) on patients with primary FSGS. Therapy with oral sparsentan (200 mg, 400 mg, or 800 mg once daily) was associated with significant reduction of proteinuria compared to oral irbesartan (300 mg, once daily), and higher proportions of patients achieved partial remission (spot Up/Uc ≤1.5 g/g and >40% reduction from baseline) without significant adverse effects.

Hypertension

Blood pressure should be measured at each visit. Pharmacotherapy is initiated with ACEi or ARB, and titrated to achieve systolic and diastolic blood pressures between 50th and 75th percentile for age and sex. Patients are advised to increase their intake of vegetables, fresh fruits, low-fat milk, legumes, and nuts, and reduce that of salt and sweets.

Dyslipidemia

Patients with persistent proteinuria show high blood levels of cholesterol, triglycerides, apolipoprotein B (apoB)-containing lipoproteins [low-density lipoprotein (LDL), very low-density lipoprotein (VLDL), and intermediate-density lipoprotein (IDL)] and lipoprotein (a). Dyslipidemia aggravates glomerulosclerosis and might contribute to progression of CKD. Patients with SRNS should be regularly screened for dyslipidemia. Patients with dyslipidemia or risk factors for cardiovascular disease are advised to reduce their intake of trans- or saturated fats and sugar, and increase their consumption of fruits, vegetables, legumes, and whole grain cereals (Cardiovascular Health Integrated Lifestyle Diets, CHILD-1 and -2). Physical activity should be increased to ensure moderate physical activity for 1–2 hr daily and vigorous physical activity at least 3 days a week, while limiting screen time to <2 hr daily. Patients with persistent dyslipidemia require therapy with statins, especially if risk factors for cardiovascular disease are present.

Other measures to retard disease progression and reduce cardiovascular risks are weight reduction to achieve body mass index (BMI) <85th centile for age, nonexposure to tobacco, and achieving target levels of lipids, fasting glucose (<100 mg/dL), and hemoglobin A1C (HbA1c); (<6%).

Patients, who have received oral corticosteroids for >2 weeks within the past 1 year, should receive additional steroid dosing during conditions associated with physiological stress, such as fever ≥38°C, inadequate oral intake, lethargy, dehydration, invasive surgery, dental surgery, trauma, and large burns.

Management of Monogenic Steroid-resistant Nephrotic Syndrome

A diagnosis of monogenic disease has important implications for management and prognosis. Patients with pathogenic or likely pathogenic variations in key podocyte genes or transcription factors do not respond to immunosuppression and progress rapidly to kidney failure. Following transplantation, the risk of disease recurrence is low. Families of patients with monogenic disease require genetic counseling, since the diagnosis has implications for prenatal testing, screening of siblings for disease, and genetic screening of potential donors for transplantation. Patients with monogenic SRNS, diagnosed at disease onset or following documentation of CNI resistance, should not be subjected to further immunosuppressive therapy.

Treatment is limited to supportive care and preparing for renal transplantation. However, some patients with a genetic cause for steroid resistance, especially those with *WT1* variants, might show partial remission following treatment with CNI. Targeted therapy is possible for specific mutations, e.g., coenzyme Q10 (CoQ10) for defect(s) in CoQ10 pathway, eplerenone for *ARHGDIA*, and corticosteroids for mutations in genes of *Rho/Rac/Cdc42* network. Principles of supportive care for patients with monogenic SRNS are similar to those outlined for congenital nephrotic syndrome (*see* later).

Approach to Management

The approach to management of childhood SRNS is summarized in **Flowchart 12.1**. Kidney biopsy is necessary, except in patients where genetic testing may obviate the need for biopsy. Patients with monogenic cause for steroid resistance should not receive immunosuppression and are managed with ACEi and supportive therapy. An immunosuppressive regimen based

Flowchart 12.1: Approach to management of steroid-resistant nephrotic syndrome (SRNS). Evaluation at baseline includes quantification of proteinuria, estimation of GFR, kidney biopsy, and in selected patients, next generation sequencing (*see footnote of Table 12.5 and text). Calcineurin inhibitors (CNI) are the mainstay of therapy of SRNS. Nonimmunosuppressive therapy with angiotensin converting enzyme (ACE) inhibitors are an important component of treatment, and the cornerstone of management of monogenic disease, in whom immunosuppression is not advisable. Patients with nongenetic SRNS who respond to immunosuppression should continue to receive CNI for 2–3 years, following which therapy is withdrawn or switched to alternative agents such as mycophenolate mofetil (MMF) or intravenous rituximab

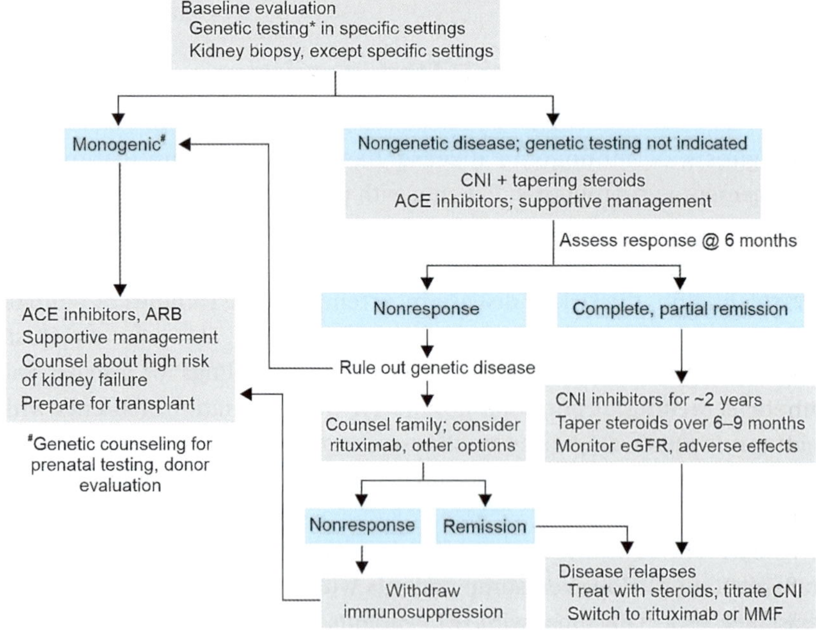

on calcineurin inhibitors, prednisone on alternate days, and ACEi is the standard of care for childhood SRNS. Lack of remission despite adequate therapy with CNI for 6 months is an indication for genetic screening, if not performed earlier. Patients with CNI-resistant disease who do not show a monogenic defect may be treated with IV rituximab or combined therapy of CNI and MMF. Immunosuppression is withdrawn in patients with continued nonresponse. Patients require regular monitoring and careful follow-up, and counseling regarding the need for compliance with medications.

OUTCOMES

Information on disease course and outcomes of SRNS is limited. Following discontinuation of CNI or alternative agents, patients with complete or partial remission of proteinuria might show sustained remission or a relapsing illness that is managed with steroid-sparing immunosuppressive regimens. In contrast, patients with nonresponse to CNI are at high risk of progression to ESKD. Patients who continue to have disease relapses or show persistent proteinuria, or decline in kidney function often require transition into care by adult nephrologists.

Pooled data from five large multicenter collaborative studies or registries, including 1,107 patients with SRNS, indicates complete remission in 27% (95% CI: 24–29%) cases, partial remission in 18% (16–21%) cases, and nonresponse in 55% (52–58%) patients. The low rates of response, compared to that reported in RCTs, might reflect real-world effectiveness of therapies. On the other hand, registry data is often inadequately phenotyped and limited by selection, information, and attrition biases.

Patients with SRNS are at high risk of kidney failure. In the PodoNet registry, the median rates of survival free of kidney failure were 74% at 5 years, 58% at 10 years, and 48% at 15 years. The etiology of disease and response to therapy are the chief determinants of long-term outcomes; histological diagnosis and type of steroid resistance might also affect the prognosis. In the above cohort, 10 years kidney survival was higher for children with complete or partial response to immunosuppression compared to those with nonresponse (94% or 72%, vs. 43%, respectively). Patients with a genetic diagnosis and those with FSGS on renal biopsy had lower 10 years kidney survival, at 29% and 52%, respectively. Pooled data from five large studies shows that patients with genetic *versus* nongenetic disease have higher risk of nonresponse [odds ratio (OR): 4.0; 95% CI: 2.5–6.5] and kidney failure (OR: 2.9; 95% CI: 2.2–3.7). In patients with undifferentiated or nongenetic SRNS, response to immunosuppression predicted kidney survival. There was a higher rate of survival free of kidney failure at 10 years in patients with complete (93%; 95% CI: 86–98%) or partial remission (73%; 65–80%), compared to nonresponse (35%; 22–49%).

Uncontrolled studies suggest that patients with MCD have higher rates of remission and better prognosis than FSGS. Patients with FSGS tip lesion tend to have a favorable prognosis, while collapsing glomerulopathy and diffuse mesangial sclerosis show lowest remission and progressive kidney failure. Compared to initial steroid resistance, patients with late resistance are more likely to have MCD, show satisfactory response to immunosuppression, and carry lower risk of progression to ESKD.

KIDNEY TRANSPLANTATION

Kidney transplantation is the optimal modality of kidney replacement therapy for patients with ESKD. FSGS ranks third among the causes of ESKD in various pediatric dialysis and transplant registries, accounting for 10–12% cases. However, the diagnosis of FSGS as the underlying etiology of ESKD has important implications in peri- and post-transplant management.

Genetic screening of the recipient is necessary, particularly for those with initial resistance or unclear diagnosis, since it stratifies the risk for allograft recurrence and helps in donor screening. In children with genetic forms of SRNS that have autosomal dominant inheritance, a parent (or sibling) with the same variant as in the recipient are not eligible to donate. Similarly, heterozygous carriers of causal variants in *COL4A3* and *COL4A4,* and female hemizygous carriers of variants in *COL4A5*, are not accepted as donors since they are at risk of kidney failure.

One of the challenges of kidney transplantation in FSGS is the risk of recurrence, which may occur within hours to days after transplant. Recurrent FSGS is also an important determinant of kidney outcome. Pooled data from multicenter reports (Europe and United States) on 581 pediatric kidney allograft recipients indicates recurrence in 39% (95% CI: 34–44%) cases. Recurrent FSGS is associated with the risk of delayed graft function, and early and late graft losses. In the North American Pediatric Renal Transplant and Collaborative Studies (NAPRTCS), patients with FSGS had 13% lower 5-year allograft survival compared to other etiologies. A meta-analysis also showed that the 5-year allograft survival in FSGS was 53% and 83% in patients with or without disease recurrence, respectively.

The chief risk factor for recurrence is the diagnosis of nongenetic disease. FSGS recurs in fewer than 5% of patients with genetic SRNS compared to 61% (95% CI: 53–69%) of nongenetic disease. Post-transplant proteinuria, observed in ~30% of patients with homozygous Fin-major mutations in *NPHS1*, is not true recurrence and is caused by *de novo* glomerulopathy associated with the generation of antinephrin antibodies in response to the allograft nephrin, which represents an immunologically foreign molecule in patients lacking nephrin expression. Patients with late steroid resistance, with presumably “circulating factor” disease, are at twice the risk of recurrence compared to those with initial steroid resistance that is a composite of immune-mediated and monogenic disease [86% vs. 42%; relative risk 1.9; 95% CI: 1.5–2.5]. Recurrence is reported more often in patients with native kidney biopsy showing MCD *versus* FSGS (75% vs. 40%; adjusted OR: 5.6; 95% CI: 1.3–23.7), and in older *versus* younger children (threshold age 6–9 years), reflecting the phenotypes of nongenetic *versus* genetic SRNS, respectively. However, the relationship with age is not definite; another study suggests higher risk in younger children. Other risk factors include rapid progression to kidney failure (<3 years from disease onset), mesangial proliferation on native biopsy, native kidney nephrectomy, Caucasian race, and living related (vs. deceased) donor transplantation. The rate of recurrence has not changed, despite changes in post-transplant immunosuppressive regimens. Disease recurrence in the first allograft confers very high (>80%) risk of recurrence in subsequent allografts.

Box 12.1 summarizes guidelines on evaluation and management of recurrent FSGS. Pretransplant counseling should include an assessment of risk of recurrence. NGS to diagnose monogenic SRNS helps ascertain the possibility of disease recurrence, and guides donor selection. Quantification of baseline proteinuria is essential prior to transplantation. Preventive strategies, including B cell depletion and plasma exchanges, have a limited role in reducing the risk of recurrence, particularly for the first transplant.

Patients with nonmonogenic disease require close monitoring of proteinuria in the post-transplant period, particularly in the first 12 months. The diagnosis of recurrence is made in patients with proteinuria and Up/Uc ≥1 mg/mg if anuric prior to transplant or increase of ratio by ≥1 mg/mg in those with proteinuria at transplantation. Allograft biopsy showing FSGS, or widespread podocyte effacement supports the diagnosis. Management comprises a combination of plasma exchanges (or immunoadsorption), high doses of cyclosporine, with or without 1–2 doses of rituximab **(Box 12.1)**. Additional strategies include therapy with ACEi or ARB, high-dose corticosteroid pulses, LDL apheresis, and ofatumumab. Prompt detection and management of recurrent FSGS leads to partial or complete remission of proteinuria in 60–75% cases.

CONGENITAL NEPHROTIC SYNDROME

The term congenital nephrotic syndrome refers to patients with nephrotic syndrome within the first 3 months of life. These infants are typically born preterm, with large placenta. Massive proteinuria leads to hypoalbuminemia and anasarca, usually within the first month of life. Antenatal ultrasonography may show hyperechoic kidneys; amniotic fluid has high levels of α-fetoprotein. Dysmorphism is uncommon and associated with specific monogenic syndromes (Pierson and Galloway Mowat).

Almost 70–85% patients with congenital nephrotic syndrome have monogenic disease. Mutations in *NPHS1* account for over three-fourths

BOX 12.1: Management of allograft recurrence of nephrotic syndrome

Monitoring

Urine protein to creatinine (Up/Uc) ratio: Performed daily for 1 week; weekly for 4 weeks; monthly for 1 year; then every 3–6 months

Blood albumin level; renal biopsy, especially if low grade proteinuria or graft dysfunction

Diagnosis

Up/Uc ≥1 mg/mg if anuric before transplant; or increase in Up/Uc by ≥1 mg/mg, if proteinuric at time of transplant

Management

Plasma exchange (PEX)

Membrane filtration or centrifugation based, heparin or citrate anticoagulation

Replacement fluid: 5% albumin; fresh frozen plasma (prefer latter if fibrinogen is low)

Schedule: Exchange 1.5 times plasma volume (60–75 mL/kg) per session daily for 3 days, then on alternate days for 2 weeks; subsequently based on degree of proteinuria; terminate after remission (proteinuria <0.5–1 g/m^2/day) for days to weeks

Immunoadsorption (IA)

Preferred in patients who cannot tolerate PEX or are PEX-refractory

2.5–3 plasma volumes, daily for 1 week; alternate days for 2 weeks; and twice a week for 2 weeks (≥12 sessions)

Medications

Intravenous (IV) methylprednisolone 250 mg/m^2/day for 3 days; taper to previous dose of oral prednisolone

Calcineurin inhibitors: Increase dose; tacrolimus trough 8–12 ng/mL; cyclosporine 150–200 ng/mL

Mycophenolate mofetil (MMF) 600 mg/m^2 PO q12 hr

Rituximab 375 mg/m^2 two-four doses, 1 week apart (avoid PEX/IA for 48 hr after rituximab)

Add angiotensin converting enzyme inhibitor, once allograft function established and stable estimated glomerular filtration rate (eGFR)

Alternate strategies: Lipid apheresis; cyclophosphamide (instead of MMF); belatacept or abatacept; ofatumumab; mesenchymal stem cells (limited data)

of cases worldwide. Fin-major and Fin-minor deletions are uncommon, except in patients with Scandinavian ancestry. Three mutations in *NPHS1* (c.2600G>A; c.1099C>T; and c.3478C>T) account for a high proportion of cases from India. Less commonly implicated genes include *WT1*, *LAMB2*, *PLCE1*, and *NPHS2*. Rarely, the condition is secondary to intrauterine infections with cytomegalovirus, rubella, toxoplasma, and syphilis. A rare etiology is neonatal membranous nephropathy due to *in situ* deposition of immune complexes of neural endopeptidase, a podocyte membrane-bound zinc metalloproteinase, and placentally transferred maternal antibodies, generated in pregnant women who lack the enzyme and are alloimmunized due to exposure to paternally derived fetal antigen.

BOX 12.2: Evaluation of patients with congenital nephrotic syndrome

Extrarenal features: Dysmorphic features, eye, urogenital abnormalities; large placenta

Evaluation

Urinalysis; urine protein to creatinine ratio
Complete blood counts
Blood creatinine, protein, albumin, electrolytes, calcium, phosphate
Transaminases, alkaline phosphatase, 25-hydroxyvitamin D
Lipid profile, free thyroxine, thyroid stimulating hormone
Renal ultrasonography
Kidney biopsy is not necessary, except if a genetic diagnosis is not established

Identifying the cause

Exome sequencing
Serology for intrauterine infections [*Toxoplasma gondii*, rubella, cytomegalovirus, and herpes simplex virus (TORCH)], syphilis, hepatitis B and C, human immunodeficiency virus (HIV)
Karyotyping (infants with ambiguous genitalia, extrarenal features)

Evaluation is directed at confirming the diagnosis, determining the etiology, and identifying complications **(Box 12.2)**. NGS focusing on the panel of genes for SRNS **(Annexure 9.4, p 845)** is recommended, and the results have implications for counseling in later pregnancies. Intrauterine infections should be excluded. The role of kidney biopsy is limited to patients in whom a genetic diagnosis is not established. Complications include poor growth, hypothyroidism, systemic infections, and thromboembolism. Infants with *WT1* variants require monitoring for Wilms tumor by ultrasonography every 3-6 months.

Guidelines on management advise symptomatic therapy, with steps to reduce anasaraca while maintaining euvolemia and optimizing nutrition. An adequate intake of energy (110-120 Cal/kg) and protein (3-3.5 g/kg/d) is ensured, orally or by feeding gastrostomy. Supplements of thyroxine, vitamin D, and calcium are necessary. IV albumin infusions (0.5-1.0 g/kg) are indicated in patients with hypovolemia or anasarca. Most guidelines do not recommend regular use of IV albumin; an individualized decision-making is based on the balance of benefits (maintains euvolemia; enables growth; and prevents hypovolemia and anasarca) and risks of regular infusions (central-line associated thrombosis or infections; infusion reactions). Therapy with ACEi reduces proteinuria, but is avoided in the neonatal period. Prostaglandin inhibitors (indomethacin and celecoxib) may be considered in refractory cases. All primary immunizations should be completed, with additional vaccines, as necessary, to protect against pneumococcal infections, influenza, and varicella. Bacterial infections should be treated promptly. Patients with a history of thrombosis require therapy with anticoagulants in the long term. Unilateral or bilateral nephrectomies may be considered in patients with repeated episodes of hypovolemia or refractory edema, persistent nephrotic range proteinuria, thrombosis, and malnutrition. Bilateral nephrectomy is required before kidney transplantation in patients with *WT1* mutations.

The chief causes of mortality are infections and progression to ESKD. Most patients develop kidney failure between 2 and 8 years of age. While kidney transplantation is the treatment of choice, it has multiple ethical, technical, and immunologic challenges.

BIBLIOGRAPHY

1. Ahn W, Bomback AS. Approach to diagnosis and management of primary glomerular diseases due to podocytopathies in adults: Core curriculum 2020. Am J Kidney Dis. 2020;75:955-64.
2. Burke GW 3rd, Mitrofanova A, Fontanella A, et al. The podocyte: Glomerular sentinel at the crossroads of innate and adaptive immunity. Front Immunol. 2023;14:1201619.
3. Campbell RE, Thurman JM. The immune system and idiopathic nephrotic syndrome. Clin J Am Soc Nephrol. 2022;17:1823-34.
4. Chanchlani R, Parekh RS. Ethnic differences in childhood nephrotic syndrome. Front Pediatr. 2016;4:39.
5. Churg J, Habib R, White RH. Pathology of the nephrotic syndrome in children. A report for the International Study of Kidney Disease in Children. Lancet. 1970;760:1299-302.
6. Corwin HL, Schwartz MM, Lewis EJ. The importance of sample size in the interpretation of the renal biopsy. Am J Nephrol. 1988;8:85-89.
7. D'Agati V, Fogo A, Bruijn J, et al. Pathologic classification of focal segmental glomerulosclerosis: A working proposal. Am J Kidney Dis. 2004;43:368-82.
8. De Vriese AS, Sethi S, Nath KA, et al. Differentiating primary, genetic, and secondary FSGS in adults: A clinicopathologic approach. J Am Soc Nephrol. 2018;29:759-74.
9. Ding WY, Koziell A, McCarthy HJ, et al. Initial steroid sensitivity in children with steroid-resistant nephrotic syndrome predicts post-transplant recurrence. J Am Soc Nephrol. 2014;25:1342-48.
10. Fogo AB. Causes and pathogenesis of focal segmental glomerulosclerosis. Nat Rev Nephrol. 2015;11:76-87.
11. Kamei K, Ishikura K, Sako M, et al. Rituximab therapy for refractory steroid-resistant nephrotic syndrome in children. Pediatr Nephrol. 2020;35:17-24.
12. Kidney Disease: Improving Global Outcomes (KDIGO) Glomerular Diseases Work Group. KDIGO 2021 Clinical Practice Guideline for the Management of Glomerular Diseases. Kidney Int. 2021;100:S1-S276.
13. Koh LJ, Martz K, Blydt-Hansen TD, NAPRTCS Registry Investigators. Risk factors associated with allograft failure in pediatric kidney transplant recipients with focal segmental glomerulosclerosis. Pediatr Transplant. 2019;23:e13469.
14. Königshausen E, Sellin L. Circulating permeability factors in primary focal segmental glomerulosclerosis: A review of proposed candidates. Biomed Res Int. 2016;2016:3765608.
15. Kopp JB, Anders HJ, Susztak K, et al. Podocytopathies. Nat Rev Dis Primers. 2020;6:68.

16. Lee JM, Kronbichler A, Shin JI, et al. Current understandings in treating children with steroid-resistant nephrotic syndrome. Pediatr Nephrol. 2021;36:747-61.
17. Lipska-Ziętkiewicz BS. Genetic steroid-resistant nephrotic syndrome overview. In: Adam MP, Feldman J, Mirzaa GM, Pagon RA, Wallace SE, Bean LJH, et al., (Eds). GeneReviews® [Internet]. Seattle (WA): University of Washington, Seattle;1993-2024.
18. Liu F, Mao JH. Calcineurin inhibitors and nephrotoxicity in children. World J Pediatr. 2018;14:121-26.
19. Liu ID, Willis NS, Craig JC, et al. Interventions for idiopathic steroid-resistant nephrotic syndrome in children. Cochrane Database Syst Rev. 2019;2019:CD003594.
20. Morello W, Proverbio E, Puccio G, et al. A systematic review and meta-analysis of the rate and risk factors for post-transplant disease recurrence in children with steroid resistant nephrotic syndrome. Kidney Int Rep. 2022;8:254-64.
21. Raina R, Jothi S, Haffner D, et al. Post-transplant recurrence of focal segmental glomerular sclerosis: Consensus statements. Kidney Int. 2024;105:450-63.
22. Ravaglia F, Melica ME, Angelotti ML, et al. The pathology lesion patterns of podocytopathies: How and why? Front Cell Dev Biol. 2022;10:838272.
23. Salfi G, Casiraghi F, Remuzzi G. Current understanding of the molecular mechanisms of circulating permeability factor in focal segmental glomerulosclerosis. Front Immunol. 2023;14:1247606.
24. Sinha A, Mathew G, Arushi A, et al. Sequential rituximab therapy sustains remission of nephrotic syndrome but carries high risk of adverse effects. Nephrol Dial Transplant. 2023;38:939-49.
25. Trautmann A, Vivarelli M, Samuel S, et al.; International Pediatric Nephrology Association. IPNA clinical practice recommendations for the diagnosis and management of children with steroid-resistant nephrotic syndrome. Pediatr Nephrol. 2020;35:1529-61.
26. Troost JP, Trachtman H, Spino C, et al. Proteinuria reduction and kidney survival in focal segmental glomerulosclerosis. Am J Kidney Dis. 2021;77:216-25.
27. Tullus K, Webb H, Bagga A. Management of steroid-resistant nephrotic syndrome in children and adolescents. Lancet Child Adolesc Health. 2018;2:880-90.
28. Vasudevan A, Thergaonkar R, Mantan M, et al.; Expert group of Indian Society of Pediatric Nephrology. Consensus guidelines on management of steroid-resistant nephrotic syndrome. Indian Pediatr. 2021;58:650-66.
28. Vivarelli M, Gibson K, Sinha A, et al. Childhood nephrotic syndrome. Lancet 2023;402:809-24.
29. Watanabe A, Feltran LS, Sampson MG. Genetics of nephrotic syndrome presenting in childhood: Core curriculum 2019. Am J Kidney Dis. 2019;74:549-57.
30. Weber LT, Tönshoff B, Grenda R, et al. Clinical practice recommendations for recurrence of focal and segmental glomerulosclerosis/ steroid-resistant nephrotic syndrome. Pediatr Transplant. 2021;25:e13955.

C3 Glomerulopathy and Membranous Nephropathy

Arvind Bagga, Aditi Sinha

MEMBRANOPROLIFERATIVE GLOMERULONEPHRITIS AND C3 GLOMERULOPATHY

The membranoproliferative pattern of glomerulonephritis (MPGN) is characterized by mesangial matrix expansion and hypercellularity, endocapillary proliferation, and diffuse thickening of the glomerular basement membrane (GBM). This pattern of injury is found in many unrelated disorders, and their identification is important for management.

A pathophysiology-based classification relies on immunofluorescence examination, deposits being defined as primary immunoglobulin and complement, primarily complement, or immunofluorescence negative. Patients that show light microscopic appearance of MPGN and immunofluorescent deposits of C3 and immunoglobulins are classified as immune-complex MPGN (IC-MPGN) **(Figs. 13.1A to D)**. Many conditions may result in IC-MPGN **(Box 13.1)**. C3 glomerulopathy (C3G) is a rare entity defined by C3-dominant glomerulonephritis (proliferative lesion with C3 deposits at least 2 orders of magnitude greater than any other immune reactant) on immunofluorescence. This condition is chiefly associated with dysregulation of the alternate complement pathway. Based on electron microscopy findings, C3G includes: (*i*) dense deposit disease (DDD) with electron-dense deposits in the lamina densa of the GBM, and (*ii*) C3 glomerulonephritis (C3GN) with deposits in subendothelial, subepithelial, and/or mesangial localization. Rarely, the MPGN pattern may be seen without immune complexes, as in sickle cell nephropathy, chronic thrombotic microangiopathy, and transplant glomerulopathy.

Histopathology

C3 Glomerulopathy

There are four major light microscopy patterns seen in DDD and C3GN including a mesangial proliferative pattern, a membranoproliferative pattern **(Fig. 13.2)**, a crescentic pattern, and an acute proliferative and exudative pattern **(Fig. 13.3)**. Immunofluorescence shows positive staining for C3 in the GBM and mesangial regions **(Fig. 13.2C)**. Similar deposits may be seen along the tubular basement membrane and the Bowman capsule in patients

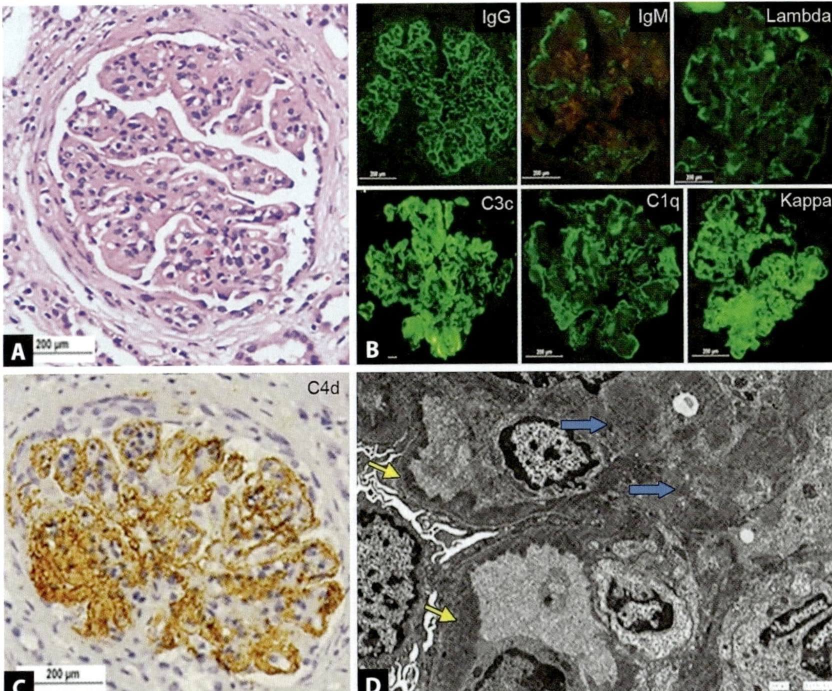

Figs. 13.1A to D: Immune complex-mediated membranoproliferative glomerulonephritis. (A) Membranoproliferative pattern of injury on light microscopy (hematoxylin–eosin, original magnification ×20); (B) Direct immunofluorescence demonstrates coarse capillary wall granular and mesangial granular staining of IgG (2+), IgM (1+), C3c (3+), C1q (2+), kappa (3+), and lambda (2+) on a scale of 0 to 3+ (fluorescein isothiocyanate-labeled antibodies, original magnification ×20); (C) Immunohistochemistry for C4d displays intense coarse granular capillary wall staining along with mesangial staining (C4d immunohistochemistry, original magnification ×20). At low-power examination, the diffuse staining of the glomeruli is noted (C4d immunohistochemistry, original magnification ×4); (D) Transmission electron microscopic images show subendothelial (yellow arrows) and large mesangial deposits (blue arrows) with widespread podocyte effacement (uranyl acetate–lead citrate, original magnification ×1550)

with DDD **(Fig. 13.3B)**. Pronase-digested paraffin immunofluorescence may reveal the presence of significant immunoglobulin deposits, which rules out C3GN. On electron microscopy, DDD shows segmental and patchy or diffuse electron dense transformation of the GBM **(Fig. 13.3C)**. Subepithelial and mesangial electron dense deposits are not uncommon. Electron microscopy in C3GN shows deposits located in the subendothelial space and mesangium, with occasional subepithelial deposits **(Fig. 13.2D)**.

Immune-complex MPGN (IC-MPGN)

The IC-MPGN is defined in patients who show MPGN pattern on light microscopy **(Fig. 13.1A)**, with C3 and immunoglobulin deposits on

BOX 13.1: Causes of membranoproliferative glomerulonephritis (MPGN)

Immune complexes detected

Infectious diseases

Hepatitis B, hepatitis C, hepatitis E, Ebstein–Barr virus, HIV
Endocarditis, shunt nephritis, visceral abscess
Tuberculosis, leprosy, brucellosis
Malaria; onchocerciasis; filariasis

Systemic immune diseases

Cryoglobulinemia, Sjögren syndrome
Systemic lupus erythematosus, rheumatoid arthritis
IgA vasculitis; hypocomplementemic urticarial vasculitis

Neoplasms/dysproteinemias

Plasma cell dyscrasia
Monoclonal gammopathy of unknown significance
Proliferative glomerulonephritis with monoclonal immune deposits
Light-chain and/or heavy-chain deposit disease
Fibrillary glomerulopathy; immunotactoid glomerulonephritis
Leukemia, lymphoma; Wilms' tumor

Other

Alpha-1-antitrypsin deficiency; celiac disease
Idiopathic

No immune complexes

Thrombotic microangiopathy, including drug-induced forms
Sickle-cell disease
Transplant glomerulopathy

immunofluorescence **(Fig. 13.1B)**. The majority of cases are secondary **(Box 13.1)** and the presence of immunoglobulins and light chains is an important clue to the underlying condition. Occasionally, evolution of IC-MPGN to C3GN or DDD is reported.

Pathogenesis

C3G is considered a complement-mediated disease, with defective control of alternate pathway. Patients with C3G show significant variations in genes of the alternate pathway and presence of C3 nephritic factor (C3NeF) in ~20 and ~80% cases, respectively.

Autoimmunity

C3NeF is an IgG antibody that binds to a neoepitope of the AP complement, C3 convertase (C3bBb) enhancing its stability and function. C3NeF was detected in 86% of DDD, 46% of C3GN, and ~50% of patients with IC-MPGN, respectively. Additional autoantibodies prolong the half-life of alternate/classical pathway C3 or C5 convertases.

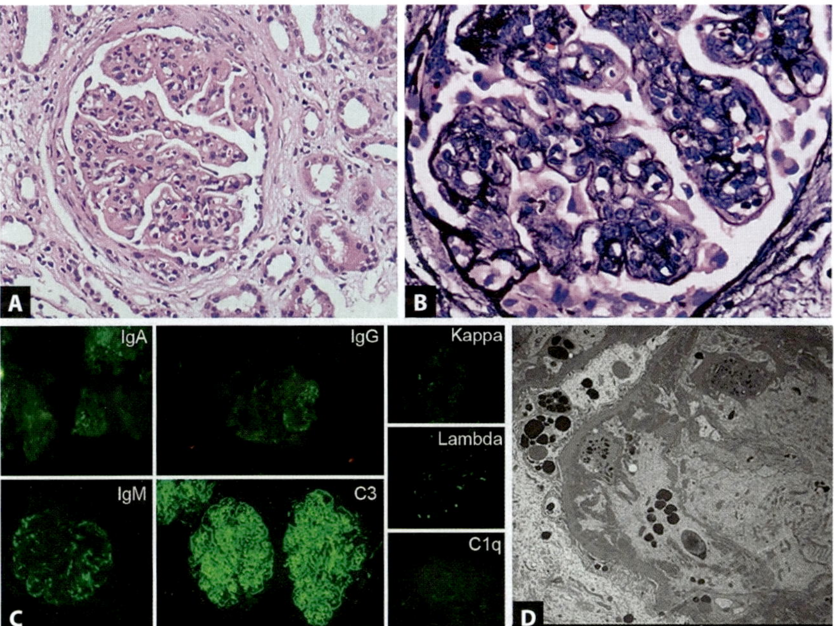

Figs. 13.2A to D: C3 glomerulonephritis in an 8-year-old girl presenting with acute nephritic syndrome, nephrotic range proteinuria, and low complement C3. (A) Hematoxylin and eosin stained glomerulus shows lobular accentuation, diffuse mesangial expansion, and endocapillary proliferation; (B) Silver methenamine-stained glomerulus indicates thickened basement membrane without double contours; (C) Immunofluorescence microscopy reveals predominantly complement C3 deposits; (D) Electron microscopy shows deposits in subendothelium and mesangium

Genetic Basis

Approximately 20–25% patients with C3G have significant variants in complement genes. Genetic causes are more common in C3G than DDD and are less likely in patients with IC-MPGN. Mutations are reported in *CFH, CFHR5, CFI, MCP, C3,* and *CFB.* Additional variations or rearrangements in genes encoding FH-related proteins (*CFHR*), formation of hybrid genes, and risk haplotypes are reported. *CFH* mutations associated with C3G are located in the N-terminal region, or affect cysteine residues throughout the FH protein.

C3G has been associated with a duplication in *CFHR5* in adult patients from Cyprus. It is proposed that dimeric forms of FHR1, FHR2, and FHR5 compete with FH for C3b binding, and protect C3b from inactivation and C3 convertase from decay. This process was increased in patients with *CFHR* hybrids or *CFHR5* mutations. Homozygous mutations in *DGKE,* a lipid kinase that modulates phosphoinositol signaling in cells, are associated with thrombotic microangiopathy as well as renal histology that mimics MPGN.

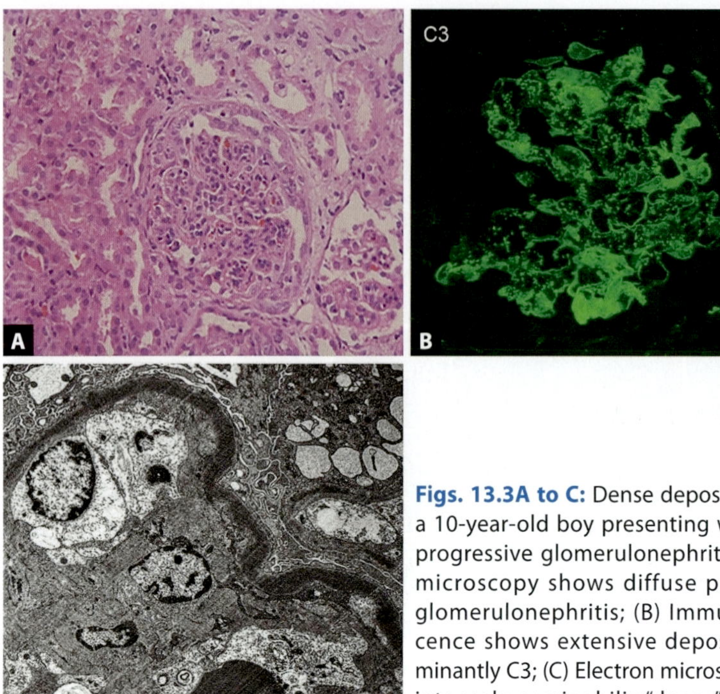

Figs. 13.3A to C: Dense deposit disease in a 10-year-old boy presenting with rapidly progressive glomerulonephritis. (A) Light microscopy shows diffuse proliferative glomerulonephritis; (B) Immunofluorescence shows extensive deposits, predominantly C3; (C) Electron microscopy shows intensely osmiophilic "dense" intramembranous deposits

Clinical Features

Almost 40–50% patients with C3G and MGPN are <18 years at diagnosis. DDD tends to present at a younger age, with 70% of patients diagnosed before 15 years. Clinical features of IC-MPGN, DDD, and C3GN show overlap, and include nephrotic syndrome in 30–65%, microscopic hematuria in 40–75%, gross hematuria in 10–20%, acute nephritic syndrome in 20–30%, and non-nephrotic proteinuria in 30–40%. Although uncommon, rapidly progressive GN has been reported in IC-MPGN, DDD, and C3GN. *CFHR5*-associated C3GN presents in children with persistent microscopic hematuria, synpharyngitic gross hematuria, and a strong family history of end-stage kidney disease (ESKD); most cases are related to Cypriot ancestry.

Hypocomplementemia is documented in a variable proportion of patients. Low levels of C3 are reported in 40–45% patients with IC-MPGN, 60–80% with DDD, and 40–50% with C3GN. Low levels of C4 are present in IC-MPGN; these levels are normal in DDD and C3GN. *Extrarenal manifestations* in C3G include acquired partial lipodystrophy and ocular C3 deposits, similar to soft drusen seen in age-related macular degeneration. These drusen consist of C3 split products and FH. Acquired lipodystrophy, due to dysregulation of complement on leukocytes, usually precedes the diagnosis of MPGN and is associated with low C3 and C3NeF.

Diagnosis

Diagnosis relies chiefly on kidney biopsy. While light microscopy in C3G may show proliferative GN of varying intensity, the diagnostic feature is intense and dominant C3 staining. Electron microscopy allows distinction between DDD and C3GN, based on the nature and location of the deposits. IC-MPGN is characterized by intense and dominant or codominant immunoglobulin deposition. As described above, in some cases, an initial biopsy can show both IgG and C3, while a subsequent biopsy may reveal a C3-dominant pattern, as seen in classic C3G. When proliferative GN due to impaired regulation of the complement AP is suspected, a detailed workup should be done **(Table 13.1)**.

Differential Diagnosis

Conditions such as systemic lupus erythematosus (SLE) and essential cryoglobulinemia should be excluded. Some patients with IC-MPGN have low C3 and C4 levels **(Box 13.1)**. Diseases presenting with low C3 and normal C4 levels are mainly infection-related glomerulonephritis (IRGN), other forms of IC-MPGN and C3G. Isolated low C3 and proliferative nephritis can be due to chronic bacteremia or shunt nephritis. *The presence of normal complement levels does not rule out C3G.*

It may be difficult to initially distinguish IRGN from C3G, since the clinical, laboratory, and histology features are similar. Kidney biopsy in poststreptococcal GN may just show acute proliferative and exudative GN;

TABLE 13.1: Diagnostic work-up for patients with MPGN and C3G

History	Family history of hematuria, proteinuria, glomerulonephritis, kidney failure Episodes of gross hematuria; frothy urine; reduced urine output
Examination	Anthropometry, BMI, blood pressure, partial lipodystrophy, retinal drusen Features of nephrotic syndrome, acute nephritic syndrome
Laboratory	Urinalysis (protein, hematuria, casts); 24-hr proteinuria, creatinine Complete blood count, urea, creatinine, protein, albumin, IgG Antinuclear antibody, anti-double-stranded DNA antibody Serology for hepatitis C and B virus *Suspected MGUS:* Serum protein electrophoresis
Complement studies	Blood C3, C4, anti-FH antibodies *If feasible:* Soluble C5b-9, total hemolytic complement (CH50); C3 nephritic factor; anti-FB antibodies, anti-C3b antibodies If feasible next-generation sequencing and MLPA: *C3, CFH, CFI, CFB, MCP, DGKE, CFHR1-5*

BMI: body mass index; MGUS: monoclonal gammopathy of undetermined significance; MLPA: multiplex ligation-dependent probe amplification; MPGN: membranoproliferative glomerulonephritis; C3G: C3 glomerulopathy

IF shows both C3 and IgG deposits, and EM shows subepithelial humps. Elevated antistreptolysin O (ASO) titers, classically associated with IRGN, can be found in ~30% patients with C3G. Transient anti-FB antibodies are often observed in patients with acute IRGN, while they are infrequent in C3G. The clinical course usually reveals whether the patient has an acute, self-limiting condition such as IRGN or a chronic disease such as C3G. The diagnosis of DDD or C3GN should be considered if the C3 level does not return to normal within 8–12 weeks of presentation, or if patients continue to show features suggestive of nephritis for more than 8–12 weeks.

Therapy

There is no evidence-based therapy for patients with IC-MPGN or C3G. Treatment advice is based on small studies and expert opinion.

Supportive Therapy

All patients with IC-MPGN or C3G should receive renin–angiotensin system inhibition (RASi) with angiotensin-converting enzyme inhibitors (ACEi) or angiotensin II receptor antagonists. Low-salt diet is advised, particularly for patients with persistent edema.

Immunosuppressive Therapy

Multiple studies in MPGN/C3G show partial to complete remission of proteinuria using long-term low-dose steroids. Prednisolone is given at a dose of 60 mg/m^2 for 4 weeks, followed by 40 mg/m^2 on alternate days for another 4 weeks, and then tapered for a total of 6–12 months. Initial therapy with IV methylprednisolone (1,000 mg/1.73 m^2 for 3 doses) may be used for patients with proteinuria exceeding 2 g/24 hr, biopsy showing intense inflammation with or without crescents, or if renal function is impaired.

Mycophenolate mofetil (MMF) has been administered alone or in combination with prednisone in idiopathic MPGN/C3G with satisfactory results. Therapy is associated with partial or complete remission in 60–70% patients. The KDIGO (Kidney Disease: Improving Global Outcomes) recommends that patients with C3G/MPGN be treated with a combination of prednisone and MMF. Therapy with prednisone is tapered and discontinued in 6–9 months; MMF monotherapy is continued for 12–18 months. The risk of nonresponse to therapy is higher in patients with low C3 levels, heavy baseline proteinuria, and in DDD.

Complement Targeting Therapy

While there is increasing evidence on the role of dysregulation of the alternate complement pathway in IC-MPGN and in C3G, case series have shown an unsatisfactory response to plasma therapy (plasma infusions, plasma exchange). C5 blockade, with eculizumab (or ravulizumab), has shown a rather variable response with benefit seen in ~30% patients. Patients with rapidly progressive disease, extracapillary proliferation, elevated sC5b9, recent disease onset, and/or clinical features overlapping with atypical hemolytic anemia syndrome, are more likely to respond to complement blockade. Other complement inhibitors, some of which target the complement pathway upstream at the level of C3 convertase (e.g., iptacopan), are being investigated.

Outcomes

Previous reports showed that progression to ESKD occurs in 40–50% of patients at 10 years, regardless of the MPGN type. Data on long-term outcomes, with the new classification, suggests similar 10 years renal survival of ~65%, with no difference between IC-MPGN, C3GN, and DDD. The presence of glomerular crescents or DDD by biopsy is independent predictor of disease progression; children show better outcomes than adults.

Disease recurrence of MPGN and DDD in transplants is frequent, with post-transplant recurrence rates of ~40% and 60%, respectively. Children with DDD are at greater risk of graft loss from disease recurrence. Several case series also suggest an increased risk of disease recurrence for C3GN and adverse impact on allograft survival.

MEMBRANOUS NEPHROPATHY

Membranous glomerulopathy or nephropathy (MN) is a histological diagnosis, characterized by stiffening of the glomerular capillary walls due to formation of immune complexes, visible as "spikes and craters" in the GBM on special stains, linear IgG deposits on immunofluorescence, and subepithelial deposits on electron microscopy. Idiopathic MN chiefly affects adults, in whom it constitutes a leading cause of nephrotic syndrome. In childhood, the condition is chiefly seen in adolescence. In 75–80% of cases, the condition is considered "primary", while the remainder are "secondary" to, or associated with, systemic diseases such as lupus, hepatitis B virus infection, medications, and malignancies **(Table 13.2)**.

Pathogenesis

Primary MN is a renal-limited autoimmune disease in which the immune deposits form *in situ* from circulating autoantibodies and the endogenous podocyte surface antigen against which they are directed. Over the past two decades, several target antigens and their associated autoantibodies have been identified that are associated with primary or secondary MN

TABLE 13.2: Etiology of secondary membranous nephropathy

Infection	Hepatitis B (most common); hepatitis C, CMV, EBV Syphilis (congenital, acquired) Malaria Tuberculosis, leprosy Bacterial endocarditis (*Streptococcus, Enterococcus* sp.) Infestations (hydatid cyst, schistosomiasis, filariasis)
Autoimmune diseases	Systemic lupus erythematosus (type V lupus nephritis) (most common) Sjögren syndrome; systemic scleroderma; mixed connective tissue disease; dermatomyositis; rheumatoid arthritis; ankylosing spondylitis Graves' disease; Hashimoto disease Ulcerative colitis; Crohn's disease; celiac disease; autoimmune hepatitis; primary biliary cirrhosis Idiopathic thrombocytopenia; type 1 diabetes; sarcoidosis; pemphigus Immune dysregulation, polyendocrinopathy, enteropathy, X-linked (IPEX) syndrome
Drugs	Gold, mercury Penicillamine, captopril, tiopronin NSAIDs Infliximab, etanercept; immune check point inhibitors (see also **Table 7.7**)
Neoplasia	Neuroblastoma, histiocytoma, Wilms' tumor, gonadoblastoma
Alloimmune and other antigens	*Fetomaternal:* Maternal homozygous/compound heterozygous *MME* variants *Cow milk:* Anti-bovine serum antigen (BSA) antibodies Enzyme replacement therapy for mucopolysaccharidoses type 6 and Pompe disease
Other causes	*De novo* post-renal transplant After hematopoietic stem cell transplant Sickle cell disease IgA deficiency

CMV: cytomegalovirus; EBV: Epstein-Barr virus; MME: membrane metalloendopeptidase (neutral endopeptidase); NSAID: nonsteroidal anti-inflammatory drug

(Table 13.3). The target antigen has been identified as the M-type phospholipase A2 receptor (PLA2R) in 70–80% of cases. Semaphorin 3B (SEMA3B) is a target antigen in MN with onset in young childhood. Neonatal MN is reported secondary to congenitally transmitted antibodies to neural endopeptidase (NEP), associated with alloimmunization in fetuses of NEP-deficient women. Top-fed infants following exposure to bovine serum albumin, and children receiving enzyme replacement with recombinant human arylsulfatase B (mucopolysaccharidosis type 6) or α-glucosidase (Pompe disease) may develop MN.

Certain autoantigens are associated with specific secondary forms of MN, e.g., antibodies to neural epidermal growth factor-like 1 (NELL1) and thrombospondin type 1 domain-containing 7A (THSD7A) are observed in association with malignancies, antibodies to exostosin (EXT1 and EXT2) or neural cell adhesion molecule 1 (NCAM1) are associated with type V lupus nephritis, and those against protocadherin FAT1 are seen in patients with hematopoietic stem cell transplant.

Clinical Features

Patients with MN present with progressive edema; laboratory testing confirms nephrotic syndrome, usually with preserved kidney function. The presentation of the illness is insidious, compared to that in patients with minimal change or focal segmental glomerulosclerosis (FSGS), and the disease occur in adolescence more often than childhood. Microscopic hematuria is more common in pediatric then adult onset MN. Thrombosis of the lower extremity, pulmonary, and renal veins, which are described in ~25% adult patients (particularly those with persistent hypoalbuminemia), are uncommon in childhood. Among patients with childhood-onset MN, secondary etiologies, including lupus, hepatitis B, various autoimmune diseases, or medications **(Table 13.2)**, are particularly important.

Diagnosis

Kidney Biopsy (Figs. 13.4 and 13.5)

The diagnosis of MN is made on kidney biopsy, with characteristic subepithelial immune deposits that alter the glomerular capillary wall, accompanied by intervening "spikes" of GBM extending between the immune deposits in advanced cases **(Figs. 13.4A and B)**. Immunofluorescence reveals linear fine granular staining for IgG along the GBM **(Fig. 13.4C)**. Electron microscopy confirms subepithelial deposits **(Fig. 13.4E)**. The biopsy can be stained for the PLA2R antigen **(Fig. 13.4D)**, which has a higher sensitivity (>80%) than anti-PLA2R antibody testing in the serum.

Membranous nephropathy may be staged from I to IV based on electron microscopy findings such as immune deposits and GBM thickness. Features suggestive of secondary MN include mesangial and endocapillary hypercellularity, full-house pattern on immunofluorescence, endothelial tubuloreticular inclusions, and subendothelial or mesangial deposits **(Figs. 13.5A to D)**. Detailed morphologic features should be described, including segmental lesions, mesangial, subendothelial and/or extraglomerular deposits, complement deposits, secondary FSGS, extent of glomerulosclerosis, interstitial fibrosis/tubular atrophy, and vascular disease.

TABLE 13.3: Antigens and autoantibodies associated with membranous nephropathy (MN)[1]

Antigen	*Frequency in MN*	*Location, site of origin*	*Location of IgG deposits*	*IgG subclass*	*Clinical association; comments*
Phospholipase 2 receptor (PLA2R)	70–85%	Podocyte	Subepithelial	IgG4	Primary MN
Thrombospondin type-1 domain-containing protein 7A (THSD7A)	2–5%	Podocyte	Subepithelial	IgG4	Primary MN, malignancy
Semaphorin 3B (SEMA3B)	<1%	GBM	Subepithelial	IgG1, IgG3	Children, young adults, women
Neural epidermal growth factor-like protein 1 (NELL1)	3–4%	Osteoblasts, tubular cells	Subepithelial	IgG1, IgG3	Primary MN; malignancy, lipoic acid supplement, indigenous agents, mercury, autoimmune diseases
Protocadherin-7 (PCDH7)	1–3%	GBM	Subepithelial	IgG1, IgG4	Primary MN; older age, spontaneous remission
Neural cell adhesion molecule 1 (NCAM1)	2% (MN), 6.6% (SLE)	Glomerular capillary, TBM	Subepithelial	IgG4	Primary MN; lupus, autoimmune diseases
Exostosin 1, 2 (EXT1, EXT2)	30% in SLE	GBM	Subepithelial, subendothelial, mesangial	IgG1, IgG2	Lupus, other autoimmune diseases
Transforming growth factor-β receptor type 3 (TGFBR3)	5–10% SLE MN	GBM, glomerular capillary	Subepithelial, subendothelial, mesangial	Variable	Women, lupus, other autoimmune diseases

Contd...

Contd...

Antigen	*Frequency in MN*	*Location, site of origin*	*Location of IgG deposits*	*IgG subclass*	*Clinical association; comments*
High-temperature requirement A serine peptidase 1 (HTRA1)	1%	Podocyte	Subepithelial	IgG4	Primary MN
Netrin G1 (NTNG1)	Uncommon	Podocyte	Subepithelial	IgG4	Primary MN
Contactin 1 (CNTN1)	Uncommon	GBM	Subepithelial	IgG4	Primary MN; CIDP
Protocadherin FAT1 (FAT1)	Uncommon	GBM, TBM	Subepithelial	IgG4, IgG2	Hematopoietic stem cell transplantation
Neuron-derived neurotrophic factor (NDNF)	Uncommon	GBM	Subepithelial	IgG1	Syphilis; young males
Proprotein convertase subtilisin/kexin type 6 (PCSK6)	Uncommon	GBM	Subepithelial	IgG1, IgG4	Prolonged NSAID use

[1]A 7-antigen panel, comprising of PLA2R, THSD7A, SEMA3B, NELL-1, PCDH7, EXT1/EXT2, and NCAM-1, is advised; other antigens are tested in septuple-negative cases

CIDP: chronic inflammatory demyelinating polyneuropathy; GBM: glomerular basement membrane; HS: heparan sulfate; IgG: immunoglobulin G; NS: nervous system; SLE: systemic lupus erythematosus; TBM: tubular basement membrane; NSAID: nonsteroidal anti-inflammatory drug

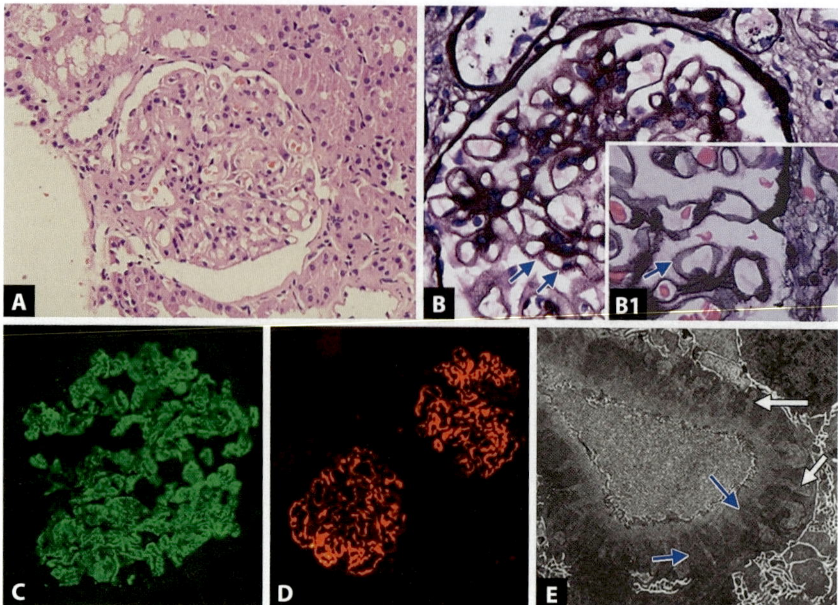

Figs. 13.4A to E: Morphologic findings in membranous nephropathy in a 14-year-old boy with serum PLA2R antibodies. (A) Hematoxylin and eosin-stained glomerulus shows prominent glomerular basement membrane with stiff capillary walls; (B) Silver methenamine-stained glomerulus indicates appearance of "spikes" (arrows) and numerous pinpoint "holes" (arrows in the inset B1) in tangential section, caused by the projections of basement membrane matrix toward the urinary space; (C) Intense, diffuse, finely granular positivity for IgG along the glomerular capillary walls and tubular basement membranes (immunofluorescence microscopy, 40×); (D) Immunofluorescence for phospholipase A2 receptor demonstrating strong and diffuse capillary wall granular staining (20×); (E) Electron-dense deposits and thickening of the basement membrane with spikes at the subepithelial aspect of the glomerular capillary wall: the blue arrows indicate subepithelial electron-dense deposits, and white arrows the relatively lucent basement membrane projections enveloping the deposits (electron microscopy, 7000×)

Serology

The availability of serologic testing for anti-PLA2R antibodies has enabled noninvasive diagnosis of primary MN in adult patients with preserved kidney function and absence of MN-associated conditions (e.g., lupus, hepatitis, and malignancy) or diabetes. KDIGO guidelines suggest that a diagnosis of MN can be made in an adult with nephrotic syndrome and positive PLA2R antibody test without kidney biopsy; biopsy may be done to determine prognosis and guide treatment decisions. A negative PLA2R antibody test does not rule out PLA2R-associated MN, as circulating antibodies are absent in early disease, when positive glomerular staining for PLA2R enables the diagnosis. While anti-PLA2R antibodies distinguish primary from secondary forms of MN,

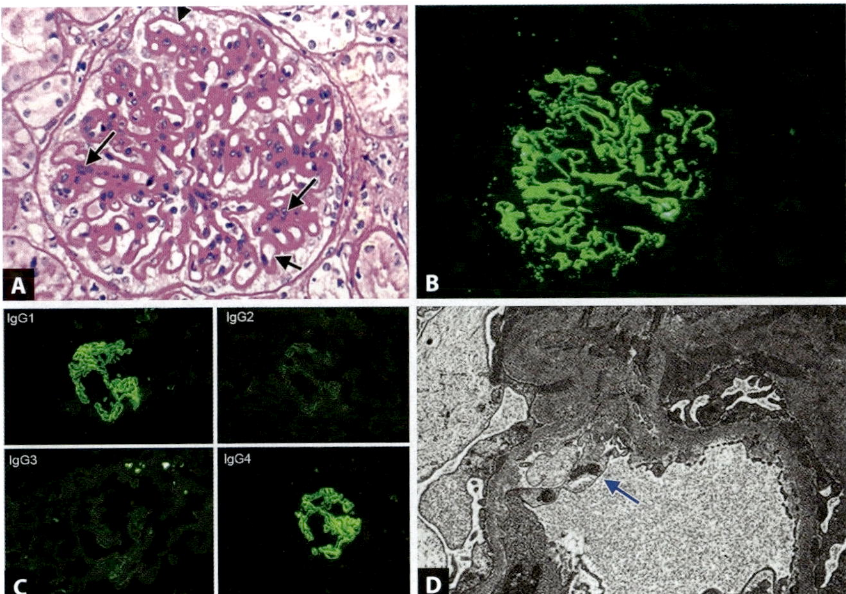

Figs. 13.5A to D: Membranous nephropathy secondary to systemic lupus erythematosus. (A) Periodic acid–Schiff-stained glomerulus indicates stiff peripheral capillary loops and mesangial proliferation (black arrows); (B) Immunofluorescence microscopy reveals diffuse global granular capillary loop and mesangial staining for IgG. IgG was dominant in an otherwise full-house pattern of granular capillary loop and mesangial pattern of staining; (C) IgG subclasses showed co-dominant staining for IgG4 and IgG1; (D) Electron microscopy reveals a tubuloreticular inclusion within endothelial cell (blue arrow)

it is still advisable to screen for secondary causes. This is important since certain secondary causes require specific management (hepatitis B, lupus, and malignancy) or confer adverse prognosis (malignancy).

Detailed evaluation is expected to yield a target antigen in >80% of cases. With the discovery of additional target antigens, experts propose a two-step antigen-based classification of MN. The first step is to identify the target antigen, using a combination of serology, staining of the kidney biopsy by immunofluorescence or immunohistochemistry, and/or mass spectrometry **(Table 13.2)**. A stepwise approach may be followed, prioritizing screening for antibodies against PLA2R and NELL1 ahead of testing for THSD7A, PCDH7, SEMA3B, and EXT1/2, followed by other antigens. The second step is the evaluation for underlying disease or associated condition, such as infections, systemic diseases, malignancies, certain drugs (NSAIDs), or nutritional supplements (lipoic acid).

Approach in Pediatric Patients

The role of serologic testing for noninvasive diagnosis of MN is limited in pediatric patients, since the probability of finding MN and/or anti-PLA2R antibodies is far lower than in adult patients. Since MN secondary to lupus, other autoimmune conditions, and hepatitis B is fairly common in childhood and adolescence, these conditions should be excluded, especially if histopathology favors secondary MN. Unless a disease association is apparent on history, physical examination, or investigations, tissue staining for PLA2R and serological testing for anti-PLA2R antibodies must be performed in patients with MN. In PLA2R-negative cases, additional testing for other antigens is considered, especially for SEMA3B, NELL1, and THSD7A.

Management

Adult patients with newly diagnosed primary MN are managed conservatively for at least 6 months on RASi (ACEi and ARB). Management of edema, hyperlipidemia, and hypertension is necessary, especially in patients with persistent nephrotic-range proteinuria. Patients with MN and marked hypoalbuminemia (albumin <2.5 g/dL) are at risk of arterial and venous thromboembolism, and are advised adequate precautions.

In adult patients, trends in anti-PLA2R antibodies as well as clinical response to conservative management guide decisions on immunosuppression. Thus, falling anti-PLA2R antibody titers or occurrence of spontaneous remission while on conservative management allows decision to continue conservative management even beyond 6 months. In contrast, a rising titer or persistent nephrotic state beyond 6 months of initial conservative management prompts consideration of immunosuppression.

Unlike adult patients, children with MN are usually treated with immunosuppressive agents and RASi. There are multiple options of first-line immunosuppressive regimens. KDIGO guidelines propose the use of clinical and laboratory criteria to assess the risk of progressive loss of kidney function, which dictates choice of immunosuppression **(Table 13.4)**. Options include: (*i*) a combination of oral and IV steroids with cyclophosphamide, which achieves remission in ~75–80% patients within 12 months; (*ii*) calcineurin inhibitors (CNI, cyclosporine, or tacrolimus), which are associated with remission rates of 70–75% in the 1st year of therapy, but have risk of relapse on discontinuation; and (*iii*) rituximab, which has similar rates of remission as CNI but with lower relapse rates over long-term follow-up. Patients with MN and at least one risk factor for disease progression are offered these regimens with the choice of therapy dictated by the risk of progression, efficacy and adverse effects, and costs of care **(Table 13.4)**.

Immunological response precedes clinical response by several months. In patients with PLA2R antibody-associated MN, monitoring of antibody titers after start of therapy allows evaluation of treatment response and provides guidance for treatment. Anti-PLA2R antibody levels should be rechecked at 6 months after start of therapy, followed by longitudinal monitoring in order to evaluate response to treatment and guide adjustments to therapy.

TABLE 13.4: Risk stratification-based management strategy for primary membranous nephropathy (adapted for children, from KDIGO 2021)

Risk category	*Criteria for definition*				*Management*
	eGFR, mL/min/1.73 m²	*Proteinuria, g/day*	*Serum albumin, g/dL*	*Additional factors*	
Low	Normal (≥60)	<3.5 g/day	>3	None	Rituximab and prednisolone,[1] or CNI and prednisolone[2]
Moderate	Normal (≥60)	3.5–8.0 g/day	</>3		
High	Low (<60)	>8.0	Any	None	Rituximab and prednisolone,[1] or Cyclophosphamide and steroids,[3] or Rituximab and CNI + prednisolone[1,2]
	Normal (≥60)	>3.5	<2.5	None	
	Normal (≥60)	>3.5	Any	Anti-PLA2R antibodies >50 RU/L; selectivity index >0.20	
Very high	Any	Any	Any	Life-threatening nephrotic syndrome Unexplained rapid decline in eGFR	Cyclophosphamide and steroids[3]

[1]Either of two dosing regimens is used for rituximab: (a) 1 g/1.73 m² 2-weeks apart; or (b) 375 mg/m² once a weeks for 1–4 doses; targeting B cell depletion

[2]Either of two agents is used for 12 months: (a) Tacrolimus, at a dose of 0.05–0.1 mg/kg/day in two divided doses (target trough 3–8 ng/mL); (b) cyclosporine, 3.5–5 mg/kg/day in two divided doses (target trough 125–225 ng/mL)

[3]Either of two regimens, (a) or (b) is used in adult patients, while most experts advise approach (c) for pediatric patients:

(a) *Cyclical cyclophosphamide*: IV methylprednisolone, at a dose of 1 g/1.73 m² daily for 3 days at start of months 1, 3, and 5; with oral prednisolone 0.5 mg/kg daily during months 1, 3, and 5; and oral cyclophosphamide 2.5 mg/kg daily during months 2, 4, and 6

(b) *Continuous cyclophosphamide*: IV methylprednisolone, 1 g/1.73 m² daily for 3 days at start of months 1, 3, and 5; oral prednisolone 0.5 mg/kg on alternate days during months 1–6 (followed by taper); and oral cyclophosphamide 1.5 mg/kg daily during months 1–6

(c) *Protocol for children*: Oral cyclophosphamide 2.5 mg/kg daily for 12 weeks, with prednisolone 1–1.5 mg/kg on alternate days for 12 weeks, followed by 0.5–1 mg/kg on alternate days during months 4–6

Partial remission, defined by decline in proteinuria and normalization of serum albumin, is an acceptable response to therapy and not an indicator of active MN particularly in patients with immunological remission. KDIGO guidelines suggest that persistence of antibodies should be considered as evidence for resistant disease. If nephrotic range proteinuria persists despite immunological response, secondary FSGS should be excluded by kidney biopsy. Relapse is defined based on urine protein to creatinine ratio, serum albumin, as well as anti-PLA2R antibody level. Trends in anti-PLA2R antibodies are important, and precede the clinical course by weeks to months.

Second-line therapy depends on the rate of decline of estimated glomerular filtration rate (eGFR). Rituximab and/or CNI are suitable options in patients with stable eGFR; the combination of cyclophosphamide and steroids is preferred in those with eGFR decline. Lack of clinical response after more than one line of therapy indicates resistant disease that requires individualized decision-making. Experimental therapies include bortezomib, daratumumab, and belimumab, or a higher dose of conventional immunosuppression. Treatment of secondary MN is directed at the underlying etiology, e.g., resection of tumor in malignancy-associated MN, and treatment of hepatitis B in viral-associated MN.

Outcomes

Progression to ESKD depends on remission of proteinuria. The incidence of ESKD at 10 years in patients with complete or partial remission ranges from 0 to 10%, compared with >50% for patients with persistent nephrotic-range proteinuria. Post-transplant recurrent MN is more likely in patients who have detectable anti-PLA2R antibodies at transplantation. In patients with PLA2R-associated MN, serological monitoring for anti-PLA2R antibodies and proteinuria should be performed at 1–3 months' intervals after transplant. Therapy for recurrent MN includes RASi blockade and rituximab. De novo cases of MN in the allograft tend to be PLA2R-negative, and might be associated with concurrent antibody-mediated rejection and reduced graft survival.

BIBLIOGRAPHY

Complement 3 Glomerulopathy and Membranoproliferative Glomerulonephritis

1. Caravaca-Fontán F, Lucientes L, Cavero T, Praga M. Update on C3 glomerulopathy: A complement-mediated disease. Nephron. 2020;144:272-80.
2. Estebanez BT, Bomback AS. C3 glomerulopathy: Novel treatment paradigms. Kidney Int Rep. 2023;9:569-79.
3. Khandelwal P, Bhardwaj S, Singh G, Sinha A, Hari P, Bagga A. Therapy and outcomes of C3 glomerulopathy and immune-complex membranoproliferative glomerulonephritis. Pediatr Nephrol. 2021;36:591-600.

4. Ponticelli C, Calatroni M, Moroni G. C3 glomerulopathies: Dense deposit disease and C3 glomerulonephritis. Front Med (Lausanne). 2023;10:1289812.
5. Vivarelli M, van de Kar N, Labbadia R, Diomedi-Camassei F, Thurman JM. A clinical approach to children with C3 glomerulopathy. Pediatr Nephrol. 2022;37:521-35.
6. Wada Y, Kamata M, Miyasaka R, et al. Clinico-pathogenic similarities and differences between infection-related glomerulonephritis and C3 glomerulopathy. Int J Mol Sci. 2023;24:8432.
7. Wong E, Nester C, Cavero T, et al. Efficacy and safety of iptacopan in patients with C3 glomerulopathy. Kidney Int Rep. 2023;8:2754-64.
8. Wong EKS, Marchbank KJ, Lomax-Browne H, et al. MPGN/DDD/C3 Glomerulopathy Rare Disease Group. C3 glomerulopathy and related disorders in children: Etiology-phenotype correlation and outcomes. Clin J Am Soc Nephrol. 2021;16:1639-51.

Membranous Nephropathy

1. Alsharhan L, Beck LH Jr. Membranous nephropathy: Core curriculum 2021. Am J Kidney Dis. 2021;77:440-53.
2. Dantas M, Silva LBB, Pontes BTM, Dos Reis MA, de Lima PSN, Moysés Neto M. Membranous nephropathy. J Bras Nefrol. 2023;45:229-43.
3. Kidney Disease: Improving Global Outcomes (KDIGO) Glomerular Diseases Work Group. KDIGO 2021 Clinical Practice Guideline for the Management of Glomerular Diseases. Kidney Int. 2021;100:S1-S27.
4. Lusco MA, Fogo AB, Najafian B, Alpers CE. AJKD Atlas of Renal Pathology: Membranous lupus nephritis, ISN/RPS class V. Am J Kidney Dis. 2017;70:e13-5.
5. Moroni G, Ponticelli C. Secondary membranous nephropathy. A narrative review. Front Med (Lausanne). 2020;7:611317.
6. Rojas-Rivera JE, Ortiz A, Fervenza FC. Novel treatments paradigms: Membranous nephropathy. Kidney Int Rep. 2023;8:419-31.
7. Sethi S, Beck LH Jr, Glassock RJ, et al. Mayo Clinic consensus report on membranous nephropathy: Proposal for a novel classification. Kidney Int. 2023;104:1092-102.
8. Tomas NM, Huber TB, Hoxha E. Perspectives in membranous nephropathy. Cell Tissue Res. 2021;385:405-22.

Acute Kidney Injury

Sudarsan Krishnasamy, Arvind Bagga

Acute kidney injury (AKI) is a clinical syndrome characterized by rapid deterioration of kidney function resulting in retention of nitrogenous wastes and inability of the kidney to regulate fluid and electrolyte homeostasis. It includes a spectrum of changes ranging from mildly elevated serum creatinine to the most severe forms with anuria and the need for kidney support therapy (KST). In this chapter, we will discuss the definition and classification, epidemiology, etiology, clinical features, evaluation including diagnostic and prognostic biomarkers, and nondialytic management of AKI. KST is discussed in a separate chapter.

DEFINITIONS AND CLASSIFICATION

The classification criteria for AKI have undergone major revisions over the last few decades with an aim to capture the spectrum of AKI and standardize the definition across various populations. Staging of AKI based on the commonly used classification criteria are shown in **Table 14.1**.

According to the KDIGO (Kidney Disease Improving Global Outcomes) criteria, AKI is defined as:

- Increase in serum creatinine by ≥0.3 mg/dL within 48 hr; or
- Increase in serum creatinine to ≥1.5 times the baseline value, which is known or presumed to have occurred within the prior 7 days; or
- Urine volume <0.5 mL/kg/hr for 6 hr

The KDIGO criteria are currently most often used in practice. The pROCK (Pediatric Reference change value Optimized Criterion for AKI) criteria, which takes into account an absolute serum creatinine increase (to account for biologic and analytical variability), and a relative proportional increase from the baseline, have been recently proposed for children.

Neonatal AKI is more difficult to define given the dynamic changes in serum creatinine with each passing day, reflection of maternal serum creatinine levels, tubular immaturity, and the difficulty in measuring urinary volumes in neonates. Proposed KDIGO criteria for neonates are given in **Table 14.2**.

TABLE 14.1: Acute kidney injury (AKI) classification criteria in children

	Stage 1	*Stage 2*	*Stage 3*
Serum creatinine criteria[@]			
Pediatric RIFLE, pRIFLE[#]	eGFR decrease by 25% (Risk)	eGFR decrease by 50% (Injury)	eGFR decrease by 75% (Failure)
Acute Kidney Injury Network (AKIN)	Increase by ≥0.3 mg/dL within 48 hr; or ≥1.5 times the baseline	Increase to 2–3 times the baseline	>3 times the baseline; or ≥4 mg/dL with acute rise of ≥0.5 mg/dL; or initiation of KST
Kidney Disease Improving Global Outcomes (KDIGO)	Increase by ≥0.3 mg/dL within 48 hr; or ≥1.5–1.9 times baseline within 7 days	Increase 2–2.9 times the baseline within 7 days	Increase >3 times the baseline; or ≥4 mg/dL; or initiation of KST
Pediatric Reference change value Optimized Criterion for AKI (pROCK)	Increase by ≥20 µmol/L (0.23 mg/dL); relative increase by ≥30% within 7 days	Increase by ≥40 µmol/L (0.45 mg/dL); relative increase by ≥60% within 7 days	Increase by ≥80 µmol/L (0.91 mg/dL); relative increase by ≥120% within 7 days
Urine output criteria			
pRIFLE	<0.5 mL/kg/hr for ≥8 hr (Risk)	<0.5 mL/kg/hr for ≥16 hr (Injury)	<0.3 mL/kg/hr for ≥24 hr; or anuria for ≥12 hr (Failure)
AKIN	<0.5 mL/kg/hr for ≥6 hr	<0.5 mL/kg/hr for ≥12 hr	<0.3 mL/kg/hr for ≥24 hr; or anuria for ≥12 hr
KDIGO	<0.5 mL/kg/hr for 6–12 hr	<0.5 mL/kg/hr for ≥12 hr	<0.3 mL/kg/hr for ≥24 hr; or anuria for ≥12 hr
pROCK	Not defined		

[@]Only pRIFLE criteria use eGFR change; others use change in serum creatinine
[#]Failure stage of AKI persisting for >4 weeks and >3 months are termed "loss" and "end-stage", respectively in pRIFLE criteria
eGFR: estimated glomerular filtration rate; hr: hour; KST: kidney support therapy; pRIFLE: Pediatric Risk, Injury, Failure, Loss, End Stage Renal Disease

EPIDEMIOLOGY

There is wide variation in the epidemiology of AKI due to use of varying definitions [pRIFLE, acute kidney injury network (AKIN), and KDIGO], and diverse clinical profiles (ill patients in the intensive care units, stable inpatients, surgical or nonsurgical, and comorbidities like malignancy, post-transplant). The international multicenter AWARE (Assessment of Worldwide AKI, Renal

TABLE 14.2: KDIGO criteria for neonatal AKI

Stage	*Serum creatinine*	*Urine output over 24 hr*
0	No change or rise <0.3 mg/dL	>1 mL/kg/hr
1	Increase by 0.3 mg/dL or more within 48 hr; or ≥1.5–1.9 times the reference* within 7 days	0.5–1 mL/kg/hr
2	Increase to 2–2.9 times the reference within 7 days	0.3–0.5 mL/kg/hr
3	≥3 times the reference; ≥2.5 mg/dL^; or receipt of dialysis	≤0.3 mL/kg/hr

*Reference creatinine refers to the lowest prior serum creatinine
^Serum creatinine of 2.5 mg/dL in neonates corresponds to glomerular filtration rate (GFR) of <10 mL/1.73 m^2/minute
AKI: acute kidney injury; KDIGO: Kidney Disease Improving Global Outcomes

Angina, and Epidemiology in children) study reported AKI incidence of 26.9% in critically-ill children, with severe AKI (KDIGO stages 2 and 3) in 11.6%. Studies from India have reported an incidence of 5–9% in hospitalized inpatients and 25–36% in critically-ill children. In neonates, the AWAKEN (Assessment of Worldwide Acute Kidney injury Epidemiology in Neonates) study reported an overall AKI incidence of 29.9%, with highest incidence (47.9%) in those born <29-weeks' gestation. The incidence of AKI is high in the surgical population (postcardiac surgery), where rates as high as 64–86% are reported.

ETIOLOGY

Traditionally, the causes of AKI are classified into prerenal or functional, renal or intrinsic, and postrenal or obstructive etiologies. **Box 14.1** lists the common causes of AKI.

AKI in neonates is often caused by multiple factors such as systemic hypoperfusion due to decreased placental blood flow, diarrheal dehydration or third-space losses, excessive insensible water losses (e.g., very low birth weight neonates, neonates on phototherapy), birth asphyxia, necrotizing enterocolitis, congenital heart disease and cardiac surgery, and nephrotoxic medications.

PATHOGENESIS

Phases of Acute Kidney Injury

Clinically, AKI is divided into four phases based on cellular events, namely the *initiation*, *extension*, *maintenance*, and *recovery* phases **(Fig. 14.1)**. The initiation phase begins with reduction in renal blood flow leading to depletion of adenosine triphosphate (ATP) and tubular damage.

BOX 14.1: Common causes of acute kidney injury

Prerenal: Acute gastroenteritis, blood loss, shock, heart failure, nephrotic syndrome

Renal

Acute tubular necrosis: Prolongation of prerenal insult, sepsis, dengue, malaria, leptospirosis, scrub typhus, nephrotoxic agents, multiorgan failure, intravascular hemolysis, rhabdomyolysis, snakebite, other envenomations

Glomerular: Acute glomerulonephritis (postinfectious), crescentic glomerulonephritis (GN), systemic lupus erythematosus, immunoglobulin A (IgA) vasculitis, polyarteritis nodosa, other vasculitis

Vascular: Renal vein or arterial thrombosis, hemolytic uremic syndrome

Acute tubulointerstitial nephritis

Postrenal

Obstructive uropathy (calculi, stricture, phimosis, malignancy, and blood clots)

Neurogenic bladder

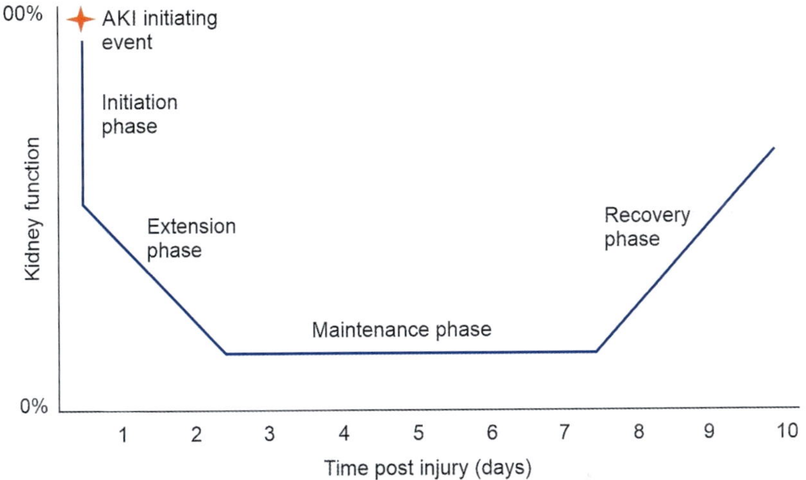

Fig. 14.1: Phases of acute kidney injury

Endothelial cells and vascular smooth muscle cells are also affected. The extent of tubular damage is determined by the severity and duration of ischemic insult. The extension phase is characterized by cellular hypoxia and the attendant inflammatory response. These events are more pronounced in the outer medullary region and corticomedullary junction. While tubular cells in the outer medulla undergo apoptosis due to the severe injury, cells in the outer cortex undergo repair following restoration of blood flow. The inflammatory cascade continues to propagate damage. During the maintenance phase, cells undergo repair and proliferation with some damaged cells undergoing apoptosis. The glomerular filtration rate (GFR) starts improving and cellular homeostasis gets restored. The recovery phase is marked by proliferation, migration, and re-establishment of cell polarity leading to normal cellular and organ function.

Renal Hemodynamics

Injury to the tubular epithelium leads to release of vasoactive compounds such as angiotensin, adenosine, endothelin, and arachidonic acid metabolites, which reduce the GFR by causing vasoconstriction of the afferent and efferent arterioles. Several experimental studies in animals have shown improvement in AKI upon application of drugs that antagonize these vasoactive compounds. Alterations of the renal microvasculature play an important role in initiation and extension of AKI.

Alterations in Microvasculature and Tubules

Endothelial damage with alteration in structure of the actin cytoskeleton and loss of glycocalyx play a key role in initiation and extension of AKI. Increased endothelial expression of adhesion molecules (intercellular adhesion molecule-1, P-selectin, and E-selectin) recruit leukocytes and inflammatory cytokines, alter platelet aggregation and the coagulation cascade, and obstruct peritubular capillaries, leading to further damage.

The proximal tubule is more vulnerable to ischemia and loses ATP quickly compared to distal tubules. Alterations to the S3 segment of the proximal tubule with changes in the brush border, blebbing and internalization of the luminal membrane, cellular swelling, mitochondrial condensation, and disruption of cell organelles have been identified. These alterations lead to intratubular obstruction and back leak.

Inflammatory Response

The inflammatory cascade is initiated and propagated by the damaged vascular endothelium and ischemic tubules. Proinflammatory cytokines [interleukin (IL)-1β, tumor necrosis factor alpha (TNF-α), transforming growth factor beta (TGF-β), IL-6, and IL-17], chemotactic cytokines [monocyte chemoattractant protein-1 (MCP-1), IL-8, CXC motif chemokine ligand 1 (CXCL1), CXCL8], and toll-like receptors (TLR-2 and TLR-4) are activated, which recruit more inflammatory response and lead to tissue damage. Progress in understanding the inflammatory response has enabled examination of novel targets (TLR-2 blockade, IL-10/Treg stimulation), for prevention and treatment of AKI.

Cellular and Metabolic Alterations in Acute Kidney Injury

Adenine Nucleotide Metabolism

Energy depletion and restoration following reperfusion contribute significantly to tubular and epithelial cell injury. Animal studies have shown that ~90% of ATP consumption in the kidneys happens within 5–10 minutes of ischemia. During reperfusion, there is rapid but incomplete recovery of ATP (~50–70% within few minutes) from the left-over adenine nucleotide pool, while the remaining happens over hours from purine nucleotide degradation products, salvage pathways, and precursors mobilized during reperfusion. Alterations in adenine nucleotide metabolism have several ramifications including epithelial damage, release of reactive oxygen species, activation of phospholipases, and increased intracellular calcium, which perpetuate AKI.

Reactive Oxygen Species

Reactive oxygen species (ROS), e.g., hydrogen peroxide, superoxide, hypochlorous acid, and hydroxyl radicals are generated during kidney reperfusion from the metabolism of adenine nucleotides to adenosine, inosine, and hypoxanthine. The damaged mitochondria leak the ROS that are produced through the electron transport system. Further, the respiratory burst and myeloperoxidase released from the activated neutrophils, iron release which donates electrons to form hydroxyl radicals, and prostaglandin metabolism lead to ROS generation, which causes multipronged damage: oxidation of intracellular proteins, and their conformational change, loss of enzyme activity, lipid peroxidation leading to membrane damage, and damage to DNA.

Intracellular Calcium

Reduction in ATP following ischemia leads to defective functioning of the Na^+/K^+-ATPase that in turn affects the Na^+/Ca^{2+} transporter. Coupled with calcium release from intracellular organelles, this leads to rise in intracellular calcium that activates multiple enzymes (proteases, phospholipases, and calpain) resulting in structural damage, inhibition of mitochondrial oxidative phosphorylation, and reduction in cellular energy stores.

Repair Mechanisms

Mechanisms involved in the repair process are: (*i*) Recovery of sublethally injured cells, (*ii*) proliferation of surviving tubular epithelial cells, and (*iii*) regeneration of tubular cells from stem cells. Heat shock proteins (Hsp70 and Hsp 25/27) are central to the repair process. Several growth factors such as epidermal growth factor (EGF), insulin-like growth factor 1 (IGF-1), hepatocyte growth factor (HGF), and fibroblast growth factor-23 (FGF-23) contribute to proliferation and redifferentiation of tubular epithelial cells. While mechanisms of regeneration are still unclear, proliferation of surviving intrinsic kidney cells play a major role, compared to bone marrow-derived or exogenous stem cells.

Sepsis-induced Acute Kidney Injury

Multiple factors lead to sepsis-induced AKI (s-AKI). Macrocirculatory and microcirculatory changes are important in pathogenesis. Systemic sepsis results in dysregulated immune response, with activation of complement system, cell death pathways, innate immunity, and cytokine storms. Damage-associated molecular patterns (DAMPs) and pathogen-associated molecular patterns (PAMPs) bind to toll-like receptors on the cell surface and promote release of proinflammatory cytokines. Cytoplasmic nucleotide oligomerization domain (NOD)-like receptor protein 3 (NLRP3) inflammasome that activates caspase-1, also contributes to the inflammatory response.

There is evidence that micro RNA (miRNA) has an important role in s-AKI. Several miRNAs (miR-4321, 4270, 15a-5p, 15b-5p) have been identified to regulate mammalian target of rapamycin (mTOR), mitogen-activated protein kinase 3 (MEKK3), and other pathways. Extracellular vesicles, autophagosome complex, efferocytosis, immunomodulation, metabolic reprogramming, and mitochondrial homeostasis have an important role in pathogenesis of s-AKI **(Fig. 14.2)**.

Acute Kidney Injury in Cancer Patients

Factors contributing to AKI in patients with cancer are: (*i*) Tumor infiltration of kidneys, (*ii*) tumor lysis syndrome, (*iii*) hypercalcemia, (*iv*) vascular occlusion, (*v*) obstructive uropathy, (*vi*) glomerular diseases [membranous nephropathy, amyloidosis, and immunotactoid or fibrillary glomerulonephritis], (*vii*) tubulointerstitial nephritis, (*viii*) thrombotic microangiopathy, (*ix*) hemophagocytic lymphohistiocytosis, (*x*) lysozymuria, (*xi*) volume depletion, (*xii*) sepsis and septic shock, (*xiii*) cast nephropathy

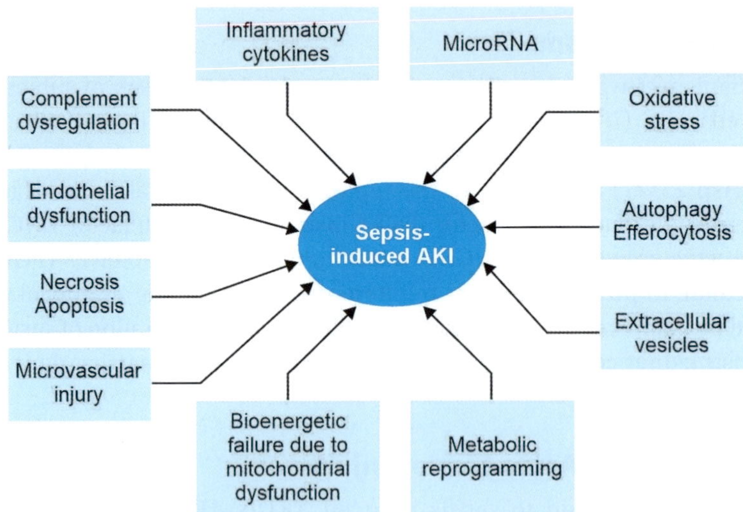

Fig. 14.2: Pathophysiology of sepsis-induced acute kidney injury (s-AKI)

(myeloma casts and drugs), (*xiv*) nephrotoxicity due to chemotherapy, radiocontrast agents, antibiotics, nonsteroidal anti-inflammatory drugs (NSAIDs), angiotensin-converting enzyme (ACE) inhibitors, and (*xv*) hematopoietic stem-cell transplantation.

CLINICAL FEATURES

Symptoms and signs of AKI depend on the severity and rapidity of accumulation of uremic substances in the blood. Uremia and hypertension may both lead to altered sensorium and seizures. Breathing may be rapid due to severe metabolic acidosis or pulmonary edema. Anasarca is noted once there is oligoanuria. Patients show progressive pallor and easy fatigability if there is severe anemia.

Focused history and meticulous examination are performed to identify the etiology and evaluate for extent of impairment and complications. Features that suggest an underlying cause include history of diarrhea, fluid or blood loss leading to severe dehydration [acute tubular necrosis (ATN)]; gross hematuria, edema, and hypertension (GN); dysentery, pallor, and petechiae [hemolytic uremic syndrome (HUS)]; or passage of dark red urine, pallor, and jaundice (intravascular hemolysis). A history of interrupted urinary stream and palpable urinary bladder or kidney(s) suggests obstructive uropathy, and that of abdominal colic, hematuria, and dysuria indicates urinary tract infection or calculi. Anuria may occur with urinary tract obstruction, cortical necrosis, bilateral vascular occlusion, severe glomerulonephritis, or vasculitis. Nonoliguric kidney failure is seen in ATN following the use of nephrotoxic agents and radiocontrast agents. Polyuria may occur in partial ureteral obstruction, AKI with preexisting tubular disorders such as diabetes insipidus, solute diuresis secondary to hyperglycemia, or mannitol infusion, or in patients receiving a large protein load. Occasionally, AKI may be superimposed on chronic kidney disease (CKD). Features such as growth retardation, short stature, pallor, rickets, and hypertension indicate underlying CKD.

LABORATORY EVALUATION

In prerenal AKI, renal blood flow and GFR decline, but tubular reabsorption of salt and water continues leading to oliguria with low urine sodium, high urine osmolality, increased blood urea nitrogen/creatinine ratio, and low fractional excretion of sodium. In intrinsic AKI, there is diminished tubular function with high urine sodium and dilute urine. Indices, which help to differentiate prerenal from intrinsic AKI are detailed in **Table 14.3**.

Of these indices, fractional excretion of sodium (FENa) is most sensitive, and is calculated as follows:

$$\text{Fractional excretion of sodium (FENa\%)} = \frac{\text{Urine sodium} \times \text{Serum creatinine}}{\text{Serum sodium} \times \text{Urine creatinine}} \times 100$$

TABLE 14.3: Indices to differentiate prerenal from intrinsic acute kidney injury (AKI)

Parameter	*Prerenal*	*Intrinsic AKI*
Urinary sodium (mEq/L)	<20	>40
Urinary osmolality (mOsm/kg)	>500	<300
Blood urea nitrogen to creatinine ratio	>20:1	<20:1
Urine to plasma osmolality ratio	>1.5	<0.8–1.2
Urine specific gravity	>1.020	<1.012
Fractional excretion of sodium (%)	<1	>1

These indices are not useful in patients with nonoliguric kidney failure and those receiving diuretics. In such patients, fractional excretion of urea may be useful, since urea is chiefly absorbed from the proximal tubule and inner medulla, segments that are relatively unaffected by loop and thiazide diuretics. Fractional excretion of urea <35% suggests prerenal AKI; it is >50% in intrinsic renal AKI.

Evaluation required for patients with AKI is summarized in **Box 14.2**. Blood, urine, and radiological investigations are done in all patients. Certain investigations, based on clinical features, are done to ascertain the etiology of AKI.

Indications for kidney biopsy are listed in **Box 14.3**. Common histopathological findings in patients undergoing kidney biopsy for AKI are shown in **Figures 14.3A to F**.

RISK STRATIFICATION AND BIOMARKERS

Over the past decade, numerous biomarkers and risk stratification methods for AKI have been developed.

Fluid Overload

Fluid overload is an important and independent predictor of mortality in critically-ill children. It is calculated as follows:

$$\text{Fluid overload\%} = \frac{\text{Fluid in (L)} - \text{Fluid out (L)}}{\text{Weight at ICU entry (kg)}} \times 100$$

The following formula is used if weight measurement is available:

$$\text{Fluid overload\%} = \frac{\text{Weight at evaluation (kg)} - \text{Weight at ICU admission (kg)}}{\text{Weight at ICU admission (kg)}} \times 100$$

Various meta-analyses confirm that fluid overload is an independent predictor of adverse outcomes, and fluid overload >10–15% is harmful. The odds of mortality increase by 6% for every 1% increase in fluid overload.

Fluid overload leads to hemodilution and masking creatinine increments; this might result in delayed diagnosis of AKI in critically-ill patients.

BOX 14.2: Initial evaluation in patients with acute kidney injury

Blood
Complete blood counts
Urea, creatinine, electrolytes*, calcium, phosphate, urate, pH, bicarbonate

Urine
Urinalysis and microscopy
Urine culture if suspicion for urinary tract infection
Osmolality, sodium, fractional excretion of sodium (FENa)

Radiology
Chest X-ray (fluid overload and cardiomegaly)
Ultrasound kidneys and urinary tract (urinary tract dilation, kidney size, echogenicity, and corticomedullary differentiation)

Investigations to determine cause
Peripheral smear; platelets and reticulocyte count; C3, lactate dehydrogenase (LDH), and haptoglobin; stool polymerase chain reaction (PCR) and Shiga toxin (for hemolytic uremic syndrome)
Malarial parasite; serology for leptospirosis, typhoid, rickettsial infection, dengue hemorrhagic fever (for tropical infections)
Blood antistreptolysin O, C3, antinuclear antibody, antineutrophil cytoplasmic antibody (for acute or rapidly progressive glomerulonephritis)
Creatinine kinase (for rhabdomyolysis)
Doppler ultrasonography (for arterial, venous thrombosis)
Kidney biopsy **(Box 14.3)**

*Electrocardiogram is done in patients with hypo- or hyperkalemia

BOX 14.3: Indications for kidney biopsy in acute kidney injury

Rapidly progressive glomerulonephritis
Presence of gross hematuria, nephrotic range proteinuria (suggests glomerulonephritis)
Features of systemic disease [lupus, immunoglobulin A (IgA) vasculitis]
Suspected acute tubulointerstitial nephritis
Unexplained or persistent AKI (identify cause, determine prognosis)
Kidney allograft dysfunction

Adjustment of serum creatinine for fluid balance is suggested using the following formula:

$$\text{Adjusted serum creatinine} = \text{measured creatinine} \times \left[1 + \frac{\text{Cumulative fluid balance (L)}}{\text{Total body water (TBW)}}\right]$$

Total body water (TBW) is calculated based on age: $k \times$ *body weight* (where k is 0.8, 0.7, and 0.6 in children <1 year, 1–2 years, and ≥2 years, respectively).

Renal Angina Index

The concept of renal angina, analogous to troponin estimation in cardiac angina, was proposed to direct biomarker assessment to a subset of critically-ill patients at high risk of AKI, to avoid indiscriminate use of biomarkers in all

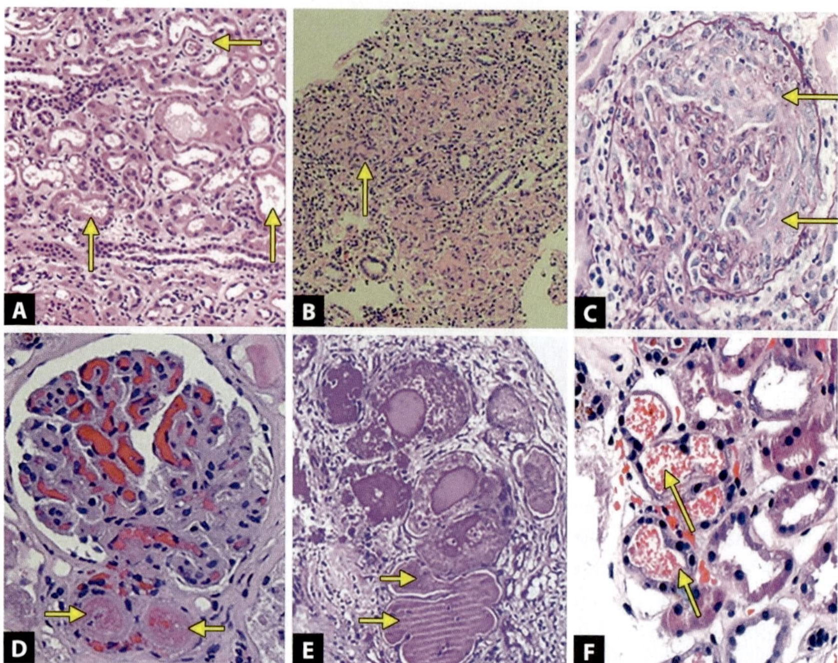

Figs. 14.3A to F: Histological findings in patients with acute kidney injury: (A) Acute tubular injury with tubular dilation, thinned tubular epithelium, and interstitial edema (yellow arrows); (B) Granulomatous interstitial nephritis with diffuse interstitial lymphocytic infiltrates and granuloma (arrow); (C) Fibrocellular crescent with multiple cell layers (arrows) chiefly of parietal epithelial cells in crescentic glomerulonephritis; (D) Thrombi (arrows) occluding the lumen of an arteriole in atypical hemolytic uremic syndrome; (E) Intraluminal casts (arrows) distending tubules in patient with light chain cast nephropathy; and (F) Pigmented granular cast (arrows) in hemoglobin cast nephropathy

critically-ill patients, given the absence of reliable signs and symptoms of AKI. The components of renal angina index (RAI) are described in **Table 14.4**. RAI is assessed 12 hr after pediatric intensive care unit (PICU) admission; a value ≥8 is predictive of severe AKI (stage 2 or 3 AKI) within the next 72 hr.

Furosemide Stress Test

Furosemide stress test (FST) has become an important AKI prediction tool in adults. The test involves administration of intravenous (IV) furosemide at 1 mg/kg (1.5 mg/kg if the patient has received furosemide in the preceding 7 days) to critically ill euvolemic patients in stage 1 AKI, followed by assessment of urine output. A urine output of <200 mL over 2 hr (100 mL/hr) after furosemide injection is predictive of stage 3 AKI, with reasonable sensitivity and specificity. Recent studies have confirmed the utility of FST as a satisfactory biomarker in children.

TABLE 14.4: Components of the renal angina index

Risk score	*Score*
ICU admission	1
Bone marrow or solid organ transplantation	3
Ventilation and inotrope use	5
Injury score	
Fluid overload <5%; or no change in eGFR	1
Fluid overload 5–9%; or decrease in eGFR by 0–24%	2
Fluid overload 10–15%; or decrease in eGFR by 25–49%	4
Fluid overload >15%; or decrease in eGFR by >50%	8

Renal angina index is the product of risk score and injury score.
eGFR: estimated glomerular filtration rate

Biomarkers

Serum creatinine is not an ideal biomarker of AKI; levels rise late following AKI (~50% nephron loss needed for creatinine to rise), tubular secretion, and interference from multiple nonrenal factors including nutritional status, muscle mass, and fluid overload affect its performance. Numerous blood and urine biomarkers **(Table 14.5)** have been identified over the past years.

Biomarkers are classified as *markers of damage* [molecules emanating from the injured kidney: neutrophil gelatinase-associated lipocalin (NGAL), kidney injury molecule-1 (KIM-1), liver-type fatty acid-binding protein (L-FABP), and IL-18], and *markers of dysfunction* [molecules upregulated in response to injury, or products that are filtered, reabsorbed or secreted by kidneys: cystatin, creatinine, and proenkephalin]. Damage markers define patients with *subclinical AKI* who manifest kidney damage without any functional change, while elevated dysfunction markers without increased damage markers represent *functional AKI.*

Electronic Alerts

The nephrotoxic injury negated by just-in time action (NINJA), which sends automatic electronic alerts to the treating physician on patients with excessive exposure to nephrotoxic medications (≥3 toxic agents given on the same day, or aminoglycoside use for ≥3 days), has been associated with significant reduction in medication-associated AKI **(Box 14.4)**.

MANAGEMENT

The principles of management include supportive care including maintenance of fluid and electrolyte balance, nutritional support, specific management of underlying disorders **(Table 14.6)**, and treatment of life-threatening complications. Patients with urinary tract obstruction need

TABLE 14.5: Biomarkers in acute kidney injury (AKI)

Biomarker	*Origin*	*Specimen*	*Detection post-AKI*	*Cut-off*
NGAL	Epithelial cells, neutrophils, distal tubule	Urine, plasma	2–4 hr	50–150 ng/mL
KIM-1	Proximal tubule	Urine	12–24 hr	50–100 pg/mL
L-FABP	Proximal tubule, other organs	Urine	1–4 hr	200–500 ng/mg creatinine
IL-18	Proximal tubule	Urine, plasma	6–24 hr	70–125 pg/mL
Cystatin C	Nucleated cells; catabolized proximally; not normally found in urine	Urine, serum	12–24 hr	0.5–1.3 mg/L
TIMP-2 × IGFBP7 Nephrocheck®	Metalloproteinases released during cell-cycle arrest	Urine	4–12 hr	0.3 (high sensitivity) and 2 (high specificity) $(ng/mL)^2/1,000$
Proenkephalin (PENK)	Surrogate for endogenous enkephalins; filtered across glomerulus	Blood	Unclear	100–500 pmol/L

NGAL and Nephrocheck® are available as point-of-care tests

hr: hours; IGFBP7: insulin-like growth factor-binding protein 7; IL-18: interleukin-18; KIM-1: kidney injury molecule-1; L-FABP: liver-type fatty acid-binding protein; NGAL: neutrophil gelatinase-associated lipocalin; TIMP-2: tissue inhibitor of metalloproteinases 2

prompt management, and definitive surgery after complications of AKI have been treated. Close monitoring, with attention to input-output, weight, and blood pressure records is necessary to improve patient outcomes.

Life-threatening Complications

In a child with AKI and oligoanuria, immediate attention is directed towards detection and management of life-threatening complications such as hyperkalemia, pulmonary edema, hypertensive emergencies, severe metabolic acidosis, and anemia **(Table 14.7)**. Urgent estimation of blood levels of hemoglobin, urea, creatinine, electrolytes and bicarbonate, electrocardiogram, and X-ray chest for pulmonary edema is required.

Supportive care is crucial to improve outcomes in AKI. Management is based on close attention to intake of fluid and electrolytes, provision of proper nutrition, prevention and treatment of infections, careful monitoring, and dialysis.

BOX 14.4: Commonly used nephrotoxic medications

Antimicrobials: Acyclovir, aminoglycosides, amphotericin B, β-lactams, cefotaxime, ceftazidime, cefuroxime, cidofovir, colistin, dapsone, foscarnet, ganciclovir, indinavir, interferon-α, pentamidine, piperacillin/tazobactam, puromycin, quinine, quinolones, rifampicin, sulfonamides, tetracycline, ticarcillin, tobramycin, vancomycin

Analgesics: Nonsteroidal anti-inflammatory drugs (NSAIDs)

Antiepileptics: Phenytoin, topiramate, zonisamide

Antihypertensives: Angiotensin-converting enzyme (ACE) inhibitors, angiotensin receptor blockers

Antineoplastic agents: Carboplatin, cisplatin, ifosfamide, mitomycin C

Immunosuppressives: Cyclophosphamide, cyclosporine, methotrexate, mesalamine, sulfasalazine, sirolimus, tacrolimus

Radiocontrast agents: High osmolar agents (diatrizoate, iothalamate, and ioxitalamate) have highest risk of nephrotoxicity. Iso-osmolar (iodixanol, ioxaglate, and iotrolan) and low osmolar agents (iohexol, ioxaglate, iomeprol, iopamidol, and ioversol) have lower risk of nephrotoxicity

Miscellaneous: Acetazolamide, allopurinol, amitriptyline, aspirin, chlorpropamide, cimetidine, clopidogrel, furosemide, haloperidol, intravenous immunoglobulin, lithium, pamidronate, proton pump inhibitors, ranitidine, thiazides

TABLE 14.6: Specific management of conditions causing acute kidney injury

Condition	*Management*
Prerenal AKI	Administer crystalloids; stop therapy with diuretics, nonsteroidal anti-inflammatory drugs and angiotensin-converting enzyme inhibitors; careful use of inotropes, antibiotics
Acute tubular necrosis	Discontinue nephrotoxic agents or toxin; careful use of antibiotics; manage hypotension, circulatory failure
Glomerulonephritis (GN)	Antibiotics (for shunt, endocarditis-related GN); immunosuppressive agents with/without plasma exchanges (rapidly progressive GN, IgA nephropathy)
Hemolytic uremic syndrome	Eculizumab; plasma exchanges or plasma infusions; immunosuppressive agents
Vasculitis	Immunosuppressive medications; plasma exchanges
Interstitial nephritis	Discontinue offending drug; corticosteroids
Renal artery, vein occlusion	Anticoagulation; thrombolysis or surgery
Intrarenal obstruction	Discontinue offending agent; alkaline diuresis (rhabdomyolysis, hemoglobinuria, urate nephropathy)
Urinary tract obstruction	Bladder catheter or nephrostomy; radiologic or surgical treatment of obstruction

TABLE 14.7: Management of complications of acute kidney injury (AKI)

Complication	*Management*
Fluid overload	Fluid restriction (400 mL/m^2 in anuric patients; 5% dextrose for insensible losses; normal saline or N/2 saline for urine output); prefer oral to IV fluids; frusemide trial; consider kidney support therapy if fluid overload >10–15%
Pulmonary edema	Oxygen; positive airway pressure (PEEP/NIV/mechanical ventilation); frusemide 2–4 mg/kg IV; fluid restriction; dialysis if not responding to above
Hypertensive emergency	Sodium nitroprusside: 0.5–10 µg/kg/min in 5% dextrose, or Labetalol infusion: 0.25–3 mg/kg/hr Add frusemide if fluid overload One-third of desired blood pressure reduction should be achieved during the first 6–8 hr; one-third in next 12–24 hr; and one-third over 2 days. Oral medications are initiated early; IV medications are tapered over 12–24 hr
Asymptomatic hypertension	Amlodipine (0.2–0.6 mg/kg/day), metoprolol (1–2 mg/kg/day), or prazosin (100–500 µg/kg/day) Blood pressure target is 90th centile; 50–75th centile on follow-up
Anemia (<6 g/dL)	Packed red cells 5–10 mL/kg during dialysis Monitor blood pressure, watch for fluid overload, hyperkalemia Add erythropoietin and iron, if known CKD stage 3–5
Metabolic acidosis	Sodium bicarbonate (IV, oral) based on severity of acidosis; consider dialysis if acidosis refractory; watch for fluid overload and hypernatremia
Hyperkalemia	Calcium gluconate (10%) 0.5–1 mL/kg (maximum 20 mL) over 10–15 minutes; repeat after 10 minutes if needed Salbutamol 2.5–5 mg nebulization q 1–2 hr; effect in 20–30 minutes Glucose (10%) 5 mL/kg with insulin 0.1 units/kg (maximum 10 U) insulin; effect in 20–30 minutes Sodium bicarbonate (7.5%) 1 mL/kg over 10 minutes; effect in 15 minutes Calcium resonium (K-Bind) 1 g/kg/dose q 8 hr orally or rectally; effect within 1–2 hr Dialysis if refractory hyperkalemia (hemodialysis is preferred)
Hyponatremia	Hyponatremia chiefly due to excess fluids; restrict fluid intake if sensorial alteration or seizures: 3% saline 3–6 mL/kg over 30–90 minutes (6 mL/kg 3% saline raises sodium by 5 mEq/L)
Hyperuricemia (tumor lysis)	Hyperhydration (2–3 L/m^2); allopurinol, and/or rasburicase If not improving, oliguria or severe AKI: Consider hemodialysis
High phosphate	Phosphate binders (calcium carbonate/acetate; sevelamer); dietary phosphorus restriction

Fluid and Electrolyte Balance

Maintaining proper fluid and electrolyte balance is crucial. The daily fluid requirement amounts to insensible water losses (400 mL/m^2), urine output, and extrarenal fluid losses. While insensible fluid losses are replaced with 10% dextrose, urinary and extrarenal losses are replaced with half-normal saline. Potassium containing fluids should be avoided. It is preferable to administer the required amounts of fluid orally, and resort to IV route in case of persistent vomiting, poor intake, or altered sensorium.

Ongoing treatment is guided by intake-output assessment, daily weight, physical examination, and serum sodium. Rapid weight loss and increasing serum sodium levels suggest inadequate free water replacement, whereas absence of weight loss, hypertension, and low serum sodium indicate excessive water intake. With improvement in kidney function, electrolyte disturbances resolve quickly.

Diet

Patients with AKI have increased metabolic needs and are usually catabolic. Adequate nutritional support is desirable with maximization of caloric intake but limited by the volume restriction necessary during the oliguric phase. Enteral nutrition is preferred and should begin as soon as feasible, targeting calories at 120–130% of basal metabolic needs, and protein at 2–3 g/kg/day. Energy composition should be obtained 20–25% from carbohydrates, 30–40% from lipids, and the remaining 35–50% from proteins. Once dialysis is initiated, dietary protein, fluid, and electrolyte intake can be carefully increased. If oral intake is poor, nasogastric feeding should be considered. Frequent review of dietary prescription, reassessing anthropometry, and monitoring blood levels of urea, electrolytes, glucose, and lipids help achieve nutrition goals. Routine vitamin and micronutrient supplementation is not necessary.

Management of Infections

Patients with AKI are susceptible to developing infections because of depressed immunity induced by azotemia, loss of protective antibodies in urine, prolonged hospital stay, concomitant malnutrition, and multiple invasive procedures. Infections (sepsis, pneumonia, peritonitis, and urinary tract infection) are the immediate cause of death. All procedures should be performed under aseptic techniques and devitalized tissue and collections should be removed. Prolonged bladder catheterization is avoided. The patient is frequently examined for infections; broad-spectrum antibiotics are commenced upon clinical suspicion of sepsis.

Drug Dosing in Acute Kidney Injury

Medications that accentuate kidney damage or delay recovery, e.g., aminoglycosides, radiocontrast media, NSAIDs, and amphotericin B, should be avoided. The dose and interval of antibiotic administration should be modified depending on the medication used and the severity of kidney injury to avoid toxic accumulation of drugs and their metabolites **(*see* Annexures 6 and 7)**. When GFR is <50% of normal, most drugs excreted by the kidneys will require modification in dose, interval, or both. Several medications are cleared by dialytic therapies, with clearance varying among the various modalities.

There is no evidence that diuretics improve kidney function or hasten the recovery. Diuretics may improve urine output but not the GFR. They may be useful in instances where a high urine flow is required to prevent intratubular precipitation, as with intravascular hemolysis, hyperuricemia, and myoglobinuria. Furosemide can cause ototoxicity, interstitial nephritis, hypotension, and persistent patent ductus arteriosus in the newborn, and should be used with caution. Similarly, low dose dopamine, calcium channel blockers, antioxidants, and thyroxin do not have a role in management of AKI.

DIALYSIS

Indications for dialysis in AKI are listed in **Table 14.8**.

All dialyses modalities, viz., peritoneal dialysis (PD), intermittent hemodialysis (IHD), sustained low efficiency daily dialysis (SLEDD), and continuous kidney replacement therapy (CKRT) are equally effective in the management of AKI. The choice of procedure depends on (*i*) age and size of the patient, (*ii*) hemodynamic status, (*iii*) availability of vascular access, (*iv*) integrity of abdominal cavity and peritoneal membrane, and (*v*) technical expertise. In patients who are hemodynamically stable, intermittent therapies are preferred, while in patients who are hemodynamically unstable, CKRT is the modality of choice. Most children with AKI who need dialysis are treated with PD in many centers, as it is easier to perform and requires minimal equipment and infrastructure. The same has been endorsed by the *0 by 25 initiative* with the goal that no patient should die from preventable or untreated AKI in low-resource areas by 2025.

An algorithmic approach involving a combination of RAI, structural and functional biomarkers to risk stratify critically-ill patients for AKI and tailor the management is suggested in **Flowchart 14.1**.

PREVENTION OF ACUTE KIDNEY INJURY

Several conditions that cause AKI can be prevented. Important measures include prompt rehydration therapy in acute diarrhea, maintenance of hydration for patients undergoing diagnostic procedures with radiocontrast media, timely diagnosis and management of sepsis, judicious use of nephrotoxic drugs, and using electronic alerts to prevent nephrotoxic

TABLE 14.8: Indications for kidney support therapy in acute kidney injury (AKI)

Indication	*Feature*
Uremia	Altered sensorium, abnormal behavior, seizures; blood urea >200–250 mg/dL
Refractory hyperkalemia	Potassium level persistently >6.0 mEq/L; electrocardiogram (ECG) changes
Refractory hyponatremia	Sodium level persistently <120 mEq/L, especially if symptomatic and refractory to fluid restriction
Fluid overload	Pulmonary edema; fluid overload (>10–15%) resistant to diuretics; cardiac failure
Refractory metabolic acidosis	pH <7.2 despite bicarbonate therapy; unable to use bicarbonate due to fluid overload or hypernatremia
Tumor lysis syndrome	Oligoanuria with severe hyperuricemia, hyperkalemia, hyperphosphatemia, azotemia; obstructive uropathy
Non-AKI indications for kidney support therapy	
Hyperammonemia, inborn errors of metabolism	Recurrent vomiting, severe metabolic acidosis, altered sensorium, seizures
Poisoning, intoxications	Paraquat poisoning; lithium, salicylate, valproate, metformin intoxication

Flowchart 14.1: Risk stratification and individualized management of critically-ill patients with acute kidney injury (AKI). eGFR: estimated glomerular filtration rate; FST: furosemide stress test; NGAL: neutrophil gelatinase-associated lipocalin

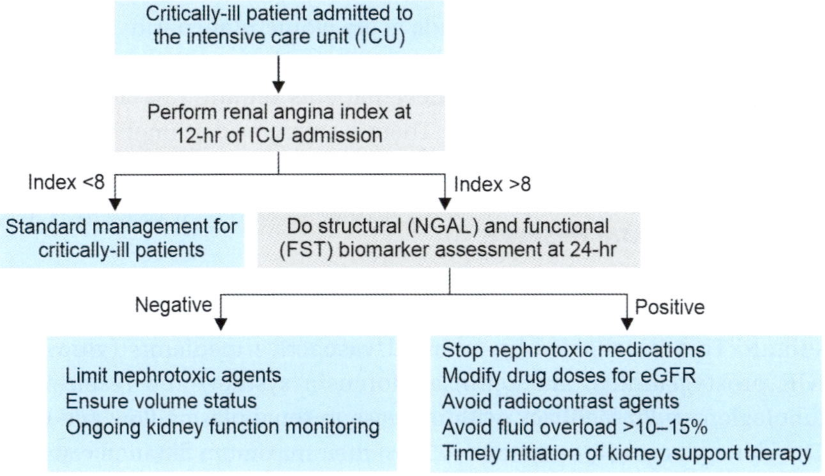

medication-induced AKI. Forced diuresis with use of allopurinol and/or rasburicase prevents AKI in patients with tumor lysis syndrome. Theophylline (single dose of 5 mg/kg within first hour of life) and caffeine (20 mg/kg loading; 5 mg/kg maintenance) have been shown to prevent AKI in neonates with perinatal asphyxia.

OUTCOMES

Optimal supportive care, coupled with prompt treatment of the underlying condition and dialysis (in severe cases) can reverse the derangements caused by AKI. The outcome depends chiefly upon the underlying condition. The prognosis is favorable in ATN from volume depletion, intravascular hemolysis, diarrhea-related HUS, acute interstitial nephritis, and drug or toxin-related AKI, when complicating factors are absent. The outcome is less satisfactory in patients with crescentic glomerulonephritis (GN), atypical HUS, and AKI associated with sepsis, cardiac surgery, and multiorgan failure. In the past, mortality due to AKI was high (30–50%) as patients were referred late with serious complications. Recent data from multiple centers report mortality rates of ~10%. Improvement in mortality is chiefly attributed to early identification and better supportive care.

Acute Kidney Disease

Acute kidney disease (AKD) is defined as "acute or subacute damage and/or loss of kidney function for a duration of between 7 and 90 days after exposure to an AKI initiating event". Kidney damage is assessed not only by serum creatinine and estimated GFR but also by albuminuria, hematuria, or leukocyturia. The relationship between AKI, AKD, and CKD is depicted in **Figure 14.4**.

Common causes for AKD include acute glomerulonephritis, hemolytic uremic syndrome, sepsis-associated acute tubular injury, and snake envenomation. Roughly half of these patients require KST acutely and 10–15% progress to CKD in 90 days. There is emerging data implicating AKD with adverse long-term kidney outcomes.

Renal Functional Reserve

Renal functional reserve (RFR) refers to the capacity of the kidney to increase its GFR in response to physiological (protein load) or pathological (AKI) stimuli. This is achieved by humoral/vasoactive mediators (glucagon, IGF, prostaglandins, and renin angiotensin system) and resetting of tubuloglomerular feedback, with increase in renal plasma flow and GFR. The kidneys normally operate at ~75% of their maximum filtration capacity. Following an episode of AKI leading to loss of nephrons, glomerular hyperfiltration ensues to maintain GFR in the normal range, however, the RFR

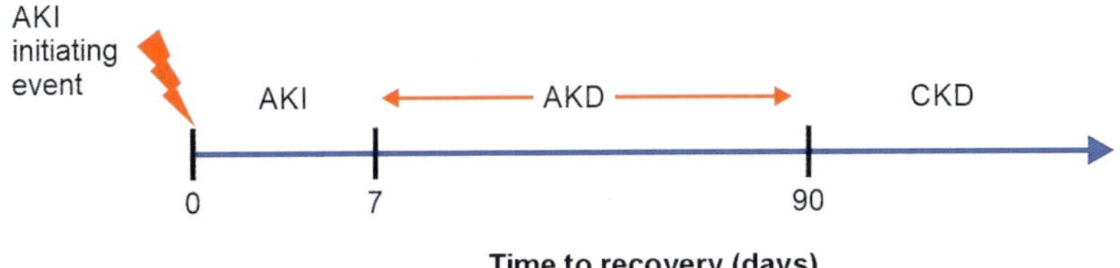

Fig. 14.4: The continuum of acute kidney injury (AKI), acute kidney disease (AKD), and chronic kidney disease (CKD) based on time to recovery of kidney function

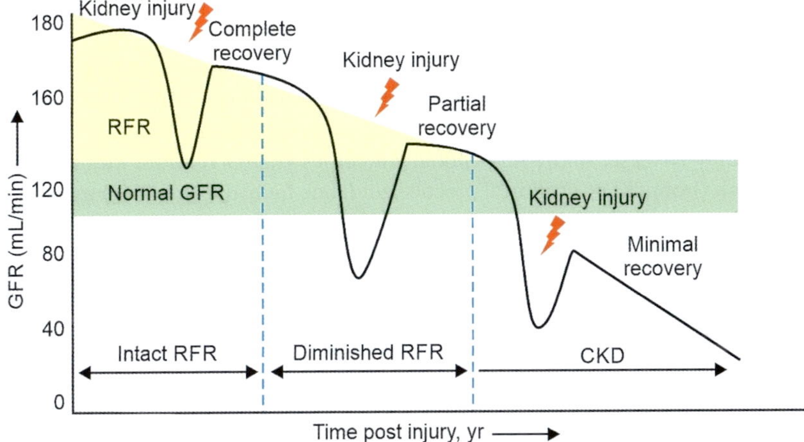

Fig. 14.5: Relationship between renal functional reserve (RFR), acute kidney injury (AKI), and chronic kidney disease (CKD)
Source: Modified from Sharma, et al. Nephron Clini Pract 2014

is reduced. Subsequent AKI episodes lead to further reduction in RFR, while the kidneys try to maintain GFR at the expense of glomerular hyperfiltration. Recent studies have shown that assessing RFR may help predict the trajectory of GFR decline over time. A hypothetical construct explaining this concept is depicted in **Figure 14.5**.

Long-term Outcome

Although complete recovery usually occurs in uncomplicated AKI, many patients (e.g., those with Shiga-toxin associated HUS, toxins, perinatal hypoxia) have significant risk of developing CKD and/or hypertension, and therefore need careful monitoring. Patients with AKI, especially those requiring kidney support therapy, should be observed for several years with regular monitoring of blood pressure, urinalysis, and estimation of blood levels of creatinine.

Acute kidney injury is common in critically-ill children and preterm neonates. Careful evaluation is warranted to identify the etiology and assess the prognosis. Recent risk stratification methods including structural and functional biomarker assessments have improved AKI prediction in children. Timely initiation of dialysis with prompt supportive care improves outcomes. Long term follow-up of all patients with AKI is recommended.

BIBLIOGRAPHY

1. Coleman C, Tambay Perez A, Selewski DT, et al. Neonatal acute kidney injury. Front Pediatr. 2022;10:842544.
2. Jetton JG, Boohaker LJ, Sethi SK, et al; Neonatal Kidney Collaborative. Incidence and outcomes of neonatal acute kidney injury (AWAKEN): a multicenter, multinational, observational cohort study. Lancet Child Adolesc Health. 2017;1(3):184-94.
3. Kaddourah A, Basu RK, Bagshaw SM, et al, AWARE Investigators. Epidemiology of acute kidney injury in critically ill children and young adults. N Engl J Med. 2017;376(1):11-20.
4. Kidney Disease: Improving Global Outcomes (KDIGO) Acute Kidney Injury Work Group. KDIGO clinical practice guideline for acute kidney injury. Kidney Int Suppl. 2012;2(1):1-138.
5. Krishnasamy S, Sinha A, Bagga A. Management of acute kidney injury in critically ill children. Indian J Pediatr. 2023;90(5):481-91.
6. Kuwabara S, Goggins E, Okusa MD. The pathophysiology of sepsis-associated AKI. Clin J Am Soc Nephrol. 2022;17(7):1050-69.
7. Macedo E, Cerdá J, Hingorani S, et al. Recognition and management of acute kidney injury in children: The ISN 0by25 Global Snapshot study. PLoS One. 2018;13(5):e0196586.
8. Menon S, Symons JM, Selewski DT. Acute kidney injury. Pediatr Rev. 2023;44(5):265-79.
9. Pistolesi V, Morabito S, Di MF, et al. A guide to understanding antimicrobial drug dosing in critically ill patients on renal replacement therapy. Antimicrob Agents Chemother. 2019;63(8):e00583-19.
10. Ruas AFL, Lébeis GM, de Castro NB, et al. Acute kidney injury in pediatrics: an overview focusing on pathophysiology. Pediatr Nephrol. 2022;37(9):2037-52.
11. Sandokji I, Greenberg JH. Novel biomarkers of acute kidney injury in children: an update on recent findings. Curr Opin Pediatr. 2020;32(3):354-9.
12. Sethi SK, Maxvold N, Bunchman T, et al. Nutritional management in the critically ill child with acute kidney injury: a review. Pediatr Nephrol. 2017;32(4):589-601.
13. Starr MC, Menon S. Neonatal acute kidney injury: a case-based approach. Pediatr Nephrol. 2021;36(11):3607-19.
14. Uber AM, Sutherland SM. Acute kidney injury in hospitalized children: consequences and outcomes. Pediatr Nephrol. 2020;35(2):213-20.

Thrombotic Microangiopathy

Mini Michael, Arvind Bagga

Thrombotic microangiopathy (TMA) is a heterogeneous group of disorders characterized by the triad of nonimmune microangiopathic hemolytic anemia, thrombocytopenia, and acute kidney injury (AKI). The unifying feature of this disease is endothelial damage, which leads to the formation of microthrombi in vascular beds in multiple organs resulting in the common pathology termed TMA. TMA includes chiefly two disorders—hemolytic uremic syndrome (HUS) and thrombotic thrombocytopenic purpura (TTP). HUS is an important cause of AKI in children, and the chief cause of children requiring acute dialysis.

ETIOLOGIC CLASSIFICATION

Hemolytic uremic syndrome (HUS) can be due to multiple etiologies **(Box 15.1)**. Shiga toxin-producing *Escherichia coli* HUS (STEC-HUS) is the most common cause of HUS. HUS associated with *Streptococcus pneumoniae* infection is a less common, but an easily distinguishable cause. The term atypical HUS (aHUS) or complement-mediated TMA defines patients in whom the illness is attributed to a disorder of the alternate complement pathway (either a mutation in a complement gene, or presence of anti-factor H antibodies). Other causes of aHUS that are not mediated by complement include metabolism-associated TMA (cobalamin C disease) and TMA associated with mutations in *DGKE* or *WT1*. The term secondary TMA implies another underlying cause for disease, such as malignant hypertension, other infections, or complement-amplifying conditions such as systemic lupus, scleroderma, and antiphospholipid syndrome. Secondary TMA can be associated with coexisting conditions such as pregnancy, malignancy, stem-cell and solid organ transplantation, and use of certain medications (calcineurin inhibitors, oral contraceptives, and quinine).

TTP presents with features similar to HUS, but with more consistent and severe thrombocytopenia and, at times, neurologic manifestations. TTP results from either congenital or acquired deficiency of von Willebrand proteasae, ADAMTS13 (a disintegrin and metalloproteinase with thrombospondin type 1 motifs, member 13).

BOX 15.1: Etiological classification of thrombotic microangiopathy (TMA)

Shiga toxin-producing *Escherichia coli* HUS
Streptococcus pneumoniae-associated HUS

Complement-mediated TMA*
Hereditary: Significant variants in *CFH, CFI, C3, CFB, MCP*; hybrid genes involving *CFH/CFHR1-5*
Acquired: Factor H antibody-associated HUS**

Noncomplement-mediated TMA
Significant variants in *DGKE, WT1; PLG, THBD*
Metabolism-associated: Cobalamin C (cblC) disease, methionine synthase (cblG) deficiency

Secondary TMA
Malignant hypertension
Drug induced: Quinine, mitomycin, ticlopidine, clopidogrel, calcineurin inhibitors, contraceptives
Pregnancy associated
Infection associated: Bartonella, Coxsackie virus, echovirus, influenza, varicella, HIV, EB virus
Transplant associated
Malignancy associated
Complement-amplifying disorders: Systemic lupus, antiphospholipid syndrome, scleroderma

Thrombotic thrombocytopenic purpura (TTP)
Inherited deficiency of ADAMTS13 (Upshaw–Schulman syndrome; congenital TTP)
Acquired deficiency: Autoantibodies to ADAMTS13 (immune-mediated TTP)

*For complete list of implicated genes and risk alleles, ***see* Annexure 9.5, p 845**
**Strongly associated with homozygous deletions in *CFHR1/3*
ADAMTS13: a metalloproteinase with thrombospondin motifs 13; CFB: complement factor B; CFH: complement factor H; CFHR: complement factor H related; CFI: complement factor I; DGKE: diacylglycerol kinase epsilon; MCP: membrane cofactor protein; PLG: plasminogen; THBD: thrombomodulin; WT1: Wilms tumor 1

Shiga Toxin Producing *E. coli*-associated Hemolytic Uremic Syndrome

Diarrhea or dysentery due to Shiga toxin producing *E. coli* (STEC) is the most common cause of HUS across the world. Rarely, other Shiga toxin-producing bacteria including *Shigella dysenteriae, S. flexneri, S. sonnei,* and *Citrobacter* species are isolated. Enteric infections due to Shiga toxin-producing enteropathogens are followed by HUS in 5–15% cases, a proportion that can reach 20–30% during outbreaks. During 1970–1990, *S. dysenteriae* was the chief cause of dysentery in children in south Asia. Multiple case series on shigella-associated HUS were reported from Bangladesh, Vellore, Chennai, and Delhi. Significantly reduced circulation of *S. dysenteriae* has resulted in considerable decline in patients with shigella-associated HUS.

The predominant STEC serotype causing HUS is O157:H7, responsible for ~2,000 cases annually worldwide. The most common non-O157 serogroups in Europe include O145, O146, O91, O103, and O26, and in the USA, O121, O45, O26, O111, O103, and O145. STEC-HUS is mostly sporadic, the incidence being highest in children younger than 5 years. The reason for its lower incidence in adults might be due to the acquired presence of anti-Shiga toxin (Stx) antibodies or to higher glomerular expression of the globotriaosylceramide 3 (Gb3) Stx receptor in children.

STEC produce two main types of Shiga toxins (Stx) known as Stx1 and Stx2, encoded by *stx1* and *stx2*. The majority of STEC O157 harbor *stx2*. Stx2 is considered more virulent than Stx1, with higher risk of causing HUS. Stx produced by bacterial infection of the large intestine binds the enterocyte, and crosses the brush border to enter the circulation. The binding of Stx, or Stx associated with microvesicles, to Gb3-expressing endothelial cells is followed by docking and release of toxin, which results in the production of cytokines and expression of adhesion molecules that trigger coagulation, fibrin deposition, and sequestration of red cells and platelets.

Streptococcus pneumoniae-associated Hemolytic Uremic Syndrome

Streptococcus pneumoniae-associated HUS (Sp-HUS), comprising 5% of cases, is a serious complication of invasive pneumococcal disease. The incidence of HUS after invasive pneumococcal disease is 0.4–0.6%. Pneumococcal neuraminidase cleaves terminal N-acetylneuraminic acid (sialic acid) from glycoproteins present on erythrocytes, glomerular endothelial cells, renal epithelial cells, and platelets, exposing the normally hidden Thomsen-Friedenreich (T) antigen. Preformed IgM antibodies react to the exposed T antigen on these cells, with a cascade of events resulting in Sp-HUS. A heavy bacterial load leads to increased production of neuraminidase, increasing the risk for Sp-HUS.

Complement-mediated TMA (aHUS)

Complement-mediated TMA or aHUS is an ultra-rare condition (prevalence 2–7 per million children) with a chronic and relapsing course, and high morbidity and mortality without treatment. While aHUS can occur at any age, onset during childhood is more frequent than in adulthood. aHUS accounts for ~10% of cases of TMA in children and the majority of cases of HUS in adults. Dysregulation of the alternative pathway can arise from loss-of-function variants in genes that encode regulators of complement activation or gain-of-function variants in genes that encode complement activation proteins **(Fig. 15.1 and Table 15.1)**. Thus, approximately 30–50% patients with aHUS carry such variants in genes encoding proteins essential for alternative pathway function: factor H (*CFH*), factor I (*CFI*), membrane cofactor protein (*MCP*, CD46), *C3*, and factor B (*CFB*). Not everyone with a significant variant develops aHUS and even in the presence of complement dysregulation,

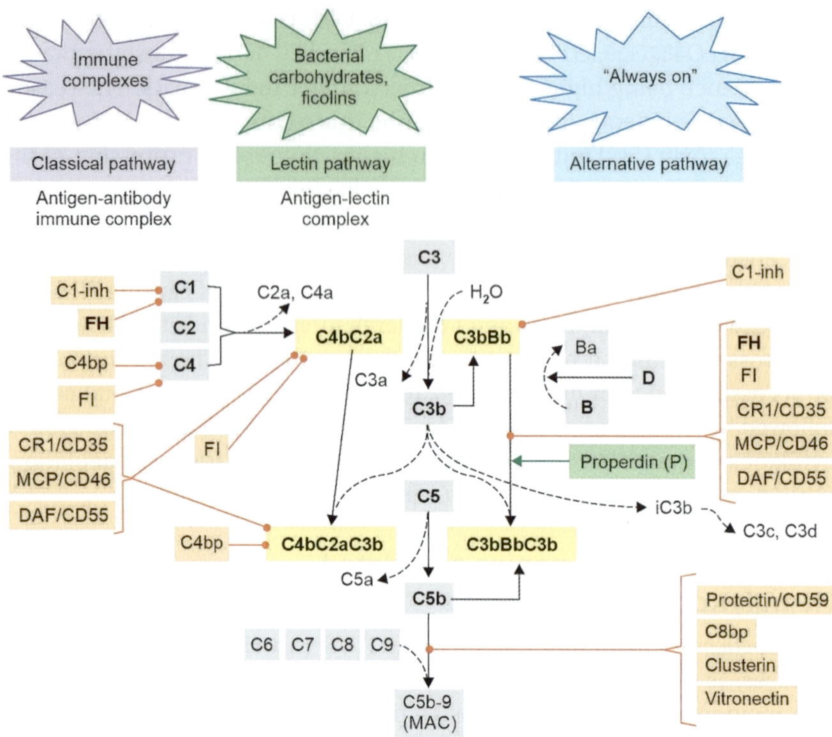

Fig. 15.1: Complement system. Activation of complement cascade through antigen (classical and lectin pathways) or spontaneous hydrolysis (alternative pathway) leads to the formation of C3 convertase (C4bC2a in classical and lectin pathways, and C3bBb in alternative pathway), followed by the C5 convertase (C4b2a3b in classical and lectin pathways, and C3bBbC3b in alternative pathway), and eventually, the membrane attack complex (MAC). The alternative pathway is self-amplifying; cleaved C3 and C5 components produce C3 and C5 convertases, which cleave further C3 and C5 molecules. Several cleavage products generated in these cascades mediate inflammation (anaphylatoxins, C3a and C5a) and cell-mediated immunity (C3a, C3c, C3d and C5a). The complement system is regulated by several proteins. Factor H (FH) is the most important regulator of the alternative pathway and acts both in solution and on the cell-surface. It accelerates the decay of the C3 convertase (C3bBb), and functions as a cofactor for factor I (FI) in cleaving C3b and C4b components. Properdin (P) is the only positive regulator of the alternative pathway, stabilizing C3 convertase and promoting its association with C3b. The C1-inhibitor (C1-inh) is a negative regulator of all three pathways. CD46 (membrane cofactor protein, MCP), CD55 (decay-accelerating factor, DAF), and CD59 (protectin) are expressed widely on cell membranes, protecting the cell from complement deposition. C8-binding protein (C8bp), clusterin, and vitronectin are soluble proteins that prevent assembly of MAC. Orange lines indicate inhibition, while green lines indicate activation

TABLE 15.1: Regulatory proteins and their mutations in complement-mediated TMA

Factor	*Function*	*% of aHUS**	*Low C3, %*	*ESKF, %*	*Relapses, %*	*Allograft recurrence, %*
Factor H (FH)	Inhibits C3b binding; accelerates decay of C3 convertase; cofactor for FI	20–30	30–50	50–70	50	75–90
Factor I (FI)	Inactivates C3b, C4b in presence of cofactors: FH, MCP, THBD	4–10	20–30	50	10–30	60–80
Membrane cofactor protein (CD46)	Cofactor for FI to cleave C3b, C4b	5–15	0–27	0–10	70–90	<20
C3	Generates C3a, C3b: Constitute C3 convertase and C5 convertase	2–10	70–80	60	50	40–70
Factor B	Binds to C3; forms C3 convertase	1–4	100	50	Common	100
Anti-FH antibodies	Binds FH; reduces cell surface regulatory activity	6–50	40–60	30–40	20–50	Low
Diacylglycerol kinase epsilon	Not linked to complement; leads to prothrombotic state	5–15	Rare	80–100	Yes	NA

*No abnormality detected in ~30% cases

ESKF: end-stage kidney failure; NA: not available; THBD: thrombomodulin

an initiating trigger such as pregnancy, infection, or medication use, is the rule rather than exception. About 15–50% of patients presenting with aHUS in childhood have FH-autoantibodies, which impair the complement regulatory functions of FH **(Table 15.1)**.

Other Causes of Hemolytic Uremic Syndrome

Noncomplement-mediated HUS, including that caused by *DGKE* and *WT1* mutations, should be considered when HUS presents during infancy, and in patients that are resistant to complement inhibitor therapy. DGKE (diacylglycerol kinase epsilon) is an intracellular lipid kinase that phosphorylates active diacylglycerol (DAG) to its inactive metabolite. Accumulation of active DAG leads to activation of protein kinase C, which in turn induces a prothrombotic state.

The pathogenesis of aHUS in patients with *WT1* mutations is not understood; reports suggest that podocyte dysfunction leads to decreased vascular endothelial growth factor (VEGF) and development of renal TMA. Glucose-6-phosphate dehydrogenase (G6PD) deficiency, an X-linked recessive disease, may mimic the diagnosis of HUS. Inborn error of vitamin B12 metabolism that is inherited as an autosomal recessive disorder, including cobalamin C (cblC) deficiency (mutation in *MMACHC*) and, less commonly, cobalamin G (cblG) deficiency (mutation in *MTR*), may present with features of HUS. Early diagnosis is important as specific therapy is available, and eculizumab is not effective. Eculizumab-refractory TMA has occasionally been reported in association with pathogenic variants in certain genes associated with nephrotic syndrome *(INF2, LMX1B, NPHS2, and ACTN4)*, apparent mineralocorticoid excess *(HSD11B2)* or primary hyperoxaluria type 1 *(AGXT)*, and significant variants in RNA processing genes leading to pontocerebellar hypoplasia type 1B (EXOSC3 pontocerebellar hypoplasia; *EXOCS3*), cerebellar ataxia, brain abnormalities, and cardiac conduction defects (CABAC syndrome; *EXOCS5*), TSEN2-related aHUS, craniofacial malformations and kidney failure (TSEN2-TRACK syndrome; *TSEN2*), and Pol III-related leukodystrophy [hypomyelination, hypodontia and hypogonadotropic hypogonadism (4H) leukodystrophy; *POLR3B*].

CLINICAL FEATURES

STEC-HUS: Within a week after consuming contaminated food, 90% of patients develop profuse and usually bloody diarrhea (hemorrhagic colitis) with abdominal pain and painful defecation. After a median duration of 7 days, when diarrhea is resolving, about 5–15% of patients develop symptoms of HUS, which include fatigue, pallor and oligoanuria, with or without fluid overload, hypertension and edema. Most patients have mild disease that is managed by optimized fluid balance, nutrition support, and control of hypertension.

Severe illness with anuria often requires dialysis; some patients also show signs of extrarenal involvement, chiefly brain and pancreas, and uncommonly liver or heart. Cerebral involvement manifests as irritability, altered consciousness, and seizures in 10–25% of cases. Shigellosis-associated HUS is usually a more severe illness, with persistent dysentery, marked kidney injury and neurologic illness, and less satisfactory outcomes.

Sp-HUS: Compared with STEC-HUS, children affected by Sp-HUS are younger (<2 years) with severe kidney and hematological disease, and are more likely to have persistent kidney dysfunction due to cortical necrosis. Approximately 25% patients have extrarenal complications, including impaired liver function.

Complement-mediated TMA (aHUS): Following a mild triggering event, these patients show acute onset of anemia, thrombocytopenia, and kidney dysfunction. Some have an insidious onset with anemia, fluctuating thrombocytopenia, preserved kidney function, and nonspecific symptoms such as malaise, fatigue, and anorexia. Extrarenal manifestations occur in about 20% patients. The age at onset of illness in patients with anti-FH-associated HUS is rather unique, being limited to 5–15 years.

DIAGNOSIS

Patients with HUS show some or all of the following features: microangiopathic hemolytic anemia fragmented red cells on peripheral smear (schistocytes ≥2%) **(Fig. 15.2)**, increased lactate dehydrogenase or undetectable haptoglobin, thrombocytopenia, and AKI. Early identification of the underlying cause is

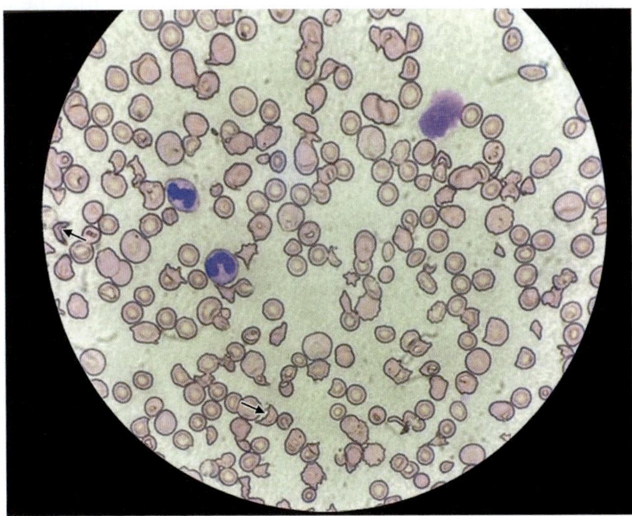

Fig. 15.2: Peripheral smear showing presence of schistocytes (arrows) and reduced platelets

important, as delay in diagnosis and initiation of therapy may lead to chronic morbidity. It is also important to rule out conditions that might mimic HUS. A direct Coombs test helps to differentiate HUS from other causes of immune-mediated hemolysis, but might be positive in Sp-HUS. A systematic approach is necessary to evaluate all patients with suspected TMA, with exclusion of systemic sepsis with or without consumptive coagulopathy. Infections such as malaria, dengue fever, typhus, and leptospirosis should be excluded. Patients with TTP also show features of TMA and can be diagnosed by testing for ADAMTS13 activity. Complement-mediated TMA (aHUS) is a diagnosis of exclusion and, therefore, all potential causes of HUS and TMA should be considered when evaluating a patient in the acute setting. A diagnostic approach for a patient with suspected TMA or HUS is shown in **Flowchart 15.1**. Investigations necessary for the diagnosis and evaluation of TMA are shown in **Box 15.2**.

Several patients with aHUS show low levels of complement C3 suggesting complement dysregulation; these patients require detailed analysis of components and regulators of the complement pathway. However, 30–50% patients with complement dysregulation may have normal C3 levels. Samples for complement studies, homocysteine, and ADAMTS13 activity should be taken before plasmapheresis or infusing blood products.

Histology: Histological features include intimal hyperplasia with thickening of arterioles and capillaries, endothelial swelling and detachment, subendothelial widening due to accumulation of cell debris, thrombi in vessel lumina and mesangiolysis **(Figs. 15.3A to F)**. Patchy or extensive renal cortical necrosis may be seen. The lesions progress to glomerular sclerosis, interstitial fibrosis, and tubular atrophy. Similar changes may be present in the brain, heart, pancreas, and gastrointestinal tract.

MANAGEMENT

General management focuses on supportive care. This includes attention to fluid and electrolyte balance, management of hypertension, monitoring for extrarenal involvement, nutritional support, and provision of kidney support therapy as required. Most children develop severe AKI and approximately two-thirds require dialytic support. Patients with severe anemia may need packed red cells. Platelet transfusions are rarely necessary, and limited to children with active bleeding, since they might increase the risk of microthrombi.

Shiga Toxin-producing *E. coli-associated* HUS

There is no specific treatment for STEC-HUS; management focuses on best supportive therapy. Epidemiological data has shown an association between dehydration and adverse outcomes in patients with STEC infection. Therefore, early use of isotonic fluids is recommended in patients with dysentery,

Flowchart 15.1: Approach to patients with thrombotic microangiopathy (TMA)
*See Box 15.2 for evaluating patients with HUS, including storing and processing of samples
**Also consider atypical HUS if positive non-synchronous family history or recurrent disease
ADAMTS13: a disintegrin and metalloproteinase with a thrombospondin type 1 motif, member 13; CD46: membrane cofactor protein; DIC: disseminated intravascular coagulation; LDH: lactate dehydrogenase
Source: Modified from Bagga A, et al. 2019

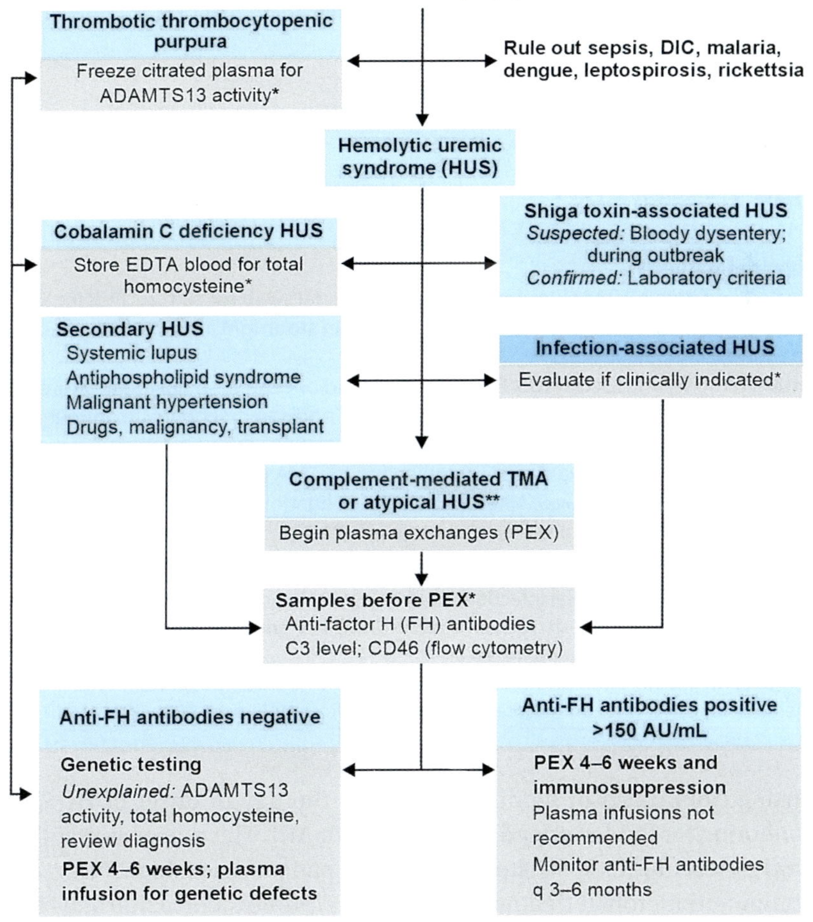

BOX 15.2: Evaluation in patients with thrombotic microangiopathy (TMA) or hemolytic uremic syndrome (HUS)

Diagnosis

Complete blood counts; peripheral smear for schistocytes; reticulocyte count[a]
Lactate dehydrogenase, haptoglobin[a]
Direct Coombs test[b]
Blood: Creatinine, electrolytes, transaminases, bilirubin, complement C3[a]
Urinalysis
Rapid test for malaria, dengue; IgM antibodies for dengue, leptospirosis (if suspected)
Coagulation profile[a] (suspected systemic sepsis)
Ultrasound abdomen
If clinical features present: Echocardiogram, neuroimaging, amylase, troponin T

Determining cause of HUS

Essential

Investigate for infection-associated or secondary HUS, if clinically suspected
Anti-factor H antibodies (ELISA)[a]; antinuclear antibodies
CD46 expression on neutrophils (flow cytometry)
ADAMTS13 activity assay[a,c]
Total homocysteine[a,c]

Selected patients

Suspected Shiga toxin-associated HUS: Stool or rectal swab for culture; PCR for Shiga toxin genes (*stx*1, *stx2*); ELISA for free Shiga toxin in stool; IgM antibodies to specific lipopolysaccharide(s)
Suspected pneumococcal HUS: Blood, pleural fluid or cerebrospinal fluid culture, PCR or ELISA; peanut lectin agglutination assay (Thomsen–Friedenreich antigen detection)
Anti-FH antibody negative disease: Sequencing for TMA genes, including *CFH, CFI, CFB, C3, CD46, DGKE, PLG, MMACHC;* multiplex ligation-dependent probe amplification (for copy number variations in *CFHR1*-5)

[a]Blood samples should be drawn before plasma exchanges or infusion
[b]Positive with pneumococcal infection, lupus; test prior to administering blood products
[c]Plasma separated from fresh citrated blood (ADAMTS13) and EDTA blood (homocysteine) within 1 hour of collection and frozen at –20 to –70°C
ADAMTS13: a disintegrin and metalloproteinase with a thrombospondin type 1 motif, member 13; *CD46:* membrane cofactor protein; *CFHR:* complement factor H related

starting from onset of bloody diarrhea to the day of onset of HUS, and monitoring for fluid overload in patients with AKI. The role of antibiotics in STEC gastroenteritis is debated. Conversely, patients with shigellosis require prompt antimicrobial treatment (with oral ciprofloxacin, azithromycin, or cefixime for 5 days) to reduce the risk of mortality and complications.

While plasma exchanges (PEX) have been used anecdotally in patients with refractory illness and severe neurological symptoms, current evidence does not support their role. Data from the German STEC-HUS registry did not show benefit of eculizumab, a humanized monoclonal anti-C5 antibody that blocks the terminal complement complex, although early treatment was

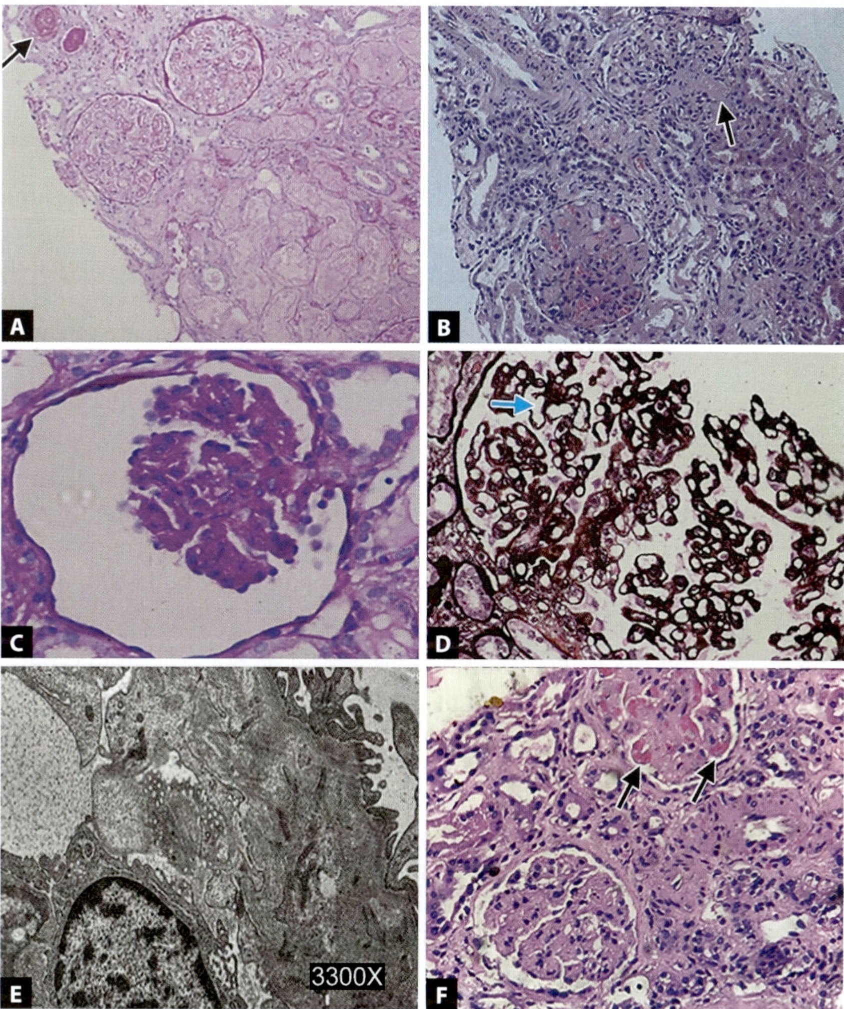

Figs. 15.3A to F: Spectrum of thrombotic microangiopathy (TMA): (A) Patchy acute cortical necrosis with necrosed glomeruli and adjacent tubules, with an arteriole at the border zone of the necrotic and viable areas showing an intraluminal fibrin thrombus occluding the lumen (arrow), and fibrin within lumina of glomerular capillaries in a 6-year-old girl with TMA associated with *Plasmodium vivax* malaria (Periodic acid Schiff, ×100 original magnification). (B) Extensive mesangiolysis associated with fibrin deposits within glomerular capillary lumina and occlusion of the feeding arteriole (arrow) in a 11-year-old boy with atypical HUS secondary to antibodies to factor H (hematoxylin eosin, 150×). (C) Glomerulus showing tuft shrinkage in chronic thrombotic microangiopathy due to homozygous *CFH* pathogenic variant (periodic acid–Schiff, 250×). (D) Glomerulus showing extensive capillary wall reduplication (arrow) (Jone's silver methenamine 400×). (E) Capillary wall showing mesangial cytoplasmic interposition in the subendothelial region, without any electron dense deposits (uranyl acetate-lead citrate 3,300×) in a 10-year-old boy with DGKE nephropathy secondary to a homozygous pathogenic *DGKE* variant. (F) Glomeruli with mesangiolysis and capillary lumina occluded with fibrin in a 15-year-old boy with post-transplant TMA and no defects in complement or cobalamin pathway (hematoxylin eosin, 100×). *Courtesy:* Professor Geetika Singh, AIIMS, New Delhi

useful in children with neurological involvement. Plasma infusions, heparin, urokinase, dipyridamole, antimotility agents, glucocorticoids, and Shiga toxin binders do not ameliorate the disease course.

Streptococcus pneumoniae-associated HUS

The principles of supportive care, including dialytic support, remain the same for all types of HUS. Patients with invasive pneumococcal disease require appropriate antibiotics. Since there is evidence of complement dysfunction in these patients, early use of C5 complement blockers may be considered in severe cases. Alternatively, patients may receive PEX, which are replaced partly by IV albumin.

Complement-mediated TMA

The standard of care for patients with complement-mediated TMA is complement blockade with eculizumab. Until recently, this therapy was not available in India and most developing countries. In absence of anti-complement therapies, intensive PEX is less than ideal, but used to be the only alternative.

Complement blockade: Eculizumab is preferred as the first-line therapy, particularly for disease that is not associated with anti-FH antibodies. Eculizumab should also be considered in patients with unsatisfactory response to 3–5 days' PEX or inability to perform PEX, due to difficult vascular access or other complications. Prospective studies have shown its efficacy in achieving 88–90% sustained hematological remission and improving kidney function. On medium term follow-up, progression to end-stage kidney disease (ESKD) or death occurred in fewer patients (6–15%), compared to those managed with plasma therapy. Prevention of meningococcal infection is crucial in eculizumab-treated patients and requires timely vaccination and antibiotic prophylaxis. Eculizumab is not indicated for therapy of non-complement disorders, e.g., *DGKE* or *MMACHC* mutations. The medication is infused once every 2–3 weeks. Discontinuation of treatment results in relapses in 40–60% patients with inherited genetic defect in complement regulation, but in ~10% with no identified defect, withdrawal of therapy is possible. A long-acting second-generation C5 inhibitor, ravulizumab, has been recently approved. Other agents blocking the complement cascade at different sites are being examined.

Plasmapheresis (plasma exchange, PEX): For our country, timely institution of PEX (60–75 mL/kg; fresh frozen plasma as exchange fluid to replace absent or mutated complement regulators) has been most appropriate for patients with suspected aHUS. PEX should begin as soon as possible, preferably within 24 hr of the diagnosis of aHUS, without awaiting biopsy diagnosis or results of complement studies. PEX is administered daily until hematological remission (platelets >100,000/μL, schistocytes <2%, LDH less than upper limit of normal for 2 consecutive days) and then tapered over 3–4 weeks. Maintenance therapy with plasma infusions is advised every 10–14 days for patients with mutations in complement genes, especially *CFH*. Adverse reactions to plasma or filter, complications of catheter insertion, infection or thrombosis, and blood-borne infections might occur in ~10% patients. The outcome of aHUS from large cohorts managed with plasma therapy alone is unsatisfactory, with 30–50% patients progressing to ESKF at 5 years' follow-up. Patients with pathogenic variants in *CD46* and *DGKE* do not show benefit with PEX.

Anti-FH Antibody-associated Hemolytic Uremic Syndrome

Since the aim of therapy for patients with anti-FH-associated HUS is reduction of antibody titers, intensive PEX is most appropriate to achieve this goal. Plasma infusions alone do not remove antibodies, and are not a substitute for PEX. A combination of PEX and immunosuppressive therapy is most useful to improve long-term outcomes. The latter consists of daily prednisolone (1 mg/kg/day for 4 weeks), followed by tapering over 6 months, and IV cyclophosphamide (500 mg/m^2 q 4 weeks) for 3–6 doses. Maintenance therapy with mycophenolate mofetil or azathioprine for 12–24 months reduces the risk of relapses.

About 15–30% patients relapse; high anti-FH titers during remission may predict relapses. Antibody titers should be sequentially estimated, especially in the first 12–24 months' follow-up. Most centers in developed countries initiate empiric therapy with eculizumab, pending anti-FH antibody results. Therapy with eculizumab is continued until anti-FH levels decline (below 1,000 AU/mL). Concomitant immunosuppressive therapy is advised to reduce the risk of relapses.

Outcome and Monitoring

Patients should be monitored for hematological remission and for renal dysfunction, proteinuria, and hypertension.

STEC-HUS: Short-term outcome of STEC-HUS is satisfactory, with resolution of renal impairment over a few weeks. On the long-term, 20–30% cases have renal sequelae, including proteinuria, hypertension, and deranged kidney function; progressive loss of kidney function is seen in ~10–12%. Oligoanuria persisting for >4 weeks, cerebral involvement, and cortical necrosis are associated with adverse prognosis.

Complement-mediated TMA (atypical HUS): The outcome of aHUS chiefly depends on the underlying mutation. Mortality is estimated at 8–14% in children at 3–5 years' follow-up. Progressive kidney dysfunction, in the absence of effective treatment, occurs in one-half of the patients, especially those with inherited genetic defects. Those with anti-FH antibodies respond to PEX and immunosuppression; progression to ESKF occurs in 15–20% patients. Patients, particularly those with abnormalities in *CD46*, should be monitored for relapses, especially following infections **(Table 15.1)**.

Allograft Recurrence

Risk of recurrence is very high up to 50–80% in the allograft after renal transplantation in patients with ESKF due to aHUS. The risk is highest (~80%) in patients with mutations in *CFH*, *C3* and *CFB*, 50% for mutations in *CFI*, 20% for those without an identifiable defect, and <10% for isolated mutations in *CD46*. Prophylactic and when eculizumab is not accessible, combined liver kidney transplantation is recommended in patients at high risk of recurrence. Patients with anti-FH-associated aHUS with high antibody levels might need PEXs before and following transplantation.

THROMBOTIC THROMBOCYTOPENIA PURPURA

Etiology and Pathophysiology

Thrombotic thrombocytopenia purpura (TTP) is associated with abnormalities of von Willebrand factor (vWF)-cleaving protease activity (ADAMTS13). TTP is rare in children; these patients have very low levels of ADAMTS13 activity, typically <10% of normal. ADAMTS13 prevents the emergence and persistence of unusually large multimers of vWF by cleaving multimeric vWF from the endothelium and platelets into smaller multimers. Patients with TTP have unusually large multimeric forms of vWF in their plasma, which are able to agglutinate platelets under high sheer stress.

The *ADAMTS13* gene is encoded on chromosome 9q34; patients with the hereditary form (congenital TTP; Upshaw-shulman syndrome) show mutations throughout the gene. Acquired (or immune-mediated) TTP is due to IgG autoantibodies that are intermittently and sometimes transiently expressed; acquired TTP can be transient or recurrent in some patients.

Clinical Features

The onset of symptoms in TTP may be gradual or sudden and can fluctuate and relapse. Neurologic involvement is central to the clinical features. Investigations show microangiopathic anemia, persistent thrombocytopenia, and AKI. However, AKI is rarely severe. The PLASMIC score, comprised of 7 components, is used to stratify patients into low-risk (0–4), intermediate-risk (5), and high-risk (6–7) of TTP. The components include (*i*) platelet count <30,000/mm^3; (*ii*) serum creatinine <2 mg/dL; (*iii*) evidence of hemolysis (reticulocyte count >2.5%, undetectable haptoglobin, bilirubin >2 mg/dL);

(*iv*) no active cancer; (*v*) no history of solid-organ or hematopoietic stem cell transplant; (*vi*) international normalized ratio (INR) <1.5; and (*vii*) mean corpuscular volume <90 fL. However, many patients with aHUS also meet these criteria.

TTP is either inherited due to *ADAMTS13* mutations or acquired due to anti-ADAMTS13 autoantibodies. When TTP is inherited (congenital TTP or Upshaw-Schulman syndrome), symptoms begin in the newborn period. Patients with anti-ADAMTS13 antibodies might present in childhood or as adults **(Table 15.2)**.

Management

Thrombotic thrombocytopenia purpura can be ruled out if ADAMTS13 activity is normal (>10%). Early diagnosis avoids the high morbidity and mortality from delayed treatment. Genetic forms of TTP are treated with infusions of fresh frozen plasma or cryoprecipitate poor plasma to provide the missing ADAMTS13. The acute episodes are typically treated with 10–15 mL/kg daily plasma until there is a response; later infusions are given at 2–4 week intervals to prevent recurrences. Acquired forms of TTP respond to removal of the autoantibodies by plasmapheresis. Additional immunosuppressive therapy, with corticosteroids and rituximab, is recommended in these patients. Recently, the use of recombinant ADAMTS13 has been shown effective and safe. Parenteral therapy with caplacizumab, a nanobody that targets the vWF A1 domain, hastens recovery of platelet count and reduces the risk of recurrence. The use of these agents is effective in both inherited and acquired forms of TTP.

Thrombotic microangiopathy (TMA) is a heterogeneous group of disorders that clinically present as HUS or TTP and characterized by the triad of nonimmune microangiopathic hemolytic anemia, thrombocytopenia, and acute kidney injury (AKI). Although the classification of HUS is constantly evolving, one based on etiology is commonly used. The most common type of HUS, especially in children younger than 5 years, is STEC-HUS, treatment of which is supportive. Complement-mediated HUS is extremely rare and carries very high morbidity and mortality, however, treatment with anti-complement therapies has made ESKD and death unusual in high-income countries. There are many other causes of HUS, including those associated with mutations in non-complement genes and HUS that develops in association with a primary disease process. For many of the rare forms of HUS, our understanding of the underlying pathophysiology is incomplete and anti-complement therapy is either not indicated or its role in treatment remains to be defined.

TABLE 15.2: Clinical features in various forms of pediatric thrombotic microangiopathy (TMA)

Feature	*Shiga toxin-associated HUS*	*Complement-mediated TMA (atypical HUS)*	*Thrombotic thrombocytopenic purpura*
Age at onset	65% 6–36 months; 5% <6 months	55% <2 years; 45% 2–15 years	*Congenital:* ≥75% in neonatal period *Immune-mediated:* 62% >9 years; 16% 2–9 years; 22% <2 years
Family history	Uncommon; synchronous if >1 family member infected	~15%; chiefly asynchronous	*Congenital:* Autosomal recessive *Immune-mediated:* Unlikely
Diarrhea at onset	95% (bloody in >80%)	20%	Possible
Platelet count	>30,000/μL	>30,000/μL	<30,000/μL
Acute kidney injury	85%; ~60% require dialysis	95%; ~60% require dialysis	Uncommon and mild[a]; rarely dialysis
Neurological symptoms	Marked with *S. dysenteriae*; overall ~20%	~20%	*Congenital:* ~35% *Immune-mediated:* ~70%
Relapses	No	20–80%	*Congenital:* ≥80% (without plasma infusions) *Immune-mediated:* ~30% if treated
Therapy	Supportive care	Eculizumab (limited availability) or plasma exchanges; immunosuppression if autoantibodies; supportive care	*Congenital:* Plasma infusion; recombinant ADAMTS13; supportive care *Immune-mediated:* Plasma exchanges; prednisone; rituximab; caplacizumab; supportive care

ADAMTS13: a disintegrin and metalloproteinase with a thrombospondin type 1 motif, member 13; HUS: hemolytic uremic syndrome

[a]Transient hematuria, hemoglobinuria; proteinuria; normal or slightly high serum creatinine

BIBLIOGRAPHY

1. Bagga A, Khandelwal P, Mishra K, et al. Hemolytic uremic syndrome in a developing country: Consensus guidelines. Pediatr Nephrol. 2019;34:1465-82.
2. Fakhouri F, Frémeaux-Bacchi V. Thrombotic microangiopathy in aHUS and beyond: Clinical clues from complement genetics. Nat Rev Nephrol. 2021;17:543-53.
3. Fakhouri F, Hourmant M, Campistol JM, et al. Terminal complement inhibitor eculizumab in adult patients with atypical hemolytic uremic syndrome: A single-arm, open-label trial. Am J Kidney Dis. 2016;68:84-93.
4. Goodship TH, Cook HT, Fakhouri F, et al. Atypical hemolytic uremic syndrome and C3 glomerulopathy: conclusions from a "Kidney Disease: Improving Global Outcomes" (KDIGO) Controversies Conference. Kidney Int. 2017;91:539-51.
5. Huemer M, Diodato D, Schwahn B, et al. Guidelines for diagnosis and management of the cobalamin-related remethylation disorders cblC, cblD, cblE, cblF, cblG, cblJ and MTHFR deficiency. J Inherit Metab Dis. 2017;40:21-48.
6. Joseph A, Cointe A, Mariani Kurkdjian P, Rafat C, Hertig A. Shiga toxin-associated hemolytic uremic syndrome: A narrative review. Toxins (Basel). 2020;12:67.
7. Liszewski M, Atkinson JP. Complement regulators in human disease: lessons from modern genetics. J Intern Med. 2015;277:294-305.
8. Loirat C, Fakhouri F, Ariceta G, et al.; HUS International. An international consensus approach to the management of atypical hemolytic uremic syndrome in children. Pediatr Nephrol. 2016;31:15-39.
9. Michael M, Bagga A, Sartain SE, Smith RJH. Hemolytic uremic syndrome. Lancet. 2022;400(10364):1722-40.
10. Muff-Luett M, Sanderson KR, Engen RM, et al. Eculizumab exposure in children and young adults: indications, practice patterns, and outcomes - A Pediatric Nephrology Research Consortium study. Pediatr Nephrol. 2021;36:2349-60.
11. Nester CM, Feldman DL, Burwick R, et al. An expert discussion on atypical HUS nomenclature. Kidney Int. 2024;106:326-36.
12. Scobell RR, Kaplan BS, Copelovitch L. New insights into the pathogenesis of Streptococcus pneumoniae-associated hemolytic uremic syndrome. Pediatr Nephrol. 2020;35:1585-91.

CHAPTER 16

Kidney Support Therapy for Acute Kidney Injury

Shina Menon

INTRODUCTION

Renal replacement therapy (RRT), recently termed kidney support therapy (KST) to indicate its role in providing support to a transiently dysfunctional organ system, is a life-saving procedure that may be needed when conservative measures to manage complications of acute kidney injury (AKI) have failed or are unlikely to be sufficient. These complications include refractory acidosis, fluid overload, hyperkalemia, uremia (typically blood urea nitrogen (BUN) >100 mg/dL or symptomatic), or an inability to provide adequate nutrition secondary to fluid restriction **(Box 16.1)**. Fluid accumulation and pathologic fluid overload in the setting of AKI is one of the most common indications for KST in children. Several forms of KST are available, including peritoneal dialysis (PD), intermittent hemodialysis (iHD), and continuous renal replacement therapy (CRRT). There are no data regarding the superiority of one modality over another with respect to outcomes in AKI. The decision regarding the choice of modality depends on patient characteristics, institutional resources, and expertise of the medical team. Each modality has advantages and disadvantages, as discussed in **Table 16.1**.

Historically, PD has been the most used KST modality in AKI. Infants and young children face unique challenges with extracorporeal therapies (CRRT and iHD), including lack of pediatric, especially neonatal-specific, KST devices and catheters, and a higher risk of hemodynamic instability due to large extracorporeal circuit volume (ECV) relative to the patient size and total

BOX 16.1: Indications for renal replacement therapy

Acute kidney injury

Electrolyte abnormalities refractory to medical therapy: Hyperkalemia, hyponatremia, hypernatremia, hyperphosphatemia, and metabolic acidosis

Uremic complications: Pericarditis, encephalopathy, and bleeding

Fluid overload >10%; diuretic resistant pulmonary edema or severe hypertension

Prevention of fluid overload; prolonged oligo/anuria necessitating fluid restriction

Non-acute kidney injury

Dialyzable toxins: Lithium, toxic alcohols, and salicylates

Inborn errors of metabolism

Hyperammonemia in fulminant hepatic failure

TABLE 16.1: Comparison of different dialysis modalities

	Peritoneal dialysis (PD)	*Intermittent hemodialysis (iHD)*	*Continuous renal replacement therapy (CRRT)*	*Prolonged intermittent renal replacement therapy (PIRRT)*
Principle	Diffusion and convection	Diffusion	Convection, diffusion, or both	Convection, diffusion, or both
Efficiency	Slow clearance; ultrafiltration is accurate or controlled	Most rapid clearance; suitable for drug toxicity, tumor lysis syndrome, hyperammonemia; provides accurate ultrafiltration	Slower clearance; suitable for removal of toxins, drugs requiring continuous convective clearance; accurate and gentle ultrafiltration	Rapid clearance; suitable for emergent situations or transition from CRRT; accurate ultrafiltration
Fluid and solute balance	Least hemodynamic compromise and fluctuations in solutes	Hypotension in small or critically-ill children; large fluctuations in solutes	Suitable for hemodynamically unstable patients and those intolerant to fluctuations in fluid balance	Lower risk of fluid and solute shifts than iHD
Access	Peritoneal catheter	Vascular access	Vascular access	Vascular access
Need for systemic anticoagulation	Not required	Usually required	Required	Usually required
Complexity; cost	Minimum equipment and training needs; feasible in small infants; inexpensive	Simpler and less labor intensive procedure than CRRT; need facility for dialysis water; expensive	Complex and labor intensive; no requirement for dialysis water; expensive	Simpler and less expensive procedure than CRRT; requires iHD facilities
Disadvantages	Risk of peritonitis, increased abdominal pressure, peritoneal fluid leakage, catheter block, protein losses	Vascular access thrombosis, stenosis, infection; risk of hemodynamic instability, bleeding	Vascular access thrombosis, stenosis, infection; bleeding; hypothermia in small children	Vascular access thrombosis, stenosis, infection; bleeding; lack of continuous or adequate clearance

blood volume (TBV). Furthermore, devices for extracorporeal therapies are not available universally, creating additional barriers to their use. However, the use of these therapies, particularly CRRT; has been increasing with the recent availability of machines, filters, and catheters for small children. Optimal KST can reverse the derangements caused by AKI. Despite advances in dialysis techniques, morbidity and mortality in resource limited settings is high.

KST involves transfer of solutes and fluid across a semipermeable membrane. Solute removal in all modalities of dialysis, be it PD, iHD, or CRRT, is governed by the physical principles of molecular movement. In PD and iHD, solute transfer is through diffusion. In CRRT, this may occur via diffusion, convection, or a combination of the two. Fluid removal (ultrafiltration) is driven by hydrostatic pressure across the membrane.

TIMING OF KIDNEY SUPPORT THERAPY

The timing of initiation of KST is obvious in the presence of severe complications of AKI, including metabolic derangements and fluid overload. However, there has been a long-standing debate whether an earlier start, prior to the onset of severe complications, would improve the outcomes. The multicenter, randomized controlled trial, Standard versus Accelerated Initiation of Renal-Replacement Therapy in Acute Kidney Injury (STARRT-AKI), which compared an accelerated strategy (within 12 hr) versus standard (based on prespecified indication) strategy of KST initiation, showed no difference in mortality at 90 days between the two groups. However, patients in the accelerated group had a higher dependence on KST and more adverse events. Except form the small tropic center ELAIM study conducted in a surgical ICU, findings from various multicenter RCTs, conducted in adult patients in medical ICUs, such as the AKIKI, AKIKI-2, IDEAL-ICU, JAMALE and BOULAM, suggest no difference in outcomes between patients indicated on KST 'early' versus; late', in absence of pressing indications **(Box 16.1)**. A multicenter prospective study showed that children with 20% or greater fluid overload at CRRT initiation had eight times higher mortality than those with less fluid overload.

PERITONEAL DIALYSIS

PD remains the most common KST modality, particularly for neonates and infants with AKI. In some centers, it is used prophylactically to prevent fluid overload after pediatric cardiac surgery, where it may have some advantages over conventional diuresis and other KST modalities. Early use of PD in this setting is shown to result in shorter time to negative fluid balance, shorter duration of mechanical ventilation, and shorter time to chest closure.

PD requires an intra-abdominal catheter, an intact peritoneum, and a dialysis solution. The International Society of Peritoneal Dialysis (ISPD) guidelines on the use of PD for AKI **(Box 16.2)** suggest the use of flexible peritoneal catheters where resources and expertise are available. Rigid stylet catheters or improvised catheters may be lifesaving in some situations **(Figs. 16.1A to D and Table 16.2)**. Tunneling of the catheter is recommended to reduce risks of peritonitis and pericatheter leaks. Depending on the size of the patient, a manual or automated set up may be used **(Fig. 16.2)**.

BOX 16.2: Key guidelines for peritoneal dialysis (PD) in children from the International Society for Peritoneal Dialysis

General guidelines

Access

Tenckhoff catheter inserted by a surgeon in the operating room is recommended

Catheters placed using Seldinger technique with an insertion kit, or those placed combining ultrasound and fluoroscopy are acceptable alternatives

Rigid catheters placed should only be used when soft catheters are not available, and their use limited to <3 days to minimize the risk of complications. Improvised PD catheters should only be used when standard options are not available

Prophylactic antibiotic one dose of intravenous vancomycin [10 mg/kg, 30 minutes prior to insertion] is recommended prior to PD catheter insertion, as following 10 mg/kg, 30 minutes prior to insertion

System

A closed delivery system with a Y connection should be used

In resource limited settings, an open system with spiking of bags may be used

Automated peritoneal dialysis is suitable based on the size of the patient and fill volume

PD solutions

Should include dextrose to achieve the target ultrafiltration

Add potassium to the dialysate once serum potassium levels fall below 4 mEq/L

Bicarbonate based solutions are preferred in hepatic dysfunction, hemodynamic instability, and persistent metabolic acidosis

Commercially prepared dialysis solutions are preferred when available. In resource limited settings, locally prepared fluids, made using sterile procedures, may be used

Acute peritoneal dialysis prescription

The initial fill volume should be limited to 10–20 mL/kg to minimize the risk of dialysate leakage

It may be gradually increased to approximately 30–40 mL/kg (800–1,100 mL/m^2), as tolerated

Each cycle may last 30–60 minutes (5–10 minutes inflow, 20–40 minutes dwell, and 5–10 minutes drain). The dwell may be gradually prolonged, as fluid and solute removal targets are achieved

Acute PD should be continuous throughout the full 24-hr period for the initial 1–3 days of therapy

TABLE 16.2: Options for peritoneal dialysis catheters and vascular access for acute dialysis based on size of patient

Peritoneal dialysis catheters	*Patient age, weight*
Cook multipurpose drainage pigtail catheters	
5 Fr	Premature infant
6 Fr	Neonate
8.5 Fr	1 month to 1 year
10.2 Fr	6 months to 2 years
12 Fr	1–5 years
Peritoneal dialysis straight catheter	
8 Fr; 5 cm length	
Tenckhoff catheter size 15 Fr	
31–32 cm	<6 months
37–38 cm	6 months to 5 years
40–42 cm	Older than 5 years
Rigid stylet PD catheter	
Child (Perforations up to 50 mm; markings till 170 mm)	<20 kg
Adult (Perforations up to 100 mm; markings till 270 mm)	>20 kg
Vascular catheters for iHD and CRRT	*Patient age, weight*
6 Fr Power PICC 7 Fr × 7 cm (Medcomp) 7 Fr × 10 cm (Medcomp) 8 Fr × 10 cm (Medcomp/Hemocath)	<5 kg
8 Fr × 10 cm (Medcomp)	5–10 kg
9 Fr × 12 cm (Medcomp)	10–20 kg
9 Fr × 12 cm (Medcomp) 11.5 Fr × 15 cm (Medcomp)	20–40 kg
11.5 Fr × 15 cm (Medcomp) 12.5 Fr × 20 cm (Covidien/Mahurkar) 12 Fr × 13 cm Triple lumen (Covidien/Mahurkar)	40–60 kg
12.5 Fr × 20 cm (Covidien) 12 Fr × 20 cm Triple lumen (Covidien/Mahurkar)	>60 kg

CRRT: continuous renal replacement therapy; iHD: intermittent hemodialysis; PD: peritoneal dialysis; PICC: peripherally inserted central catheter

For neonates and infants, the setup is typically manual and gravity based. Once the infant can tolerate a fill volume of ~100–150 mL, a PD cycler can be used for automated PD. For older children, one may use an automated cycler from the beginning. However, there is no evidence that automated PD is safer than manual exchanges.

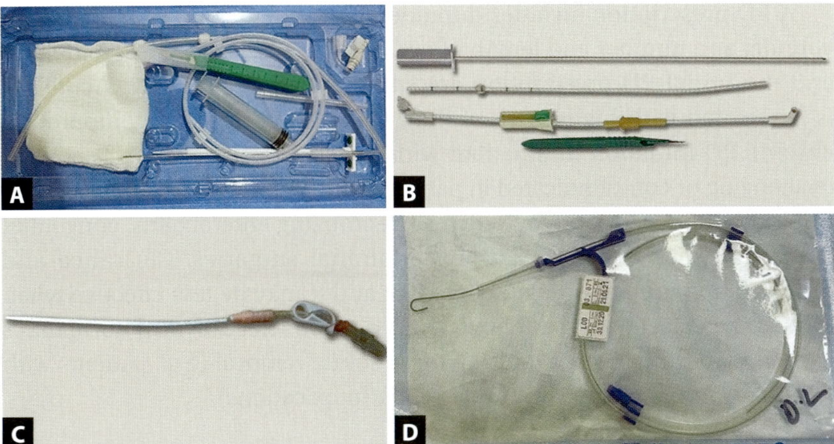

Figs. 16.1A to D: Catheters for peritoneal dialysis (PD). (A) Cuffed PD catheter (Tenckhoff) with instruments for insertion; (B) Rigid PD catheter with stylet and instruments for insertion; (C) Single-lumen hemodialysis catheter; (D) with guidewire; the latter (C and D) can be repurposed as a rigid PD catheter in neonates

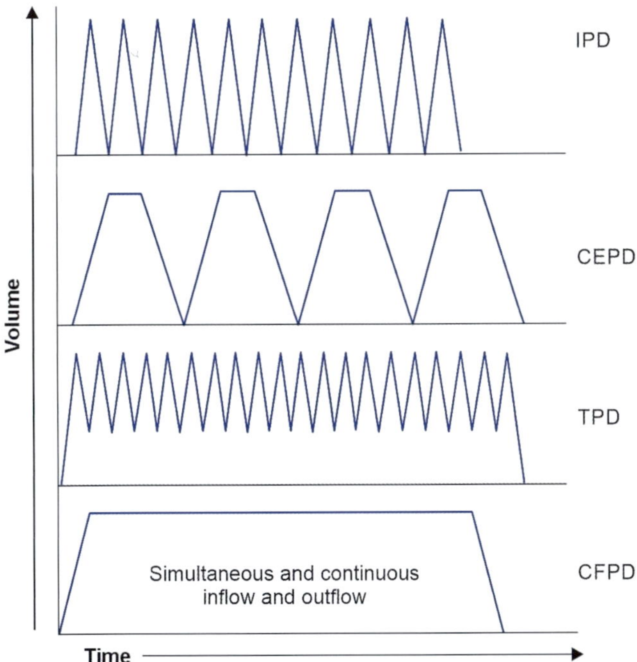

Fig. 16.2: Modalities of peritoneal dialysis. High volume peritoneal dialysis (HVPD) is similar to IPD but uses higher volumes and is repetitive. CEPD: continuous equilibrated peritoneal dialysis; CFPD: continuous flow peritoneal dialysis; IPD: intermittent peritoneal dialysis; TPD: tidal peritoneal dialysis

A PD prescription includes duration of treatment, type of dialysate, fill volume, and number and length of cycles **(Fig. 16.2)**. Key ISPD guidelines and the initial PD prescription are summarized in **Box 16.2**. Acute PD is associated with higher risk of fluid leak and peritonitis, compared to chronic PD initiation in a patient with a well-healed catheter. It may be challenging or contraindicated in patients with abdominal wall defects and/or intra-abdominal pathology such as necrotizing enterocolitis, congenital diaphragmatic hernia, or recent abdominal surgeries. Clearance and ultrafiltration are not predictable in PD, and it may be less effective when immediate correction of fluid overload or severe electrolyte abnormalities is desired, or in patients requiring rapid solute removal (e.g., patients with inborn errors of metabolism or ingestions/intoxications).

INTERMITTENT HEMODIALYSIS (iHD)

iHD is a highly efficient modality that can provide rapid clearance of toxins, e.g., in patients with inborn errors of metabolism or intoxication, or with hyperkalemia. It requires placement of a double lumen central venous catheter that supports adequate blood flow rate, availability of a dialysis machine, and trained specialized nursing staff **(Fig. 16.3)**. The blood flow and dialysate rates are much higher compared to CRRT, and the treatment generally lasts 3–4 hr. iHD is more suitable for older children, and those who are hemodynamically stable, although it has been used successfully in neonates and infants with intoxication and hyperammonemia.

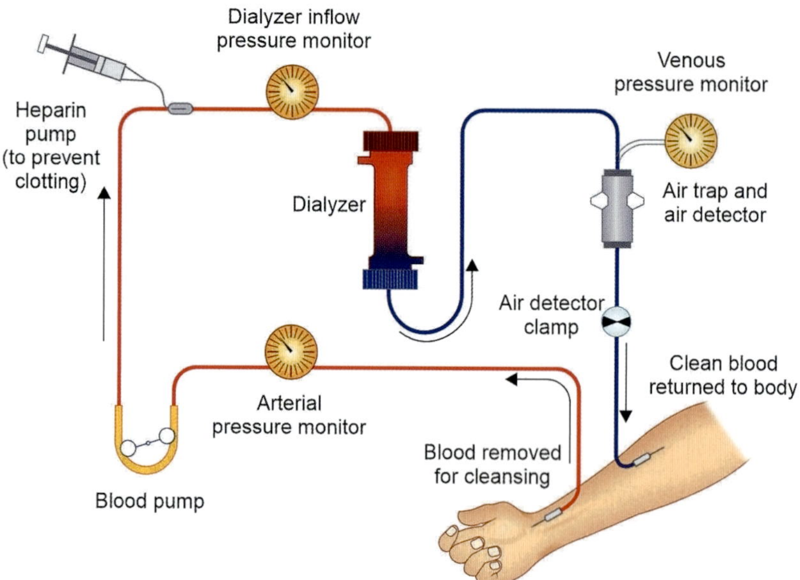

Fig. 16.3: Hemodialysis circuit

CONTINUOUS RENAL REPLACEMENT THERAPY (CRRT)

CRRT is an option for patients with AKI who are hemodynamically unstable. Like PD, it allows maintenance of electrolyte balance and fluid homeostasis in a slow continuous fashion without rapid solute or fluid shifts. The nomenclature for the various subcategories of CRRT is based on the primary method of solute clearance (convection, diffusion or both) **(Figs. 16.4A to D)**. Continuous venovenous hemofiltration (CVVH) relies on convection and requires a substitution fluid to replace part or all the ultrafiltrate. The composition of the replacement fluid varies based on the patient's requirement and can be infused pre- or postfilter. Continuous venovenous hemodialysis (CVVHD) uses diffusive clearance. Finally, continuous venovenous hemodiafiltration (CVVHDF) uses both dialysis fluid and substitution fluids for combined diffusion and high-grade convection. Chief components of a CRRT prescription are summarized in **Box 16.3**.

Unlike iHD which uses an online dialysate production system, CRRT uses previously prepared and packaged fluids. Bicarbonate based fluids are considered the standard of care, though many of the commercially available preparations may contain a small, clinically insignificant amount of lactate to improve stability. In addition to a buffer, CRRT solutions also contain varying amounts of sodium, potassium, chloride, glucose, phosphate, calcium, and magnesium. **Box 16.4** summarizes common complications of extracorporeal therapy.

CRRT in Neonates and Infants

CRRT in neonates and infants is more challenging than in older children. The devices commonly used (e.g., Prismaflex™, NxStage™) are designed for adults, have larger filters necessitating higher blood flow rates, and hence require larger catheters (minimum 7 Fr or 8 Fr double-lumen catheter) **(Table 16.3)**. The smallest filters available worldwide include CAR-125 with Renaflo II (NxStage Medical, Inc., Lawrence, MA) with an ECV of 83 mL, and M60 and HF-20 (Baxter Healthcare, Deerfield, Illinois, USA) with ECV of 93 mL and 60 mL, respectively. Even the smallest of these (HF-20) is relatively large for most neonates (e.g., for a 3 kg baby with TBV of 240 mL, the ECV/TBV ratio is 25%, versus a recommended ratio of <10%.

The Aquadex™ FlexFlow system (Nuwellis, Eden Prairie, MN) was originally designed for adults with diuretic resistant heart failure and fluid overload. The ECV (33 mL) and blood flow rate (5–40 mL/min) are relatively low compared to iHD and conventional CRRT (e.g., Prismaflex™, NxStage™), making it more suitable for neonates and infants. The system was adapted by Askenazi et al. to provide CVVH by adding prefilter replacement fluid to achieve convective clearance. This has been well tolerated with infants showing minimal hemodynamic changes during circuit initiation, and only minor complications reported.

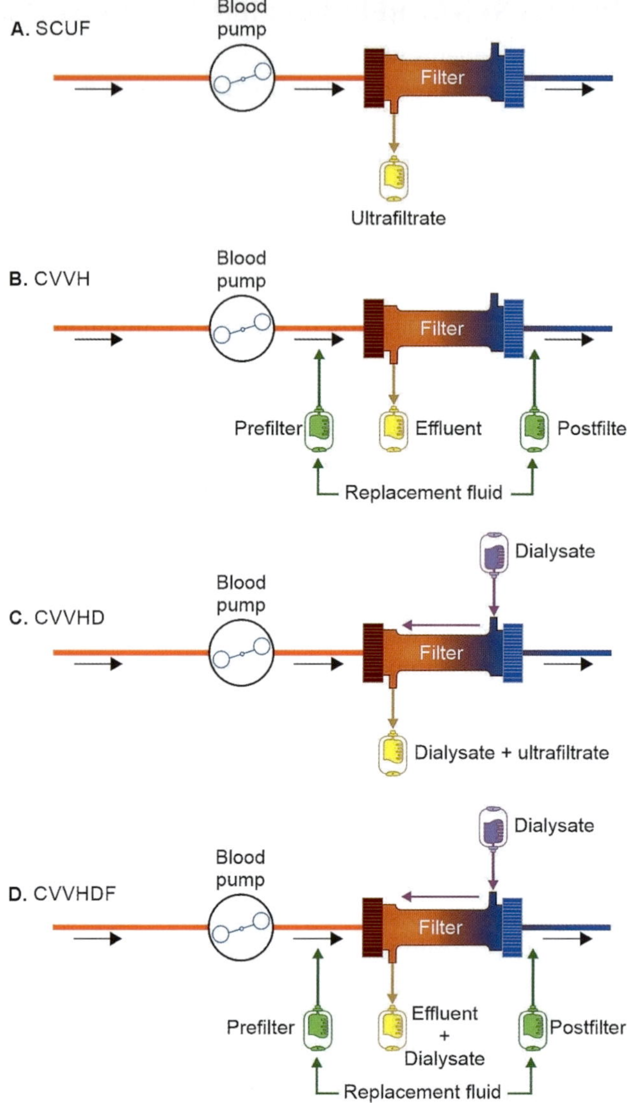

Figs. 16.4A to D: Circuit diagrams for modalities of continuous kidney replacement therapy (CKRT). Blood flows from left to right from the patient to the blood pump and then to the filter from which it is returned to the patient. (A) *Slow continuous ultrafiltration (SCUF)*: In this modality, there is no diffusive clearance and only ultrafiltrate (UF) is generated across the filter; this method is preferred for isolated UF removal when kidney function is normal; (B) *Continuous venovenous hemofiltration (CVVH):* Replacement fluid is run either pre- or postfilter in a volume to replace the effluent; excess effluent is removed to ensure UF desired for negative fluid balance; clearance is convective rather than diffusive; (C) *Continuous venovenous hemodialysis (CVVHD):* Blood flows across the filter in a countercurrent fashion with the dialysate fluid and the effluent predominantly consisting of dialysate fluid with minimal, if any, UF, as in intermittent hemodialysis; (D) *Continuous venovenous hemodiafiltration (CVVHDF):* This modality combines CVVH with CVVHD, such that the blood and dialysis fluid run in countercurrent directions, the replacement fluid is either pre- or postfilter, and the effluent comprises of the dialysate and replacement fluids

BOX 16.3: Components of prescription of continuous renal replacement therapy (CRRT) for acute kidney injury (AKI)

Continuous venovenous hemofiltration (CVVH), continuous venovenous hemodialysis, or continuous venovenous hemodiafiltration (CVVHDF) may be used

Access

Double lumen dialysis catheter

Internal jugular vein is preferred; femoral vein may be used if other access is not available

Size depends on patient size and device **(Table 16.2)**

Blood flow rate (BFR)

Depends on patient size, catheter, and device flow requirements

May range from 3–12 mL/kg/min based on these factors

Clearance is not dependent on BFR, hence high rates are not needed

Anticoagulation

Regional: Regional citrate anticoagulation, epoprostenol

Systemic: Heparin, bivalirudin

Clearance

Prescribed at 2,000 mL/1.73 m^2/h or 25–30 mL/kg/h. This is divided between dialysate and replacement fluid, based on which treatment modality is chosen.

A higher dose may be needed initially based on underlying disease (liver failure) or laboratory parameters

Fluids: Usually commercially available fluids used based on the device used

Ultrafiltration: Depends on patient clinical status and blood pressure; may range between 1 and 3 mL/kg/h

Carpediem™ (Medtronic, Minneapolis, MN) is a miniaturized CRRT device designed specifically for neonates and infants that has been available for use in Europe since 2013. It has filters with ECV of 27, 32, and 41 mL, can run at lower blood flow rates (2–50 mL/min) and has precise ultrafiltration control. Initial studies reported use of double lumen central venous catheters of 4 Fr, 5 Fr, and 6.5 Fr as well as umbilical catheters for access. It can provide CVVH or CVVHD and is well tolerated by neonates and infants.

Newcastle Infant Dialysis and Ultrafiltration System (NIDUS) is an automated, syringe-driven system that repeatedly withdraws 5–12.5 mL aliquots of blood from a single-lumen central venous line, passes and returns it across a dialysis filter, and then returns the dialyzed blood back to the baby.

CRRT in Patients Treated with Extracorporeal Membrane Oxygenation

AKI is common in patients treated with extracorporeal membrane oxygenation (ECMO). Infants treated with ECMO can have CRRT performed via connection of a hemofilter in-line with ECMO or adding a CRRT machine to the extracorporeal ECMO circuit. The type of KST used in patients treated with ECMO varies among institutions.

BOX 16.4: Common complications of extracorporeal therapies

Associated with vascular access
Bleeding
Thrombosis
Hemothorax, pneumothorax
Pericardial tamponade
Arrhythmia
Air embolism
Central line associated bloodstream infection
Exit site infection

Associated with anticoagulation
Bleeding
Heparin induced thrombocytopenia
Associated with citrate: Hypocalcemia, hypernatremia, metabolic alkalosis, metabolic acidosis

Associated with extracorporeal circuit
Air embolism
Filter clotting and blood loss
Hypothermia
Anaphylaxis
Bradykinin release reaction

Other
Hemodynamic instability
Electrolyte disturbances: Hypocalcemia, hypokalemia, hypophosphatemia, hyper- and hyponatremia
Loss of amino acids and micronutrients
Inadequate dosing of drugs

TABLE 16.3: Continuous renal replacement therapy devices available for neonates and infants

Machine	*Extra-corporeal volume (mL)*	*Filter (m^2)*	*Blood flow (mL/min)*	*Ultra-filtration (mL/h)*	*Modalities*
Prismaflex™	60 93	0.2 0.6	10–100 (±2) 50–200 (±10)	0–500	CVVH, CVVHD CVVHDF, SCUF
Aquadex™	33	0.12	10–40 (±5)	0–500	CVVH, SCUF
NIDUS™	<17	0.045	5 (single lumen)	0–60	CVVHD, SCUF
CARPEDIEM™	27 32 41	0.075 0.15 0.25	2–50 (±1)	0–150 0–240 0–600	CVVH, CVVHD SCUF

CARPEDIEM: Cardio-Renal Pediatric Dialysis Emergency Machine; CVVH: continuous venovenous hemofiltration; CVVHD: continuous venovenous hemodialysis; CVVHDF: continuous venovenous hemodiafiltration; NIDUS: Newcastle Infant Dialysis and Ultrafiltration System; SCUF: slow continuous ultrafiltration

PROLONGED INTERMITTENT RENAL REPLACEMENT THERAPY

Any extracorporeal mode of KST performed intermittently over a prolonged session (i.e., ≥6 hr) can be defined as prolonged intermittent renal replacement therapy (PIRRT). Such prolonged and intermittent sessions are useful if the patient's overall healthcare goals require multiple sessions or hours of continuous therapy. The chief modality is sustained low efficiency dialysis (SLED), which uses slower flow rates and longer treatment sessions than iHD with gentler ultrafiltration, and allows for greater mobilization, rehabilitation, and parental bonding since the patient is not connected to the machine all the time, unlike with CRRT. It is usually performed daily, termed sustained low efficiency daily dialysis (SLEDD), to offer a transition modality from continuous inpatient to intermittent outpatient therapies. The addition of convective clearance (SLEDD-F) using replacement fluid that is removed as efficient similar to CVVHOF in CRRT, allerease for improved clearances.

Either iHD or CRRT devices may be used for this purpose. With a conventional iHD device, longer sessions and lower dialysate and blood flow rates are used. In neonates and infants, CRRT machines are more commonly used.

TABLE 16.4: Prescription for various extracorporeal dialysis modalities

	Intermittent hemodialysis (HD)	*PIRRT using HD machine (without hemofiltration)*	*PIRRT using CRRT machine*	*Continuous renal replacement therapy (CRRT)*
Modality	Diffusion	Usually diffusion	Can be diffusion or convection or both	
Blood flow rate (mL/min)	150–300	100–150	30–150, depending on the machine	
Duration (hr)	2–4	6–8	6–18	Continuous
Dialysate rate	300–800 mL/min	100–300 mL/min (≤twice BFR)	Usually 25–30 mL/kg/h, split between dialysate and replacement based on modality used PIRRT may need higher rate, based on clinical parameters	
Replacement rate	Not applicable	Not applicable		
Anticoagulation	Heparin	Heparin	Regional or systemic	

BFR: blood flow rate; CRRT: continuous renal replacement therapy; HD: hemodialysis; PIRRT: prolonged intermittent renal replacement therapy

KST ACCESS AND PRESCRIPTION

Table 16.4 highlights similarities and difference in KST prescriptions using HD, CRRT, and PIRRT. **Table 16.2** shows available peritoneal dialysis catheters and vascular access for acute KST.

Several forms of kidney support therapy are available for patients with AKI. One may consider patient clinical factors, available resources, and the risk benefit profile to make the decision.

BIBLIOGRAPHY

1. de Galasso L, Picca S, Guzzo I. Dialysis modalities for the management of pediatric acute kidney injury. Pediatr Nephrol. 2020;35:753-65.
2. Goldstein SL, Vidal E, Ricci Z, et al. Survival of infants treated with CKRT: Comparing adapted adult platforms with the Carpediem™. Pediatr Nephrol. 2022;37:667-75.
3. Jeong R, Wald R, Bagshaw SM. Timing of renal-replacement therapy in intensive care unit-related acute kidney injury. Curr Opin Crit Care. 2021;27:573-81.
4. Kedarnath M, Alexander EC, Deep A. Safety and efficacy of continuous renal replacement therapy for children less than 10 kg using standard adult machines. Eur J Pediatr. 2023;182:3619-29.
5. Khwaja A. KDIGO clinical practice guidelines for acute kidney injury. Nephron Clin Pract. 2012;120:c179-84.
6. Krishnasamy S, Sinha A, Bagga A. Management of acute kidney injury in critically ill children. Indian J Pediatr. 2023;90:481-91.
7. Menon S, Broderick J, Munshi R, et al. Kidney support in children using an ultrafiltration device: A multicenter, retrospective study. Clin J Am Soc Nephrol. 2019;14:1432-40.
8. Nourse P, Cullis B, Finkelstein F, et al. ISPD guidelines for peritoneal dialysis in acute kidney injury: 2020 Update (paediatrics). Perit Dial Int. 2021;41:139-57.
9. Raina R, Vijayaraghavan P, Kapur G, et al. Hemodialysis in neonates and infants: A systematic review. Semin Dial. 2018;31:289-99.
10. Sanderson KR, Harshman LA. Renal replacement therapies for infants and children in the ICU. Curr Opin Pediatr. 2020;32:360-6.
11. Selewski DT, Goldstein SL. The role of fluid overload in the prediction of outcome in acute kidney injury. Pediatr Nephrol. 2018;33:13-24.
12. Sethi SK, Mittal A, Nair N, et al. Pediatric Continuous Renal Replacement Therapy (PCRRT) expert committee recommendation on prescribing prolonged intermittent renal replacement therapy (PIRRT) in critically ill children. Hemodial Int. 2020;24:237-51.
13. Spector BL, Misurac JM. Renal replacement therapy in neonates. Neoreviews. 2019;20:e697-710.
14. Vasudevan A, Phadke K, Yap HK. Peritoneal dialysis for the management of pediatric patients with acute kidney injury. Pediatr Nephrol. 2017;32:1145-56.

CHAPTER 17

Urinary Tract Infections and Vesicoureteric Reflux

Jitendra Meena, Pankaj Hari

URINARY TRACT INFECTION

Urinary tract infections (UTIs) constitute a common cause of morbidity in infants and children. When associated with abnormalities of the urinary tract, they may lead to long-term complications including renal scarring, loss of function, and hypertension. Prompt detection and treatment of UTI and any complicating factors are important.

Epidemiology

Urinary tract infection is associated with nonspecific signs and symptoms in infants. The usual age for occurrence of the first symptomatic UTI is the 1st year of life, particularly in boys, when it mainly affects the upper urinary tract. The incidence of UTI in term neonate is approximately 1% and in the preterm 3%, both with male preponderance. During infancy, the risk of developing UTI is equal in boys and girls, and thereafter higher in girls. Population-based studies show that 2% of boys and 7–8% of girls had at least one UTI by 7 years of age. Probability of having UTI in a febrile infant is approximately 5–7%. The risk is higher in children with malnutrition and chronic diarrhea. Awareness of the likelihood of UTI in a young child presenting with fever is necessary for prompt diagnosis, evaluation, and treatment. Obstructive lesions may be found in 5–10% of boys investigated for UTI; overall 20–30% patients show the presence of primary vesicoureteric reflux (VUR). Delay in starting treatment, presence of dilating VUR, and presence of obstruction are risk factors for renal scarring.

Etiology

About 90% of the first symptomatic UTIs and 70% of recurrent infections are due to *Escherichia coli*. Other organisms including *Klebsiella, Staphylococcus saprophyticus*, and *Streptococcus faecalis* may occasionally be responsible. *Proteus* and *Pseudomonas* are associated with recurrent UTI, instrumentation, urolithiasis, and nosocomial infections. Pathogens of low virulence and fungi may be causative in the immunocompromised. *Candida albicans* infections are relatively common in preterm infants, immunocompromised children, and following prolonged antibiotic therapy.

Periurethral Bacterial Flora

Normal periurethral flora consisting of commensal *Lactobacilli* prevents epithelial attachment by virulent organisms. Elimination of protective flora by broad-spectrum antibiotics or colonization with uropathogenic enteric organisms predisposes to UTI.

Pathogenesis

In the neonatal period, renal parenchymal infection is due to hematogenous spread. Beyond the neonatal period, most UTIs are caused by ascending infection. Uropathogenic bacteria are generally enteric organisms derived from fecal flora, which initially colonize the periurethral area. Direct extension of infection can occur in the presence of fistula from vagina or intestine to the urinary tract.

Predisposing Factors

Conditions that predispose to UTI include bladder bowel dysfunction (BBD), VUR, obstructive uropathy, and stones in the urinary tract. There is a cause-and-effect relationship between functional constipation and recurrent UTI and VUR. UTI is ten times more common in noncircumcised infants, with colonization of the prepuce being contributory. The increased incidence of UTI in girls may be related to their short urethra, which permits easy entry of bacteria into the bladder. Babies born to mothers with bacteriuria during pregnancy develop colonization by uropathogens and show higher incidence of UTI. Broad-spectrum antibiotic therapy may abolish the normal bacterial flora of perineum and allow infection by virulent organisms, predisposing to UTI.

Host Defense

Symptomatic UTI occurs when local defense mechanisms are overcome by virulence of uropathogens. Most bacteria that reach the urinary bladder are expelled with micturition. A small number may persist and are destroyed by bladder epithelial cells. Other defense mechanisms include secretory IgA in urine and blood group antigens in urothelial secretions. Breastfeeding has been found to protect infants against UTI during the first 6 months of life. Human milk provides antiadhesive factors in the urine and stabilizes intestinal flora with less pathogenic enteropathogens. Whenever bladder emptying is incomplete and there is urinary stasis due to structure obstruction or bladder dysfunction, the risk of developing UTI is increased. Primary disturbances of bladder function with incomplete evacuation are often present in children with recurrent UTI in whom no anatomical abnormalities of the urinary tract or VUR can be demonstrated.

Bacterial Virulence

Colonization and adhesion of bacteria to the epithelial cells is crucial step in pathogenesis of UTI. Through these processes, uropathogens multiply and induce inflammation in urinary tract. Bacterial adhesion to epithelial cell surface is mediated by bacterial fimbriae (pili) that are hair-like appendages containing adhesins at the tip **(Fig. 17.1)**. Type 1 fimbriae bind to various proteins on urothelial surface which are mannosylated. These host proteins (uroplakin 1a, Tamm–Horsfall glycoprotein, and β1 and α3 integrins) play key roles in pathogenesis of UTI caused by *E. coli.* Pathogenic strains of *E. coli* which cause pyelonephritis also have additional P fimbriae which aid in evading the host immune response. Adherence of *E. coli* to glycosphingolipid receptors recruits toll-like receptors (TLRs) on the urothelial cells. Activation of TLR triggers a cytokine cascade which induces production of adhesion molecules and chemotaxis of leukocytes causing local inflammation. Bacterial adherence to the uroepithelium helps in ascending into the kidney, even in children without vesicoureteral reflux (VUR).

Virulent strains of *E. coli* that cause pyelonephritis have an adhesin on their fimbriae that agglutinates red blood cells of the P1 blood group, hence called P-fimbriated *E. coli.* The O antigen (lipopolysaccharide, endotoxin) of

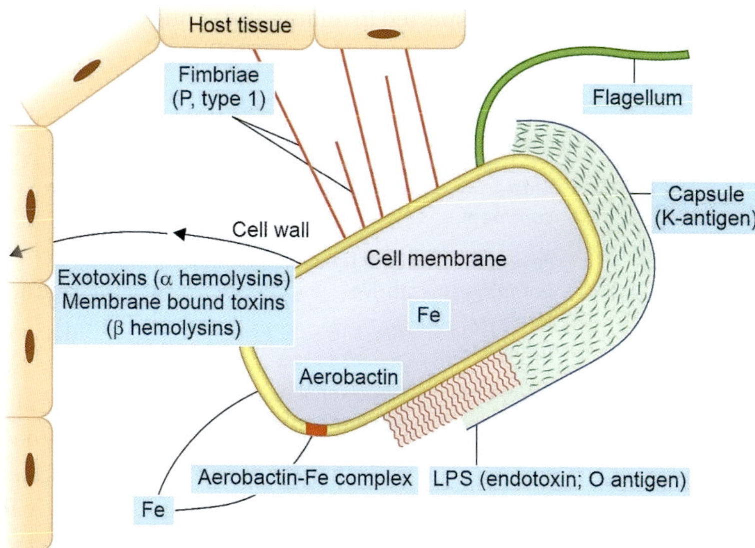

Fig. 17.1: Virulence determinants of *Escherichia coli* include flagellum for motility, P-fimbriae for adhesion to uroepithelium, hemolysin for lysis of host cells, and siderophore (aerobactin) for scavenging iron from these cells. Type 1 fimbriae also provide a supplementary mechanism for adherence. The capsular K-1 antigen decreases ability of antibody and/or complement to bind to the bacterial surface and the ability of phagocytes to engulf bacterial cells. LPS: lipopolysaccharide

E. coli is responsible for inducing inflammation and fever, and the capsular K antigen, for resistance to phagocytosis and bactericidal effect of serum. Virulent bacteria also produce a hemolysin that damages the uroepithelium, and aerobactin that scavenges iron from the urine that is needed for their metabolism **(Fig. 17.1)**. Persistence and multiplication of bacteria depend upon production of glycocalyx polymers forming biofilm on epithelial surface. Such films form on uroepithelial surfaces, surfaces of indwelling catheters, and fibers of infant diapers. Bacteria on the surface of the biofilm are killed by antibiotics, but those in deeper layers resist treatment.

Clinical Features

The manifestations of UTI are related to the patient age, stage in toilet training, location of infection in the urinary tract, and severity of the infection **(Table 17.1)**.

Neonates and Infants

In neonates, acute pyelonephritis presents with features of sepsis such as lethargy, seizures, shock, unstable temperature, and persistence of physiological jaundice. Other symptoms include failure to thrive, vomiting, and diarrhea. In infants, unexplained fever may be the only symptom of acute pyelonephritis. UTI should be suspected in infants and young children below 2 years of age having unexplained fever.

TABLE 17.1: Symptoms and signs of urinary tract infection

Age		*Most common*	*Less common*	*Uncommon*
Infants <3 months		Fever, vomiting, lethargy, irritability	Poor feeding; failure to thrive	Abdominal pain, jaundice, hematuria
Infants >3 months; older children	*Preverbal*	Fever	Abdominal pain, loin tenderness; vomiting, poor feeding	Lethargy, irritability, hematuria, failure to thrive
	Verbal	Frequency, dysuria	Dysfunctional voiding, incontinence, pain abdomen, loin tenderness	Fever, malaise, vomiting, hematuria

Adapted from National Collaborating Centre for Women's and Children's Health (UK). NICE guidelines: Urinary tract infection in children: diagnosis, treatment and long-term management. London: RCOG Press; 2007

Older Children

Dribbling, prolonged voiding, straining, crying during micturition, and poor urinary stream indicate an abnormality of the distal urinary tract. Diurnal incontinence, urgency, frequency, and squatting suggest voiding dysfunction. Dysuria, frequent voiding, and hypogastric pain suggest cystitis. Fever, chills and rigor, and flank pain indicate renal parenchymal involvement (pyelonephritis). Turbid or foul-smelling urine also suggests UTI. Gross hematuria may occasionally be present.

It is difficult to clinically differentiate between UTI involving kidney parenchyma (pyelonephritis) from that confined to the bladder and urethra. Febrile UTI in young children is, therefore, assumed to involve the upper tract.

Recurrent Urinary Tract Infection

Recurrence after the first UTI is observed in 30–50% of children. Of these, the majority occur within 3 months of the initial episode; *E. coli* is the most common organism. Girls in the school age group with an anatomically and functionally normal urinary tract may develop recurrent lower tract afebrile UTI. Many of these children may have bladder bowel dysfunction and symptoms of bladder instability, such as urge incontinence. Boys rarely have recurrent UTI in the absence of underlying complicating factors.

Diagnosis

The diagnosis of UTI is confirmed based on a positive urine culture. While urinalysis is helpful in making a presumptive diagnosis, a properly collected specimen for urine culture is obtained before starting empirical treatment. Evaluation of clinical features is important, since culture may be negative if antibiotics are recently administered, or an antiseptic solution is used for local cleansing.

Urine Specimen Collection

Urine specimen should be obtained carefully to prevent contamination by commensal flora, especially in girls. A clean catch midstream specimen is most widely used in toilet trained children. In girls, parents should be instructed to part the labia and clean with water. While cumbersome and time-consuming clean catch midstream collection can be attempted to obtain urine specimen in nontoilet trained children. Time to urine collection can be shortened by voiding stimulation strategies such as *Quick-Wee* method. If clean catch midstream fails or patients is critically ill, catheterization or suprapubic aspiration should be used for collecting urine. Suprapubic aspiration can be performed safely under ultrasound guidance using a 21-gauge needle, inserted 1–2 cm above the pubic symphysis. Fullness of the bladder is ensured prior to suprapubic aspiration.

Bag specimens have unacceptably high contamination rate and are not recommended. In children with indwelling catheters, preferred method is to insert a new catheter and collect urine specimens. However, if not feasible, urine can be aspirated from the catheter using a sterile needle and syringe. Obtaining urine specimen for culture is difficult in patients with ureterostomy or vesicostomy.

The specimen should be transported to laboratory as early as possible, or stored at 4°C. It is examined microscopically, and cultured.

Urine Microscopy

Urinalysis is a useful screening test in clinically suspected UTI for starting antibiotic therapy. Microscopy is performed on a freshly voided specimen (within 1 hour after voiding) or on a refrigerated specimen (within 4 hr after voiding). The presence of >10 leukocytes/mm^3 in an uncentrifuged specimen or >5 leukocytes per high-power field in a centrifuged specimen is significant. UTI should *not* be diagnosed on finding isolated leukocyturia, which is not uncommon in a child having fever and in girls from vaginal contamination. Leukocytes may lyse rapidly in dilute or alkaline urine or if microscopy is delayed. White cell casts in urine indicate renal parenchymal involvement. The finding of bacteria on a Gram-stained urine specimen has a high sensitivity and specificity for predicting a diagnosis of UTI.

Rapid Diagnostic Dipstick Tests

Urinary bacteria convert nitrate to nitrite, detected by color change on chemically coated paper strips. The intensity of color change is proportional to the number of bacteria in the urine. The diagnostic utility of the nitrite test is limited as it can be falsely negative in infants with urinary frequency resulting in insufficient time for incubation of bacteria in urine, or during infection with bacteria that lack nitrate reductase, e.g., *Streptococcus*. Production of esterase by neutrophils in the urine can be detected by chemical methods. Positive dipstick tests for nitrite and for leukocyte esterase have satisfactory sensitivity and specificity for diagnosis of UTI **(Table 17.2)**.

While bacteriuria evaluation for bacteriuria, based on microscopic examination of freshly voided urine, shows best combination of sensitivity and specificity in making a presumptive diagnosis, its feasibility in clinical practice is limited. Adding leukocyturia to bacteriuria does not improve diagnostic accuracy. The combination of dipstick-based nitrite and leukocyte esterase provides satisfactory diagnostic accuracy and it is easy to perform bedside. Hence, recent guidelines suggest using urine dipstick test for making a presumptive diagnosis of UTI and for initiating empirical antibiotic therapy.

TABLE 17.2: Sensitivity and specificity of urinalysis

Test	*Sensitivity, % (95% CI)*	*Specificity, % (95% CI)*
Leukocyte esterase test positive	79 (72–84)	90 (86–94)
Nitrite test positive	47 (40–54)	98 (98–99)
Leukocyte esterase or nitrite test positive	84 (80–88)	88 (81–93)
Leukocyte esterase and nitrite test positive	64 (42–82)	98 (95–99)
Leukocyturia on microscopy	76 (68–83)	90 (85–94)
Bacteriuria on microscopy	86 (78–91)	94 (89–97)
Leukocyturia and bacteriuria	89 (75–96)	83 (64–93)

Source: Hari P, et al. 2024

Urine Culture

Definitions of positive or negative cultures are dependent on the method of urine collection. Specific threshold for significant bacterial growth in urine culture is to differentiate between true infection and contamination by periurethral flora. In urine specimens collected by suprapubic aspiration, risk of contamination is lowest hence any bacterial growth (equivalent to colony count of 10^3/mL) is considered significant and evidence of true UTI. For catheterized specimen, growth of $\geq 10^4$ colony-forming unit is considered significant. Traditionally, a colony count of $>10^5$/mL organisms of a single species of bacteria isolated in a midstream clean catch urine sample is considered significant bacteriuria. Infants have smaller bladder capacity and void frequently and may show lower colony counts. This concept is also supported by some studies which suggest that taking a specific cutoff of 10^5 colony-forming unit may miss true UTI in almost 10–25% children. Hence for urine specimen collected by midstream clean catch, a colony count of 10^{4-5}/mL can be considered significant growth in appropriate clinical context.

The diagnosis of UTI is confirmed in the presence of both significant bacterial growth on culture and symptoms of UTI. Leukocyturia is not mandatory for diagnosis of UTI as it can be observed in other conditions such as febrile illness and acute glomerulonephritis. A considerable proportion of children may have UTI with leukocyturia.

The colony counts may be low if urine is very dilute or antibiotic therapy has been started.

Laboratory Investigations

Blood culture should be done in neonates and infants. Acute pyelonephritis is suggested by neutrophilic leukocytosis and raised levels of inflammatory markers [erythrocyte sedimentation rate (ESR), C-reactive protein (CRP), and procalcitonin]. Other abnormalities such as presence of antibody-coated bacteria in urine and increased levels of lactic dehydrogenase isoenzyme V have been used to diagnose pyelonephritis but are of little utility.

Treatment

The diagnosis of UTI is suspected based on clinical evaluation and urine dipstick or microscopy. Antibiotic therapy should be initiated promptly (within 48–72 hr of onset of fever) to prevent kidney scarring. An appropriate empirical antibiotic should be started after obtaining sample for urine culture. The choice of initial antibiotic is based on local antibiotic susceptibility pattern of the uropathogens. Other factors which can influence the choice of initial antibiotics are age at presentation, severity of illness, and localization of infection (acute pyelonephritis vs. cystitis).

A third-generation cephalosporin (cefotaxime or ceftriaxone) is administered parenterally **(Table 17.3)**. Preferred oral agents include

TABLE 17.3: Antibiotics for treatment and prophylaxis of urinary tract infections (UTI)*

Medication	*Dose (mg/kg/day)*	*Remarks*
Oral		
Amoxicillin, co-amoxiclav	30–50, in 2–3 divided doses	Choice for uncomplicated UTI; risk of resistance
Cephalexin Cefadroxil	30–50, in 3 divided doses 30–40, in 2 divided doses	Uncomplicated UTI, not effective against *Proteus* spp.
Cefixime	10, in 2 divided doses	Broad-spectrum agent
Ciprofloxacin	10–20, in 2 divided doses	*Avoid:* <3 months and G6PD deficiency; risk of seizures
Parenteral		
Gentamicin Amikacin	5–6, in 1–2 divided doses 10–15, in 1–2 divided doses	Once daily dosing is effective
Cefotaxime Ceftriaxone	100, in 2–3 divided doses 75–100, in 1–2 divided doses	Safe and convenient as single medication
Prophylaxis		
Cotrimoxazole, trimethoprim	1–2, of trimethoprim	Fluid intake; avoid in infants <6 weeks and G6PD deficiency
Nitrofurantoin	1–2	GI upset; avoid in G6PD deficiency, infants <3 months, renal dysfunction; resistance rare
Cephalexin Cefadroxil Cefaclor	10 3–5 5–10	Used in young infants when use of nitrofurantoin and cotrimoxazole is restricted

*Dosage of drugs requires adjustment in renal failure
G6PD: glucose-6-phosphate dehydrogenase; GI: gastrointestinal

co-amoxiclav, cefixime, and cefaclor. Emerging resistance of *E. coli* to ampicillin and cotrimoxazole has rendered them less effective. Cephalexin has no activity against *P. vulgaris* and *Pseudomonas*. Norfloxacin and ciprofloxacin are broad-spectrum fluoroquinolones that are active against *E. coli, K. pneumoniae, P. mirabilis,* and *Pseudomonas aeruginosa*. They are not used as first-line agents and reserved for serious infections. Since nalidixic acid and nitrofurantoin are excreted in the urine without achieving therapeutic systemic concentrations in renal parenchyma, they should not be used to treat febrile children, where pyelonephritis cannot be excluded.

Usually, a single antimicrobial should be used in community-acquired infections and combinations are reserved for sick patients. For adolescents with cystitis, first-generation cephalosporins or co-amoxiclav can be used as initial empirical antibiotic therapy. Therapy with oral antibiotics has been found to be as effective as parenteral antibiotics in treatment of UTI. Hence, all patients with symptomatic UTI can be managed with oral antibiotic except patients with septicemia, poor oral intake, and infant age <2 months. Even in these patients, oral antibiotics may be administered after 48–72 hr of parenteral therapy once the patient is less toxic and can accept orally.

Most patients with UTI show clinical resolution of symptoms in 48–72 hr. Unsatisfactory response raises the suspicion of antimicrobial resistance or complication such as pyonephrosis. If the expected clinical response does not occur with 2 days of antimicrobial therapy, another urine specimen should be cultured, and ultrasonography performed to exclude complicating factors. Antibiotic treatment can be modified based on bacterial sensitivity if clinical response is unsatisfactory. However, it is not mandatory to change the antibiotic after culture sensitivity report as there is a considerable discordance between in vivo clinical response and in vitro susceptibility pattern.

Duration of Treatment

The duration of therapy is 7–10 days for children with symptomatic UTI. There is insufficient evidence for benefit of short (<5 days) course of antibiotics for treatment of acute pyelonephritis, and children are more likely to eliminate bacteria with the 7–10 days course. Older children and adolescents, where diagnosis of cystitis can be established, may be treated with shorter duration of antibiotics, lasting 3–5 days.

General Measures and Urinary Tract Infection Surveillance

General measures consist of increasing fluid intake, regular bowel habits with avoidance of constipation, and complete bladder emptying. The wiping action in girls should be in an anterior to posterior direction to avoid periurethral soiling with fecal matter. The child should not delay emptying the bladder. Urgency, wetting of pants, holding maneuvers, hesitancy, and frequency suggest bladder bowel dysfunction, which should be managed appropriately.

Parents should be explained about UTI, proper collection of urine samples, and general measures in the management. The importance of compliance with therapy and follow-up visits should be emphasized. Urine should be promptly examined if there are symptoms suggestive of UTI or unexplained fever in young children or those with risk factors. Children with VUR and history of UTI in past are considered to be at risk of UTI. All patients with one or more episodes of UTI with fever should have appropriate imaging studies to detect abnormalities of the kidney and urinary tract.

Imaging Studies

Approximately one-third of children presenting with symptomatic UTI have underlying abnormalities of kidney and urinary tract, hence traditionally it was considered necessary to perform detailed imaging studies. Ultrasonography, dimercaptosuccinic acid (DMSA) scan, and micturating cystourethrography (MCU) are the imaging modalities most commonly employed.

Ultrasonography

Ultrasonography is not associated with radiation exposure, but is operator dependent. The anatomy of the kidneys and urinary tract is examined. Kidney size and pelvic diameters are measured and calyceal and ureteral dilatation noted. Kidney, ureteric or bladder calculi can be diagnosed. Ultrasonography has mostly replaced plain X-ray of abdomen for diagnosis of urolithiasis. A high postvoid residue (>20 mL in children aged 4–6 years; >10 mL in those >7 years) suggests BBD. Similarly, increased bladder wall thickness in an adequately filled bladder also suggests BBD. Experienced radiologists can also help to diagnose constipation based on the transverse rectal diameter. While ultrasonography may not diagnose all abnormalities, it does provide important clues. Hence, it should be performed in all children following a UTI.

Micturating Cystourethrogram

Micturating cystourethrogram is useful for delineating the anatomy of urinary tract. Following urethral catheterization, the contrast medium is filled in the bladder, and images obtained during bladder filling and voiding. Since the procedure requires catheterization, there is increased risk of UTI if aseptic precautions are not followed. Some centers recommend the use of antibiotic prophylaxis to minimize the risk. Oral amoxicillin (one dose 1 hour before MCU, and second dose 6 hr later) can be used. MCU can be performed any time following treatment of the episode of UTI.

While MCU is associated with discomfort and radiation exposure, it is the gold standard for detecting and grading VUR. MCU also provides information on filling and emptying of bladder and presence of residual urine.

Intravenous Pyelography

Intravenous pyelography (IVP) provides sharp anatomic details (duplex kidneys; abnormalities at pelviureteric junction) and is a satisfactory indicator of kidney function. However, it involves high dose of radiation and hazards of the contrast agent, and is rarely used in the current era.

Direct Radionuclide Cystourethrogram

A radionuclide dye is introduced into the bladder. While the procedure is adequate for detecting VUR, it does not provide its detailed grading. Since it exposes the patient to less radiation, it can be employed for follow-up studies in patients with VUR.

Dimercaptosuccinic Acid Scan

Dimercaptosuccinic acid scan is the gold standard for diagnosis of parenchymal kidney scarring. DMSA scanning also detects acute pyelonephritis, when decreased areas of tracer uptake are seen without distortion of normal kidney outline. Hence, it is recommended that DMSA scan should be performed 4–6 months following the episode of UTI to detect permanent kidney scarring. Due to poor diagnostic accuracy in detecting high-grade VUR, acute phase DMSA scan is not useful. It also does not assist in decision making for acute management of UTI.

Urologic Evaluation Following Urinary Tract Infection

Primary VUR and BBD are the two most common abnormalities associated with recurrence of UTI. Existing interventions for VUR have limited efficacy in preventing recurrent UTI and do not reduce the risk of kidney scarring. Considering the balance of exposing every child to radiation and with limited interventions to change the outcomes, most guidelines recommend less aggressive and restrictive imaging following UTI in children **(Flowchart 17.1)**. The current approach is, therefore, focused on detecting high-grade VUR and kidney scarring in specific subgroups.

All children with recurrent UTI should be evaluated with an MCU study and DMSA scintigraphy irrespective of ultrasonography findings. In children with single episode of UTI, MCU is considered only if ultrasonography shows abnormalities. Recent studies suggest that children in whom UTI is caused by uropathogens other *E. coli* have high likelihood of underlying high-grade VUR. Hence, the MCU may also be considered in children <2 years old with

Flowchart 17.1: Evaluation following urinary tract infection (UTI). DMSA: dimercaptosuccinic acid scan; MCU: micturating cystourethrogram; USG: ultrasonography; VUR: vesicoureteric reflux

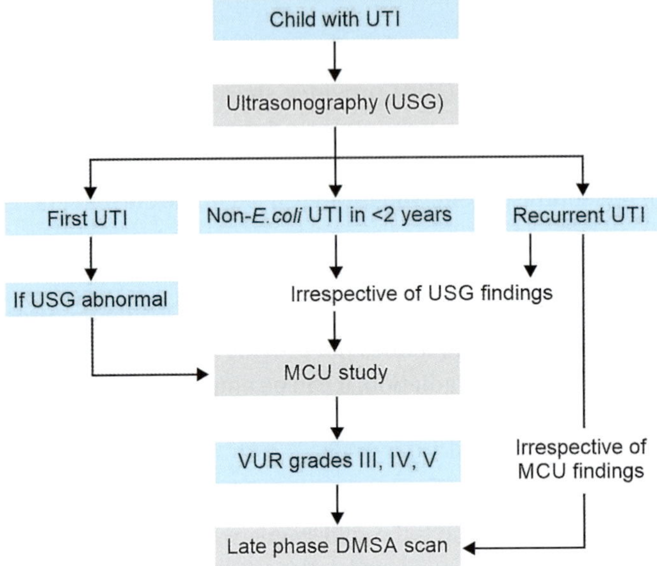

non-*E. coli* UTI. Since the risk of recurrent UTI and acquired kidney scars is more with high-grade VUR, late DMSA scans should perhaps be limited to children with recurrent UTI and high-grade VUR. This less aggressive evaluation avoids unnecessary radiation exposure to many patients, while detecting kidney scarring where it is essential.

Asymptomatic Bacteriuria

Asymptomatic bacteriuria refers to the presence of significant bacteriuria on repeated examination without symptoms of UTI. Its frequency is about 0.5% in girls and 0.37% in boys aged <19 years. Failure to thrive, abdominal pain, fever, and abnormal micturition are absent. Lack of symptoms and normal blood levels of C-reactive protein support the benign nature of asymptomatic bacteriuria. Up to half of the children with asymptomatic bacteriuria can have leukocyturia. The causative organisms, mostly *E. coli,* are of low virulence and lack the characteristics of invasive strains that cause pyelonephritis. It is proposed that these organisms prevent colonization by virulent strains. Unnecessary use of antibiotics in asymptomatic patients may lead to clearance of these organisms with low virulence and superinfection with virulent bacteria.

Asymptomatic bacteriuria should not be treated except in pregnancy and patients who are planned for invasive instrumentation in urinary tract. There is no evidence to support the treatment of asymptomatic bacteriuria in children with abnormal urinary tract or those with immunodeficiency. Bacteriuria may persist for few months, but tends to resolve with time.

Risk Factors and Prevention of Urinary Tract Infection

Identification of risk factors that predispose to kidney scarring and progressive renal deterioration is important especially in children below the age of 1 year.

Genital Hygiene

It is important to encourage proper hygiene and voiding habits, especially in girls. General measures for prevention of UTI include a liberal fluid intake, regular and complete bladder emptying.

Bladder Bowel Dysfunction and Recurrent Urinary Tract Infection

Bladder bowel dysfunction is characterized by lower urinary tract symptoms accompanied by constipation or encopresis. It is an important risk factor for recurrence of UTI with or without VUR. Initial diagnosis of BBD is based on clinical evaluation, and voiding diary. Patients should be asked about history of lower urinary tract symptoms such as incontinence, urgency, hesitancy, frequency, voiding postponement, and voiding posture. Validated questionnaire tools such as dysfunctional voiding symptom score (DVSS) aid in diagnosis of BBD. Rome IV criteria and Bristol Stool Form Scale can be used for diagnosis of constipation. Imaging modalities such abdomen X-ray and ultrasonography can be used to diagnose BBD in non-toilet trained children. Invasive methods such urodynamic studies are usually reserved for children not responding to initial treatment or in those with suspected neurological defects.

It is suggested that all children with UTI should be evaluated for BBD and managed appropriately with urotherapy. Studies have shown that risk of recurrence of UTI can be reduced significantly following optimal management of BBD. Urotherapy includes adequate hydration, frequent voiding, double voiding, adequate toilet training, and treatment of constipation with laxatives. Pharmacotherapy such as oxybutynin, mirabegron, or tamsulosin may be used in children not responding to 4–6 months of urotherapy.

Foreskin and Urinary Tract Infection

Several epidemiological studies have found a significant association between an intact foreskin and UTI, especially in infants. Evidence suggests that circumcision significantly reduces the risk of recurrent UTI. In children at high risk of UTI, the benefits outweigh the risk associated with the surgery. Hence, circumcision may be considered for preventing UTI in infants with high-grade VUR and recurrent UTI.

Screening for VUR and Urinary Tract Abnormalities

Antenatal ultrasonography allows detection of various underlying renal anomalies. These require prompt investigations and appropriate management. Screening of children at high risk of VUR (siblings of patients with reflux), patients with renal anomalies (duplex collecting system, renal ectopia, multicystic kidney, and horseshoe kidney), and UTI surveillance will facilitate management of UTI.

VESICOURETERIC REFLUX (VUR)

VUR is the retrograde passage of urine into the upper urinary tract during detrusor contraction during micturition. Normally, the long submucosal and intravesical segment of the ureter at the vesicoureteric junction acts as an effective valve mechanism, which closes when the bladder contracts, preventing the return of bladder urine into the ureter. Incompetence of the vesicoureteric junction due to shortening and a lack of obliquity of the submucosal and intravesical segments results in VUR **(Fig. 17.2)**.

In VUR, retrograde flow of urine from the ureter into papillary collecting ducts and renal tubules can occur. Intrarenal reflux provides a mechanism whereby pathogenic organisms that might be present in the bladder gain access to kidney parenchyma and initiate inflammation and scarring.

There is a strong inheritance pattern for primary VUR. The risk of a sibling of a child with VUR having reflux is about 25–30%. If one of the parents had VUR, there is 25–50% increased risk of reflux in offspring. A genetic basis for VUR is evident from its familial clustering in predominantly autosomal dominant, but also autosomal recessive, X-linked, and polygenic patterns. VUR associated with developmental malformations of other organs such as eye, ear, and face is termed *syndromic VUR*. Several genes have been identified for this form of VUR. Candidate genes associated with primary nonsyndromic VUR include *ROBO2, SOX17, RET, PAX2, SLIT2, UPK3A*, and

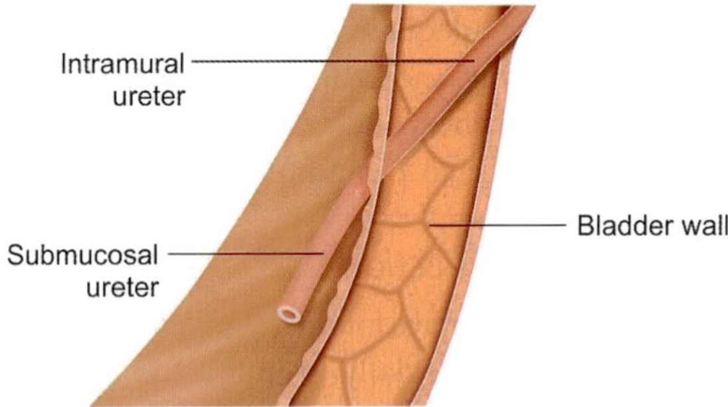

Fig. 17.2: Normal ureterovesical junctions. Refluxing ureterovesical junction has same anatomic features as nonrefluxing orifice, except for inadequate length of intravesical submucosal ureter. The orifice may be situated more medially and caudally. Some orifices with borderline submucosal tunnels reflux intermittently

AGTR2. VUR may occur in association with other abnormalities, such as megacystis megaureter, duplex systems, posterior urethral valve and ectopic ureters, and an acquired defect in neuropathic bladder (secondary VUR).

The precise population prevalence of VUR is not known, and ranges from ~1 to 10%. About 20–30% of children and 40–50% of neonates with UTI have VUR. About 20–30% children with UTI and VUR develop renal scarring, of which 5–10% show progressive kidney failure. Gross VUR during infancy is mostly seen in boys and is usually bilateral. In older children, girls are often affected and have milder grades of VUR.

Intrarenal Reflux

Reflux of urine from the calyces into parenchyma (termed intrarenal reflux) does not occur at every papilla. Papillae situated at the poles of the kidney are fused together as compound structures and present a flat or concave surface to the calyx. Their papillary ducts have wide orifices opening directly to the area cribrosa and allow free reflux. Other papillae, usually situated at the mid-zone of the kidney, are simple conical structures. In these papillae, the papillary ducts have slit-like orifices, which close when the pelvic pressure rises so that reflux does not occur. These observations explain the chiefly polar distribution of wedge-shaped reflux scarring that is demarcated from adjacent unscarred parenchyma. The calyceal clubbing that accompanies reflux-associated scars is a result of papillary distortion and retraction following scar contraction.

About 30% children have only nonrefluxing papillae and are probably protected from intrarenal reflux and scarring even with repeated UTI. The intramural ureteric length is 0.5 cm in the neonate, which increases to 1.3 cm in the adult. The elongation of the tunnel along with an increase in bladder wall muscle and adrenergic tone are chiefly responsible for spontaneous resolution of VUR.

VUR and Kidney Scarring

Along with intrarenal reflux, bacterial virulence and the host inflammatory response influence the scarring process. Patients with secondary severe VUR (e.g., in posterior urethral obstruction, neurogenic bladder) without urinary infection have experimentally been shown to produce kidney scarring and may be important in neonates and infants. However, in setting of primary VUR, most reflux-associated acquired kidney scarring is the result of parenchymal infection introduced by intrarenal reflux. Recent evidence suggests that inflammation plays central role in developing kidney scarring in children with acute pyelonephritis. Incidence of developing new kidney scarring following an episode of febrile UTI is almost 10–15%. *Recurrent UTI, high-grade VUR, and delay in initiation of antimicrobial therapy are important risk factors for kidney scarring.* Risk of scarring following UTI increases with number of febrile UTI.

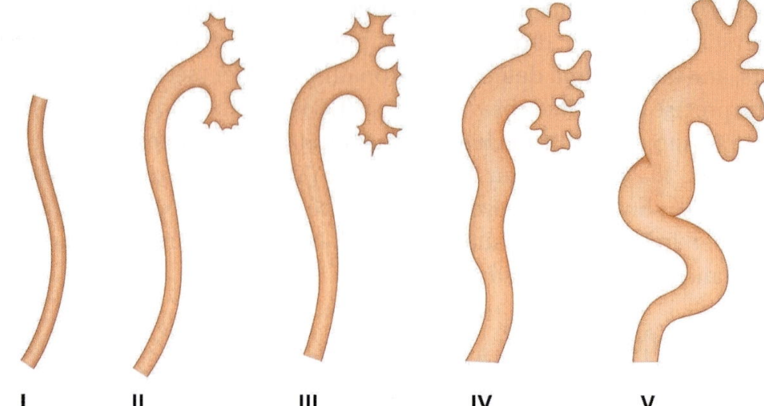

Fig. 17.3: Grading of vesicoureteric reflux on micturating cystourethrogram. Grade I: Reflux into the nondilated distal ureter; grade II: Reflux into the upper collecting system in nondilated ureter; grade III: Reflux into dilated ureter; grade IV: Reflux into grossly dilated ureter; grade V: Massive reflux with ureteral dilation and tortuosity and effacement of calyceal details

VUR and Hypodysplasia

Antenatal ultrasonography often detects hydronephrosis with varying enlargement of kidney in the fetus. In about 10–20% of boys with severe VUR (grade IV–V), the kidneys are small with smooth outline, without history of UTI. Such kidneys probably represent renal maldevelopment occurring *in utero* and show histological evidence of dysplasia. Severe grades of VUR and renal dysplasia are uncommon in girls. Patients with primary VUR and hypodysplasia progress to chronic kidney disease (CKD), rather those with acquired kidney scarring following UTI.

Diagnosis

VUR is diagnosed and graded on a radiocontrast MCU. A standard reflux grading system is widely used **(Fig. 17.3)**. Mild-to-moderate grades (I–III) include increasing severity of reflux without calyceal blunting; in severe (IV–V) VUR, there are marked dilatation and tortuosity of ureter, gross dilatation of calyces, and intrarenal reflux **(Fig. 17.4)**. Direct radionuclide cystography (DRCG), that is more sensitive and has less radiation exposure than MCU, is preferred for follow-up evaluation.

Bladder Bowel Dysfunction and VUR

Voiding dysfunction is present in a large proportion of children with higher grades of VUR that persist beyond the age of 2–3 years. Detrusor sphincter dyssynergia, unstable bladder, and discoordinated bladder have

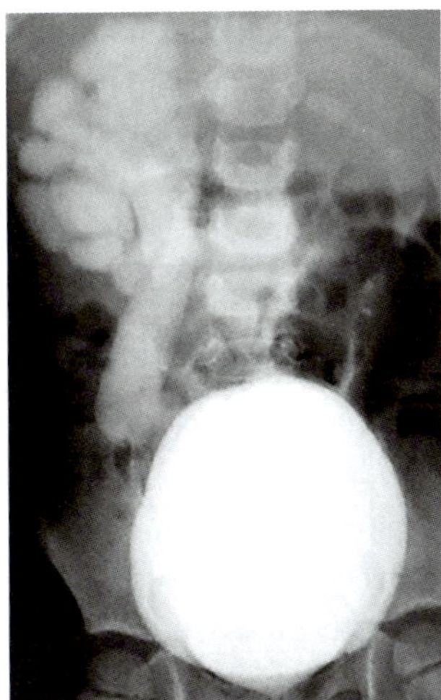

Fig. 17.4: Micturating cystourethrogram showing dilation of pelvicalyceal system and ureter on right side, indicating grade V vesicoureteric reflux

been observed in such cases (Chapter 19). Such abnormalities should be appropriately managed especially if surgical correction chemically coated paper strips is being considered.

Familial VUR

Siblings of children with VUR, especially those below 36 months old, are investigated for reflux. If ultrasonographic evaluation shows dilated pelvicalyceal system, DRCG or MCU is considered.

Spontaneous Resolution of VUR

Primary VUR tends to resolve by the age of 6–10 years. Grades I–III VUR are more likely to disappear than grades IV–V, resolution rates being 70–90% and 10–35%, respectively. The higher the grade of VUR, the longer it takes to resolve. Data from a large study suggests that median time to resolution was 38, 98, and 156 months in grades I–II, III, and IV–V VUR, respectively. Therefore, persistence of VUR beyond 12–18 months should not invariably be regarded as an indication for surgical correction. VUR occurring at all levels of intravesical pressure is less likely to resolve than that seen only at peak pressures.

Management

The management of VUR remains controversial. Evidence for improvement in long-term outcome from treating VUR is limited, and reflux may be self-limiting in considerable proportion of the patients. Most of the kidney parenchyma damage progressing to kidney failure is likely to be due to congenital dysplasia, and is not amenable to current treatment strategies.

The objective of treatment is to prevent recurrence of UTI and kidney scarring from pyelonephritis. Treatment options include antibiotic prophylaxis with close surveillance for UTI, surgical reimplantation, and submucosal endoscopic injection of *Deflux*. Parental preference should be given consideration while deciding therapy.

Antibiotic prophylaxis, while awaiting spontaneous resolution of VUR, is the first choice in most children. Such treatment prevents bacterial colonization, chiefly by *Enterobacteriaceae,* at the urethral orifice thus reduces the incidence of ascending infection. While antibiotic prophylaxis has been shown to reduce the risk of recurrent febrile UTI, it does not prevent kidney scarring and is associated with increased risk of antimicrobial resistance. Pooled data from clinical trials has shown that antibiotic prophylaxis is not effective in children with recurrent UTI without VUR, and in those with low-grade VUR. Antibiotic prophylaxis should, therefore, be used judiciously in specific groups of children.

Guidelines for management of VUR by the Indian Society of Pediatric Nephrology are outlined in **Table 17.4**. Patients with high-grade VUR and those with BBD should initially receive antibiotic prophylaxis, while awaiting spontaneous resolution of VUR. Close surveillance for UTI is necessary. Antibiotic prophylaxis may be stopped if the patient is toilet-trained, there is no recurrence of UTI in last 1 year, and BBD is optimally managed. Associated BBD should be treated, as it may interfere with resolution of VUR. Surgical treatment is considered for patients with grades III–V reflux if there are recurrent breakthrough febrile UTIs.

The antibiotic used should be effective against coliform bacteria and achieve a high urinary concentration with minimal alteration of bowel flora. The preferred agents are nitrofurantoin and cotrimoxazole **(Table 17.3)**, given as a single bedtime dose. Trimethoprim alone is as effective as cotrimoxazole. Breakthrough UTI may result from noncompliance or

TABLE 17.4: Management of vesicoureteric reflux (VUR)

Strategy	*Indications*
Antibiotic prophylaxis	*Recommended:* High-grade VUR, recurrent UTI in patients with BBD irrespective of VUR severity *Consider*: Infants with low-grade VUR
Surgical reimplantation	Recurrent febrile UTI despite antibiotic prophylaxis and optimal management of BBD
Circumcision	Option for children with high-grade VUR and recurrent UTI

BBD: bladder bowel dysfunction; UTI: urinary tract infection

development of bacterial resistance, mainly to trimethoprim. Nitrofurantoin may cause nausea and vomiting that may result in discontinuation of therapy in a proportion of patients. Cephalexin or cefixime is preferred in young infants and those with deficiency of the enzyme, glucose-6-phosphate-dehydrogenase. Amoxicillin and quinolones are unsuitable for prophylaxis because intestinal colonization with *E. coli* resistant to these agents develops rapidly. Reinfection of the urinary tract with resistant bacteria may then occur. Breakthrough UTI should be promptly treated.

The child is trained to void again a few minutes after initial bladder evacuation (double voiding), so that the refluxed urine entering the bladder is expelled. Regular timed voiding, every 4–5 hr, is advised. Compliance with long-term therapy is crucial.

Surgical Treatment

Ureteric reimplantation or endoscopic submucosal injection of Deflux is considered for patients with recurrent breakthrough UTI and grade IV–V VUR. Surgery should be delayed until 2–3 years of age since the chances of spontaneous resolution are significant, and reimplantation of a dilated ureter into the small bladder of an infant is technically challenging. Surgery is also advised in patients with: (*i*) noncompliance with medical management; and (*ii*) parental preference for surgery. Ureteric reimplantation procedures suggested by Lich-Gregoir, Politano-Leadbetter, and Cohen have been used with success rates of over 95%.

Endoscopic injection of dextranomer/hyaluronic acid copolymer (Deflux) beneath the intramural segment of ureter has increasingly been used to prevent VUR. The success of this technique depends upon the grade of reflux, absence of bladder dysfunction, mound configuration, and surgical expertise. Although success rates of 60–90% are reported, recurrence of VUR may occur in a significant proportion. The results are less satisfactory with higher grades of reflux, duplex collecting system, and in patients with dysfunctional voiding or neuropathic bladder.

Bladder function is evaluated by urodynamic studies before surgery. High-pressure bladder is appropriately managed. Chemoprophylaxis is continued for 6 months after surgery. MCU/DRCG to document resolution of reflux can be done 3–6 months after surgery. Since obstruction may develop at the vesicoureteric junction (and rarely at pelviureteric junction), ultrasonography is performed on follow-up annually for 5 years.

Subsequent Monitoring

Urine cultures are not necessary in asymptomatic patients. Asymptomatic bacteriuria is not treated. Patients with UTI with symptoms should be promptly managed. Blood pressure, height, weight, proteinuria, and serum creatinine level are recorded every 6–12 months. Voiding cystography (DRCG or MCU) may be performed 3–5 years after the initial diagnosis to document resolution of reflux **(Figs. 17.5A to C)**. Ultrasonography (USG) can be done every year to monitor renal growth and cortical scarring. Follow-up DMSA scans are limited to children having breakthrough UTI.

Reflux Nephropathy

Reflux nephropathy is the term used to describe kidney scarring associated with primary VUR. The lesions are asymmetric and involve one or both kidneys. They are wedge-shaped with cortical thinning and dilatation and distortion of the underlying calyces; intervening areas are normal and show compensatory hypertrophy. The scars result from passage of infected urine into the renal parenchyma through intrarenal reflux. However, high-pressure sterile VUR, as in posterior urethral obstruction and neurogenic bladder, may occasionally cause renal scarring. Extravasation of infected urine into interstitium leads to periductal fibrosis and destruction of microvasculature. Scarring is usually sublobar in distribution and results from injury and disruption of single collecting duct that subtends several thousand nephrons. The kidneys are small with segmental atrophic areas, with loss of all parenchymal elements **(Fig. 17.6)**. The incidence of scarring is related to the severity of VUR; 85% patients with grade V VUR have renal scars.

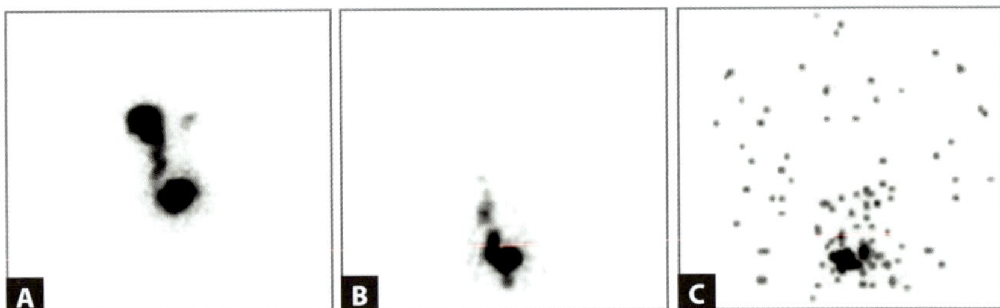

Figs. 17.5A to C: Sequential radionuclide cystography in a boy with right vesicoureteric reflux. Note the significant reflux with dilated ureter and pelvis (A), which has reduced on repeat studies done after 12 months (B) and 36 months (C)

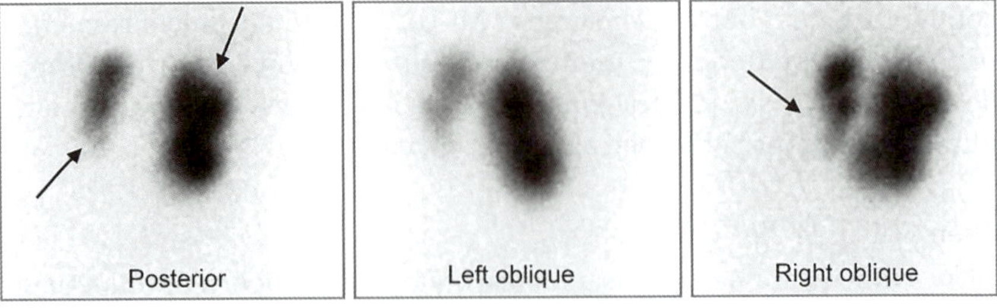

Fig. 17.6: Dimercaptosuccinic acid scan showing irregular renal outlines (arrows) suggestive of renal scarring in both kidneys

Clinical Features

Clinical features associated with reflux nephropathy include pyelonephritis, hypertension, and progressive loss of kidney function. In late stages, renal tubular acidosis, hyperkalemia, anemia, and mineral bone disease develop. Persistent VUR and UTI may lead to complications during pregnancy. The risk of CKD and hypertension in children with renal scarring is variable and depends on the severity of scarring. Such consequences are more common when VUR is accompanied by congenital hypodysplasia.

Course

In patients with severe kidney scarring, damage may continue to increase even after VUR has disappeared (by surgical treatment or spontaneously). Hyperfiltration glomerular injury and immune mechanisms may be involved in the pathogenesis. Appearance of albuminuria indicates glomerular injury, characterized by focal segmental glomerulosclerosis.

Reflux Nephropathy and Pregnancy

Reflux nephropathy may not be uncommon in women of childbearing age. Pregnancy-related complications are higher in women with reflux nephropathy. It is frequently associated with UTI and hypertension, and an increased rate of fetal loss. A majority of acute episodes of pyelonephritis occur in patients in whom VUR is still present at the time of conception, whereas upper UTI rarely occurs if VUR has been corrected. The presence of hypertension (associated with impaired renal function) adversely affects fetal outcome.

Management

Administration of angiotensin-converting enzyme (ACE) inhibitors is effective in maintenance of normal blood pressure and reduction of proteinuria, thereby retarding the progression of renal injury. There is no role of surgical repair of VUR in patients with reflux nephropathy and advanced kidney dysfunction, as this intervention does not improve long-term outcomes in these patients.

FUNGAL INFECTIONS

Fungal UTIs are commonly encountered in infants and children who receive immunosuppressive agents and broad-spectrum antibiotic therapy and when IV lines or bladder catheters are kept in situ for prolonged periods. The incidence is particularly high in intensive care units. Lower tract fungal UTIs are caused by the ascending route whereas renal involvement may, in addition, take place by disseminated hematogenous infection. Fungal accretion or bezoar formation may occur and cause obstruction and occasionally acute kidney injury. The possibility of fungal UTI should be considered whenever predisposing factors are present. The most common organism is *Candida albicans*; other *Candida* species and rarely *Aspergillus* or *Cryptococcus* may be isolated.

Persistent fever is a common clinical feature. Fungal UTI is indicated by the presence of pseudohyphae in the urinary sediment. Special stains, e.g., Grotto's methenamine silver, should be used. Candiduria can be consequence of candidemia or represent a fungal UTI. Differentiation of contamination from true infection is challenging. If candiduria is detected, it is confirmed on a repeat culture obtained by a clean-catch mid-stream specimen, or by bladder catheterization. An indwelling bladder catheter is often heavily colonized. Ultrasonography and other imaging studies may be necessary to detect upper tract involvement.

Bladder catheters should be removed since eradication of fungus in presence of catheters and stents is difficult. If systemic features are absent and fungal cultures from other body fluids are negative, bladder irrigation with amphotericin B may be sufficient. Oral fluconazole is useful in the treatment of *Candida* cystitis. With features of upper tract involvement, therapy with IV amphotericin B (0.7–1 mg/kg) or fluconazole (5–10 mg/kg) for up to 3 weeks is necessary. Occasionally, the addition of oral flucytosine is required. Surgical measures are required if features of obstruction are present.

RENAL TUBERCULOSIS

Tuberculosis of the kidney and urinary tract is uncommon in children, since such involvement usually takes place 5–15 years after the primary infection. The diagnosis of renal tuberculosis is often delayed. In patients with disseminated tuberculosis, kidneys often show histological abnormalities but mostly there are no symptoms. Renal infection takes place by spread from the primary pulmonary lesion that seeds the cortex. Cortical granuloma can remain dormant for years and then reactivate. Caseating lesions may discharge debris and tubercle bacilli into the renal pelvis, ureter, and bladder where the disease can get established. Healing by fibrosis can lead to strictures. Caseation progresses from the medullary lesions to involve the papilla. The medullary abscess may replace the pyramid or discharge into the draining calyx. The lesions may advance to cause extensive kidney damage. Focal or more diffuse calcification is usual.

Renal tuberculosis can manifest with abdominal pain, flank pain abdominal mass, dysuria, frequency of micturition, and occasionally gross hematuria may be the presenting features. Ureteric colic may occur from passage of clots or debris. Urinalysis shows mild proteinuria, hematuria, and leukocyturia. Sterile acid pyuria is regarded as characteristic of tuberculosis.

Tuberculin test is positive. The finding of acid-fast bacilli on direct smear examination is not reliable, since *Mycobacterium smegmatis* is also acid fast. Tubercle bacilluria may be intermittent and, therefore, 3–5 specimens should be cultured. Urine cultures require 6–8 weeks in LJ medium, and the sensitivity ranges between 80 and 97%. Newer culture methods (BACTEC, MGIT-based) and polymerase chain reaction (PCR) for *M. tuberculosis* may be of diagnostic help. PCR is highly sensitive (96%) and specific (98%). The Xpert MTB/RIF is a cartridge-based nucleic acid amplification test for rapid diagnosis of *Mycobacterium species* in the urine, as well as providing information on rifampicin sensitivity. The lateral flow assay is a rapid diagnostic test that detects the mycobacterial cell wall glycolipid lipoarabinomannan.

Excretory urogram or CT scan shows abnormalities depending upon the extent and pattern of renal involvement. Imaging findings include kidney scarring and calcification, distorted pelvicalyceal system, ureteric strictures, stenosis, outflow obstruction, hydroureteronephrosis, and small capacity bladder. Cystoscopy is rarely indicated for diagnostic purposes.

Genitourinary tuberculosis is a severe form of disease with relatively high bacterial load. Antitubercular therapy is instituted and compliance treatment with ensured. Short-course antituberculous therapy is effective, comprising 2 months' intensive therapy with rifampicin, isoniazid, pyrazinamide, and ethambutol, followed by 4 months continuation phase with rifampicin, isoniazid, and ethambutol. Longer duration of therapy, for 9–12 months, is necessary in case of recurrence of the disease, immunosuppression, and concomitant HIV infection. Most experts recommend 10 years follow-up after pharmacologic treatment because of the risk of late relapse.

BIBLIOGRAPHY

Urinary Tract Infection

1. Al Lawati H, Blair BM, Larnard J. Urinary tract infections: Core curriculum 2024. Am J Kidney Dis. 2024;83:90-100.
2. Hari P, Meena J, Kumar M, et al. Evidence-based clinical practice guideline for management of urinary tract infection and primary vesicoureteric reflux. Pediatr Nephrol. 2024;39:1639-68.
3. Kaufman J, Temple-Smith M, Sanci L. Urinary tract infections in children: an overview of diagnosis and management. BMJ Paediatr Open. 2019;3:e000487.
4. Klein RD, Hultgren SJ. Urinary tract infections: microbial pathogenesis, host-pathogen interactions and new treatment strategies. Nat Rev Microbiol. 2020;18:211-26.
5. Schwartz L, de Dios Ruiz-Rosado J, Stonebrook E, et al. Uropathogen and host responses in pyelonephritis. Nat Rev Nephrol. 2023;19:658-71.
6. Tullus K, Shaikh N. Urinary tract infections in children. Lancet. 2020;395:1659-68.
7. Williams G, Craig JC. Long-term antibiotics for preventing recurrent urinary tract infection in children. Cochrane Database Syst Rev. 2019;4:CD001534.

8. Yang S, Gill PJ, Anwar MR, et al.; Canadian Pediatric Inpatient Research Network. Kidney ultrasonography after first febrile urinary tract infection in children: A systematic review and meta-analysis. JAMA Pediatr. 2023;177:764-73.

Vesicoureteric Reflux

1. Bortnick EM, Nelson CP. Vesicoureteral reflux: Current care trends and future possibilities. Urol Clin North Am. 2023;50:391-402.
2. Cajigas-Loyola SC, Chow JS, Hayatghaibi S, et al. Imaging of vesicoureteral reflux: Expert panel narrative review. Am J Roentgenol; 2024. 1-9.
3. Gnech M, 't Hoen L, Zachou A, et al. Update and summary of the European Association of Urology/European Society of Pediatric Urology Pediatric Guidelines on Vesicoureteral Reflux in Children. Eur Urol. 2024;85:433-44.2
4. Mattoo TK, Mohammad D. Primary vesicoureteral reflux and renal scarring. Pediatr Clin North Am. 2022;69:1115-29.
5. Williams G, Hodson EM, Craig JC. Interventions for primary vesicoureteric reflux. Cochrane Database Syst Rev. 2019;2:CD001532.

Tubercular and Fungal Urinary Tract Infection

1. Bagga A. Genitourinary tuberculosis. In: Lodha R, Kabra SK, Seth V (Eds). Essentials of Tuberculosis in Children, 5th edn. New Delhi: Jaypee Brothers Medical Publisher; 2022. pp. 181-4.
2. Behzadi P, Behzadi E, Ranjbar R. Urinary tract infections and *Candida albicans*. Cent European J Urol. 2015;68:96-101.
3. Kauffman CA. Diagnosis and management of fungal urinary tract infection. Infect Dis Clin North Am. 2014;28:61-74.
4. Muneer A, Macrae B, Krishnamoorthy S, et al. Urogenital tuberculosis: epidemiology, pathogenesis and clinical features. Nat Rev Urol. 2019;16:573-98.

CHAPTER 18

Obstructive Uropathy

M Srinivas

Urinary tract obstruction is defined as restriction to the urinary outflow that if not managed satisfactorily, leads to progressive renal damage. Obstructive uropathy is an important cause of end stage renal disease requiring kidney replacement therapy.

Antenatal ultrasonography (USG) detects hydronephrosis in about 1 in 100 fetuses, the prevalence ranging from 0.6 to 5.4% depending on diagnostic criteria. The condition is bilateral in 17–54% and additional abnormalities are occasionally associated. Hydronephrosis may be secondary to obstruction at various sites, from renal pelvis to the tip of urethra, being most common at pelviureteric junction. The ureter can get obstructed by external compression or kinks at any site along its course in the retroperitoneum. Similarly, the urethra is vulnerable to obstructive pathology at the internal and external meatus. The abnormalities causing obstructive uropathy can be congenital or acquired, the former being more common **(Box 18.1)**.

Pathophysiology

The urinary tract serves as a reservoir as well as conduit for transporting urine produced by the kidneys. Onset and the duration of obstruction correlate with kidney development and thereby kidney function. Obstruction to the flow of urine causes stasis, increased pressure and dilatation of the proximal structures, and an increased risk of infection. Complete reversal of the effects of obstruction can be achieved by early treatment but prolonged obstruction leads to changes that are irreversible or only partially reversible.

BOX 18.1: Causes of obstructive uropathy

Renal calyx: Infundibular stenosis, tuberculosis, calculi
Pelviureteric junction: Congenital obstruction, kinks, bands, adhesions, aberrant vessels
Ureter: Stricture, calculi, primary megaureter, vascular obstruction
Ureterovesical junction: Ureterocele, congenital obstruction
Bladder: Calculi, diverticulum, bladder neck hypertrophy, neurogenic bladder
Anterior urethra: Diverticulum, stricture, valves, polyps
Posterior urethra: Posterior urethral valves, diverticulum, stricture, polyps
Meatus: Meatal stenosis, preputial adhesions, phimosis

Acute obstruction (e.g., from a calculus) produces severe symptoms and may lead to rapid decline in renal function. Obstruction in the urethra, the most distal part of the urinary tract, results in dilatation of the proximal urethra. The bladder, in an attempt to overcome the obstruction, undergoes compensatory hypertrophy, manifesting with thickened bladder wall with trabeculations and sacculations, and hypertrophy of the bladder neck. Intravesical pressure increases, causing decreased emptying of the ureter into the bladder and vesicoureteric reflux. The thickened bladder wall can pinch the intramural portion of the ureter, resulting in obstruction and dilatation of the ureter, hydronephrosis, and thinned renal parenchyma. Stasis of urine in the dilated tract predisposes to infections.

At the cellular level, obstruction causes tubular dilatation and stretch induced apoptosis, resulting in epithelial cell to mesenchymal transformation. Ureteral obstruction also recruits inflammatory cells that release interleukins and chemokines leading to fibroblast proliferation and interstitial fibrosis. The combination of stasis, repeated infections, and high intraluminal pressure causes scarring and progressive chronic kidney disease (CKD), suggested by proteinuria and hypertension that is due to alteration in glomerular hemodynamics and reduced glomerular perfusion/filtration. Unrelieved obstruction results in myogenic failure and exhaustion of ureteric and bladder musculature. Obstructive uropathy during the intrauterine period causes varying degrees of renal dysplasia that can be detected on dimercaptosuccinic acid (DMSA) scintigraphy in the neonatal period. Severe dysplasia may be progressive even after obstruction is relieved.

Clinical Features

A dilated urinary system may be detected on antenatal USG. Infant may present with dribbling or poor stream of urine, pain during micturition, fever, urinary tract infection (UTI), or features suggestive of sepsis. The kidneys and/or the bladder may be palpable.

Investigations

Imaging and radionuclide procedures are necessary to evaluate for obstructive uropathy. These include USG, radiocontrast studies, magnetic resonance (MR) imaging and MR urography, and radionuclide scintigraphy. Cystoscopy can be diagnostic as well therapeutic in some situations [e.g., posterior urethral valve (PUV)]. The indications and role of various imaging modalities are summarized in **Box 18.2**.

The application of routine antenatal USG has advanced the understanding and recognition of obstructive uropathy in early infancy. It allows prompt investigations and appropriate management in the neonatal period. Antenatal hydronephrosis has been defined by measuring anteroposterior diameter of the pelvis at different periods of pregnancy.

BOX 18.2: Modalities for evaluation of obstructive uropathy

Ultrasonography: Urinary tract dilatation, renal cortical thickness, calyceal size, pelvic anteroposterior diameter, ureter dilation, thickness of bladder, mass, calculi
Doppler ultrasound: Renal blood flow, aberrant vessels, resistive index

Radiocontrast studies
Intravenous pyelography: Hydrocalyx, hydronephrosis, calculi, ureterocele
Micturating cystourethrography: Bladder and urethral obstruction, vesicoureteric reflux
Retrograde urethrography: Urethral obstruction
Retrograde, antegrade ureteropyelography: Ureteral and pelviureteric junction obstruction
CT, MRI scans: Complex congenital anomalies, duplex system, poorly functioning kidney

Radionuclide studies
DTPA, LLEC scan: Upper tract function, obstruction, split renal function, GFR assessment
DMSA, MAG3, GHA scan: Renal scarring
Radionuclide cystogram: Vesicoureteric reflux, bladder outlet obstruction
Endoscopy: Direct visualization (e.g., posterior urethral valves), therapy (valves, ureterocoele)

CT: computed tomography; DMSA: dimercaptosuccinic acid; DTPA: diethylenetriamine pentaacetic acid; GFR: glomerular filtration rate; GHA: glucoheptonate; LLEC: L,L-ethylenedicysteine; MAG3: mercaptoacetyltriglycine-3; MRI: magnetic resonance imaging

Although USG detects dilatation, it provides little information about the functional status of the kidney. A radionuclide dynamic renogram [with diethylenetriamine pentaacetic acid (DTPA) or L,L-ethylenedicysteine (LLEC)] is necessary for evaluating obstruction and determining individual kidney function. A glomerular agent provides information about the glomerular filtration rate (GFR) and renal tracer uptake, whereas a glomerular/tubular agent about the renal uptake, split renal function, and pattern of drainage pattern. The intravenous urogram (IVU), although providing superior anatomic details, is carried out if facilities for radionuclide scintigraphy are not available.

CONDITIONS CAUSING OBSTRUCTIVE UROPATHY

Preputial Adhesions, Phimosis, and Meatal Stenosis

At birth, glans penis is covered with prepuce, the meatus is not easily visible, and the prepuce is not retractable, due to normal preputial adhesions that bind preputial skin to glans. Separation of the prepuce occurs due to keratinization of the subpreputial epithelium. Ballooning of prepuce occurs during micturition, which is responsible for normal developmental process of separating prepuce from the glans. At the end of first year of life, retraction of the foreskin behind the glandular sulcus is possible in about 50% and in 90% by 3 years. If there is a delay in this process and the child has difficulty or pain during micturition, release of preputial adhesions is indicated. True phimosis is uncommon and occurs from scarring due to recurrent balanoposthitis. It is rarely diagnosed in children below the age of 3 years unless prepucial scarring is present. Congenital preputial adhesions and true phimosis predispose to smegma collection, which may cause recurrent balanoposthitis. If physiological phimosis does not resolve by 3 years or the child has dysuria, preputial dilatation and release of preputial adhesions are carried out.

True phimosis causes the prepuce to balloon up with the child straining during micturition, which results in back pressure effects on the bladder and upper tract. In such cases circumcision may be indicated. Some experts recommend making a dorsal slit in the prepuce with preputioplasty.

Meatal stenosis can result in urinary tract obstruction. The usual causes are inappropriate instrumentation and ammoniacal meatitis in circumcised boys. Children with myelomeningocele and paraplegia with anesthesia in saddle area are particularly at risk. Congenital meatal stenosis is rare, but boys with hypospadias may have a stenosed meatus. Ritual circumcision by untrained personnel may also be complicated by meatal stenosis. The symptoms include thin urine stream, straining at micturition, frequency, and dysuria. Urethritis and UTI may occur and stone formation may be seen. Urethra proximal to stenosis is dilated and the effects of back pressure may rarely extend to the bladder and upper tracts. The treatment consists of regular meatal dilatation, which can be explained to the parents for carrying out at home. If it fails, meatotomy or meatoplasty is performed.

Anterior Urethral Diverticulum

These are encountered on the ventral aspect of the anterior urethra as a fluctuant ventral penile swelling. The abnormality is caused by a weakness of the corpus spongiosum, which allows the affected segment of the urethra to form a diverticulum **(Fig. 18.1)**. Although both the proximal and distal lips of the diverticulum consist of attenuated tissue, the distal lip acts like a flap valve when it is full and causes obstruction. The diverticulum may be wide or narrow mouthed, with more complications with the latter.

Patients present with dribbling of urine but there may be dysuria, straining, thin stream, recurrent UTIs, and a swelling in the perineum, which becomes prominent when the child attempts to void. Pressure on the diverticulum may increase the urine flow and improve the stream by preventing valvar action of the distal lip. Multiple calculi may form in the diverticulum. The diagnosis is confirmed by retrograde urethrography. There are three ways to treat anterior urethral diverticulum: (*i*) Endoscopic division of the distal lip, (*ii*) excision of the diverticulum with multilayered urethroplasty and

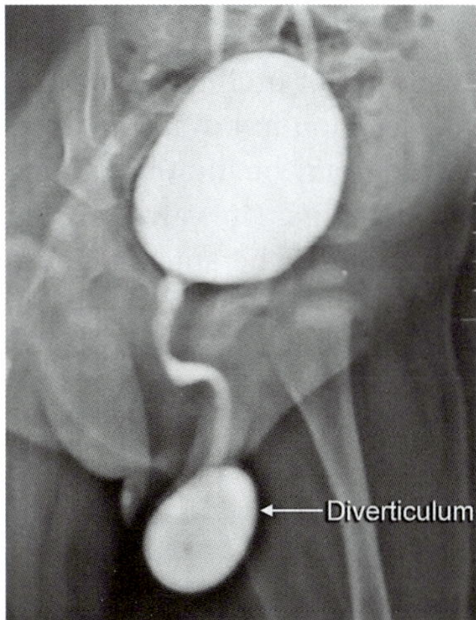

Fig. 18.1: Anterior urethral diverticulum. Micturating cystourethrogram shows saccular outpouching from the ventral aspect of the bulbar urethra

(*iii*) marsupialization with staged repair. Large diverticuli require multilayered urethroplasty.

Urethral Strictures

Strictures of the urethra can be congenital or acquired. They can be situated anteriorly or posteriorly and the narrow segment may be long or short. Congenital strictures are not common, seen almost always in boys and usually located in the membranous urethra. They present with dribbling of urine or thin urinary stream associated with straining, palpable bladder, and sometimes palpable kidneys. There may be an inability to catheterize the bladder. The level and the length of stricture can be examined by a retrograde urethrogram and micturating cystourethrogram (MCU) **(Fig. 18.2)**.

The MCU shows features similar to those found in PUVs. The diagnosis is confirmed by cystoscopy during which internal urethrotomy can be performed using laser or diathermy. This is done using a resectoscope by incising the stricture at 12 o'clock position. If internal urethrotomy is not possible, the stricture needs to be excised and urethral continuity restored with or without proximal urinary diversion as single stage or multistage procedure.

Acquired strictures are more common and can follow traumatic rupture associated with pelvic fractures, inappropriate instrumentation, prolonged indwelling catheters, and surgical procedures on the urethra, e.g., fulguration of PUV and urethroplasty. Some strictures respond to dilatation or internal urethrotomy while others need complicated single or multistage operative procedures. The back pressure effects of urethral stricture, the degree of upper tract dilatation, and the resulting renal dysfunction are variable.

Posterior Urethral Valves

Congenital valves in the posterior urethra (PUV) constitute the chief cause of lower urinary tract obstruction in boys, with an estimated incidence of 1:8,000 births. The condition may be life-threatening in neonates and can lead to CKD in up to 30% patients. The valves are located just distal to the verumontanum at the junction of the anterior and posterior urethra. The valves were classified by Young et al., based on their location and explain their physiological effects **(Fig. 18.3)**. In the most common form (type I, 95% of all PUV), they appear to radiate distally from the verumontanum and merge to form an anterior commissure just proximal to the external urethral sphincter.

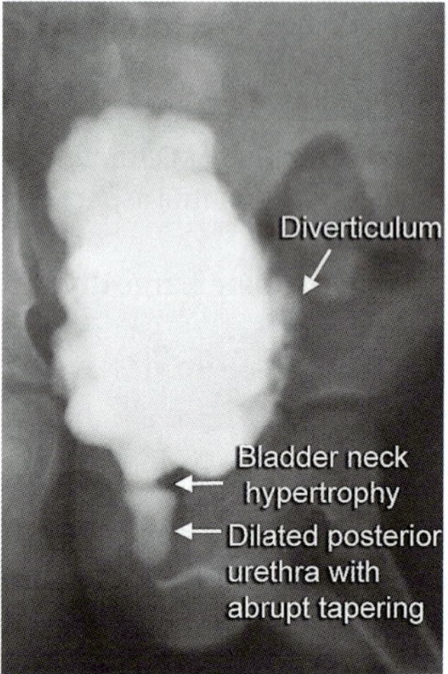

Fig. 18.2: Urethral stricture. Micturating cystourethrography shows the dilated posterior urethra, bladder neck hypertrophy, and bladder diverticuli in a 10-year-old boy who developed urethral stricture following fulguration of posterior urethral valves

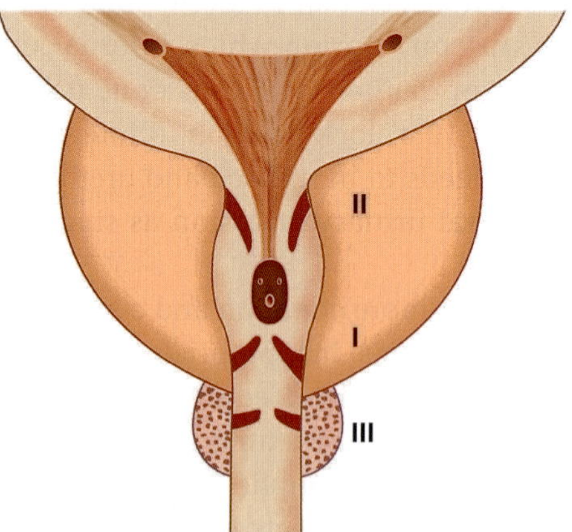

Fig. 18.3: Young classification of posterior urethral valve

These produce bilateral cusps with a slit-like opening between them, which causes obstruction to the flow of urine by a ballooning effect. Retrograde passage of a catheter may or may not meet any resistance. Catheterization of bladder may be difficult in some cases as the catheter might be coiled up in the dilated urethra. PUV type II are extremely rare and often undetected, because the valves spread proximally and may not obstruct the flow of urine. Type III valves are less common (5% of all PUV) and consist of a diaphragm with a central hole within the prostatic urethra, either above or below the verumontanum, which often gets treated when retrograde catheterization tears the valves. Obstruction to the flow of urine during organogenesis can have profound impact on kidney and bladder function. It causes dilatation of the posterior urethra and hypertrophy of the bladder neck. The bladder wall thickens and shows trabeculations or sacculations, with varying grades of vesicoureteral reflux (VUR). Recurrent infections result in renal scarring (reflux nephropathy) and CKD.

Clinical Features

Clinical features vary based on the degree of obstruction and the timing of clinical manifestation. Antenatally, PUV should be suspected in a fetus with bilateral hydronephrosis and hydroureter, and a thick-walled bladder. Oligohydramnios and renal dysplasia indicate impaired fetal renal function and can present with Potter sequence. The infant presents with features of obstruction such as dribbling of urine, poor urinary stream, straining, retention, and palpable bladder. Recurrent UTI, vomiting, and failure to thrive may be present. Renal function is impaired to a varying degree. In later ages, they can manifest with urge incontinence and small frequent voids.

Diagnosis

Prenatal diagnosis is usually made on antenatal USG. The clues on USG include bilateral hydronephrosis, keyhole sign (dilated posterior urethra), a dilated bladder with thick bladder wall (>3 mm), and oligohydramnios. Rare findings include bladder diverticula, perirenal urinoma, and urinary ascites with or without hyperechogenic kidneys. The diagnosis is confirmed by MCU, which shows a dilated posterior urethra, poor flow into the distal urethra, and abnormalities of the bladder (thickened wall, trabeculations, and sacculations) (**Fig. 3.19**). There can be presence of bilateral or unilateral severe VUR or bladder diverticulum, which might provide some protection to upper urinary tract.

Management

Antenatal management: Intrauterine obstruction and impaired renal function lead to decreased urine output and oligohydramnios. Amniotic fluid is necessary for normal development of the lung and its reduced volume causes pulmonary hypoplasia. Antenatal interventions have been attempted to relieve the obstruction, with limited benefits. Placing of a vesicoamniotic shunt has been suggested to preserve amniotic fluid and allow pulmonary development. Fetal surgery is hazardous and considered only at specialized centers.

Postnatal treatment: In a boy with suspected PUV, a multidisciplinary approach is necessary, including stabilization of vitals in children who are very sick, urgent MCU to enable diagnosis, definitive management, and subsequent follow up of kidney and bladder function.

Urological management: The initial goal in management is bladder drainage by catheterization using 6F infant feeding tube (without a balloon). If the catheter gets coiled up in the posterior urethra and does not enter the bladder, a suprapubic puncture might be required for imaging and drainage. Once the baby is stable and there is no infection, endoscopic incision or resection of the valves is done **(Flowchart 18.1)**. An appropriate sized resectoscope is used to resect the valves at 5, 7, and 12 o'clock positions. Valve incision is done with a 9Fr resectoscope for term, normal weight babies. If the urethral meatus is small, the miniature fiber cystourethroscope 0° angle of view with instrument channel 2.4 Fr is used. This is a 4.5–6 Fr panendoscope, which can be used

Flowchart 18.1: Management of a neonate with posterior urethral valves (PUV)
KUB: kidney, ureter, urinary bladder; MCU: micturating cystourethrography; USG: ultrasonography; UTI: urinary tract infection

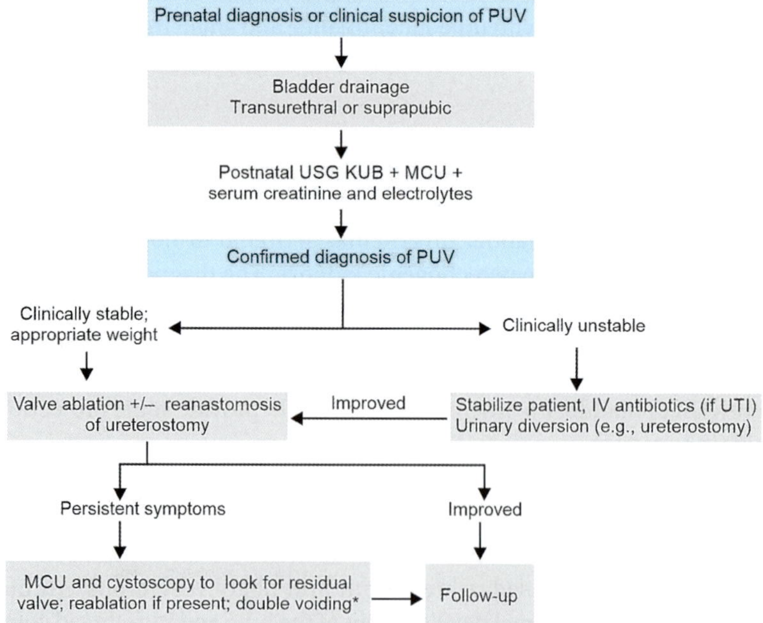

even in small newborns for electrofulguration of PUV. The techniques of valve ablation vary according to practical expertise: Incision with electrocautery or cold-knife, laser incision/fulguration. Extensive electrocoagulation might result in urethral stricture formation. Bladder drainage through vesicostomy is necessary only if the necessary expertise is not available. However, a definitive surgical procedure should be carried out at the earliest.

Urinary diversion: In clinically unstable or very low birth weight neonates, urinary diversion by vesicostomy is still in practice. It is however discouraged, since it can alter bladder dynamics. High urinary diversion (high loop ureterostomy) is necessary if there is no improvement in renal function even after valve ablation, progressive decline in kidney function (secondary to vesicoureteric junction obstruction due to thickened bladder wall, or high grade vesicoureteric reflux) or recurrent urinary infections. This helps in draining and thereby decompressing the upper urinary tract. The valves are later fulgurated, and ureterostomies closed.

Complications include recurrent UTI, vesicoureteric reflux and reflux nephropathy, progressive kidney failure, and valve bladder syndrome. Valve bladder syndrome is a poorly compliant, small capacity bladder. Polyuria, residual urine volume, and bladder insensitivity synergistically decrease functional bladder capacity resulting in increased bladder pressure. This can be initially managed by frequent voiding, and use of anticholinergic medications.

Follow-up: Long-term prognosis depends on kidney and bladder status at the time of diagnosis. Certain parameters are predictive of long-term outcomes **(Table 18.1)**. Voiding history, blood pressure, serum creatinine, electrolytes, and bicarbonate levels need to be monitored at regular intervals. Significant vesicoureteric reflux is seen in up to 80% cases and is bilateral in 30%. VUR is managed conservatively in view of poor bladder compliance. Long term observation is important, as bladder dysfunction and delayed continence are major problems. Serial USG is done to monitor the size of kidneys, screen for asymmetric growth and dilated urinary tract, and postvoid residual urine. Uroflowmetry and urodynamic evaluation is necessary in some patients

TABLE 18.1: Factors suggesting outcome in patients with posterior urethral valves

Good prognostic markers	*Poor prognostic markers*
Serum creatinine <0.8 mg/dL at 1-year Satisfactory corticomedullary differentiation Presence of pop-off mechanism (massive reflux to nonfunctioning kidney, urinary ascites, or bladder diverticulum)	Prenatal diagnosis before 24 weeks Respiratory distress at birth Bilateral vesicoureteric reflux Persistent incontinence after 5 years Serum creatinine >1 mg/dL after initial therapy Proteinuria and hypertension

to assess bladder dynamics. About 30–50% patients show progressive deterioration of kidney function and require renal replacement therapy. Management of bladder dysfunction may be required in the pre- and post-transplant periods.

Bladder Diverticulum

Bladder diverticulum represents an outpouching of the bladder mucosa through the bladder wall and may be a congenital or acquired defect. Important causes include bladder outlet obstruction, neuropathic bladder, prune belly syndrome, Ehlers-Danlos syndrome, and postsurgical procedures such as ureteric reimplantation. They are also reported as a protective pop-off mechanism in children with PUV. A diverticulum arising from the region of the bladder neck can track behind the posterior urethra and cause obstruction to flow of urine. Such patients present with features of distal urinary tract obstruction similar to those in PUV. Paraureteric diverticulum manifests with features of VUR or obstruction at the vesicoureteric junction. Bladder diverticula need to be excised, and with paraureteric diverticulum, the ureter reimplanted.

Ureterocele

This is a congenital anomaly in which the terminal part of the ureter distends within the bladder to form a sac. The basis for their formation is abnormal development of the bladder trigone leading to abnormal ureteric insertion. Ureretoceles may be intravesical or ectopic in nature; these may be a single system or associated with a duplex system. In the latter, the upper moiety is usually involved. The site of obstruction is the ureteric orifice, which is usually ectopic; back pressure effects result in hydroureteronephrosis. Occasionally, the ureterocele may descend into the posterior urethra and cause bladder outlet obstruction and result in vesicoureteric reflux on the contralateral side.

They can present as antenatal hydronephrosis and postnatally with recurrent UTI, and intermittent pelvic pain. The classic description of cobra head appearance **(Fig. 18.4A)** on an IVU is diagnostic, but this procedure is seldom required. On USG, ureterocele appears as a hypoechoic impression at the ureterovesicle junction **(Fig. 18.4B)**. MCU helps in identifying the associated vesicoureteric reflux. Overdistension of the bladder may cause the ureterocele to collapse, while an empty bladder may allow a large ureterocele to enlarge, giving the impression of a partially full but normal bladder. Ectopic ureters can sometimes displace the bladder and mimic an ureterocele (pseudoureterocele). Treatment consists of endoscopic deroofing. Secondary VUR may require reimplantation of the ureter(s). Ureteroceles that produce bladder outlet obstruction are managed by excision and ureteric reimplantation.

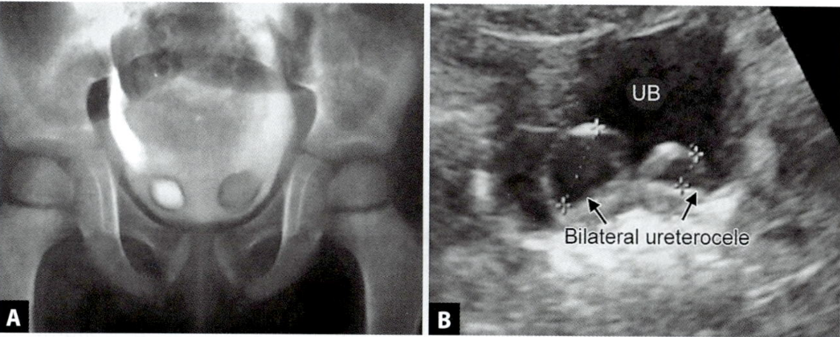

Figs. 18.4A and B: Bilateral ureterocele. (A) Intravenous urography shows "cobra head" appearance of bilateral ureters; (B) Ultrasound shows dilated hypoechoic impression near the urinary bladder (UB)

Megaureter

Megaureters are dilated ureters with a luminal diameter of >7 mm in fetus >30 weeks gestation till 12 years of age. The condition is bilateral in 25%, and the contralateral kidney is absent or dysplastic in 10–15%. Primary megaureter is due to an aperistaltic (adynamic) juxtavesical segment that effectively causes obstruction to urine flow. Megaureters can also be classified based on the presence of obstruction alone, reflux alone, or in combination. Nonrefluxing nonobstructed megaureter is also called as primary dilated megaureter. Refluxing nonobstructed is associated with high grade VUR and a dilated ureter. Obstructed and nonrefluxing is associated with ectopic ureter opening mostly in duplex system.

Secondary obstructive megaureter represents an obstructive process due to elevated bladder pressure. Common causes include PUV, spina bifida, tethered spinal cord, prune belly syndrome, and neurogenic bladder. The detrusor pressure may rise to over 40 cmH_2O and result in hydronephrosis. Non-neurogenic voiding dysfunction, if severe enough to elevate bladder pressure above the safe range, may produce similar changes. Other anatomic causes of secondary distal ureteral obstruction include ureterocele, ectopic ureter, bladder diverticula, periureteral fibrosis, and external compression by retroperitoneal tumor, masses, or aberrant vessels. The ureter tends to dilate from its distal end upwards. They can be detected antenatally on routine USG or postnatally present with UTIs, abdominal mass, or groin pain, and occasionally hematuria. Calculus formation may occur. They can also be associated with renal [ipsilateral pelviureteric junction obstruction (PUJO), contralateral VUR, and renal hypodysplasia] or extrarenal (ear tags, tracheomalacia, and undescended testes) anomalies. DTPA renogram and MCU are performed to determine the type of megaureter; MR urography may be necessary. Management depends on the type of megaureter. Surgical treatment consists of excision of the obstructing lower segment of the ureter and its reimplantation, and is required in all obstructed megaureters. Nephroureterectomy is necessary if the split renal function of the same side is poor (<5–10%).

Pelviureteric Junction Obstruction

Obstruction at the pelviureteric junction (PUJ) is one of the most frequent causes for hydronephrosis comprising 10–30% of antenatally detected hydronephrosis. The condition is more common on the left side, and in boys; bilateral obstruction is rare.

The obstruction is most commonly intrinsic due to an adynamic segment; extrinsic factors, such as an abnormally crossing vessel, adhesive bands, arteriovenous malformation, and ureteral folds are less common. PUJO may also occur due to high grade vesicoureteric reflux or renal calculi. Infants with antenatally detected hydronephrosis are usually asymptomatic. Older children may present with abdominal pain (dull constant pain or severe spasmodic pain), abdominal lump or with UTI. Gross hematuria may occur following minor abdominal trauma. Pain and an abdominal mass that resolves with passage of a large amount of urine (Dietl crisis) are uncommon.

Management

The principles of management of antenatal hydronephrosis are discussed in Chapter 31. Patients where hydronephrosis is diagnosed on incidental evaluation, should undergo renal scintigraphy to confirm the presence and severity of obstruction, and to determine differential function **(Fig. 4.5)**. Patients with no impairment of renal function and slow drainage (>10 minutes) are managed conservatively. Those with a palpable lump and pain, reduction in split renal function (<40%), and *t*½ greater than 20 minutes, and showing >10% fall in differential kidney function are considered for surgery.

The most frequently utilized reconstruction technique is dismembered pyeloplasty that can be performed using an extraperitoneal approach. Success rates in providing drainage are high although it is not invariably reflected in improvement in spilt renal function. Patients managed conservatively require close follow-up and early surgical intervention if functional deterioration is noted. Unilateral nephrectomy may rarely be required in patients with extremely poor renal function (<10%), particularly in the presence of systemic hypertension. Rarely, a drainage procedure (percutaneous nephrostomy) may be done to examine if renal function recovers, before deciding for nephrectomy.

Ureterovesical Junction Obstruction

Ureterovesical junction obstruction (UVJO) is characterized by obstruction at the distal end of the ureter, where it meets the bladder and results in megaureter (primary obstructive megaureter). UVJO is typically caused by an adynamic segment of the distal ureter. UVJO is seen more often in boys and is unilateral with more left sided involvement. The condition is often detected prenatally; recurrent UTI is also a frequent clinical presentation. The diagnosis is made using a combination of USG, dynamic scintigraphy and MR urography. The management, as in PUJO, is conservative since most vesicoureteric junction obstruction (VUJO) resolve spontaneously. Patients require to be followed by frequent ultrasonographic assessment. Surgery is required in ~10% and comprises either of primary reimplantation or temporary diversion by cutaneous ureterostomy to enable maturation and retonization of the distal ureter.

Prune Belly Syndrome

This rare lower urinary tract malformation is defined by the triad of partial or complete lack of abdominal wall musculature with a dry prune like wrinkly skin appearance of the abdomen, variable dilatation of the upper and lower urinary tract, and bilateral cryptorchidism. The majority of patients are males. Mutations in *HNF1*β and *CHRM3* genes have been described.

COMPLICATIONS OF OBSTRUCTION

Apart from obstructing the flow of urine, obstructive uropathy has multiple effects on the kidneys and urinary tract.

Urinary Tract Infections

Urinary stasis, stones, and foreign bodies (stents, catheters) predispose to UTI. Attempts to sterilize the urinary tract when obstruction or foreign bodies are present are usually not successful.

Bladder Dysfunction

The stretch injury in obstructive uropathy becomes irreversible as the cellular and extracellular characteristics of the bladder wall alter. Bladder dysfunction (valve bladder syndrome) develops in patients with PUVs. Features of this syndrome are persistent dilation of the upper urinary tracts, thick-walled noncompliant urinary bladder, urinary incontinence, and polyuria (due to distal tubular damage).

Hypertension and Proteinuria

Hypertension is common in patients with reflux nephropathy. It occurs due to alteration in glomerular vasculature, affecting perfusion and filtration. Hypertension and retrograde glomerular injury can cause sclerosis and podocyte injury and result in proteinuria. Angiotensin-converting enzyme

(ACE) inhibitors controls hypertension and have an impact on proteinuria reduction as well. Calcium channel blockers and β-blockers are also effective in controlling hypertension.

Stones

Magnesium ammonium phosphate (struvite) and calcium phosphate stones form in the presence of infected urine. The infecting organism in most cases is *Proteus* species.

Tubular Dysfunction

Significant tubular injury may be present in patients with obstructive uropathy. Polyuria and nocturia may occur due to poor urinary concentration. Some patients show a tendency to salt wasting that requires sodium chloride supplementation. Children with unilateral or bilateral hydronephrosis often show systemic acidosis due to inadequate urinary acidification [distal renal tubular acidosis (RTA)]. Patients undergoing urinary diversions (ureterosigmoidostomy) have high bicarbonate loss in stools, which further worsens metabolic acidosis. Large doses of alkali supplements may be required to maintain serum bicarbonate in the normal range. Other features of CKD (mineral bone disease and anemia) should be looked for and appropriately managed.

BIBLIOGRAPHY

1. Arredondo MJ, Pérez RBP, Rico JM, et al. Pop-off mechanisms as renoprotective mediators in children with posterior urethral valves: A systematic review and meta-analysis. J Pediatr Urol. 2024;20(1):57-66.
2. Buder K, Opherk K, Mazzi S, Rohner K, Weitz M. Non-surgical management in children with non-refluxing primary megaureter: a systematic review and meta-analysis. Pediatr Nephrol. 2023;38(11):3549-58.
3. Farrugia MK, Hitchcock R, Radford A, et al. British Association of Pediatric Urologists. Consensus statement on management of primary obstructive megaureter. J Pediatr Urol. 2014;10(1):26-33.
4. Herthelius M. Antenatally detected urinary tract dilatation: long-term outcome. Pediatr Nephrol. 2023;38(10):3221-7.
5. Khondker A, Chan JY, Malik S, et al. Primary ablation versus urinary diversion in posterior urethral valve: Systematic review and meta-analysis. J Pediatr Urol. 2023;19(4):408-17.
6. Kurtz MP. Prenatal diagnoses and intervention. Urol Clin North Am. 2023;50(3):351-9.
7. Lange-Sperandio B, Rosenblum ND. Pediatric obstructive uropathy. In: Emma F, Goldstein S, Bagga A, Bates CM, Shroff R (Eds). Pediatric Nephrology, 8th edn. Springer Nature, New York; 2022. pp. 1369-98.
8. Lombel RM, Brakeman PR, Sack BS, Butani L. Urologic considerations in pediatric chronic kidney disease. Adv Chronic Kidney Dis. 2022;29(3):308-17.

9. Melo FF, Mak RH, Simões E Silva AC, et al. Evaluation of urinary tract dilation classification system for prediction of long-term outcomes in isolated antenatal hydronephrosis: A cohort study. J Urol. 2021;206(4):1022-30.
10. Meneghesso D, Bertazza PN, Spagnol R, et al. Nadir creatinine as a predictor of renal outcomes in PUVs: A systematic review and meta-analysis. Front Pediatr. 2023;11:1085143.
11. Morris RK, Malin GL, Quinlan-Jones E, et al. The Percutaneous shunting in Lower Urinary Tract Obstruction (PLUTO) study: evaluation of the effectiveness, cost-effectiveness and acceptability of percutaneous vesicoamniotic shunting for lower urinary tract obstruction. Health Technol Assess. 2013;17(59):1-232.
12. Pohl HG. Embryology, treatment, and outcomes of ureteroceles in children. Urol Clin North Am. 2023;50(3):371-89.
13. Rai A, Hsieh A, Smith A. Contemporary diagnosis and management of pelviureteric junction obstruction. BJU Int. 2022;130(3):285-90.
14. Rivetti G, Marzuillo P, Guarino S, et al. Primary non-refluxing megaureter: Natural history, follow-up and treatment. Eur J Pediatr. 2024;183:2029-36.
15. Sinha A, Bagga A, Krishna A, et al. Revised guidelines on management of antenatal hydronephrosis. Indian Pediatr. 2013;50(2):215-31.
16. Vincent K, Murphy HJ, Twombley KE. Urinary tract dilation in the fetus and neonate. Neoreviews. 2022;23(3):e159-e174.

Voiding Disorders

Jyoti Sharma, Madhuri Kanitkar

Voiding disorders are functional, abnormal patterns of micturition that occur due to abnormalities in the storage or voiding phase of the urinary bladder in the absence of a neurological or anatomic lesion. This chapter provides a brief description of the anatomy and physiology of the bladder, followed by an outline of approach to voiding disorders.

APPLIED ANATOMY AND PHYSIOLOGY

The urinary bladder is located partly in the lower abdomen in children and descends completely into the pelvis during puberty. Its unique innervation as well as arrangement of smooth and striated muscle fibers, allow the bladder to store urine at low pressure, sense appropriately when it is filled with adequate urine, and void completely by a coordinated contraction of the detrusor muscle and relaxation of the sphincters at a socially appropriate time and place **(Figs. 19.1 to 19.4)**.

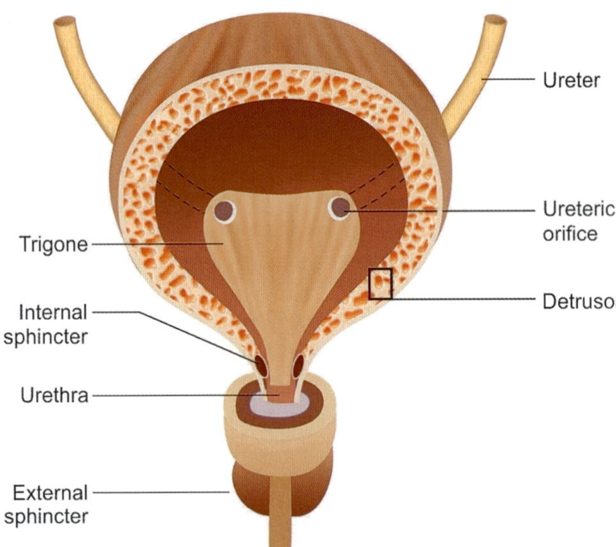

Fig. 19.1: Anatomy of the urinary bladder highlighting the three muscles: the detrusor, internal sphincter, and external sphincter. The trigone is an area bound by the two ureteric openings and the internal urethral orifice

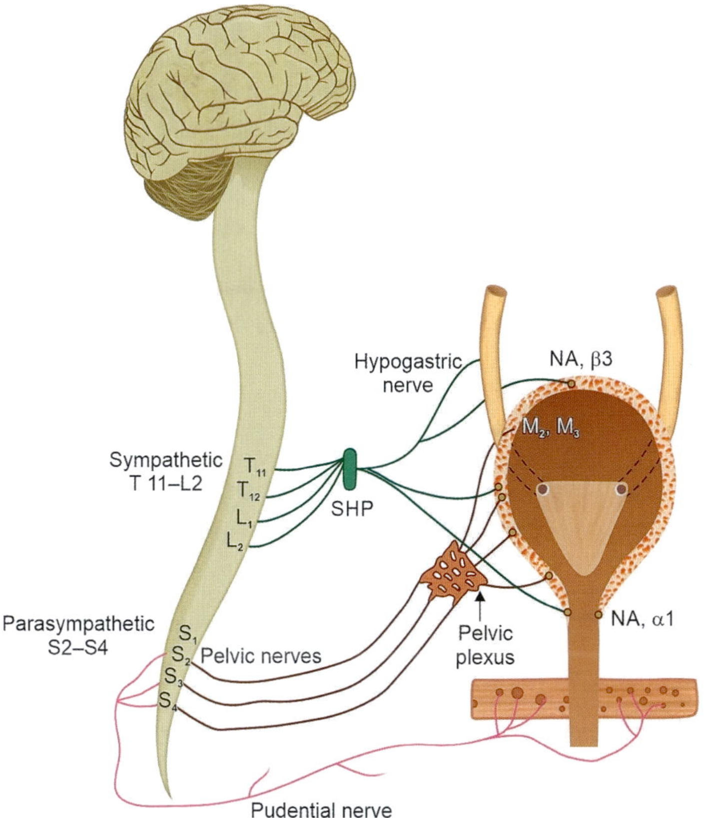

Fig. 19.2: Thoracolumbar spinal cord segments thoracic 11 to lumbar 2 (T11–L2) give rise to fibers (green) that travel to the thoracolumbar sympathetic ganglia and then to the superior hypogastric plexus (SHP). Nerves from the plexus coalesce to form the right and left hypogastric nerves that innervate the ureter, detrusor, the base of the bladder, and the urethra. They provide noradrenergic (NA) excitatory stimulation of the β_3 receptors of the detrusor and facilitate storage of urine by relaxation of the bladder body with simultaneous contraction of the bladder outlet and urethra via action on α_1 receptors of the bladder neck and proximal urethra. Parasympathetic preganglionic (brown) fibers travel in sacral roots and pelvic nerves to ganglia in the pelvic plexus (PP) and intramural in the bladder wall; they supply parasympathetic fibers to the detrusor (M2, M3 receptors) and bladder neck (nicotinic receptors). Somatic motor fibers (magenta) arise from motor neurons of S2–S4 cord segments and supply the striated muscles via the pudendal nerve. All nerves to the bladder also carry sensory afferent fibers from the bladder

The lower urinary tract remains in "storage" mode during bladder filling, maintained in this state by the sympathetic system. During this phase the external urethral sphincter must remain contracted and the detrusor muscle relaxed as urine pours down the ureters. Regions in the brain, which are not completely delineated, are active in "storage" not only to maintain these

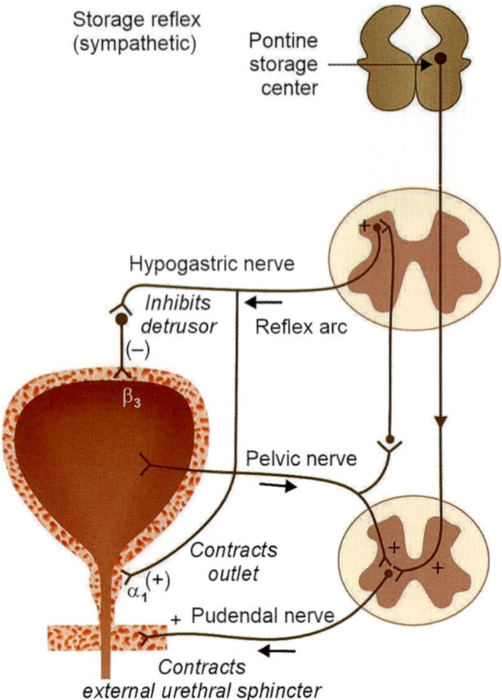

Fig. 19.3: Storage reflex. Bladder filling and distension cause low-level firing of Aδ-fibers carried via the pelvic nerve. Sympathetic firing from the lumbar region, is transmitted via hypogastric nerve to stimulate β_3-adrenoceptors leading to relaxation of the bladder wall and α_1-adrenoceptors at bladder neck and proximal urethra to maintain them in contracted state (reflex arc). Afferent pelvic nerve impulses also stimulate the pudendal (somatic) outflow to the external sphincter. Sphincter afferents also inhibit parasympathetic activity keeping the bladder relaxed (not shown in the figure). Voluntary control of micturition is mediated through signaling from the pontine storage center to the external sphincter through the somatic fibers of the pudendal nerve

properties of the detrusor and sphincter, but also to monitor the progression of bladder filling. When the bladder is full, there is "switch" to voiding mode (at pontine micturition center) in which the sphincters relax and the detrusor muscle contracts, mediated by the parasympathetic system. Though previously believed that voiding in neonates is entirely a spinal reflex activity, there is certainly some central nervous system neuronal activity. Sleeping neonates exhibit limb movements, grimace, cry, or even wake up when they void, suggesting that higher brain centers are involved in the process of micturition.

The bowel and bladder have a common embryological origin, share common neural pathways, and lie in proximity in the bony pelvis; hence their function is often reciprocally affected. The rectum is designed to serve as a passage and a signal organ. However, if a child is chronically constipated,

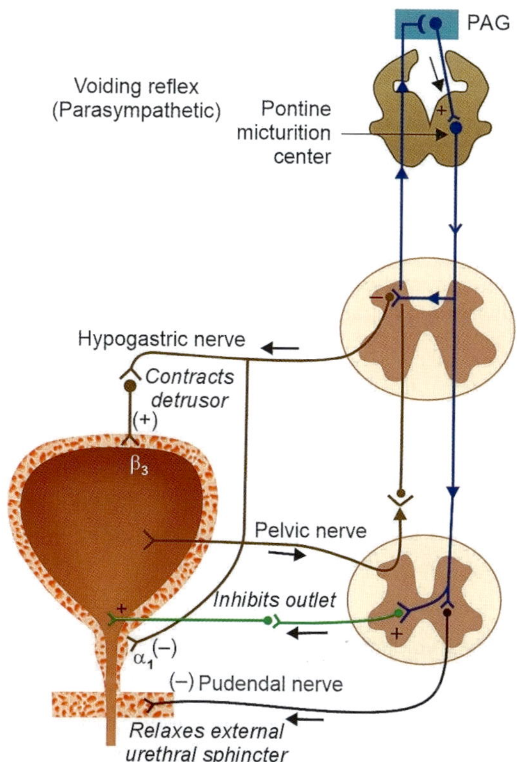

Fig. 19.4: Voiding reflex. At initiation of voiding, bladder afferent activity via the pelvic nerve increases. Ascending afferent input from the spinal cord passes through relay neurons in the periaqueductal grey (PAG) matter before reaching the pontine micturition center (PMC). The PMC is the switch in the voiding pathway since it stimulates the parasympathetic outflow to the bladder and bladder neck through the hypogastric nerve which leads to contraction of the detrusor and relaxation of the internal sphincter. It also stimulates urethral smooth muscle through the pelvic splanchnic nerve (shown in green) and inhibits the spinal guarding reflexes, which are conducted via the pudendal nerve, resulting in relaxation of the external sphincter

the distended rectum may exert pressure on the bladder, cause incomplete bladder emptying and recurrent urinary tract infections (UTI) or frequent voiding that may be associated with incontinence. Children with voiding postponement may also habitually ignore bowel signals, resulting in constipation and increasing the risk of UTI.

Developmental Changes in Voiding

After the first 48 hr of life, neonates pass urine almost every hour; the frequency decreases at 6 months to about 10–15 times per day. After the first year the frequency of voiding reduces to 8–10 times per day, and gradually to the frequency of 4–7 times a day seen in older children and adults.

TABLE 19.1: Expected bladder capacity at different ages

Age	*Expected bladder capacity (EBC), mL*
Neonate	30
Children up to 2 years	7 × weight (in kg)
>2 years	(Age in years + 1) × 30 (range is 65–150% EBC)

TABLE 19.2: Terminology of the International Children's Continence Society (ICCS) for some important lower urinary tract symptoms (LUTS)

Term	*Description*
Storage symptoms	
Incontinence	Involuntary leakage of urine; may be continuous or intermittent
Enuresis	Intermittent incontinence during sleep
Urgency	Sudden, unexpected, and compelling need to void
Increased frequency of voiding	≥8 times a day
Decreased frequency of voiding	≤3 times a day
Voiding symptoms	
Dysuria	Burning or discomfort during micturition
Intermittency	Micturition during which there are several stops and starts
Terms like hesitancy, straining, weak stream are self-explanatory	
Holding maneuvers	Strategies to: (*i*) postpone voiding; (*ii*) suppress urgency associated with overactive bladder, e.g., crossing of legs, or pressing the heel against the perineum

Between 2 and 4 years of age, a child becomes developmentally ready to be toilet trained. By 5 years, 90–95% are dry by day and 85% by night. The expected bladder capacity at different ages is shown in **Table 19.1**.

APPROACH TO A CHILD WITH A VOIDING DISORDER

To establish uniformity in the description of lower urinary tract symptoms and disorders, the International Children's Continence Society (ICCS) has established a nomenclature with standard definitions **(Table 19.2)**.

The age of reference at which lower urinary tract symptoms get recognized is 5 years; however, cognizance may be given to them earlier for children who become toilet trained at a younger age. Children with voiding disorders are brought to attention with history of incontinence or recurrent UTI. On specific questioning, details of increased or decreased frequency or urgency may be elicited. An important aspect of history and clinical examination of these children is to rule out systemic disease or a neurological or structural abnormality. History of continuous incontinence suggests an anatomical abnormality such as an ectopic ureter or a neurogenic bladder. It is important to elicit a history of failure to thrive, polydipsia, and polyuria to exclude tubular disorder, chronic kidney disease (CKD), or diabetes mellitus. On clinical examination, well-developed abdominal muscles (which may be used for voiding), renal mass (hydronephrosis), fecoliths, or a palpable bladder are looked for. Careful examination should be performed for midline spinal stigmata (occult spinal cord defect), neurological defects in the lower limbs, specifically sensory deficit in perineal area, and inner aspect of thighs. Girls must be examined for vulval synechia or labial adhesions **(Fig. 19.5)**.

Having established the presence of a voiding disorder, the diagnosis of the type of disorder is based on clinical parameters and noninvasive urodynamics, i.e., a *voiding diary* and *uroflowmetry* with electromyography (EMG). Parents are asked to maintain a voiding diary or a frequency volume chart in which they document the volume of each void for at least 48 hr **(Fig. 19.6)**. They need to record the fluid intake over 48 hr as well. This helps understand the intake pattern especially if most of the fluid is consumed in the evening. Smart phone applications are available to make diary recording easier for families.

Simultaneously, history regarding bowel movements is recorded. The Indian Society of Pediatric Gastroenterology, Hepatology and Nutrition Committee, and the Indian Academy of Pediatrics have defined constipation as a delay or difficulty in defecation sufficient to cause significant distress to a child and is chronic when it has persisted for 4 weeks or longer. In addition, diagnostic criteria have been laid down for the diagnosis of

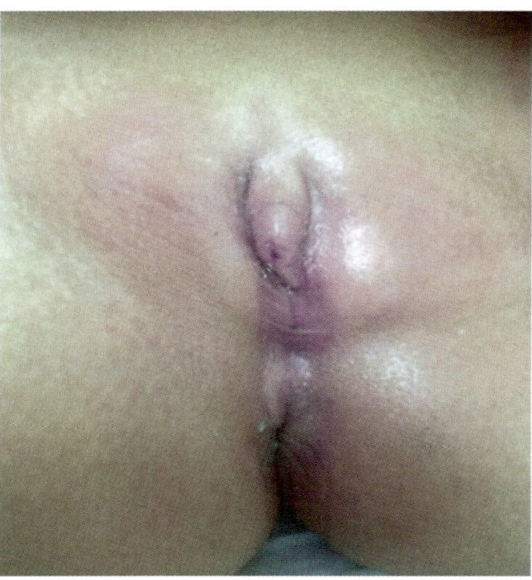

Fig. 19.5: Labial adhesions

Date

Time	Drink type & volume of fluid	Time	Voided volume	Enuresis +/–	Comments: day time accident

Incontinence frequency

Bowel movements for 2 weeks

Normal number of voids: 4–7/day

Expected bladder capacity (EBC): (Age in years +1) x 30 mL

Maximum voided volume (MVV): the largest volume of voided urine measured over a 24-hr period (excluding the first morning void)

Bladder capacity too small if MVV <65% EBC

Bladder capacity too large if MVV >150% EBC

Nocturnal polyuria: if overnight voided volume and volume of first morning void >130% of EBC

Fig. 19.6: Sample drink and voiding diary, detailing information that needs to be collected. The adjacent text describes the interpretation of a voiding diary

BOX 19.1: Diagnosis of constipation

Presence of ≥2 of the following for >4 weeks

i. Defecation frequency ≤2 times per week*
ii. Fecal incontinence once per week, after acquisition of toileting skills
iii. History of excessive stool retention
iv. History of painful or hard bowel movements
v. Presence of a large mass in the rectum or on per abdomen examination
vi. History of large-diameter stools that may obstruct the toilet

Other manifestations in the form of irritability, decreased appetite, and/or early satiety may be observed, which improve after defecation.

*Based on the normal stool frequency of >1/day in Indian children older than 2 years

Source: Yachcha, et al. Indian Pediatrics 2018

constipation **(Box 19.1)**. The Bristol stool chart is a useful pictorial tool that helps the child and parents to identify the type of stool and substantiate the presence or absence of constipation. Rectal diameter >3 mm seen posterior to the bladder on ultrasonography of kidneys, ureter, and bladder, and visualization of a loaded colon in the scout film of micturating sonography corroborates the presence of constipation **(Figs. 19.7A and B)**. The Dysfunctional Voiding Score System (DVSS), is used as a voiding scoring system in some clinics. It provides both qualitative and quantitative evaluation of bladder and bowel symptoms. Children with constipation and a voiding disorder need simultaneous attention to management of constipation as well as treatment of the voiding disorder as described subsequently.

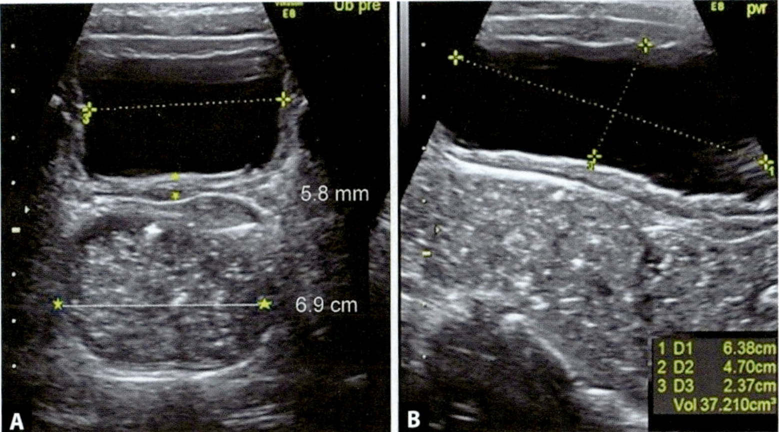

Figs. 19.7A and B: Ultrasonography in a 7-year-old girl who presented with a febrile UTI and history of holding maneuvers. (A) Thick-walled bladder (5.8 mm), fecal-loaded rectum with diameter of 6.9 cm; (B) Postvoid urine volume 37 mL

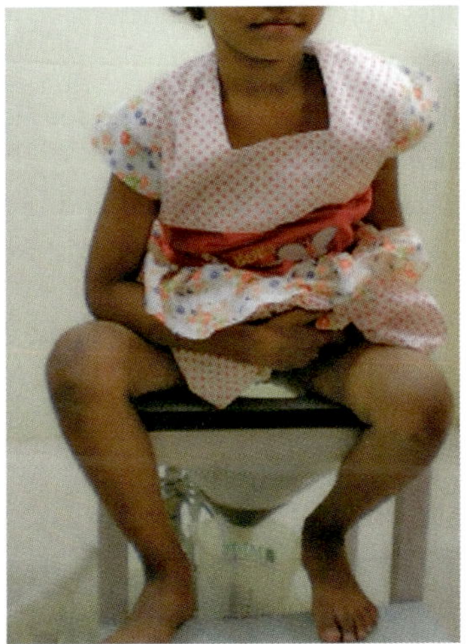

Fig. 19.8: Uroflowmetry

Uroflowmetry is a simple procedure in which a toilet trained child is asked to wait till she/he has the urge to void, and then asked to void in a jar connected to a transducer **(Fig. 19.8)**. The urine flow is recorded as a volume curve generated over time (in seconds) on *X*-axis and flow rate in milliliter per second on *Y*-axis. It gives information regarding the total volume of urine voided, maximum flow rate in milliliter per second, total voiding time, and flow time. The shape of the flow curve correlates with specific patterns of bladder behavior **(Fig. 19.9)**. It is useful for the diagnosis of an overactive bladder (OAB), underactive bladder, and bladder outlet obstruction. When used with perineal surface EMG electrodes, additional information can be obtained about the pelvic floor relaxation, or the lack of it, during voiding.

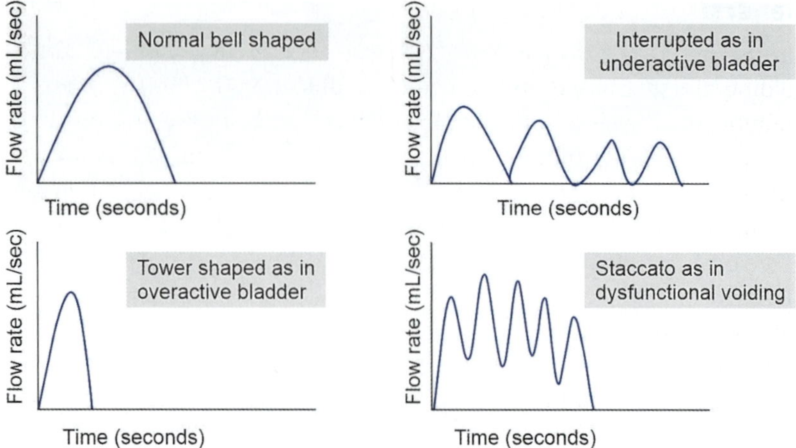

Fig. 19.9: Uroflowmetry patterns. These urine flow rate to time curves provide useful information regarding voided volume and maximum flow rate. Characteristic patterns aid in identifying the disorder, especially when used as adjunct with a voiding diary and ultrasonography of the kidneys, ureters, and bladder

TABLE 19.3: Ultrasound findings of significance (also ***see*** **Figs. 19.7A and B**)

Parameter	*Significant finding*
Thickened bladder wall	≥2.0 mm when distended, and ≥3.0 mm when empty
Postvoid residue	4–6 years: >30 mL or >21% of the expected bladder capacity
	7–12 years: >20 mL or 15% of the expected bladder capacity
Rectal distension	>3.0 cm correlates with the presence of stool in the rectum

The amount of residual urine in the bladder is assessed immediately after voiding via an ultrasound device.

A *urodynamic study* is an invasive procedure in which pressure is measured in the bladder (vesical pressure) and rectum (abdominal pressure) during the filling as well as voiding phases, with simultaneous perineal EMG electrodes. Detrusor pressure is calculated by subtracting abdominal pressure from the vesical pressure. This evaluation is mainly indicated when the history, physical examination, and/or noninvasive investigation suggests the possibility of neurogenic bladder, or when there is a need to determine detrusor pressure to assess the safety of the bladder prior to kidney transplantation. Urodynamic evaluation may also be required in a child with a voiding disorder refractory to therapy.

Urinalysis and the ratio of urine calcium to creatinine is advised in patients with frequent voiding to screen for UTI (cystitis) or hypercalciuria, respectively. Ultrasonography of the kidneys, ureters, and bladder is done in patients with previous UTI **(Table 19.3) (Figs. 19.7A and B)**.

General Management

Urotherapy is the nonsurgical, nonpharmacological management of a voiding disorder based on behavioral modification, for lower urinary tract malfunction as well as constipation and fecal incontinence. It is the first line therapy used in all children with these disorders and is classified as standard and specific. *Standard urotherapy* begins with creating a rapport with parents and the child and educating them regarding the normal functioning of the urinary tract in a simplified manner. It includes an explanation for the likely cause for the condition, and advice regarding behavioral modification with respect to ensuring adequate fluid intake and a balanced diet, timed and complete voiding, avoidance of holding maneuvers, and regular bowel emptying. A record of fluid intake and a voiding diary are useful since they help the family to objectively register the symptoms. Support and encouragement via regular follow-ups are imperative. Star charts are a useful aid, where a reward is given for positive behavior modification, rather than achieving dryness. *Specific urotherapy* refers to use of the alarm, biofeedback for pelvic floor muscle relaxation techniques, and clean intermittent catheterization. *Transcutaneous electric nerve stimulation (TENS)*, over posterior tibial region at the ankle, by surface electrodes that deliver stimuli at a frequency between 10 and 25 Hz, has been found useful in the management of children with an overactive bladder.

COMMON VOIDING DISORDERS

Enuresis

Enuresis is defined as intermittent incontinence that occurs during sleep in a child who is 5 years or older, and is considered for treatment if it occurs more than once in a month for 3 months. It is classified as *primary,* if the child has never been dry, or *secondary* if the child has been dry for at least 6 months before the onset of enuresis. A more relevant classification is *monosymptomatic enuresis (MNE)* when the child suffers from bed wetting alone, and *nonmonosymptomatic (NMNE)*, when enuresis is associated with daytime symptoms. The daytime symptoms may be: (*i*) daytime incontinence, (*ii*) urgency (sudden, unexpected, and imperative urge to void), (*iii*) voiding difficulties (poor stream, hesitancy, and need to strain to void), and (*iv*) abnormally low or high daytime voiding frequency (voiding <4 or >7 times per day). The history for daytime symptoms must be elicited proactively since often it is not forthcoming, and management of children with NMNE differs from that of MNE. Very often the voiding diary helps diagnose the daytime symptoms when history is not elicited.

Enuresis is believed to occur due to one or a combination of the following factors, namely low secretion of antidiuretic hormone resulting in nocturnal polyuria, a small nocturnal bladder capacity, and high arousal threshold from sleep. In addition, certain comorbid factors associated with enuresis are constipation, behavioral disorders such as attention deficit hyperactivity disorder (ADHD) and sleep disordered breathing as seen in children with adenotonsillar hypertrophy **(Fig. 19.10)**.

The ICCS recommends that a child with enuresis who is older than 6 years should receive appropriate management. Enuresis is a cause of embarrassment, anxiety, and low self-esteem for children. It might also result in unsatisfactory school performance and inferior quality of life. Despite their high threshold for arousal from sleep, the quality of their sleep is poor, leading to poor daytime performance. These children are at risk for emotional and physical abuse by parents or caregivers who are overwhelmed by daily handling of wet bedclothes or the economic strain of having to use disposable ones. Lastly, untreated, 0.5–1% adults continue to suffer from enuresis.

As in other voiding disorders, pathological causes of enuresis need to be excluded. Usually, detailed history and meticulous examination are adequate to rule out pathological causes of polyuria that manifest as enuresis, i.e., tubular disorders, chronic kidney disease, and diabetes mellitus **(Fig. 19.11)**.

Daytime symptoms (as in NMNE), and comorbid conditions must be managed before or concurrently with the management of enuresis to achieve success in the management. Hence, a voiding diary is advised in all children being evaluated for enuresis. As an example of NMNE, constipation and fecal impaction may cause bladder overactivity and enuresis. Treatment of constipation, along with other measures of urotherapy, are likely to result in resolution of enuresis. Similarly, enuresis is known to resolve in 50% of the children who undergo adenoidectomy for sleep disordered breathing.

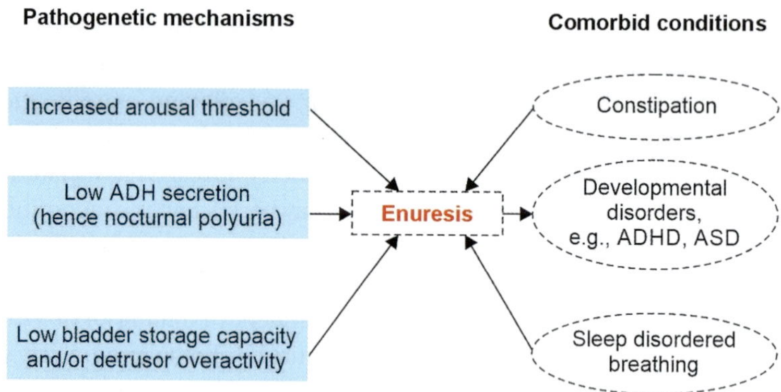

Fig. 19.10: Proposed pathogenesis of enuresis and comorbid conditions that may aggravate enuresis. There is a mismatch between the bladder capacity and the urine output because a child may have low nocturnal antidiuretic hormone (ADH) secretion, polyuria, and a small bladder capacity. Management of comorbid conditions prior to, or simultaneously are essential to the success of management of enuresis. ADHD: attention deficit hyperactivity disorder; ASD: autism spectrum disorder

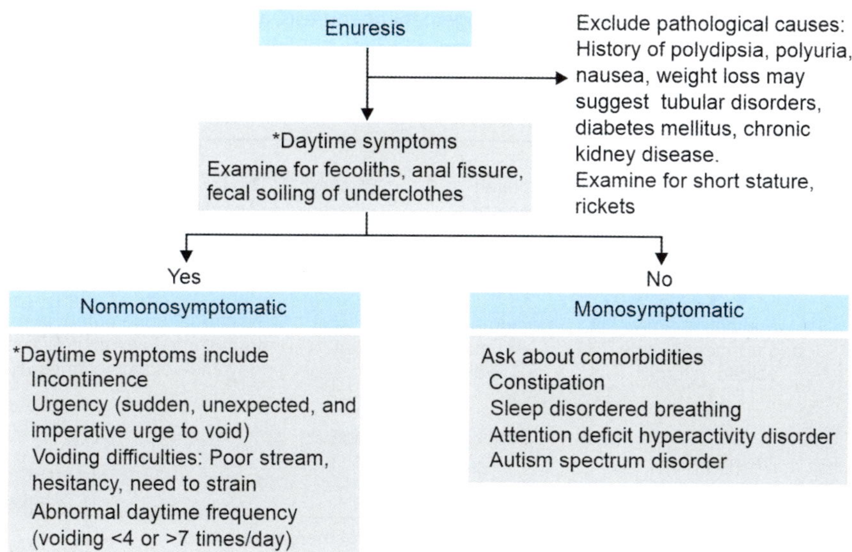

Fig. 19.11: Approach to a child with enuresis

Management of enuresis is difficult in children with conditions like autism spectrum disorder or ADHD, and is necessarily carried out simultaneously. Urotherapy has an important role to play in the management of all children, especially in those who have NMNE. The child and the parents should understand that enuresis is not the child's fault, that some of his peers are also likely to be suffering from the condition and that there are means of overcoming it. The general advice regarding adequate fluid intake during the day, timed voiding, regularizing bowel habits is relevant for all children before starting any specific therapy. Registration of symptoms by maintenance of a voiding diary is useful in the assessment of the capacity of a child's bladder, how it compares to the expected bladder capacity for her/his age and whether there is nocturnal polyuria **(Fig. 19.6)**. This information is used to plan the management **(Flowchart 19.1)**.

The enuresis alarm is a form of behavioral therapy that conditions the child to awaken to the sensation of a full bladder. It consists of a moisture sensor that is placed in the clothes of the child. Initially the alarm goes off when the child voids and the parents have to rouse the child to take him to the toilet. Gradually, the child learns to wake up to bladder fullness due to the conditioning effects on arousal and/or by increasing the nocturnal storage volume of the bladder. It takes 4–6 weeks for the alarm to show some effect. For the alarm to be a success, the family and the child should be motivated, since the first few weeks require perseverance. If there is no improvement in 1 month, it is advisable to discontinue therapy. The success rate is 50–70%, and the alarm has the lowest relapse rate. Once a child has been consistently

Flowchart 19.1: Algorithm of management of enuresis, as per the International Children's Continence Society Guidelines

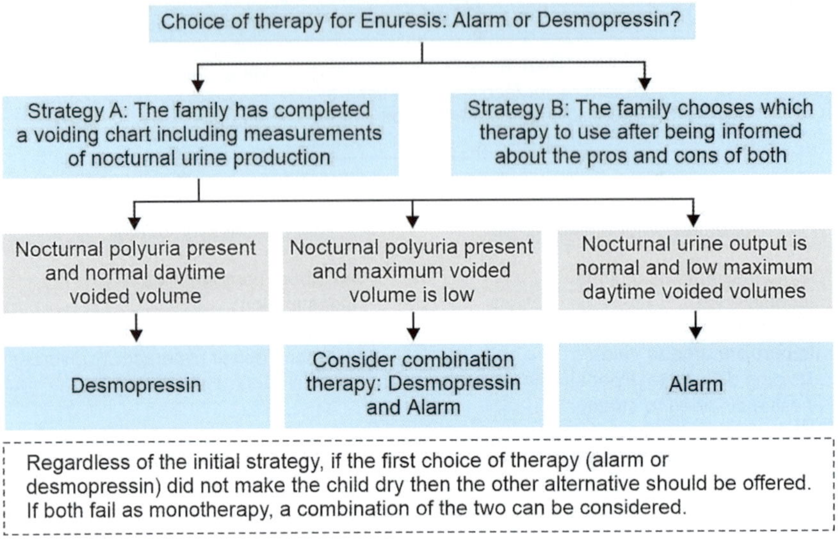

Choice of therapy for Enuresis: Alarm or Desmopressin?

- Strategy A: The family has completed a voiding chart including measurements of nocturnal urine production
- Strategy B: The family chooses which therapy to use after being informed about the pros and cons of both

Nocturnal polyuria present and normal daytime voided volume	Nocturnal polyuria present and maximum voided volume is low	Nocturnal urine output is normal and low maximum daytime voided volumes
↓	↓	↓
Desmopressin	Consider combination therapy: Desmopressin and Alarm	Alarm

Regardless of the initial strategy, if the first choice of therapy (alarm or desmopressin) did not make the child dry then the other alternative should be offered. If both fail as monotherapy, a combination of the two can be considered.

dry for 14 days, alarm use can be discontinued in a structured fashion. Dry bed training refers to "over training" beyond achieving dryness, once success has been achieved with the alarm. The child is encouraged to drink more water before bedtime and continue to use the alarm till she/he is dry.

Desmopressin is a synthetic vasopressin analogue that is the management of choice when nocturnal polyuria is present, alarm therapy alone fails, or when alarm is not acceptable. It is also the most advisable form of treatment for special occasions such as for stayovers and camps. It may be of special use during menstruation in girls who have attained menarche. There is a risk of hyponatremia associated with use of the drug; hence, fluid restriction after evening is advised when desmopressin is prescribed. For this reason, it is preferable to use the lyophilisate (MELT) tablet, of 120 and 240 µg, instead of the intranasal spray, which carries risk of inadvertent overdosing. The parents are advised to give a tablet an hour before bedtime; evening fluid should be restricted to <200 mL and the last drink should be consumed 1 hr before giving desmopressin. A response is seen within 1–2 weeks. In case there is no response in 2 weeks, desmopressin should be discontinued. For those who become dry, treatment should be continued for 6–24 months with 1 week interruption every 3 months to see if enuresis has resolved.

Children who do not respond to either alarm or desmopressin should be reevaluated for any missed primary disorder, e.g., a neurological cause and for comorbid factors that might need to be treated. If these are ruled out or treated and the child continues to be symptomatic, the child has therapy resistant enuresis that requires treatment and evaluation by experts.

Anticholinergics (oxybutynin or tolterodine) are second line agents, that might be considered when there is evidence of bladder overactivity causing or contributing to enuresis, or as an adjunct to desmopressin. Constipation must be treated prior to starting these medications. Children on anticholinergic medications need to be evaluated for increasing postvoid residue (PVR) by ultrasonography of the bladder every 3–6 months. In case of side effects, other medications such as mirabegron may be used.

The third line drug imipramine has serotonergic, anticholinergic, and noradrenergic actions on the bladder; it decreases urine production and improves arousal. The chief side effect is cardiotoxicity. The medication should be used under supervision, and only if there is failure of, or contraindication to use of, first- and second-line drugs. The recommended dose is 25 mg for children 6–9 years of age, and 50 mg for older children. Response is usually seen after 1 month. If found effective, drug free periods of 1–2 weeks are recommended to prevent development of tolerance. Finally, the drug must be tapered gradually before stopping.

Overactive Bladder

It is the most common of all voiding disorders seen in children, characterized by small, frequent voids with urgency and daytime incontinence with or without enuresis. Patients exhibit holding maneuvers, more to prevent accidents rather than to postpone voiding. They may also complain of suprapubic and perineal pain, and constipation. History and voiding diary are adequate for diagnosis **(Table 19.4)**. Acute cystitis and hypercalciuria

TABLE 19.4: Voiding diary of an 8-year-old boy shows that he voids 11 times/day (increased frequency). While the expected bladder capacity (EBC) is 270 (175–405) mL, the maximum voided volume (first morning void being excluded) is 100 mL (low volume voids). During daytime, he shows one episode of urge incontinence, suggesting an overactive bladder

Drink volume	*Time*	*Voided volume*	*Remarks*
200 mL milk	7.30 AM	130 mL	
250 mL	10.45 AM	50 mL	
	11.30 AM	60 mL	
	1.15 PM	100 mL	
260 mL	3.30 PM	60 mL	
	5 PM	80 mL	Urgency; wet
100 mL tea	6 PM	60 mL	
	7.30 PM	100 mL	
180 mL	8.45 PM	80 mL	
100 mL	10.30 PM	60 mL	
	11.00 PM	50 mL	

can mimic overactive bladder (OAB), but in these conditions the patient is uncomfortable due to dysuria and fever. Although not necessary for diagnosis, uroflowmetry shows a "tower shaped" curve **(Fig. 19.9)**. Management involves treatment of constipation and urotherapy. The anticholinergic medication, oxybutynin, is given at a dose of 0.3 mg/kg/day in two divided doses. Its effect should be evaluated 6–8 weeks later; side effects include constipation and an increased PVR. For children who do not improve, dual anticholinergic therapy or treatment with mirabegron, an adrenergic receptor stimulant may be considered. Idiopathic OAB is a self-limited condition, and a trial of discontinuing medications should be attempted after 3 months. As mentioned earlier, TENS has been used for OAB.

Underactive Bladder

A child with an underactive bladder, is often brought to attention due to recurrent UTI, daytime dribbling, incontinence, and voiding three or fewer times/day **(Table 19.5)**. Due to incomplete emptying, the bladder becomes large and the mucosal proprioception decreases, setting up a vicious circle. The child may also give a history of having to strain (and recruit the abdominal muscles), i.e., use the Valsalva maneuver to void. Ultrasonography shows large PVR, and uroflowmetry demonstrates an interrupted pattern or a flat prolonged curve **(Fig. 19.9)**.

Management includes treatment of UTI and constipation, if present. The child with recurrent UTI may be initiated on uroprophylaxis till the voiding frequency and volume improve and PVR decreases. Urotherapy includes instructions for timed voiding (every 2–3 hr) and double voiding to empty the bladder of the PVR. Those who present late and continue to have large residues, may require clean intermittent catheterization. Others who can empty their bladder with double or triple voiding during the day, may need an overnight bladder catheter drainage in case there is deterioration of renal functions, upper tract dilatation or recurrent UTI.

Dysfunctional Voiding

This term is used for the abnormal, simultaneous contraction of the urethral sphincter even as the detrusor contracts during voiding **(Figs. 19.12A and B)**.

TABLE 19.5: Voiding diary of a 10-year-old boy with an underactive bladder. The expected bladder capacity is 330 mL (range 214–430 mL); but the child shows relatively large bladder volumes and voids infrequently (<4 times)

Time	*Voided volume*
7 AM	500
2 PM	600
11 PM	550

This results in a high pressure in the bladder and incomplete voiding, predisposing these children to vesicoureteric reflux and pyelonephritis. The patient, usually a girl, is brought to attention with UTI and may have a history of holding maneuvers and constipation. Ultrasonography shows a variable combination of hydroureteronephrosis, increased PVR, and a thickened bladder wall, with perhaps a loaded colon. The characteristic finding on uroflowmetry is a staccato curve with simultaneous pelvic floor activity on EMG. Micturating cystourethrography (MCU) shows lack of opening of the bladder neck during the voiding phase, and in girls a dilated urethra described as a "spinning top appearance" **(Fig. 19.13)**. The clinical features might raise a suspicion of a neurogenic bladder. Magnetic resonance imaging (MRI) of lumbosacral spine helps differentiate a neurogenic cause

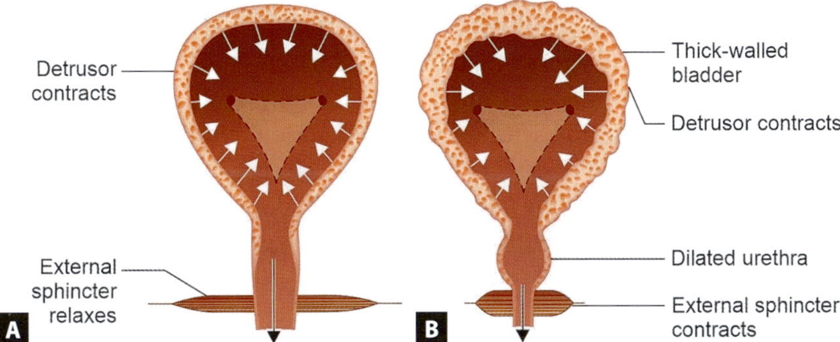

Figs. 19.12A and B: Detrusor sphincter dyssynergia. (A) During normal voiding, when the detrusor contracts, the sphincter(s) relaxes to allow urine to flow freely; (B) In children with dysfunctional voiding, when the detrusor contracts, the sphincter also contracts, resulting in incomplete voiding, residual urine, and urinary tract infections. Over time, patients may develop a thick-walled bladder and dilated urethra

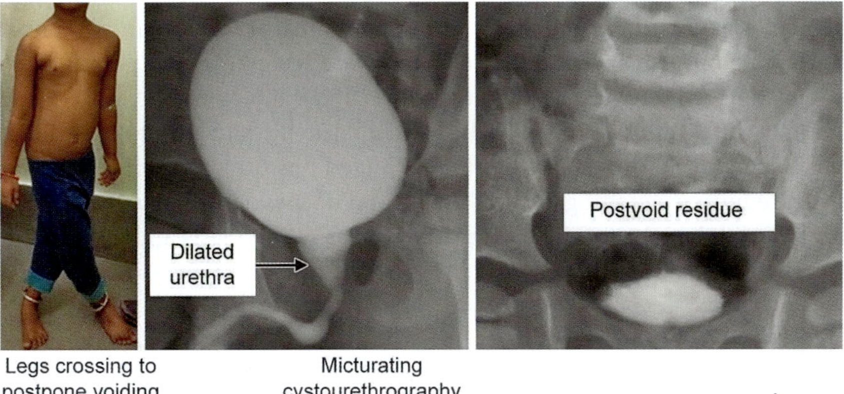

Fig. 19.13: A 6-year-old girl with dyfunctional voiding, crossing her legs to postpone voiding. The voiding film of her micturating cystourethrography shows "spinning top" appearance of the dilated urethra, and postvoid film shows significant residual volume

such as a tethered chord from idiopathic dysfunctional voiding. If the patient is a male, a close differential diagnosis is bladder outlet obstruction and cystoscopy may therefore be required. Management entails treatment of the UTI, followed by uroprophylaxis till the time that the voiding pattern improves and there is minimal or no PVR. Treatment of constipation, and all the measures of urotherapy should be instituted. These children benefit from the use of α blockers (tamsulosin 0.4–0.8 mg/day; terazosin 0.5 mg/day, increase if required up to 2 mg/day) and pelvic floor muscle rehabilitation, especially animated biofeedback. For resistant cases, TENS of the tibial nerve or injection of botulinum toxin into the external sphincter have been used.

Extraordinary Daytime Frequency Syndrome (Pollakiuria)

Usually a toilet trained child, otherwise in good health, presents with acute onset of passing small volume (10–15% expected bladder capacity) and frequent voids (almost every 10–15 minutes). There is no associated incontinence, dysuria, abdominal or flank pain, or change in bowel habits, and no night-time symptoms like increased frequency or enuresis. A differential diagnosis of cystitis and hypercalciuria should be considered. The condition is self-limiting and resolves within days to weeks. The parents may be encouraged to identify an emotional trigger, if any. Management entails reassurance of the parents and the child.

Vaginal Reflux

This condition is typically seen in overweight toilet-trained girls, who experience incontinence immediately upon standing up after voiding using a *western style* toilet. They usually do not have other lower urinary tract symptoms. These girls have a habit of voiding with their legs closely adducted. This results in vaginal reflux of urine that dribbles out as soon as the child is upright. Diagnosis is based upon history and demonstrating a lack of incontinence if the child voids in the correct posture, i.e., completely removing her underpants, so that the legs are abducted while voiding. The parents can be advised that initially the child can be made to sit on the toilet seat facing backwards to ensure the abducted posture or use of the Indian toilet requiring squatting. Vaginal reflux and postvoid dribbling is also seen in girls with labial adhesions **(Fig. 19.5)**; these require lysis and application of estrogen cream.

Giggle Incontinence

This refers to large volume incontinence seen during or immediately after giggling or laughing and is seen in 7–15 years old girls. Patients show normal cystometry between episodes. A possible centrally mediated pathogenesis is postulated. Management is by pelvic floor muscle retraining. Some patients respond to therapy with methylphenidate at a dose of 0.2–0.5 mg/kg/day in three divided doses.

Bladder Bowel Dysfunction

Bladder bowel dysfunction (BBD), previously referred to as dysfunctional elimination syndrome, refers to coexistence of any of the voiding disorders with constipation or fecal incontinence. Most children who present with bladder symptoms have concurrent bowel disorders which are missed unless looked for. The likely reasons for the concurrence have been discussed in the introduction. Success with the management of a voiding disorder is unlikely if coexisting constipation is not addressed earlier or concomitantly. Treatment of constipation alone at times can resolve the voiding disorder. It is important to treat constipation adequately and over a longer duration of time to yield results. Autism spectrum disorder and ADHD may often be associated conditions. Children with BBD suffer from low self-esteem, shame, isolation, and poor school performance, especially if they have episodes of urinary or fecal incontinence. Management is directed at management of constipation and of the specific voiding disorder.

Management of Constipation

Management begins with explaining to the parents and the child regarding the close connection between the bowel and the bladder. To take advantage

TABLE 19.6: Drugs used for the treatment of constipation

Drug	*Dose*	*Side effects*
Disimpaction		
Oral polyethylene glycol	1.5–2 g/kg/d PO, in two divided doses for 3–6 days	Loose stools, bloating, flatulence, nausea, vomiting
Rectal phosphate enema	2–18 years: 2.5 mL/kg, maximum 133 mL/dose	Hyperphosphatemia, hypocalcemia
Maintenance		
Osmotic agents		
Polyethylene glycol (PEG 3350)	>1 year: 4.25–17 g/d	Bloating, flatulence, nausea, vomiting
Lactulose	1–3 mL/kg OD or BD	Abdominal distension
Lactitol monohydrate	250–400 mg/kg/d (10 mg/15 mL)	
Stimulants		
Senna	3–10 years: 5 mg/d >10 years: 10 mg/d	Abdominal pain, diarrhea
Bisacodyl	5 mg every other day, can increase to 10 mg daily	Abdominal pain, diarrhea

of the gastrocolic response, the parents are advised to make the child sit in the toilet, 2–3 times a day, for 5–10 minutes after each meal. If using an English toilet/potty seat, it is important to have appropriate angulation of knees so that thighs are parallel to the floor and feet are resting on either the floor or on a stool. This comfortable posture helps ensure complete bowel emptying. Here too, a star chart (positive reinforcement) for agreed upon behavior is useful. Though not evidence based, a high fiber diet containing cereals, whole pulses with bran, vegetables, and fruits is recommended along with adequate water intake. Children who have chronic constipation often have palpable fecoliths. These will need disimpaction and occasionally enemas prior to treating the constipation. Thereafter all children with constipation require maintenance therapy with osmotic agents, with or without stimulants **(Table 19.6)**. Maintenance therapy should be continued for 3–6 months and tapered gradually to ensure sustained effects especially with the bowel evacuation routine.

BIBLIOGRAPHY

1. Austin PF, Bauer SB, Bower W, et al. The standardization of terminology of lower urinary tract function in children and adolescents: Update report from the standardization committee of the International Children's Continence Society (ICCS). Neurourol Urodyn. 2016;35:471-81.
2. Middleton T, Ellsworth P. Pharmacologic therapies for the management of non-neurogenic urinary incontinence in children. Expert Opin Pharmacother. 2019;20:2335-52.
3. Neveus T, Estrada CR, Austin PF. Bladder disorders. In: Emma F, Goldstein SL, Bagga A, Bates CM, Shroff R, eds. Pediatric Nephrology, 8th edn. Switzerland: Springer, Switzerland; 2022. pp. 1400-08.
4. Nevéus T, Fonseca E, Franco I, et al. Management and treatment of nocturnal enuresis. J Pediatr Urol. 2020;16:10-19.
5. Nieuwhof-Leppink AJ, Hussong J, Chase J, et al. Definitions, indications and practice of urotherapy in children and adolescents. J Pediatr Urol. 2021;17:172-81.
6. Yachha SK, Srivastava A, Mohan N, et al; Indian Society of Pediatric Gastroenterology, Hepatology and Nutrition. Management of childhood functional constipation. Indian Pediatr. 2018;55:885-92.

CHAPTER 20

Tubular Diseases

Aditi Sinha, Arvind Bagga

INTRODUCTION

Prompt diagnosis of tubular disorders is important since appropriate management is possible and delayed treatment might lead to irreversible growth delay and other complications. The diagnosis of a primary tubular disorder implies that there is no significant impairment of glomerular filtration or tubulointerstitial inflammation. Thus, tubular dysfunction observed in glomerular (e.g., focal segmental glomerulosclerosis) and cystic diseases is regarded as secondary. A tubular disorder may be congenital or acquired. It may involve a single function of the tubule [e.g., renal glucosuria, nephrogenic diabetes insipidus (NDI)] or multiple functions (e.g., Fanconi syndrome). A primary tubulopathy is usually congenital and hereditary, and often involves a single tubular function. Secondary derangement of tubular function is usually acquired due to endogenous or exogenous toxic substances and involves multiple functions.

The most common symptom of tubular disorders is poor growth or failure to thrive. Other clinical features include delayed motor milestones, polyuria, excessive thirst, recurrent episodes of dehydration, vomiting or fever, rickets, bone pains, weakness, constipation, and craving for salt and savory foods. Most disorders are diagnosed based on simple and readily available urine and plasma biochemical tests (*see* Chapter 2). This involves estimation of glomerular filtration rate (GFR), renal ultrasound, and quantitative determinations of various substances in the blood and urine. Plasma levels of inorganic phosphate and amino acids may fluctuate during the day, due to several factors including dietary intake. The normal values and ranges of various substances and their renal handling are related to age.

RENAL TUBULAR ACIDOSIS

Renal tubular acidosis (RTA) comprises a group of tubular transport defects characterized by inability to appropriately acidify the urine with resultant metabolic acidosis. The underlying abnormality is an impaired bicarbonate reabsorption or excretion of H^+ ions or their combination, occurring in absence of or out of proportion to impairment in the GFR.

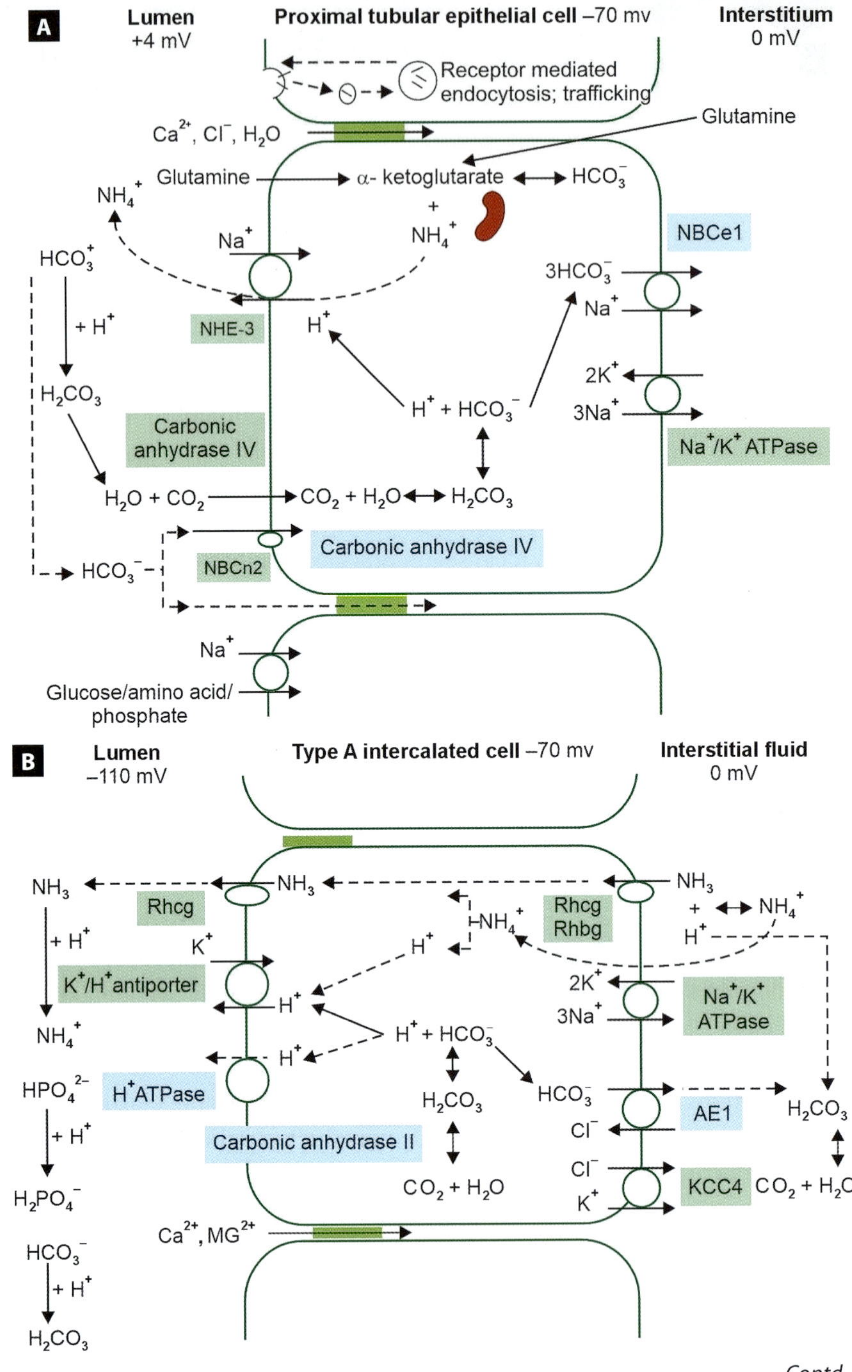
A
Lumen
+4 mV
Proximal tubular epithelial cell –70 mv
Interstitium
0 mV
Receptor mediated endocytosis; trafficking
Glutamine
Ca2+, Cl–, H2O
Glutamine
α- ketoglutarate
HCO3–
NH4+
+
NH4+
Na+
NBCe1
HCO3–
3HCO3–
Na+
+ H+
NHE-3
H+
2K+
H2CO3
H+ + HCO3–
3Na+
Carbonic anhydrase IV
Na+/K+ ATPase
H2O + CO2
CO2 + H2O
H2CO3
Carbonic anhydrase IV
HCO3–
NBCn2
Na+
Glucose/amino acid/ phosphate
B
Lumen
–110 mV
Type A intercalated cell –70 mv
Interstitial fluid
0 mV
NH3
Rhcg
NH3
NH3
Rhcg
Rhbg
NH4+
+
NH4+
H+
+ H+
K+
H+
K+/H+ antiporter
H+
2K+
3Na+
Na+/K+ ATPase
NH4+
H+ + HCO3–
H+
HPO42–
H+ATPase
H2CO3
HCO3–
AE1
H2CO3
+ H+
Cl–
Carbonic anhydrase II
Cl–
H2PO4–
CO2 + H2O
K+
KCC4
CO2 + H2O
Ca2+, MG2+
HCO3–
+ H+
H2CO3

Contd...

Contd...

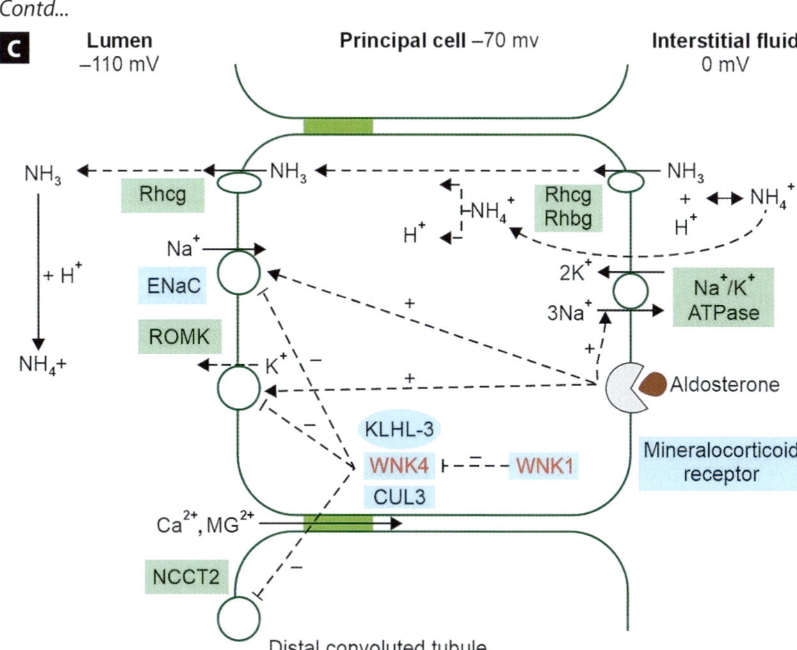

Figs. 20.1A to C: Mechanisms of acid base homeostasis in the kidney. Blue colored text boxes indicate the channels or proteins affected in patients with renal tubular acidosis (RTA). *(A) Bicarbonate absorption and ammoniagenesis in proximal tubule.* H^+ is secreted into the lumen by the sodium (Na^+)-exchanger-3 (NHE-3). Secreted H^+ combines with filtered luminal HCO_3^- to form H_2CO_3, which dissociates to H_2O and CO_2. These diffuse into the cell to form H_2CO_3. HCO_3^- and Na^+ cross the basolateral membrane using Na^+/HCO_3^- cotransporter/exchanger 1 (NBCe1). Na^+ exits the cell via active transport by Na^+/K^+ ATPase. Electrogenic H^+ secretion generates a small lumen-positive voltage promoting paracellular flow of cations. NH_4^+ is generated in the mitochondria and utilizes NHE-3 for exit to the luminal aspect. Luminal NH_4^+ is partly reabsorbed in the thick ascending limb of Henle and accumulates in the interstitium. Proximal tubular cells are also the site of Na^+ coupled reabsorption of glucose, amino acids and PO_4^{3-}. (B) *Distal acidification in cortical collecting ducts.* α-intercalated cells actively secrete H^+, through the H^+ ATPase and H^+/K^+ antiporter. HCO_3^- ions generated intracellularly exit the cell by the HCO_3^-/Cl^- exchanger (anion exchanger 1, AE1). Ammonia (NH_3) enters the intercalated and principal cells through Rhesus glycoproteins (Rhbg, Rhcg) and is secreted into the lumen through Rhcg. Secreted H^+ is buffered by HPO_4^{2-} to $H_2PO_4^-$ (titratable acidity) and by luminal ammonia to NH_4^+. *(C) H^+ and K^+ secretion in collecting ducts.* Principal cells mediate Na^+ absorption and K^+ secretion. The apical membrane has the amiloride sensitive epithelial sodium channel (ENaC); Na^+ exits basolaterally via Na^+/K^+ ATPase. Aldosterone binding to its receptor (MR) enhances Na^+ absorption by ENaC and basolateral exchange by Na^+/K^+ ATPase, K^+ secretion through renal outer medullary potassium (ROMK) channels, and H^+ secretion by H^+ ATPase. WNK-kinase 4 interacts with sodium chloride symporter (NCC), ENaC, and ROMK channels in an inhibitory manner; WNK-kinase 1 further inhibits WNK-kinase 4. Kelch-like 3 (KLHL3) and cullin 3 (CUL3) proteins promote degradation of WNK-kinase 4. Aldosterone synthesis is stimulated by hyperkalemia and by hypovolemia-induced increase in angiotensin II. Angiotensin II directly stimulates ENaC (and also enhances sodium reabsorption elsewhere, proximally by the Na^+/H^+ antiporter, and distally by the sodium chloride cotransporter, NCCT) but inhibits ROMK mediated K^+ secretion. Hence, hypovolemia is associated with maximal Na^+ reabsorption and conservation of K^+ while hyperkalemia is associated with increased Na^+ absorption by the ENaC and coupled secretion of K^+ through the ROMK

Normal Physiology

Approximately 60% of the filtered sodium (Na^+) is reabsorbed in the proximal segments, along with water, potassium (K^+), bicarbonate (HCO_3^-), phosphate, amino acids, and low molecular weight proteins. Several distinct transport mechanisms exist for reabsorption of different substances, carriers often mediating the transfer of solutes across the cell membrane. In contrast, the distal tubule has important roles in the fine adjustment of sodium reabsorption, excretion of potassium, maximum urinary acidification, and urinary concentration. **Figures 20.1A to C** illustrate the mechanisms of proximal bicarbonate absorption and distal tubular proton and potassium excretion. Sodium transport by principal cells creates a lumen negative transepithelial potential that promotes proton (H^+) secretion by intercalated cells.

The renin angiotensin aldosterone system (RAS) increases renal Na^+ retention during hypovolemia and K^+ secretion during hyperkalemia **(Figs. 20.1 and 20.2)**. Angiotensin II increases sodium reabsorption by the sodium/hydrogen exchanger 3 in the proximal tubule but also enhances distal sodium absorption by sodium chloride cotransporter (NCCT) in distal convoluted tubules and epithelial sodium channel (ENaC) in the late distal convoluted tubules and cortical collecting ducts. Aldosterone stimulates sodium uptake by NCCT and ENaC and increases potassium secretion by the renal outer medullary potassium channel (ROMK) along the entire distal nephron. Aldosterone also influences H^+ secretion by the intercalated cells of the cortical collecting duct, both directly by increased expression of H^+ ATPase and carbonic anhydrase and indirectly by enhanced lumen electronegativity through Na^+ reabsorption.

Etiology of Renal Tubular Acidosis

Two major varieties of RTA are observed in children, distal RTA (dRTA, type I) and proximal RTA (pRTA, type II); a third form (type IV) characterized by hypoaldosteronism and hyperkalemia is rare. **Table 20.1** lists inherited conditions associated with RTA, while acquired causes of RTA are listed in **Table 20.2**.

Type I (Distal) Renal Tubular Acidosis

This is characterized by metabolic acidosis secondary to decreased secretion of H^+ ions, resulting in lower values for titrable acidity and NH_4^+ secretion than required to keep pace with daily acid production. In *hypokalemic dRTA* (classic RTA or type I RTA), urine pH cannot reach maximal acidity (i.e., remains >5.3) despite systemic acidemia indicating low H^+ concentration in the collecting duct. The condition is secondary to either a secretory (rate) defect or a gradient (permeability) defect. In the former, the rate of secretion

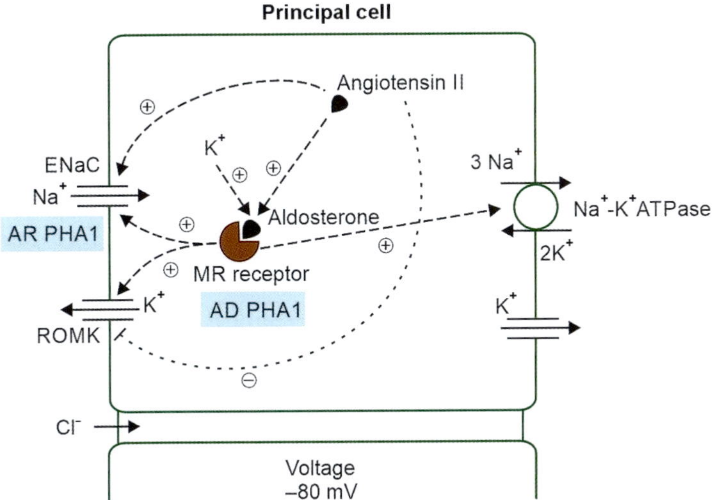

Fig. 20.2: Mechanism of mineralocorticoid action. Principal cells mediate sodium (Na^+) absorption and potassium (K^+) transport. The apical membrane contains an amiloride sensitive Na^+ channel (epithelial sodium channel, ENaC); Na^+ exits basolaterally via Na^+/K^+ ATPase. Sodium transport creates a lumen negative transepithelial potential that increases the rate of H^+ secretion by intercalated cells. Aldosterone secretion is stimulated by hypovolemia induced increase in angiotensin II and by hyperkalemia. Its binding to the mineralocorticoid receptor (MR) enhances Na^+ absorption by the ENaC, basolateral exchange by the Na^+/K^+ ATPase, and increases expression of renal outer medullary potassium (ROMK) channels that mediate K^+ secretion. Further, angiotensin II directly stimulates ENaC (in addition to increasing proximal tubular absorption of Na^+ by the Na^+/H^+ antiporter and distal convoluted tubule Na^+ chloride cotransporter, NCCT) but inhibits ROMK mediated K^+ excretion. Hence, hypovolemia is associated with maximal Na^+ reabsorption and conservation of K^+, while hyperkalemia is associated with increased Na^+ delivery to the collecting duct, increased absorption by the ENaC, and coupled secretion of K^+ through the ROMK. Textboxes indicate the channel/ receptor affected in patients with autosomal dominant (AD) and autosomal recessive (AR) forms of pseudohypoaldosteronism type 1 (PHA1)

of H^+ is low for the degree of acidosis, e.g., secondary to defective function of H^+ ATPase, H^+/K^+ ATPase, or the Cl^-/HCO_3^- exchanger **(Fig. 20.1)**. The gradient (permeability) defect is characterized by an appropriate rate of H^+ secretion but an increased backleak, resulting in dissipation of the pH gradient. Hypokalemia is attributed to increased tubular losses of potassium that are enhanced by RAS stimulation following urinary Na^+ losses and volume contraction. Hypercalciuria and hyperphosphaturia occur due to the release of calcium phosphate from bone in order to buffer excess H^+ during acidosis, acidosis-induced downregulation of renal Ca^{2+} transport proteins and increased distal sodium delivery. Hypocitraturia results from citrate utilization in proximal tubular cells, and due to the high luminal pH favoring conversion of citrate^{3-} to the readily reabsorbable citrate^{1-}. Persistent acidosis and hypercalciuria lead to nephrocalcinosis.

TABLE 20.1: Inherited forms of renal tubular acidosis (RTA)

Gene[#]	*Protein*	*Nonrenal manifestation or syndrome*
TYPE 1 (distal)		
SCL4A1[#1]	Anion exchanger 1 (AE1)	AD: none; AR: hemolytic anemia (Southeast Asian ovalocytosis, spherocytosis type 4)
ATP6V1B1	B1 subunit of H^+-ATPase	Early onset deafness
ATP6V0A4	A4 subunit of H^+-ATPase	Normal hearing or delayed hearing loss
ATP6V1C2	C2 subunit of H^+-ATPase	Normal hearing
FOXI1	Forkhead box I1	Early onset deafness
WDR72	Tryptophan-aspartate repeat domain 72	Amelogenesis imperfecta
TYPE 2 (proximal)		
SCL4A4	Sodium bicarbonate cotransporter 1 (NBC1)	Band keratopathy, cataract; defective enamel; intellectual disability, basal ganglia calcification
Fanconi syndrome		
SLC2A2	Glucose transporter GLUT2	Fanconi Bickel syndrome: hypo-/hyperglycemia, diabetes; hepatomegaly; rickets
GATM[#4,$]	Glycine amidinotransferase	Fanconi renotubular syndrome type 1; rickets^
SLC34A1	Sodium-dependent phosphate transporter 2A	Fanconi renotubular syndrome type 2; rickets^
EHHADH[#4]	Enoyl-CoA hydratase; hydroxyacyl dehydrogenase	Fanconi renotubular syndrome type 3; rickets
HNF4A	Hepatocyte nuclear factor 4A	Fanconi renotubular syndrome type 4; maturity onset diabetes type 1; macrosomia
NDUFAF6	NADH: ubiquinone oxidoreductase complex assembly factor 6	Fanconi renotubular syndrome type 5; pulmonary interstitial fibrosis
CLCN5[#2]	Renal chloride channel	Dent disease: night blindness; nephrocalcinosis; rickets^
OCRL1[#2]	Phosphatidyl inositol bisphosphate phosphatase	Lowe syndrome: cataracts, seizures, cryptorchidism ^
CTNS	Cystinosin	Cystinosis: photophobia; hypothyroidism; hypogonadism; pancreas deficiency; cerebral atrophy^

Contd...

Contd...

Gene[#]	*Protein*	*Nonrenal manifestation or syndrome*
FAH	Fumarylacetoacetate hydrolase	Tyrosinemia type 1: chronic liver disease; rickets
ATP7B	ATPase, Cu^{2+}-transporting polypeptide	Wilson disease: chronic liver disease; neurological manifestations
GALT	Galactose-1-phosphate uridylyltransferase	Galactosemia: chronic liver disease; cataract; hypoglycemia; hypotonia
ALDOB	Fructose-1-phosphate aldolase	Hereditary fructose intolerance: chronic liver disease; hypoglycemia
G6PC	Glucose-6-phosphatase-α	Glycogen storage disease type I a
SLC37A4	Glucose 6 phosphate translocase	Glycogen storage disease type II b
VPS33B	Vacuolar protein sorting	ARC syndrome type 1: arthrogryposis; cholestasis; microcephaly; DI
VIPAS39	VPS33B-interacting protein, SPE39 homolog	ARC syndrome type 2: arthrogryposis; cholestasis; microcephaly; DI
Multiple[*#3]	Multiple defects described	Mitochondrial disorders
TYPE 3 (combined)		
CA2	Carbonic anhydrase type II (CAII)	Osteopetrosis, blindness, deafness, mental retardation
TYPE 4 (hyperkalemic)		
MR (NR3C2)[#4]	Mineralocorticoid receptor (MR)	Pseudohypoaldosteronism type 1
SCNN1B	Epithelial sodium channel (ENaC)	Pseudohypoaldosteronism type 1
WNK4[#4,$]; *WNK1*[#4]; *KLHL3*[#1]; *CUL3*[#4]	Serine threonine (lysine deficient) protein kinases; Kelch-like protein-3, Cullin-3	Pseudohypoaldosteronism type 2, Gordon syndrome
CYP21 *CYP11B2*	21-hydroxylase Aldosterone synthase (11-β hydroxylase)	Congenital adrenal hyperplasia Congenital adrenal hyperplasia

[#]Defects are inherited in autosomal recessive manner, except as [1]autosomal dominant (AD) or autosomal recessive (AR); [2]X-linked; [3]maternal or sporadic; and [4]autosomal dominant. For list of all relevant genes, please see **Annexure 9.2**

*Examples include: *BCS1L*, *SURF1*, *COX10*, *TMEM70*, *SARS2*, *MRPS22*, *TSFM*, *C10orf2*, and *RRM2B*

[$]Defects that are caused by gain-of-function variations

[^]Defects that are associated with a high rate of progression to kidney failure

ARC: arthrogryposis, renal dysfunction, cholestasis; DI: diabetes insipidus; NADH: nicotinamide adenine dinucleotide, reduced (H) form

TABLE 20.2: Acquired defects causing renal tubular acidosis (RTA)

Type 1 (distal)	*Type 2 (proximal)*	*Type 4*
Systemic disease *Autoimmune:* Sjögren syndrome, systemic lupus, erythematosus, autoimmune hepatitis, primary biliary cirrhosis, autoimmune thyroiditis, rheumatoid arthritis *Others:* Sarcoidosis, Wilson disease, vitamin D toxicity, hyperparathyroidism, idiopathic hypercalciuria, medullary sponge kidney; post kidney transplant *Medications* Amphotericin B, ibuprofen, tacrolimus ***Voltage defects (hyperkalemic distal RTA)*** Obstructive uropathy; postobstructive state; sickle cell disease; systemic lupus; erythematosus; lithium, allograft rejection	*Medications and toxins* *Anticancer:* Ifosfamide, cisplatin, oxaliplatin, streptozocin *Anticonvulsants:* Valproate, topiramate *Antivirals*: Tenofovir, adefovir, didanosine, lamivudine, stavudine, cidofovir *Antibiotics*: Aminoglycosides, expired tetracyclines *Others:* Deferasirox, lenalidomide, heavy metals, acetazolamide, ranitidine, zoledronic acid, apremilast; L-lysine and L-arginine; aristolochic acid (Chinese herb nephropathy); fumaric acid; suramin; paraquat *Systemic disease:* Amyloidosis; post kidney transplant; focal glomerulosclerosis; metachromatic leukodystrophy; cyanotic heart disease; vitamin D deficiency, hyperparathyroidism; multiple myeloma, light chain disease; paroxysmal nocturnal hemoglobinuria	***Reduced aldosterone production*** Primary adrenal insufficiency; critical illness *Medications:* NSAIDs, ACE inhibitors, angiotensin receptor blockers; heparin; β blockers; CNI *Hyporeninemic hypoaldosteronism:* Interstitial nephritis, diabetic nephropathy ***Aldosterone resistance*** *Systemic:* Sickle cell disease, systemic lupus *Medications:* Spironolactone, eplerenone; amiloride, triamterene, trimethoprim, pentamidine; CNI *Pseudohypoaldosteronism type 3* *Transient:* Infants with urinary tract infection; after relief of obstruction in obstructive uropathy

ACE: angiotensin converting enzyme; CNI: calcineurin inhibitors; NSAID: nonsteroidal anti-inflammatory drugs

Incomplete dRTA refers to milder variants in which defective tubular H^+ secretion does not lead to systemic acidosis since daily acid excretion is enabled by enhanced ammoniagenesis.

Distal RTA with hyperkalemia may occur due either to (*i*) voltage defect caused by insufficient negative intratubular potential at the level of cortical collecting duct leading to failure to generate and/or maintain an appropriate electrical gradient to favor H^+ secretion (hyperkalemic dRTA); or (*ii*) rate defect due to aldosterone deficiency or resistance (type IV RTA). The voltage defect leads to reduced secretion of H^+ and K^+, decreased trapping and excretion of NH_4^+ and hyper- or normokalemia. Apart from the latter finding, the voltage defect resembles classic dRTA.

Type II (Proximal) Renal Tubular Acidosis

The primary defect is bicarbonaturia due to reduced renal threshold for HCO_3^- excretion. Thus, at normal plasma bicarbonate level, 15% or more of filtered bicarbonate is excreted in urine. The distal acidification mechanism is intact. Once the plasma bicarbonate falls, the proximal tubule can reabsorb most of the filtered bicarbonate. Thus, in steady state, the daily acid loads are successfully excreted and these children do not progressively accumulate acid, unlike in dRTA. Primary isolated pRTA secondary to defective bicarbonate reabsorption is rare and occurs sporadically or as an autosomal recessive or dominant trait. Proposed mechanisms include deficient carbonic anhydrase on the brush border and defective pump secretion or function of the Na^+/HCO_3^- cotransporter, H^+ ATPase, Na^+/H^+ antiporter, and Na^+/K^+ ATPase **(Table 20.1; Fig. 20.1)**.

Proximal RTA is more commonly a part of generalized proximal tubular dysfunction, termed Fanconi syndrome, characterized by global dysfunction of proximal tubules, with tubular proteinuria, aminoaciduria, and variable degrees of bicarbonaturia, phosphaturia, electrolyte wasting, and glucosuria. There is, in addition, impaired reabsorption of water, bicarbonate, sodium, potassium, and organic acids. Plasma concentrations of glucose and amino acids are normal, but those of phosphate are low. Sporadic Fanconi syndrome is more common than autosomal recessive, autosomal dominant, and X linked recessive (Dent syndrome) forms. Among inherited conditions, cystinosis is common **(Table 20.1)**. Ifosfamide, used in the treatment of solid tumors, can lead to proximal tubular dysfunction in over 50% patients **(Table 20.2)**.

Type III Renal Tubular Acidosis

This term was suggested for a group of patients described earlier as having features of both pRTA and dRTA. Many patients with dRTA show transient features of proximal tubular dysfunction that recovers following correction of systemic acidosis. The criteria for type III RTA have been met in a group of patients with RTA, osteopetrosis, cerebral calcifications, and variable mental retardation secondary to mutations in *CAII* (located at 8q22) encoding isoform II of the enzyme carbonic anhydrase (Guibaud-Vainsel syndrome).

Type IV Renal Tubular Acidosis

This condition is characterized by hyperkalemic acidosis and intact ability to lower urine pH, and is caused by aldosterone resistance or deficiency **(Tables 20.1 and 20.2)**. Aldosterone increases urinary K^+ losses by enhancing its membrane permeability, increases Na^+ absorption resulting in a negative intratubular potential, stimulates basolateral Na^+/K^+/ATPase and directly stimulates the proton pump **(Fig. 20.2)**. Aldosterone deficiency or resistance thus causes hyperkalemic metabolic acidosis. Net H^+ excretion is decreased due to inhibition of ammoniagenesis by hyperkalemia. Although maximally acidic urine (pH <5.3) is formed, indicating the ability to establish a maximal H^+ gradient, ammonium excretion is low resulting in a positive anion gap.

Clinical Features

Distal RTA: The chief features, in infancy and early childhood, include marked failure to thrive, weakness, polyuria, and polydipsia. Later rachitic manifestations or osteomalacia is prominent. Hypokalemia is common and severe and may lead to muscle weakness, neck flop, and occasionally transient paralysis. Hypercalciuria, hypocitraturia, and high urine pH contribute to occurrence of nephrocalcinosis and stones. Incomplete forms of dRTA are suspected in patients presenting with nephrocalcinosis or nephrolithiasis without systemic acidosis; diagnosis is made on demonstrating hypercalciuria and inability to lower urinary pH when acidosis is induced pharmacologically.

In children, dRTA is almost always primary; presentation in later childhood should prompt evaluation for systemic lupus or Sjögren syndrome. The majority of patients with autosomal recessive dRTA have sensorineural deafness; ovalocytosis and hemolytic anemia may be seen in patients from South Asia. Patients with autosomal dominant dRTA present at an older age or during adulthood with milder disease.

Proximal RTA: Failure to thrive (growth retardation) is the chief clinical feature. Irritability, anorexia, and listlessness are present. Rachitic deformities are rare in isolated pRTA but striking in Fanconi syndrome. Nephrocalcinosis is uncommon except with Dent and Lowe syndrome. While symptoms related to hypokalemia (e.g., weakness, paralysis) are uncommon, hypokalemia and consequent polyuria are seen in Fanconi syndrome. Patients with Fanconi syndrome show glucosuria, aminoaciduria, citraturia, phosphate wasting with rickets or osteomalacia, tubular proteinuria, hypokalemia with polyuria, and uricosuria with hypouricemia. During infancy, polyuria, polydipsia, and recurrent episodes of dehydration and fever are common. Factors responsible for polyuria include osmotic diuresis due to presence of excessive amounts of solutes in the tubular fluids and impaired urinary concentration due to persistent hypokalemia.

Type IV RTA: Findings of the underlying disease (hypoaldosteronism or resistance to action of aldosterone) predominate over features of tubular acidosis. There is nephrocalcinosis or urolithiasis and bone disease is rare. Advanced tubulointerstitial diseases leading to mineralocorticoid resistance should be suspected, particularly in older children. Aldosterone unresponsiveness, associated with obstructive uropathy, is the most common cause of type IV RTA in children. Inherited causes, particularly congenital adrenal hyperplasia (CAH) secondary to 21-hydroxylase deficiency and the autosomal recessive form of pseudohypoaldosteronism (PHA type 1), should be considered in infants presenting with salt loss, hypotension, metabolic acidosis, and hyperkalemia; levels of plasma renin and aldosterone are high. The autosomal dominant form of PHA type 1 is less severe; symptoms improve with age.

Differential Diagnosis

Metabolic acidosis may result from extrarenal processes, which result in either increased endogenous acid synthesis (e.g., ketoacidosis) or enhanced bicarbonate losses. Intestinal and pancreatic secretions and bile have high quantities of HCO_3^-, therefore conditions such as diarrhea, removal of pancreatic or intestinal secretions or bile by tube drainage or fistula lead to loss of HCO_3^- and metabolic acidosis.

Hyperchloremic acidosis may also result from ureterosigmoidostomy due to presence in the colon of an anion exchange pump that absorbs luminal Cl^- (of urinary origin) and exchanges it for HCO_3^-, and due to colonic absorption of NH_4^+ (of urinary origin) that releases H^+ when metabolized in the liver. Cholestyramine causes metabolic acidosis by acting as anion exchange resins, where colonic luminal bile acids are exchanged for Cl^- released by the resin, resulting in bile acid complexes being excreted fecally.

Laboratory Findings

Evaluation in patients with metabolic acidosis and suspected RTA requires consecutive tests as follows.

Plasma anion gap: All types of RTA are associated with hyperchloremic normal anion gap metabolic acidosis. Assessment of the anion gap [serum $Na^+ - (Cl^- + HCO_3^-)$; normal: 8–12 mEq/L] helps distinguish RTA and diarrhea, that cause hyperchloremic acidosis with normal anion gap, from diabetic ketoacidosis, lactic acidosis, and other causes of wide anion gap acidosis (see Chapter 6). While advanced chronic kidney disease (CKD) with estimated glomerular filtration rate (eGFR) below 15 mL/min is associated with metabolic acidosis and elevated anion gap, patients with eGFR 20–50 mL/min often show normal anion gap acidosis.

Urinary ammonium excretion and urine anion gap (urine net charge): Regeneration of HCO_3^- consumed in the neutralization of nonvolatile acids is an important component of urinary acidification and involves excretion of titrable acid and ammonium (NH_4^+) ions. During chronic acidosis, NH_4^+ excretion is more important and may increase several folds (in adults, from 35–40 mmol/day to 200–300 mmol/day). Urinary NH_4^+ excretion is increased in the presence of an exogenous or endogenous acid load, or with extrarenal losses of HCO_3^-, as in diarrhea. In patients with RTA, urinary NH_4^+ remains low despite systemic acidosis. Hence, estimating urinary NH^+ excretion is important when evaluating patients with metabolic acidosis.

The difference between the sum of urinary Na^+ and K^+ and urinary Cl^-, termed urine anion gap (UAG), indirectly estimates NH_4^+ excretion. Unless the urine is very alkaline (pH >7.5), contribution of HCO_3^- to urinary anions is negligible. Since the sum of charges on urinary cations and anions is equal, and the difference between urinary unmeasured anions (sulfates, phosphates, and organic anions) and cations (calcium, magnesium) is fairly constant at about 80 mEq/L, hence:

$Na^+ + K^+ + NH_4^+ + \text{unmeasured cations} = Cl^- + \text{unmeasured anions}$

$NH_4^+ = (\text{unmeasured anions} - \text{unmeasured cations}) - (Na^+ + K^+ - Cl^-)$

$NH_4^+ = 80 - \text{Urine anion gap; or Urine anion gap} = 80 - NH_4^+$

Normally, the UAG is positive, about 30–35 mEq/L, due to the presence of dissolved anions. Patients with systemic acidosis from extrarenal HCO_3^- losses (e.g., diarrhea) have intact mechanisms of renal acidification resulting in enhanced NH_4^+ synthesis and excretion with Cl^- ions, causing the UAG to become negative. A positive UAG indicates inappropriately low renal NH_4^+ excretion, as seen in all forms of RTA.

The application of UAG as an index of urinary NH_4^+ excretion has some caveats. First, the UAG approximates NH_4^+ excretion only in patients with chronic, not acute, hyperchloremic metabolic acidosis. The validity of UAG is limited if the urine pH is >6.5, since HCO_3^- is then a significant urinary anion, which is not included in calculation of UAG. Here, the measurement of urine osmolal gap is more useful in estimating urinary NH_4^+ excretion. Finally, UAG might depend significantly on diet, since plant-based diets contain a lower net-acid load than animal-based diets.

Urine pH: Urine pH measures the concentration of free H^+ and assesses the integrity of distal H^+ secretion. In presence of systemic acidosis, urine pH is normally <5.3; pH >5.3 suggests defective distal urinary acidification.

Patients with acidosis (plasma HCO_3^- <15 mEq/L) due to pRTA or type IV RTA are able to acidify urine to achieve urine pH <5.3. It should, however, be understood that urine pH measures the concentration of free H^+ in the urine, which constitutes <1% of the total amount of H^+ secreted in the distal nephron. The use of urine pH alone for the diagnosis of dRTA in patients with systemic acidosis is not recommended, since most protons are excreted as NH_4^+ and as titrable acids.

The pH should be measured electrometrically on fresh voided specimen, as dipsticks are unreliable; urine left standing might get contaminated with urea splitting organisms, resulting in high urine pH.

Induced systemic acidosis: If systemic acidosis is absent, an oral load of ammonium chloride is given, followed by the measurement of urine pH and NH_4^+ excretion. A decline in plasma CO_2 content by 3–5 mEq/L is accompanied by fall in urine pH to <5.3. The *ammonium chloride test,* used chiefly to unmask the defect in renal acidification in patients with incomplete or partial dRTA and compensated systemic acidosis, is difficult to administer in children as ammonium chloride is unpalatable. Instead, the combination of furosemide (1 mg/kg) and fludrocortisone (0.025 mg/kg) is proposed as a suitable alternative (*fludrocortisone furosemide test*). An inability to lower urine pH below 5.3 during 6-hr following early morning oral administration of the combination suggests impaired distal acidification. Healthy individuals and patients with type IV RTA and pRTA show low urine pH (<5.3) and increase in K^+ excretion. In patients with hypokalemic dRTA, the urine pH does not fall but the K^+ excretion increases, indicating intact function of principal cells. Patients with hyperkalemic dRTA with defects in cortical Na^+ reabsorption do not show increase in H^+ or K^+ excretion since luminal electronegativity is not enhanced.

Bicarbonate loading test: Sodium bicarbonate is given orally or as an intravenous (IV) infusion, while measuring urine pH in timed samples collected under mineral oil. Loading is continued till consecutive samples show urine pH >7.5 and plasma HCO_3^- >22–24 mEq/L. The fractional excretion of HCO_3^- and urine to blood (U–B) CO_2 gradient are measured to enable characterization of RTA.

- *Fractional excretion of bicarbonate:* Proximal tubules normally reabsorb almost all filtered HCO_3^-. Following alkalization to normalize serum HCO_3^- (>22 mEq/L), $FEHCO_3$ provides a useful assessment of proximal tubular handling of HCO_3^-. While values >15% indicate pRTA, levels are in the normal range (<5%) in distal and type IV RTA.
- *Urine to blood CO_2 gradient:* Loading with sodium bicarbonate makes luminal HCO_3^- available to combine with H^+ secreted by distal tubules. Carbonic acid dehydrates to form CO_2 that is trapped in the tubular

lumen. In presence of urine pH >7.5 and normal plasma HCO_3^-, the urine pCO_2 should exceed 70 mm Hg and U–B pCO_2 gradient is >20 mm Hg if distal acidification is intact. Patients with decreased rates of tubular H^+ secretion (dRTA) show urine pCO_2 <50 mm Hg and U–B pCO_2 <10 mm Hg. Patients with other forms of RTA show normal urinary pCO_2 values.

Interpretation of Findings and Further Testing

The interpretation of the earlier mentioned tests is summarized in **Table 20.3** and **Flowchart 20.1**. Based on initial evaluation, additional tests may be useful.

Distal RTA: There usually is severe metabolic acidosis with blood pH below 7.2 and bicarbonate below 15 mEq/L. Serum potassium levels are decreased,

TABLE 20.3: Investigations to differentiate types of renal tubular acidosis (RTA)

	Proximal RTA	*Distal RTA*		*Type 4 RTA*
		Classic	*Hyperkalemic (voltage defect)*	
Plasma potassium	Normal/low	Low	High	High
Serum bicarbonate, mEq/L	12–20	Usually <12	Usually >17	Usually >17
Urine pH	<5.3	>5.3[1]	>5.3	<5.3
Urine anion gap	Positive	Positive	Positive	Positive
Urine ammonium	Low	Low	Low	Low
Fractional bicarbonate excretion	>10–15%	<5%[2]	<5%	>5–10%
U-B PCO_2, mm Hg	>20	<20[3]	</>20	>20
Urine calcium	Normal	High	High/normal	Normal/low
Other tubular defects (phosphaturia; low molecular weight proteinuria, generalized aminoaciduria, glucosuria)	Often present	Absent[2]	Absent	Absent
Nephrocalcinosis	Absent[4]	Present	Present/absent	Absent
Rickets	Common	Usually present	Uncommon	Absent

[1]Urine pH can be lowered below 5.3 in patients with mild rate-dependent defects
[2]Proximal tubular dysfunction might be present with severe acidosis, particularly in patients with *ATPV0A4* defects
[3]Urine to blood PCO_2 gradient (U-B PCO_2) might be >20 mm Hg in gradient (back-leak) defect
[4]Nephrocalcinosis might be present in certain forms of Fanconi syndrome, e.g., Dent syndrome, cystinosis, Lowe syndrome, and Fanconi Bickel syndrome

Flowchart 20.1: Evaluation of a patient with renal tubular acidosis (RTA). $FEHCO_3$: fractional excretion of bicarbonate; TTKG: transtubular potassium gradient; U–B CO_2: urine to blood CO_2 gradient

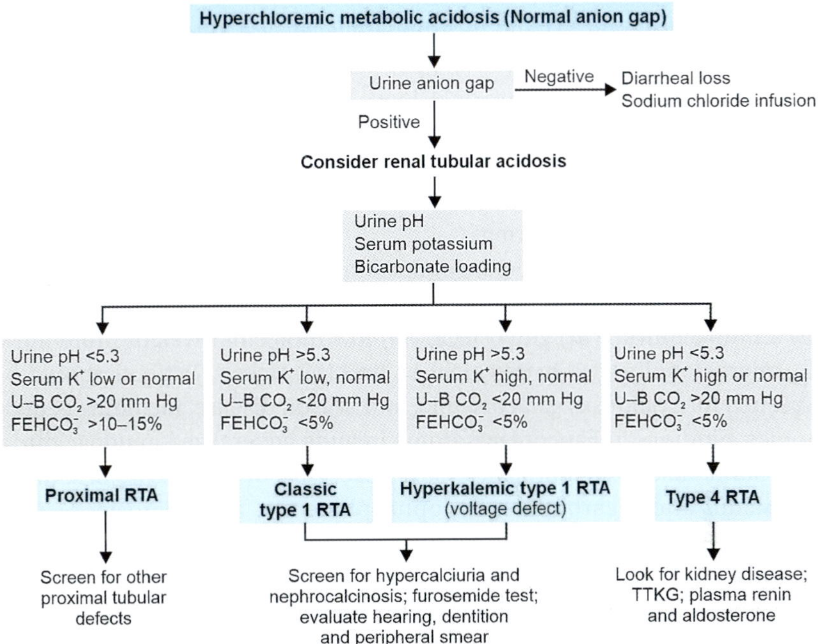

often below 3 mEq/L. Urine pH is >6. The proximal tubular reabsorption of bicarbonate is normal, but renal bicarbonate excretion may be 5–15% during infancy and in young children.

X-ray films usually show rickets. Most patients with untreated dRTA show hypercalciuria, defined as urinary calcium excretion >4 mg/kg/day or urine calcium/creatinine ratio >0.2 (beyond infancy). Hypocitraturia is difficult to document due to nonavailability of the test at many centers and lack of established normative values in children. High urine pH, hypercalciuria, and hypocitraturia favor the deposition of calcium in renal parenchyma resulting in renal calculi and/or nephrocalcinosis, detected on ultrasonography. All patients should undergo hearing evaluation. Evaluation for lupus, osteopetrosis, Sjögren syndrome, and chronic hepatitis is done in patients presenting at an older age. In patients with incomplete dRTA, failure of urinary acidification should be demonstrated pharmacologically using the fludrocortisone furosemide test.

Genetic testing should be offered to all patients with suspected inherited dRTA **(Annexure 9.2, p 845)**. Causative (pathogenic or likely pathogenic) variations are identified in 60–80% of patients with diagnosis of primary dRTA. Early presentation, especially in the first decade of life, is suggestive of inherited form of dRTA. A positive family history with dominant inheritance suggests *SLC4A1*; hemolytic anemia points to variations in anion exchanger;

sensorineural hearing loss suggests variations in either one of the H^+ pump subunits, or the transcription factor *FOXI1*; while an enamel disorder suggests variations in *WDR72*.

Proximal RTA: Blood pH and bicarbonate levels are low and the urine pH is relatively alkaline. However, the pH falls below 5.3 if systemic acidosis is induced by an exogenous acid load. The diagnosis is confirmed by determining the fractional excretion of bicarbonate. Following bicarbonate loading, >15% of filtered bicarbonate is excreted in urine. The difference between urine and blood pCO_2 is >20 mm Hg in this state. Urinary calcium and citrate excretion are normal.

All children with pRTA require evaluation for Fanconi syndrome, including secondary forms. These include assessment of (*i*) phosphate excretion, (*ii*) aminoaciduria, (*iii*) glucosuria, (*iv*) low molecular weight proteinuria (β_2-microglobulin), (*v*) hypercalciuria, and (*vi*) rickets. Patients should be screened for cystinosis, galactosemia, and Wilson disease, including genetic studies. Findings in Fanconi syndrome include generalized aminoaciduria, glucosuria, mild proteinuria, uricosuria, excessive urinary losses of sodium, potassium and bicarbonate, hypophosphatemia, and acidosis. As with isolated pRTA, excessive losses of bicarbonate are absent during sustained acidosis.

Hypophosphatemia secondary to impaired proximal tubular reabsorption is an important feature in Fanconi syndrome. Rickets is due to the combination of low levels of 1,25 $(OH)_2$ D, hypophosphatemia and acidosis. The fractional excretion of phosphate is determined on a timed (6-hr, 12-hr, or 24-hr) urine specimen and is normally <5–12%. The tubular reabsorption of phosphate (TRP, 100 – fractional excretion) is 88–95%. Since TRP varies with dietary phosphate intake, plasma phosphate levels and GFR, the tubular maximum for phosphate, corrected for GFR (TmP/GFR) is recommended as a sensitive tool of phosphate reabsorption. The normal value of TmP/GFR in adults is 2.2–4.2 mg/dL and varies by age. **Annexure 6 (p 823)** provides the Walter and Bijvoet nomogram, used to estimate tubular maximum reabsorption of phosphate (TmP)/GFR in adults and the thresholds provided by Brodehl, which are preferred in children.

Increased delivery of sodium to the distal tubule leads to enhanced exchange of sodium for potassium, adding to urinary potassium losses. Persistent hypokalemia leads to tubular dysfunction and impaired urinary concentration. The losses of amino acids and glucose in Fanconi syndrome are of no clinical significance. Normally 1–6 mg/kg of amino acids are excreted daily, of which 98% is reabsorbed in the proximal tubule. Glucosuria is due to a lowered renal tubular threshold; tubular maximum reabsorption for glucose is usually normal. Tubular proteinuria is mild, consisting of low molecular weight proteins (enzymes, hormones, and light chain immunoglobulin) and is of no clinical significance.

Type IV RTA: Patients with RTA, hyperkalemia, and ability to appropriately acidify urine are labeled as type IV RTA. Acidosis is mild in proportion to hyperkalemia. Ammonia excretion in these patients is low, but it is unclear whether this is due to direct inhibition of ammoniagenesis or secondary to hyperkalemia. Sodium excretion is increased, with or without consequent volume contraction.

Workup includes evaluation for obstructive uropathy or tubulointerstitial disease. Measurement of plasma renin activity and aldosterone levels are useful. The *transtubular potassium gradient* (TTKG) is useful in diagnosing type IV RTA and in conjunction with mineralocorticoid challenge helps distinguish deficiency from aldosterone resistance. This test is an index of K^+ gradient in the distal tubular lumen and interstitium and provides an accurate assessment of aldosterone effect on late distal and cortical collecting tubules in patients with hyperkalemia and normal renal function. Normal individuals have TTKG between 6 and 12; in presence of hyperkalemia, TTKG should rise to >10. Inappropriately low TTKG (<8) suggests hypoaldosteronism or tubular resistance to aldosterone; subsequent rise in TTKG to >7 upon administering fludrocortisone suggests hypoaldosteronism.

Management

Distal RTA: Hypokalemia should be treated before correction of acidosis. Acidosis can be corrected by administration of alkali solution (Uriliser, Shohl solution; see **Annexure 5, p 820**). The initial dose of alkali is 2–3 mEq/kg/day and is increased until the blood bicarbonate levels become normal. The initial amount of bicarbonate required for maintaining acid base status might be high at 5–10 mEq/kg/day; alkali requirements decrease after the age of 5 years but are required lifelong. The use of sodium bicarbonate, as an alkali supplement, should be avoided since high urinary sodium excretion worsens hypercalciuria. With adequate correction of acidosis, renal potassium losses are reduced but some patients require prolonged potassium supplements.

Subclinical acidosis results in bone demineralization and osteoporosis. If there is severe rickets and osteopenia, small doses of vitamin D may be given cautiously. Correction of acidosis results in a striking increase in the growth velocity. The growth velocity in infants increases within a few weeks but may take several months in older children. Early treatment leads to reduction of hypercalciuria and increase in urinary citrate excretion, preventing nephrocalcinosis. Urinary calcium excretion should be monitored; if hypercalciuria persists despite correction of acidosis, cautious administration of thiazides (hydrochlorothiazide 1–2 mg/kg/day) may be considered. Thiazides cause contraction of extracellular fluid volume and increase proximal HCO_3^- reabsorption. Hydrochlorothiazide increases K^+ excretion and, therefore, a part of the alkali should be administered as potassium citrate.

A high proportion of patients with defects in the H^+ATPase or *FOXI1* dRTA suffer from hearing loss, which requires monitoring during childhood, and is usually progressive. Hearing loss is not reversed with alkali therapy, and most patients will require hearing aids and/or cochlear implants. **Box 20.1** summarizes key recommendations of the European Rare Kidney Disease Reference network and European Society for Pediatric Nephrology on management of dRTA. Attention to extrarenal disease is important, e.g., patients with variations in H^+ ATPase subunits require screening for and management of hearing loss.

BOX 20.1: Summary of recommendations on the management of distal renal tubular acidosis (RTA)

Diagnosis

Patients with features suggestive of distal RTA should be comprehensively evaluated to ascertain the underlying diagnosis

Genetic studies should be done in all patients with suspected primary distal RTA

Patients who do not show a genetic cause should be revaluated to confirm the diagnosis, including results of genetic studies

Considering the difficulties in interpreting dual energy X-ray absorptiometry (DEXA) results in children, experts do not advise routine assessment of bone mineral density in children with distal RTA. For adults, assessment by DEXA (every 2–3 years) may be helpful in assessing fracture risk and treatment adequacy

Patients with nephrocalcinosis/lithiasis and borderline low bicarbonate levels should be screened for RTA by assessing urinary acidification, by ammonium chloride loading or the frusemide-fludrocortisone test. Similarly, patients with Sjögren syndrome and urolithiasis or hypokalemia should be assessed for RTA

Therapy

Patients with distal RTA should be treated with alkali supplements. Patients with persistent hypokalemia require additional potassium supplements

The aim of therapy is to maintain plasma bicarbonate, chloride and potassium, and urinary calcium excretion within age-appropriate range

The use of thiazides in routine treatment of patients with distal RTA is not recommended. Similarly, growth hormone therapy is not advised, unless there is persistent stunting despite adequate metabolic control

Monitoring

Patients with distal RTA should be cared for at centers with experience in long-term management of such patients

These patients should be regularly assessed, clinically and biochemically. All patients should have renal tract ultrasonography performed at diagnosis, and at regular intervals of follow-up

Patients with RTA with mutations in *ATP6V1B1*, *ATP6V0A4*, or *FOXI1* require early and developmentally appropriate hearing screening, including at least once by 24–30 months of age. Patients with sensorineural hearing loss require audiological follow-up. Patients with variations in *WDR72* should undergo dental assessment for amelogenesis imperfecta. Some patients with specific variations in *SLC4A1* show associated hemolytic anemia

Source: Adapted from Trepiccione F, et al. 2021

Proximal RTA: The correction of acidosis requires administration of 5–20 mEq/kg/day of alkali. Since large amounts of alkali are lost in urine as HCO_3^-, it is prudent to give modest amount of sodium bicarbonate (5–8 mEq/kg/day). Restriction of dietary sodium and administration of hydrochlorothiazide (1.5–2 mg/kg/day) help by causing contraction of extracellular fluid volume that increases HCO_3^- reabsorption. Since thiazides enhance K^+ excretion, part of the alkali should be given as potassium citrate. Correction of acidosis results in improved growth velocity.

Patients with Fanconi syndrome require management of the underlying condition. Sick patients need IV rehydration (0.9% saline), usually with added potassium. Urinary losses of sodium, potassium, bicarbonate, and phosphate should be replaced orally. Adequate fluid intake is particularly important during infancy. Rickets can be healed by providing phosphate (50–100 mg/kg/day as neutral salt; see **Annexure 5, p 820**), correction of acidosis, and administration of moderate doses of vitamin D.

Type IV RTA: While hyperkalemia requires potassium restriction regardless of etiology, therapy is directed toward specific cause. Mineralocorticoid supplementation as fludrocortisone is useful in patients with CAH and Addison disease. Patients with autosomal recessive PHA type 1 require large amounts of salt supplements throughout life. Therapy with thiazides corrects the abnormalities noted in patients with PHA type 2.

Outcomes

Patients with all forms of RTA require long-term follow-up for monitoring of growth and kidney function. Most patients with dRTA show satisfactory catchup growth if diagnosed early and managed appropriately. Despite adequate supplements, growth failure often persists in patients with Fanconi syndrome, and final height is often unsatisfactory. About one-third of patients with dRTA followed beyond puberty show declining kidney function. Reasons for renal dysfunction include recurrent episodes of acute kidney disease associated with volume depletion, and interstitial fibrosis associated with nephrocalcinosis and/or hypokalemia.

Long-term outcomes in Fanconi syndrome are also influenced by extrarenal features, e.g., liver (tyrosinemia, Wilson disease, galactosemia, and hereditary fructose intolerance) or central nervous system (Lowe syndrome, Wilson disease) disease. Untreated patients with Fanconi–Bickel syndrome are at risk of hypoglycemia, and later hepatocellular carcinoma. Patients with cystinosis and Dent disease show progressive decline in kidney function by the first and third decade, respectively.

CONDITIONS WITH FANCONI SYNDROME

Cystinosis

Cystinosis is an autosomal recessive inherited condition characterized by deposition of cystine crystals in the cornea, conjunctiva, bone marrow, leukocytes, lymph nodes, and other organs. The affected gene *CTNS*, located on 17p, encodes for cystinosin, a ubiquitous lysosomal proton-driven cystine transporter working in parallel with the vacuolar H^+ATPase **(Fig. 20.3A)**. In patients with cystinosis, the loss of function of cystinosin impairs transport of cystine from lysosomes to cytosol, leading to very high levels of free cystine within the lysosomes. Cystinosin may have an important role in regulating lysosomal kinetics and exocytosis; absence of cystinosin is associated with decreased expression of the multiligand receptors megalin and cubilin in the proximal tubule apical surfaces, cell dedifferentiation, and segmental proximal tubular atrophy. Tubular handling of cystine is normal and there is no cystinuria.

Three clinical forms are recognized. The most severe form, affecting 95% patients, is termed infantile nephropathic cystinosis and is caused by severe truncating mutations affecting both alleles of *CTNS*. Patients with juvenile or late-onset nephropathic cystinosis present in late childhood or adolescence with mild forms of renal Fanconi syndrome or isolated proteinuria and slow progression of renal disease. The ocular or adult form is diagnosed in adulthood when evaluated for corneal cystine deposits; deposits may also be seen in bone marrow and leukocytes but not the kidneys. Juvenile and ocular cystinosis are caused by milder variants in at least one allele of *CTNS*.

Patients with infantile nephropathic cystinosis present at 4–6 months of age with polyuria, polydipsia, failure to thrive, vomiting, constipation, dehydration, growth retardation, and severe rickets. Biochemical evidence of proximal tubular dysfunction includes electrolyte losses, glucosuria, low molecular weight proteinuria, severe acidosis, and hypophosphatemia. In absence of therapy, renal injury progresses to end stage renal disease by 10–12 years. With development of renal insufficiency, the manifestations of tubular dysfunction become less prominent, and polyuria and polydipsia decrease.

Photophobia may be a striking feature in some cases, noted by 3 years of age, and progressing to blepharospasm, superficial punctate keratopathy, and recurrent corneal erosions. Cystine deposits in other organs result in: (*i*) hypothyroidism (noted in 75% by 10 years); (*ii*) hypergonadotropic hypogonadism with delayed puberty and/or infertility; (*iii*) insulin-dependent diabetes mellitus (during second or third decade); (*iv*) hepatosplenomegaly (in 33% patients by 15 years); and (*v*) generalized muscle atrophy with distal muscle weakness (by young adulthood), severe exercise intolerance, and respiratory failure. Subtle neurological defects may be noted, particularly learning difficulties and fine motor incoordination.

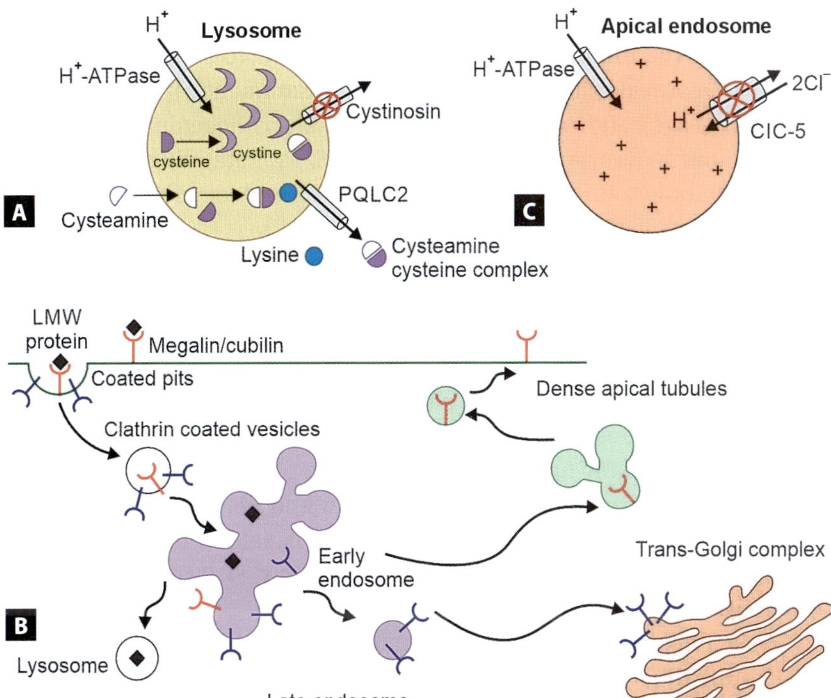

Figs. 20.3A to C: Defects in three inherited forms of Fanconi syndrome. (A) Cystinosin is a lysosomal proton-driven cystine transporter that works in parallel with the vacuolar H^+-ATPase to export cystine, the oxidized form of cysteine. Loss of function of cystinosin in patients with cystinosis results in lysosomal accumulation of cystine. Cysteamine enters lysosomes and forms a cysteamine–cysteine complex, which resembles lysine and can be exported by the amino acid transporter, PQLC2. (B) Low molecular-weight (LMW) proteins, including lipids, vitamins, nutrients and hormones bind to receptors megalin or cubilin in proximal tubular cells and are endocytosed into clathrin coated pits. Following internalization the receptor ligand complexes dissociate inside endosomes. Subsequently, megalin and cubilin receptors are recycled in dense apical tubules to the luminal membrane, whereas the ligand is directed to lysosomes for degradation or released in cytosol before being returned to circulation. The OCRL1 protein (inositol polyphosphate 5 phosphatase) interacts with clathrin to regulate its trafficking between endosomes and the Golgi network. Patients with mutations in *OCRL1* gene show impaired expression and trafficking of megalin and cubilin receptors leading to Fanconi syndrome. (C) Vesicular acidification is mediated by the vacuolar H^+-ATPase, which requires a net Cl^- conductance to dissipate the positive charge gradient. The electrogenic chloride-proton antiporter ClC-5, encoded by *CLCN5* gene, mediates Cl^- conductance to facilitate acidification. Loss of function of ClC-5 in Dent disease leads to accumulation of positive charges within the endosome, impairing its acidification and preventing endocytosis of ligand-receptor complexes leading to multiple trafficking defects in proximal tubules, including loss of megalin and cubilin and low-molecular-weight proteinuria

The diagnosis is confirmed by demonstrating (*i*) elevated levels of cystine in leukocytes (>2 nmol cystine/mg protein; normal <0.2 nmol cystine/mg protein); (*ii*) corneal cystine crystals on slit lamp examination (present beyond 18 months of age); and/or (*iii*) pathogenic or likely pathogenic, homozygous or compound heterozygous variants in *CTNS*. Prenatal diagnosis can be made by demonstrating such variants in *CTNS* in deoxyribonucleic acid (DNA) from amniocytes or chorionic villi.

The management of Fanconi syndrome requires supplementation of electrolytes, phosphate, and fluid losses, and provision of adequate calories. While useful in increasing salt reabsorption and reducing polyuria, there is no consensus on the use of indomethacin in patients with nephropathic cystinosis; if used, the agent should be discontinued when the patient is dehydrated, hypotensive, or shows fall in renal function. Early nasogastric, jejunal, or gastrostomy tube placement and use of proton pump inhibitors help achieve dietary intakes. Hypothyroidism and diabetes are managed. Therapy with recombinant growth hormone is safe and effective, and is initiated early to achieve adult height of around –2.0 to –2.5 standard deviation scores.

Specific therapy with cysteamine enables cystine depletion **(Fig. 20.3A)** and should thus be initiated early and continued lifelong. The most commonly used preparation is cysteamine bitartrate (Cystagon®). Therapy is given in four divided doses, initiated at one-sixth of the target dose and increased in 4–6 weeks to 1.3 g/m^2/day of free base (2 g/m^2/day for children >12-year-old or >50 kg), not exceeding 1.95 g/m^2/day. The dose is titrated to achieve leukocyte cystine <0.2 nmol cystine/mg protein. Adverse effects include acrid sulfur body and breath odor (reduced by concomitant use of riboflavin or chlorophyll tablets), and diarrhea. Rare complications include elbow angioendotheliomas, *striae rubrae*, bony deformities, and neurological symptoms. A novel enteric-coated delayed release formulation of cysteamine bitartrate (Procysbi®) enables twice daily administration and has fewer gastrointestinal adverse effects. While not curative, specific therapy delays progressive kidney failure by 6–10 years, and prevents late nonrenal complications of cystinosis. Since oral cysteamine therapy has no effect on corneal cystine crystals, cysteamine hydrochloride eye drops are administered 6–10 times a day to dissolve crystals; available preparations include 0.44% cysteamine ophthalmic solution (Cystaran®) and 0.55% gel (Cystadrops®).

Renal transplantation is successful but does not correct the systemic disorder and cystine continues to accumulate in nonrenal tissues, resulting in multisystem dysfunction. Transplantation of allogeneic or genetically-modified autologous hematogenous stem cells has shown promise in delaying renal and extrarenal complications of cystinosis and is currently being tested in a Food and Drug Administration (FDA)-approved clinical trial.

Fanconi–Bickel Syndrome

This autosomal recessive disorder of monosaccharide transport is caused by variations in *SLC2A2* (3q26.2), encoding the glucose transporter, GLUT2. Patients present in the first year of life with doll-like faces, hepatomegaly, large kidneys, and severe Fanconi syndrome with rickets. Hypoglycemia and glucose and galactose intolerance are common; early onset cataract is uncommon. Compared to other conditions, patients with Fanconi–Bickel syndrome have severe glucosuria and galactosuria. Genetic analysis of *SLC2A2* is confirmatory.

Treatment includes frequent meals and management of the Fanconi syndrome. Frequent night-time feeding helps prevent hypoglycemia and improve growth. Uncooked cornstarch and nocturnal enteric nutrition decrease the frequency of hypoglycemia and improve growth. Patients require long-term monitoring in view of risk of hepatocellular carcinoma.

Lowe Syndrome

Lowe syndrome (oculocerebrorenal syndrome of Lowe, OCRL) is a rare condition with a prevalence of 1 in 500,000 is characterized by anomalies of the eyes, nervous system, and kidneys. Ocular abnormalities include bilateral congenital cataract, strabismus, infantile onset glaucoma, and cheloids. Neurological involvement manifests as hypotonia with hyporeflexia at birth, severe psychomotor retardation evident in early childhood, and behavioral abnormalities (temper tantrums, stereotypes, aggressiveness, and obsessive compulsive behavior) that appear later. Seizures, including febrile convulsions, are common. Fanconi syndrome, with pRTA, phosphaturia, hypercalciuria, and generalized aminoaciduria, is noted during early infancy. Aminoaciduria may decrease later as glomerular filtration falls during the second decade of life. Low molecular weight proteinuria is often severe; some patients show albuminuria and nephrotic syndrome. Facial dysmorphism includes frontal bossing, deep-set eyes, chubby cheeks, and fair complexion.

The disease is transmitted as an X-linked recessive condition, caused by mutations in *OCRL1* localized at Xq26.1, encoding the enzyme phosphatidylinositol (4,5) bisphosphate 5 phosphatase in the Golgi network. The disease manifestations are secondary to accumulation of the enzyme substrate, phosphatidylinositol bisphosphate, which causes changes in protein trafficking, defective actin cytoskeleton polymerization, and altered cell signaling for endocytosis **(Fig. 20.3B)**. *De novo* mutations are noted in 30% affected individuals.

The diagnosis is clinical, but enzymatic and molecular testing for *OCRL* mutations are available for confirmation of the diagnosis and for prenatal detection of the disease. Most mothers carrying the pathogenic mutation are detected by molecular testing or by slit-lamp examination (punctuate white to gray radial opacities in lenticular cortex). Low molecular weight proteinuria may help with antenatal diagnosis. Treatment is symptomatic, including cataract extraction, glaucoma control, physical and speech therapy, and medications for behavioral problems. Appropriate therapy is given for the RTA and bone disease, comprising citrates and bicarbonate (base requirement 3–8 mEq/kg/day), phosphate, potassium, and water. Rickets is treated with oral phosphate supplements and vitamin D. The life span of patients rarely exceeds 40 years. Most deaths are related to respiratory illness, seizures, or renal failure.

Dent Disease

Dent disease is a proximal tubulopathy characterized by low molecular weight proteinuria, hypercalciuria, nephrocalcinosis, nephrolithiasis, and progressive kidney failure. Proximal tubular dysfunction suggestive of Fanconi syndrome is common, including aminoaciduria, glucosuria, hyperphosphaturia, kaliuresis, and uricosuria. Excretion of β2-microglobulin, α1-microglobulin, or retinol-binding protein is increased 100–1000-fold but is usually asymptomatic except for recurrent night blindness. Rickets or osteomalacia is noted in up to one-third patients. Hypercalciuria, noted in the range of 4–14 mg/kg/day, leads to nephrocalcinosis by late childhood and adolescence, and renal failure in the third to fifth decade of life. Renal biopsy may show focal segmental glomerulosclerosis, tubular atrophy, and interstitial fibrosis.

The disease is inherited in an X-linked recessive manner, affecting mainly boys with female carriers being generally asymptomatic or presenting with low molecular weight proteinuria and hypercalciuria without nephrocalcinosis or progressive disease. In over 60% cases, termed Dent 1, the disease is caused by mutations in the *CLCN5* gene, encoding the electrogenic chloride/proton exchanger ClC-5. Patients with Dent 2 disease, comprising 15% of all cases, have mutations in *OCRL1*, the gene associated with the oculocerebrorenal syndrome of Lowe. Patients with Dent 2 disease may additionally show mild intellectual disability and cataracts. **Figures 20.3B and C** outline the functional relevance of ClC-5 and *OCRL1* in the endocytic pathway for reabsorption of low molecular weight proteins and other molecules in the proximal tubule. The diagnosis of Dent disease is suspected based on criteria listed in **Box 20.2**. The diagnosis is established in a male proband with the identification of hemizygous pathogenic or likely pathogenic variation in either *CLCN5* or *OCRL1* by molecular genetic testing.

Management is supportive with supplementation of fluid and electrolyte losses, and use of thiazides to reduce urinary calcium excretion. Therapy with vitamin D may worsen hypercalciuria. Renal transplantation is safe as the disease does not recur in the allograft.

BOX 20.2: Diagnostic criteria for Dent disease

Low molecular weight proteinuria (ß2-microglobulin, retinol binding protein, and/or α1-microglobulin)
Hypercalciuria: >4 mg/kg/24-h; calcium: creatinine ratio*
At least one of the following:
- Nephrocalcinosis
- Nephrolithiasis
- Microscopic or gross hematuria
- Hypophosphatemia
- Estimated glomerular filtration rate below normal for the age
- Family history consistent with X-linked inheritance

Increased calcium to creatinine (mg/mg): 0–1 years >0.81; 1–3 years >0.56; 3–5 years >0.41; 5–7 years >0.30; 7–18 years >0.25
Source: *Matos V, et al. 1997

Hereditary Tyrosinemia

Hereditary tyrosinemia type 1 is an autosomal recessive disorder, with elevated levels of tyrosine. Mutations in *FAH* (15q25.1), which encodes the enzyme, fumarylacetoacetate hydrolase (FAH), result in impaired metabolism of L-tyrosine. Raised levels of succinylacetone is characteristic. Most patients present in early infancy with acute liver failure, or later with a subacute presentation including failure to thrive, hepatosplenomegaly, and coagulopathy. These patients are at risk of hepatocellular carcinoma, with high blood levels of α-fetoprotein.

Kidney manifestations include the spectrum of findings seen in Fanconi syndrome; enlarged kidneys and nephrocalcinosis may be seen, and kidney failure is uncommon. Neurological features include porphyria-like crises, often precipitated by intercurrent infections, and characterized by acute abdominal pain, limb weakness, and transient hypertension; and acute progressive ascending motor neuropathy that might require assisted ventilation.

The diagnosis is made in presence of high succinylacetone and confirmed by genetic studies. While urinary testing for succinylacetone is widely available, plasma levels are preferred for diagnosis as well as monitoring response to therapy. Ultrasonography of liver and kidneys is performed at baseline and regular intervals; magnetic resonance imaging (MRI) is indicated in presence of nodules in the liver.

Management includes dietary restriction of tyrosine and phenylalanine and administration of 2-nitro-4-trifluoromethylbenzoyl-1, 3-cyclohexanedione, or nitisinone (NTBC), Orfadin® (1 mg/kg once daily) to block the tyrosine pathway. Common adverse effects include cytopenias, ocular complications, and learning difficulty. Fanconi syndrome improves following therapy with NTBC, and after liver transplantation.

OTHER TUBULAR DISORDERS

Renal Glucosuria

Renal glucosuria is a benign disorder characterized by presence of large amounts of glucose in the urine, with normal blood glucose levels. There is no other defect of proximal tubular function. Normally, the filtered glucose is completely reabsorbed by the proximal tubule until the tubular maximum is exceeded. Two types of abnormalities are commonly present. In type A, the tubular maximum is low, and the capacity of all tubules to reabsorb glucose is reduced. In type B, the tubular maximum is normal, but there is a wide variation in the resorptive capacity of individual nephrons and those with reduced capacity are easily saturated. The unreabsorbed glucose is excreted. In the rare type O, there is virtually no tubular reabsorption of glucose. The inheritance pattern is usually autosomal recessive; dominant inheritance is occasionally reported. Significant variants in the gene encoding SGLT2, *SLC5A2*, cause type A or type O glucosuria. Defects in SGLT1 (*SLC5A1*) are associated with type B glucosuria. No treatment is necessary.

Cystinuria

This is a relatively common inherited renal tubular disorder characterized by a defect in the transport of the four dibasic amino acids cystine, lysine, ornithine, and arginine. The inheritance is autosomal recessive. Cystine has low solubility in urine and its high levels lead to calculus formation. Excessive excretion of cystine is due to an impairment of brush border membrane transport (defect in *SLC3A1*, on chromosome 2p), present in the kidneys as well as the intestine. Pathogenic or likely pathogenic variants in *SLC7A9* (locus 19q13.1) are also reported. Contiguous deletion involving the *SLC3A1* and *PREPL* lead to the rarely described cystinuria-hypotonia syndrome, characterized by congenital hypotonia, lactic acidosis, and failure to thrive.

Cystine crystals, typically flat hexagonal, may be found in a freshly voided morning urine specimen. The urinary cyanide-nitroprusside test gives a magenta red color. Affected patients show increased cystine concentration on a 24-h urine specimen (>310 mg cystine/g creatinine). The four amino acids can be identified on paper chromatography. The most important aspect of treatment is to ensure a high fluid intake. Other measures include increased fluid intake (3–4 liters daily), urinary alkalization (urine pH 7–8), dietary salt restriction, and use of more specific agents such as penicillamine, tiopronin, and captopril. Urological intervention is indicated in patients with obstructed stones.

Mitochondrial Cytopathies

Mitochondrial cytopathies are diverse disorders with abnormalities in mitochondrial DNA causing multiorgan dysfunction. Impaired respiratory chain activity causes accumulation of reduced NADH (nicotinamide adenine dinucleotide, reduced (H) form), promoting conversion of acetoacetic acid into 3-hydroxybutyrate in mitochondria and pyruvate into lactate in cytosol. Patients present with neurological symptoms (apnea, hypotonia, lethargy, stroke like episodes, developmental delay, seizures, mycoclonus, polyneuropathy, myopathy, or hypotonia), but cardiac (cardiomyopathy, arrhythmias, and heart block), endocrine and hematological (sideroblastic anemia, neutropenia, and thrombocytopenia) involvement is common. Renal features include proximal tubular defects including Fanconi syndrome, tubulointerstitial nephritis, cystic renal disease, and glomerulopathies. Tubulopathy is frequently associated with Pearson and Kearns-Sayre syndromes.

Diagnosis is suggested by presence of tubulopathy, proteinuria or hematuria along with neurological symptoms, and high serum or cerebrospinal fluid lactate, with increased ratio of lactate to pyruvate. Investigations include magnetic resonance spectroscopy (elevated cerebral lactate), gas chromatography/mass spectrometry (elevated urinary organic acids), and genetic studies. Renal biopsy shows chronic tubulointerstitial changes with damaged proximal tubules; electron microscopy shows proliferation of abnormal mitochondria. Most inherited conditions are fatal. Apart from bicarbonate and phosphate supplements, oral coenzyme Q10 (CoQ10) supplementation may be useful.

Nephrogenic Diabetes Insipidus

Primary NDI, recently renamed "arginine vasopressin (AVP) resistance", is a rare condition characterized by tubular unresponsiveness to the antidiuretic hormone (ADH, vasopressin). In 90% cases, the disease is inherited in an X-linked recessive pattern and caused by significant variants at Xp28, the locus for the gene encoding the arginine vasopressin V2 receptor (*AVPR2*) in the collecting duct **(Fig. 20.4)**. Through cyclic adenosine monophosphate (cAMP)-adenylate cyclase mediated activation of protein kinase, *AVPR2* mediates the phosphorylation of the intracellular water channels aquaporin 2, which translocate to the luminal surface, to absorb water. Most commonly the variants are missense mutations, causing entrapment of functional *AVPR2* within the endoplasmic reticulum. In 10% cases, disease transmission may be in an autosomal recessive or autosomal dominant manner, in which case variants in the gene encoding aquaporin 2 (chromosome 12q) have been identified. NDI may also occur due to acquired insensitivity to the action of vasopressin, as in conditions listed in **Box 20.3**.

Secondary nephrogenic DI is diagnosed in the setting of polyuria and polydipsia that is not merely due to decreased solute and fluid reabsorption (isosthenuria, due to lack of generation of the medullary interstitial concentration gradient), after demonstration of hyposthenuria (low urine

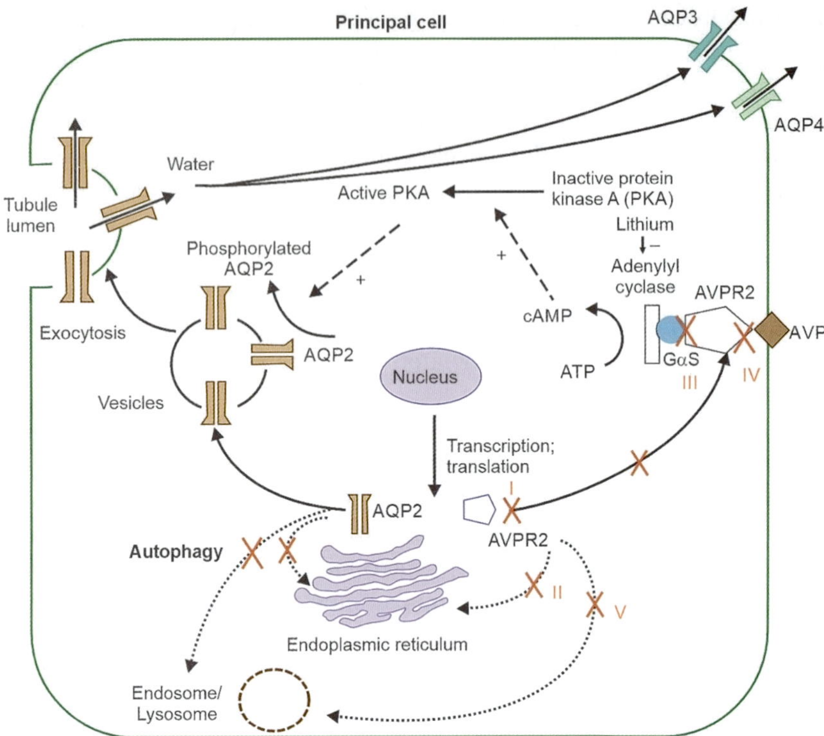

Fig. 20.4: Nephrogenic diabetes insipidus (NDI). Arginine vasopressin (AVP) binds to vasopressin receptor type 2 (AVPR2) on the basolateral side of principal cells of the collecting duct. Activation of cytosolic G protein (GαS) activates adenylyl cyclase, leading to increased cyclic adenosine monophosphate (AMP), protein kinase A (PKA) activation, phosphorylation of water channel aquaporin-2 (AQP2), and movement of vesicles containing the channels to the apical surface. The functional form of AQP2 is a homotetramer, with each monomer containing a water pore. At the apical plasma membrane, AQP2 mediates water reabsorption along an osmotic gradient. Water entering the principal cell via AQP2 exits via AQP3 and AQP4 in the basolateral plasma membrane. Mutations in *AVPR2*, underlying X-linked recessive NDI, most commonly cause misfolding of the receptor and its retention in the endoplasmic reticulum (type II defect), but may also affect receptor expression (type I defect), its interaction with vasopressin (type IV) or the G protein ligand (type III), or its trafficking to another cellular compartment (type V defect), indicated by "X". Some pathogenic variants are associated with a partial phenotype. Homozygous or compound heterozygous variants in *AQP2*, underlying autosomal recessive NDI, usually lead to the retention of misfolded AQP2 in the endoplasmic reticulum; less often, the mutant AQP2 is trafficked into the endosome or lysosome, or degraded rapidly (indicated by "X"). Patients with autosomal dominant (AD) NDI carry heterotetramers of AQP2, containing both wildtype and mutated proteins. These heterotetramers are either retained in the Golgi apparatus or are misrouted to late endosomes, lysosomes, or basolateral membrane. Polyuria in patients treated with lithium is secondary to inhibition of adenylate cyclase, which decreases *AQP2* transcription. Hypercalciuria might act through the calcium sensing receptor (CaSR), expressed on apical surface of medullary collecting ducts, which inhibits cAMP formation. The mechanism by which hypokalemia reduces AQP2 expression on cell surface is unclear

BOX 20.3: Causes of nephrogenic diabetes insipidus (arginine vasopressin resistance)

Primary
Defect in vasopressin receptor, AVPR2: X-linked recessive
Defect in water channel aquaporin 2, AQP2
Autosomal recessive: Defective cellular processing and/or function of AQP2
Autosomal dominant: Mutant *AQP2* prevents plasma membrane targeting of wild type AQP2

Secondary^
Bartter syndrome type 1 (*SLC12A1*) and 2 (*KCNJ1*)
Apparent mineralocorticoid excess (*HSD11B2*)
Fanconi syndrome: primary; secondary
Distal renal tubular acidosis
Cystic kidney diseases: Nephronophthisis; Bardet–Biedl syndrome; polycystic kidney disease
Drugs: Lithium, demeclocycline, cyclophosphamide, ifosfamide, vincristine, cidofovir, tenofovir, didanosine, foscarnet
Hypokalemia: Inhibition of AQP2 expression through unclear mechanism
Hypercalciuria, hypercalcemia: Stimulate calcium sensing receptor; inhibits cyclic AMP, inhibits AQP2 expression
Obstructive uropathy

^See text for diagnostic criteria

osmolality despite relatively high serum osmolality), and lack of response to desmopressin (DDAVP). **Box 20.3** lists conditions associated with secondary DI).

Clinical Features

The severity is variable. Polyuria and polydipsia are striking features and usually present in neonatal period. Irritability, poor feeding, and recurrent episodes of dehydration and fever are common. History of polyhydramnios is lacking and birth weight is normal, but postnatally the child fails to thrive. High fluid intake results in reduced intake of solid foods and malnutrition; bone age is normal. Fever is often mistakenly believed to be of infective origin and extensive laboratory investigations are carried out to find the cause. Polyuria continues even when dehydration is present. Constipation is common. Older children may present with nocturia or nocturnal enuresis. Symptoms may be delayed in exclusively breastfed infants since breast milk provides a lower osmolal load than cow milk.

Repeated episodes of hypernatremia and dehydration, with risks of cerebral edema due to rapid rehydration, may lead to neurological abnormalities including psychomotor retardation, intracranial calcification, and sequelae of hemorrhage and necrosis. Many patients manifest attention deficit, hyperactivity, and restlessness. Rarely, seizures are noted, usually during therapy, particularly if correction of dehydration is rapid.

Persistent polyuria in patients with NDI might cause hydronephrosis, and even megacystis, hydroureter, and a large capacity hypotonic urinary bladder.

Some heterozygous females with *AVPR2* mutations may manifest a mild disease phenotype, putatively due to skewed inactivation of X chromosome in the kidneys. Milder mutations that cause partial stimulation of adenylyl cyclase lead to a less severe phenotype, with later age at onset and mild growth retardation. The manifestations of the disease do not differ between the X-linked and autosomal forms of the disease; patients with acquired NDI have delayed onset and milder features.

Laboratory Findings

Urinary osmolality is usually below 150 mOsm/kg. Serum sodium levels are high, often above 170 mEq/L, with corresponding increase in serum chloride and osmolality. Urinary sodium concentration is low. With persistent polyuria, the urinary tract may dilate to accommodate large volumes of urine. During dehydration, the blood urea and creatinine levels may be raised but with hydration these return to normal. The diagnosis is confirmed by failure of the urinary osmolality to rise following either water deprivation or administration of DDAVP (see Chapter 2; **Box 20.4** and **Fig. 20.4**). The period of water deprivation should not exceed 4 hr in infants and 7–8 hr in older children, following which, in normal children, the ratio of urine to plasma osmolality should exceed 1.5. In patients with NDI, the urine osmolality does not rise above 200 mOsm/ kg, and urine output is not reduced during the 6 hr following administration of 10–20 μg of intranasal DDVAP.

Copeptin, which is secreted in an equimolar amount to AVP, can easily be measured in plasma or serum by immunoassay. Its levels are highly correlated with plasma levels of AVP that is unstable ex vivo, and is measured unreliably. Baseline plasma copeptin levels above 21.4 pmol/L strongly suggest the diagnosis of NDI. In contrast, low plasma copeptin levels at baseline (threshold value <4.9 pmol/L), after overnight water deprivation (threshold <2.6 pmol/L), or stimulation of AVP secretion by infusion of arginine (threshold <3.8 pmol/L), or by hypertonic saline (<4.9 pmol/L) indicate central diabetes insipidus (DI).

Treatment

A large intake of water is necessary to compensate for the urinary losses, but difficult to ensure in infants. The parents need clear instructions to that effect. Restriction of dietary sodium to 1 mEq/kg/day will reduce the osmolar load and the need for associated water excretion. A low protein diet, recommended for the same purpose, is not advised since it may interfere with growth. Administration of hydrochlorothiazide at a dose of 2–3 mg/kg/day, when combined with sodium restriction, can lead to a significant reduction of urine volume. Amiloride at 20 mg/1.73 m^2/day has an additive effect, since both agents have different sites of action in the tubule (the former in the early distal tubule and the latter in the cortical and medullary collecting duct). Combination of the two agents also reduces the risk of hypokalemia.

Diuretics increase sodium excretion resulting in contraction of extracellular sodium content that leads to an increase in proximal tubular reabsorption of sodium and water. Thiazides probably also increase expression of the *AQP2* protein. Chronic thiazide therapy is associated with dyslipidemia, hyperglycemia, and hyperuricemia.

Younger children tolerate indomethacin (2 mg/kg/day) better than amiloride, but its prolonged use is not recommended since it may reduce GFR and cause gastrointestinal side effects. Future therapies for NDI focus on enabling trafficking of functional *AVPR2*/*AQP2* protein trapped in endoplasmic reticulum to their site of action, through chemical or pharmacological chaperones.

Bartter Syndrome

Bartter syndrome is a rare salt-losing kidney disorder characterized by secondary hyperaldosteronism with hypokalemia, metabolic alkalosis, and low to normal blood pressure. While the disorder is uncommon, the diagnosis is often missed. Children present in infancy with polyuria, polydipsia, vomiting, constipation, and failure to thrive. Recurrent episodes of dehydration, muscle weakness, and cramps are prominent in older children. The blood pressure is low normal for age. Laboratory findings include severe hypokalemia (serum K^+ 1.5–2.5 mEq/L), hypochloremia, and metabolic alkalosis. Urinary chloride concentration is usually >20–30 mEq/L. Hyperuricemia and hyponatremia may be present. The fractional excretion of K^+, Na^+, and Cl^- is increased. Urinary calcium excretion is normal or high. Kidney biopsy, if it were to be performed, shows hyperplasia of the juxtaglomerular apparatus.

Etiology

The molecular basis of Bartter syndrome is an inability to reabsorb chloride and sodium in the thick ascending limb of Henle due to defects in ion transporters **(Table 20.4 and Fig. 20.5)**. Increased delivery of sodium chloride to distal parts of the nephron leads to salt wasting, hypokalemia, polyuria, volume contraction, and stimulation of the renin-angiotensin-aldosterone axis. While urinary sodium is recovered by an increase in aldosterone mediated activity of the ENaC, loss of chloride with ammonium or potassium results in hypochloremic metabolic alkalosis and hypokalemia. Hypokalemia, volume contraction, and elevated angiotensin increase intrarenal prostaglandin E2 synthesis, which stimulates the renin-angiotensin-aldosterone axis.

BOX 20.4: Water deprivation test in polyuria

Indications and prerequisites

Polyuria: Urine output >2 L/m^2/d or >6 mL/kg/h at any age; >150 mL/kg/d at birth, >100–110 mL/kg/day till <2-year-old; >40–50 mL/kg/d in older children and adults

Normal kidney function tests, potassium, calcium and blood sugar

Hypotonic urine: Urine osmolality <300 mOsm/kg

Blood osmolality >270 and <300 mOsm/kg

Contraindications

Hypernatremia (blood sodium >145 mEq/L)

Dehydration

Procedure

Following overnight fast, the test is begun early morning (6 AM), under close monitoring over 4–8 hr (4-hr for infants, 7–8 hr for older children; up to 12–14 hr in primary polydipsia)

Fluids and food are restricted; patient is advised to remain semirecumbent, except for voiding urine

Blood sampling for serum sodium and osmolality is performed hourly, through a wide bore cannula with free flow of blood

Urine voids are collected every hour from the patient and one control (e.g., parent) for urine osmolality and specific gravity

Patient is monitored closely for evidence of hypovolemia or dehydration, both for patient safety and to avoid nonosmotic stimulation of vasopressin secretion, such as postural hypotension, vasovagal syncope, or episodes of nausea or hypotension

End points

Any one of the following:

1. Blood osmolality >295 mOsm/kg, or serum sodium >145 mEq/L
2. Urine osmolality >300 mOsm/kg; in infants and young children >450 mOsm/kg; or urine-to-serum osmolality ≥1.5
3. Plateau urine osmolality (<10% increase in urine osmolality in three consecutive samples)
4. Weight loss >5% or any features of dehydration (dry mucous membranes; reduced skin turgor); tachycardia or orthostatic hypotension (>10 mm fall in systolic blood pressure, increase in pulse rate >10 bpm on standing)

Interpretation[1]

When (2) occurs earlier than (1): Continue water deprivation for the designated time

- Urine osmolality >750 mOsm/kg: Suggests *psychogenic polydipsia*
- Urine osmolality between 300 and 750 mOsm/kg: *Consider (a) and (b) below*

When (1) occurs earlier than (2): Pitressin test: Administer desmopressin at a dose of 5–10 µg intravenous (IV) or subcutaneously, or 2–4 µg of pitressin intranasally; interpret as follows:

- Urine osmolality after 1–2 hr is >150% of the value before the challenge: Consider *complete central diabetes insipidus (DI)*
- Urine osmolality after 2 hr is <110% of the value before the challenge: *Complete nephrogenic DI*
- Urine osmolality after 2 hr is 110–150% of the value before the challenge: *Consider (a) and (b) below*

Contd...

Contd...

a. *T-1 weighted MRI brain:* A hyperintense signal (bright spot) at the location of the posterior pituitary gland indicates normal state, nephrogenic DI, or primary polydipsia; and its absence suggests central DI

b. *Therapeutic trial:* Therapeutic doses of desmopressin (dDAVP) (10–20 µg intranasally) or pitressin (5 units IV) are given daily for 4–7 days along with *ad lib* fluid intake, while monitoring as an inpatient for thirst, urine output, urine osmolality, body weight, and blood sodium. Interpretation is as follows:
   - Features of water intoxication within 24 hr: Suggests *primary polydipsia*
   - Prompt and complete abolition of polyuria, increase in urine osmolality, no or delayed impact on thirst and polydipsia, occurrence of hyponatremia: Suggests *primary polydipsia*
   - Prompt and complete abolition of thirst, polydipsia and polyuria, increase in urine osmolality by 110–150%, no hyponatremia: Suggests *partial central DI*
   - No change in variables in 48 hr (change in urine osmolality <110%): Suggests *partial nephrogenic DI*

Precautions and caveats of water deprivation test and pitressin challenge

Nonosmotic stimuli can increase arginine vasopressin (AVP) release, e.g., hypotension and nausea

The bladder should be completely emptied during each collection

Calibrate the osmometer against standard solutions of 290, 100, and 500 mOsm/kg

Estimate blood sodium concentration simultaneously to confirm the accuracy of osmolality readings

Incomplete response to dDAVP might occur in infants, long-standing disease, and incomplete DDAVP absorption

[1]The preferred terms for central and nephrogenic DI are AVP deficiency and AVP resistance, respectively

Presentation and Classification

Several subtypes of Bartter syndrome are now recognized **(Table 20.4)** that differ from each other in the underlying defect, age of onset, severity of symptoms, presence of urinary concentrating defect, other electrolyte abnormalities (including hypomagnesemia), and urinary calcium excretion. Defects in sodium chloride reabsorption by the furosemide-sensitive sodium-potassium-chloride cotransporter (NKCC2, type I) or return of potassium to the tubular lumen by the channel ROMK (type II) often present antenatally with polyhydramnios and severe neonatal manifestations. Since potassium recycling also drives paracellular calcium and magnesium reabsorption, these patients have significant hypermagnesiuria and hypercalciuria. Newborns with Bartter syndrome type II may present with transient acidosis and hyperkalemia due to impaired potassium secretion in the cortical collecting duct.

Type III or classic Bartter syndrome, caused by impaired cellular exit of chloride in the thick ascending limb through the basolateral chloride channel ClC-Kb, typically has milder phenotype, possibly since cellular exit of chloride through other channels, e.g., ClC-Ka, continues to occur. The clinical features in type III disease are similar to Gitelman syndrome.

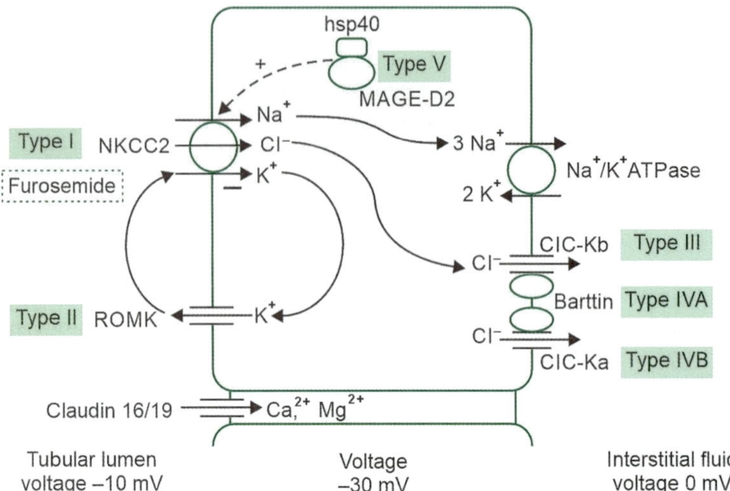

Fig. 20.5: Pathophysiology of Bartter syndrome. Transepithelial sodium chloride absorption in thick ascending limb of loop of Henle is facilitated by coordinated activity of the apical furosemide-sensitive sodium (Na^+) potassium (K^+) chloride (Cl^-) cotransporter (NKCC2), renal outer membrane potassium (ROMK) channel, basolateral Na^+/K^+-ATPase, and basolateral ClC-Kb (in the thick ascending limb and distal convoluted tubule) or ClC-Ka (in the thin and thick ascending limbs). While the NKCC2 is the predominant channel for sodium chloride reabsorption, the luminal exit of potassium through apical ROMK channels is essential to replenish urinary potassium to ensure activity of the NKCC2, and provides the driving force for paracellular absorption of calcium and magnesium. The exit of chloride from the basolateral side is mediated through Cl^- channels ClC-Ka and ClC-Kb, which require a functioning beta subunit called Barttin for their proper membrane localization. The binding of melanoma-associated antigen D2 (MAGE-D2) to its cytoplasmic chaperone, heat shock protein 40 (hsp40 or DNAJB1), protects NKCC2 (in the thick ascending limb of the loop of Henle) and sodium chloride cotransporter (NCCT, in the distal convoluted tubules) from intracellular degradation, and stimulates their apical expression (see also **Table 20.8**)

Sensorineural deafness may be associated in subtype IV, caused by defective expression of the chloride channel ClC-Ka or the barttin subunit of ClC-K, since complexes of ClC-Ka/ClC-Kb and Barttin are critical for potassium recycling in the inner ear. Unlike subtypes I–IV that are autosomal recessive conditions, subtype V is inherited in an X-linked manner, with very early presentation but spontaneous resolution of symptoms after birth.

Differential Diagnosis

Conditions that need to be distinguished from Bartter syndrome are listed in **Table 20.5**. Patients with Bartter syndrome are differentiated from those with nonrenal causes of chloride loss, e.g., chronic vomiting, chloride diarrhea, laxative abuse, dietary deficiency, and cystic fibrosis. In these conditions, the urinary chloride concentration is <10 mEq/L. Bartter syndrome types I, II, IV, and V may cause maternal polyhydramnios and preterm labor.

TABLE 20.4: Tubular disorders with hypokalemic metabolic alkalosis and normal or low blood pressure

Disorder	Protein	Location	Gene, location	Inheritance	Presentation
Bartter syndrome (BS)					
Type 1 (antenatal BS)	Bumetanide sensitive sodium potassium chloride cotransporter-2 (NKCC2)	Luminal membrane of thick ascending limb (TAL)	*SLC12A1*; 15q15-q21.1	Autosomal recessive (AR)	Antenatal; polyhydramnios; prematurity; failure to thrive; hypokalemic metabolic alkalosis; hypercalciuria; nephrocalcinosis
Type 2 (antenatal BS)	Inwardly rectifying renal outer medullary potassium channel (Kir1.1, ROMK1)	Luminal membrane of TAL and cortical collecting duct	*KCNJI*; 11q24	AR	Antenatal; polyhydramnios; prematurity; failure to thrive; transient neonatal hyperkalemia; hypercalciuria; nephrocalcinosis
Type 3 (classic BS)	Chloride channel, kidney, B (ClC-Ka)	Basolateral membrane of TAL and distal collecting duct (DCT)	*CLCNKB*; 1p36	AR	Growth retardation; hypochloremic metabolic alkalosis; less/no hypercalciuria; no nephrocalcinosis; mild hypomagnesemia
Type 4 (antenatal BS with sensorineural deafness)	4A: Barttin, beta subunit of chloride channel, kidney (ClC-K)	Basolateral membrane of thin ascending limb, TAL and DCT	*BSND* deletion; 1p31	AR	Antenatal; polyhydramnios; prematurity; polyuria; marked hypokalemic metabolic alkalosis; sensorineural deafness; transient hypercalciuria, no nephrocalcinosis; chronic kidney disease
	4B: Chloride channel, kidney, A (ClC-Ka)	Basolateral membrane of thin ascending limb, TAL	*CLCNKA-CLCNKB*; 1p36	AR	
Type 5 (antenatal BS)	Melanoma-associated antigen D2 (MAGE-D2)	Luminal membrane of TAL and DCT	*MAGED2*; Xp11.21	X linked	Antenatal: severe polyhydramnios; large for gestational age; transient disease in most cases
Gitelman syndrome	Thiazide sensitive sodium chloride cotransporter	Luminal membrane of DCT	*SLC12A3*; 16q13	AR	Hypokalemic metabolic alkalosis; hypocalciuria; hypomagnesemia; chondrocalcinosis
EAST/SeSAME syndrome	Inwardly rectifying potassium channel Kir4.1	Basolateral membrane of DCT and cortical collecting duct	*KCNJ10*; 1q23	AR	Metabolic alkalosis; hypocalciuria; hypomagnesemia; epilepsy; ataxia; mental retardation; sensorineural deafness

EAST epilepsy, ataxia, sensorineural deafness and salt-wasting tubulopathy; SeSAME seizures, sensorineural deafness, ataxia, mental retardation, and electrolyte imbalance

TABLE 20.5: Differential diagnosis of Bartter syndrome

Disorder	*Distinguishing feature*
Pseudo-Bartter syndrome, e.g., cystic fibrosis	Low urinary chloride
Congenital chloride diarrhea	Low urinary chloride
Surreptitious vomiting, laxative use	Low urinary chloride
Gitelman syndrome	Hypocalciuria, hypomagnesemia
HNF1 β nephropathy	Renal malformation, cysts; hypomagnesemia, maturity onset diabetes
EAST/SeSAME syndrome	Ataxia, seizures, deafness, developmental delay
HELIX syndrome	Hypermagnesemia, hypocalciuria, hypohidrosis, lacrimal gland dysfunction, icthyosis, xerostomia
Primary hyperaldosteronism	Hypertension, low renin
Apparent mineralocorticoid excess; Liddle syndrome	Hypertension, low renin, and aldosterone
Autosomal dominant hypocalcemia	Hypocalcemia, seizures

The diagnosis is suggested by high amniotic fluid chloride, postnatal polyuria (>15 mL/kg/day), low urine osmolality (<300 mOsm/kg), and increased urinary prostaglandin E2 (PGE2). Hypercalciuria and nephrocalcinosis are seen in types I and II. Neonates with defect in the ROMK channel (type II) presenting with hyperkalemia and hyponatremia may be misdiagnosed as mineralocorticoid deficiency or PHA type I. Polyuria caused by NDI is not associated with hyponatremia. Patients with the EAST (epilepsy, ataxia, sensorineural deafness, and tubulopathy) syndrome have severe neurological features **(Tables 20.4 and 20.7)**. Genetic testing, with the use of a gene panel, is recommended for all patients with suspected Bartter syndrome, to confirm the diagnosis and enable genetic counseling **(Table 20.6; Annexure 9.2, p 845)**.

The presentation in patients with Gitelman syndrome **(Tables 20.4 and 20.7)** may resemble that for classic Bartter syndrome. However, the former has milder renal salt wasting with metabolic alkalosis, and low to normal chloride levels, hypokalemia, hypomagnesemia, and hypocalciuria. Fractional excretion of chloride, reflecting distal chloride reabsorption, before and after administration of a thiazide diuretic or during hypotonic saline diuresis, do not reliably distinguish these patients from classic Bartter syndrome.

Other causes of dysfunction of salt transport in the distal tubule include Sjögren syndrome, Dent disease, sarcoidosis, Kearns–Sayre syndrome and cystinosis, and therapy with aminoglycosides, prostaglandins, or cytotoxic

TABLE 20.6: Gene panel for evaluating patients with suspected Bartter syndrome[1]

Gene	*Disorder*
SLC12A1	Bartter syndrome I
KCNJ1	Bartter syndrome II
CLCNKB	Bartter syndrome III
CLCNKA	Bartter syndrome IV b
BSND	Bartter syndrome IV a
MAGED2	Bartter syndrome V
SLC12A3	Gitelman syndrome
CASR	Autosomal dominant hypocalcemia
KCNJ10	EAST/SeSAME syndrome
SLC26A3	Congenital chloride diarrhea
CLDN10	HELIX syndrome
SCNN1A	Pseudohypoaldosteronism type 1B, multisystem form
SCNN1B	Pseudohypoaldosteronism type 1B, multisystem form; Liddle syndrome
SCNN1G	Pseudohypoaldosteronism type 1B, multisystem form
NR3C2	Pseudohypoaldosteronism type 1A, renal-limited
HSD11B2	Apparent mineralocorticoid excess
CYP11B1, CLCN2, KCNJ5, CACNA1H	Familial hypoaldosteronism

[1]See **Annexure 9.2 (p 845)** for the list of genes to be screened

drugs (e.g., cisplatin). Chronic administration of diuretics may mimic the metabolic abnormalities seen with Bartter or Gitelman syndromes.

Management

Therapy in Bartter syndrome is directed toward replacing losses, by fluid, sodium, potassium, and chloride supplementation. The principles of management are summarized in **Box 20.5**.

Outcomes

Growth failure, recurrent dehydration, and dyselectrolytemia are common. In contrast to Bartter type I and II that are severe during the perinatal period and show improved growth with aggressive therapy, patients with classic and type IV disorders may worsen in adulthood. Hypokalemia and hypomagnesemia predispose to cardiac arrhythmias and QT prolongation. Metabolic derangements also potentiate the effect of anesthetic agents. Patients with chronic volume contraction and those with type IV disease are at risk of CKD. A few cases are reported to have undergone kidney transplantation.

TABLE 20.7: Magnesium wasting diseases

Disorder	*Protein*	*Location*	*Gene, Locus*	*Inheritance*	*Presentation*
Familial hypomagnesemia with secondary hypocalcemia (hypomagnesemia 1: reduced intestinal absorption; renal leak)	Transient receptor potential cation channel, melastatin related, member 6 (TRPM6)	DCT; intestinal epithelia	*TRPM6*, 9q21.3	AR	Severe hypomagnesemia, secondary parathyroid resistance, hypocalcemia; infantile seizures and tetany; calcinosis (myocardium, kidneys, cerebral arteries)
Isolated dominant hypomagnesemia (hypomagnesemia 2)	γ subunit of sodium potassium ATPase	DCT	*FXYD2*, 11q23	AD	Hypomagnesemia, hypocalciuria; seizures, muscle cramps
Familial hypomagnesemia, hypercalciuria, nephrocalcinosis (FHHNC; hypomagnesemia 3)	Paracellin-1 (claudin-16), paracellular tight junction protein	TAL	*CLDN16*, 3q28	AR	Severe hypomagnesemia, hypercalciuria, nephrocalcinosis, hyperuricemia, neonatal seizures, sensorineural deafness, kidney failure within first two decades
Isolated recessive hypomagnesemia (hypomagnesemia 4)	Epidermal growth factor	DCT	*EGF*, 4q25	AR	Infantile onset; seizures, neurodevelopmental delay; hypomagnesemia, normal calcium excretion
FHHNC with ocular involvement (hypomagnesemia 5)	Claudin-19, paracellular tight junction protein	TAL	*CLDN19*, 1p34	AR	Severe myopia, nystagmus or macular coloboma in addition to symptoms described for FHHNC
Renal hypomagnesemia 6	Ancient conserved domain protein 2 (cyclin M2)	DCT, TAL	*CNNM2*, 10q24	AD/AR	Variable age at presentation; intellectual disability; obesity

Contd...

Contd...

Disorder	***Protein***	***Location***	***Gene, Locus***	***Inheritance***	***Presentation***
Renal hypomagnesemia with myokymia	Potassium channel Kv1.1	DCT	*KCNA1*, 12p13	AD	Episodic progressive ataxia; myokymia; recurrent cramps; tetany
Renal cysts and diabetes syndrome	Hepatocyte nuclear factor 1	DCT, CCD	*HNF1B*, 17q12	AR	Maturity onset diabetes; hypocalciuria, hyperuricemia, hypermagnesuria; cystic dysplasia, renal agenesis, glomerulocystic kidney disease
Hypomagnesemia and metabolic syndrome	Mitochondrial-coded Trna (isoleucine)	DCT	Mitochondrial coded isoleucine t-RNA *(MTTI)*	Maternal	Hypomagnesemia, hypermagnesuria, hypocalciuria; hypercholesterolemia; hypertension
AD hypoparathyroidism	Calcium magnesium sensing receptor (CaSR)	TAL, DCT	Activating mutation of *CASR*; 3q13	AD	Onset in childhood; seizures, carpopedal spasms; hypocalcemia, hypomagnesemia; low PTH
Gitelman syndrome	Thiazide sensitive sodium chloride cotransporter (NCCT)	DCT	*SLC12A3*,16q13	AR	Hypokalemic metabolic alkalosis, hypocalciuria, hypomagnesemia; chondrocalcinosis
EAST/SeSAME syndrome	Potassium channel Kir4.1	DCT	*KCNJ10*; 1q23	AR	Hypomagnesemia, hypocalciuria; epilepsy, ataxia, sensorineural deafness; tubulopathy

AD: autosomal dominant; AR: autosomal recessive; CCD: cortical collecting duct; DCT: distal convoluted tubule; PTH: parathyroid hormone; TAL: thick ascending limb

BOX 20.5: Management of Bartter syndrome

Therapy

Sodium chloride (5–10 mEq/kg/day) supports extracellular volume and improves electrolyte abnormalities. Occasional patients with type I or type II Bartter syndrome who shows secondary nephrogenic diabetes insipidus are not administered sodium supplements

Potassium chloride (1–3 mEq/kg/d) for treating hypokalemia; aim to target ~3 mEq/L

Magnesium supplementation, chiefly in type III disease: Organic salts (aspartate, citrate, and lactate) have higher bioavailability than magnesium oxide or hydroxide **(Annexure 5)** target serum magnesium ~1.45 mg/dL

Administer supplements in divided doses throughout the day

NSAIDs

Therapy with nonsteroidal anti-inflammatory drugs (NSAIDs) suppresses prostaglandin formation, with improved growth and electrolyte profile

Agents: Indomethacin (1–4 mg/kg/d divided in 3–4 doses); ibuprofen (15–30 mg/kg/d in three divided doses); celecoxib (2–10 mg/kg/d in two doses)

Euvolemia should be achieved prior to using NSAIDs, to avoid potential nephrotoxicity

Long-term therapy may be associated with gastrointestinal and renal adverse effects. Interventions for gastric acid suppression may be necessary; small risk of hypomagnesemia

Supportive therapy

Maximize caloric intake to facilitate optimal growth. Tube feeding or gastrostomy may be required

Therapy with potassium sparing agents, angiotensin-converting enzyme inhibitors, and angiotensin receptor blockers are not routinely indicated

Therapy for hypercalciuria with thiazide diuretics is not routinely advised

Follow-up

Follow-up visits: Anthropometry, pubertal development; creatinine, electrolytes, magnesium, pH, bicarbonate; urine calcium excretion; ultrasound abdomen

DISORDERS WITH RENAL MAGNESIUM WASTING

Magnesium is a major cation whose deficiency manifests as enhanced neuromuscular excitability (tetany, carpopedal spasms), hypocalcemia, and cardiac arrhythmias. Magnesium homeostasis depends on the balance between intestinal uptake and renal excretion. Intestinal absorption involves active transcellular transport, mediated by the channels transient receptor potential melastatin related type 6 (TRPM6) or TRPM7, and a passive paracellular pathway. Only 15% of filtered Mg^{2+} is absorbed proximally; 70% in the thick ascending limb, and 15% in the distal convoluted tubule, leaving 3–5% to be excreted in the urine. In the thick ascending limb, passive paracellular reabsorption of magnesium is mediated by claudin-16 and -19 **(Fig. 20.6)**, and depends on the active reabsorption of sodium mediated by NKCC, recycling of potassium into the lumen via ROMK, and efflux of sodium and chloride via the Na^+K^+-ATPase and ClC-K, respectively.

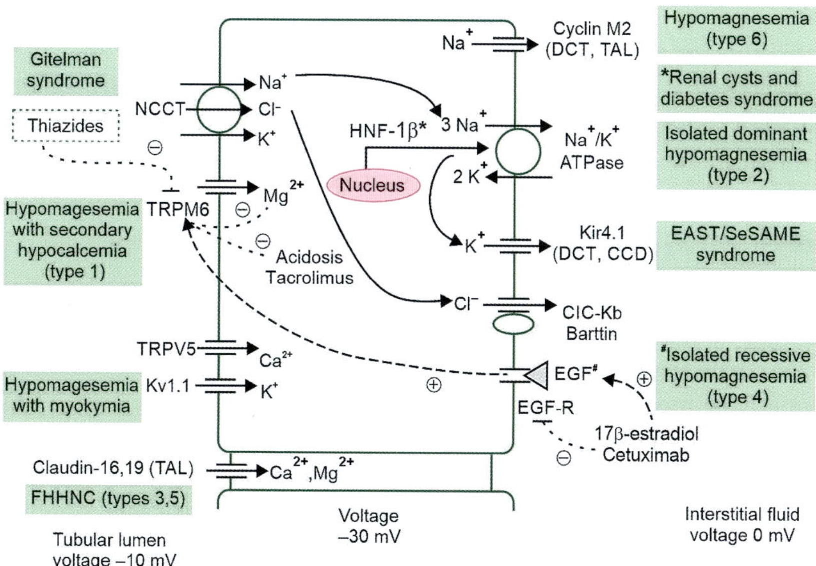

Fig. 20.6: Absorption of sodium, chloride, and magnesium ions in the distal convoluted tubule (DCT). Transepithelial sodium chloride absorption is mediated by the electroneutral thiazide-sensitive sodium chloride cotransporter (NCCT) with basolateral exit via the Na^+/K^+-ATPase and ClC-Kb/Barttin. Unlike the thick ascending limb (TAL), there is no active participation in luminal transport of potassium; however, the Kir4.1 channel in the basolateral membrane allows for recycling of potassium ions entering the tubular cells and counters movement of the extruded sodium. More distal parts of the DCT express the epithelial sodium channel (ENaC) as the main pathway for apical sodium reabsorption. Reabsorption of magnesium and calcium in the DCT is active and transcellular in nature, consisting of uptake through selective ion channels (TRPM6 and TRPV5, respectively), unlike in the TAL, where the passive paracellular absorption of these cations through the claudin 16 and 19 channels is influenced by renal outer membrane potassium (ROMK) activity **(Fig. 20.5)**. Textboxes indicate various disorders associated magnesium wasting **(*see* Table 20.7)**. CCD: cortical collecting duct; EAST syndrome: epilepsy, ataxia, sensorineural deafness and tubulopathy; EGF: epidermal growth factor; EGF-R: EGF receptor; FHHNC: familial hypomagnesemia with hypercalciuria and nephrocalcinosis

The Ca^{2+} sensing receptor (CaSR) inhibits ROMK and prevents paracellular Ca^{2+} and Mg^{2+} reabsorption. In the distal convoluted tubule, Mg^{2+} is absorbed by active transport through TRPM6, the activity of which is influenced by its intracellular concentration, pH, and other factors **(Fig. 20.6)**.

Etiology

Hypomagnesemia is commonly the result of poor enteral intake and malabsorption, but may be secondary to renal wasting in acquired tubular diseases (chronic pyelonephritis, interstitial nephritis, postobstructive diuresis, and acute tubular necrosis) or occur as an adverse effect of therapy with osmotic or thiazide diuretics, cisplatin, carboplatin, calcineurin inhibitors, or aminoglycosides. Magnesium wasting may also be seen in patients with Gitelman syndrome, EAST syndrome, and classic and antenatal Bartter syndrome with sensorineural deafness. Disorders associated with hypomagnesemia and hypermagnesuria are summarized in **Table 20.7**.

Gitelman Syndrome

Gitelman syndrome, also known as familial hypokalemic hypomagnesemia, is a rare autosomal recessive salt-losing tubulopathy characterized by hypokalemic metabolic alkalosis, hypomagnesemia, and hypocalciuria. The underlying mechanism is a defect in the apical thiazide-sensitive, NCCT in the distal tubule. The majority of patients with Gitelman syndrome are compound heterozygous for two significant variants in *SLC12A3*, which encodes NCCT. Most of these are missense variants. A significant proportion of patients only have a heterozygous variant in *SLC12A3*; an additional deep intronic variant or gene rearrangement might be responsible for the phenotype in such patients.

Clinical and biochemical manifestations mimic classic Bartter syndrome, including metabolic alkalosis and hypomagnesemia. However, the symptoms are generally milder and usually appear in older school going children and adults. Variability is reported in age at presentation, severity of symptoms, and biochemical abnormalities. Patients may be detected following the incidental finding of hypokalemia, or when evaluated for growth retardation, constipation, or enuresis. There are episodes of muscular weakness, cramps and fatigue, vomiting, abdominal pain, and tetany; polyuria and growth retardation are mild. Uncommon manifestations include chondrocalcinosis and sclerochoroidal calcifications (associated with hypomagnesemia), cardiac arrhythmias, autoimmune disorders (chiefly of the thyroid), and vertigo. Case series describe an increased risk of mild hypertension and type 2 diabetes mellitus.

Urinary calcium excretion is low, due to increase in paracellular calcium reabsorption in the proximal tubule (parallel to sodium reabsorption, secondary to volume depletion). The diagnostic features of Gitelman syndrome are shown in **Box 20.6**. Features in Gitelman syndrome mimic chronic thiazide administration, including normal or low blood pressure, hypokalemic metabolic acidosis, hypomagnesemia, and hypocalciuria. The combination of hypocalciuria with renal magnesium wasting distinguishes Gitelman from Bartter syndrome and most magnesium losing states **(Tables 20.4, 20.5 and 20.7)**. Patients with Gitelman syndrome require long-term use of oral potassium and magnesium supplements.

BOX 20.6: Gitelman syndrome: Diagnosis and management

Diagnosis

Chronic hypokalemia (<3.5 mEq/L) with concomitant potassium wasting (spot urine potassium to creatinine ratio >18 mEq/g) in absence of potassium lowering medications

Metabolic alkalosis

Hypomagnesemia (<1.70 mg/dL) with inappropriate magnesium wasting (fractional excretion <4%)

Hypocalciuria (spot urine, calcium to creatinine ratio <0.07 mg/mg)

High renin (activity or plasma levels)

Fractional excretion of chloride >0.5%

Normal or low blood pressure

Normal kidney ultrasound; no abnormalities or nephrocalcinosis

Confirmation

High throughput sequencing to diagnose mutations; screen for genes that phenocopy Gitelman syndrome

Therapy

Salt supplementation

Magnesium supplements: 5 mg/kg/dose given 3–4 times daily; prefer chloride, lactate or aspartate salt

Potassium supplements: 1–3 mEq/kg/day (oral potassium chloride)

Spironolactone, eplerenone or amiloride in refractory cases

Indomethacin, rofecoxib (cyclooxygenase-2 inhibitor) are less often indicated

EAST Syndrome

Mutations in the gene *KCNJ10* encoding the K^+ channel Kir4.1 cause a rare autosomal recessive disorder characterized by epilepsy, ataxia, sensorineural deafness and salt-wasting tubulopathy, termed EAST or SeSAME (seizures, sensorineural deafness, ataxia, mental retardation, and electrolyte imbalance) syndrome. *KNCJ10* (Kir4.1) is expressed in the brain, inner ear, eye, and kidneys. The renal salt-wasting is caused by transport defects in the distal convoluted tubule, where *KCNJ10* plays an important role as a basolateral K^+ channel **(Fig. 20.6)**, with K^+ recycling across the basolateral membrane enabling normal activity of Na^+-K^+-ATPase. Renal abnormalities mimic findings in Gitelman syndrome, including urinary Na^+ loss, activation of renin-angiotensin-aldosterone axis, hypokalemic metabolic alkalosis, hypomagnesemia, and hypocalciuria.

Management of Magnesium Deficiency

Intravenous infusions are required in symptomatic patients. The initial dose is 20–50 mg/kg body weight of magnesium sulfate, given over 20 minutes; doses may be repeated every 6–8 hr. Asymptomatic hypomagnesemia or chronic magnesium deficiency is treated with oral magnesium (10–20 mg/kg q 6–8 hr). Intestinal absorption and bioavailability is superior for organic magnesium (citrate, aspartate) salts. Potassium sparing diuretics and aldosterone antagonists are effective in reducing magnesium excretion.

HYPOKALEMIC METABOLIC ALKALOSIS AND HYPERTENSION

Hypertension in childhood may rarely be secondary to single gene mutations, inherited in an autosomal dominant or recessive fashion that leads to increased epithelial sodium or chloride reabsorption, high urinary potassium secretion, suppression of plasma renin activity (PRA) and/or excessive mineralocorticoid action with hypokalemic metabolic alkalosis (Chapter 25).

PSEUDOHYPOALDOSTERONISM

Pseudohypoaldosteronism comprises a heterogeneous group of disorders characterized by an apparent state of renal tubular unresponsiveness or resistance to the action of aldosterone, manifest as hyperkalemia and metabolic acidosis with normal GFR. The disorder is classified into PHA type 1, the classic form, and PHA type 2, also termed Gordon or chloride shunt syndrome **(Table 20.8)**. PHA type 1 is characterized by lack of renal response to aldosterone leading to salt wasting and potassium retention. PHA type 2 is characterized by defect in potassium excretion in response to mineralocorticoids while sodium and chloride reabsorption are unchanged or enhanced.

The PHA type 1 includes two entities with isolated renal or multiple target organ defects, inherited in autosomal dominant and recessive forms, respectively. In addition, transient forms of PHA are described in neonates and infants following pyelonephritis with or without underlying obstructive uropathy, and after renal vein thrombosis.

Pseudohypoaldosteronism type 2 is caused by mutations in genes regulating the sodium potassium cotransporter (NCCT) and ROMK potassium channels, most commonly mutations in serine threonine kinases, *WNK1* or *WNK4* **(Fig. 20.1; Tables 20.1 and 20.8)**. *WNK4* normally inhibits NCCT and ROMK channels to decrease sodium reabsorption and potassium secretion. Mutations in *WNK4* lead to an abnormal protein that no longer inhibits sodium channels but inhibits potassium channels more strongly. *WNK1* blocks inhibition of NCCT by *WNK4*, thereby increasing sodium reabsorption, but independently inhibits potassium channels with decrease in potassium secretion. Gain in function mutations of *WNK1* or loss of function mutations in *WNK4* lead to increased sodium reabsorption and decreased potassium secretion, resulting in hypertension and hyperkalemia.

TABLE 20.8: Causes of pseudohypoaldosteronism (PHA). Hyperkalemic metabolic acidosis is common to all types

Disorder	*PHA type 1*		*PHA type 2*	
Subtype	Renal limited (classic PHA of infancy; Cheek and Perry syndrome)	Multiple target organ (autosomal recessive PHA 1)	Gordon syndrome (chloride shunt syndrome, mineralocorticoid resistant hyperkalemia)	Spitzer–Weinstein syndrome
Cause	Inactivation of mineralocorticoid receptor	Inactivation of epithelial sodium channel (ENaC)	Gain of function of sodium chloride cotransporter and paracellular chloride reabsorption; volume overload	
Inheritance	Autosomal dominant	Autosomal recessive	Autosomal dominant	Not known
Gene; chromosome	*NR3C2* encoding mineralocorticoid receptor; 4q31	*SCNN1A, SCNN1B* or *SCNN1G* encoding, α, β, or γ subunit of ENaC;12p13.3; 16p12.2; 16p12.2	PHA 2A: unknown, 1q31-42 PHA 2B: *WNK4*, 17q21 PHA 2C: *WNK1*, 12p13 PHA 2D: *KLHL3*, 5q31 PHA 2E: *CUL3*, 2q36	Not known
Organs affected	Kidney	Kidney, sweat and salivary glands, colon	Kidney	Kidney
Age at presentation	Neonatal period or infancy	Neonatal period or infancy	Adulthood; PHA 2E and recessive forms of PHA 2D present in infancy	Adolescence
Key features	Salt wasting	Salt wasting; respiratory tract infections; eczematoid rash	Hypertension; PHA 2E most severe, PHA 2C mildest	Hypertension uncommon; short stature
Duration of symptoms	Outgrow by two years	Lifelong	Lifelong	Lifelong
Plasma renin; aldosterone	High; high	High; high	Low; normal to high	Low; normal to high
Serum sodium	Low or normal	Low to normal; high sodium in sweat and saliva	Normal	Normal
Hypercalciuria	May be present	Absent	Present (especially in PHA 2B)	Present
Therapy	Sodium supplements (3–20 mEq/kg of Na^+ daily, as NaCl and $NaHCO_3$; potassium binding resins	Sodium supplements (usually >20 mEq/kg of Na^+ daily); potassium binding resins; thiazides	Thiazides; salt restriction	Thiazides; salt restriction

CUL3: Cullin 3; KLH3: Kelch-like 3; WNK: with no lysine (K) kinases

BIBLIOGRAPHY

1. Alonso-Varela M, Gil-Peña H, Santos F. Incomplete distal renal tubular acidosis in children. Acta Paediatr. 2020;109:2243-50.
2. Bagga A, Sinha A. Renal tubular acidosis. Indian J Pediatr. 2020;87:733-44.
3. Blanchard A, Bockenhauer D, Bolignano D, et al. Gitelman syndrome: Consensus and guidance from a Kidney Disease: Improving Global Outcomes (KDIGO) Controversies Conference. Kidney Int. 2017;91:24-33.
4. Bockenhauer D, Bichet DG. Inherited secondary nephrogenic diabetes insipidus: concentrating on humans. Am J Physiol Renal Physiol. 2013;304:F1037-42.
5. Chinsky JM, Singh R, Ficicioglu C, et al. Diagnosis and treatment of tyrosinemia type I: US and Canadian consensus group review and recommendations. Genet Med. 2017;19. PMID: 28771246.
6. Choi N, Kang HG. Bartter syndrome: Perspectives of a pediatric nephrologist. Electrolyte Blood Press. 2022;20:49-56.
7. Ehlayel AM, Copelovitch L. Update on Dent disease. Pediatr Clin North Am. 2019;66:169-78.
8. Emma F, Nesterova G, Langman C, et al. Nephropathic cystinosis: An international consensus document. Nephrol Dial Transplant. 2014;29: iv87-94.
9. Foreman JW. Fanconi syndrome. Pediatr Clin North Am. 2019;66:159-67.
10. Fulchiero R, Seo-Mayer P. Bartter syndrome and Gitelman syndrome. Pediatr Clin North Am. 2019;66:121-34.
11. Giglio S, Montini G, Trepiccione F, et al. Distal renal tubular acidosis: A systematic approach from diagnosis to treatment. J Nephrol. 2021;34:2073-83.
12. Hureaux M, Vargas-Poussou R. Genetic basis of nephrogenic diabetes insipidus. Mol Cell Endocrinol. 2023;560:111825.
13. Jin YY, Huang LM, Quan XF, et al. Dent disease: Classification, heterogeneity and diagnosis. World J Pediatr. 2021;17:52-7.
14. Kashoor I, Batlle D. Proximal renal tubular acidosis with and without Fanconi syndrome. Kidney Res Clin Pract. 2019;38:267-81.
15. Kavanagh C, Uy NS. Nephrogenic diabetes insipidus. Pediatr Clin North Am. 2019;66:227-34.
16. Konrad M, Nijenhuis T, Ariceta G, et al. Diagnosis and management of Bartter syndrome: Executive summary of the consensus and recommendations from the European Rare Kidney Disease Reference Network Working Group for Tubular Disorders. Kidney Int. 2021;99:324-35.
17. Laghmani K, Beck BB, Yang S-S, et al. Polyhydramnios, transient antenatal Bartter syndrome and MAGED2 mutations. N Engl J Med. 2016;374:1853-63.
18. Nozu K, Yamamura T, Horinouchi T, et al. Inherited salt-losing tubulopathy: An old condition but a new category of tubulopathy. Pediatr Int. 2020;62:428-37.
19. Palmer BF, Kelepouris E, Clegg DJ. Renal tubular acidosis and management strategies: A narrative review. Adv Ther. 2021;38:949-68.
20. Refardt J. Diagnosis and differential diagnosis of diabetes insipidus: Update. Best Pract Res Clin Endocrinol Metab. 2020;34:101398.
21. Trepiccione F, Walsh SB, Ariceta G, et al. Distal renal tubular acidosis: ERKNet/ESPN clinical practice points. Nephrol Dial Transplant. 2021;36:1585-96.
22. Vaz de Castro PAS, Bitencourt L, de Oliveira Campos JL, et al. Nephrogenic diabetes insipidus: a comprehensive overview. J Pediatr Endocrinol Metab. 2022;35:421-34.
23. Veys KR, Elmonem MA, Arcolino FO, et al. Nephropathic cystinosis: An update. Curr Opin Pediatr. 2017;29:168-78.

CHAPTER 21

Tubulointerstitial Diseases

Aditi Sinha, Arvind Bagga

ACUTE INTERSTITIAL NEPHRITIS

Acute interstitial nephritis (AIN) is an immune-mediated injury to tubulointerstitial compartment of kidneys with relative sparing of glomeruli. The condition may account for ~10% pediatric patients with acute kidney injury (AKI).

Etiology

Medications, infections, and systemic disorders [systemic lupus erythematosus (SLE) and Sjögren syndrome] are the common etiologies in children **(Table 21.1)**. Medications incriminated include antibiotics (ampicillin, ciprofloxacin, methicillin, and rifampicin), proton-pump inhibitors, and nonsteroidal anti-inflammatory drugs (NSAIDs) **(Table 21.2)**. Drug-induced AIN is usually a delayed T-cell-mediated hypersensitivity reaction that is triggered by either: (*i*) a drug or its metabolite (hapten)

TABLE 21.1: Etiology of tubulointerstitial nephritis (TIN)

Etiology	*Examples*
Drugs	See **Table 21.2**
Infections	
Viral	Cytomegalovirus, hepatitis, HIV, Epstein–Barr virus, hantavirus, BK polyomavirus
Bacterial	*Salmonella, Streptococcus, Yersinia, Brucella, Leptospirosis*
	Acute pyelonephritis (Focal TIN)
Fungal	Histoplasmosis
Parasitic	Leishmania, toxoplasma
Immune-mediated	Sarcoidosis, systemic lupus erythematosus, Sjögren disease, inflammatory bowel disease
Granulomatous TIN	Medications **(Table 21.3)**; sarcoidosis; tuberculosis; bacterial/fungal infections; granulomatosis with polyangiitis
TIN with uveitis	
Idiopathic	

TABLE 21.2: Drugs associated with tubulointerstitial nephritis	
Analgesics	NSAIDs (ibuprofen and ketorolac), selective cyclooxygenase-2 inhibitors
Antibiotics	Beta-lactams, cephalosporins, sulfonamides, nitrofurantoin, chloramphenicol, fluoroquinolones (ciprofloxacin), doxycycline, erythromycin, vancomycin, minocycline, and gentamicin
Antitubercular therapy	Rifampin, ethambutol, and isoniazid
Antivirals	Acyclovir, abacavir, and indinavir
Antiepileptics	Phenytoin, carbamazepine, phenobarbital, lamotrigine and levetiracetam
Antacids	Proton pump inhibitors, histamine receptor antagonists
Diuretics	Furosemide, thiazide diuretics, amiloride, and triamterene
Immunosuppression	Cyclosporine, azathioprine, and sulfasalazine
Other	Allopurinol, alendronate, lithium, and chlorpropamide

NSAIDs: nonsteroidal anti-inflammatory drugs

interacting with a carrier protein (haptenization); or (*ii*) direct interaction of the drug with a specific host protein (direct pharmacological interaction of drugs with immune receptors), wherein the core structural component of each drug is the antigen and similar drug structures from various classes may cause cross-reactivity.

Clinical Features

The classic triad of fever, rash, and eosinophilia, occurring within a few days of the initiation of a medication, is seen in only 10% of patients. Presenting features are nonspecific, and include fatigue, weight loss, headache and flank pain.

Diagnosis

While AIN is obvious in patients presenting with the classic triad, more often than not, the diagnosis is not straight-forward. Few patients manifest oliguric AKI; nonoliguric AKI or an insidious decline in kidney function not meeting AKI criteria is more common. Urinalysis reveals leukocyturia (sterile pyuria) and leukocyte casts **(Fig. 2.1B)**. Eosinophiluria (>1% of leukocytes) and hematuria are uncommon. Patients may show evidence of Fanconi syndrome (normal anion gap metabolic acidosis, glucosuria, and aminoaciduria). Tubular proteinuria is seen in 90% cases of drug-induced AIN. Urinary biomarkers such as α1-microglobulin and β2-microglobulin may help to diagnose and monitor disease activity.

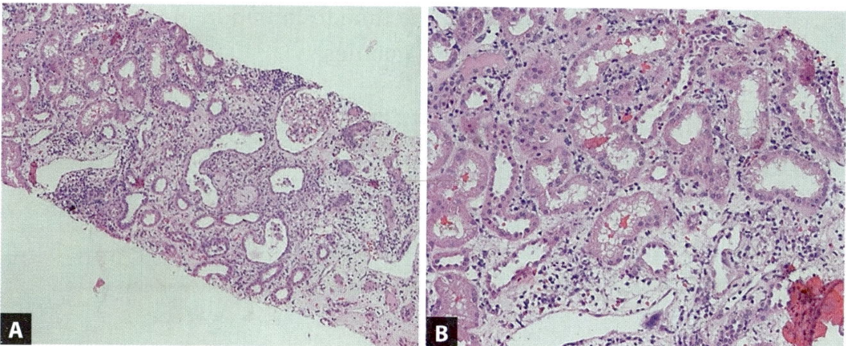

Figs. 21.1A and B: Acute interstitial nephritis. (A) Light microscopy shows moderate to dense tubulointerstitial lymphomononuclear inflammation with edema and acute tubular injury; the glomeruli are unremarkable; (H&E 100×). (B) High-power view shows inflammatory infiltrate rich in lymphocytes, plasma cells and occasional eosinophils, with associated tubulitis and interstitial edema (H&E 200×)

Kidney biopsy is the gold standard for diagnosis. Histology shows interstitial inflammatory abnormalities with damage to tubular cells **(Figs. 21.1A and B)**. Inflammation with T cells, monocytes, macrophages, plasma cells, and eosinophils is patchy, mostly in the deep cortex and outer medulla. Tubulitis represents the extension of the inflammatory infiltrate into tubules. Immunofluorescence is unremarkable, except for C3 deposition in anti-glomerular basement membrane (GBM) disease and IgG deposits in the tubular basement membrane in IgG4-related kidney diseases.

Management

Management of drug-induced AIN involves anticipation (vigilance), diagnosis (timely detection), treatment, and prevention. Treatment is based on the underlying etiology. Removal of the offending agents results in spontaneous resolution in most cases. Corticosteroids are advised in patients with persistently impaired kidney function (beyond 5–7 days of discontinuing the offending agent) and/or severe AIN. Corticosteroids inhibit the activation and proliferation of T lymphocytes and eosinophils that are implicated in the development of AIN. Prednisolone is given at the dose of 0.8–1.0 mg/kg daily for 3–4 weeks and then tapered and discontinued over 5–6 weeks. Maintenance therapy with mycophenolate mofetil (MMF) is not required, except in patients with systemic disease.

Outcomes

Delay in diagnosis of AIN leads to ongoing inflammation, which results in interstitial fibrosis and tubular atrophy. The risk of incomplete recovery from AIN and occurrence of chronic kidney disease (CKD) is as high as 40–60% in certain forms of drug-induced AIN. The time to initiation of corticosteroids appears to have an impact on kidney outcomes.

TUBULOINTERSTITIAL NEPHRITIS AND UVEITIS SYNDROME

This rare entity is characterized by concomitant or consecutive occurrence of acute idiopathic interstitial nephritis and bilateral anterior uveitis.

Epidemiology

Tubulointerstitial nephritis and uveitis (TINU) does not show any geographic or racial predilection. The condition is common in adolescent girls (female to male ratio of 3:1; median age 15 years); affected boys are younger. Estimates suggest that TINU might account for a significant proportion of pediatric and adult patients with TIN. Some patients might initially present with acute nongranulomatous anterior uveitis.

Etiopathogenesis

TINU is believed to be an immune-mediated process. Reported associations include human leukocyte antigen (HLA) types (HLA-DQA1*01, HLA-DQB1*05, HLA-DRB1*01, and HLA-DRB1*0102), exposure to medications (NSAIDs, antibiotics), infections (*Chlamydia trachomatis*, Epstein–Barr virus, *Mycobacterium tuberculosis*, *Toxoplasma gondii*, and varicella zoster), and systemic disease (hypoparathyroidism, hyperthyroidism, IgG4-related disease, and rheumatoid arthritis). The condition might result from hypersensitivity reaction or hapten-induced cytokine production and immune response. Alternatively, it is caused by targeted disruption or dysfunction of similar proteins in the kidney tubule and ciliary epithelium in the eyes. The detection of autoantibodies against modified C-reactive protein in kidneys and eyes suggests roles for target autoantigen(s) and humoral immunity.

Clinical Features

TINU should be suspected in patients with unexplained AKI and/or progressive decline in estimated glomerular filtration rate (eGFR). Initial symptoms are nonspecific, including fever, malaise, fatigue, and flank pain. Since TIN usually precedes uveitis, the history of malaise presents before ocular symptoms; TIN and uveitis can occasionally present concurrently, or uveitis may precede TIN. TIN is usually more severe in older patients.

Features of anterior uveitis include acute onset of eye pain, redness, decreased vision, and photophobia. Uveitis is usually unilateral to begin with, and progressively becomes chronic and bilateral. In 80% of cases, physical examination reveals bilateral nongranulomatous anterior uveitis. Up to 20% of patients show intermediate uveitis, posterior uveitis, or panuveitis. Additional findings include posterior synechiae (a common complication), cells in the vitreous, optic disk swelling, macular edema, chorioretinal scar, cataracts, and glaucoma.

Diagnosis

The diagnosis is made on careful eye examination, serum biochemistry and urinalysis, with or without kidney biopsy. The classification criteria proposed by the Standardization of Uveitis Nomenclature Working Group (2021) require demonstrating the presence of both anterior uveitis (with or without intermediate or posterior chamber involvement) and TIN, and the exclusion of syphilis and sarcoidosis.

Anterior uveitis is diagnosed if there are cells in the anterior chamber, regardless of presence or absence of vitritis, choroiditis, or retinal vascular changes. The diagnosis of TIN is confirmed on kidney biopsy, or suggested by abnormal kidney function tests, abnormal urinalysis (tubular proteinuria, glucosuria, eosinophiluria, sterile pyuria, and casts of white cells with/without red cells), or elevated urine β2 microglobulin. Kidney biopsy shows interstitial edema and inflammatory cell infiltrate comprising eosinophils, lymphocytes, neutrophils, plasma cells and histiocytes, tubular injury and edema, and epithelial cell degeneration. The glomeruli and blood vessels are spared. Immunofluorescence does not reveal immune deposits.

Patients may show normochromic, normocytic anemia, elevated erythrocyte sedimentation rate, hypergammaglobulinemia, and elevated C-reactive protein.

Differential Diagnosis

Tubulointerstitial nephritis and uveitis is a diagnosis of exclusion. Conditions that present with kidney involvement and uveitis should be excluded, including sarcoidosis, Sjögren syndrome, SLE, syphilis, granulomatosis with polyangiitis, Behçet disease, IgG4-related renal disease, infectious mononucleosis, tuberculosis, toxoplasmosis, brucellosis, and histoplasmosis.

Management

Most patients with TIN are initiated on oral therapy with prednisolone that is continued for weeks to months. Patients with persistently impaired kidney functions may receive three pulses of IV methylprednisolone, followed by a short course of oral prednisolone. MMF or azathioprine is preferred in patients with nephritis that is refractory to therapy with corticosteroids, or in those with persistently impaired kidney function or relapses.

Anterior uveitis is managed with topical steroids and cycloplegic drugs. Up to 80% of patients need systemic corticosteroids at the onset. On the long term, up to 70% of patients with anterior uveitis have corticosteroid-refractory disease or recurrent symptoms for which they are considered for steroid-sparing immunomodulatory therapy, including MMF, azathioprine or methotrexate, and rarely, adalimumab. Given the risks of relapses and sequelae of inflammation, therapy with topical steroids and steroid-sparing therapy is continued for 1–2 years of remission.

Monitoring

Since uveitis is often recurrent, long-term therapy and monitoring is recommended. Ophthalmological screening and serum and urine biochemistry are repeated once every 3 months up to 1 year. Urine β2 microglobulin correlates with uveitis and nephritis, and is a useful biomarker for asymptomatic inflammation.

Outcomes

Nephritis often resolves spontaneously and recurs less often than uveitis. Adverse kidney outcomes are uncommon. However, in one series, up to 70% patients progressed to advanced CKD within 1 year. Early treatment with corticosteroids is a key predictor of long-term kidney function. Ocular inflammation tends to be resistant and chronic, has complications in up to 20% cases, and recurs in 40–70% cases. Most recurrences occur within the first few months of stopping therapy. However, most patients have satisfactory visual outcomes.

CHRONIC TUBULOINTERSTITIAL NEPHRITIS

Chronic tubulointerstitial nephritis (TIN) is a nonspecific pattern of kidney injury that may occur following exposure to drugs, heavy metals, or toxins, in association with vesicoureteric reflux, obstructive uropathy, nephrolithiasis, or chronic ischemia, or as part of systemic immunologic or inherited disease. Chronic TIN is a consequence of AIN of any etiology. Drug-induced AIN is the chief etiology, typically observed in elderly subjects who chronically use NSAIDs. Chronic TIN is also reported following sustained environmental exposure to toxins, e.g., lead, cadmium, and mercury; toxins in complementary and alternate medicine, e.g., aristolochic acid in traditional Chinese medicine herbs; and prolonged low-dose exposure to ochratoxin A (a mycotoxin), polycyclic aromatic hydrocarbons (local coals such as lignite), or aristolochic acid (*Aristolochia clematitis* plant) in Balkan endemic nephropathy. In childhood, the condition may be drug-induced or associated with TINU, systemic inflammation (sarcoidosis, lupus, Sjögren syndrome, and IgG4 disease), or inherited defects (autosomal dominant tubulointerstitial kidney disease).

Presentation is nonspecific or varies by the underlying disease; a history of AIN inciting the injury may not be recalled. Investigations reveal low-grade proteinuria, relatively bland urinary sediment, and slowly progressive decline in glomerular filtration rate. Some patients show Fanconi syndrome with glucosuria and aminoaciduria. Kidney biopsy reveals chronic interstitial nephritis with scattered tubulitis. The lymphoplasmacytic infiltration is out of proportion to the degree of interstitial fibrosis and tubular atrophy. In advanced stages, the glomerular and vascular compartments are secondarily involved with periglomerular fibrosis, ischemic wrinkling of GBM, glomerulosclerosis, vascular sclerosis, and hyalinosis. Management is conservative unless the underlying systemic disease is amenable to immunosuppression (see below). There is limited data on the outcomes of chronic TIN, particularly in children.

Chronic Interstitial Nephritis in Agricultural Communities

Chronic interstitial nephritis in agricultural communities (CINAC) not associated with traditional risk factors predominantly affects young male farmers between the third and fifth decades of life in countries in Central America (Nicaragua, El Salvador, Guatemala, and Costa Rica), Asia (Sri Lanka and Andhra Pradesh in India), and Africa (Egypt). Other names for this entity include CKD of unknown or uncertain origin (CKDu), agrochemical nephropathy, and by region, Central American nephropathy, Salvadoran agricultural nephropathy, Mesoamerican endemic nephropathy, chronic tubulointerstitial kidney disease of Central America, Uddanam endemic nephropathy, or Sri Lankan agricultural nephropathy. The prevalence of CINAC is as high as 15–21% in farming communities in these regions. Less often, CINAC affects women, children, and adolescents in these communities.

Various occupational, environmental, and genetic risk factors are proposed to explain the pathophysiology of CINAC in different communities, include exposure to agrochemicals (pesticides or herbicides, e.g., paraquat, glyphosate, methamidophos, and methyl parathion) and contaminated water (cadmium and arsenic) or soil (volcanic soil, arsenic, and natural contaminants), repeated episodes of dehydration with heat stress in hot humid weather, and underlying genetic predisposition. Unconfirmed risk factors include snake bites, infections, and abuse of NSAIDs.

Diagnostic criteria for CINAC include eGFR <60 mL/min/1.73 m^2, tubular proteinuria, nil or minimal albuminuria, belonging to agricultural community in CINAC endemic area, and lack of other known causes for CKD (diabetes, hypertension, and glomerulopathies). Ultrasound shows small kidneys with irregular contours. Kidney biopsy shows chronic tubulointerstitial nephritis, glomerulosclerosis, and mild chronic vascular injury of varying severity.

Sarcoidosis

Sarcoidosis is a multisystem disorder that can affect almost any organ system with characteristic noncaseating granulomas. Pulmonary sarcoidosis is the most common manifestation, followed by skin, ocular, cardiac, and central nervous system involvement. Kidney disease is relatively uncommon, but can progress to advanced CKD.

Epidemiology

The incidence of sarcoidosis varies by region, from 3.7 per 100,000 in Japan to 10–11 per 100,000 in Northern Sweden and United States, and 28.2 per 100,000 population in Finland. The highest incidence is in Afro-Americans women (39.1) and men (29.8 per 100,000 Afro-Americans). Kidney involvement is reported in 0–30% cases. Isolated renal sarcoidosis without systemic disease has been reported occasionally.

Kidney Disease

The most common kidney disease in patients with sarcoidosis is hypercalciuric nephrolithiasis with or without nephrocalcinosis. In sarcoidosis, pulmonary macrophages autonomously overexpress 1α-hydroxylase, leading to overproduction of 1,25-$(OH)_2$ vitamin D, which causes hypercalcemia and/or hypercalciuria, leading to kidney stones or nephrocalcinosis.

The term renal sarcoidosis refers to the granulomatous interstitial nephritis seen in this condition **(Figs. 21.2A to C)**. Others have defined renal sarcoidosis as treatment-responsive kidney failure from granulomatous and nongranulomatous interstitial nephritis related to sarcoidosis. Approximately 20% of patients with systemic sarcoidosis develop granulomatous interstitial nephritis. These granulomas are composed of macrophages, epithelioid cells, mononuclear cells, and CD4+ cells, with few CD8+ cells in the peripheral zone. The likelihood of granulomatous inflammation is higher in patients with advanced CKD.

Glomerular disease is also reported, with diverse manifestations. The most common histological diagnoses includes IgA nephropathy and membranous nephropathy, and rarely minimal change disease, focal segmental glomerulosclerosis, membranoproliferative glomerulonephritis, and proliferative or crescentic glomerulonephritis with or without antineutrophil cytoplasmic antibody (ANCA) positivity. Systemic sarcoidosis may be associated with secondary (or AA) amyloidosis (see Chapter 7).

Clinical Features and Diagnosis

Patients present with clinical features of interstitial lung disease, including low-grade fever, malaise, dry cough, dyspnea, and reduced exercise capacity. Diagnosis of sarcoidosis requires the presence of noncaseating granuloma

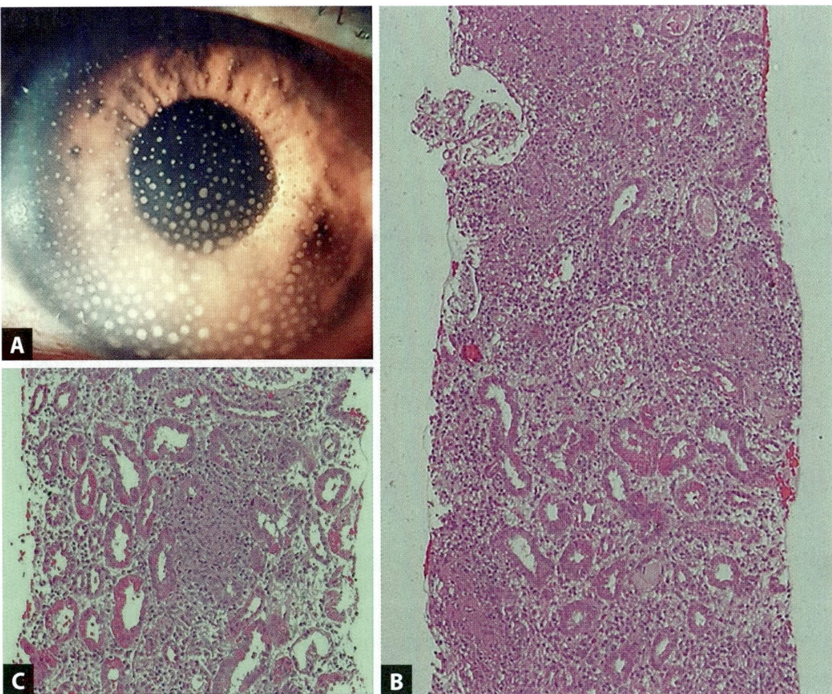

Figs. 21.2A to C: Sarcoidosis in a 4-year-old girl presenting with acute kidney injury, polyuria, dehydration, and hypercalcemia. (A) Ophthalmoscopic evaluation by slit lamp reveals multiple mutton fat keratic precipitates, suggestive of chronic anterior granulomatous uveitis; (B) Kidney biopsy low power view in light microscopy shows dense tubulointerstitial lymphomononuclear inflammation with interspersed multiple epithelioid cell granulomas, suggesting chronic granulomatous interstitial nephritis; the glomeruli are uninvolved (H&E 100×). (C) High power view shows presence of a non-necrotizing epithelioid cell granuloma with adjacent lymphomononuclear interstitial infiltrate (H&E 200×)

and compatible presentations after exclusion of other identifiable causes. The diagnosis of pulmonary sarcoidosis is based on suggestive findings on pulmonary function tests, chest radiography and high-resolution computed tomography, elevated calcium, low parathyroid hormone, elevated 1,25-$(OH)_2$ vitamin D, and increased levels of angiotensin-converting enzyme (ACE). Where feasible, tissue diagnosis should be performed.

Evaluation for kidney disease includes assessment of kidney function (creatinine and estimated GFR), quantification of proteinuria, and urinalysis. Serum levels of calcium and 1,25-$(OH)_2$ vitamin D are measured along with 24-hour urine calcium excretion. An ultrasound of the kidneys is done for nephrolithiasis or nephrocalcinosis. Kidney biopsy is advised in patients with confirmed or suspected sarcoidosis with low eGFR, abnormal urinalysis, proteinuria, and/or abnormal ultrasound findings. Histopathological findings help to confirm the diagnosis. Granulomas are rare in patients with isolated interstitial nephritis or TINU, and their presence in a setting of TIN suggests sarcoidosis **(Table 21.3)**. This is particularly true if there is evidence of systemic granulomatous disease **(Fig. 21.2)**.

Management

Kidney disease related to nephrolithiasis and nephrocalcinosis is managed with alkalization of urine and correction of hypercalcemia with hyperhydration and immunosuppression. Kidney manifestations secondary to altered calcium homeostasis have satisfactory prognosis since steroid therapy normalizes calcium levels and reduces risk of nephrolithiasis.

Patients with renal sarcoidosis with granulomatous interstitial nephritis with or without glomerular lesions have been treated with immunosuppression. Glucocorticoids are the mainstay of management. Therapy with prednisone is initiated at 0.5–1 mg/kg/day for 4 weeks, followed

TABLE 21.3: Etiology of granulomatous interstitial nephritis

Medications	
Analgesics	NSAIDs (ibuprofen and ketorolac)
Antibiotics	Penicillin, cephalosporin, fluoroquinolones, rifampicin, and nitrofurantoin
Antivirals	Indinavir
Antiepileptics	Carbamazepine
Antacids	Proton pump inhibitors
Diuretics	Furosemide and thiazide diuretics
Antihypertensive drugs	Captopril and valsartan
Biological therapies	Immune checkpoint inhibitors (ipilimumab and nivolumab)
Others	Allopurinol, alendronate, and mesalamine
Infections	
Mycobacteria	*Mycobacterium tuberculosis* and atypical mycobacteria
Fungi	Histoplasmosis, candidiasis, and cryptococcosis
Others	Toxoplasmosis and Epstein–Barr virus
Systemic diseases	
Autoimmune	Sarcoidosis, systemic lupus erythematosus, and Sjögren syndrome
Vasculitis	Granulomatosis with polyangiitis, eosinophilic granulomatosis with polyangiitis
Others	Immunoglobulin G4-related disease, common variable immune deficiency
Idiopathic	Tubulointerstitial nephritis with uveitis syndrome

by tapering over 6–12 months to 5 mg/day, which is continued for another 6–12 months. Most patients show significant improvement in kidney function with steroids alone. Glucocorticoids are required on the long-term in patients who show decline of eGFR following discontinuation of steroid therapy.

Relapses are treated by increasing the dose of steroids to the last effective dose. Additional use of azathioprine (1–2 mg/kg daily), MMF (1,200 mg/m^2 daily in two divided doses), or leflunomide (loading dose 100 mg for 1–3 days, followed by 10–20 mg daily or on alternate days) with or without hydroxychloroquine (4–5 mg/kg daily) is considered in patients with refractory disease or those with steroid toxicity. Patients with refractory disease may benefit from use of tumor necrosis factor-α (TNF-α) inhibitors, especially infliximab (3–5 mg/kg per dose, q 2–6 weeks).

Outcomes

Relapse of symptomatic sarcoidosis is noted in 20–80% of patients upon withdrawal of steroid therapy. Patients experience low quality of life due to dyspnea, chest pain, cough, malaise, fatigue, and arthralgia. While renal sarcoidosis responds satisfactorily to treatment, 60–80% patients show CKD 3–5 on follow-up. Factors that influence outcomes are the level of creatinine at diagnosis, kidney histology, the presence of tubulointerstitial fibrosis, and response to treatment. A high renal burden of granulomas is associated with unsatisfactory outcomes compared to nongranulomatous nephritis. Early treatment is crucial, with maximum benefit in kidney function seen in the first 4–6 weeks.

Sjögren Syndrome

Sjögren syndrome is characterized by a chronic inflammatory cell infiltration of the exocrine salivary and lacrimal glands and is associated with the "sicca complex" of xerostomia and xerophthalmia. Systemic manifestations occur in approximately one-third of patients, and include involvement of the kidneys, lungs, esophagus, thyroid, stomach, and pancreas. Other patients have features of connective tissue disease, most commonly rheumatoid arthritis, and less frequently SLE, scleroderma, polymyositis, or mixed connective tissue disease. Chronic active hepatitis, primary biliary cirrhosis, Crohn disease, and fibrosing alveolitis, lymphoma or Waldenström macroglobulinemia are also described.

The 2016 ACR/EULAR classification criteria are used to diagnose Sjögren syndrome based on the weighed sum of the following clinical parameters or laboratory results: (*i*) anti-Ro/SSA positivity (3 points); (*ii*) focal lymphocytic sialadenitis on labial salivary gland biopsy with focus score ≥1 foci/4 mm^2 (3 points); ocular dryness, as suggested by either (*iii*) positive Schirmer test (≤5 mm per 5 minutes; 1 point); and/or (*iv*) ocular staining score ≥5 (1 point);

and (5) oral dryness, as suggested by unstimulated whole saliva flow rate ≤0.1 mL/min (1 point). A score of≥4 points in an individual with either ocular or oral dryness is considered diagnostic.

Only 5% patients with Sjögren syndrome have overt evidence of kidney disease. Kidney manifestations usually relate to tubulointerstitial involvement with tubular defects such as distal renal tubular acidosis, impaired concentrating ability, hypercalciuria, and, less frequently, Fanconi syndrome, Gitelman syndrome, nephrogenic diabetes insipidus or nephrolithiasis. Kidney biopsy shows chronic interstitial inflammation with variable interstitial fibrosis and tubular atrophy. In 15% cases, kidney involvement is in the form of glomerular disease secondary to immune-complex deposition, ranging from mesangioproliferative GN to focal proliferative or diffuse proliferative GN, and membranous nephropathy.

Hypokalemia with or without distal renal tubular acidosis is the chief finding, seen in 30–50% and 5–70% patients, respectively, with kidney involvement. Conversely, Sjögren syndrome is the most likely diagnosis in patients with distal renal tubular acidosis in adolescence or adulthood. Patients with Sjögren syndrome with preserved eGFR and tubular dysfunction are assumed to have TIN, and do not require kidney biopsy. Kidney biopsy is performed in patients with impaired kidney function and/or abnormal urinalysis.

Most patients with tubulointerstitial disease respond to therapy with corticosteroids. Patients with immune-complex GN associated with Sjögren syndrome are usually treated in a manner similar to lupus nephritis.

Immunoglobulin G4-related Disease

This systemic fibroinflammatory condition is characterized by high serum IgG4 and histopathological evidence of a lymphoplasmacytic infiltrate predominantly comprising of IgG4+ plasma cells (IgG4+ to IgG+ plasma cells ≥40%), storiform pattern of fibrosis ("cartwheel" appearance), and obliterative phlebitis. While immunoglobulin G4-related disease (IgG4-RD) most commonly presents with autoimmune pancreatitis, other manifestations, including chronic sclerosing sialadenitis, lymphadenopathy, dacryoadenitis, and orbital pseudotumor mimic autoimmune, malignant and rheumatologic conditions. Renal manifestations, seen in approximately 15% cases of IgG4-RD, are usually in the form of IgG4-related TIN. Less often, there is urinary tract obstruction due to IgG4-related retroperitoneal fibrosis. While glomeruli are usually spared, membranous nephropathy, membranoproliferative glomerulonephritis, IgA nephropathy, minimal change disease, and amyloidosis are reported.

Blood levels of IgG and IgG4 are elevated. Other findings include low complement C3 (60%), peripheral eosinophilia (40%), and antinuclear antibodies (30%). Kidney biopsy shows a dense lymphoplasmacytic infiltrate, ranging from diffuse TIN to tumor-like masses, often associated with storiform fibrosis and infiltrating eosinophils, but without obliterative phlebitis. Common patterns include an acute TIN with minimal interstitial fibrosis, chronic TIN with expansive interstitial fibrosis, and advanced sclerosing pattern. Immunohistochemical staining reveals IgG4+ plasma cells. Immunofluorescence shows granular IgG and C3 deposits along the tubular basement membrane. Electron microscopy may reveal electron dense deposits in the tubular basement membranes. Corticosteroid therapy leads to marked improvement. Other medications, such as azathioprine, MMF, and cyclophosphamide, are used in combination with steroids in relapsing or refractory disease.

AUTOSOMAL DOMINANT TUBULOINTERSTITIAL KIDNEY DISEASE

The term autosomal dominant tubulointerstitial kidney disease (ADTKD) is used for rare familial conditions characterized by progressive CKD, tubulointerstitial fibrosis without significant glomerular lesions, and bland urinary sediment, with or without overt kidney cysts. Progression to end-stage kidney disease (ESKD) occurs at 25–70 years of age. In the past, ADTKD was described as medullary cystic kidney disease (MCKD), a condition similar to nephronophthisis.

Improved understanding of the genetic basis of ADTKD has led to the identification of six subtypes, named after the incriminated genes that show overlapping clinical phenotypes, namely, ADTKD-UMOD, ADKTD-MUC1, ADTKD-REN, ADTK-HNF1B, ADTKD-SEC61A1, and ADTKD-DNAJB11 **(Table 21.4)**. ADTKD-UMOD and ADTKD-MUC1 are the most common types.

Etiopathogenesis

All implicated genes are expressed in tubular cells of the intermediate and/or distal nephron, and in the case of *UMOD*, exclusively in the thick ascending limb of Henle. Disease pathogenesis is similar across the different subtypes, except *HNF1B*, and is explained by a "gain-of-function" mechanism. Except for HNF1B mutations, the disease is confined to kidneys and follows misfolding of encoded proteins, leading to cellular stress and cytotoxicity. Disease-causing variants lead to impaired secretion and intracellular accumulation of the defective protein in the cytosol, endoplasmic reticulum, and/or Golgi complex, leading to endoplasmic reticulum stress, induction of "unfolded protein response", or interference with polymerization of wild-type protein. *HNF1B* is a transcription factor whose haploinsufficiency, due to gene deletion or pathogenic mutation, alters transcriptional activation of its target genes.

TABLE 21.4: Types of autosomal tubulointerstitial kidney disease (ADTKD)

Entity	*Age at presentation*	*Renal imaging*	*Investigations*[1]	*Extrarenal findings; comments*	*Age at ESKD*
ADTKD-UMOD	*Adulthood:* Rarely, gout in childhood	Occasional cysts (not medullary)	Early hyperuricemia, low fractional excretion of urate; low urinary uromodulin	*Gout:* Frequent, early onset (for age and CKD stage) Most common ADTKD	Median 50 (range 20–75) years
ADTKD-MUC1	Adulthood	Occasional cysts (not medullary)	–	Gout less frequent; no extra-renal features	Earlier, at 45 (16–80) years
ADTKD-REN	Anemia at 1–3 year; CKD by 3–4 year	Normal to small sized kidneys	Hyperkalemia; acidosis; low urinary uromodulin; low renin	Hypoproliferative anemia; hypotension; high risk of AKI	Usually >35–50 years
ADTKD-HNF1B	Childhood or adulthood	Bilateral renal cysts; CAKUT (cystic hypodysplasia, VUR, MCDK); echogenic	Hypokalemia; hypomagnesemia; hyperglycemia	Hypoplastic pancreas; maturity-onset diabetes; developmental delay; genital abnormalities	Varies by phenotype
ADTKD-DNAJB11[2]	Adulthood	Enlarged cystic kidneys	–	Liver cysts; phenotype of ADPKD and ADTKD; very rare	60–70 years
ADTKD-SEC61A1[2]	Early onset	Small cystic dysplastic kidneys	–	Neutropenia, respiratory tract infections; abscess formation; hypogammaglobulinemia	50–70 years
ADTKD-NOS	Adulthood	No specific finding	–	No specific finding	Not available

[1]All types have hyperuricemia, but this is most common and earliest in ADTKD-UMOD
[2]These genes were recognized beyond the KDIGO Consensus report of 2015, and were previously included under ADTKD—not otherwise specified (NOS)
CAKUT: congenital abnormalities of kidneys and urinary tract; HNF1B: hepatocyte nuclear factor 1β; MCDK: multicystic dysplastic kidney; MUC1: mucin 1; REN: renin; UMOD: uromodulin; VUR: vesicoureteric reflux

Clinical Features

Features common to all subtypes of ADTKD include: (*i*) insidiously progressive CKD, (*ii*) autosomal dominant inheritance, (*iii*) no exposure to drugs that cause tubulointerstitial nephritis, and (*iv*) lack of significant hypertension in the early stages. Patients with childhood onset ADTKD might report nocturia or nocturnal enuresis. Despite 100% penetrance (except in *HNF1B* variants), family history may be lacking in ADTKD because of *de novo* mutations (seen in 30–50% cases of HNF1B nephropathy) or inter-individual variation in age at onset and severity of CKD within families. Gout is common, especially in men, but it is not pathognomonic of ADTKD.

Table 21.4 outlines the features specific to various subtypes. ADTKD-REN presents in childhood, ADTKD-HNF1B and ADPKD-SEC61A1 may present in childhood or adulthood, and the other subtypes are diagnosed in adulthood. Gout in childhood or early adulthood and/or a strong family history of gout suggests the UMOD subtype. Lack of preprorenin expression in the REN variant is associated with reduced erythropoietin production, leading to transient childhood-onset anemia that resolves after puberty, and an inability to regulate volume, which predisposes to hypovolemia and AKI.

The *HNF1B* mutations have pleomorphic phenotypes and extrarenal features, summarized by the acronym MAGIC-LUCID, for hypo*m*agnesemia, *a*utosomal dominant, *g*ynecologic abnormalities (bicornuate uterus), *i*ncomplete penetrance, *c*ystic kidneys and other kidney malformations, *l*iver test abnormalities, hyper*u*ricemia and gout, *C*KD, *i*ntellectual disability (in patients with 17q12 deletion), and maturity onset *d*iabetes of youth. Usually, childhood-onset HNF1B nephropathy manifests with congenital anomalies of the urinary tract (CAKUT), while ADTKD as a presentation is observed in adults. Other phenotypes of HNF1B nephropathy in childhood or adolescence include Fanconi renotubular syndrome and maturity onset diabetes.

Evaluation

Urinalysis indicates a bland urinary sediment and no or mild albuminuria or proteinuria. Ultrasound reveals normal or small-sized kidneys. While hyperuricemia is out of proportion to the stage of CKD (most prominently in the UMOD variant), it is not specific to ADTKD. Kidney cysts of varying number and size can be noted, particularly in advanced CKD. However, cysts are not present consistently, and their frequency is similar to that in noncystic CKD.

Histology indicates interstitial fibrosis, tubular atrophy, thickening and lamellation of tubular basement membranes, with or without tubular dilatation (microcysts); glomerular and vascular compartments are preserved. Reduced renin staining is shown in the cells of the juxtaglomerular apparatus in ADTKD-REN. Electron microscopy does not provide additional diagnostic information, apart from occasional demonstration of mutant uromodulin in the endoplasmic reticulum of cells in the thick ascending limb (ADTKD-UMOD), or mucin-1 in distal tubules (ADTKD-MUC1).

Next-generation sequencing enables the diagnosis in patients with unknown CKD with or without family history of kidney disease. Most variants in *UMOD* (16p12.3) are located in exons 3 and 4, and those in *REN* (1q32.1) in exon 1. Next-generation or direct sequencing may miss whole gene deletion of *HNF1B* (17q12), responsible for 40% cases of HNF1B nephropathy (occurring as part of 17q12 recurrent deletion syndrome); copy number variations require testing by multiplex ligation-dependent probe amplification or quantitative PCR. Genetic testing for *MUC1* (1q22) is challenging because the pathogenic variants (nucleotide deletions, insertions, and duplications that invariably produce the same frameshift *MUC1* variant) are always located within a variable tandem repeat sequence (VNTR) in its open reading frame. The location of the variant (commonly insertion of a single cytosine within a 60 bp repeat unit of the VNTR) varies by the mutation, i.e., occurs in a different unit of the repeat in each family. Hence, ADTKD-MUC1 cannot be diagnosed through commercial laboratories; research laboratories may diagnose cases through targeted mutation analysis for known familial mutations or genetic linkage analysis in large families with multiple affected members.

Differential Diagnosis

Autosomal dominant tubulointerstitial kidney disease was previously considered a disorder related to nephronophthisis, despite differences in inheritance (autosomal dominant vs. recessive), age at presentation (adulthood vs. childhood), and differing extrarenal phenotype (gout vs. retinitis pigmentosa, congenital hepatic fibrosis). ADTKD is readily distinguished from other familial CKD based on clinical phenotype, e.g., AD polycystic kidney disease (enlarged kidneys with multiple cysts, liver cysts, and/or intracranial aneurysms); Alport syndrome (microscopic hematuria and proteinuria, sensorineural deafness, lenticonus or macular flecks); Alagille syndrome (cholestatic jaundice, vesicoureteric reflux, cardiac abnormalities, butterfly-shaped vertebrae, prominent forehead, deep set eyes); Townes-Brocks syndrome (solitary and/or dysplastic kidneys, vesicoureteric reflux, imperforate anus, dysplastic ears, thumb, hand and ear abnormalities); and hypoparathyroidism deafness renal (HDR) syndrome.

Diagnosis

KDIGO criteria for establishing the diagnosis of ADTKD are: (*i*) family history compatible with autosomal dominant inheritance of CKD, which fulfils the clinical features listed earlier, and compatible histology in at least one affected family member; or (*ii*) mutation in one of the genes in the affected individual or a family member. The term ADTKD-HNF1B is reserved for cases where tubulointerstitial fibrosis is the chief explanation for the clinical presentation.

Management

The management of CKD follows standard guidelines (Chapter 26). Affected individuals should undergo annual testing of kidney function, maintain a healthy lifestyle to control other risk factors for progression of CKD, e.g., hypertension, diabetes, obesity, and smoking, and avoid dehydration and exposure to radiocontrast and nephrotoxic drugs. AKI following NSAIDs is likely in patients with ADTKD-REN. Allopurinol or febuxostat is used in patients with gout and/or persistent hyperuricemia. Diuretics are avoided given their potential to aggravate hyperuricemia and hypovolemia. Low-salt diet is not preferred, particularly in ADTKD-UMOD and ADTKD-REN in whom it may worsen hyperuricemia and hypovolemia, respectively. Patients with ADTKD-REN may require therapy with erythropoiesis stimulating agents and/or fludrocortisone for anemia and symptomatic hypotension, respectively.

Decisions on kidney function tests and genetic testing in asymptomatic family members are guided by individualized counseling. This is true for children with UMOD- or MUC1-related ADTKD, who are likely to have uncomplicated childhood course, in contrast to patients with REN, HNF1B, and SEC61A1 related disease that requires referral to pediatric nephrologists. Genetic testing is mandatory when screening living related donors in families with ADTKD.

Outcomes

The rate of decline of eGFR is highly variable, even among individuals in a family with the same mutation. Patients may progress to ESKD between 20 and 80 years of age, but most often do so at 30–50 years of age. Patients with gout appear to progress earlier.

BIBLIOGRAPHY

1. Aiyegbusi O, McGregor L, McGeoch L, et al. Renal disease in primary Sjögren's syndrome. Rheumatol Ther. 2021;8:63-80.
2. Amaro D, Carreño E, Steeples LR, et al. Tubulointerstitial nephritis and uveitis (TINU) syndrome: A review. Br J Ophthalmol. 2020;104:742-47.
3. Baughman RP, Valeyre D, Korsten P, et al. ERS clinical practice guidelines on treatment of sarcoidosis. Eur Respir J. 2021;58:2004079.
4. Bergner R, Löffler C. Renal sarcoidosis: Approach to diagnosis and management. Curr Opin Pulm Med. 2018;24:513-20.
5. Bleyer AJ, Wolf MT, Kidd KO, et al. Autosomal dominant tubulointerstitial kidney disease: More than just HNF1β. Pediatr Nephrol. 2021;37:933-46.

6. Eckardt KU, Alper SL, Antignac C, et al.; Kidney Disease: Improving Global Outcomes. Autosomal dominant tubulointerstitial kidney disease: diagnosis, classification, and management: A KDIGO consensus report. Kidney Int. 2015;88:676-83.
7. Econimo L, Schaeffer C, Zeni L, et al. Autosomal dominant tubulointerstitial kidney disease: An emerging cause of genetic CKD. Kidney Int Rep. 2022;7: 2332-44.
8. Eddy AA. Drug-induced tubulointerstitial nephritis: Hypersensitivity and necroinflammatory pathways. Pediatr Nephrol. 2020;35:547-54.
9. Fogo AB, Lusco MA, Najafian B, et al. AJKD atlas of renal pathology: Chronic interstitial nephritis. Am J Kidney Dis. 2017;70:e1-e2.
10. Janetos TM, Lee PHA, Goldstein DA. Tubulointerstitial nephritis and uveitis syndrome in pediatric patients. Ocul Immunol Inflamm. 2023;31:1955-64.
11. Jayasumana C, Orantes C, Herrera R, et al. Chronic interstitial nephritis in agricultural communities: Worldwide epidemic with social, occupational and environmental determinants. Nephrol Dial Transplant. 2017;32:234-41.
12. Joyce E, Glasner P, Ranganathan S, et al. Tubulointerstitial nephritis: Diagnosis, treatment, and monitoring. Pediatr Nephrol. 2017;32:577-87.
13. Orantes-Navarro CM, Herrera-Valdés R, Almaguer-López M, et al. Toward a comprehensive hypothesis of chronic interstitial nephritis in agricultural communities. Adv Chronic Kidney Dis. 2017;24:101-06.
14. Pakzad-Vaezi K, Pepple KL. Tubulointerstitial nephritis and uveitis. Curr Opin Ophthalmol. 2017;28:629-35.
15. Ruebner RL, Fadrowski JJ. Tubulointerstitial nephritis. Pediatr Clin North Am. 2019;66:111-19.
16. Salvadori M, Tsalouchos A. Immunoglobulin G4-related kidney diseases: An updated review. World J Nephrol. 2018;7:29-40.
17. Sanchez-Quiros J, Giralt L, Fonollosa A, et al. Diagnostic and management strategies of tubulointerstitial nephritis and uveitis syndrome. Clin Ophthalmol. 2023;17:2625-30.
18. Southgate G, Clarke P, Harmer MJ. Renal outcomes in tubulointerstitial nephritis and uveitis (TINU) syndrome: A systematic review and meta-analysis. J Nephrol. 2023;36:507-19.
19. Ungprasert P, Ryu JH, Matteson EL. Clinical manifestations, diagnosis, and treatment of sarcoidosis. Mayo Clin Proc Innov Qual Outcomes. 2019;3:358-75.
20. Živná M, Kidd KO, Barešová V, et al. Autosomal dominant tubulointerstitial kidney disease. Am J Med Genet C Semin Med Genet. 2022;190:309-24.

CHAPTER 22

Vitamin D Refractory Rickets

Amita Sharma, Ashley A Sharma, Marie McGourty

Rickets is failure of apoptosis of unossified cartilage in the growth plate because of impaired mineralization. This leads to prolonged cartilage proliferation. Bone growth begins with chondrocytes undergoing sequential longitudinal alignment, vascularization, and apoptosis, forming a scaffold (primary spongiosa) for mineralization. Both calcium and phosphorus are essential for mineralization. X-ray examination can both diagnose and estimate severity of rickets.

Calcipenic rickets is due to vitamin D deficiency, failure of activation of vitamin D, or resistance to the action of vitamin D. Rarely, insufficient calcium intake or absorption may be causal. Calcipenic rickets cause secondary hyperparathyroidism, which increases bone resorption and osteopenia, and decreases bone mass. Associated hypocalcemia, if severe, may cause irritability, tetany, and seizures.

Phosphopenic rickets is characterized by low serum levels of phosphorus, usually caused by renal phosphate wasting and, less commonly, by nutritional phosphorus deficiency. Unlike calcipenic rickets, there is increased under-mineralized osteoid. Osteopenia is not seen because of lack of secondary hyperparathyroidism.

Refractory rickets presents a significant diagnostic challenge, especially in areas where nutritional rickets is common. When a child with suspected nutritional rickets shows no improvement with vitamin D supplementation, a diagnosis of vitamin D refractory rickets should be considered.

VITAMIN D METABOLISM

Vitamin D plays a crucial role in mineralization by promoting hydroxyapatite deposition. Vitamin D_2 (ergocalciferol) is derived from plant and fungal sources. Vitamin D_3 (cholecalciferol) can be obtained from natural dietary sources such as oily fish, liver, and eggs, or following conversion of cholesterol via 7-dehydrocholesterol pathway aided by sunlight.

Both vitamins D_2 and D_3 are hydroxylated in the liver by CYP27A1 to 25(OH) vitamin D_2 (ercalcidol) and 25(OH) vitamin D_3 (calcidol), which are together termed as 25(OH) vitamin D. 25(OH) vitamin D has a half-life of approximately 3 weeks and is thus an ideal measure for vitamin D sufficiency. Vitamin D levels are defined as insufficient, deficient and severely deficient at levels below 20 ng/mL, 12 ng/mL and 5 ng/mL, respectively. One hundred units of either ergocalciferol or cholecalciferol increase 25(OH) vitamin D levels by 1 ng/mL. Optimal calcium absorption occurs when 25(OH) vitamin D levels range from 20 to 30 ng/mL **(Fig. 22.1)**.

25(OH) vitamin D is converted by 1-α hydroxylase (CYP27B1) in the kidney to 1,25 dihydroxycholecalciferol (calcitriol). Calcitriol has a circulatory half-life of 24 hr, and it is maintained at a low level of about 0.1% of 25(OH) vitamin D. Thus, it is not an indicator of vitamin D stores. Calcitriol is not routinely measured. Compared to vitamin D_3, 25(OH)D is ten-fold, and calcitriol is 1,000-fold, metabolically more potent. Calcitriol increases TRPV5 and TRPV6 abundance and activity in the intestine and kidney, thus increasing gut and tubular calcium reabsorption, respectively. Calcitriol inhibits *PTH* expression by binding to the VDR in the parathyroid gland, thus decreasing PTH cell proliferation. Vitamin D works synergistically with PTH to activate osteoclasts.

RICKETS

Vitamin D deficiency remains prevalent in special populations, including breastfed infants, children with limited sun exposure, vegans, and individuals with malabsorptive diseases, such as celiac disease. Liver disease can hinder the hydroxylation process to 25(OH) vitamin D, while drugs inducing cytochrome P450, such as barbiturates, stimulate the conversion of 25(OH) vitamin D to inactive metabolites. Congenital nephrotic syndrome may lead to decreased levels of 25(OH) vitamin D due to urinary protein loss, and kidney function loss in chronic kidney disease (CKD) results in deficiency of calcitriol due to impaired 1-α hydroxylation. Genetic studies have revealed rare deficiencies in cytochrome enzymes that cause hereditary pseudovitamin D deficiency rickets, more commonly termed vitamin D dependent rickets (VDDR).

Vitamin D deficiency rickets usually respond to standard doses of vitamin D, while few patients may require moderate doses. Nutritional rickets is usually treated with a daily dose of 2,000 IU of ergocalciferol or cholecalciferol along with oral calcium for at least 3 months. This combined treatment supports skeletal remineralization, prevents hypocalcemia, and normalizes serum calcium and phosphate levels within 3 weeks. Treatment duration is individually tailored, and ongoing adequate nutritional vitamin D intake (at least 600 IU/day after 12 months) is crucial post-treatment. A higher and sustained intake of vitamin D might result in hypercalcemia. The earliest response to vitamin D is a rise in serum phosphate concentration followed by decreasing PTH levels. Alkaline phosphatase levels initially rise but normalize in 3–6 months. In malnourished children with zinc deficiency, alkaline phosphatase levels might remain normal. The provisional zone of calcification becomes visible on X-rays within 3–4 weeks.

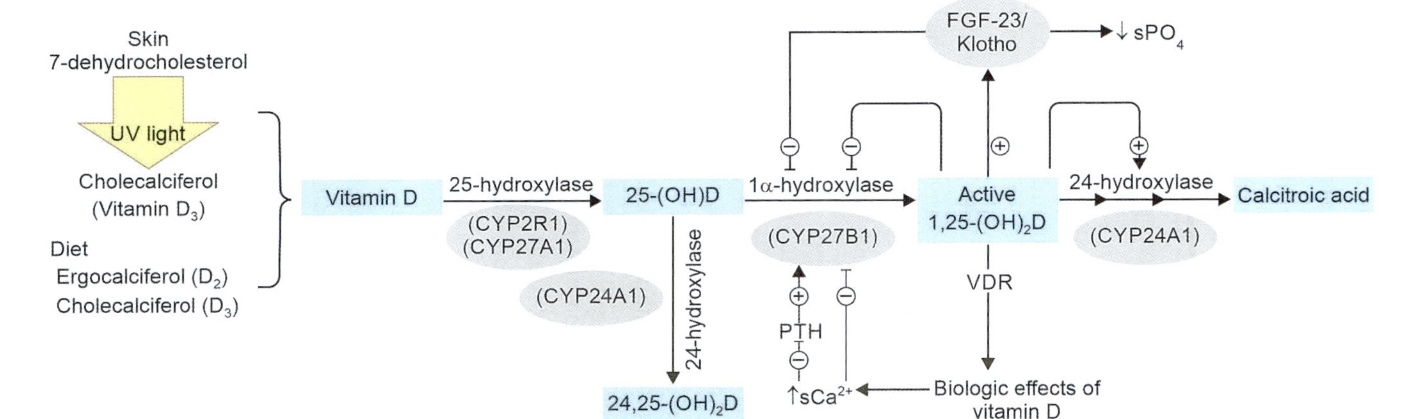

Fig. 22.1: Vitamin D metabolism. Dermal photochemical synthesis of vitamin D_3 (cholecalciferol) occurs from 7-dehydrocholesterol in response to ultraviolet (UV) B light exposure. Vitamin D_2 (ergocalciferol) and D_3 (cholecalciferol) can also be obtained from diet. Both vitamin D_2 and vitamin D_3 are transported to the liver, where they are converted to 25(OH) vitamin D by 25-hydroxylase (first step of activation). 25(OH) vitamin D is converted to 1,25$(OH)_2$ vitamin D (calcitriol) by 1-α hydroxylase (second step of vitamin D activation) in the kidney. This conversion is regulated by many factors, including serum levels of calcium (sCa^{2+}), phosphorus (sPO_4), fibroblast growth factor 23 (FGF23) and parathyroid hormone (PTH). Calcitriol is also metabolized to inactive metabolites, such as 24,25-dihydroxyvitamin D. Respective cytochrome enzymes are indicated in parentheses in gray ovals. Vitamin D-dependent rickets (VDDR) type 1 results from enzymatic defects in the synthesis of calcitriol, whereas VDDR type 2 results from defects in the vitamin D receptor (VDR)

The human body stores approximately 90% of its total phosphorus in the skeleton as calcium/phosphate crystals, primarily hydroxyapatite. Phosphorus is crucial for hydroxyapatite synthesis, and its deficiency impairs skeletal mineralization. Phosphorus homeostasis involves absorption, reabsorption, and bone deposition/mobilization, regulated by factors such as vitamin D, PTH, and fibroblast growth factor 23 (FGF23) acting on the kidney, intestines, and bone. PTH and 1,25$(OH)_2$D increase calcium reabsorption in distal renal tubules via TRPV5 channel upregulation and activation. Osteocyte-secreted FGF23 binds Klotho coreceptor, activating *FGFR1*. This activation triggers internalization and degradation of NaPi2a and NaPi2c, suppresses renal 1-α hydroxylase, and stimulates 24-hydroxylase, leading to reduced proximal tubular Pi reabsorption and decrease in circulating calcitriol levels.

Calcipenic rickets is caused by disorders of vitamin D metabolism and end organ resistance to vitamin D. VDR defect associated with alopecia is a severe phenotype. Causes of phosphopenic rickets include phosphate deficiency, FGF23-driven renal phosphate loss, and tubular phosphate wasting independent of FGF23. X-linked hypophosphatemia (XLH) is the prototypical disorder, presenting with growth failure, bone deformities, dental abscesses, and hearing loss; other forms include autosomal dominant and autosomal recessive hypophosphatemic rickets, tumor-induced osteomalacia, fibrous dysplasia (FD), and rare genetic disorders affecting phosphate metabolism.

Hypophosphatemia is a potent stimulus for renal synthesis of 1,25$(OH)_2$D. The resulting increase in calcitriol stimulates intestinal absorption of phosphorus and calcium, and their mobilization from the bone. Elevated plasma calcium levels lead to the suppression of PTH, reduced phosphorus excretion, and increased calcium excretion. These changes result in an increase in serum phosphorus with minor change in serum calcium **(Fig. 22.2A to C)**. Secondary hyperparathyroidism in vitamin D deficiency leads to increased renal phosphorus loss. Therefore, tubular phosphate reabsorption needs to be estimated, along with levels of PTH and vitamin D.

Like phosphate metabolism, calcium homeostasis relies on the intricate interplay among the three major organ systems: bone, intestines, and kidneys. The primary regulators are PTH and calcitriol, with calcitonin playing a secondary role. PTH responds to hypocalcemia by influencing the kidneys to: (*i*) reduce calcium excretion; (*ii*) increase phosphate excretion; and (*iii*) enhance the synthesis of 1,25$(OH)_2$ vitamin D. Consequently, the elevated 1,25$(OH)_2$ vitamin D levels stimulate the absorption of phosphorus and calcium in the intestines, along with their release from the bone **(Table 22.1)**.

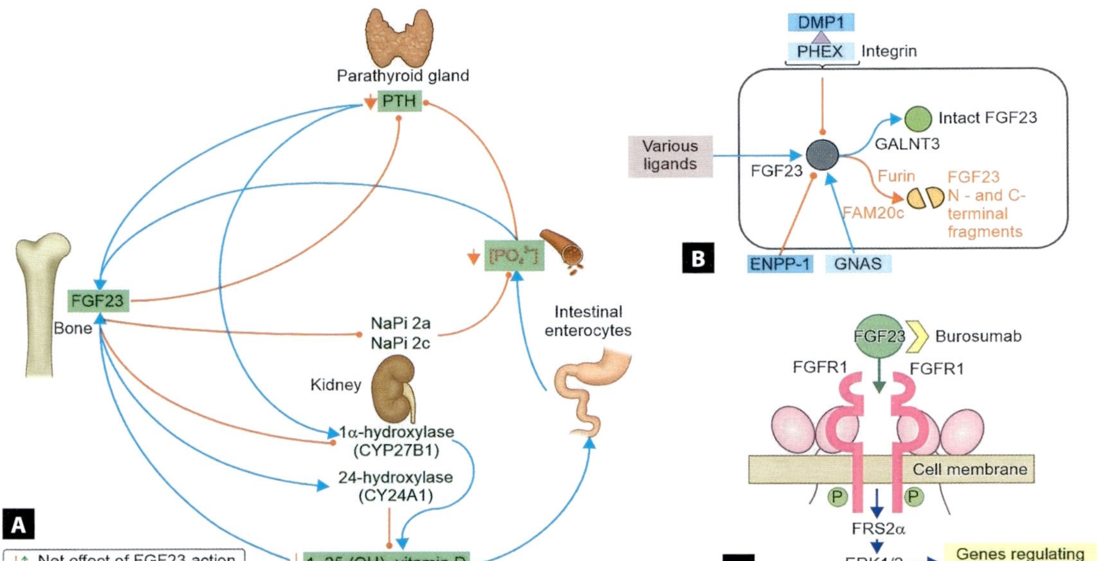

Figs. 22.2A to C: Regulation of serum phosphate and fibroblast growth factor 23 (FGF23). Red and blue lines indicate inhibitory and stimulatory effects. **(A)** FGF23, synthesized in the bone, acts on the proximal tubule to inhibit sodium/phosphate cotransporters NaPi2a and NaPi2c and, thereby renal phosphate reabsorption. FGF23 also inhibits the renal enzyme, 1α-hydroxylase and stimulates 24-hydroxylase leading to reduced serum calcitriol and decrease in intestinal phosphate absorption. FGF23 inhibits parathyroid hormone (PTH) synthesis and secretion, whereas PTH stimulates FGF23 production. FGF23 is stimulated by serum calcitriol and an increase in serum phosphate or dietary phosphate intake. **(B)** FGF23 is synthesized by early osteocytes and late osteoblasts in bones. Its expression is inhibited by dentin matrix protein 1 (DMP1). DMP1 binds to PHEX via an acidic serine- and aspartate-rich MEPE-associated (ASARM) motif (triangle) and to an integrin to downregulate FGF23 expression. The mechanisms whereby ectonucleotide pyrophosphatase/phosphodiesterase 1 (ENPP1) and α-subunit of the Gs G protein-coupled receptor (GNAS) influence FGF23 levels, are unclear. Posttranslational modifications of FGF23 influence its biological activity. When glycosylated by N-acetylgalactosaminyltransferase 3 (GALNT3), it remains intact (intact, iFGF23), and binds to the FGFR1 receptor and α-klotho in the kidney epithelium. When phosphorylated by Family with sequence similarity 20, member C (FAM20c), FGF23 is cleaved by a furin leading to the release of N and C-terminal fragments. FGF23 transcription is upregulated by high PTH (binding to PTH receptor activates protein kinase A and nuclear receptor related-1 (Nurr1) signaling]; 1,25-dihydroxyvitamin D (vitamin D receptor/retinoid X receptor heterodimer translocates to nucleus to activate vitamin D response elements in *FGF23*); calcium [calcium-dependent nuclear factor of activated T cells (NFAT) signals to NFAT response elements in FGF23 promotor]; iron deficiency and inflammation [stabilize hypoxia-inducible factor (HIF) 1α that binds to HIF-binding sites in the FGF23 promotor]; erythropoietin (enhances FGF23 transcription); and CKD-related inflammatory factors [stimulate nuclear factor kappa-light-chain-enhancer of activated B cells (NF-kB), which enhances FGF23 transcription through the calcium channel Orai1). High serum phosphate induces GALNT3, which stabilizes intact FGF23, while HIF1α mediates the cleavage of FGF23. **(C)** Fibroblast growth factor (FGF) signaling. FGF23 signals through the FGF23 receptor, which consists of a homodimer of tyrosine kinase FGF receptors (FGFRs) (types 1c, 3c, or 4) and the αKlotho coreceptor. This signaling is commonly through the mitogen-activated protein kinase (MAPK) pathway extracellular signal-regulated kinases 1 and 2 (ERK1/2), which are activated by phosphorylation of FGFR substrate-2α (FRS2α). Burosumab is an anti-FGF23 antibody that blocks the binding of FGF23 to the FGFR1/Klotho receptor

TABLE 22.1: Action of various hormones involved in causing rickets

Hormone	*Main stimulus*	*Actions*	
		Stimulating effects	*Inhibitory effects*
Parathyroid hormone (PTH)	Hypocalcemia	Bone resorption; 1-α hydroxylase; phosphaturia	24-hydroxylase
Fibroblast growth factor 23 (FGF23)	1,25$(OH)_2$ vitamin D, phosphorus	24-hydroxylase; phosphaturia	1,25$(OH)_2$ vitamin D; PTH
1,25$(OH)_2$ vitamin D	PTH, hypocalcemia, hypophosphatemia	Gut calcium and phosphorus absorption; FGF23; 24-hydroxylase	PTH; phosphaturia

REFRACTORY RICKETS

Coined by Albright in 1937, the term "vitamin D refractory rickets" describes a condition first observed in a patient with X-linked hypophosphatemic rickets, with no response to ergocalciferol or cholecalciferol.

Lack of response to vitamin D therapy is termed vitamin D resistant/ refractory rickets. Findings of short stature, alopecia, poor dentition, bone abnormalities, similar findings in other family members, and parental consanguinity are suggestive of refractory rickets. Timely diagnosis is imperative for the initiation of therapy and the prevention of complications. These disorders are categorized based on the primary mineral deficiency, whether phosphate or calcium **(Table 22.2)**.

CALCIPENIC RICKETS

Vitamin D-dependent rickets (VDDR) are rare, inherited defects caused by loss of 1-α hydroxylase or 25-hydroxylase (VDDR1), or impaired calcitriol signaling (VDDR2)**(Table 22.2)**. VDDR and nutritional rickets have similar clinical and biochemical characteristics. Vitamin D-dependent rickets type 3 (VDDR3), a recently identified form, arises from gain-of-function mutations in *CYP3A4* (24-hydroxylase), which causes increased vitamin D inactivation, therefore requiring lifelong treatment with high-dose cholecalciferol or active vitamin D.

Common principles of management of various forms of VDDR include calcium and activated form of vitamin D supplementation to address hypocalcemia at presentation and prevent further hypocalcemia during remineralization, while monitoring for hyperparathyroidism. Regular biochemical monitoring is crucial for optimal treatment.

Vitamin D-dependent rickets type IA [VDDR IA; Online Mendelian Inheritance in Man (OMIM) 264700] is caused by loss of function of

CYP27B1, which encodes 1-α hydroxylase, a mitochondrial P450 enzyme on chromosome 12. Splice site mutations and insertions are common that inactivate the enzyme by disrupting the function of heme binding domain. The disease is frequent in certain populations and has an autosomal recessive inheritance.

Children present by 3–6 months with signs of severe rickets. Additional symptoms due to hypocalcemia include failure to thrive, hypotonia, congestive heart failure, respiratory compromise, irritability, tetany, seizures, and fractures. Since clinical features resemble nutritional rickets but are not corrected by 25(OH) vitamin D or vitamin D_2/D_3, VDDR 1A is also known as pseudovitamin D deficiency rickets.

Laboratory results resemble vitamin D-deficient rickets. Serum levels of calcium and phosphorus are low, while those of alkaline phosphatase and PTH are very high. The distinguishing feature is exceptionally low blood level of $1,25(OH)_2$ vitamin D and normal 25(OH) vitamin D.

Management involves lifelong administration of either calcitriol, given twice daily (because of short half-life), or alphacalcidiol, given once daily. During the initial 3–6 months, higher doses of vitamin D and oral calcium are necessary to meet the increased skeletal demands. It is recommended to aim for calcium levels in the low-normal range, with PTH levels in the high-normal range, to prevent hypercalciuria and nephrocalcinosis.

Vitamin D dependent rickets type 1B (VDDR IB; OMIM 600081) arises from loss of function mutation in *CYP2R1*, affecting hepatic 25-hydroxylation, leading to deficiency of 25(OH) vitamin D, and therefore, calcitriol. The disorder exhibits autosomal recessive inheritance.

Clinical features of VDDR IB may include bone pains, restricted physical activity, bowing of lower limbs, hypocalcemia, hypophosphatemia, and elevated levels of PTH and alkaline phosphatase.

VDDR1B is treated with: (*i*) calcidiol [25(OH) vitamin D]; (*ii*) pharmacological dosages of vitamin D_2 or D_3; or (*iii*) physiological doses of calcitriol, along with calcium supplementation. Calcidiol restores low 25(OH)D, enabling PTH-controlled conversion to calcitriol. Drug doses must be adjusted to keep mid-normal calcium and PTH levels.

Vitamin D-dependent rickets type 2A (VDDR 2A; OMIM 277440) arises from *VDR* mutations which impair receptor signaling and thus cause end organ resistance. *VDR* belongs to the steroid-thyroid-retinoid receptor gene superfamily. The gene located on chromosome 12 has 14 exons. It features a conserved deoxyribonucleic acid (DNA) binding domain at the N terminal and a variable ligand binding domain at the C terminal. The molecular basis of the disease is heterogeneous. Nonsense mutations, missense mutations in the DNA binding domains, and mutations interfering with retinoid X receptor (RXR) dimerization are associated with severe phenotype and alopecia, whereas ligand binding domain mutations are less severe.

TABLE 22.2: Etiology of refractory rickets

Disorder (OMIM ID, if any)	*Gene*	*Mechanism/pathogenesis*
Calcipenic rickets and/or osteomalacia (low or normal serum calcium, high PTH)		
Nutritional rickets (vitamin D and/or calcium deficiency)	NA	Vitamin D deficiency
Vitamin D dependent rickets type 1A (VDDR1A; 264700)	*CYP27B1*	Impaired synthesis of 1,25 $(OH)_2$ D in kidney
Vitamin D dependent rickets type 1B (VDDR1B; 600081)	*CYP2R1*	Impaired synthesis of 25(OH)D in liver
Vitamin D dependent rickets type 2A (VDDR2A; 277440)	*VDR*	Impaired signaling of the VDR
Vitamin D dependent rickets type 2B (VDDR2B; 164020)	*HNRNPC*	Impaired signaling of the VDR
Vitamin D dependent rickets type 3 (VDDR3; 619073)	*CYP3A4*	Increased inactivation of 1,25$(OH)_2$ D
Phosphopenic rickets and/or osteomalacia with reduced dietary intake of phosphate (normal or low TmP/GFR, serum FGF23 and PTH)		
Breastfed very low birthweight infants	Not applicable	Dietary phosphate deficiency or impaired bioavailability
Use of elemental or hypoallergenic formula diet or parental nutrition		
Excessive use of phosphate binders		
Gastrointestinal surgery or disorders		
Phosphopenic rickets and/or osteomalacia with renal tubular phosphate wasting due to elevated FGF23 levels and/or signaling (low TmP/GFR, high or normal serum FGF23, normal or low PTH)		
X-linked hypophosphatemia (XLH; 307800)	*PHEX*	Increased expression and impaired cleavage of FGF23 in bone
Autosomal dominant hypophosphatemic rickets (ADHR; 193100)	*FGF23*	FGF23 protein resistant to degradation

Contd...

Contd...

Disorder (OMIM ID, if any)	***Gene***	***Mechanism/pathogenesis***
Autosomal recessive hypophosphatemic rickets 1 (ARHR1; 241520)	*DMP1*	Increased expression of FGF23 in bone
Autosomal recessive hypophosphatemic rickets 2 (ARHR2; 613312)	*ENPP1*	
Raine syndrome associated (ARHR3; 259775)	*FAM20C*	
Fibrous dysplasia (174800)	*GNAS*	
Tumour-induced osteomalacia (TIO)	Not applicable	Increased FGF23 expression in tumor cells
Cutaneous skeletal hypophosphatemia syndrome (SFM; 163200)	*RAS*	Unknown
Osteoglophonic dysplasia (OGD; 166250)	*FGFR1*	Increased FGF23 expression in bone
Hypophosphatemic rickets and hyperparathyroidism (612089)	*KLOTHO*	Unknown; translocation of the KLOTHO promoter
Phosphopenic rickets and/or osteomalacia with renal tubular phosphate wasting independent of FGF23 (low TmP/GFR and low or normal FGF23 and PTH)		
Hereditary hypophosphatemic rickets with hypercalciuria (HHRH; 241530)	*SLC34A3*	Loss of function of NaPi2c in the proximal tubule
X-linked recessive hypophosphatemic rickets; Dent disease (300554; 300009)	*CLCN5*	Loss of function of CLCN5 in the proximal tubule
Hypophosphatemia and nephrocalcinosis (612286); Fanconi reno-tubular syndrome type 2 (613388)	*SLC34A1*	Loss of function of NaPi2a in the proximal tubule
Cystinosis (219800) â	*CTNS*	Cysteine accumulation in the proximal tubule
Other inherited forms of Fanconi syndrome **(*see* Table 20.1)**	Multiple genes	
Iatrogenic proximal tubulopathy	Not applicable	Drug toxicity

VDDR 2 is an autosomal recessive disease with males and females equally affected. Heterozygous carriers, usually parents of affected patients, are asymptomatic with normal bone development. VDDR 2, if associated with alopecia, usually presents at 3–6 months of age, and is associated with severe hypocalcemia requiring intravenous calcium.

Treating VDDR 2A is particularly challenging due to vitamin D resistance. Hypocalcemia usually requires high doses of oral calcium and 25(OH)D or 1,25$(OH)_2$D supplements. Infusions of intravenous calcium, if required, may be associated with side effects of cardiac arrhythmias and nephrolithiasis. At puberty, patients with VDDR 2A often experience improved intestinal calcium absorption for unknown reasons, achieving stable normocalcemia with moderate oral calcium doses.

Vitamin D-dependent rickets type 2B (VDDR 2B) is caused by mutations in *HNRNPC*, resulting in impaired signaling of the vitamin D receptor **(Table 22.2)**. VDDR 3 is a new entity due to mutation in *CYP3A4*, which causes increased inactivation of calcitriol.

PHOSPHOPENIC RICKETS

Hypophosphatemic rickets can be classified based on etiology as (*i*) dietary phosphate deficiency or impaired bioavailability, (*ii*) FGF23-mediated renal phosphate wasting, and (*iii*) primary or acquired tubular phosphate wasting. The laboratory abnormalities are shown in **Table 22.3**.

Lack of Dietary Phosphate or Limited Availability

Phosphate-deficient diets are uncommon; nutritional rickets mostly stem from low calcium intake or lack of vitamin D. However, special populations, such as very low birth weight infants with inadequate phosphorus supplementation, children on special low phosphorus formulas, decreased absorption, i.e., short bowel syndrome, and excessive phosphate binder use, may develop hypophosphatemia. Severe, persistent low serum phosphorus may lead to myopathy, hemolysis, and rhabdomyolysis.

FGF23-mediated Disorders

FGF23-mediated renal phosphate wasting is caused by either increased FGF23 synthesis or reduced degradation.

X-linked hypophosphatemia is the most frequent cause of hypophosphatemic rickets, with a prevalence of 4–5/100,000 children, and accounting for approximately 80% of cases of refractory rickets. Renal phosphate wasting, hypophosphatemia, and inappropriately normal concentrations of 1,25$(OH)_2$D are the characteristic findings. XLH, an X-linked dominant disorder, is primarily caused by *PHEX* mutations, impacting FGF23 expression in bone and teeth.

TABLE 22.3: Biochemical investigations in various forms of rickets

Disorder	*Calcium*	*Phosphate*	*Parathyroid hormone*	*25(OH) vitamin D*	*1,25(OH)$_2$ vitamin D*	*Urine phosphate*	*Alkaline phosphatase*
Vitamin D deficiency	N, ↓	↓	↑	↓	↓, N, ↑	↑	↑
Vitamin D-dependent rickets type 1	↓	↓	↑↑	N	↓	↑	↑
Vitamin D-dependent rickets type 2	↓	↓	↑↑	N	↑↑	↑	↑
X-linked hypophosphatemia	N	↓	N, ↑	N	IN	↑	↑
Autosomal dominant hypophosphatemic rickets	N	↓	N	N	IN	↑	↑
Hypophosphatemic rickets with hypercalciuria	N	↓	N	N	IN	↑	↑
Tumor-induced osteomalacia	N	↓	N	N	IN	↑	↑
Fanconi syndrome	N	↓	N	N	IN	↑	↑

IN: inappropriately normal for level of phosphate

Hypophosphatemia, arising from reduced tubular reabsorption of phosphate (TRP), is the defining feature. TRP is calculated as follows:

$$TRP = 1 - \frac{\text{Urine phosphorus} \times \text{Serum creatinine}}{\text{Serum phosphorus} \times \text{Urine creatinine}}$$

In the absence of family history, diagnosis is often delayed as serum phosphorous levels are high in infancy and may go unrecognized. Children with XLH usually have significant deformities of lower limbs, disproportionate short stature, and under-mineralized dentin, leading to enamel weakening and abscess formation. Rare complications include Chiari malformation type 1 and syringomyelia. Diagnosis delay is common in adults, especially with mild symptoms and no family history. Adults may suffer from periodontitis, enthesopathies, osteoarthritis, and pseudofractures, causing pain, reduced quality of life, and immobility.

The treatment approach for XLH involves either treatment with oral phosphate supplements and calcitriol or the use of burosumab, a recently approved alternative **(Fig. 22.2)**. Conventional therapy requires adjustment of phosphate and active vitamin D doses to mitigate side effects, which continue until adult height is reached. Nephrocalcinosis, a common complication, lacks clear pathogenesis. Regularly monitoring PTH and urinary calcium excretion, alongside screening for nephrocalcinosis using renal ultrasound, is vital.

Burosumab, while more effective and convenient, is costly and not licensed for children under 12 months. Monitoring and adjunctive therapies, such as growth hormone for persistent short stature and surgical interventions for leg bowing, are considered based on individual patient needs. Additionally, dental care and management of neurosurgical complications are crucial aspects of comprehensive XLH multidisciplinary care.

Autosomal-dominant hypophosphatemic rickets (ADHR) is a rare condition caused by activating mutations in *FGF23* on chromosome 12p12.3. These mutations render the protein resistant to cleavage, leading to elevated FGF23 levels in the blood and similar clinical effects seen in other FGF23-related disorders.

The disease has an incomplete penetrance with highly variable phenotype. Adults may exhibit weakness, fatigue, bone pain, and pseudo-fractures. Tumor-induced osteomalacia (TIO) is an important differential diagnosis. Iron levels play a significant role in regulating FGF23 pathways, and iron deficiency increases the likelihood of clinical symptoms in ADHR patients.

The principles of management of ADHR are similar to XLH with oral phosphate and active vitamin D supplements, in addition to correction of iron deficiency.

Autosomal-recessive hypophosphatemic rickets (ARHR1, ARHR2) result from mutations in either the dentine matrix acidic phosphoprotein 1 (*DMP1*) gene on chromosome 4q22.1 or the ectonucleotide pyrophosphatase/ phosphodiesterase 1 (*ENPP1*) gene on chromosome 6q23.2, both active in bone and teeth **(Table 22.2)**. Clinical manifestations mimic those of XLH.

The DMP1 is crucial for bone, cartilage, and teeth development, while ENPP1 regulates bone mineralization and tissue calcification by producing inorganic pyrophosphate (PPi). Initially found in infantile arterial calcification, *ENPP1* mutations show high phenotypic variability with family members exhibiting diverse clinical presentations despite sharing the same biallelic variants, such as enthesopathy and primary hyperparathyroidism.

Managing patients with ARHR2 is challenging since ENPP1 deficiency not only leads to hypophosphatemic rickets but can also cause arterial, cardiac, or articular calcification, or present with infantile generalized arterial calcification. Phosphate supplements and active vitamin D typically resolve rickets and normalize alkaline phosphatase in ARHR1 patients with *DMP1* mutations. Those with biallelic *ENPP1* mutations may develop hyperparathyroidism necessitating partial parathyroidectomy. ENPP1 enzyme replacement shows promise for future treatment.

Autosomal-recessive forms of hypophosphatemic rickets 3 (ARHR3), or Raine syndrome, results from mutations in *FAM20C* (7q22.3), a key regulator of osteoblasts and osteocytes, which is involved in FGF23 cleavage **(Fig. 22.2)**. Patients rarely survive infancy. Nonlethal forms rarely present with rickets; instead, they show generalized osteosclerosis and varying dysmorphism. Bone mineralization may improve in nonlethal Raine syndrome, as shown in preliminary data in FAM20C-deficient mice.

Tumor-induced osteomalacia stems from excess FGF23 and other phosphaturic factors produced by benign, slow-growing mesenchymal tumors. Although rare in children, it is a significant consideration for adults with bone pain, weakness, fatigue, and pseudofractures, along with hypophosphatemia and elevated FGF23 levels. Total tumor removal is the preferred treatment, quickly restoring normal FGF23 and phosphate levels, although complete bone recovery may take a year. Burosumab could be an alternative if complete tumor removal is not achievable.

Fibrous dysplasia arises from activating *GNAS* mutations on chromosome 20q13.3, seen in McCune-Albright syndrome, causing increased FGF23 production in bone. Mild hypophosphatemia, linked to phosphate wasting, can lead to fractures and bone pain. Rare skin disorders with FGF23 excess include epidermal nevi, congenital melanocytic nevi, and Schimmelpenning–Feuerstein–Mims syndrome. Therapy with bisphosphonates, burosumab, oral phosphate, and active vitamin D supplements have been used with variable results.

Osteoglophonic dysplasia (OD) is due to *FGFR1* mutation on chromosome 8p11.23, leading to increased FGF23 expression in bones. Similarly, Klotho mutation may cause hypophosphatemic rickets with hyperparathyroidism **(Table 22.2)**.

Hypophosphatemic Conditions with Normal or Inhibited FGF23 Function

Hereditary hypophosphatemic rickets with hypercalciuria (HHRH) was initially identified in a highly consanguineous Bedouin tribe. It results from mutations in *SLC34A3*, which encodes NaPi2C. HHRH shares similarities with XLH, such as hypophosphatemia, renal phosphate loss, and elevated alkaline phosphatase, but differs with hypercalciuria, suppressed PTH, and increased 1,25$(OH)_2$D levels (an appropriate response to low phosphorus). Elevated 1,25$(OH)_2$D enhances calcium absorption, leading to hypercalciuria. Skeletal manifestations include osteopenia and osteomalacia, with varied clinical features such as idiopathic infantile hypercalcemia, nephrolithiasis, and rickets from renal phosphate loss.

Oral phosphorus supplements are used for treatment, thereby boosting serum phosphate levels, reducing 1,25$(OH)_2$D concentration, and improving calcium absorption in the gut, thus leading to decreased hypercalciuria and osteopenia improvement. Long-term safety of phosphorus supplements is not known, and careful monitoring for hypercalciuria and nephrocalcinosis is necessary. Adjunctive measures include increased fluid intake and salt restriction; therapy with thiazides may improve hypercalciuria.

Hypophosphatemia and nephrocalcinosis might also be seen with defect in another sodium-phosphorus transporter NaPi2a (encoded by *SLC34A1*) that results in similar biochemical profile as HHRH with only nephrocalcinosis. Response to phosphate supplements is rapid.

Renal Fanconi syndrome causes renal phosphate wasting due to generalized proximal tubular dysfunction. It leads to polyuria, hypophosphatemia, and metabolic acidosis, resulting in malnutrition, rickets, and growth failure. Nephropathic cystinosis, caused by *CTNS* mutations, is a lysosomal storage disorder leading to cystine buildup in the proximal tubule, causing Fanconi syndrome and eventual kidney failure. The clinical features may be ameliorated by therapy with cysteamine, and phosphorus and bicarbonate supplements. Recent trials with stem cells appear promising. Other uncommon causes of Fanconi syndrome include Dent disease characterized by loss of function of *CLCN5* in the proximal tubule, Fanconi Bickel (*GLUT2* mutation), and Fanconi renotubular syndromes **(*see* Chapter 20)**.

CHRONIC KIDNEY DISEASE

In patients with CKD, bone pathology, particularly renal osteodystrophy is common due to persistent overstimulation of the parathyroid glands.

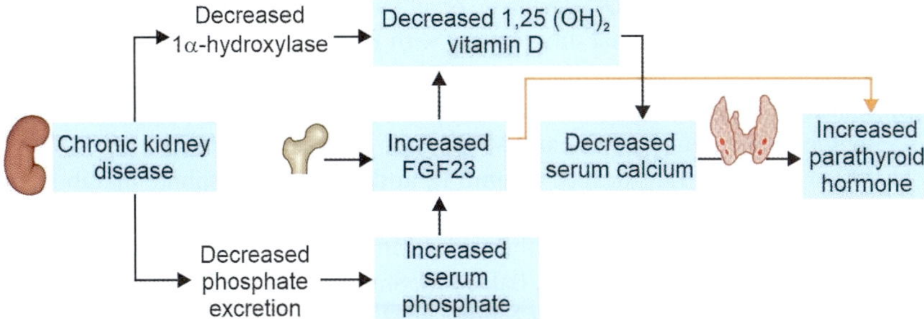

Fig. 22.3: Factors affecting blood levels of parathyroid hormone (PTH) in patients with chronic kidney disease (CKD). The levels of fibroblast growth factor 23 (FGF23) are increased due to its limited renal clearance and increased production by bone in response to hyperphosphatemia, caused by decreased renal clearance of phosphate. 1-α hydroxylase activity is decreased by elevated FGF23 levels, and due to reduced renal function. In CKD, the elevated levels of FGF23 paradoxically lead to an increase in PTH due to downregulation of FGF23 receptor expression. Chronic overstimulation of the parathyroid glands thus drives features of renal osteodystrophy

Impaired kidney function leads to inadequate phosphate excretion; hyperphosphatemia directly stimulates the parathyroid glands and triggers FGF23 production from the osteocytes. Further, patients with CKD show downregulated FGF23 receptors and reduced 1-α hydroxylase which causes decrease in $1,25(OH)_2$ vitamin D synthesis and low blood levels of calcium, leading to secondary hyperparathyroidism. Elevated PTH levels induce a state of high bone turnover, culminating in renal osteodystrophy **(Fig. 22.3)**. Importantly, the same factors driving renal osteodystrophy, namely elevated serum phosphorus and FGF23 levels, also contribute to cardiovascular morbidity in patients with CKD. Therapy for mineral bone disease associated with CKD [mineral bone disorder (MBD)-CKD] is discussed in Chapter 26.

BIBLIOGRAPHY

1. Chanchlani R, Nemer P, Sinha R, et al. An overview of rickets in children. Kidney Int Rep. 2020;5:980-90.
2. Friedman A. A brief history of rickets. Pediatr Nephrol. 2020;35(10):1835-41.
3. Govindarajan S, Khandelwal P, Sharma S, et al. Clinical features and genetic sequencing of children with Fanconi-Bickel syndrome. Indian J Pediatr. 2023;90:178-80.
4. Haffner D, Leifheit-Nestler M, Grund A, et al. Rickets Guidance: Part I-Diagnostic workup. Pediatr Nephrol. 2022;37:2013-36.
5. Haffner D, Leifheit-Nestler M, Grund A, et al. Rickets Guidance: Part II-Management. Pediatr Nephrol. 2022;37:2289-302.
6. Haffner D, Linglart A. Renal hypophosphatemia. In: Emma F, Goldstein S, Bagga A, Bates CM, Shroff R (Eds). Pediatric Nephrology, 8th edition. New York: Springer Nature; 2022. pp. 957-86.

7. Mannstadt M, Magen D, Segawa H, et al. Fanconi-Bickel syndrome and autosomal recessive proximal tubulopathy with hypercalciuria (ARPTH) are allelic variants caused by GLUT2 mutations. J Clin Endocrinol Metab. 2012;97:1978-86.
8. Marik B, Bagga A, Sinha A, et al. Genetic and clinical profile of patients with hypophosphatemic rickets. Eur J Med Genet. 2022;65:104540.
9. Miller WL, Imel EA. Rickets, vitamin D, and calcium/phosphate metabolism. Horm Res Paediatr. 2022;95:579-92.
10. Schlingmann KP, Konrad M. Inherited disorders of renal calcium handling. In: Emma F, Goldstein S, Bagga A, Bates CM, Shroff R (Eds). Pediatric Nephrology, 8th edition. New York: Springer Nature; 2022. pp. 1047-62.
11. Wagner CA, Rubio-Aliaga I, Hernando N. Renal phosphate handling and inherited disorders of phosphate reabsorption: an update. Pediatr Nephrol. 2019;34:549-59.
12. Yamazaki M, Michigami T. Osteocytes, and the pathogenesis of hypophosphatemic rickets. Front Endocrinol (Lausanne). 2022;13:1005189.
13. Yu Y, Sanderson SR, Reyes M, et al. Novel NAPI-IIC mutations causing HHRH and idiopathic hypercalciuria in several unrelated families: Long-term follow-up in one kindred. Bone. 2012;50:1100-6.

Nephrolithiasis and Nephrocalcinosis

Aditi Sinha, Arvind Bagga

Renal calculi (nephrolithiasis) are uncommon in children, although they are detected frequently. An underlying metabolic cause is identified in a significant proportion of cases.

PATHOGENESIS

Crystallization and calculus formation depends upon a number of factors. The point at which urine is saturated with a solute is called its "solubility product," which refers to the molar concentration at saturation. The point at which the solute can no longer remain in solution is termed the "formation product." Between these two indices, there is a metastable zone in which the existing crystals grow but precipitation does not occur. At the formation product, spontaneous nucleation takes place. Cellular debris and other particles provide nuclei for secondary nucleation. A damaged uroepithelium following urinary tract infections (UTIs) may provide a nidus for crystal growth (heterogeneous nucleation).

The role of inhibitors of calculus formation is poorly understood. Substances such as magnesium, citrate, pyrophosphate, uropontin, nephrocalcin, ribonucleic acid, and zinc have been suggested to inhibit formation of calcium crystals. The pH of urine influences the solubility. An acidic pH (<6) increases the solubility of calcium phosphate, and pH between 6 and 7 that of uric acid. An alkaline pH (>7.4) helps to keep cystine in solution. The formation of calcium oxalate crystals is not affected by changes in urinary pH. Citrate forms soluble complexes with calcium and reduces its free ion concentration. Of various factors, increased excretion of solutes, low urinary citrate and abnormal pH are important in calculus formation. Urinary infection with urea-splitting organisms such as *Proteus* is also an important cause.

RENAL CALCULI

Etiology

Renal stones are generally composed of calcium salts (70%), uric acid, magnesium ammonium phosphate, or cystine. Conditions that predispose to renal calculi are listed in **Table 23.1**. An underlying risk factor is identified

TABLE 23.1: Metabolic abnormalities and conditions associated with nephrolithiasis or nephrocalcinosis

Disorder (most common stone type)	*Gene(s) implicated, if any*[1]
Hypercalciuria with hypercalcemia (calcium oxalate, calcium phosphate)	
Infantile hypercalcemia or vitamin D hypersensitivity (24-D hydroxylase deficiency)	*CYP24A1* (including polymorphisms)
Infantile hypercalcemia type 2 or hypophosphatemic nephrolithiasis/osteoporosis type 1 (sodium phosphate cotransporter, NaPi, IIa defect)[2]	*SLC34A1*
Williams–Beuren syndrome	Deletion at 7q11.23 (including *ELN, LIMK1*)
Primary hyperparathyroidism	*MEN1, HRPT2, SAC, CASR*[3a]
Vitamin D overdose	
Production of parathyroid hormone (PTH) related peptide (malignancy, sarcoidosis)	
Hypercalciuria with normal serum calcium with or without hypocitraturia[4] *(calcium oxalate, calcium phosphate)*	
Idiopathic (absorptive) hypercalciuria	*ADCY10 (SAC), VDR*
Hereditary hypophosphatemic rickets with hypercalciuria (NaPi IIc defect)	*SLC34A3*
Hypophosphatemic nephrolithiasis/osteoporosis type 2 [defective sodium-hydrogen exchanger 3 (NHE3) channel]	*SLC9A3R1*
Hypophosphatemic rickets, on therapy with phosphate and calcitriol	*PHEX, FGF23, DMP1, ENPP1, FAM20C*
Distal renal tubular acidosis	*ATP6V0A4, ATPV1B1, SLC4A1, WDR72, FOXI1*
Bartter syndrome types 1 and 2	*SCL12A1, KCNJ1*
Dent disease	*CLCN5*
Autosomal dominant hypocalcemia with hypercalciuria	*CASR*[3b]
Familial hypomagnesemia with hypercalciuria and nephrocalcinosis	*CLDN16, CLDN19*
Lowe syndrome	*OCRL1*
Enamel renal (MacGibbon–Lubinsky) syndrome	*FAM20A, WDR72*
Atypical dominant Fanconi syndrome with young onset diabetes	*HNF4A*
Apparent mineralocorticoid excess	*HSD11B2*
Osteopetrosis with distal or proximal renal tubular acidosis	*CA2*
Glycogenosis type 1a, type 1b[5]	*SCL37A4 (G6PC)*

Contd...

Contd...

Disorder (most common stone type)	***Gene(s) implicated, if any***[1]
Pseudohypoaldosteronism	*WNK1, WNK4*
Frusemide use	
Hyperoxaluria (calcium oxalate)	
Primary hyperoxaluria, types 1, 2, and 3	*AGXT, GRHPR, HOGA1*
Enteric hyperoxaluria	*SLC26A1, SLC26A6*
Dietary hyperoxaluria	
Abnormal purine, pyrimidine metabolism (uric acid)	
Lesch–Nyhan syndrome	*HPRT1*
Partial HPRT deficiency (Kelley–Seegmiller syndrome)	*HPRT1*
Renal hypouricemia (familial hypouricemic hyperuricosuria) types 1, 2, and 3	*SLC22A12, SLC2A9, URAT1*
Hartnup disease (Pellagra-like dermatosis)	*SLC6A19*
Xanthinuria types 1 and 2	*XDH, MOCOS*
Glycogenosis type 1a, 1b[5]	*SCL37A4 (G6PC)*
Others	
Wilson disease	*ATP7B*
Inflammatory bowel disease; ileostomy	
Adenine phosphoribosyl transferase deficiency (dihydroxyadenine)	*APRT*
Cystinuria (cystine)	*SLC3A1, SLC7A9*
AD polycystic kidney disease (calcium oxalate or uric acid)	*PKD1, PKD2*
Medullary sponge kidney	*GDNF, RET*
Melamine toxicity (melamine with cyanuric acid)[6]	
Milk-alkali syndrome	
Urinary tract anomalies and infection (magnesium ammonium phosphate or carbonate apatite)	
Ketogenic diet (uric acid and/or calcium phosphate)	
Tumor lysis syndrome	
Metabolic syndrome	

[1]Variants of uromodulin and fetuin seem to be protective
[2]Nephrolithiasis and nephrocalcinosis are uncommon in Bartter syndrome types 3 (*CLCNKB*) and 4 (*BSND*)
[3]Caused by *CASR* mutations that cause [a]loss or [b]gain of function; inherited in autosomal recessive and dominant pattern, respectively
[4]Postulated to be secondary to hypokalemia and potassium depletion
[5]Both hypercalciuria and hyperuricemia are described
[6]Reported following contamination of melamine in powdered infant formula
AD: autosomal dominant; HPRT: hypoxanthine guanine-phosphoribosyl transferase

in 75–85% children with renal stones. Predisposing conditions include a metabolic abnormality (40–50%), infection or structural anomaly of the urinary tract (10–25%).

Clinical Features

The symptoms are recurrent flank pain, renal colic, repeated attacks of UTIs, and gross or microscopic hematuria. Pain is a common symptom in adolescents and school-aged children, but present in only one-half of children below 6 years of age. The child may pass gravel or a small stone. Occasionally, the stone may be "silent" and lead to obstructive uropathy. A stone in the urethra or in both ureters may precipitate acute kidney injury. Unexplained sterile pyuria, recurrent UTI, or gross hematuria should raise the suspicion for renal stones.

Imaging

A plain X-ray film of abdomen will show radiopaque stones but might miss small calculi and does not inform about possible obstruction **(Fig. 23.1)**. Ultrasonography is convenient and not associated with radiation exposure but can only image the kidney and proximal ureter and is less sensitive for detecting stones smaller than 3 mm. Ultrasonography is a good initial choice, and in uncomplicated situations, all that is required. Calyceal deposits of Tamm–Horsfall protein are harmless, but mimic nephrocalcinosis in preterm neonates.

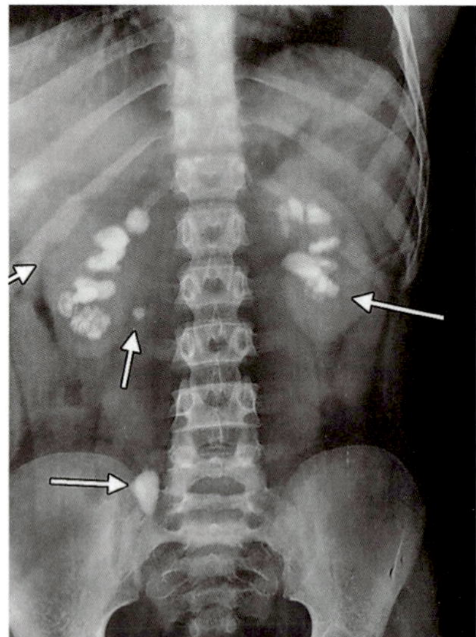

Fig. 23.1: X-ray abdomen showing nephrocalcinosis in a child with primary hyperoxaluria type 1

BOX 23.1: Investigations in urolithiasis

Imaging: Plain X-ray, ultrasonography, intravenous pyelogram (IVP), computed tomography (CT) abdomen
Blood: Urea, creatinine, electrolytes, pH, bicarbonate, calcium, phosphorus, uric acid, magnesium, alkaline phosphatase, parathyroid hormone
Urine: Urinalysis (including pH, specific gravity), culture
Spot specimens: Calcium, protein, uric acid, oxalate, citrate, magnesium, creatinine
24-hour urine: Volume, protein, creatinine, sodium, calcium, phosphorus, magnesium, oxalate, uric acid, citrate, cystine
Sodium nitroprusside test (or amino acid screen) for cystine
Stone analysis
Next generation sequencing: Bioinformatics targeted to cover genes (listed in **Table 23.1 and Annexure 9.7, p 845**)

Intravenous pyelography is useful to demonstrate an anomaly of the kidney or urinary tract and changes secondary to obstruction. There is, however, a risk of radiocontrast infusion and contrast mediated acute kidney injury. Pure uric acid stones are radiolucent and may be detected on ultrasonography or as a filling defect on intravenous pyelogram (IVP). Helical computed tomography (CT) without contrast is the most sensitive and specific radiological technique for diagnosing renal calculi. It has advantages over other imaging studies: It does not require the use of radiocontrast, shows the distal ureters, can detect radiolucent and even small radiopaque stones as small as 1–2 mm, provides accurate stone sizing, and demonstrates hydronephrosis. In order to keep the exposure to radiation "ALARA" (as low as reasonably achievable), most experts recommend ultrasonography as the preferred modality for initial screening as well as follow-up monitoring in children.

Etiologic Evaluation

A list of laboratory investigations is given in **Box 23.1**. Chief metabolic abnormalities identified are hypercalciuria, hyperoxaluria, and hypocitraturia. Infection may be the primary cause of nephrolithiasis; or occur concomitantly with a metabolic or structural abnormality. The likelihood of finding a metabolic cause is increased if there is a positive family history of stones, nephrocalcinosis, sterile urine, recurrent stone disease, and other features such as failure to thrive, polyuria, and rickets.

Careful, accurate studies are needed to reach a diagnosis. The cornerstone of evaluation is an accurate 24-hour urine collection. Since urinary constituents are influenced by dietary intake, 24-hour urine collections (to exclude diurnal fluctuations related to intake of food and beverages) provide useful information and an assessment of the patient's daily fluid intake. Urine sampling should be avoided in patients receiving parenteral infusions, during UTIs and following lithotripsy or relief of urinary tract obstruction. Stones in situ may diminish the excretion of urinary lithogenic material, as these may concurrently be absorbed by the stone.

Two or three 24-hour collections are recommended. The reliability of urine collection is estimated from the urinary creatinine excretion. In children with stable renal function, urinary creatinine excretion is 10–20 mg/kg per day. In specific cases, blood analyses for parathyroid hormone (PTH), vitamin A or D metabolites, oxalate and genetic testing shall be necessary. Timed urine samples for oxalate, glycolate, and glycerate are collected in containers with hydrochloric acid as a preservative.

Ratios are more prone to error than timed samples and should be interpreted with respect to daytime, relation to meals, medication, age, and regional differences. Metabolic urinalysis should be performed on multiple 24-hour urine collections.

Table 23.2 shows the normal values for urinary excretion of various substances. If the calculus is removed, its composition should be determined by infrared spectroscopy or X-ray diffraction. Chemical stone analysis is less accurate.

SPECIFIC ENTITIES AND MANAGEMENT

Medical management focuses on ensuring adequate urinary volumes, avoiding hypercalciuria, restriction of sodium, and correction of hypocitraturia. Principles of management of common metabolic etiologies are summarized in **Table 23.3**. Definitive treatment is possible in certain conditions. Important underlying conditions are discussed.

Hypercalciuria

Idiopathic hypercalciuria, characterized by normal concentration of serum calcium but excess urinary calcium, is the most common cause of renal calculi. The condition may be a familial, autosomal dominant condition. An increased intestinal absorption of calcium is responsible in most cases. It leads to rise in plasma calcium, which suppresses PTH, and results in reduced renal tubular reabsorption of calcium and hypercalciuria.

Idiopathic hypercalciuria is often detected in children with recurrent gross hematuria or microscopic hematuria. It may also be associated with the "frequency dysuria" syndrome. Chronic negative calcium balance may lead to osteoporosis and bone fractures. Siblings should be examined for hypercalciuria, and other disorders that cause hypercalciuria should be excluded **(Table 23.1)**. These include primary hyperparathyroidism, prolonged immobilization, Cushing syndrome, hyperthyroidism, hypervitaminosis D, and distal renal tubular acidosis.

TABLE 23.2: Normal values for urinary excretion of solutes (spot urine solute/creatinine ratio; 24-hour excretion)

Age group	*Calcium*		*Oxalate*		*Uric acid**		*Cystine*		*Citrate***	
	mg/mg	*mg/kg/day*	*mg/mg*	*mg/1.73 m^2/day*	*mg/mg*	*mg/kg/day*	*mg/mg*	*mg/1.73 m^2/day*	*mg/mg*	*mg/1.73 m^2/day*
0–1 month	<0.81	<4	<0.29	<45	<2.2	<13		<13	>0.42	Boys ≥180 Girls ≥250
1–6 months			<0.18		<2.4		<121		>0.18	
6–12 months			<0.14		<2.3					
1–2 years	<0.56		<0.10		<2.1	<11	<32	<50		
2–3 years	<0.50		<0.08		<1.93					
3–5 years	<0.41		<0.06		<1.64		<31			
5–7 years	<0.30		<0.06		<0.19	<9	<13.5			
7–10 years	<0.25		<0.05		<0.83					
10–14 years	<0.24				<0.65		<25	<50		
>14 years	<0.20		<0.05		<0.59					

Urinary solute excretion values must be confirmed with at least 2 sets of timed collection reports, or with one timed collection with separate solute-to-creatinine ratio

Values in empty cells are the same as the value in cell above

24-hour urine collection: (1) Container needs to contain either thymol 5% in isopropanol, or 2N HCl before collection starts; (2) Adequacy is assessed by the creatinine content, which is 8–10 mg/kg/day in neonates, 10–15 mg/kg/day in prepubertal children, and 15–24 mg/kg/day in older children

*If <2-yr-old: <815 mg/1.73 m^2

**Calcium: citrate is normally <0.33 mg/mg

TABLE 23.3: Principles of management of conditions associated with nephrocalcinosis

Abnormality	*Targeted therapy*
Hypercalciuria	Increased fluid intake; moderate salt restriction (1–1.5 mEq/kg/day); relative restriction of animal proteins; potassium citrate (1–2 mEq/kg/day base reduces calcium excretion and crystallization); hydrochlorothiazide (1–2 mg/kg/day; risks of hypokalemia, dyslipidemia, and hyperuricemia)
Hypocitraturia	Potassium citrate (1–2 mEq/kg/day)
Bartter syndrome	Potassium supplements, potassium sparing diuretics, prostaglandin inhibitors (indomethacin, ibuprofen)
Distal renal tubular acidosis	Potassium and alkali supplements (typically as potassium citrate; 3–5 mEq/kg of base)
Hypomagnesemia	Oral magnesium supplements (50–100 mg/kg/day; as magnesium lactate or oxide)
Primary hyperoxaluria	Increased fluid intake; pyridoxine (3–5 mg/kg) in selected mutations; restrict dietary oxalate (spinach, peanuts, and cocoa); combined liver and kidney transplantation; therapy based on RNA interference (if feasible)
Cystinuria	Increased fluid intake (urine output >2 L/m^2 BSA to achieve specific gravity <1.005); restrict dietary salt (1–1.5 mEq/kg/day) and methionine (<1,200–1,400 mg/day in adults); potassium citrate (1–3 mEq/kg/day; 60–80 mEq/m^2 BSA to achieve urine pH >7.5); tiopronin (α-mercaptopropionyl glycine, 15–40 mg/kg/day), D-penicillamine (20–40 mg/kg/day; maximum 1.2 g/day), or captopril (1–2 mg/kg/day) to achieve urinary cystine <300 mg/day

BSA: body surface area; RNA: ribonucleic acid

Management

The treatment of idiopathic hypercalciuria consists of ensuring a high fluid intake and avoiding periods of dehydration **(Table 23.3)**. The urinary excretion of sodium and calcium is closely interrelated. Dietary sodium loading increases urinary calcium excretion while a low sodium diet has the opposite effect. Moderate salt restriction is therefore useful. Recommended dietary allowances for protein and calcium should be provided. A high-protein diet (animal protein) should be avoided. Although dietary excess of calcium should be avoided, dietary calcium is not restricted. Low calcium diets result in negative systemic balance and osteoporosis and are accompanied by higher urinary oxalate excretion.

Citrate supplements: Administration of potassium citrate (1.5–2 mEq/kg/day) results in reduction of calcium excretion and an increase of urinary citrate and potassium.

Thiazides: Long-acting thiazide diuretics (hydrochlorothiazide 1–2 mg/kg/day) increase calcium reabsorption in the distal convoluted tubule, reducing its excretion. It is proposed that thiazide diuretics be used if dietary measures over 3–6 months fail to reduce urinary calcium levels. Patients receiving thiazide diuretics should be monitored for hypokalemia, and if necessary, supplemented with potassium or a potassium sparing diuretic (e.g., amiloride). Since thiazides may adversely affect lipid metabolism and lead to hyperuricemia, their long-term use is restricted.

Renal Tubular Acidosis

Approximately two-thirds of patients with distal (type 1) renal tubular acidosis (RTA) have nephrocalcinosis or nephrolithiasis. The stones are generally composed of calcium phosphate. Stone formation occurs because of increased urine calcium and phosphate excretion, a high urine pH, and decreased citrate excretion. Some patients with distal RTA have hyperoxaluria, secondary to a defect in tubular oxalate transporters. Alkali administration reduces nephrocalcinosis and nephrolithiasis by decreasing calcium and increasing citrate excretion, despite maintenance of a high urine pH.

Hyperoxaluria

Primary hyperoxaluria (PH) is an inborn error of glyoxylate metabolism characterized by increased urinary excretion of oxalate. About 15% of urinary oxalate is derived from diet and the remainder from the metabolism of glyoxylate and ascorbic acid. **Figure 23.2** depicts the pathways of glyoxylate and oxalate metabolism in the liver, in relation to the defects underlying various types of PH. The three forms of PH differ in genetic basis and clinical and biochemical features, as shown in **Table 23.4**.

In most common, PH type 1 (PH1), there is deficiency of the peroxisomal hepatic enzyme, alanine: glyoxylate aminotransferase (AGT), which converts glyoxylate to glycine **(Fig. 23.2)**, and is encoded by *AGXT* (2q37.3). Homozygous mutations of the gene result in deficiency of AGT leading to accumulation of glyoxylate and glycolate, and subsequent conversion to oxalate. Genetic heterogeneity may explain differences in clinical features, including variable age of onset and severity. Recurrent stone formation and nephrocalcinosis start in early childhood and lead to end-stage kidney disease (ESKD) by early adult life. Irregular, spiky stones form and give rise to pain, colic, hematuria, and obstruction. The renal injury is due to obstruction, infection, and

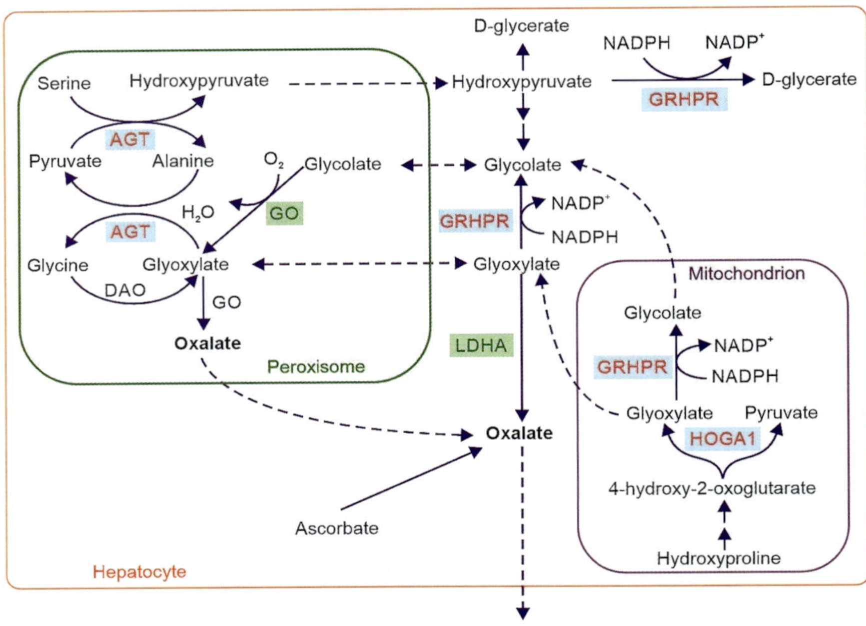

Fig. 23.2: Pathogenesis of primary hyperoxaluria (PH). In hepatocytes, the glyoxylate pathway has a key role in gluconeogenesis and ureagenesis. Glyoxylate is metabolized to glycine in the peroxisome by alanine:glyoxylate aminotransferase (AGT), or glycolate in the cytosol by glyoxylate reductase/hydropyruvate reductase (GRHPR). Glyoxylate is also generated in the mitochondria by collagen breakdown, the final step of which is catalyzed by 4-hydroxy-2-oxoglutarate aldolase (HOGA). Inability to metabolize glyoxylate leads to its oxidation into oxalate, by the glycolate oxidase (GO) in the peroxisome, and L-lactate dehydrogenase (LDHA) in the cytosol. Oxalate exits the cell to be excreted by the kidneys. The hepatic enzymes whose deficiency leads to the three types of PH are shown in maroon, namely, AGT (type 1), GRHPR (type 2), and HOGA (type 3). RNA interference by lumasiran blocks GO, while that by nedosiran blocks LDHA. Given their sites of action, lumasiran is specific therapy for PH type 1, while nedosiran is expected to benefit all three types of the disease. DAO: D-amino acid oxidase; NADP: nicotinamide adenine dinucleotide phosphate; NADPH: nicotinamide adenine dinucleotide phosphate hydrogen

TABLE 23.4: Key characteristics of the three types of primary hyperoxaluria (PH)

Feature	*PH1*	*PH2*	*PH3*
Gene	*AGT*	*GRHPR*	*HOGA1*
Frequency	80% of cases	<10% of cases	>10% of cases
Variants common in Asia	c.33dupC; c.302T >C	c.494 G>A; c.404+3_404+6del	c.834_834+1GG>TT
Presentation	Recurrent kidney stones or nephrocalcinosis with onset in childhood; UTI; hematuria; failure to thrive	Kidney stones; UTI; hematuria	Kidney stones; UTI; hematuria
Nephrocalcinosis	Common; severe	Less common; less severe	Uncommon; rarely severe
Presentation in infancy	10–20%	No	No
End-stage kidney failure	>50–100%	~25%	Rare; chronic kidney disease <20%
Systemic oxalosis	Common	Reported	Uncommon
Degree of hyperoxaluria	+++	++	++
Increased urinary metabolites	Glycolate[1]	L-glycerate[1]	4-hydroxy-2-oxoglutarate[1], 4-hydroxyglutamate, 2,4-dihydroxyglutarate

[1]Elevated urinary levels support the diagnosis; however, levels may be in normal range
AGT: alanine:glyoxylate aminotransferase; GRHPR: glyoxylate reductase/hydropyruvate reductase; HOGA: 4-hydroxy-2-oxoglutarate aldolase; UTI: urinary tract infection

extensive deposition of calcium oxalate in the renal parenchyma. About 50% of patients develop ESKD by 5 years of age. Infantile oxalosis, characterized by diffuse nephrocalcinosis and ESKD within the first year of life, may be suspected based on oxalate deposits in the bone marrow and retina **(Figs. 23.3A to D)**. Once kidney function declines, there is increase in plasma levels of oxalate (>30 mmol/L). In later stages, there is oxalate deposition in the eyes, bones, muscles, blood vessels, and heart (systemic oxalosis). Since serious morbidity can result from systemic oxalosis, it is recommended that renal replacement with intensive dialysis followed by transplantation be initiated early in these patients. The diagnosis is suggested by marked hyperoxaluria (usually >100 mg/1.73 m^2 per day). Confirmation of the diagnosis is done by sequencing of *AGXT*.

Until recently, there was no definite treatment. Following advances in management, especially using therapies based on interference with

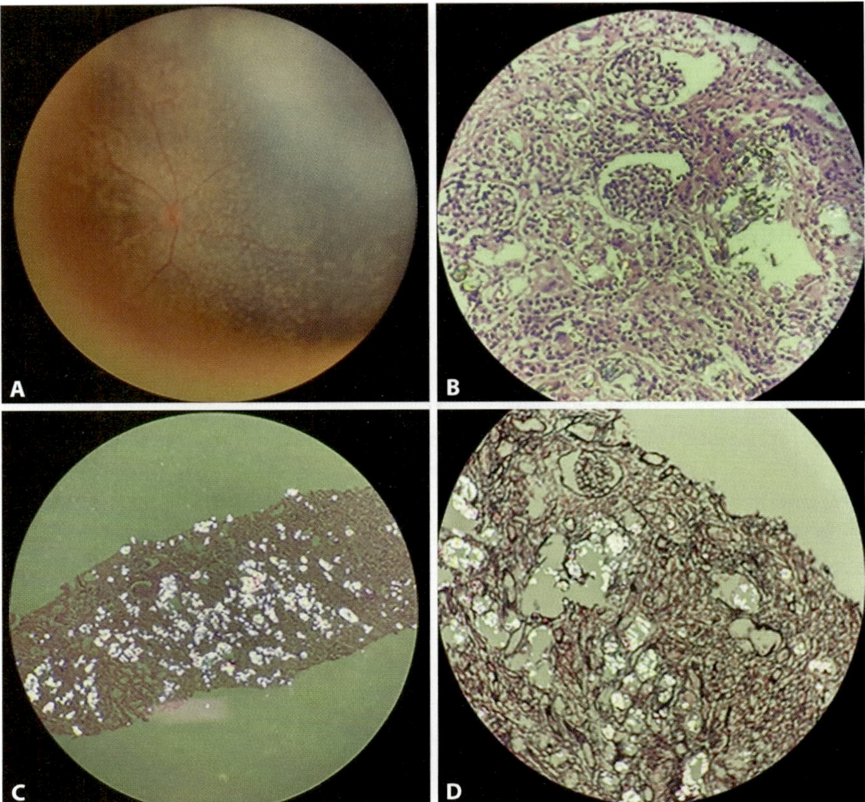

Figs. 23.3A to D: Infantile hyperoxaluria. (A) Retinoscopy showing extensive oxalate deposition in the central and peripheral retina; (B) Kidney biopsy specimen shows calcium oxalate crystals on light microscopy by hematoxylin and eosin, and (C) on polarized light; (D) Deposits were seen clearly on silver methenamine staining. *Courtesy:* Prof. Iftikhar Ijaz and Dr. Humaira Nazir, King Edward Medical University, Lahore

ribonucleic acid (RNA) synthesis of hepatic enzymes, the ERKNet, and OxalEurope have developed consensus clinical practice guidelines for evaluation and management of PH. The principles of management are summarized in **Box 23.2**. Two RNA-interference based oxalate-lowering therapies, lumasiran and nedosiran are now available, which are approved by the Food and Drug Administration (FDA) for therapy of PH1. Nedosiran is being examined for its efficacy in patients with PH type 2 (PH2) and PH type 3 (PH3). Supportive measures include increasing fluid intake, reducing dietary salt intake, avoiding excessive intake of food items rich in oxalate (spinach, peanuts, and cocoa), and alkalinization of urine **(Table 23.3 and Box 23.2)**. Since 30% patients with PH1 (chiefly those with homozygous p.Gly170Arg or p.Phe125Ile mutations, less so with other nontruncating genotypes, e.g., p.Gly41Arg) show reduced urinary oxalate secretion with

BOX 23.2: Summary of ERKNet and OxalEurope 2023 recommendations on management of primary hyperoxaluria (PH)

Offer genetic testing to all patients with strong clinical or biochemical suspicion of PH.

Assess urinary oxalate and creatinine in 24-hr urine; if not feasible, use first morning spot urine oxalate-to-creatinine ratio, interpreted in relation to age-appropriate thresholds **(Table 23.3)**. Collect urine specimen in container with 2N HCl to reduce urine pH to ≤2.0; alternatively, store the sample at 4°C and acidify in lab within 24 hr.

Hyperoxaluria is present if urine oxalate is higher than the upper reference limit, at least twice.

If feasible, assess urinary calcium oxalate crystal volume (>200 pure whewellite crystals/mm^3 of urinary sediment suggest PH1); also measure urine metabolites glycolate, l-glycerate, 4-hydroxy-2-oxoglutarate (HOG), and 2,4-dihydroxyglutarate (DHG) **(Table 23.4)**.

Measure plasma oxalate levels only in patients with chronic kidney disease (CKD) stage 4 or 5 and interpret them based on reference values that account for the eGFR.

Therapy for patients with suspected PH and preserved kidney function:
(*i*) Hyperhydration (3.5–4 L/day in adults; 2–3 L/m^2 in children; consumed over 24 hr, (*ii*) potassium citrate (0.1–0.15 g/kg/day in divided doses), and *(iii)* balanced diet; avoid foods with extremely high oxalate (spinach, rhubarb, chocolate, and nuts)

Test all patients with PH1 for response to pyridoxine, and titrate its dose based on urinary oxalate excretion.

When surgical management is required, prefer percutaneous nephrolithotomy (PCNL) and ureteroscopy to extracorporeal shockwave lithotripsy (ESWL)

Perform follow-up ultrasound imaging annually, lifelong.

Perform eye examination and echocardiography at diagnosis in patients with infantile oxalosis (PH associated CKD 5D before 1-year-old); repeat annually

In patients with PH1, consider kidney replacement therapy earlier than kidney failure if they are at high risk of systemic oxalosis, suggested by high plasma oxalate and comorbidities. In absence of access to RNAi therapy, initiate intensified hemodialysis, using a high-flux hemodialyzer (>1 m^2 capillary surface per m^2 BSA) with maximal blood flow (>150–200 cm^3/min/m^2 BSA). Titrate the dialysis dose, as tolerated, to achieve clinical response and plasma oxalate levels in the range of values for patients with kidney failure without PH.

Consider either sequential or combined transplant in pyridoxine-unresponsive patients with PH1 lacking access to RNAi therapy, based on surgeon's preference and clinical situation. Combined transplant is preferred at eGFR <30 mL/min/1.73 m^2. During liver transplantation, the native liver is removed completely.

Consider isolated kidney transplantation in patients with PH1 and CKD 5D with pyridoxine-responsive mutations. Isolated liver transplantation is suggested in patients with PH2 and eGFR <30 mL/min/1.73 m^2.

Where feasible, consider RNAi therapy in patients with genetically proven PH1 who are unresponsive or only partially responsive to pyridoxine, or have a mutation consistent with pyridoxine-unresponsiveness, and have urinary oxalate >1.5 times the reference value (or in CKD 5D, elevated plasma oxalate), with active stones, nephrocalcinosis or advanced CKD.

Monitor urinary and plasma oxalate levels at least q6 months after liver transplantation until normal at least thrice. Similarly, monitor levels after kidney transplant in patients receiving pyridoxine and/or RNAi therapy until levels normalize, and at least annually afterwards.

BSA: body surface area; eGFR: estimated glomerular filtration rate; RNAi: RNA interference-based oxalate lowering therapy (currently, lumasiran, and nedosiran for PH1)

pyridoxine supplements, 3-6 months' trial with the agent (3–5 mg/kg/day) is recommended. Most patients with PH1 and end-stage kidney failure (ESKF) require combined liver and kidney transplantation to correct the metabolic defect and restore kidney function. Otherwise, there is a high risk of recurrence of oxalosis in the allograft.

The PH2 results due to homozygous mutations in the gene, *GRHPR* (9q12), which encodes the enzyme glyoxylate and hydroxypyruvate reductase (GR/HPR). Compared to PH1, the illness is less common and the clinical course less severe **(Table 23.4)**. Patients with PH2 have less active stone formation, rarely show nephrocalcinosis and progression to ESKD. Since the enzyme GR/HPR is also involved in conversion of beta-hydroxypyruvate to D-glycerate, these patients excrete L-glyceric acid in the urine. The diagnosis is suggested by elevated levels of urinary oxalate and L-glyceric acid. These patients do not benefit from pyridoxine, nor do they require liver transplantation.

The PH3, which is uncommon (5%), occurs due to mutations of *HOGA1*, encoding mitochondrial 4-hydroxy-2-oxoglutarate aldolase that catalyzes cleavage of 4-hydroxy-2-oxoglutarate (produced from hydroxyproline) to pyruvate and glyoxylate. Patients with PH3 present early with nephrolithiaisis. Recurrent stones are uncommon, and these patients do not show progressive ESKF.

Enteric Hyperoxaluria

The absorption of oxalate occurs chiefly in the duodenum and colon and is influenced by dietary constituents. Normally, dietary calcium binds to ingested oxalate, reducing its absorption. Dietary calcium deficiency, therefore, enhances oxalate absorption from the gut. Similarly, chronic small bowel or pancreatic disease, which are both associated with fat malabsorption, result in enhanced colonic absorption of oxalate (enteric hyperoxaluria). Patients with enteric hyperoxaluria show moderate amounts of 24-hour urinary oxalate excretion, in the range of 40–100 mg/1.73 m^2. At risk variants and polymorphisms are described in two genes encoding intestinal or renal anion transporters, namely *SLC26A1* and *SLC26A6.* Management includes intake of low oxalate, low fat diet with calcium carbonate, or citrate administered with meals to bind dietary oxalate. Administration of cholestyramine (that binds fatty and bile acids) may be useful. The use of *Oxalobacter formigenes,* a gram negative aerobic bacterium that metabolizes oxalate, holds promise.

Hyperuricosuria

Excessive excretion of uric acid may occur in conditions such as leukemia and lymphoma, especially after cytotoxic therapy **(*see* Table 1)**. Uric acid calculi may occur in patients with the metabolic syndrome, primary gout, and Lesch–Nyhan syndrome. Below a urine pH of 5.6, uric acid exists in unionized form, which is relatively insoluble and precipitates. Uric acid gravel may cause obstruction and acute renal failure. Alkalization with bicarbonate or citrate should be aimed at maintaining a urine pH between 6 and 7. Uric acid levels are effectively reduced with medications such as allopurinol and recombinant urate oxidase (rasburicase).

Infection-associated Stones

Recurrent urinary infection with *Proteus* (rarely *Providencia, Klebsiella pneumoniae*, and *Serratia marcescens*) such as in patients with obstructive uropathy or urinary stasis may cause stone formation. Bacterial urease activity leads to formation of ammonium from urea, which raises the urine pH causing precipitation of calcium phosphate-carbonate (carbonate apatite), and magnesium ammonium phosphate (struvite). The carbonate apatite is found within the struvite calculi, resulting in formation of triple-phosphate stones. These amorphous stones mould easily into the renal calyces, grow rapidly, and fill the renal collecting system with staghorn calculi. Surgical stone removal is difficult and recurrence of stone formation is common. Percutaneous nephrolithotomy (PCNL) is employed to completely remove struvite calculi, but some patients require open surgery to repair associated renal anomalies. Acetohydroxamic acid, that reversibly inhibits the enzyme urease, has been proposed as an adjunct to antimicrobial therapy in patients with chronic urea splitting urine infection.

Cystine Stones

Cystinuria is the most common genetic cause of nephrolithiasis in children. Cystine stones comprise approximately 5% of renal stones in children and adolescents. Cystinuria is an autosomal recessively transmitted disorder characterized by lack of reabsorption of dibasic amino acids (cystine, ornithine, lysine, and arginine) along the luminal border of the proximal renal tubule. While high concentrations of the other three amino acids do not cause any problems, cystine that is much less soluble at low urine pH tends to form stones. Patients show homozygous inactivating mutations in either *SLC3A1* (type A cystinuria) or *SLC7A9* (type B cystinuria), encoding for the two subunits of the heterodimeric amino acid transporter. Heterozygous carriers of significant variants in *SLC7A9*, and less often, specific mutations of *SLC3A1*, often have increased urinary cystine concentrations, but no nephrolithiasis. Hence, the condition is increasingly considered an autosomal dominant disorder with incomplete penetrance for nephrolithiasis. Large deletions and duplications are common in both genes; hence, if conventional sequencing fails to detect the causative variant, multiplex ligation-dependent probe amplification (MLPA) should be performed to detect copy number variations. The hypotonia cystinuria syndrome is caused by homozygous

2p21 deletion in which at least two genes are deleted, namely, *SLC3A1* and *PREPL*, which causes congenital myasthenia.

The clinical features of this condition are solely related to nephrolithiasis. While the diagnosis is usually made during childhood or adolescence (median age at presentation is 12 years), patients may occasionally present in infancy or late adulthood. Cystine calculi are radiopaque and usually multiple, yellow brown in color; occasionally patients may have large branched (staghorn) calculi. Patients have conventionally been screened for cystinuria by the cyanide-nitroprusside test; a positive test indicates urinary cystine concentration >75 mg/L. Recently, the attenuated total reflection—Fourier transform infrared spectroscopy (ATR-FTIR) was shown to be a cost-effective screening test for cystinuria with high specificity and sensitivity. Urinalysis reveals pathognomonic flat hexagonal crystals in approximately 25% cases. Confirmation of diagnosis is possible following stone analysis and genetic testing. Measurement of urinary cystine excretion is useful for diagnosis and follow-up. The spot cystine to creatinine ratio is elevated above age-appropriate threshold **(Table 23.2)**, corresponding to >400 mg/day of cystine excretion.

The goal of therapy is to reduce excretion and increase the solubility of cystine. Patients with cystine calculi are advised an increased fluid intake and modest reductions in sodium and methionine intake. The urine output is maintained at >2 L/m^2 body surface area (ensuring urine specific gravity <1.005) and therapy with potassium citrate or potassium bicarbonate advised to maintain urine pH >7.5; together, these measures ensure that the cystine excretion remains <243 mg/L and cystine supersaturation is <1. Home monitoring of urine pH is useful to titrate therapy to ensure urinary alkalinization as well as avoid a very high urine pH, which increases the risk of calcium phosphate stones. If conservative measures are unable to adequately reduce the urinary cystine concentration, or stones recur, therapy with a thiol-containing, cystine-binding drug, such as D-penicillamine or tiopronin, is initiated that cleave disulfide bonds of cystine to form cysteine homodimers **(Table 23.3)**. Patients prescribed D-penicillamine are monitored closely for adverse effects, such as mucocutaneus lesions, altered taste, neutropenia, thrombocytopenia, gastrointestinal symptoms, raised transaminases, and proteinuria. While tiopronin has fewer and less severe effects, it is not easily available. Proteinuria, including nephrotic syndrome, is reported during therapy with tiopronin. Therapy with captopril is recommended if tiopronin is not available or unsuccessful. Response to and adherence with therapy is monitored by 24-hour urine collection to assess volume, and to measure cystine, urine pH, creatinine, sodium, and calcium. Medical interventions are often insufficient, and patients undergo several surgical procedures to treat recurrent nephrolithiasis. Other therapies include inhibitors of crystal growth, e.g., cystine dimethyl ester and α-lipoic acid, measures to alkalinize urine (ADV7103; potassium citrate with potassium bicarbonate), or increase urine output, e.g., tolvaptan.

Melamine Calculi

Melamine, a synthetic non-nutritive substance containing nitrogen, can falsely elevate measures of protein content in foodstuffs. During 2007–2008, there were reports that several manufacturers of powdered infant formula in China apparently added melamine to raise the measured protein content and thereby exposed infants and young children to very high levels of melamine. Such exposure resulted in cases of acute kidney failure and nephrolithiasis. Composed of crystals of melamine and cyanuric acid, these stones were not uniformly radiopaque, but were detected on ultrasound or CT scans. Some stones were loose and soft, resulting in urine that was cloudy and turbid. Patients did not show persistence of calculi or renal dysfunction on follow-up. Food safety regulations are necessary to prevent similar accidents.

Idiopathic Calculi

Even after extensive evaluation, there is a group of patients in whom an etiology for stone formation is not found. Excretion of calcium, oxalate, and uric acid is normal. The results of stone analysis are an important guide to therapy. These patients are advised to increase fluid intake (>2–2.5 L/1.73 m^2) and decrease animal protein and salt intake **(Table 23.3)**. Long-term therapy with potassium citrate (2 mEq/kg/day) results in decreased stone formation; citrate binds to urinary calcium forming a soluble complex and reducing precipitation of calcium with other anions. Compliance is ensured by regularly measuring the urine pH. There is limited data on the efficacy and long-term safety of therapy with magnesium and/or phosphate supplements in children with recurrent stones.

Surgical Treatment of Stones

Appropriate therapy depends on the site, size, and composition of the stone, and anatomy of the urinary tract. Ureteric stones below 5 mm are likely to pass spontaneously and do not require specific therapy. Renal ultrasonography is used to monitor stone movement and passage. *If a stone is retrieved, its composition is determined.*

Chief indications for surgical intervention include stones unlikely to pass spontaneously due to their large size; urolithiasis causing obstruction; pain despite adequate analgesia; decreased renal function either due to kidney failure, solitary kidney, or bilateral obstruction; and struvite stones.

Table 23.5 summarizes the choice of procedure for surgical management of stones based on their size and location. Small stones (<20 mm diameter) are

TABLE 23.5: Indications and types of surgical procedures according to site and size of kidney stones[1]

Location	*Size*	*Intervention*
Kidney		
Upper pole, middle calyces or renal pelvis	<10 mm	Extracorporeal shockwave lithotripsy (ESWL) or ureteroscopy If fails, consider percutaneous nephrolithotomy (PCNL)
	≥10–<20 mm	Ureterostomy, PCNL or ESWL (AUA does not advocate PCNL)
	≥20 mm	PCNL preferred to ureterostomy or ESWL
Lower pole	<10 mm	ESWL or ureteroscopy If fails, consider PCNL
	≥10–<20 mm	PCNL or ureterostomy preferred over ESWL in patients with factors unfavorable for ESWL[2] ESWL may be considered in the absence of these factors (AUA considers ESWL second-line)
	≥20 mm	PCNL preferred to ureterostomy or ESWL
Proximal ureter	<10 mm	ESWL or ureteroscopy
	≥10 mm	Ureteroscopy preferred to ESWL (AUA suggests either option)
Distal ureter	<10 mm	Medical expulsive therapy with tamsulosin for 4–6 weeks if stones >5 mm (<10 mm, according to AUA)[3]; if fails, consider ESWL or ureteroscopy (ureteroscopy preferred by AUA)
	≥10 mm	Ureteroscopy preferred to ESWL
Bladder	Not applicable	Transurethral cystolithotripsy preferred to percutaneous cystolithotripsy Large stones require open cystolithotomy

[1]Recommendations according to European League of Urology. Where the American Urology Association (AUA) differs, their opinion is provided in parenthesis
[2]Factors unfavorable for ESWL include narrow infundibulum, a long skin to stone distance, a long calyx, stones that are shock-wave-resistant (calcium oxalate monohydrate, brushite, and cystine), and a steep infundibular-pelvic angle
[3]Tamsulosin use is off label in children and may be associated with adverse effects

treated by extracorporeal shockwave lithotripsy (ESWL), in which shock waves are focused at the stone, resulting in its fragmentation. Stone free rates after ESWL in children range between 60 and 90%. Calculi composed of uric acid and calcium oxalate disintegrate easily, but cystine and calcium phosphate, that are comparatively harder, do not. ESWL is suitable for radiopaque stones in the renal pelvis and upper ureter but has lower success rates for stones in the lower renal calyces, stones located in calyceal diverticuli or in patients with complex renal anatomy. Passing stone fragments can cause renal colic;

other complications include hematuria, perirenal hematoma, and local bruising. ESWL is a relatively safe procedure with no long-term influence on renal growth or function.

The PCNL is preferred in patients with stones that are large (>20 mm), in the lower pole or in calyceal diverticuli, cystine calculi (relatively resistant to ESWL), contraindications to ESWL (bleeding diathesis, oliguric renal failure, and urinary tract obstruction), and anatomic abnormalities (horseshoe kidney, ureteropelvic junction obstruction). Stone fragmentation is achieved using pneumatic LithoClast probes, ultrasound probes or holmium-yttrium aluminum garnet (Ho:YAG) laser probes. Stone fragments are collected through wire baskets or graspers, inserted through the instrument. The availability of miniaturized ureteroscopic endoscopes (4.5–5F) has enabled the application of ureterorenoscopy (URS) in children. URS is suited for calculi in the mid- and distal ureter but has also been used for removing calculi in the proximal ureter or kidney. Open surgery is preferred for removing large stones (staghorn calculi) or associated with anatomical abnormalities (pelviureteric junction obstruction, obstructive megaureters).

Vesical Calculi

Bladder calculi account for ~5% of urinary calculi. They usually occur in patients with foreign bodies, obstruction, or infection of the bladder, typically following pelvic surgery, and in patients with indwelling urinary catheters. Patients who undergo bladder augmentation using a vascularized gastric patch (gastrocystoplasty) are protected from vesical stones, while those in whom intestinal segment is used (ileum, colon) tend to develop stones following colonization by urease-producing organisms, producing an alkaline pH. Children at risk for bladder stones include those with uncorrected anatomic abnormalities, such as posterior urethral valves and vesicoureteral reflux. Management entails relieving obstruction, eliminating infection, and surgical removal of stone.

Endemic Vesical Calculi

Primary bladder calculi were reported to account for up to 15–40% of calculi in children in developing countries, where the major source of dietary proteins are cereals. With improving nutritional status, the incidence of these calculi has declined to 3–15%. In India, they remain common in western Uttar Pradesh, Delhi, Punjab, parts of Gujarat and Maharashtra.

Epidemiological and clinical studies reveal that these children eat mainly a cereal-based diet, lacking in animal protein, calcium, and phosphate. The urine has relatively high content of ammonium and urate ions, with formation of ammonium acid urate crystals and stones. Increased uric acid saturation is proposed to block the action of mucopolysaccharide inhibitors of stone formation. Urinary oxalate excretion is increased in patients with a high intake of oxalate from leaves and vegetables; ammonium acid urate stones therefore also contain calcium oxalate. The risk of stone formation is compounded by low urine volumes due to limited water intake, recurrent episodes of diarrhea, and high ambient temperatures. No overt signs of protein energy malnutrition or deficiency of micronutrients is seen.

Vesical stones usually affect boys between 1 and 5 years of age, with peak incidence around 3 years. Unlike renal stones, recurrence of vesical stones in children is extremely rare. Symptoms are caused by mechanical obstruction or associated cystitis. Vague abdominal pain, dysuria, frequency of micturition, interruption of urinary stream, and pulling and rubbing of penis are common symptoms. Suprapubic pain and dribbling of urine may be present. Plain X-ray film of the abdomen and ultrasonography show the bladder calculus. In a few cases, hydronephrosis, hydroureter, and bladder diverticuli are seen. On X-ray diffraction, ammonium acid urate and calcium oxalate are present in the majority of the stones, often in concentric layers. The overall composition of vesical stones shows preponderance of uric acid over its ammonium salt.

Small stones may be expelled spontaneously but suprapubic cystolithotomy is required in most cases. A systematic review of 1,034 pediatric patients with vesical calculi reported in eight studies, concluded that open cystolithotomy, transurethral cystolithotripsy, and percutaneous cystolithotripsy have similar stone-free rates during follow up, while ESWL appeared to be less effective for treating vesical stones in children. A mixed cereal diet with milk supplements is useful in prevention of vesical stones. Such a diet increases phosphate and decreases oxalate excretion, reducing the incidence of vesical stones.

NEPHROCALCINOSIS

Nephrocalcinosis implies deposition of calcium in renal parenchyma. Nephrocalcinosis is less common than urinary tract calculi, although both may occur together. Focal deposition of calcium (dystrophic calcification) may be seen in an area of previously damaged parenchyma, but diffuse nephrocalcinosis usually results from a metabolic disorder.

Calcium content of the renal parenchyma must substantially increase before nephrocalcinosis is visible on X-ray. For detection and monitoring of nephrocalcinosis, high-resolution ultrasonography is preferred. Nephrocalcinosis associated with various metabolic diseases is most prominent at the corticomedullary junction **(Figs. 23.4A to D)**. Common causes include hypercalciuria, RTA, and hyperoxaluria **(Table 23.6)**. Hyperoxaluria causes a coarse and diffuse nephrocalcinosis involving both cortex and the medulla **(Figs. 23.4A to D)**; in infants it may cause renal failure without stone formation. Hyperparathyroidism is not a common cause in

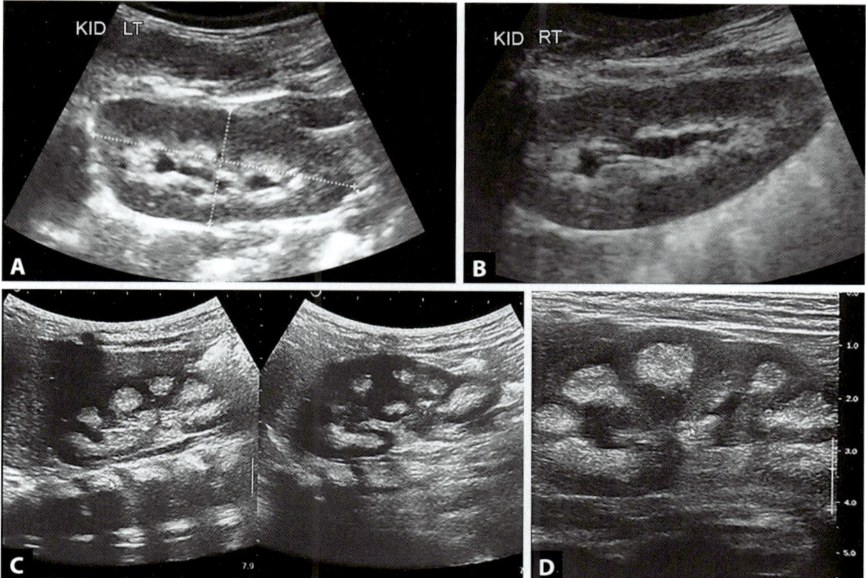

Figs. 23.4A to D: Ultrasonography showing nephrocalcinosis. (A and B) Grade 2 nephrocalcinosis in siblings with hypophosphatemic nephrolithiasis/osteoporosis type 1 (sodium phosphate cotransporter, NaPi and IIa defect), and (C and D) severe (grade 3) nephrocalcinosis in an infant with distal renal tubular acidosis with homozygous anion exchanger (*SLC4A1*) defect

TABLE 23.6: Causes of nephrocalcinosis

Common	
Distal renal tubular acidosis	
Primary hyperoxaluria type 1	
Idiopathic hypercalciuria	
Uncommon	
Primary hyperparathyroidism	Hyperthyroidism or hypothyroidism
Prematurity	Furosemide treatment in neonates
Bartter syndrome types 1 and 2	X-linked hypercalciuria (Dent disease)
Familial hypomagnesemia with hypercalciuria and nephrocalcinosis	Idiopathic hypercalcemia
Vitamin D or A intoxication	Cushing syndrome
Sarcoidosis	Medullary sponge kidney
Infantile hypercalcemia types 1 and 2	Hypophosphatemic rickets with hypercalciuria
William-Beuren syndrome	Congenital chloride diarrhea
Cortical necrosis*	Chronic glomerulonephritis*
Following trauma*	Renal tuberculosis*

*Predominantly cortical nephrocalcinosis

children, though important in adults. Nephrocalcinosis may be seen in very low birth weight infants receiving therapy with furosemide or acetazolamide. Unlike most renal tubular disorders, nephrocalcinosis in preterm neonates resolves with time and stoppage of diuretic therapy. Occasionally, transient deposition of Tamm–Horsfall protein within the renal in preterm neonates may mimic the ultrasonographic appearance of nephrocalcinosis. Nephrocalcinosis should be distinguished from the punctate calcification seen in medullary sponge kidney, a condition more often seen in adults.

Patients with nephrocalcinosis are advised a liberal fluid intake. Those with nephrocalcinosis and hypercalciuria are advised modest restriction of animal protein and sodium intake. Potassium citrate is administered to achieve a urine pH around 7. The prognosis of nephrocalcinosis depends on the underlying cause. While most patients do not progress to ESKD, patients with PH, hypomagnesemia with hypercalciuria, and Dent disease show deteriorating kidney function.

BIBLIOGRAPHY

1. Akram M, Jahrreiss V, Skolarikos A, et al. Urological guidelines for kidney stones: Overview and comprehensive update. J Clin Med. 2024;13:1114.
2. Daga A, Majmundar AJ, Braun DA, et al. Whole exome sequencing frequently detects a monogenic cause in early onset nephrolithiasis and nephrocalcinosis. Kidney Int. 2018;93:204-13.
3. D'Ambrosio V, Capolongo G, Goldfarb D, et al. Cystinuria: an update on pathophysiology, genetics, and clinical management. Pediatr Nephrol. 2022;37:1705-11.
4. Davis NF, Donaldson JF, Shepherd R, et al. Treatment outcomes of bladder stones in children with intact bladders in developing countries: A systematic review of >1,000 cases on behalf of the European Association of Urology Bladder Stones Guideline panel. J Pediatr Urol. 2022;18:132-40.
5. Groothoff JW, Metry E, Deesker L, et al. Clinical practice recommendations for primary hyperoxaluria: An expert consensus statement from ERKNet and OxalEurope. Nat Rev Nephrol. 2023;19:194-211.
6. Hoppe B, Martin-Higueras C. Improving treatment options for primary hyperoxaluria. Drugs. 2022;82:1077-94.
7. Jiang P, Xie L, Arada R, et al. Qualitative review of clinical guidelines for medical and surgical management of urolithiasis: Consensus and controversy 2020. J Urol. 2021;205:999-1008.
8. Lu P, Wang Z, Song R, et al. Clinical efficacy of extracorpoeal shock wave lithotripsy in pediatric urolithiasis: Systematic review and meta-analysis. Urolithiasis. 2015;43:199-206.
9. Mandal A, Khandelwal P, Geetha TS, et al. Metabolic and genetic evaluation in children with nephrolithiasis. Indian J Pediatr. 2022;89:1243-50.
10. Münch J, Goodyer PR, Wagner CA. Tubular diseases and stones seen from pediatric and adult nephrology perspectives. Semin Nephrol. 2023;43:151437.
11. Shastri S, Patel J, Sambandam KK, et al. Kidney stone pathophysiology, evaluation and management: Core curriculum 2023. Am J Kidney Dis. 2023;82:617-34.

12. Spivacow FR, Del Valle EE, Boailchuk JA, et al. Metabolic risk factors in children with kidney stone disease: An update. Pediatr Nephrol. 2020;35:2107-12.
13. Taguchi K, Yasui T, Milliner DS, et al. Genetic risk factors for idiopathic urolithiasis: A systematic review of the literature and causal network analysis. Eur Urol Focus. 2017;3:72-81.
14. Tekgül S, Stein R, Bogaert G, et al. European Association of Urology and European Society for Pediatric Urology Guidelines on Pediatric Urinary Stone Disease. Eur Urol Focus. 2022;8:833-9.
15. Tzelves L, Türk C, Skolarikos A. European Association of Urology Urolithiasis Guidelines: Where are we going? Eur Urol Focus. 2021;7:34-8.
16. Zeng G, Zhao Z, Mazzon G, et al. European Association of Urology Section of Urolithiasis and International Alliance of Urolithiasis Joint Consensus on retrograde intrarenal surgery for the management of renal stones. Eur Urol Focus. 2022;8:1461-8.

Cystic Kidney Disease

Ashima Gulati, Helen Liapis, Paul Winyard

Kidney cysts in children can present at any age, ranging from the perinatal period to adolescence. Bilateral cystic kidneys are often a manifestation of an inherited kidney condition with an identifiable single gene cause. Of these, polycystic kidney disease (PKD) and various nephronophthisis (NPHP) syndromes are specific conditions, each with a unique genetic defect and distinct yet potentially interconnected pathophysiology in terms of their mechanistic relationship to the cilium-centrosome complex. More importantly, different forms of PKD and NPHP may have overlapping radiological presentations. Imaging, specifically ultrasonography, is the chief modality that brings these conditions to clinical attention. It is imperative to consider many of these cystic kidney conditions as differential diagnosis, but also to recognize them individually given their variable disease course, prognosis, and options for management. Kidney cysts presenting as part of congenital anomalies of the kidneys and urinary tract (CAKUT) are mostly sporadic and less often due to a single gene cause, as discussed in Chapter 5.

Of note, cystic kidney disease is a major contributor to chronic kidney disease (CKD) and end stage kidney disease (ESKD) in children and young adolescents. A hallmark of PKD is the formation of cysts from various regions of the nephron (depending on the type of PKD) leading to destruction of the adjacent normal renal tissues. A key distinction between different cystic conditions is whether the cysts arise during kidney development *in utero* or after the full nephron complement has been reached at ~32–36 weeks' gestation. Examples of the former group are autosomal recessive polycystic kidney disease (ARPKD) and cystic dysplastic syndromes. These conditions disrupt nephrogenesis, leading to a reduced number of nephrons from the start, hence predisposing to CKD at a young age. The latter includes conditions such as typical autosomal dominant polycystic kidney disease (ADPKD) and NPHP, which start with relatively normal nephron numbers and develop CKD at later ages.

This chapter focuses on the two major forms of PKD in children, ADPKD and ARPKD, and other syndromic cystic kidney conditions **(Table 24.1)**, including NPHP that are mostly inherited in an autosomal recessive pattern and can collectively be termed as ciliopathies due to their underlying pathogenetic mechanisms relating to defects in the primary cilia **(*see* Annexure 9.6, p 845)**.

POLYCYSTIC KIDNEY DISEASE

Polycystic kidney disease is a monogenic form of cystic kidney disease, inherited in either an autosomal dominant or recessive manner (ADPKD or ARPKD, respectively) that presents in varied age groups ranging from perinatal/neonatal period to adulthood. ADPKD has an incidence of 1 in 1000 live births, making it the most common cause of inherited kidney disease worldwide. ARPKD is less common with an incidence of 1 in 26500 live births. Though ARPKD is more likely to present early with antenatal/perinatal and childhood onset, it is also recognized that ~2% of clinically significant ADPKD can present in the perinatal to early childhood period with early progression to CKD. Similarly, milder ARPKD cases can rarely present in adulthood, thus allowing for considerable overlap in the age at presentation in PKD.

Autosomal Dominant Polycystic Kidney Disease

The ADPKD is the most common single gene disorder causing kidney failure worldwide. The lifetime risk estimate of 1 in 1000 from epidemiologic studies is consistent with the more recent genetic prevalence estimate of ADPKD based on large general population sequence databases. ADPKD is the fourth leading cause of ESKD in the United States after diabetes, hypertension, and glomerulonephritis, and typically results in ESKD by 50–70 years of age depending on the underlying genetic mutation. These statistics iterate the global impact of ADPKD and are significant to note since this is an important disease without a cure.

Clinical Features

Childhood onset ADPKD is diagnosed in several ways: (*i*) incidental finding in asymptomatic children having investigations for kidney or abdominal issues, but with true (de novo) or false negative family history; (*ii*) screening of asymptomatic at-risk children with positive family history; and (*iii*) symptomatic severe early presentation with hypertension, kidney pain, infections and/or CKD.

It is important to recognize the substantial clinical and subclinical morbidity impact of ADPKD in children with implications on long-term management and contribution to adult disease. The early presentation of ADPKD is important to recognize for several reasons. Severe perinatal forms may result in perinatal demise with clear implications for genetic counseling. Early presenting ADPKD is relevant to the differential diagnosis of large echogenic kidneys in the antenatal period and infancy.

Recognizing childhood involvement provides an opportunity to monitor hypertension and its sequelae, proteinuria, gross hematuria, nephrolithiasis and risk factors for rapid progression, and management of early complications.

TABLE 24.1: Syndromes with kidney cysts

Syndromes	*Inheritance*	*Genes**	*Clinical features*
Autosomal dominant polycystic kidney disease (ADPKD)	Autosomal dominant	*PKD1, PKD2* *GANAB, DNAJB11, IFT140* *ALG9* (predominantly liver cysts)	Bilateral kidney cysts often in the setting of a positive family history of PKD Extrarenal features: Liver cysts; cysts in spleen and pancreas; intracranial aneurysms are in children *PKD1/PKD2* are two major genes; other genes listed here may phenocopy ADPKD but differ in age-related presentations and CKD progression
Autosomal recessive polycystic kidney disease (ARPKD)	Autosomal recessive	*PKHD1* (~99% cases) *DZIP1L, CYS1*	Enlarged diffusely microcystic kidneys; biliary duct plate malformation causing congenital hepatic fibrosis
Bardet–Biedl syndrome	Autosomal recessive	*BBS1-16*	Renal dysplasia with calyceal abnormalities and occasional cysts Retinopathy; digital anomalies; obesity; diabetes mellitus; male hypogonadism
Beckwith–Wiedemann syndrome	Autosomal dominant	*ICR1, KCNQ1OT1, CDKN1C*	Large dysplastic kidneys with or without cysts Brain and digital malformations; somatic overgrowth
Branchio-oto-renal syndrome	Autosomal dominant	*EYA1, SIX1, SIX5*	Renal agenesis or dysplasia with occasional cysts Deafness and branchial arch defects, e.g., cysts and fistulae in the neck, preauricular pits, external ear malformations
Ellis–van Creveld syndrome	Autosomal recessive	*EVC, EVC2*	Nephronophthisis; ectodermal dysplasia Short limbs and ribs; polydactyly; dysplastic nails and teeth; congenital heart disease

Contd...

Contd...

Syndromes	*Inheritance*	*Genes**	*Clinical features*
Jeune syndrome	Autosomal recessive	*DYNC2H1, IFT80, IFT 139–140, WDR19*	Nephronophthisis, cystic kidneys; hepatic fibrosis Asphyxiating thoracic dystrophy with respiratory insufficiency; rhizomelia, polydactyly
Meckel–Gruber	Autosomal recessive	*B9D1-2, CC2D2A, CEP290, MKS1, RPGRIP1L, TMEM216*	Cystic renal dysplasia; hepatic fibrosis Brain defects: Occipital encephalocele, hydrocephalus; polydactyly
Orofacial digital type 1	X-linked	*OFD1*	Males die before birth; females show renal cysts Orofacial: Large frenulum, cleft lip and/or palate, dental malocclusion and crowding, broad nasal root Digital abnormalities: Brachy-, syn- or polydactyly; mild mental delay; tremor
Renal cysts and diabetes	Autosomal dominant	*TCF2/HNF1 beta*	Renal dysplasia, cysts and hypoplasia; Urogenital: bicornuate uterus Maturity onset diabetes of the young; hyperuricemia; hypomagnesemia
Tuberous sclerosis	Autosomal dominant	*TSC1* and *TSC2* (adjacent to *PKD1*)	Renal cysts, angiomyolipoma, renal cell carcinoma Cutaneous: Adenoma sebaceum, ash leaf spots, café au lait spots, shagreen patch CNS: Tubers, nodules, tumors; cardiac rhabdomyoma; retinal hamartoma
Von Hippel–Lindau syndrome	Autosomal dominant	*VHL*	Renal cysts and renal cell carcinoma; retinal, cerebellar and spinal hemangiomas; malignant and benign tumors of the brain, spinal cord, pancreas and adrenals
Zellweger syndrome	Autosomal recessive	Different *PEX* genes; commonly *PEX1*	Cystic dysplastic kidneys; hepatic fibrosis; hypotonia with depressed neonatal and deep tendon reflexes Eyes: Ocular clouding, cataract, glaucoma; hearing defects

***Annexure 9.6 (p 845)** contains the list of genes to be screened for variants in patients with suspected cystic kidney disease

CKD: chronic kidney disease; CNS: central nervous system

Early use of specific interventions, such as water drinking for good hydration, low salt diet, and exercise regimens, are expected to positively impact risk factors for CKD progression, including hypertension. Thus, though ADPKD is widely recognized as an adult-onset symptomatic disease, it contributes substantially to disease burden in young children. These factors underscore the importance of recognizing early presenting "symptomatic" or "clinically significant" ADPKD and also the early presenting "asymptomatic" or "clinically silent" ADPKD. The major difference is in the manifestation of nonrenal systemic features, including liver cysts and extrarenal cysts in spleen or pancreas. Vascular aneurysmal complications, seen in adults, are extremely rare in children. These are not usually considered during evaluation, unless there is a significant family history of this complication.

Diagnostic Considerations: Family History

In ADPKD, cysts develop early in disease, however, in the absence of a specific therapy routine screening is not indicated and is most commonly guided by discussion with the family.

Recognition of early childhood ADPKD heavily relies on family history of similar disease in parents or even grandparents, in case parents are young and have not yet come to clinical attention. Screening imaging of asymptomatic parents (or grandparents if parents are younger than 40 years) may help ascertain family history and make a clinical diagnosis especially in perinatal or very early onset severe ADPKD, which can be biallelic due to hypomorphic variants inherited from each of the asymptomatic or mildly affected parent. However, absence of a positive family history does not rule out ADPKD, since 5–10% patients have a *de novo* gene defect or missed family history due to mild disease or genetic mosaicism.

Imaging

Ultrasound is the chief initial investigation for detection of kidney cysts. Ultrasound criteria to diagnose and/or exclude ADPKD have been proposed for ages ≥15 years in the presence of a positive family history.

US findings in ADPKD may range from large hyperechogenic kidneys to definite bilateral and diffusely scattered cysts in enlarged kidneys with varied preservation of intervening parenchyma **(Figs. 24.1A to D)**. Magnetic resonance imaging (MRI) (without contrast) is more sensitive in depicting kidney cysts and can be helpful in equivocal cases, or for MRI based total kidney volume (TKV) measurements for severity correlation in adults; childhood TKV ranges are not well-established. TKV increase exponentially over time, and the increase of TKV is a strong predictor of future decline of kidney function.

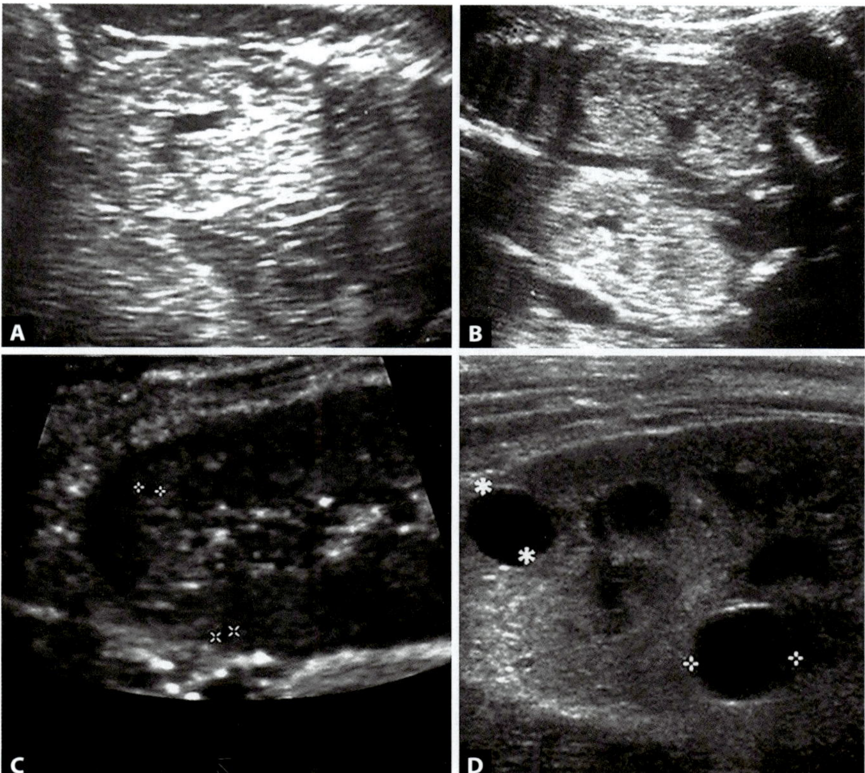

Figs. 24.1A to D: Imaging of polycystic kidney disease (PKD); (A and B) Antenatal ultrasound demonstrating nonspecific appearances of large, bright kidneys. These could be ARPKD, ADPKD, *HNF1B* associated disease or cystic dysplasia, though large size kidneys more often associate with PKD. Appearances may change during gestation; cysts may develop and prognosis is linked to amniotic fluid levels (oligohydramnios is associated with a poor prognosis); (C) Postnatal ultrasound demonstrating two small cysts which measured 0.5 cm each at the age of 6 months; (D) or 2 cm each at 12 years; both children had a family history of ADPKD. ADPKD: autosomal dominant polycystic kidney disease; ARPKD: autosomal recessive polycystic kidney disease; *HNF1B*: hepatocyte nuclear factor-1 beta

A "salt and pepper" appearance, described for enlarged kidneys with heterogeneous and increased parenchymal echogenicity due to ARPKD, can also be a manifestation of very early perinatal onset ADPKD or *HNF1B* associated kidney disease.

Genetics and Molecular Spectrum

Mutations in *PKD1* (~77% cases) [online mendelian inheritance in man (OMIM)173900] located on chromosome 16p13.3 or *PKD2* (~15% cases; (OMIM 173910) on chromosome 4q22, encoding two integral membrane proteins polycystin-1 (PC-1) and polycystin-2 (PC-2), respectively, underlie ADPKD. About 8% cases do not have these clear-cut underlying defects in *PKD1* or *PKD2* and several other genes have now been implicated in rare cases (*GANAB, DNAJB11*; **Table 24.1**). Some of the remainder may still have *PKD1/2* mutations but are missed because of the genetic complexity of these genes. In addition to this genetic heterogeneity, there is considerable locus heterogeneity with many private unique mutations in both *PKD1* and *PKD2* in ADPKD families.

Genotype-phenotype correlations associate protein-truncating *PKD1* variants with more severe kidney disease compared to *PKD1* missense and *PKD2* variants. However, these correlations are complicated, given the significant intrafamilial variability with the same underlying gene defect, thought to be due to other yet unidentified or poorly understood genetic background factors, epigenetic mechanisms, and environmental influences.

Management

The management of ADPKD is supportive with careful attention to proteinuria and blood pressure control, particularly with angiotensin converting enzyme (ACE) inhibitors. Hyperlipidemia should be managed appropriately. Restriction of dietary salt is recommended. There are several promising therapies for ADPKD in adults that target specific molecular pathways. Tolvaptan, a vasopressin antagonist, is approved for use in select adults with ADPKD and rapidly progressive kidney disease, and/or rapid rates of cyst growth (***see*** **Annexure 24.1, p 569**). Appropriate hydration is necessary to prevent thirst, dehydration and hypernatremia. Few reports have described benefits of tolvaptan rescue in children with massively enlarged ADPKD kidneys. Results of trials of tolvaptan in children are awaited (clinical trials.gov; pkdcure.org). Other agents, including octreotide, tyrosine kinase inhibitors, and micro-RNA based strategies are being examined.

Autosomal Recessive Polycystic Kidney Disease

The recessive form of PKD (ARPKD) belongs to a broad category of hepatorenal fibrocystic diseases. With an incidence of 1 in 26,500 live births, ARPKD is much less common than ADPKD but more likely to present with significant renal abnormalities before birth or in childhood. Textbooks cite a high rate of up to 21% perinatal deaths in ARPKD, but this incidence has been reduced by earlier antenatal detection and termination before birth. The overall outlook is satisfactory if babies with ARPKD do not have respiratory issues at birth, with >80% surviving into adulthood. However, marked hypertension requiring multiple medications and progression to CKD are common in childhood.

It is also increasingly recognized that a subset of ARPKD with milder forms of kidney disease can present during adolescence or even in adulthood. This subset of ARPKD usually shows prominent liver manifestations. Therefore, the older terminologies linking ARPKD as a childhood form and ADPKD as an adult form of PKD should *not* be used since many ARPKD patients can present later and ADPKD is being increasingly diagnosed in childhood because of better antenatal US and family screening.

Patients with ARPKD present *in utero* with bright, enlarged kidneys. The key prognostic indicator is the amount of amniotic fluid during early pregnancy. There is a high risk of perinatal death from immature lung development with anhydramnios, or oligohydramnios before 24-weeks' gestation. This accounts for many of the older case series that reported poor survival.

Clinical Features

ARPKD can present with kidney and/or hepatic features; renal abnormalities are common in early life, with hepatic features common in later childhood. The most frequent antenatal finding is progressively enlarging echobright kidneys, with loss of corticomedullary differentiation. Fetal kidneys often grow significantly beyond the 95th percentile, but it is rare to see overt cysts because each cyst is tiny, even though there are many of them. This contrasts with early ADPKD or cystic dysplastic kidney malformations where there are fewer, but larger, very obvious cysts. Postnatal prognosis is related to volume of amniotic fluid, worsening as volume falls below the 5th percentile with risk of dystocia and oligohydramnios or Potter sequence, and death from pulmonary hypoplasia.

Undiagnosed babies are occasionally detected because of enlarged kidneys and oliguria, but ARPKD is more likely to present with poor feeding, vomiting, or failure to thrive as children develop renal failure. Some patients do not develop these problems until their teens or later. Almost all children with ARPKD have elevated blood pressure. Hepatic complications tend to occur in older children, particularly hepatomegaly which can cause portal hypertension, splenomegaly, and esophageal varices. Suppurative cholangitis and hepatic insufficiency are rare complications.

Diagnosis

ARPKD is suggested by antenatal scans suggesting bilateral echobright kidneys with loss of corticomedullary differentiation and lack of overt cysts. These start as normal sized kidneys but grow during gestation to >95th percentile and may be accompanied by oligohydramnios. The antenatal differential diagnoses include ADPKD and glomerulocystic disease, but these may also have (or develop) frank cysts, and isolated bilateral dysplasia or dysplasia syndromes. The renal cysts and diabetes syndrome, caused by mutations of the gene encoding hepatocyte nuclear factor 1 beta (*HNF1B*), is an important cause of bright kidneys antenatally. Meckel-Gruber and Beckwith-Wiedemann syndromes have characteristic extrarenal findings such as encephalocele or fetal overgrowth, respectively. Postnatally, the kidneys are symmetrically enlarged and echogenic, and individual cysts may become visible; these are rarely larger than 2 cm. High resolution ultrasound, contrast enhanced CT or MRI scans are useful for assessing the kidneys. Liver findings are less consistent but may show increased echogenicity and cystic dilation of the intrahepatic biliary tree.

Genetics and Molecular Spectrum

Mutations in the polycystic kidney and hepatic disease 1 gene (*PKHD1*) cause ~99% of ARPKD cases; this is located on chromosome 6p21 and encodes a protein named fibrocystin (or polyductin). There are a large number of known mutations spread throughout the gene, and the majority of patients are compound heterozygotes. There is a high risk of fetal presentation and neonatal death if the child carries two truncating mutations. Linkage can be used in informative families, particularly if there are issues of potentially affected fetus. It is important to ensure that pathology is obtained if pregnancy is terminated, in order to confirm the diagnosis for future pregnancies. Less than 1% of cases with ARPKD presentation have been recently described due to variants in *DZIP1L* and *CYS1* **(Annexure 9.6)**.

Management

The management of ARPKD is supportive. There are no known antenatal interventions to reduce progression, and termination should be discussed when there is oligohydramnios before 24-weeks' gestation. Infants need temporary respiratory support if they do have sufficient lung function to survive and will then need management of renal insufficiency. Rarely, the kidneys get so large that they compromise breathing and feeding; nephrectomy should be considered, although utility is controversial. Patients with ARPKD can have severe systemic hypertension and require multiple antihypertensive agents. Portal hypertension and its complications usually arise later, and variceal bleeding can be life-threatening.

Pathophysiology of Cyst Formation

The mechanisms operating in PKD cause cystogenesis as a unifying morphology, with an interplay of several signaling pathways with an underlying crucial role of the primary cilium/centrosome complex. The precise and detailed function of the polycystin proteins is not fully understood. *PKD1* encodes polycystin-1, a 4304 amino acid protein, that functions as nonkinase membrane receptor; *PKD2* encodes polycystin-2, a 968 amino acid, nonselective cation permeable channel. Both are complex proteins that interact to form a complex in the primary cilium and function in complex signaling pathways. The ARPKD protein that is *PKHD1* encoded, i.e., fibrocystin, also localizes to the cilia.

Pathologic Considerations

Pathology of PKD affected kidneys is mostly available on autopsy specimens **(Figs. 24.2A to F)**. The site of cyst origin along the nephron is an important differentiator between ADPKD and ARPKD. In ADPKD, cysts can arise from all parts of the nephron including glomerular and tubular segments. These cysts then eventually pinch off or disconnect from the tubular lumen. It is important to note that very early onset, perinatally presenting, severe ADPKD demonstrates glomerulocystic kidney disease (GCKD) pathology **(Fig. 24.2C)**.

In ARPKD, kidneys show diffuse microcysts, giving them a sponge-like appearance **(Figs. 24.2E and F)**. Cysts only arise from collecting ducts and stay attached to their nephron of origin, eventually generating cylindrical cysts extending from medulla to cortex. These elongated cysts explain the linear streakiness seen on pyelography and on ultrasonography. In the liver, there is a ductal plate abnormality with bile duct proliferation and abnormal branching, associated with periportal hepatic fibrosis **(Fig. 24.2F)**.

IMAGING IN CYSTIC KIDNEY DISEASES

Renal ultrasound is the mainstay imaging modality used for initial detection and follow up of cystic kidney disease in infants and children. It provides clinically useful information with reasonable capacity to delineate disease-specific findings, such that this information, combined with the clinical history, can help make a presumptive specific diagnosis in most cystic kidney conditions. This, combined with the advantage of technical ease without need for sedation, and avoidance of radiation or contrast exposure, makes ultrasonography the chief modality for detection, characterization, and follow up of cystic kidney disease. Fetal MRI is being increasingly used in conjunction with abnormal prenatal ultrasound findings, mostly to look at other nonkidney syndromic findings that are usually associated with other syndromic cystic conditions (e.g., NPHP) but are absent in PKD.

ARPKD: Massively enlarged kidneys are more likely to be ARPKD. The most described appearance is that of the "salt and pepper" pattern comprising enlarged kidneys with tiny microcysts due to fusiform tubular dilatation and some small detectable cysts that are randomly distributed throughout the kidneys causing enlarged kidneys with heterogeneous increased parenchymal echogenicity. Kidney involvement in ARPKD is diffuse corticomedullary with

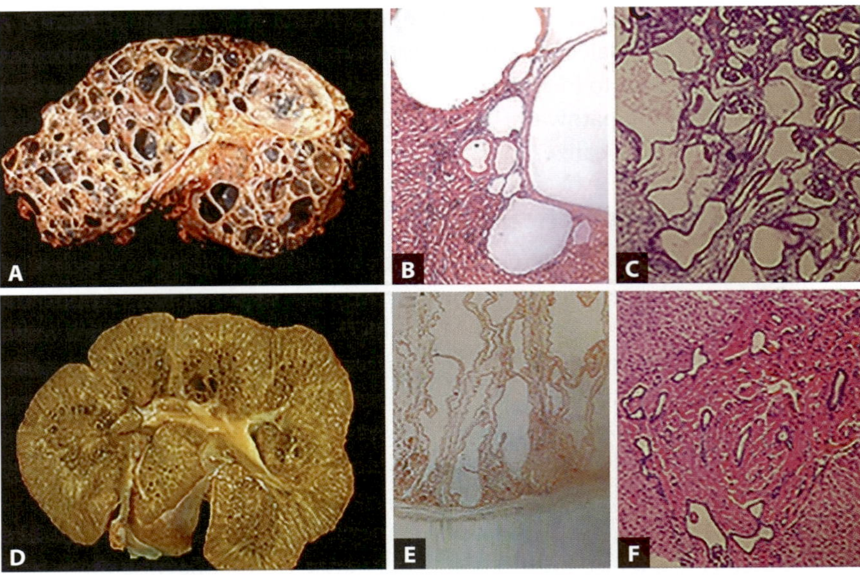

Figs. 24.2A to F: Pathology of polycystic kidney disease (PKD). Morphology and hematoxylin and eosin-stained sections in children with (A and B) autosomal dominant PKD; (C) Glomerulocystic kidney disease; (D to F) Autosomal recessive PKD. (A) Cross-section of ADPKD kidney demonstrates a number of prominent cysts that can be counted; (B) Several large cysts, including one glomerular cyst, surrounded by relatively well preserved normal glomeruli and tubules; (C) Severe glomerulocystic kidney disease presenting antenatally, associated with renal dysplasia. Almost every cyst contains a glomerular tuft; (D) Cross-section of ARPKD kidney demonstrates multiple tiny cysts, too numerous to count easily; occasional larger cysts as disease progresses; (E) Linear nature of some ARPKD cysts, which extend from medulla to cortex; these give rise to a "streaky" appearance on ultrasound and contrast enhanced CT; (F) Characteristic appearance of ductal plate abnormality in liver of ARPKD with proliferation of circumferential, ectatic bile ducts and ductules. ADPKD: autosomal dominant polycystic kidney disease; ARPKD: autosomal recessive polycystic kidney disease

loss of corticomedullary distinction in patients with kidney-predominant early-onset ARPKD, *versus* predominant medullary disease with ductal dilation confined to the medulla, especially in patients with late-onset kidney involvement and liver-predominant ARPKD.

ADPKD: Kidneys show well-defined cysts, which might mimic the homogenous appearance of ARPKD, especially in the initial pathogenesis of very early onset severe forms. Mostly, children with ADPKD have enlarged or normal sized kidneys with hyperechoic cortex and some subcentimetric cysts in both kidneys. Rarely, the imaging findings can be variable, with severe neonatal presentation that mimics the ARPKD salt and pepper pattern.

HNF1β related cysts: Kidney size may be normal to moderately large. Commonly all patients have bilateral kidney cysts of varying size and location.

Infantile nephronophthisis: Kidney size is variable but mostly normal or small sized, with hyperechoic cortex and abnormal corticomedullary differentiation with or without definite localized cysts.

On follow-up imaging in both ARPKD and ADPKD, the size and number of well-defined macrocysts tends to increase. It is important to consider all above-mentioned conditions **(*see* Table 24.1)** in the differential diagnosis, since there is often an overlap of imaging findings. The "salt and pepper pattern", while characteristic of ARPKD, may be seen in early onset ADPKD, and in glomerulocystic disease related to mutations in *HNF1β*.

Another ultrasound pattern that is observed in children with NPHP and glomerulocystic disease is the presence of normal to small-sized kidneys, abnormal corticomedullary differentiation, and hyperechoic cortex with cysts varying in size, number, and location. A color comet-tail artifact may be useful when suspecting a renal ciliopathy in case of enlarged hyperechoic kidneys with no detectable microcysts on ultrasound.

Table 24.2 lists the most prominent single-gene causes of monogenic CAKUT with or without kidney cysts. The most common underlying genes during molecular investigation of PKD in the perinatal/neonatal or childhood period include *PKD1, PKD2, PKHD1, HNF1B, DZIP1L,* and *CYS1* when considering a gene panel approach **(Annexure 9.6)**. These genes can be tested as a PKD limited gene panel or as part of a comprehensive genomic approach such as whole exome sequencing. The genetic complexity of cystic kidney disease, including the molecular heterogeneity and technical challenges with *PKD1* variant detection and interpretation, often requires genetics expertise.

OTHER CILIOPATHIES, OR INHERITED CYSTIC KIDNEYS

There are many other causes of cystic kidneys, the most common being defects in kidney development such as cystic dysplastic and multicystic dysplastic kidneys (Chapter 5). There is also an important group of genetic disorders, initially thought to be unrelated but now grouped together as "ciliopathies" because of structural or molecular defects in the primary cilium. The main conditions are NPHP/medullary cystic kidney diseases (MCKD) complex characterized by corticomedullary cysts. Multiorgan syndromes such as the Bardet–Biedl syndrome feature renal cysts with dysplastic elements, in combination with abnormalities in other organ systems **(Table 24.1)**. The elements of renal dysplasia in these groups contrast with PKD where the cysts arise from and are surrounded by (at least initially) relatively normal tissues.

The primary cilium is a finger-like projection from the cell, surrounded by the cell membrane. It is stimulated by fluid flow across the cell surface and modulates intracellular calcium levels and several signaling pathways. The primary cilium has nine peripheral microtubule bundles, similar to classical motile cilia, but it lacks the two central structures, so it is termed "9+0".

TABLE 24.2: Monogenic causes of congenital anomalies of kidney and urinary tract (CAKUT) with or without kidney cysts

Gene/gene family	*CAKUT type*
Angiotensin-related (*ACE, AGT, AGTR1*)	Renal tubular dysgenesis (can also be induced by angiotensin-related medications)
BBS genes	Bardet–Biedl syndrome with tubulointerstitial and glomerular changes with or without cysts, dysplasia
BICC1	Multicystic dysplastic kidney
BMP4 or *BMP7*	Renal hypodysplasia or agenesis; flow impairment, obstruction
BNC2	CAKUT, dominant lower urinary tract obstruction
CDC5L	Renal agenesis
CDKN1C	Renal medullary dysplasia
CHD1L	CAKUT
CHD7	VACTERL
CHRM3	Functional bladder outlet obstruction; prune-belly syndrome
DNAJB11	ADPKD
DSTYK	CAKUT
EYA1	Branchio-oto-renal syndrome; renal hypoplasia
FGFR1 & *FGFR2*	Renal agenesis
FOXC1 or *FOXC2*	CAKUT
FRAS1, FREM1, FREM2, GRIP1	Fraser syndrome–associated genes, CAKUT
GANAB	ADPKD
GATA3	Vesicoureteric reflux (VUR)
GDF11	Renal agenesis
GDNF	Hirschsprung disease; VUR, renal agenesis, CAKUT
GFRA1	CAKUT (GFRA1 is the coreceptor for GDNF)
GLI3	Pallister–Hall syndrome
GPC3	Cystic and dysplastic kidneys
GREB1L	Renal agenesis, genital tract malformation/agenesis
GREM1	Renal agenesis
HNF1β	Renal hypodysplasia; renal cysts and diabetes syndrome, maturity onset diabetes of the young
HPSE2	Urofacial syndrome; Ochoa syndrome with dysmorphic, poorly emptying bladder
JAG1	Alagille syndrome

Contd...

Contd...

Gene/gene family	*CAKUT type*
KAL1	Kallmann syndrome, renal agenesis and hypodysplasia
NOTCH2	Alagille syndrome
NPHP1	Renal hypodysplasia, nephronophthisis
OFD1	Oral-facial-digital syndrome with glomerulocystic kidneys
PAX2	Renal coloboma syndrome, renal hypodysplasia, VUR
PAX8	Hypothyroidism and renal agenesis
PBX1	Renal hypoplasia
PKD1/2	ADPKD; a few large cysts arising from all nephron segments
PKHD1	ARPKD; many cysts arising from collecting ducts only
REN	Renal tubular dysgenesis
RET	Hirschsprung disease, CAKUT (*RET* is the main receptor for GDNF)
ROBO2	VUR, CAKUT
SALL1	Townes–Brocks syndrome, renal hypoplasia
SIX1; SIX2; SIX5	Branchio-oto-renal syndrome, renal hypodysplasia, CAKUT
SOX9	CAKUT
SOX17	Pelviureteric junction obstruction, VUR
TBX18	CAKUT (dominantly inherited)
UMOD	Renal hypodysplasia, occasional cysts
UPIIIA	Renal hypodysplasia
WNT4	Renal hypoplasia
WT1	Denys–Drash, WAGR, Frasier syndromes; mesangial sclerosis, Wilms tumors; urogenital abnormalities; renal agenesis
XPNPEP3	Nephronophthisis, tremor, sensorineural hearing loss, mitochondriopathy

ADPKD: Autosomal dominant polycystic kidney disease; ARPKD: Autosomal recessive polycystic kidney disease; GDNF: glial cell derived neurotrophic factor; VACTERL: vertebral anomalies, anorectal anomalies (anal atresia), cardiac anomalies, tracheoesophageal fistula or atresia, renal anomalies, and limb anomalies; WAGR: Wilms tumor, aniridia, genitourinary anomalies, and mental retardation syndrome

Defects in the primary cilium cause complex changes in its function, but these are easily integrated into a simple concept of perturbed differentiation. For example, a normal epithelial cell is relatively quiescent, has low proliferative rate, and regulates transporter proteins to specific parts of the cells. In contrast, the improperly differentiated "ciliopathy cell" is more likely to divide or die, and both balance and direction of secretion versus absorption is dysregulated. Nephrons do not properly differentiate if this occurs during nephrogenesis, and there is risk that cysts will form, and normal tissues can be destroyed.

Glomerulocystic Kidney Disease

Glomerulocystic kidney disease is a heterogeneous group of disorders that share the common feature of prominent cysts arising from Bowman space. It may be classified as a different cystic kidney disease until biopsy, when the diagnosis is confirmed if 5% or more of the glomeruli are cystic, i.e., have dilated Bowman space greater than or equal to two times the normal **(Fig. 24.2C)**. ADPKD and ARPKD are both linked to GCKD, even though cysts in ARPKD classically arise from the collecting ducts. Other primary associations are with uromodulin [termed autosomal dominant glomerulocystic kidney disease (AD GCKD)], *HNF1β* and renin mutations **(*see* Chapter 21)**, trisomy 21 or 18, Turner syndrome, orofaciodigital syndrome, glutaric aciduria type II, tuberous sclerosis, and NPHP. Secondary associations are chiefly renal dysplasia in children, particularly when linked to lower urinary tract obstruction, although ischemia and vasculitis can be complicated by GCKD later in life. Kidneys with GCKD can be of any size (enlarged, normal, or small). Clinical presentation is variable, with the condition often found when patients are evaluated for other issues.

Nephronophthisis

The NPHP family of syndromes is the most frequent genetic cause of progressive kidney failure in children and adolescents. Inheritance is autosomal recessive and mutations in over 20 genes have been described in patients with NPHP and related conditions such as Joubert, Meckel–Gruber, Senior–Loken, and Mainzer–Saldino syndromes **(Annexure 9.6)**. Aberrant function of cells carrying a "primary cilium" in other sites such as the cerebellum, liver, bone, and retina is proposed to cause extrarenal phenotypes in these conditions.

Classical juvenile NPHP is characterized by insidious loss of renal function corresponding to progressive tubulointerstitial nephritis, usually culminating in kidney failure between 8 years and adolescence. The first symptoms are increased thirst and urination, typically from around 3 years of age. These are caused by urinary concentrating defect, which occurs before kidney structure is grossly altered. The condition should be considered when presented with these symptoms and normal sized kidneys. Loss of corticomedullary differentiation is seen later, with cysts classically at the corticomedullary junction as CKD develops.

Mutations in *NPHP1* and *NPHP3–9* genes are described in juvenile NPHP. Defects in *NPHP2* cause the infantile form with cortical microcysts and kidney failure before 5 years of age. Kidneys are large in this condition; patients are hypertensive, and some show *situs inversus*. Extrarenal features in related conditions with NPHP depend on the syndrome and include retinitis pigmentosa, nystagmus, visual loss (Senior–Loken syndrome); cerebellar vermis hypoplasia, mental retardation, hypotonia, and eye movement abnormalities (Joubert syndrome); short-limbed dwarfism, postaxial polydactyly, nail dysplasia, and congenital heart defects (Ellis-van Creveld); or diminutive thorax with short ribs and multiple skeletal abnormalities (Jeune asphyxiating thoracic dystrophy).

Diagnosis

Syndromic extrarenal features should elucidate the diagnosis for many of the conditions above, whereas it is the history that points to isolated NPHP. The chief clinical features are polyuria and polydipsia. Children may also start to wet the bed many years after being dry at night. There may be a family history of the condition and parental consanguinity. Some children have renal sodium wasting and avid salt intake; hypertension is uncommon until late. Urinalysis shows low specific gravity but no other abnormalities. The insidious nature of NPHP can delay diagnosis, leading to classical signs of progressive CKD with bony deformities, failure to thrive, and severe anemia. Renal ultrasound shows normal sized kidneys at the early stage, they then get progressively smaller with loss of corticomedullary differentiation. Cysts are seen in ~50% patients by ultrasound, characteristically in the medulla or corticomedullary junction. CT or MRI scans are more sensitive at detecting these cysts. Defects in urine concentration in siblings and other family members can help establish the diagnosis.

Medullary cystic kidney disease autosomal dominant tubulointerstitial kidney disease, ADTKD) is pathologically similar to NPHP, presenting with symptoms and signs of a defect in urinary concentration and progressive interstitial fibrosis. Cysts are described in the corticomedullary junction or medulla in 40% of patients and are thus not required to make the diagnosis. There are usually no extrarenal malformations. It is an autosomal dominant condition caused by mutations in *MCKD1* on chromosome 1q21, which encodes for MUC1 (mucin protein), or *MCKD2* on 16p12 that encodes uromodulin. The latter group is also described as uromodulin-associated kidney disease or familial juvenile hyperuricemic nephropathy because of its frequent association with gout. Kidney failure occurs in adults, with median onset at 62 years and 32 years for mutations in *MCKD1* and *MCKD2*, respectively (***see* Chapter 21**).

Pathology

The pathology of NPHP and MCKD comprises a triad of tubular cysts, tubulointerstitial inflammation and fibrosis, and tubular basement

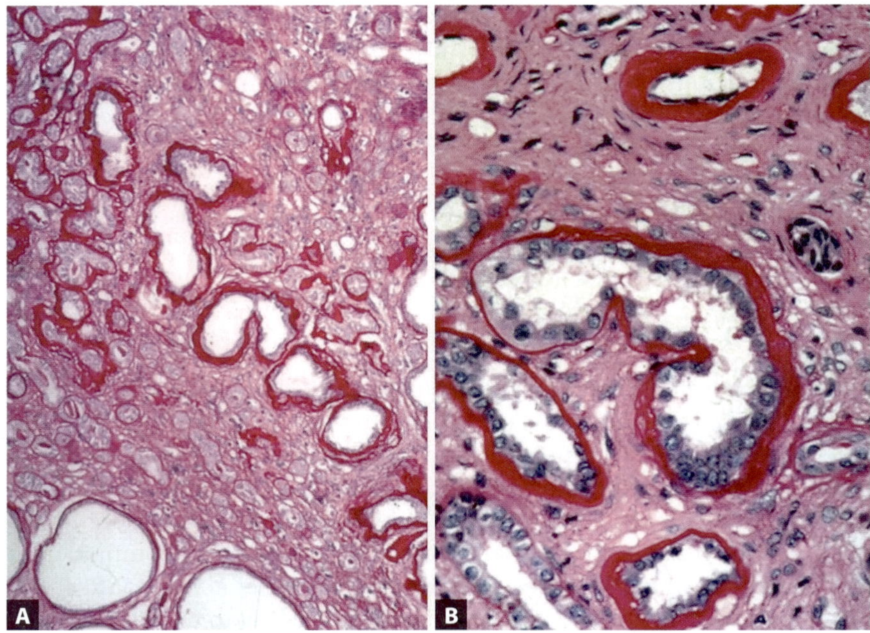

Figs. 24.3A and B: Light microscopy findings in a patient with nephronophthisis. Findings include (A) Dilatation of tubules, tubular atrophy, and tubulointerstitial fibrosis; (B) Dedifferentiation and attenuation of tubular epithelium with focal thinning of tubular basement membrane, consistent with chronic sclerosing tubulointerstitial nephropathy

membrane disruption **(Figs. 24.3A and B)**. Glomerulosclerosis is seen in 20–50% of cases. Cystic dilation involves distal tubules and collecting ducts, but does not occur in all, and is usually a late finding. Infantile NPHP is characterized by cortical microcysts and absence of medullary cysts. Dilated tubules may contain acellular material that stains with antibodies to uromodulin, the Tamm–Horsfall protein. Electron microscopy reveals dilated tubules with irregular outpouching and tubular basement membrane thickening, splitting, and replication, alternating with thin or entirely absent segments.

Management

There are no specific therapies that target the ciliopathies, and management of non-renal abnormalities may be much more difficult than the renal problems. The mainstay of treatment is supportive care to regulate blood pressure and manage complications of CKD. Blockade of the renin-angiotensin pathway using ACE inhibitors and receptor blockers is standard therapy, particularly when there is significant proteinuria. Cysts or kidneys rarely get large enough to require aspiration, deroofing, or removal.

Annexure 24.1: Online Calculator for Kidney Volume and Classification of Imaging for patients with typical ADPKD >15-yr-old (Mayo Foundation for Medical Education and Research)

https://www.mayo.edu/research/documents/pkd-center-adpkd-classification/doc-20094754

Scan the QR code below or type the following link in browser window:

BIBLIOGRAPHY

1. Gimpel C, Bergmann C, Bockenhauer D, et al. International consensus statement on the diagnosis and management of autosomal dominant polycystic kidney disease in children and young people. Nat Rev Nephrol. 2019;15:713-26.
2. Guay-Woodford LM, Bissler JJ, Braun MC, et al. Consensus expert recommendations for the diagnosis and management of autosomal recessive polycystic kidney disease: Report of an international conference. J Pediatr. 2014;165:611-7.

Imaging

1. Irazabal MV, Rangel LJ, Bergstralh EJ, et al. Imaging classification of autosomal dominant polycystic kidney disease: a simple model for selecting patients for clinical trials. J Am Soc Nephrol. 2015;26:160-72.
2. Pei Y, Hwang YH, Conklin J, et al. Imaging-based diagnosis of autosomal dominant polycystic kidney disease. J Am Soc Nephrol. 2015;26:746-53.
3. Pei Y, Obaji J, Dupuis A, et al. Unified criteria for ultrasonographic diagnosis of ADPKD. J Am Soc Nephrol. 2009;20:205-12.
4. Thomas CC, Jana M, Bagga A, et al. Ultrasound imaging of renal cysts in children. J Ultrasound Med. 2021;40: 621-35.

Genetic Studies and Pathogenesis

1. Bergmann C, Guay-Woodford LM, Harris PC, et al. Polycystic kidney disease. Nat Rev Dis Primers. 2018;4:50.
2. Burgmaier K, Brinker L, Erger F, et al.; ESCAPE group; GPN group; ARegPKD consortium. Refining genotype-phenotype correlations in 304 patients with autosomal recessive polycystic kidney disease and PKHD1 gene variants. Kidney Int. 2021;100:650-59.
3. Gambella A, Kalantari S, Cadamuro M, et al. The landscape of HNF1β deficiency: A syndrome not yet fully explored. Cells. 2023;12:307.
4. Gulati A, Dahl N, Tufro A. Inherited glomerular diseases in the gilded age of genomic advancements. Pediatr Nephrol. 2020;35:959-68.
5. Gulati A, Dahl NK, Hartung EA, et al. Hypomorphic *PKD1* alleles impact disease variability in autosomal dominant polycystic kidney disease. Kidney360. 2023;4:387-92.
6. McConnachie DJ, Stow JL, Mallett AJ. Ciliopathies and the kidney: A review. Am J Kidney Dis. 2021;77:410-19.
7. Wolf MTF, Bonsib SM, Larsen CP, et al. Nephronophthisis: A pathological and genetic perspective. Pediatr Nephrol. 2024;39:1977-2000.

Recommended Reading

1. ADPedKD. (2024). [online] Available from www.adpedkd.org. [Last accessed June, 2024].
2. ARegPKD. (2012). [online] Available from www.aregpkd.org. [Last accessed June, 2024].
3. ARPKD/CHF alliance. (2010). [online] Available from https://www.arpkdchf.org. [Last accessed June, 2024].
4. Mayo Foundation for Medical Education and Research. ADPKD Mayo imaging classification for 15-80 years. [online] Available from https://www.mayo.edu/research/documents/pkd-center-adpkd-classification/doc-20094754. [Last accessed June, 2024].
5. PKD Foundation. (2022). [online] Available from pkdcure.org. [Last accessed June, 2024].
6. PKD Foundation. Mayo ADPKD mutation database. [online] Available from https://pkdb.mayo.edu. [Last accessed June, 2024].

CHAPTER

25

Hypertension

Aditi Sinha, Arvind Bagga

INTRODUCTION

The prevalence of hypertension in children is increasing. There is a growing recognition of the association of high blood pressure with obesity and sedentary lifestyle, and the long-term consequences of hypertension. Pediatricians usually do not routinely measure blood pressure, and asymptomatic hypertension is often missed. It is important to identify childhood predictors of essential hypertension and plan intervention strategies since hypertension is associated with cardiovascular adverse events later in life. In practice, most cases of symptomatic hypertension in children are secondary and a treatable cause is identified in a large proportion.

MEASUREMENT OF BLOOD PRESSURE

Measurement of blood pressure should constitute an important part of the clinical examination **(Box 25.1)**. The child should be comfortable and preferably at rest for at least 5 minutes prior to measurement of blood pressure. The preferred method of measurement is by auscultation. While oscillometric devices are easier to use and reduce observer variation, measurements are approximately 6–9 mm Hg higher than values obtained on auscultation. Hence, oscillometric blood pressure measurements that are >90th percentile should be confirmed by auscultation during the same visit. Oscillometric devices should also be regularly calibrated. While blood pressure is conventionally measured in the upper arm, measuring blood pressure in lower extremities is useful when suspecting coarctation of the aorta. Radial or umbilical arterial pressure monitoring is used in sick patients. The width of the bladder should equal 40% of the middle upper arm circumference, and the length of the bladder should cover 80–100% of the arm circumference. **Table 25.1** provides recommended dimensions for size of the bladder of blood pressure cuff based on the size of the child. A list of oscillometric devices validated for use in children in the clinic/office, home, and for ambulatory blood pressure monitoring (ABPM) is available at www.stridebp.org.

Standardized clinic blood pressure measurement refers to readings obtained following standard procedures **(Box 25.1)**. This includes preparation of the patient as well as specifications of the setting, equipment, measurement

BOX 25.1: Standardized blood pressure measurement in clinic and at home

Site, equipment, and personnel

Blood pressure should be measured by trained healthcare workers, who are retrained annually. Training videos are available at: https://www.whleague.org/whl-resources/awareness-and-screening/new-online-bp-certification-course; https://www.stridebp.org/training; https://targetbp.org/blood-pressure-improvement-program/controlbp/measure-accurately/accurate-bp-measurement-matters/

Blood pressure is measured in a quiet room, at comfortable temperature, using a device validated for children (https://www.validatebp.org/; https://bihsoc.org/bp-monitors/; https://hypertension.ca/bpdevices; https://www.stridebp.org/; www.jpnsh.jp/com_ac_wg1.html; and www.hochdruckliga.de/betroffene/blutdruckmessgeraete-mit-pruefsiegel). Automated devices should be validated against the manual method, using aneroid sphygmomanometer

Appropriate cuff size should be used. The width of the bladder should be ≥40% of the length, and the bladder should encircle ≥80% of the circumference of the arm.

Patient preparation

Rule out caffeine, nicotine, or alcohol intake or exercise in the last 30 minutes. Allow the child to void, if required, and seat him/her comfortably for 3–5 minutes. The child should sit upright with back supported, arm bare, straight and supported, legs uncrossed, and feet flat on the floor

Blood pressure should be measured at least twice, and in more than one limb. Check for any contraindication to measuring blood pressure in a limb, e.g., arteriovenous fistula

Measurement

Wrap the cuff around the upper arm such that the center of the bladder overlies brachial artery pulsation in the antecubital fossa, and the lower end of the cuff is 2–3 cm above the antecubital fossa. The cuff should exert comparable tightness at the top and bottom edges, one finger easily slides under the cuff at its top and bottom, and the cuff should not touch the stethoscope that is placed over the brachial artery

Keep the cuff at the level of the heart and deflate the cuff by <2–3 mm Hg per second. Korotkoff phases 1 and 5 indicate systolic and diastolic blood pressures, respectively

Blood pressure should be measured in both upper limbs. Elevated values should be confirmed with a manual measurement. Interpret the average of ≥2 measurements

Interpretation

Interpret the blood pressure value based on percentiles for age and sex **(Annexure 25.1–25.2, p 616)**

If the value indicates hypertension, measure blood pressure in all four limbs using appropriate cuff sizes

Home blood pressure monitoring

Measure blood pressure before antihypertensive drug intake; on each occasion, measure twice, 2–5 minutes apart; note both values and their average

On the long-term, measure blood pressure twice a day, 1–2 times a week or month

Source: Cheung AK, et al. Am J Med 2023

TABLE 25.1: Recommended dimensions for size of bladder of blood pressure cuff

Age group	*Width, cm*	*Length, cm*	*Maximum arm circumference, cm*
Newborn	4	8	10
Infant	6	12	15
Child	9	18	22
Small adult	10	24	26
Adult	13	30	34
Large adult	16	38	44
Thigh	20	42	52

procedure, and the way in which the blood pressure readings are recorded. Standardization of the procedures is necessary, because many aspects including the physical condition, clinic environment, and equipment can result in inaccurate and unreliable values. **Box 25.1** summarizes a simplified standardized blood pressure measurement protocol, which is feasible to implement in daily practice, with minimal compromise in measurement accuracy and reliability. Training videos and online certification on standardized blood pressure measurement are available online at various sources, such as https://www.stridebp.org/training.

Ambulatory Blood Pressure Monitoring

Ambulatory blood pressure monitoring is a valuable tool in the investigation of pediatric hypertension. ABPM involves repetitive, noninvasive measurements of blood pressure using portable devices in outpatients over an entire day. Since blood pressure measurements have a circadian pattern (higher during the day and reduced by 10% during sleep) an ABPM device that provides 50–60 readings over 24 hr can be useful when evaluating children for white coat hypertension (WCH), masked hypertension, and secondary hypertension. In comparison with clinic blood pressure, ABPM is a better predictor of target organ damage in adults and is a better target for therapeutic goals in high-risk pediatric populations. While ABPM is more accurate than home blood pressure monitoring, its use is limited to children older than 5 years or taller than 120 cm (*see* later). Most recent guidelines [European Society of Hypertension (ESH) 2016; American Academy of Pediatrics (AAP) 2017; and Update on Pediatric ABPM 2022] endorse the use of ABPM in the evaluation and management of hypertension in children and adolescents. **Box 25.2** details precautions and considerations in the application and interpretation of ABPM.

BOX 25.2: Ambulatory blood pressure monitoring

Site, equipment, and personnel

Ambulatory blood pressure monitoring (ABPM) should be conducted in an office setting by personnel trained in the application of the device and interpretation of ABPM data in children

Use an oscillometric or auscultatory device that has been validated for pediatric use: https://www.validatebp.org/; https://bihsoc.org/bp-monitors/; https://hypertension.ca/bpdevices

Patient preparation and measurement

Apply the monitor to the nondominant arm, except in: (*i*) Presence of a permanent dialysis access on nondominant arm; (*ii*) Discrepancy in clinic blood pressure by >5 mm Hg between the two arms (place cuff on arm with higher blood pressure); and (*iii*) Patients with repaired coarctation aorta with normal arch anatomy (place cuff on the right arm)

Establish the usual bedtime and time of waking up: Program the devices to record blood pressure every 15–20 minutes during wake hr and every 20–30 minutes during sleep

Measure resting blood pressure with the ABPM device and check its comparability to that from the same arm by the same technique or manually

Ask the patient to record the timing and doses of antihypertensive medications, periods of physical exercise, unusual activity, and sleep and wake times in a diary

Analysis and interpretation

Consider the study optimal if it meets the following criteria: (*i*) Monitoring period spans 24 hr; ≥18 hr are accepted if sleep period is captured and the latter criteria are met; (*ii*) ≥70% of all attempted readings are successful; (*iii*) ≥40 successful readings are present over the monitoring period; and (*iv*) ≥1 blood pressure reading is present per hr, including during sleep

Program the software to edit outliers: (*i*) Individual wake and sleep blood pressure and heart rate measurements which are considerably outside the normal ranges for the patient's age; (*ii*) Systolic blood pressure <60 mm Hg or >220 mm Hg; (*iii*) Diastolic blood pressure <35 mm Hg or >120 mm Hg; (*iv*) Heart rate <40 beats/minute or >200 beats/minute; and (*v*) Pulse pressure <40 mm Hg or >120 mm Hg

Apply the appropriate thresholds according to normative data based on sex, height, and age **(Annexure 25.3–25.4, p 616)**

Inspect and report the following: (*i*) Mean ambulatory systolic and diastolic blood pressures during the entire 24-h, wake, and sleep periods; (*ii*) Blood pressure load (proportion of readings above the threshold value); and (*iii*) Extent of dipping (percent difference between mean blood pressures during awake and sleep) in systolic and diastolic blood pressures

Interpret the ABPM phenotype, as per criteria in **Table 25.2**

Source: Flynn JT, et al. Hypertension 2022

Home Blood Pressure Monitoring

Home blood pressure monitoring has been used to obtain out-of-office measurements. While this procedure is widely used in adults, pediatric guidelines differ with respect to the applicability of this technique.

Normal Blood Pressure

Blood pressure standards are based on gender, age, and height to provide a precise classification of hypertension. The 2017 AAP guidelines include updated normative pediatric thresholds based on normal-weight children **(Annexures 25.1–25.2, p 616)**. The adjustment to exclude overweight and obese children and adolescents resulted in an overall 1–4 mm Hg drop in systolic and diastolic pressure values for the 90th and 95th percentiles. Normative data for oscillometric blood pressure in Indian children was recently published but needs further validation.

DEFINITION AND CLASSIFICATION OF HYPERTENSION

The normative blood pressure percentiles based on normal-weight children (2017) **(Annexures 25.1–25.2, p 616)** are used to categorize blood pressure as normal, elevated, and stage 1 or stage 2 hypertension **(Table 25.2)**. Blood pressure thresholds for boys and girls of normal height for age are shown in **Figures 25.1A and B**. Use of these criteria more sensitively identifies children and adolescents with risk factors for cardiovascular disease, such as elevated body mass index, dyslipidemia, prediabetes, and/or presence of hypertension-related target organ damage.

A child is considered normotensive if the systolic and diastolic blood pressure is $<90^{th}$ percentile. If the blood pressure is $>90^{th}$ percentile or >120/80 mm Hg, it is repeated to verify the value. Values between the 90th and 95th percentiles indicate elevated blood pressure. Systolic or diastolic values $>95^{th}$ percentile should be repeated on two more occasions to confirm the diagnosis of hypertension. All children showing systolic or diastolic blood pressure values above the 95th percentile are considered hypertensive and need diagnostic evaluation, which is considered urgent with values 12 mm above the 95th percentile (stage 2 hypertension). The AAP guidelines use a threshold of ≥130/80 mm Hg to define hypertension in adolescents (≥13 years of age) that aligns with the updated (2017) adult hypertension guidelines by the American Heart Association (AHA) and American College of Cardiology. These recommendations differ from the ESH guidelines on high blood pressure in children, which recommend a threshold of 140/90 mm Hg for those ≥16-years-old **(Table 25.3)**.

TABLE 25.2: Definition and staging of hypertension in children

Category[1]	*Children aged 1–13 years*		*Children aged ≥13 years*	
Clinic blood pressure[2]				
Normal blood pressure	$<90^{th}$ percentile		<120/<80 mm Hg	
Elevated blood pressure	$\geq 90^{th}$ percentile to $<95^{th}$ percentile		≥120/<80 to <129/<80 mm Hg	
Stage 1 hypertension	$\geq 95^{th}$ percentile to $<95^{th}$ percentile +12 mm Hg		≥130/80–139/89 mm Hg	
Stage 2 hypertension	$\geq 95^{th}$ percentile +12 mm Hg		≥140/90 mm Hg	
Ambulatory blood pressure	*Clinic systolic or diastolic blood pressure*	*Mean ambulatory systolic or diastolic blood pressure*	*Clinic systolic or diastolic blood pressure*	*Mean ambulatory systolic or diastolic blood pressure*
Normal	$<95^{th}$ percentile	$<95^{th}$ percentile, or adolescent cut points[3]	<130/80 mm Hg	<125/75 mm Hg 24-hr, and <130/80 mm Hg when awake, and <110/65 mm Hg in sleep
White coat hypertension	$\geq 95^{th}$ percentile		≥130/80 mm Hg	
Masked hypertension	$<95^{th}$ percentile	$\geq 95^{th}$ percentile, or adolescent cut points[3]	<130/80 mm Hg	≥125/75 mm Hg 24-hr, or ≥130/80 mm Hg when awake, or ≥110/65 mm Hg in sleep
Ambulatory hypertension	$\geq 95^{th}$ percentile		≥130/80 mm Hg	

[1]Blood pressure categories and definitions are based on the 2017 Clinical Practice Guidelines of the American Academy of Pediatrics and 2022 Update of the American Heart Association on Pediatric Ambulatory Blood Pressure Monitoring. If blood pressure categories differ for systolic (SBP) and diastolic (DBP) blood pressure, the higher of the two categories is used to make a diagnosis

[2]On the basis of age, sex, and height percentiles for systolic (SBP) and diastolic blood pressure (DBP)

[3]Including 24-h, awake, and sleep blood pressure

Sources: 1. Flynn JT, et al. Pediatrics 2017

2. Flynn JT, et al. Hypertension 2022

Normative data for ABPM is available from a study on 1,141 German children. The AHA statement on ABPM in children and the ESH guidelines provide the overall 24-h, awake, and sleep values for 50th, 75th, 90th, 95th, and 99th percentiles based on sex and height **(Annexures 25.3–25.4, p 616)**. Although widely used, there are concerns with the applicability of these normative datasets, including limited data for small children (<5-years-old or <120 cm height), absence of ethnic and racial diversity, and lack of variability in diastolic pressures with increasing height.

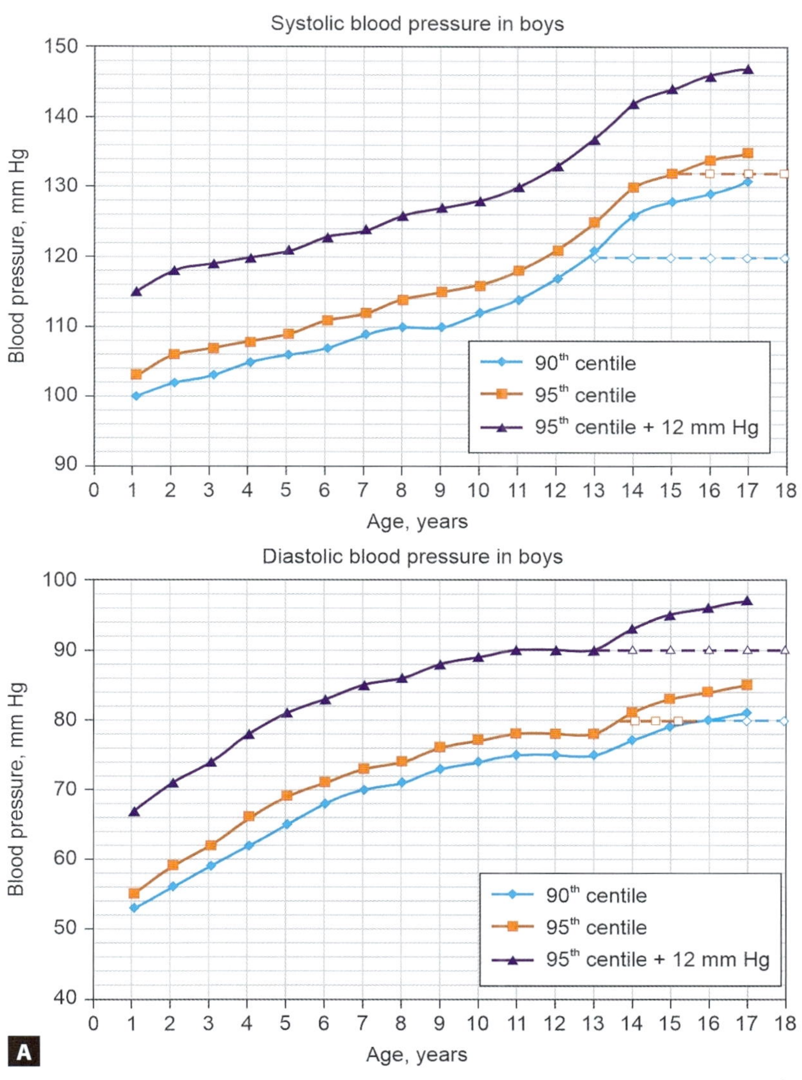

Contd...

Contd...

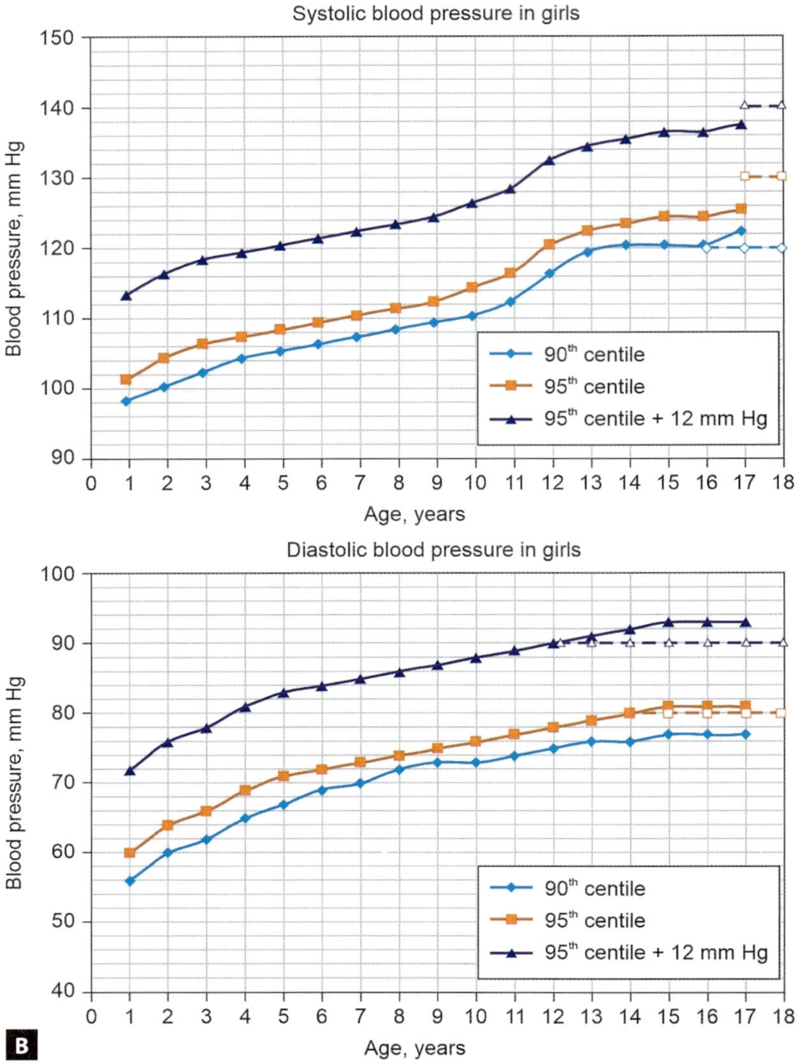

Systolic blood pressure in girls

Blood pressure, mm Hg

Age, years

90th centile
95th centile
95th centile + 12 mm Hg

Diastolic blood pressure in girls

Blood pressure, mm Hg

Age, years

90th centile
95th centile
95th centile + 12 mm Hg

B

Figs. 25.1A and B: Blood pressure percentiles for systolic and diastolic blood pressure in boys and girls of normal height for age. Blue, orange, and gray lines indicate values at the 90th percentile, 95th percentile, and 12 mm above the 95th percentile. Horizontal lines indicate static thresholds advocated for use in adolescents ≥13 years of age

Both the AHA and ESH guidelines use the 95th percentile of ambulatory blood pressure as the threshold for hypertension **(Table 25.3)**. The AHA 2022 update on pediatric ABPM recommends using a static threshold to define ambulatory hypertension in adolescents, which is consistent with adult guidelines. The ESH guidelines recommend using the adult criteria

TABLE 25.3: Differences in terminology and targets in clinical practice guidelines on management of pediatric hypertension by the European Society of Hypertension (2016) and the American Academy of Pediatrics/American Heart Association (2017)

Guidelines	*European Society of Hypertension*	*American Academy of Pediatrics/American Heart Association*
Definition of hypertension	*<16-year-old:* ≥95th centile *≥16-year-old:* ≥140/90 mm Hg	*<13-year-old:* ≥95th centile *≥13-year-old:* ≥130/80 mm Hg
Stage 2 hypertension	*<16-year-old:* ≥99th centile + 5 mm Hg	*≥13-year-old:* ≥140/90 mm Hg
Additional terms defined	High normal blood pressure Isolated systolic hypertension	Elevated blood pressure Target organ injury
Target blood pressure		
All children	<95th centile; consider <90th centile	*<13-year-old:* <90th centile *≥13-year-old:* <130/80 mm Hg
Chronic kidney disease	*Nonproteinuric CKD:* <75th centile *Proteinuric CKD:* <50th centile	*On ABPM:* 24-hr mean arterial pressure <50th centile

ABPM: ambulatory blood pressure monitoring; CKD: chronic kidney disease

once the 95th percentile exceeds adult values. The 2022 update provides a new scheme for classifying ABPM (***see* Table 25.2**), which focuses on average blood pressure instead of 'load', the percentage of times the blood pressure value exceeds the threshold value. The emphasis on load was removed since it was not shown to provide additional value over mean blood pressures in predicting left ventricular hypertrophy (LVH). With the recognition of the detrimental effects of nocturnal hypertension, the 2022 update advises assessment of both awake and sleep records, and not just the overall 24-hr average. Finally, the 2022 classification does not leave any patient 'unclassified', unlike previously. Studies suggest that utilizing these criteria will increase the prevalence of pediatric ambulatory hypertension, especially for wake records in older, taller boys and for nocturnal hypertension in children older than 8 years of age. The ABPM phenotypes defined with the new classification are superior in predicting hypertension-related target organ damage than the old paradigm. Overall, the 2022 definitions include only those criteria which predict cardiovascular outcomes, and are in alignment with adult guidelines, thus aiding in the transition of adolescents to adult care.

Table 25.2 and **Figure 25.2** provide the scheme for classification of blood pressure based on office/clinic and ABPM. **Flowchart 25.1** summarizes AAP recommendations on frequency and intensity of evaluation for hypertension in various categories.

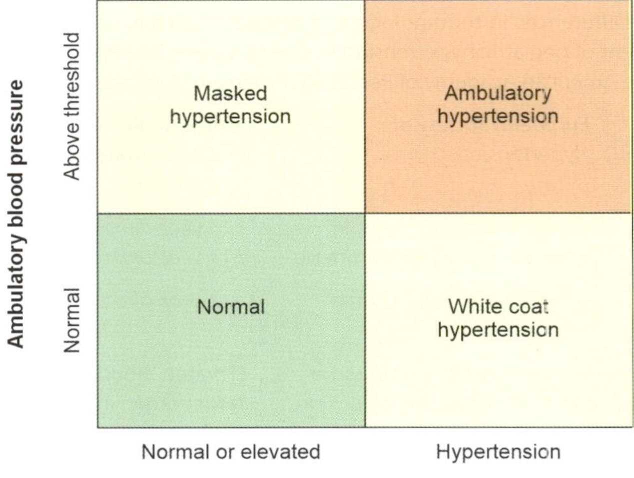

Fig. 25.2: Classification of blood pressure category based on clinic and ambulatory blood pressure thresholds provided in **Annexures 25.1–25.4 (p 616) and Table 25.2**

Flowchart 25.1: Identification and management of blood pressure in various categories following screening for hypertension

*If blood pressure is found to be normal at any point, annual screening is resumed

**Patients with hypertensive emergency require immediate referral to the emergency room or inpatient management

ABPM: ambulatory blood pressure monitoring

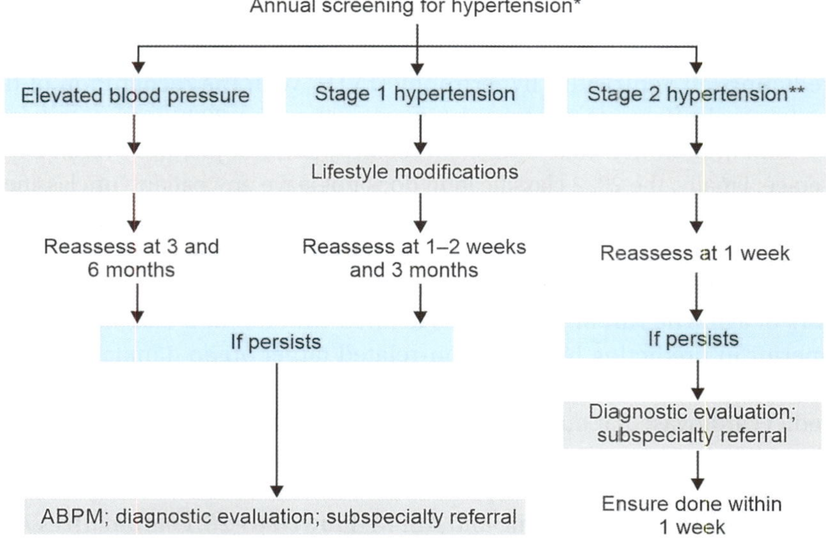

EPIDEMIOLOGY

A meta-analysis of 47 studies estimated the global prevalence of childhood hypertension at 4% (95% CI 3.3–4.8%), and that of elevated blood pressure (prehypertension) at 9.7% (7.3–12.4%). Stage 2 hypertension was present in 0.95% (0.5–1.6%) of children. The prevalence of hypertension was higher in overweight and obese children (15.3% and 5%, respectively) and in young adolescents aged 14 years (7.1–7.9%). Applying the new normative values and definitions results in 6% of North American adolescents being reclassified into a higher blood pressure stage.

The prevalence of childhood hypertension has increased longitudinally by 75–79% from 2000 to 2015. This appears to be chiefly in the form of primary hypertension, the incidence of which has risen with increased incidence of pediatric obesity. While secondary hypertension is reported as the principal cause of hypertension in childhood, its prevalence varies from 3.7 to 9.0% in primary care clinics or school-based screening, compared to 20–44% in subspecialty referral clinics.

SCREENING FOR HYPERTENSION AND AMBULATORY BLOOD PRESSURE MONITORING

Annual screening is recommended for all children and adolescents beginning at 3 years of age. **Table 25.4** lists threshold values in the outpatient that should

TABLE 25.4: Threshold blood pressure values to detect children who require screening for hypertension

Age (years)	*Boys*		*Girls*	
	Systolic (mm Hg)	*Diastolic (mm Hg)*	*Systolic (mm Hg)*	*Diastolic (mm Hg)*
1	98	52	98	54
2	100	55	101	58
3	101	58	102	60
4	102	60	103	62
5	103	63	104	64
6	105	66	105	67
7	106	68	106	68
8	107	69	107	69
9	107	70	108	71
10	108	72	109	72
11	110	74	111	74
12	113	75	114	75
≥13	120	80	120	80

The table assumes that normal height for age. Threshold values will increase or decrease by 2–3 mm Hg for higher and lower height, respectively
Source: Flynn JT, et al. Pediatrics 2017

alert a physician to the likelihood of hypertension and identifies children who require reassessment of blood pressure. Screening more frequently than annually is indicated if there are specific hypertensive risk factors listed in **Box 25.3**. If the blood pressure reading by an oscillometric device is elevated, it should be repeated with auscultation. If an auscultatory blood pressure measurement is elevated despite correct measurement technique, it should be repeated twice more at the same visit, and the average of the last two auscultatory readings is used as a final measure. A diagnosis of hypertension is made if the blood pressure is above the stage 1 hypertension threshold on three separate clinic visits. **Flowchart 25.1** summarizes recommendation of the AAP on diagnosis and frequency of reassessment for hypertension.

Compared to office measurements, ABPM is more consistent and accurate in diagnosing hypertension. ABPM is used to screen for or confirm hypertension in specific settings where hypertension is likely, such as persistently elevated blood pressure or stage 1 hypertension **(Flowchart 25.1)**, high-risk conditions where hypertension, including masked hypertension, is likely, and patients with suspected WCH **(Table 25.5)**. The indications for evaluation and management of white coat and masked hypertension are discussed in the following text.

ETIOLOGY

Acute severe hypertension may be seen in patients with infection related glomerulonephritis or hemolytic uremic syndrome. Uncommon causes

BOX 25.3: Indications for screening for hypertension at every health care contact*

Age <3 years
Prematurity (<32 weeks gestation), small for gestational age, very low birth weight, umbilical artery cannulation; other neonatal complications requiring stay in intensive care
Congenital heart disease, whether or not corrected
Known kidney disease, urinary tract malformation, recurrent urinary tract infections, hematuria; or proteinuria
Solid-organ or bone marrow transplant
Brain disease associated with increased intracranial pressure
Malignancy
Illness associated with hypertension (e.g., neurofibromatosis, tuberous sclerosis, sickle cell disease)
Therapy with drugs that elevate blood pressure (e.g., corticosteroids, oral contraceptives, stimulants)

Age ≥3 years*
Any of the above conditions
Obesity
Diabetes
History of aortic arch obstruction or coarctation

*All children older than 3 years require annual measurement of blood pressure

TABLE 25.5: Indications for ambulatory blood pressure monitoring

Setting	*Rationale*
Clinic hypertension	Confirm the diagnosis, especially before starting antihypertensive medications; rule out white coat hypertension; discriminate essential from secondary hypertension (latter suggested by nocturnal and/or diastolic hypertension; lack of dipping)
Suspected secondary hypertension	Identify masked hypertension, including nocturnal hypertension, abnormal dipping pattern
Coarctation of the aorta	Detect recurrent or masked hypertension during follow up after repair
Genetic syndromes: Neurofibromatosis type 1; Turner or William syndrome	Detect secondary hypertension, e.g., with renal artery stenosis or coarctation of aorta
Chronic kidney disease	Identify masked hypertension, including nocturnal hypertension and abnormal dipping pattern; optimize blood pressure control to retard disease progression and/or reverse target organ damage
Obesity with/without sleep-disordered breathing	
Types 1 and 2 diabetes	Identify abnormal circadian variation; optimize blood pressure control to retard kidney disease and vascular involvement
Obstructive sleep apnea	Identify masked hypertension, including nocturnal hypertension and abnormal dipping pattern
Solid organ transplant	
While on antihypertensive drugs	Assess adequacy of blood pressure control; confirm symptomatic hypotension; detect pseudoresistant hypertension
In clinical research	Objectively estimate blood pressure control; identify blood pressure patterns associated with increased cardiovascular risk

include Guillain-Barre syndrome, severe burns, and head injury. Common causes of persistent hypertension are shown in **Box 25.4** .

Although primary hypertension is a growing problem, secondary causes of hypertension should be considered in most children and adolescents diagnosed with hypertension. Renal parenchymal disease and renovascular lesions account for the majority of cases, of which chronic glomerulonephritis and reflux nephropathy are the most frequent causes. A high proportion of patients with C3 glomerulopathy and crescentic glomerulonephritis, polyarteritis nodosa, lupus nephritis, and immunoglobulin A (IgA) vasculitis have hypertension. Hypertension is frequent in dominant as well as recessive forms of polycystic kidney disease, even when glomerular function is preserved. Reduction of blood flow to one or both kidneys or its segments

BOX 25.4: Etiology of persistent hypertension in children

Renal parenchymal disease: Chronic glomerulonephritis; reflux nephropathy; obstructive uropathy; polycystic kidney disease; renal dysplasia; segmental renal hypoplasia
Renovascular disease: Idiopathic aortoarteritis (Takayasu disease); renal artery stenosis; fibromuscular dysplasia; renal artery thrombosis
Primary (essential) hypertension
Cardiovascular disease: Coarctation of aorta
Endocrine disease: Pheochromocytoma, neuroblastoma, primary hyperaldosteronism, Cushing syndrome, congenital adrenal hyperplasia
Monogenic causes of hypertension
Renal tumors: Wilms tumor, nephroblastoma, hemangiopericytoma
Substance abuse; intake of drugs containing steroids

(branch renal artery stenosis) account for 10–20% of cases. Endocrine causes of hypertension are rare.

In the neonate, renal artery occlusion following umbilical artery catheterization is an important cause. Coarctation of aorta, commonly distal to the origin of the left subclavian artery, is an important cause of sustained severe hypertension in infancy. Other important causes in infants include renal artery stenosis, bronchopulmonary dysplasia, and congenital renal anomalies. (*see* also Chapter 31).

CLINICAL FEATURES

Children with hypertension are often asymptomatic. Headache, abdominal pain, nausea, vomiting, and weight loss may be present. Severe hypertension may cause several complications, such as impairment in sensorium, visual disturbances, focal neurological deficits, seizures, and heart failure. These occur at lower blood pressure levels than those producing similar problems in adults. In acute situations, the clinical manifestations are related to the rapidity of the increase in blood pressure. In the newborn period, hypertension manifests with features suggesting sepsis, intracranial hemorrhage, or cardiorespiratory distress.

History and physical examination might provide clues to etiology. Kidney disease is suggested by history of urinary tract infections (reflux nephropathy), and/or hematuria with edema (glomerulonephritis). Joint swelling, photosensitive rash, and oral ulcers suggest systemic lupus erythematosus. History of muscle weakness suggests hypokalemia that might be associated with hyperaldosteronism or monogenic causes such as Liddle syndrome. Lower blood pressures and pulse volume in the lower limbs indicate coarctation of aorta. Tachycardia and diaphoresis might indicate hyperthyroidism, pheochromocytoma, or neuroblastoma; proptosis and goiter suggest hyperthyroidism. Growth retardation supports the diagnosis of chronic kidney disease (CKD), while overweight/obesity and acanthosis nigricans favor primary hypertension, with or without metabolic syndrome. Rapid weight gain associated with moon facies, acne, striae, and hirsutism, suggests Cushing syndrome. General physical examination might suggest a syndromic diagnosis, such as William syndrome (elfin facies, mild intellectual disability), Turner syndrome (webbed neck, short stature, widely spaced nipples, and increased carrying angle), neurofibromatosis (café au lait spots, neurofibromas), or tuberous sclerosis (adenoma sebaceum, ash-leaf macules, and shagreen patches). Other clues to diagnosis include presence of an abdominal mass (Wilms tumor, neuroblastoma, and pheochromocytoma), flank or epigastric bruit (renal artery stenosis), palpable kidneys (polycystic kidney disease, hydronephrosis), and ambiguous or virilized genitalia (congenital adrenal hyperplasia). The presence of retinopathy, apical heave with cardiac enlargement, and edema indicate sustained severe hypertension with end-organ damage that is seen in secondary hypertension.

Obstructive sleep apnea is suggested by history of frequent snoring (≥3 nights per week); labored breathing during sleep; gasps, snorting noises, or apneic episodes during sleep; sleep enuresis (especially secondary enuresis); sleeping in a seated position or with the neck hyperextended; and daytime sleepiness. Learning disability and attention deficit/hyperactivity are often associated. Physical examination may indicate overweight/obesity; tonsillar hypertrophy; adenoidal facies; micro- or retrognathia; and/or high-arched palate.

DIAGNOSTIC EVALUATION

The extent to which investigations for etiology are required depends on the persistence and severity of hypertension, which reflects the likelihood of a secondary etiology. Guidelines broadly agree on the intensity of evaluation of hypertensive children for underlying disorders. A secondary cause is particularly likely in children younger than 6 years, those with severe (stage 2) hypertension, and in presence of family history of hypertension at a young age, particularly if severe or associated with major adverse cardiovascular events (stroke, sudden cardiac death). The AAP guidelines suggest that diastolic hypertension is a better predictor of secondary cause than the severity of blood pressure elevation. In contrast, they recommend against extensive evaluation for secondary causes in obese children, those older than 6 years of age, those with family history of essential hypertension, and without signs or symptoms of an underlying cause. However, a recent study that found secondary hypertension in half of the children with traditional risk factors, overweight and obesity, indicates caution in following this advice of AAP guidelines.

Table 25.6 summarizes recommendations on initial diagnostic evaluation in children with hypertension. A careful history and physical examination

TABLE 25.6: Recommendations for initial diagnostic evaluation in children with hypertension

All children with hypertension	
Urinalysis	
24-h urine protein excretion (or first morning urine spot protein to creatinine ratio)[1a]	
Blood urea, creatinine, electrolytes, bicarbonate, uric acid, calcium	
Lipid profile (fasting): Total, LDL and HDL cholesterol, triglycerides	
Fasting blood glucose[1b]	
Retinal examination[2]	
Echocardiography[3]	
Abdominal ultrasound[1c]	
Etiology based investigations in children with suspected secondary hypertension[4]	
Etiology	*Recommended evaluation*
Chronic kidney disease	Urinalysis; renal ultrasound, DMSA scintigraphy, micturating cystourethrogram
Renovascular hypertension	Plasma renin activity, renal ultrasound and Doppler, DTPA scintigraphy, angiography (MR, CT, conventional)
Pheochromocytoma	24-hr urine and plasma catecholamines; metaiod-obenzylguanidine scan; abdominal CT, MR scan
Primary aldosteronism	Plasma renin activity, aldosterone
Cushing syndrome	Plasma cortisol, 24-hr urinary free cortisol; dexamethasone suppression test
Coarctation of aorta	Chest X-ray, echocardiography, angiography (MR, conventional)
Congenital adrenal hyperplasia	Plasma deoxycorticosterone and corticosterone, 18-hydroxycorticosterone, and deoxycorticosterone, 11-deoxycortisol
Other monogenic forms	See **Table 25.9**
Obstructive sleep apnea	Polysomnography

Based on recommendations of American Academy of Pediatrics (AAP) 2017; European Society of Hypertension (ESH) 2016 (children) and 2023 (all ages); Joint Statement of HyperChild/NET and European Academy of Pediatrics (EAP) 2023; and Hypertension Canada 2020

[1]Not recommended by AAP 2017 except in children [a]with CKD; [b]at risk of diabetes and [c]those <6-year-old or with abnormal blood chemistry or urinalysis

[2]Recommended by the ESH 2016, ESH 2023 and Joint statement of HyperChild/NET and EAP 2023 only in severe or symptomatic hypertension or in hypertensive emergency; no recommendation by AAP 2017

[3]Chest X-ray or electrocardiogram are not sensitive enough to screen for left ventricular hypertrophy (AAP 2017)

[4]Consider in specific clinical settings, and in children younger than 6 years, or those with stage 2 hypertension or diastolic hypertension

CT: computed tomography; DMSA: ^{99m}Tc-dimercaptosuccinic acid scan; DTPA: ^{99m}Tc-diethylenetriaminepentaacetic acid scan; HDL: high-density lipoproteins; LDL: low-density lipoproteins; MR: magnetic resonance

often suggest the diagnosis. If not done previously, blood pressure should be measured in all four limbs, and bruit should be auscultated for over the carotid arteries and the abdomen. The retina is examined for hypertensive retinopathy. Preliminary investigations are carried out for the etiology, the degree of target organ damage (which reflects the severity and duration of hypertension) and identify patients that need further evaluation. All patients with hypertension should undergo evaluation of serum urea and creatinine, electrolytes, and urinalysis. Most experts recommend performing ultrasound on all children and adolescents with hypertension. An electrocardiography is not considered adequate for LVH; an echocardiography should be performed.

Primary hypertension is likely in obese and adolescent children, particularly those with a family history of essential hypertension. Children with stage 2, symptomatic or diastolic hypertension, young age (<6 years), clues on history and physical examination, and/or evidence of target organ damage are most likely to have an underlying etiology. Additional investigations are limited to these patients. The choice of investigations varies by the etiology suspected **(Table 25.6)**. Measurement of the plasma renin activity (PRA) is a useful screening test for high mineralocorticoid states and in renovascular hypertension. Renal angiography is carried out to confirm renal artery stenosis.

MANAGEMENT

The therapy of secondary hypertension depends on the cause and degree of hypertension **(Flowchart 25.2)**. Guidelines for management of hypertension in children recommend a stepped-care approach to reduce blood pressure to target **(Flowchart 25.2; Table 25.3)**. Specific management is necessary in certain scenarios. Surgical treatment is indicated in coarctation of aorta, pheochromocytoma and other endocrine tumors, and most forms of renovascular hypertension. Renal artery stenosis and renal aneurysm are managed by percutaneous transluminal angioplasty or stenting of renal arteries.

Lifestyle Measures

In all cases of elevated blood pressure and confirmed stage 1 hypertension, the first step in management involves lifestyle modifications, such as exercise and dietary changes **(Box 25.5)**. These measures are tried for a period of 6–12 months and continued if pharmacotherapy is initiated.

Antihypertensive Therapy

Children presenting with symptomatic or stage 2 hypertension and those with features of target organ damage require therapy with antihypertensive medications. Pharmacotherapy is also indicated in children and adolescents

Flowchart 25.2: Suggested step-wise algorithm for management of hypertension in children and adolescents requiring pharmacotherapy
*Single-pill combinations are preferred where feasible
ABPM: ambulatory blood pressure monitoring; ACEi: angiotensin converting enzyme inhibitor; ARB: angiotensin receptor blocker; CCB: calcium channel blocker; CKD: chronic kidney disease

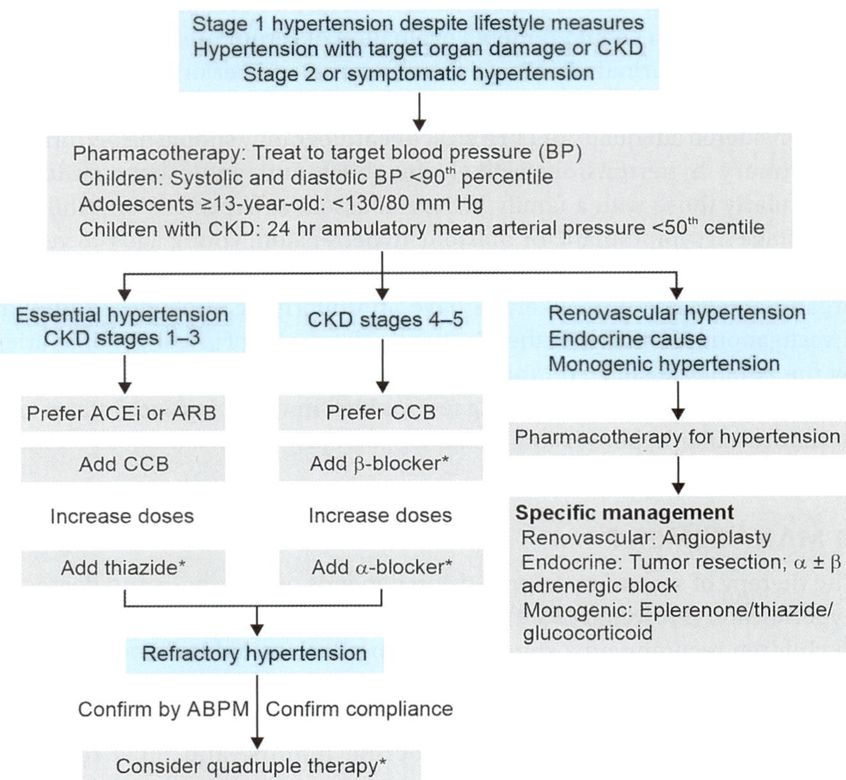

failing lifestyle modifications, and those with comorbid diabetes or CKD. Various medications used to treat hypertension include angiotensin converting enzyme inhibitors (ACEi), angiotensin receptor blockers (ARB), calcium channel blockers (CCBs), β-adrenergic blockers, α-adrenergic blockers, and diuretics and their combinations. **Table 25.7** provides details of doses and considerations in use of these medications. In the absence of contraindications, ACEi and CCBs are considered first-line therapy. As a next step, usually a β-adrenergic blocker, diuretic, α-adrenergic blocker, or direct vasodilator are added **(Flowchart 25.2)**.

Angiotensin Converting Enzyme Inhibitors

ACEi such as enalapril, ramipril, and lisinopril have been demonstrated to be safe and effective in lowering blood pressure. They are well tolerated by most

BOX 25.5: Lifestyle interventions for blood pressure reduction in children and adolescents

Diet

Dietary approaches to stop hypertension (DASH) diet involves adhering to the following number of food servings daily: (*i*) fruits and vegetables 4–5 (≥3); (*ii*) low-fat milk products ≥2; (*iii*) whole grains 6; (*iv*) fish, poultry, and lean red meats ≤2; (*v*) legumes and nuts 1; (*vi*) oils and fats 2–3; and (*vii*) added sugar and sweets (including sweet beverages) ≤1; total dietary sodium <2,300 mg/day in adolescents[1]

Fats

Diet rich in monounsaturated fat; prefer olive oil (polyphenols have cardiovascular health benefits)

Salt restriction

- Safe and adequate intake of salt in children is defined as follows: (*i*) 1,100 mg/day at 1–3 years; (*ii*) 1,300 mg/day at 4–6 years; (*iii*) 1,700 mg/day at 7–10 years; (*iv*) 2,000 mg/day at 11–17 years
- Adequate intake of salt in infants 7–11 months is 200 mg/day (based on sodium content of breast milk)

Physical activity

- Moderate to vigorous physical activity for 30–60 minutes on 3–5 days per week (AAP 2017); regular, daily physical activity, for ≥60 minutes, ≥3 times a week (ESH 2016)
- Sedentary recreational screen time limited to ≤2 hr daily

Weight

- Body mass index to be maintained at <85th percentile for age and sex
- Obese adolescents to lose weight gradually, at 1–2 kg each month, to achieve the above target

Sleep: Ensure adequate sleep duration (≥5–7 hr)

Social interactions: Engage in positive social interactions and experiences.

[1]Examples of serving sizes for a 2,000 calorie diet are in parentheses as follows: Whole grains (half cup of cooked rice), vegetables (one cup raw salad or half cup cooked vegetables), fruits (half cup of fruit juice or half an apple or pear), dairy (one cup fat-free curd or yoghurt), lean protein (one egg, 30 g lean meat, or 110 g tofu), nuts, seeds, and legumes (10 peanuts, 6 almonds or cashew nuts, or 16 pistachios), sweets (one small cupcake or cola drink 350 mL), and fats and oils (1 tablespoon peanut butter or 1 teaspoon olive oil)

patients and do not have any metabolic adverse effects. The most common adverse effect is a dry, persistent cough that is attributed to retention of bradykinins and the neurotransmitter substance P. Hyperkalemia and a reduction in the glomerular filtration rate (GFR), indicated by acute rise in serum creatinine by 20–30%, may occur. Hence, blood levels of electrolytes and creatinine should be measured 10–14 days after initiation of therapy. Recent guidelines suggest the continued use of ACEi or ARB when the estimated GFR falls below 30 mL/min/1.73 m^2, while monitoring closely for

TABLE 25.7: Drugs for treatment of hypertension

Medication	*Initial dose, per kg/day*	*Maximum dose, per kg/day (maximum adult dose)*	*Divided daily doses*	*Precautions and adverse effects (AE)*
α Adrenergic blockers				First dose hypotension common. Prazosin is available as an extended-release preparation, which must be swallowed whole, without crushing
Prazosin Doxazosin	0.05–0.1 mg 0.5–1.0 mg	0.5 mg NA (16 mg/day)	2–3 2–3	
β Adrenergic blockers				*Caution:* Avoid in asthma and heart failure. Atenolol is given at 50% dose at GFR <50 mL/min/1.73 m^2; and on alternate day at GFR <10 mL/min/1.73 m^2; atenolol is dialyzable. Labetalol is preferred in acute symptomatic or refractory hypertension, rather than routinely in chronic hypertension. Phenoxybenzamine is reserved for management of pheochromocytoma *AE:* Dyslipidemia, blunting of hypoglycemic symptoms; sleep disturbance with propranolol
Atenolol Propranolol Metoprolol succinate Labetalol Phenoxybenzamine	0.5 mg 1 mg 1 mg 1–3 mg 0.2 mg	2 mg (100 mg/day) 8 mg (640 mg/day) 2 mg (200 mg/day) 10–12 mg (1.2 g/day) 1–2 mg	1–2 3 2 2 2	
Central alpha agonist				*Caution:* Preferred in acute symptomatic or refractory hypertension. Risk of rebound hypertension on abrupt discontinuation. *AE:* First dose hypotension common; sedation (clonidine)
Clonidine Methyldopa	5–7 µg 5 mg	25 µg (900 µg/day) 40 mg (3 g/day)	3 2–3	
Calcium channel blockers				Nifedipine, available as extended-release preparation, must be swallowed whole. First dose hypotension common
Nifedipine (slow release) Amlodepine	0.2 mg 0.05–0.2 mg	3 mg (120 mg/day) 0.6 mg (10 mg/day)	1–2 1–2	
Angiotensin converting enzyme inhibitors (ACEi)				Useful in treatment of renal parenchymal disease; monitor serum potassium and creatinine periodically *Common AE:* Cough with ACEi (not ARB), headache, dizziness, asthenia *Severe AE:* hyperkalemia, AKI, angioedema, fetal toxicity; anemia and neutropenia (chiefly with ACEi)
Captopril Enalapril Lisinopril Ramipril	0.3 mg 0.0.8 mg 0.06 mg 5–6 mg/m^2/day	6 mg (450 mg/day) 0.6 mg (40 mg/day) 0.6 mg (40 mg/day) NA (20 mg/day)	3 2 1 1–2	

Contd...

Contd...

Medication	***Initial dose, per kg/day***	***Maximum dose, per kg/day (maximum adult dose)***	***Divided daily doses***	***Precautions and adverse effects (AE)***
Angiotensin receptor blockers (ARB)				*Contraindications:* Pregnancy, angioedema with ACEi; bilateral renal artery stenosis *Caution:* Avoid use at low GFR (<25 mL/min/1.73 m^2); avoid use in neonates or use minimal doses; ACEi are dialyzable
Losartan	0.6 mg	1.4 mg (100 mg/day)	2	
Valsartan	1.3 mg	2.7 mg (320 mg/day)	1	
Irbesartan	6–12 yr: 75–150 mg/day >12 yr: 150–300 mg/day	300 mg/day	1 1	
Candesartan	0.2 mg	0.4 mg (32 mg/day)	1	
Olmesartan	>6 yr, 20–35 kg: 10 mg/day >6 yr, >35 kg: 20 mg/day	>6 yr, 20-35 kg: 20 mg/day >6 yr, >35 kg: 40 mg/day	1–2	
Mineralocorticoid receptor antagonists				*Common AE:* Hyperkalemia, especially if used with ACEi or ARB or at low GFR
Eplerenone Spironolactone	>4 years: 25 mg/day 1 mg	NA (100 mg/day) 3.3 mg (100 mg/day)	1–2 1–2	
Diuretics				*Caution:* Monitor electrolytes, fluid status; thiazides may be less effective at GFR <30 mL/min/1.73 m^2 *AE:* Dehydration, hypokalemia, metabolic alkalosis; dyslipidemia, hyperuricemia, hyperglycemia, hypomagnesemia (thiazides); hypercalciuria (furosemide)
Hydrochlorthiazide Chlorthalidone Furosemide	0.5–1 mg 0.25 mg 0.5 mg	3 mg (50 mg/day) 2 mg (50 mg/day) 6 mg	2 1 1–2	
Vasodilators				Preferred for acute symptomatic or refractory hypertension. *AE:* First dose hypotension (common); headache, palpitations, fluid retention, congestive heart failure; minoxidil causes hypertrichosis and pericardial effusion
Hydralazine Minoxidil	1–2 mg 0.1–0.2 mg	5–8 mg (200 mg/day) 1 mg (50 mg/day)	3–4 1–2	

The maximum recommended adult dose (mentioned in parentheses) should not be exceeded
AKI: acute kidney injury; GFR: glomerular filtration rate

acute decline in kidney function and/or hyperkalemia. A rare adverse effect is angioedema. ACEi should be prescribed cautiously to patients with impaired kidney function, and their use avoided in those with bilateral stenosis of the renal arteries. ACEi should not be used in pregnancy, since their use has been associated with fetal and neonatal death, renal tubular dysgenesis, and defects in skeletal development.

Angiotensin Receptor Blockers

Blockade of the angiotensin II receptor achieves more specific lowering of blood pressure without associated adverse effects, e.g., cough. The indications, contraindications, and guidelines for monitoring are similar to those advised for ACEi. Although ARB (losartan, valsartan, irbesartan, and olmesartan) have been less extensively used in children, their efficacy and safety is established, and dose guidance is available.

Calcium Channel Blockers

There are three major groups of CCBs with distinct properties: phenylalkylamines (verapamil), dihydropyridines (nifedipine, nicardipine, and amlodipine), and benzothiazepines (diltiazem). Dihydropyridines have relative selectivity for arteriolar smooth muscle and are most widely used in treatment of hypertension. Availability of sustained release preparations permits once or twice daily administration. CCBs are safe and effective in lowering blood pressure. Adverse effects include tachycardia, headache, and flushing (especially with the fast-acting dihydropyridines), ankle edema and constipation (with verapamil). These agents do not have adverse metabolic effects. Amlodipine is a lipophilic dihydropyridine with a longer duration of action. The tablets can be crushed or placed in suspension. Children seem to require higher doses of amlodipine on a per kilogram body weight basis, and twice-a-day regimen of administration is more effective.

β-Adrenoceptor Blockers

β-blockers are safe and effective antihypertensive agents and widely used in children. A variety of β-blockers are available. Some are cardioselective (atenolol, metoprolol), while others have α-blocking and vasodilator properties (labetalol). Common adverse effects include bradycardia, syncope, irritability, lethargy, weakness, and depression. These drugs are contraindicated in patients with asthma, diabetes mellitus, congestive heart failure, Raynaud phenomenon, and atrioventricular conduction defects.

α-Adrenoceptor Blockers

α-Adrenoceptor blocking agents (prazosin, phenoxybenzamine, and phentolamine) are effective in lowering blood pressure. Prazosin antagonizes peripheral α1-adrenergic receptors resulting in dilatation of arteriolar resistance and venous capacitance vessels. Pediatric experience with this drug is limited. Phenoxybenzamine and phentolamine are used exclusively in the treatment of pheochromocytoma. The main adverse effect is first dose postural hypotension.

Diuretics

Compared to loop diuretics, thiazides (chlorthiazide, hydrochlorthiazide, and chlorthalidone) provide a sustained but less vigorous diuresis. Thiazides are less effective in patients with GFR <30 mL/min/1.73 m^2, although data supports its utility in adults with CKD stages 4–5. Loop diuretics are effective in patients with low GFR. Prolonged and high dose therapy might result in multiple metabolic effects, such as hypokalemia, metabolic alkalosis, hyperuricemia, and impaired glucose tolerance. Prolonged therapy with thiazide diuretics has an adverse effect on the lipid profile. These agents are valuable ancillary treatment to other antihypertensive medications. A combination of diuretics with potassium sparing drugs or ACEi prevents potassium depletion.

Others

Direct vasodilators, such as hydralazine and minoxidil, are effective in lowering blood pressure, but some of their adverse effects (tachycardia, headache, and salt and water retention) make it difficult to use them as monotherapy. Concurrent use of β-blockers or diuretics is needed. Clonidine and methyldopa inhibit central sympathetic output (through stimulation of α2-adrenergic receptors). Rebound hypertension may occur in patients who suddenly discontinue using clonidine. Other adverse effects include dry mouth, depression, sedation, and hallucinations.

Chronic Kidney Disease

Guidelines recommend that children with nondialysis dependent CKD should receive antihypertensive treatment beginning when blood pressure is consistently above the 90th percentile for age, sex, and height. An ACEi or ARB is preferred, irrespective of the level of proteinuria, unless with low GFR (<30 mL/min/1.73 m^2). The ESH recommends lowering blood pressure to below the 75th percentile for age, sex, and height percentile, in children with nonproteinuric CKD. In those with proteinuria, blood pressure should be lowered to achieve systolic and diastolic readings ≤50th percentile for age, sex, and height unless achieving these targets is limited by signs or symptoms of hypotension **(Table 25.3)**. The AAP recommends that ABPM be considered to ensure that the target blood pressure is achieved, indicated by mean ambulatory blood pressure below the 50th centile for age and height **(Flowchart 25.2)**.

Stepwise and Combination Therapy

The management of children with sustained hypertension starts with low doses of one drug and titration of the dose to therapeutically effective levels. The initial drug is usually an ACEi or ARB, but CCBs may be considered particularly in children with advanced CKD. Single agent therapy with an ACEi (enalapril, ramipril) or CCBs (nifedipine, amlodepine) may be sufficient to control moderate hypertension.

If one of the initial medications is ineffective in lowering blood pressure, it is necessary to use a drug from a different class. If therapy with a single drug is only partly effective, it is preferable to add a small dose of a drug from another class rather than increase the dose of a single drug. This permits the addition of different primary actions while minimizing homeostatic compensations that limit the fall in blood pressure. Combination therapy also reduces adverse effects by using drugs in moderate doses. An additive effect has been shown when combining a diuretic with a β-blocker, ACEi or a dihydropyridine CCB. Combinations of ACEi, ARB, and/or mineralocorticoid antagonists are contraindicated in view of additive risks of hyperkalemia and acute kidney injury. A similar effect is seen when a β-blocker is combined with α-blocker.

Treatment-resistant Hypertension

Resistant hypertension in adults is defined as persistently elevated blood pressure despite treatment with three or more antihypertensive agents of different classes, prescribed at maximally effective (and tolerated) doses, including at least one diuretic. Adherence must be ensured before labeling treatment resistance. ABPM might be performed to prevent false diagnosis and to examine for lability of blood pressure control **(Flowchart 25.2)**. Administration of multiple drugs in a small child is difficult but compliance must be ensured. In difficult situations (chronic glomerulonephritis, posttransplantation), other medications (hydralazine, clonidine, prazosin, and minoxidil) are advised.

Follow-up Care

Children and adolescents with systemic hypertension require frequent follow up to ensure adherence and adequate blood pressure control. Annual ABPM is recommended, along with screening for target organ damage. Stepwise reduction of antihypertensive medication may be possible in some patients after blood pressure has remained in the normal range for 8–12 months. Hypertensive children should avoid highly static (isometric) exercises such as weight and power lifting, gymnastics, and body building. In contrast, aerobic exercises are encouraged except in presence of left ventricular dysfunction. Children with no evidence of target organ involvement can participate in all sports once blood pressure is adequately controlled.

HYPERTENSIVE EMERGENCIES

Blood pressure levels 12 mm or more above the 95th centile or blood pressure >140/90 mm Hg in adolescents are considered "severe". Patients with severe hypertension are likely to manifest clinical features of end organ involvement and need urgent attention. The AAP defines hypertensive emergency as blood pressure measurements ≥30 mm Hg above the 95th percentile based on age, sex, and height. Other experts suggest using a cutoff of 20% above the limit of stage 2 hypertension. These patients are at risk of acute target organ damage, which can be life-threatening with serious sequelae if therapy is inadequate. A distinction is made between a hypertensive emergency and urgency, based on the presence or absence of acute target organ dysfunction/ damage; however, this demarcation is often not useful.

Clinical Features

Hypertensive emergencies are typically associated with a rapid rise in blood pressure. Chronic elevation of blood pressure is usually well tolerated with few symptoms. The child may present with features of encephalopathy. Thus, there may be headache, vomiting, ataxia, sensorial disturbances, stupor, and seizures. Focal neurological deficits such as hemiparesis, blurring, and transient loss of vision may be present.

Management

The immediate aim is to bring the blood pressure down to safe (yet still hypertensive) values followed by gradual reduction to normal over the next 48 hr. Overenthusiastic therapy with precipitous decline of blood pressure (particularly in patients with long standing hypertension) should be avoided. At the same time, supportive measures are instituted to manage various complications that may be present, such as seizures, heart failure, and airway obstruction.

Potent agents, listed in **Table 25.8**, can decrease the blood pressure within a few minutes. Patients presenting with seizures, loss of consciousness, pulmonary edema, or congestive cardiac failure should preferably receive intravenous (IV) nitroprusside or labetalol in a closely monitored, preferably intensive care, environment. The reduction of blood pressure should be achieved slowly since a precipitous fall in blood pressure can lead to neurological sequelae. Patients with long standing hypertension, renovascular disease, or those having neurological symptoms and signs are particularly susceptible to developing such complications. The patient must be closely monitored during treatment to detect hypotension. The neurological status and pupillary reaction should be frequently examined.

Approximately 25–33% of the desired reduction is made over the first 6–8 hr, with gradual lowering of the blood pressure over 24–48 hr. The target blood pressure level is the 95th centile of the systolic value for

TABLE 25.8: Treatment of hypertensive emergencies[1]

Drug	*Route: Dose*	*Onset of action*	*Duration*	*Adverse effects; caution or comments*
Sodium nitroprusside	*Intravenous (IV) infusion:* 0.5–8 µg/kg/min	<30 sec	<10 minutes	Nausea, vomiting; muscle twitching, headache, tachycardia; thiocyanate/cyanide toxicity (dizziness, confusion seizures, stiff jaw, and lactic acidosis) if used for >72 hr or with kidney failure); inactivated by light; reconstituted in 5% dextrose to achieve a concentration of 50–200 µg/mL (max. 1 mg/mL in fluid restricted patients)
Nitroglycerine	*IV infusion:* 0.1–3 µg/kg/min	1–2 minutes	5–10 minutes	Headache, tachycardia; methemoglobinemia; useful in heart failure predominantly as a vasodilator; limited data in children
Labetalol	*IV infusion (preferred):* 0.25–3 mg/kg/h, or IV bolus: 0.2–1 mg/kg; repeat in 5–10 minutes	5–10 minutes	2–6 hr	Transient nausea, pallor, bradycardia, orthostatic hypotension, abdominal pain, diarrhea; avoid in patients with asthma, congestive heart failure; diluted in 5% dextrose and given slowly
Nifedipine	*Oral or sublingual (bite and swallow):* 0.25–0.5 mg/kg (max. 10 mg)	10–30 minutes	1-6 hr	*Increased cerebral blood flow:* Flushing, headache, syncope; unpredictable hypotension; reflex tachycardia, pedal edema
Nicardipine	*IV infusion:* 1–3 µg/kg/min	1–10 minutes	10–30 minutes	Flushing, reflex tachycardia, headache, phlebitis, nausea, increased intracranial pressure; increases cyclosporin levels
Hydralazine	*Slow IV:* 0.1–0.5 mg/kg/dose; can repeat after 4 hr	5–20 minutes	4–12 hr	Tachycardia, palpitations, flushing, headache, fluid retention

Contd...

Contd...

Drug	*Route: Dose*	*Onset of action*	*Duration*	*Adverse effects; caution or comments*
Clonidine	*IV bolus (preferred):* 2–6 µg/kg per dose, or oral: 0.05–1 mg/dose, repeat q h (max. 0.8 mg total dose)	*IV:* 10 minutes *Oral:* 15–30 minutes	2-4 hr	Sedation, dry mouth, rebound hypertension
Phentolamine	*IV bolus:* 0.1–0.2 mg/kg (max 5 mg); can repeat q 2–4 hr	10 minutes	30-60 minutes	Reflex tachycardia, abdominal pain
Enalaprilat	*IV bolus:* 0.005–0.01 mg/kg per dose	15 minutes	6 hr	Contraindicated in bilateral renal artery stenosis; kidney failure
Esmolol	*IV infusion:* 100–500 µg/kg/min	<60 seconds	10-30 minutes	Bradycardia; contraindicated in asthma
Furosemide	*IV bolus:* 0.5–2 mg/kg/dose	30 minutes	2 hr	Hypotension with high doses
Urapidil	*IV bolus, followed by infusion:* 0.5–4 mg/kg bolus, then 0.2–2 mg/kg/h	1–5 minutes	3 hr	Sedation, nausea, palpitations (tachycardia, bradycardia); contraindicated with AV fistula
Isradipine	*Oral:* 0.05–0.1 mg/kg/dose (max. 0.8 mg/kg/day)	1–3 hr	>12 hr	Hypotension with higher doses
Captopril	*Oral:* 0.1–0.2 mg/kg/dose; repeat 6–24 hr	10–20 minutes	>2 hr	Contraindicated in bilateral renal artery stenosis; kidney failure
Minoxidil	*Oral:* 0.1–0.2 mg/kg/dose	5–10 minutes	2–5 days	Fluid retention; dizziness

[1]In case the blood pressure falls too rapidly or below the desired level, a bolus of 50 mL of normal saline may be administered

the age and sex. It is preferable to administer the antihypertensive drug by constant infusion with careful regulation of the dose to achieve a controlled fall in blood pressure. The risk of hypotension is greater with sublingual administration of nifedipine. Children with severe hypertension may be salt depleted on presentation and routine administration of diuretics is not recommended since volume contraction and severe hypotension may ensue. However, in presence of evidence of salt and fluid overload (e.g., in acute glomerulonephritis) and adequate kidney function, a dose of frusemide should be administered intravenously.

Sodium Nitroprusside

Blood pressure and pulse rate are monitored continuously and changes in the rate of infusion are made after constant readings of blood pressure are obtained. The infusion of sodium nitroprusside is gradually tapered once the blood pressure has been reduced to safe levels. Since sodium nitroprusside is not stable when exposed to sunlight, the bottle and infusion line should be wrapped in an aluminum foil. The drug should be used with caution in severe renal or hepatic dysfunction and impaired cerebral circulation. Thiocyanate toxicity may occur if the drug is used for >72 hr.

Labetalol

Constant infusion of labetalol is often preferred for treatment of hypertensive emergency. The dose is 1–3 mg/kg/h, titrated by incremental infusion according to the level of blood pressure. The same precautions as during the infusion of sodium nitroprusside are observed. No dosage reduction is required in renal or hepatic impairment.

Nifedipine

This drug is given at a dose of 0.25 mg/kg/dose orally or sublingually, although little absorption takes place by the latter route. Nifedipine is available in 5 and 10 mg capsules; the drug must be removed from the capsule or the patient bites through the capsule. Lowering of blood pressure is seen within few minutes. The absorption of nifedipine is erratic and the response unpredictable. The dose can be repeated, if necessary, twice at 10-minute intervals. Since the medication is sensitive to light, contents of the capsule or crushed tablets are used immediately to avoid loss in potency. Children with long standing hypertension show impaired cerebral autoregulation of blood flow and are at risk of neurologic sequelae following rapid lowering of blood pressure. It is prudent to avoid nifedipine in these circumstances. However, oral nifedipine can be safely used for treatment of acute severe hypertension.

Risk of Hypotension

Occasionally, a rapid fall in blood pressure may cause permanent neurological sequelae. The risk of such complications is high in patients with chronic, severe hypertension with end organ damage such as retinopathy and left ventricular enlargement. In such cases there is a loss of vascular elasticity and narrowing of lumina. Such vessels cannot readily react to changes in blood flow, especially during hypotension. Loss of autoregulation and rapid hypotension in the brain may lead to ischemic injury especially to the visual cortex and the optic nerve. Careful administration of medications and close monitoring are important to balance the risks of cerebral hemorrhage due to hypertension and ischemic complications from hypotension. Precipitous fall in blood pressure is corrected with rapid administration of 0.9% saline.

Subsequent Care

Once the blood pressure is brought down to safe levels, maintenance oral treatment is introduced. Medications such as nifedipine (slow release form), ACEi, and β-blockers are effective. Other agents such as hydralazine, clonidine, and prazosin may be required.

ESSENTIAL (PRIMARY) HYPERTENSION

Primary hypertension in children is conventionally considered a diagnosis of exclusion. Recent studies indicate a steep increase in the prevalence of primary hypertension paralleling the obesity epidemic. The proportion of children diagnosed with primary hypertension has been increasing, particularly in patients seen at primary rather than referral centers, and among overweight and obese older children and adolescents. Both elevated blood pressure and hypertension are commonly detected in obese children. Hypertension is also more likely to be primary in patients with type 2 diabetes, obstructive sleep apnea, or those with family history of primary hypertension. Patients with primary hypertension are likely to have asymptomatic stage 1 hypertension or elevated blood pressure, often detected incidentally. There may be a family history of hypertension.

Etiology

As in adults, the pathogenesis of primary hypertension in children is linked to aberrations in counter-regulatory natriuretic and antinatriuretic pathways that lead to impaired renal sodium handling and salt sensitivity. Examples of antinatriuretic pathways include sympathetic nervous system and renin-angiotensin-aldosterone system (RAS), while the renal autocrine/ paracrine dopamine system is an important natriuretic pathway. Primary hypertension is proposed to result from complex interactions of these two systems with dietary salt intake in relation to obesity, insulin resistance, inflammation, and oxidative stress. Insulin resistance, in obesity, leads to salt and water retention and activation of RAS, while the secretion of leptin by adipocytes leads to increased sympathetic outflow and altered vascular reactivity. Primary hypertension has also been linked to low birth weight and low nephron endowment. Genetic factors play a role in hypertension independent of diet and habitus; multiple mutations and single nucleotide polymorphisms have been identified in primary hypertension **(Annexure 9.8, p 845)**. Environmental factors such as passive smoking and a sedentary lifestyle are relevant in adolescents.

Evaluation and Management

A diagnosis of essential hypertension is rarely made below 6 years of age. Careful clinical and laboratory evaluation is required to rule out secondary cause, as discussed earlier. The goal of lifestyle measures **(Box 25.5)** is to reduce body mass index to consistently below the 85th percentile for sex and age. Reduced salt and caloric intake and adequate physical activity is necessary. Weight loss is associated with improved blood pressure and suffices to lower the blood pressure below the 90th percentile. Constant motivation of the child and family members is essential to achieve and sustain this goal. Pharmacotherapy is indicated in patients failing lifestyle measures, those with type 2 diabetes, stage 2 or symptomatic hypertension, evidence of target organ damage, and those with a family history of complications of hypertension. In such patients, initial pharmacotherapy with ACEi or ARB is preferred. Regular follow up visits are required to assess control of hypertension. After 6–12 months of treatment, antihypertensive drugs may be reduced in some patients.

MASKED HYPERTENSION

The highest prevalence of masked hypertension is in children with CKD, obesity, diabetes, and after heart transplantation. The prevalence of masked hypertension in healthy children with other risk factors for hypertension, such as prematurity, overweight, obstructive sleep apnea, or positive family history of hypertension **(Box 25.3)**, is up to 9%, compared to 0–3% in those without any of them. Most hypertension guidelines recommend to screen for masked hypertension in children with CKD, type 1 and 2 diabetes, obesity, after solid organ transplantations, and those with repaired coarctation of aorta. Experts also recommend screening healthy children for masked hypertension if they have positive family history of hypertension, elevated office blood pressure, inconsistent office records of hypertension, or hypertension mediated organ damage with normal office blood pressure. While there is modest agreement between blood pressure values by ABPM and home blood pressure monitoring, the latter is not preferred in diagnosing masked hypertension since it has lower sensitivity and lower positive predictive value than ABPM.

Masked hypertension has been consistently associated with increased left ventricular mass index and LVH in children and adolescents. Other associations include unsatisfactory performance in executive function in childhood, and early hypertensive kidney injury in studies in adults. While AAP guidelines advise only lifestyle measures **(Box 25.5)** for masked hypertension, the European guidelines also suggest pharmacotherapy, while acknowledging that evidence to support the advice is limited. Antihypertensive medications are considered in presence of hypertension-mediated organ damage, CKD, and type 2 diabetes.

WHITE COAT HYPERTENSION

An international database of adult patients shows that the frequency of WCH varied from 6 to 13% depending on whether the overall 24-h awake, sleep, or all three records were used for classification. In contrast, up to half of children referred for evaluation of elevated office blood pressures appear to have WCH. With the removal of emphasis on blood pressure 'load' in the classification scheme provided in the 2022 pediatric ABPM, the prevalence of WCH in children is expected to decline to half of the previous estimates. Overall, the prevalence of WCH is higher in obese children than children with normal weight.

In adults, WCH is associated with increased risk of future hypertension and adverse cardiovascular outcomes. This effect is pronounced for those with consistently elevated office blood pressure on consecutive measurements ('stable' WCH) than those whose office blood pressure was elevated once ('unstable' WCH). However, the cardiovascular consequences of WCH, studied chiefly as surrogate cardiovascular outcomes in children, remain unclear. While the prevalence of LVH and impaired pulse wave velocity was similar between normotensive children and those with WCH, children with WCH tend to have higher left ventricular mass index and blood pressure variability, increased carotid intima media thickness, and impaired cerebral vasoreactivity compared to healthy children. While the risk of progression of WCH to hypertension is not clear, obesity and WCH appear to confer additive risks in this regard.

The AAP and AHA recommend ABPM to detect WCH, chiefly to avoid unnecessary testing and inappropriate treatment. Hence, physicians often ignore WCH and do not advise follow-up. The appropriate clinical approach to WCH in children and adolescents is unclear. Recent studies suggest that children with WCH, particularly those with stable WCH, might progress to an abnormal ABPM phenotype, especially in the form of nocturnal hypertension. The AAP suggests that patients with WCH undergo repeat ABPM 1–2 years later.

RENAL ARTERY STENOSIS

Renal artery stenosis is an important cause of secondary hypertension in childhood. Takayasu disease (nonspecific aortoarteritis) is characterized by diffuse and variable involvement of the arch and descending aorta; the subclavian, femoral, and renal arteries and other vessels may also be involved. Absent peripheral pulses and bruit in the epigastric, subcostal region or flanks are characteristic. Renal artery stenosis may be congenital or secondary to fibromuscular dysplasia, neurofibromatosis, or collagen vascular disease. Rare causes of renovascular disease include renal artery thrombosis, aneurysms, and monogenic forms of midaortic syndrome **(Annexure 9.8, p 845)**. In each of these conditions, the lesions may be unilateral or bilateral and involve segmental or interlobar renal arteries, and the main renal artery. Activation of the RAS is the hallmark of renovascular hypertension.

Patients typically present with severe stage 2 hypertension, often with target organ injury or hypertensive emergency. Asymmetry in pulses and blood pressure and presence of neck or renal bruits point to the diagnosis of Takayasu aortoarteritis. It is not uncommon for children with unilateral renal artery stenosis to present with polyuria and hypokalemia metabolic alkalosis with hyponatremia, termed the "hyponatremic hypertension syndrome", attributed to natriuresis from the unaffected kidney in presence of excessive RAS activation.

Conventional tools to diagnose renovascular hypertension include Doppler sonography, diethylenetriamine pentaacetate (DTPA) renography, and computed tomography (CT) or magnetic resonance (MR) angiography **(Figs. 25.3A to C)**. The diagnosis of Takayasu aortoarteritis is made by conventional angiography, which also defines the extent and type or disease (see Chapter 9). Active disease is suggested by elevated erythrocyte sedimentation rate, increased carotid intima medial thickness, and evidence of arteritis on angiography. Conventional imaging has low sensitivity for the diagnosis of fibromuscular dysplasia, particularly in young children with involvement of segmental renal arteries. If clinical suspicion is high, digital subtraction angiography must be performed. Revascularization by percutaneous transluminal angioplasty can often be performed in the same session. The procedure is avoided during active inflammation in aortoarteritis, except if severe target organ damage is present and hypertension is refractory to medical measures. Patients with unilateral stenosis not amenable to intervention may be considered for therapy with ACEi or ARB, since it is the most effective pharmacotherapy, but is likely to cause decline in function of the affected kidney. Nephrectomy is considered in patients with refractory hypertension if the affected kidney contributes <10% of the global kidney function and percutaneous transluminal angioplasty has failed.

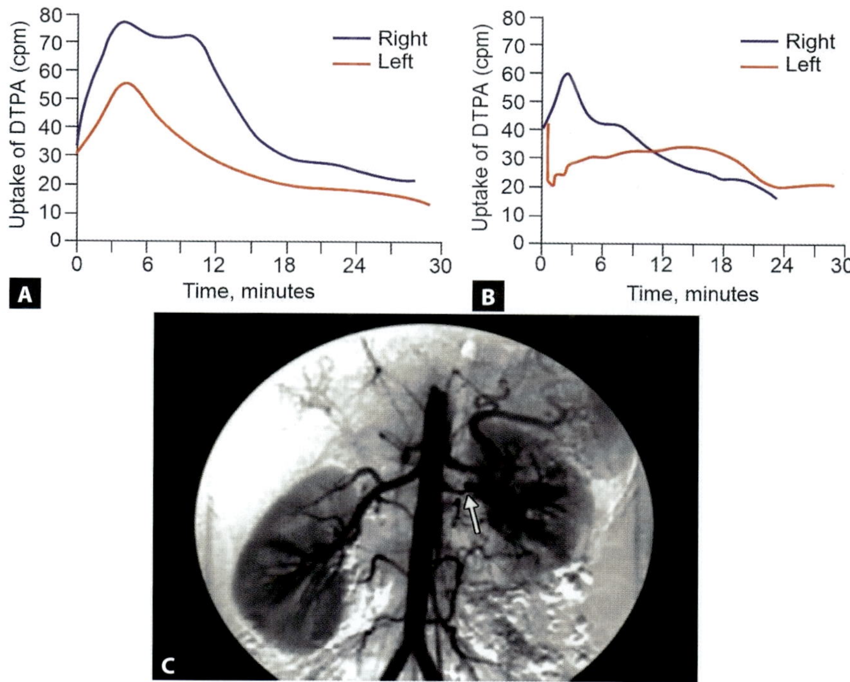

Figs. 25.3A to C: Renal artery stenosis in left kidney. Diethylenetriamine pentaacetate (DTPA) scan (A) showing reduced uptake in left kidney; (B) the uptake and excretion of the tracer is further reduced following administration of captopril; (C) angiography shows stenosis involving proximal part of left renal artery (arrow). cpm: counts per minutes

MONOGENIC HYPERTENSION

Hypertension in childhood may rarely be secondary to single gene mutations, inherited in an autosomal dominant or recessive fashion, that lead to increased epithelial sodium or chloride reabsorption, high urinary potassium secretion, suppression of PRA, and/or excessive mineralocorticoid action with hypokalemic metabolic alkalosis **(Table 25.9; Fig. 25.4; Flowchart 25.3; and Annexure 9.8, p 845)**. Findings that prompt the consideration of these entities include family history of early-onset hypertension or major adverse cardiovascular events (strokes, sudden cardiac death); abnormal potassium levels (low or high), metabolic alkalosis or acidosis and suppressed renin secretion **(Flowchart 25.3)**. Hypertension may be mild to severe and electrolyte abnormalities subtle or lacking. The hypokalemia metabolic alkalosis in monogenic hypertension is distinguished from Bartter and Gitelman syndromes by elevated blood pressure, euvolemia, and decreased levels of PRA.

TABLE 25.9: Monogenic forms of hypertension

Disease	*Defect*	*Gene; inheritance*	*Features*	*Other abnormalities*	*Treatment*
Metabolic alkalosis; low or normal potassium					
Low plasma renin and aldosterone levels					
17α-hydroxylase 17,20-lyase deficiency[1]	Congenital adrenal hyperplasia	*CYP17A1*; AR	Low cortisol, gonadal hormones; increased deoxycorticosterone and corticosterone; high progesterone relative to 17α-progesterone	Presentation in adolescence; male pseudohermaphroditism, primary amenorrhea; hypokalemia	Eplerenone, spironolactone; hydrocortisone; gonadal hormones
11β-hydroxylase deficiency[1]	Congenital adrenal hyperplasia	*CYP11B1*; AR	Increased deoxycorticosterone, 11-deoxycortisol and androgens; increased urinary 17-ketosteroids	Virilization; female pseudohermaphroditism; short stature; precocious puberty	Hydrocortisone; if required, eplerenone or spironolactone
Apparent mineralocorticoid excess	Cortisol, not deactivated by 11β-hydroxysteroid dehydrogenase, activates the mineralocorticoid receptor	*HSD11B2*; AR	Increased ratio of cortisol to cortisone metabolites (tetrahydrocortisol + allotetrahydrocortisol: tetrahydrocortisone >1); free cortisol: cortisone >0.5	Low birth weight, failure to thrive; hypercalciuria; nephrocalcinosis; osteopenia; cardiac conduction abnormalities	Eplerenone, spironolactone
Liddle syndrome	Activation of epithelial sodium channel	*SCNN1B*, *SCNN1G*, *SCNN1A*; AD	Low urinary aldosterone (<5 μg/day) or metabolites	Onset in childhood or adoles-cence; metabolic alkalosis; family history common, sudden cardiac death	Amiloride, triamterene
Familial glucocorticoid resistance (Chrousos syndrome)	End organ resistance to glucocorticoids; compensatory increase in ACTH, cortisol, androgens	*NR3C1*; AR, AD	High urinary free cortisol; cortisol >50 nmol/L after overnight DST	Adult-onset hypertension; adrenal hyperplasia; androgen excess (ambiguous genitalia; virilization; precocious puberty; baldness; oligomenorrhea); hypoglycemia	Dexamethasone; eplerenone, spironolactone

Contd...

Contd...

Disease	***Defect***	***Gene; inheritance***	***Features***	***Other abnormalities***	***Treatment***
Activating MR mutation (Geller syndrome)	Increased sensitivity of MR; altered binding to progesterone in pregnancy	*NR3C2*; AD	Spironolactone exacerbates hypertension	Early onset (<20 years) severe hypertension; worsening in pregnancy	Amiloride; finerenone
High or normal aldosterone, low renin; high aldosterone to renin ratio (ARR)					
Glucocorticoid remediable aldosteronism [familial hyperaldosteronism (FHA), type 1]	ACTH sensitive aldosterone production by adrenal zona fasciculata; unresponsive to hypokalemia	Hybrid *CYP11B1* and *CYP11B2*; AD	High urinary 18-hydroxycortisol and 18-oxocortisol; high oxotetrahydrocortisol to tetrahydroaldosterone ratio; aldosterone <4 ng/dL after DST; chimeric gene demonstrated by long-range PCR or Southern blot	Moderate to severe hypertension; hemorrhagic strokes due to ruptured aneurysms; potassium often normal	Prednisolone 2.5–5 mg or dexamethasone 0.125–0.25 mg/kg/day^2; amiloride, triamterene; spironolactone; thiazides worsen hypokalemia
FHA type 2	Depolarization of zona glomerulosa cells by chloride influx stimulates aldosterone synthase	*CLCN2;* AD	Normal adrenals	Delayed onset of hypertension; most common familial form; incomplete penetrance common; variable hypokalemia	Eplerenone, spironolactone
FHA type 3	Adrenal hyperplasia; low potassium influx increases sodium influx, depolarizing zona glomerulosa	*KCNJ5*; AD	High urinary 18-hydroxycortisol; aldosterone not suppressed by DST	Severe hypertension beginning in childhood; polyuria; metabolic alkalosis; severe hypokalemia	Eplerenone, spironolactone; bilateral adrenalectomy

Contd...

Contd...

Disease	*Defect*	*Gene; inheritance*	*Features*	*Other abnormalities*	*Treatment*
FHA type 4	Adrenal nodule or adrenal hyperplasia; depolarization of zona glomerulosa cells by calcium influx	*CACNA1H*; AD	Normal 18-hydroxycortisol; aldosterone suppressed by DST	Severe hypertension; severe hypokalemia; developmental delay or attention deficit	Eplerenone, spironolactone
Primary aldosteronism with seizures and neurological abnormalities (PASNA) syndrome		*CACNA1D*; AD		Early onset severe hypertension; cardiac defects; seizures; cerebral palsy; congenital hyperinsulinemic hypoglycemia	
Hyperchloremic metabolic acidosis; high or normal potassium; normal or high aldosterone; low renin					
Gordon syndrome or pseudohypoaldosteronism (PHA) type 2 A–E (see also **Table 20.8**)	Lack of inhibition of NCCT and ROMK channels by WNK or other proteins	Gain of function *WNK1* (2C); loss of function *WNK4* (2B), *KLHL3* (2D)*, *CUL3* (2E); and chr 1q31-42 (2A)[3]	Low fractional excretion of sodium; hypercalciuria in *WNK* mutations	Adult onset, except in PHA 2E (*CUL3*) and AR PHA 2D (*KLHL3*); PHA 2E has most severe and 2C mildest hypertension; short stature, intellectual impairment, dental abnormalities, muscle weakness	Thiazide

[1]May have high or variable plasma aldosterone

[2]Equivalent to 8–10 mg/m^2/day

[3]All are inherited autosomal dominant (AD) pattern except KLHL3 (20) which is Inherited either are AD or in autosomal recessive (AR) Manner

ACTH: adrenocorticotropic hormone; AD: autosomal dominant; AR: autosomal recessive; chr: chromosome; DHEA: dehydroepiandrosterone; DST: dexamethasone stimulation test; MR: mineralocorticoid receptor; NCCT: sodium chloride cotransporter; PCR: polymerase chain reaction; PRA: plasma renin activity; ROMK: renal outer medullary potassium; WNK: with no lysine (K) kinases

Pathophysiology

In normal conditions, aldosterone is the chief mineralocorticoid regulating electrolyte and water balance through its effects on distal tubules and cortical collecting ducts. Following its binding to a nuclear mineralocorticoid receptor (MR), aldosterone increases synthesis of various proteins, chiefly Na^+-K^+ ATPase on the basolateral surface, and epithelial sodium channels (ENaC) and renal outer medullary potassium channel (ROMK) on the luminal surface, to increase sodium reabsorption and potassium secretion in the distal tubules **(Fig. 25.4A)**. Cortisol is also a ligand for the MR and shows potent salt retaining activity. Cortisol is, however, normally metabolized by 11β-hydroxysteroid dehydrogenase to cortisone, which lacks that action.

The monogenic disorders grouped under "mineralocorticoid" hypertension include: (*i*) increased production of aldosterone (glucocorticoid remediable aldosteronism (GRA), familial hyperaldosteronism (FHA), and familial glucocorticoid resistance); (*ii*) increased production of other hormones with mineralocorticoid action (two forms of congenital adrenal hyperplasia); (*iii*) prereceptor disorder with loss of selectivity of the MR [apparent mineralocorticoid excess (AME)]; (*iv*) receptor disorder with constitutive activation of the MR (Geller syndrome); and (*v*) postreceptor disorder with enhanced function of the ENaC (Liddle syndrome) **(Fig. 25.4A)**. Except for conditions included in (*i*) above, where plasma levels of aldosterone are high and PRA low, all other conditions are characterized by low plasma aldosterone and PRA **(Flowchart 25.3)**. **Table 25.9** summarizes the genetic bases, clinical and biochemical phenotype, and therapy for these conditions **(Annexure 9.8, p 845)**. Patients with congenital adrenal hyperplasia due to deficiency of 17α-hydroxylase (*CYP17A1*) have hypertension due to accumulation of deoxycorticosterone **(Figs. 25.4A and B)**. An inability to form 17-OH-pregnenolone blocks sex hormone synthesis, leading to delayed sexual development in girls and ambiguous genitalia in boys. Deficiency of 11β-hydroxylase (*CYP11B1*) also causes accumulation of deoxycorticosterone, but androgen synthesis is increased, leading to virilization in girls and precocious puberty in boys.

Normally, cortisol is produced by the zona fasciculata via adrenocorticotropic hormone (ACTH)-mediated stimulation of *CYP11B1*, and aldosterone is produced by the zona glomerulosa via angiotensin-II-mediated stimulation of *CYP11B2* **(Figs. 25.4B and C)**. Patients with glucocorticoid remediable hypertension (GRA) or familial hyperaldosteronism type 1 (FHA-1) have a hybrid or chimeric gene on chromosome 8q that consists of the regulatory region of the 11β-hydroxylase (*CYP11B1*) gene coupled to the coding sequence of the aldosterone synthase (*CYP11B2*) gene, resulting in aldosterone synthesis in the cortisol producing region (zona fasciculata) of the adrenal gland. Hence, ectopic synthesis of aldosterone occurs in the zona fasciculata, positively regulated by ACTH and unaffected by angiotensin II

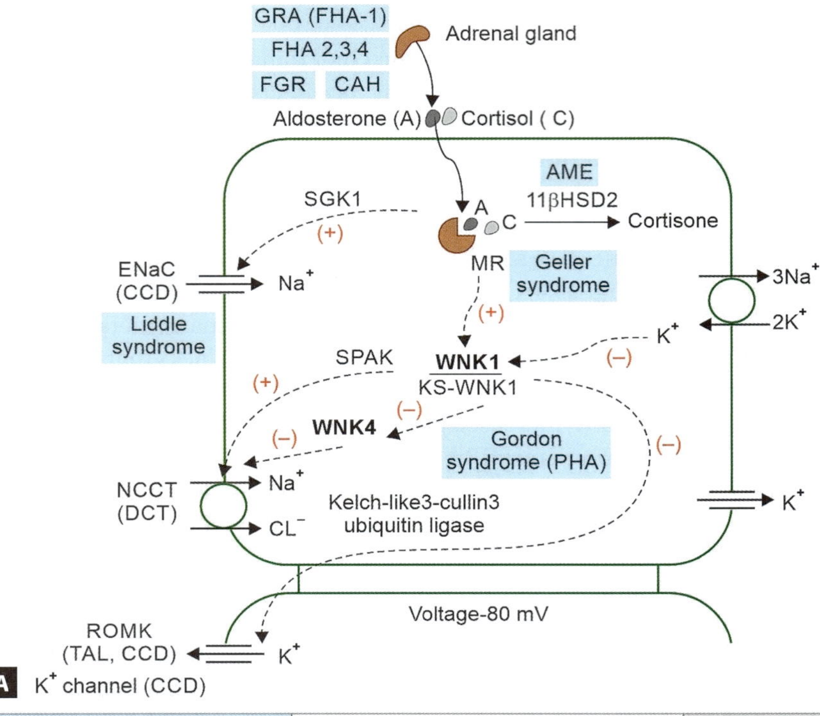
GRA (FHA-1)
FHA 2,3,4
FGR
CAH
Adrenal gland
Aldosterone (A)
Cortisol (C)
AME
11βHSD2
SGK1
A
C
Cortisone
(+)
ENaC
(CCD)
Na+
MR
Geller syndrome
3Na+
Liddle syndrome
(+)
K+
2K+
SPAK
WNK1
(–)
(+)
KS-WNK1
(–)
WNK4
Gordon syndrome (PHA)
(–)
(–)
NCCT
(DCT)
Na+
CL–
Kelch-like3-cullin3 ubiquitin ligase
K+
Voltage-80 mV
ROMK
(TAL, CCD)
K+
A
K+ channel (CCD)

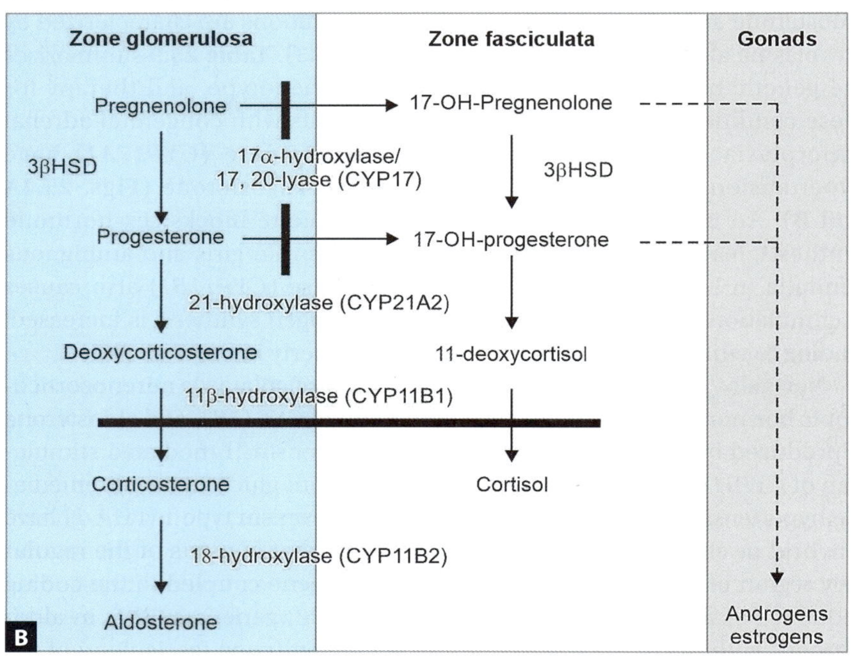
Zone glomerulosa
Zone fasciculata
Gonads
Pregnenolone
17-OH-Pregnenolone
3βHSD
17α-hydroxylase/
17, 20-lyase (CYP17)
3βHSD
Progesterone
17-OH-progesterone
21-hydroxylase (CYP21A2)
Deoxycorticosterone
11-deoxycortisol
11β-hydroxylase (CYP11B1)
Corticosterone
Cortisol
18-hydroxylase (CYP11B2)
Aldosterone
Androgens
estrogens
B

Contd...

Contd...

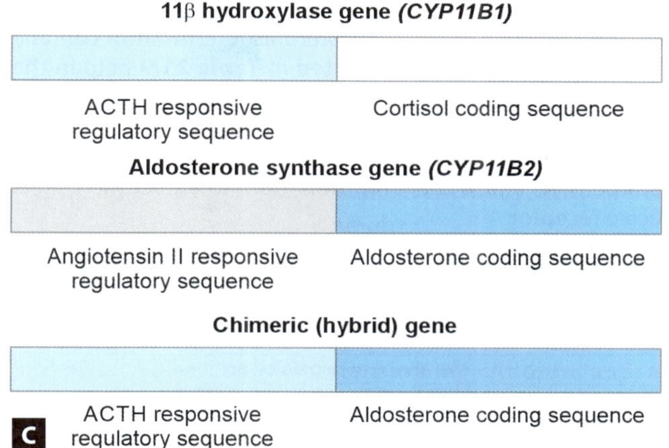

Figs. 25.4A to C: (A) Sodium (Na^+) and potassium (K^+) handling in the thick ascending limb (TAL), distal convoluted tubule (DCT) and principal or intercalated cells of the cortical collecting duct (CCD), shown figuratively in one cell, in relation to aldosterone (A) binding to the mineralocorticoid receptor (MR). The predominant apical Na^+ transporters are the thiazide-sensitive sodium chloride cotransporter (NCCT) in the DCT and the amiloride-sensitive epithelial sodium channel (ENaC) in the CCD. The respective channels for potassium recycling are the renal outer medullary potassium (ROMK) and K^+ channels. Enzyme activation and inhibition are indicated by (+) and (–), respectively. Aldosterone activates the ENaC in the CCD through serum and glucocorticoid-inducible kinase 1 (SGK1) and the NCCT in the late DCT through with-no-lysine kinase 1 (WNK1) and proline alanine-rich kinase (SPAK). Aldosterone effects on ROMK and K^+ channels vary by the stimulus (the "aldosterone paradox") and are likely mediated by the balance between WNK1 and kidney-specific (KS-)WNK1. During hypovolemia, a high WNK1/KS-WNK1 ratio inhibits ROMK to conserve potassium, and inhibits WNK4, which normally inhibits NCCT in the DCT. Thus, hypovolemia-induced hyperaldosteronism stimulates both ENaC and NCCT to conserve Na^+. Hyperkalemia decreases the WNK1/KS-WNK1 ratio, which activates ROMK, thus stimulating K^+ secretion. The low ratio also stimulates WNK4, which inhibits NCCT activation by aldosterone. During hyperkalemia, aldosterone continues to activate ENaC through SGK1, which stimulates Na^+ exchange for K^+ in CCD. Key defects in monogenic forms of hypertension are indicated by textboxes (*see* also **Table 25.9**). (B) *Adrenal steroid biosynthesis and congenital adrenal hyperplasia.* Deficiency of 17α-hydroxylase or 11β-hydroxylase leads to accumulation of deoxycorticosterone (DOC) and hypertension. Sex hormone synthesis is inhibited in patients with 17α-hydroxylase deficiency and increased in those with 11β-hydroxylase deficiency. (C) *Familial hyperaldosteronism (FHA) type 1 or glucocorticoid remediable hypertension* is caused by formation of a chimeric gene containing the regulatory region of the 11β-hydroxylase (*CYP11B1*) gene coupled to the coding sequence of the aldosterone synthase (*CYP11B2*) gene, resulting in aldosterone synthesis in the cortisol producing region (zona fasciculata) of the adrenal gland. 11βHSD: 11β-hydroxysteroid dehydrogenase; ACTH: adrenocorticotropic hormone; AME: apparent mineralocorticoid excess; CAH: congenital adrenal hyperplasia; CUL3: cullin 3; FHA: familial hyperaldosteronism; FGR: familial glucocorticoid resistance; GRA: glucocorticoid remediable aldosteronism; KLHL3: kelch like protein 3; PHA: pseudohypoaldosteronism

Flowchart 25.3: Approach to evaluation for monogenic hypertension. The combination of aldosterone and plasma renin activity **(*see* Box 25.6)** allow distinction of primary aldosteronism and rare familial hyperaldosteronism (FHA) from conditions with low renin and low aldosterone. Evaluations listed in **Table 25.9** help in the differential diagnosis. Patients with hyperaldosteronism require magnetic resonance imaging (MRI) abdomen for adrenal glands. Next generation sequencing ensuring adequate coverage of specific genes is recommended; however, FHA type 1 requires Southern blot or long-range polymerase chain reaction (PCR) to detect the chimeric gene. MR mineralocorticoid receptor

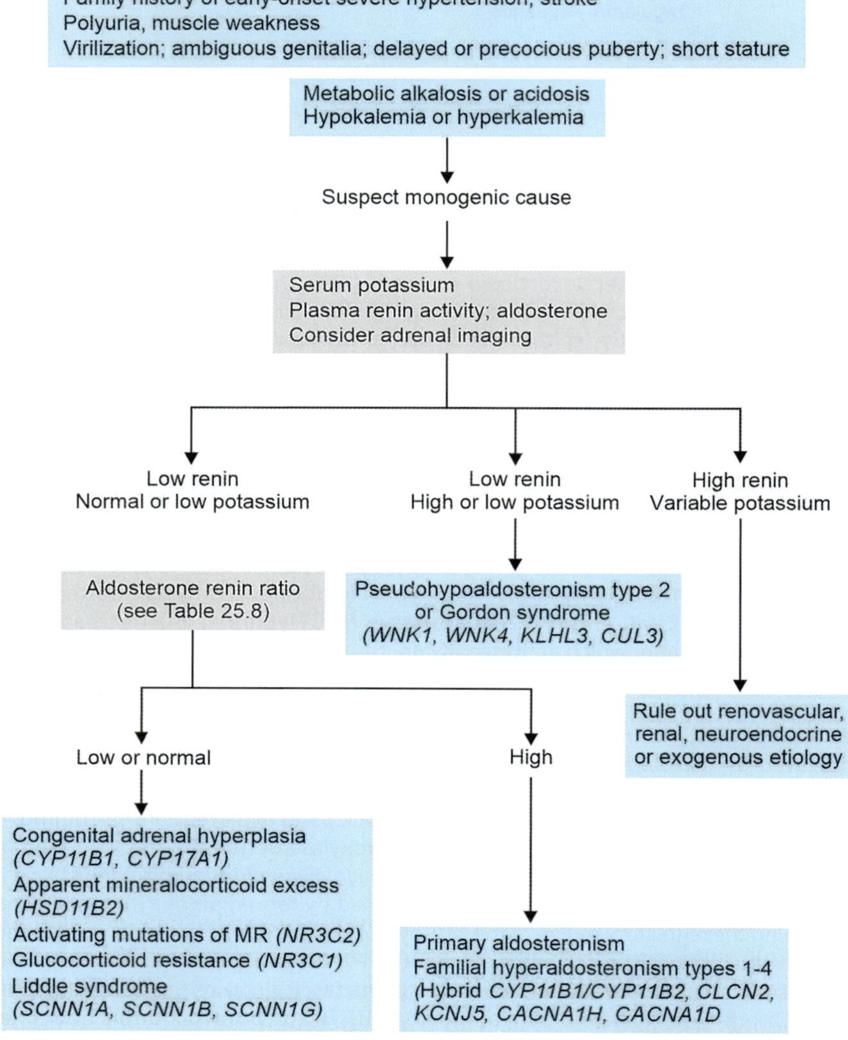

and potassium. Since the aldosterone synthase also carried out 18-hydroxylation and oxidation of the 18-methyl carbon to aldehyde, the production of 18-hydroxycorticosterone metabolites is increased.

Cortisol is a tenfold more potent activator of the MR than aldosterone. In the kidney, 11β-hydroxysteroid dehydrogenase isoform 2 (*HSD11B2*) converts cortisol to cortisone, which does not activate the receptor. In the syndrome of AME, mutations render the enzyme ineffective allowing cortisol to saturate the MR and induce hypertension and hypokalemia. Patients with Geller syndrome have an enzyme isoform with increased sensitivity to mineralocorticoids; increased avidity of binding to progesterone leads to presentation as pregnancy induced hypertension.

Patients with Liddle syndrome, considered the mirror image of pseudohypoaldosteronism type 1, have mutations in the gene encoding β, γ, or α subunits of the ENaC leading to constitutive expression and sodium retention. In Gordon syndrome (considered the mirror image of Gitelman syndrome), gain of function mutations of *WNK1* or loss of function mutations of *WNK4, KLHL3, or CUL3* result in gain in function of sodium chloride cotransporter (NCCT) and ROMK leading to sodium and chloride retention and hyperkalemia. Hyperkalemia is also secondary to loss of tubular luminal electronegativity in the collecting duct due to reduced sodium delivery, that results in decrease in H^+ and potassium absorption.

Liddle Syndrome (Pseudohyperaldosteronism)

Liddle syndrome, an autosomal dominant condition caused by gain-of-function mutations of ENaC, has features akin to hyperaldosteronism. Enhanced Na^+ reabsorption in the distal nephron causes volume expansion, hypertension, and suppressed renin and aldosterone secretion. Functional coupling of Na^+ reabsorption to K^+ and H^+ secretion in the distal nephron results in hypokalemic alkalosis. Liddle syndrome predominantly manifests in teenage children with variable polyuria, increased thirst, failure to thrive, and hypertension. Patients are at risk of cerebral hemorrhage and cardiovascular disease. Levels of urinary mineralocorticoids are within normal limits. Salt restriction or K^+ supplements do not increase aldosterone secretion. No improvement is seen after administration of the MR blocker, spironolactone. Therapy consists of restriction of salt intake and administration of K^+ supplements. Triamterene (2–4; up to 6 mg/kg/day; maximum 300 mg daily) directly inhibits ENaC, resulting in increased urinary Na^+ and decreased K^+ excretion and resolution of hypertension. Amiloride (0.1–0.2 mg/kg q12 h, maximum 10 mg daily) may also be used.

Apparent Mineralocorticoid Excess

This autosomal recessive condition occurs due to deficiency of the renal isoform of the enzyme 11β-hydroxysteroid dehydrogenase. This defect results in high intrarenal levels of cortisol, which binds to MRs resulting in Na^+ retention and urinary K^+ loss. Carbenoxolone or glycyrrhizinic acid (found in licorice compounds) are potent inhibitors of this enzyme. Consumption of these agents may therefore be associated with features similar to AME. Clinical features of this condition closely mimic those of Liddle syndrome and include polyuria, increased thirst, failure to thrive, and early onset hypertension. There is a history of intrauterine growth retardation. Marked hypokalemia and metabolic alkalosis is present. Plasma renin and aldosterone levels are low. The diagnosis is made by detecting elevated urinary levels of hydrogenated metabolites of cortisol to cortisone (tetrahydrocortisol + allotetrahydrocortisol: tetrahydrocortisone). Treatment with oral dexamethasone (10–30 µg/kg daily) suppresses cortisol secretion resulting in reduced Na^+ reabsorption and amelioration of hypertension and hypokalemia. Patients also respond to treatment with potassium supplements combined with spironolactone, triamterene, or amiloride.

Glucocorticoid Remediable Aldosteronism

The GRA (or FHA-1) has autosomal dominant inheritance with aldosterone secretion that is solely under control of ACTH, due to formation of a chimeric gene with ectopic expression of aldosterone synthase activity in zona fasciculata cells of the adrenal cortex under regulation of ACTH **(*see* Fig. 25.4C)**. Consequently, there is hyperaldosteronism and suppression of angiotensin II-stimulated aldosterone production in the zona glomerulosa. Patients present early in life with moderate to severe hypertension. A family history of hypertension, with early deaths due to cerebrovascular accidents is present.

Hypokalemia is characteristic, but serum K^+ may be normal. Levels of PRA are reduced. Although aldosterone levels are high, determination of serum aldosterone has poor sensitivity as a screening test. Hyperaldosteronism is increased by administration of corticotrophin and reduced by glucocorticoids. Following dexamethasone suppression, an aldosterone level of <4 ng/dL is strongly suggestive but lacks specificity. Increased urinary excretion of 18-oxocortisol and 18-hydroxycortisol is characteristic. Genetic testing using molecular biologic techniques for the chimeric gene is 100% sensitive and specific for the diagnosis and is preferred over the dexamethasone suppression test. Treatment with low-dose dexamethasone is useful in reducing blood pressure and correcting electrolyte disturbances. Therapy with MR antagonists is as effective and avoids disruption of the hypothalamic-pituitary-adrenal axis.

Familial forms of Hyperaldosteronism

Familial hyperaldosteronism type 2–4 are dominantly inherited condition that presents with hypertension and hypokalemia. Unlike GRA, hyperaldosteronism in these conditions is associated with gain-of-function mutations in genes encoding channels that affect the polarization of cells in the zona glomerulosa, inducing increased expression of the aldosterone synthase **(*see* Table 25.9)**. Unlike GRA, serum cortisol may not be dexamethasone suppressible. Except for type 2 FHA, patients show familial occurrence of aldosterone producing adenoma or bilateral idiopathic hyperplasia.

Adrenal Enzymatic Disorders

Inherited deficiency of 11β-hydroxylase or 17α-hydroxylase causes mineralocorticoid excess with hypertension and hypokalemic metabolic alkalosis **(*see* Table 25.9)**. Replacement with corticosteroids is beneficial.

Gordon Syndrome

This autosomal dominant disorder is characterized by hypertension, hyperkalemia, and hyperchloremic metabolic acidosis with normal GFR. Hyperkalemia may be present from birth, but as in GRA, hypertension may not develop until later in life. Some patients may have short stature, intellectual impairment, muscle weakness, hypercalciuria, and renal stones. Plasma renin and aldosterone are reduced. Administration of hydrochlorthiazide (1–2 mg/kg/day) or frusemide (1–2 mg/kg/day) results in reversal of clinical and biochemical abnormalities. Sodium bicarbonate is required to correct acidosis.

Evaluation

Monogenic causes of hypertension account for ~2–5% patients with sustained hypertension **(Flowchart 25.3)**. Precautions are necessary while sampling for and interpreting values of plasma aldosterone and renin **(Box 25.6)**. Genetic sequencing is confirmatory and has replaced biochemical investigations. However, targeted next generation sequencing (NGS) **(Annexure 9.8, p 845)** may fail to detect large deletions or duplications, or intronic changes, such as those reported in *CYP11B1, NR3C2, SCNN1B, WNK1, HSBD11B2,* and *CYP17A1.* Multiplex ligation-dependent probe amplification (MLPA) or whole genome sequencing may be necessary. The diagnosis of GRA requires testing by Southern blot or long-range polymerase chain reaction (PCR) to detect the chimeric gene. Sanger sequencing is required to confirm variants detected on NGS, screen parents to confirm segregation, and for antenatal counseling.

PRIMARY ALDOSTERONISM

Primary aldosteronism, caused by bilateral adrenal hyperplasia and adrenal adenoma, is the most common form of mineralocorticoid hypertension. Familial forms may be associated with bilateral adrenal hyperplasia and/or adenoma **(*see* Table 25.9)**. Screening for hyperaldosteronism is recommended in presence of: (*i*) Hypertension and unexplained persistent hypokalemia or diuretic-induced hypokalemia; (*ii*) Severe hypertension

BOX 25.6: Measurement of aldosterone to renin ratio (ARR)

- Correct hypokalemia, aiming to achieve potassium level >4 mEq/L
- Avoid salt restriction: Might increase renin and aldosterone, leading to false negative ARR
- Withdraw agents affecting ARR, such as potassium-wasting diuretics, spironolactone, eplerenone, amiloride, triamterene, and confectionary or chewing tobacco that contains licorice for ≥4 weeks; and β-adrenergic blockers, central α2 antagonists, angiotensin converting enzyme (ACE) inhibitors, angiotensin receptor blockers, and dihydropyridine calcium channel blockers for ≥2 weeks. Prefer to use prazosin, hydralazine, slow-release verapamil, or doxazosin
- Collect blood between 8 and 10 AM, following an upright position (sitting, standing, walking) for at least 2 hr, after seating the patient for 5–15 minutes for sample collection
- Transport sample at room temperature; freeze the plasma immediately if pending assay
- Measure aldosterone by mass spectroscopy, and renin by chemiluminescent assay [direct renin concentration (DRC)] or radioimmunoassay [plasma renin activity (PRA)]
- Base management decisions on multiple values, rather than one ratio
- Interpret the ARR using the following thresholds: >20, if aldosterone is in ng/dL and PRA in ng/mL/h (conventional values); >750, if aldosterone is in pmol/L and PRA in ng/mL/h; >2.5, if aldosterone is in ng/dL and PRA in pmol/L/min; >60, if aldosterone is in pmol/L and PRA in pmol/L/min; >3.7, if aldosterone is in ng/dL and DRC in mU/L; >68, if aldosterone is in pmol/L and DRC in mU/L; >5.7, if aldosterone is in ng/dL and DRC in ng/L; and >144, if aldosterone is in pmol/L and DRC in ng/L[1]
- The renin assay should be sufficiently sensitive to measure levels as low as 0.2–0.3 ng/mL/h of PRA or 2 mU/L of DRC. At very low renin levels (PRA <1 ng/mL/h), ARR might be nonspecifically elevated (false-positive screening), and DRC does not correlate well with PRA
- A diagnosis of primary aldosteronism is supported by an elevated level of aldosterone (usually >15 ng/dL or 416 pmol/L), in addition to elevated ARR.

[1]*Conversion factors:* Aldosterone: 1 ng/dL (conventional unit) ~=27.7 pmol/L (SI unit); PRA: 1 ng/mL/h (conventional unit) ~=12.8 pmol/L/min (SI unit); and DRC: 1 ng/L (conventional unit) ~= 1.58 mU/L (SI unit). PRA to DRC, by immunometric method: 1 ng/mL/h ~=8.2 mU/L (SI unit) or 5.2 ng/L (conventional unit) when measured by the Nichols Institute Diagnostics automated chemiluminescence immunoassay or the Bio-Rad Renin II radioimmunoassay; and 1 ng/mL/h ~= 12 mU/L (SI unit) or 7.6 ng/L (conventional unit) when measured by the Diasorin automated chemiluminescence immunoassay

Source: Funder JW, et al. 2008

that requires ≥3 medications; (*iii*) Onset of hypertension <20 years of age; (*iv*) Adrenal incidentaloma; and (*v*) Family history of hypertension at young age. The ratio of aldosterone to PRA is the method of screening, with precautions in interpretation **(*see* Box 25.6)**. A ratio >20 ng/dL per ng/mL/h (554 pmol/L per ng/mL/h) with plasma aldosterone concentration >15 ng/dL (416 pmol/L) in a morning sample from an ambulatory patient with normokalemia suggests primary aldosteronism. The diagnosis is confirmed by any of IV saline loading, oral sodium loading, fludrocortisone suppression test, and captopril suppression test. Following biochemical confirmation, high resolution adrenal CT and/or magnetic resonance imaging (MRI) should be performed. While unilateral laparoscopic adrenalectomy is recommended for adrenal adenoma or unilateral hyperplasia, patients with bilateral hyperplasia or contraindication(s) to surgery may be treated with spironolactone or eplerenone.

NEUROENDOCRINE TUMORS

Hypertension in childhood may rarely be secondary to pheochromocytoma or paraganglioma, which are tumors originating from chromaffin cells. While pheochromocytoma is localized to the adrenal gland, paragangliomas are present in other locations. Hypertension is caused by catecholamine secretion and/or pressure by tumor mass on vessels. These tumors may occur sporadically or as part of familial syndromes such as multiple endocrine type 2, neurofibromatosis type 1, von Hippel–Lindau syndrome, or familial paraganglioma syndrome.

Patients with neuroendocrine tumors present with acute severe or sustained hypertension, headaches, sweating, and palpitations. Diagnosis is based on the levels of catecholamines and their metabolites in plasma and urine. Elevated plasma metanephrines are considered most sensitive and specific; caution is necessary in collection of sample and interpretation of results in patients receiving antihypertensive agents. CT and MR are reported to have reasonable sensitivity for tumor detection. More recently, nuclear imaging with Gallium-68 DOTATATE, a form of somatostatin-receptor functional imaging, is recommended for the diagnosis. The treatment of choice is the tumor excision. The most important pre- and perioperative consideration is the management of hypertension and monitoring and management of hemodynamic lability. Patients are typically initiated on adrenergic blockade preoperatively: usually with IV phenoxybenzamine for 3 days before surgery, or phenoxybenzamine, prazosin, or other α-blockers orally for 1–3 weeks. Despite these measures, tumor manipulation during surgery often causes hypertension while tumor removal is followed by hypotension. CCBs and selective α-antagonists are useful in avoiding blood pressure lability. Repeat measurement of catecholamines after 1 week are useful to confirm tumor removal and cure. However, metachronous occurrence of multifocal pheochromocytoma is relatively common, and long term monitoring is necessary to detect recurrences. Novel therapeutic approaches, including tyrosine kinase inhibitors (sunitinib, cabozantinib) and genetically targeted therapies, are under investigation.

Annexure 25.1: Normal Values for Auscultatory Blood Pressure in Boys *Scan the QR code below or type the following link in browser window:* https://drive.google.com/file/d/1g-vM537TD9b4V431HrrGFVmybu9tNYJD/view?usp=sharing	
Annexure 25.2: Normal Values for Auscultatory Blood Pressure in Girls *Scan the QR code below or type the following link in browser window:* https://drive.google.com/file/d/1Y2WdNJKgX2ZfR3I6z6GRk72LNFnd67Nf/view?usp=sharing	
Annexure 25.3: Normal Values for Ambulatory Blood Pressure in Boys *Scan the QR code below or type the following link in browser window:* https://drive.google.com/file/d/1kSdrYzChokWariOm75oHPJhdK-1cJr5y/view?usp=sharing	
Annexure 25.4: Normal Values for Ambulatory Blood Pressure in Girls *Scan the QR code below or type the following link in browser window:* https://drive.google.com/file/d/1A4Awg4wf78oUFNsKuADuDaAUd28EenVe/view?usp=sharing	

BIBLIOGRAPHY

1. Authement C, Samuels J, Samuel JP. Antihypertensives in children and adolescents. Curr Hypertens Rep. 2022;24:581-7.
2. Cheung AK, Whelton PK, Muntner P, et al. International Consensus on Standardized Clinic Blood Pressure Measurement - A call to action. Am J Med. 2023;136:438-45.e1.
3. Daniels SR. White coat hypertension often progresses to hypertension. J Pediatr. 2022;251:220-24.
4. De Oliveira Campos JL, Bitencourt L, Silva DF, et al. Renovascular hypertension in pediatric patients: Update on diagnosis and management. Pediatr Nephrol. 2021;36:3853-68.
5. Falkner B, Gidding SS, Baker-Smith CM, et al.; American Heart Association Council on Hypertension. Pediatric primary hypertension: An underrecognized condition. Hypertension. 2023;80:e101-11.

6. Flynn JT, Kaelber DC, Baker-Smith CM, et al. Clinical practice guideline for screening and management of high blood pressure in children and adolescents. Pediatrics. 2017;140:e20171904.
7. Flynn JT, Urbina EM, Brady TM, et al.; American Heart Association. Ambulatory blood pressure monitoring in children and adolescents: A scientific statement from the American Heart Association. Hypertension. 2022;79:e114-24.
8. Funder JW, Carey RM, Fardella C, et al. Case detection, diagnosis and treatment of patients with primary aldosteronism. J Clin Endocrinol Metab. 2008;93(9):3266-81.
9. Goulas I, Evripidou K, Doundoulakis I, et al. Prevalence of masked hypertension and its association with left ventricular hypertrophy in children and young adults with chronic kidney disease: A systematic review and meta-analysis. J Hypertens. 2023;41:699-707.
10. Hanevold CD. White coat hypertension in children and adolescents. Hypertension. 2019;73:24-30.
11. Haseler E, Sinha MD. Hypertension in children and young adults. Pediatr Clin North Am. 2022;69:1165-80.
12. Khandelwal P, Deinum J. Monogenic forms of low-renin hypertension: Clinical and molecular insights. Pediatr Nephrol. 2022;37:1495-509.
13. Lurbe E, Agabiti-Rosei E, Cruickshank JK, et al. 2016 European Society of Hypertension guidelines for the management of high blood pressure in children and adolescents. J Hypertens. 2016;34:1887-920.
14. Lurbe E, Mancia G, Calpe J, et al. Joint statement for assessing and managing high blood pressure in children and adolescents. Front Pediatr. 2023;11:1140357.
15. Miyashita Y, Hanevold C, Faino A, et al. White coat hypertension persistence in children and adolescents: The Pediatric Nephrology Research Consortium Study. J Pediatr. 2022;246:154-60.e1.
16. Narang R, Saxena A, Ramakrishina S, et al. Oscillometric blood pressure in Indian school children. Indian Pediatr. 2015;52:939-45.
17. Seeman T, Hamdani G, Mitsnefes M. Hypertensive crisis in children and adolescents. Pediatr Nephrol. 2019;34:2523-37.
18. Seeman T, Šuláková T, Stabouli S. Masked hypertension in healthy children and adolescents: Who should be screened? Curr Hypertens Rep. 2023;25:231-42.
19. Siddiqi N, Shatat IF. Antihypertensive agents: A long way to safe drug prescribing in children. Pediatr Nephrol. 2020;35:2049-65.
20. Song P, Zhang Y, Yu J, et al. Global prevalence of hypertension in children: A systematic review and meta-analysis. JAMA Pediatr. 2019;173:1154-63.
21. Stabouli S, Beropouli S, Goulas I, et al. Diagnostic evaluation of the hypertensive child. Pediatr Nephrol. 2024;39:339-43.
22. Stergiou GS, Palatini P, Parati G, et al. European Society of Hypertension. European Society of Hypertension practice guidelines for office and out-of-office blood pressure measurement. J Hypertens. 2021;39:1293-302.
23. Thakkar HV, Pope A, Anpalahan M. Masked hypertension: A systematic review. Heart Lung Circ. 2020;29:102-11.
24. Wühl E, Calpe J, Drożdż D, et al. Joint statement for assessing and managing high blood pressure in children and adolescents: Chapter 2. How to manage high blood pressure in children and adolescents. Front Pediatr. 2023;11:1140617.
25. Wühl E, Witte K, Soergel M, et al. German Working Group on Hypertension. Distribution of 24-h ambulatory blood pressure in children: normalized reference values and role of body dimensions. J Hypertens. 2002;20:1995-2007.

CHAPTER 26

Chronic Kidney Disease

Aditi Sinha, Arvind Bagga

INTRODUCTION

The term chronic kidney disease (CKD) refers to structural or functional abnormalities of the kidney lasting for at least 3 months, with or without decreased glomerular filtration rate (GFR). These abnormalities include structural, pathological or functional abnormalities, detected by urinalysis, blood or urine biochemistry, histology, or imaging.

DEFINITION, DIAGNOSIS, AND STAGING

The term CKD was first proposed by the National Kidney Foundation-Kidney Disease and Outcome Quality Initiative (NKF-KDOQI) expert group to identify patients who have kidney damage and/or a GFR below 60 mL/min per 1.73 m^2 lasting for 3 months or longer. It replaced the prior nomenclature of chronic renal failure (CRF), which implied severe and irreversible loss of kidney function that eventually requires kidney replacement therapy (KRT). Similar to the 2012 guidelines, the 2024 Clinical Practice Guidelines of the Kidney Diseases Improving Global Outcomes (KDIGO) define CKD as any abnormality of kidney structure or function which has persisted for at least 3 months and has implications for health.

The KDIGO definition of CKD includes mild alterations in kidney function or structure that have implications for health and outcomes. A diagnosis of CKD is made in the presence of either of the following criteria, present for 3 months or longer—(*a*) GFR below 60 mL/min/1.73 m^2; or (*b*) one or more markers of kidney damage, including any of the following: (*i*) *albuminuria:* Albumin excretion rate >30 mg/24-hr or albumin-to-creatinine ratio >30 mg/g; (*ii*) *urine sediment abnormalities:* Isolated microscopic hematuria with dysmorphic red cells; red cell, white cell, or granular casts; oval fat bodies or fatty casts; and tubular epithelial cells; (*iii*) *electrolyte and other abnormalities due to tubular disorders:* Renal tubular acidosis, nephrogenic diabetes insipidus, potassium and magnesium wasting, Fanconi syndrome, nonalbumin proteinuria, and cystinuria; (*iv*) *abnormalities detected by histology or inferred:* Glomerular diseases [focal segmental glomerulosclerosis (FSGS), autoimmune diseases, systemic infections, drugs, and neoplasia]; vascular diseases (hypertension, ischemia, vasculitis, and thrombotic microangiopathy); tubulointerstitial diseases (urinary infections, stones, obstruction, and drug toxicity); and cystic and congenital diseases; (*v*) *structural abnormalities:* Polycystic kidneys or multiple cysts; congenital abnormalities of the kidney and urinary tract (CAKUT) such as hypodysplastic kidneys or hydronephrosis due to obstruction; cortical scarring due to infarcts, pyelonephritis, or vesicoureteral reflux; renal masses or enlarged kidneys due to infiltrative diseases; or small hyperechoic kidneys; or (*vi*) *history of kidney transplantation.*

The cutoff of 3 months to define chronicity, while arbitrary, helps differentiate CKD from acute kidney injury (AKI) and acute kidney disease (AKD). However, this threshold does not apply to patients in whom there is clear evidence of CKD, e.g., CAKUT in infants ≤3 months of age, and patients with single kidney or polycystic kidneys. In others, proof of chronicity is established by reviewing past estimates of GFR, albuminuria or proteinuria, and urine microscopy; imaging findings such as reduced kidney size or cortical thickness; findings on histopathology such as fibrosis and atrophy; history of conditions known to cause or contribute to CKD; and repeat measurements within and beyond the 3-month threshold.

Staging of Chronic Kidney Disease

The severity of CKD has conventionally been graded based on estimated GFR (eGFR). The GFR is estimated from the level of serum creatinine and height, using the modified Schwartz formula (see Chapter 2). eGFR below 60 mL/min/1.73 m^2 is considered as decreased GFR, and that below 15 mL/min/1.73 m^2 as end-stage kidney disease (ESKD). An eGFR-based classification of CKD was first proposed by the NKF-KDOQI, in which five categories with progressively lower GFR were identified. The GFR categories were retained in subsequent classifications, but the staging was modified by KDIGO in 2012 to add two elements that have implications for patient outcomes and management, namely the etiology and proteinuria. Thus, the 2012 and 2024 KDIGO guidelines use the "CGA" concept to classify CKD based on the cause (C) of CKD, stage of kidney function determined by GFR (G), and degree of albuminuria (A) **(Table 26.1 and Fig. 26.1)**. Pooled data from adult studies indicate that the risk for several important outcomes, including all-cause mortality, cardiovascular disease, and ESKD, increases incrementally both down GFR categories and across albuminuria categories, and influences prognosis. Further, the classification recognizes two subcategories of stage 3, namely G3a and G3b, based on data supporting different outcomes and risk profiles. For adults, the CGA classification helps patients and physicians to understand the disease severity, defines the indications for specialist referral, guides specific investigations and therapeutic interventions, and is a tool to study the epidemiology, natural history, and outcomes of CKD.

There are three concerns with the CGA classification. Stages G1 and G2 are better defined by associated abnormalities (proteinuria, hematuria,

TABLE 26.1: Stages of chronic kidney disease (CKD) based on Clinical Practice Guidelines of the Kidney Diseases Improving Global Outcomes (KDIGO) 2024[1]

GFR category[2]	*eGFR, mL/min/1.73 m²*	*Description*
G1	>90	Normal or high
G2	60–89	Mildly decreased
G3a	45–59	Mildly to moderately decreased
G3b	30–44	Moderately to severely decreased
G4	15–29	Severely decreased
G5	<15, or on dialysis	Kidney failure
Albuminuria category	***Albumin excretion rate, mg/day or albumin creatinine ratio, mg/g***[3]	***Description***
A1	<30	Normal to mildly increased
A2	30–300	Moderately increased
A3	>300	Severely increased

[1]CKD is classified based on three parameters, namely cause or etiology, estimated glomerular filtration rate (eGFR) and albuminuria, abbreviated as "CGA"
[2]In the absence of evidence of kidney injury (see text), categories G1 or G2 alone do not fulfil criteria for CKD
[3]Albumin creatinine ratios, measured on 24-hr urine samples, are approximately equivalent to albumin excretion rate

and structural anomalies) than by the eGFR. GFR varies with age, gender, and body size, increasing with renal maturation from infancy to reach adult values at 2 years of age; hence, CKD stages based on eGFR apply only to children >2-year-old. Unlike in the elderly, an eGFR below 90 mL/min/1.73 m^2 is alarming in childhood or adolescence since healthy children should have excellent kidney function. Finally, the prognostic utility of the CGA classification in children with CKD is unclear. Other than CGA, additional factors and events might influence the risk of progression of childhood-onset CKD, such as low nephron endowment, low birth weight, prematurity, small kidney size, genetic disease, history of AKI, and exposure to nephrotoxic drugs.

Analysis of data from the two longitudinal pediatric CKD cohorts (ESCAPE and CKiD) has been used to create six ordered stages of pediatric CKD using combinations of categories of eGFR (60–89, 45–59, 30–44, and 15–29 mL/min/1.73 m^2) and urine protein to creatinine ratio (PCR: <0.5, 0.5–2.0, and >2.0 mg/mg) which provides an incremental estimate of the time to ESKD in children, similar to the KDIGO CGA classification. Median times to ESKD range from >10 years for KDIGO CKD G3a with UPCR <0.5 mg/mg, to 0.8 years for CKD G4 and UPCR >2 mg/mg. Further, across stages, the time to ESKD was almost half for patients with glomerular compared to nonglomerular

				Albuminuria categories		
				A1	A2	A3
				Normal to mildly increased	Moderately increased	Severely increased
				<30 mg/g <3 mg/mmol	30–300 mg/g 3–30 mg/mmol	>300 mg/g >30 mg/mmol
GFR categories (mL/min/1.73 m^2)	G1	Normal or high	≥90			
	G2	Mildly decreased	60–89			
	G3a	Mildly to moderately decreased	45–59			
	G3b	Moderately to severely decreased	30–44			
	G4	Severely decreased	15–29			
	G5	Kidney failure	<15			

Fig. 26.1: Staging of CKD by glomerular filtration rate (GFR) and albuminuria categories based on the KDIGO 2024 guidelines. The combined associations of eGFR and ACR categories are presented as "heatmaps," a color-coded depiction of the associations of increased risk with worsening CKD for 10 outcomes in adult patients, including two general (all-cause mortality and all-cause hospitalization), two kidney-specific (kidney failure and AKI) and six cardiovascular (cardiovascular mortality, myocardial infarction, heart failure, stroke, atrial fibrillation, and peripheral arterial disease) outcomes. Green indicates low risk (if no other markers of kidney disease are present, considered as no CKD); yellow indicates moderately increased risk; orange indicates high risk; and red indicates very high risk. The associations between eGFR and risks are stronger when using the combined creatinine and cystatin CKD-EPI equation. These heatmaps have not been verified in pediatric cohorts. ACR: albumin creatinine ratio; AKI: acute kidney injury; CKD: chronic kidney disease; eGFR: estimated glomerular filtration rate

disease. However, this classification has not been validated across diverse pediatric CKD cohorts.

EPIDEMIOLOGY

Data from hospital-based studies suggests that the prevalence of pediatric CKD G2–G5 varies from 30 per million age-related population (pmarp) in Japan to 882 pmarp in Israel. Epidemiological studies and registry data from Europe, US, Japan, and Australasia indicate that the prevalence of CKD 2–5 or albuminuria is higher, affecting around 0.3–1% of children. This is consistent with prevalence estimates of CKD in young adults (20–29 years old), which is estimated at 1.8–2.6% globally. These estimates suggest that pediatric CKD is approximately as prevalent as childhood cancers and type 1 diabetes mellitus. Data from developing regions, including south Asia, is limited.

The incidence of ESKD in childhood was reported at 4 pmarp per year in Japan, 9 pmarp per year in Europe and Australia/New Zealand, and 13 pmarp per year in the United States. Similarly, the prevalence of ESKD ranges from 22 pmarp in Japan, to 55 pmarp in Australia and New Zealand, 60 pmarp in Europe, and 77 pmarp in USA. The incidence of children initiated on dialysis across Europe was 5.5–6.6 pmarp during 2007–2016, with the prevalence rising by 2% annually, from 26.4 pmarp in 2007 to 32.1 pmarp in 2016. The incidence and prevalence of ESKD is higher in boys, older children and African-Americans. Since most patients with ESKD in developing regions do not receive KRT, accurate estimates of ESKD in these areas in lacking.

ETIOLOGY

Important conditions causing CKD are shown in **Table 26.2**. CAKUT, such as posterior urethral valve, hypodysplasia, and reflux nephropathy, are leading causes of CKD in childhood. In older children, glomerulonephritis and FSGS are an important cause of CKD. Global registry data indicates that the leading cause of ESKD in childhood is CAKUT, followed by glomerular diseases (glomerulonephritis and FSGS). Overall, the proportion of CAKUT decreases with advancing age, and that of glomerular diseases increases. However, in sub-Saharan Africa, primary glomerular diseases appear to account for 50% of childhood-onset ESKD initiated on dialysis. Important causes in infancy include obstructive uropathy, renal cortical necrosis, infantile polycystic kidney disease, and renal hypoplasia. The etiology of CKD remains unknown in a fair proportion of patients with CKD. With availability of genetic testing, several patients are identified to have hereditary nephropathies and ciliopathies as underlying causes of CKD in childhood.

Disorders that increase risk for CKD are listed in **Box 26.1**. Children with these conditions merit regular follow-up to detect CKD timely. Patients with AKI are at considerable risk of CKD on the long term, especially if AKI is severe. The risk of development of inherited glomerulopathies (e.g., Alport syndrome and MYH9-related disease) and cystic kidney disease (polycystic kidneys and nephronophthisis) is determined by the inheritance pattern. Overall, almost 10% of patients with CKD, regardless of family history and age at presentation, have been observed to carry pathogenic and likely pathogenic variant(s) that represent a plausible genetic basis for the causation or progression of CKD.

PATHOPHYSIOLOGY OF CHRONIC KIDNEY DISEASE AND ITS PROGRESSION

Compensatory Mechanisms

The kidneys maintain chemical homeostasis despite loss of nephrons through changes in the remnant glomerular and tubular function and structure. Important functional changes include: (*i*) *Increase in single nephron GFR*:

TABLE 26.2: Etiology of chronic kidney disease (CKD) in childhood

Etiology	*Usual % (range)*	
	CKD 2–5[1a]	*CKD 5/5D*[1b]
Glomerular diseases: *Glomerulonephritis:* Idiopathic; with systemic diseases[2] Focal segmental glomerulosclerosis Alport syndrome Congenital nephrotic syndrome Amyloidosis	9–21 (5–47)	18–29
Congenital anomalies of the kidney and urinary tract:	41–61 (34–64)	29–40
Obstructive uropathy: Posterior urethral valves[3]	8–20 (4–26)	
Hypodysplasia with/without vesicoureteric reflux	17–49 (9–58)	
Reflux nephropathy with/without hypodysplasia	6–12 (0–26)	
Cystic kidney diseases: Autosomal recessive polycystic kidney disease Nephronophthisis	11–19 (6–26)	10–22
Tubulointerstitial disease: *Inherited defects:* Cystinosis, primary hyperoxaluria, Dent disease, Bartter syndrome, and hypomagnesemia with hypercalciuria *Acquired:* Nephrolithiasis and sickle cell disease		
Acute kidney injury: Acute cortical necrosis Hemolytic uremic syndrome	1–3 (0–8)	19–32
Unknown[4]		

[1]Based on data from [a]11 and [b]4 large international registries across the world
[2]*Examples:* Systemic lupus, IgA vasculitis, polyarteritis nodosa, microscopic polyarteritis; hepatitis B or C; HIV
[3]Less common causes are bilateral pelviureteric or ureterovesical junction obstruction
[4]Might include etiologies from other categories, if evaluated late in disease course

BOX 26.1: Risk factors for chronic kidney disease in children

Congenital anomalies of the kidney and urinary tract (CAKUT)
- Vesicoureteric reflux associated with recurrent urinary infections and kidney scar(s)
- Obstructive uropathy
- Renal dysplasia or hypoplasia
- Solitary functional kidney

History of acute nephritis or IgA vasculitis
Systemic lupus erythematosus or vasculitis
Nephrotic syndrome
History of acute kidney injury, especially if severe or in neonatal period
Family history of polycystic kidneys or inherited kidney disease
Low birth weight; prematurity
Presence of diabetes and hypertension

An increase in glomerular blood flow to the remaining functional nephrons, through relatively greater dilatation of the afferent versus the efferent arterioles, increases the transcapillary hydraulic pressure and single nephron GFR, and therefore augments the total GFR; (*ii*) *tubuloglomerular balance*: Increased filtration from normal glomeruli is associated with a proportionate increase in reabsorption of sodium, glucose, and amino acids from the corresponding tubule, as well as increase in tubular secretion of fixed acids and potassium, such that these tubular functions increase to compensate for the decline in the number of tubules, and the urine output remains relatively unchanged, despite increase in GFR. Corresponding structural changes include (*i*) an increase in glomerular volume, secondary to a hemodynamically mediated increase in capillary lumen volume, hypertrophy of glomerular cells, and increase in mesangial matrix; and (*ii*) an increase in tubule size and volume, predominantly affecting proximal tubules.

Mechanisms of progressive kidney injury regardless of the etiology of CKD, once there is a critical loss of nephron mass, kidney failure is progressive. **Figures 26.2A to C** demonstrates important pathways that determine progressive kidney injury in patients with CKD. When a proportion of nephrons is damaged, the remaining compensate for the loss of renal function by hyperperfusion and hyperfiltration, which gradually leads to glomerular injury and sclerosis and indirectly, to tubulointerstitial inflammation and fibrosis. While glomerular inflammation and glomerulosclerosis are most pronounced in glomerular diseases **(Fig. 26.2A)**, inflammatory pathways are also activated in patients with acute tubular injury **(Fig. 26.2B)**, and nonspecifically following activation of renin-angiotensin-aldosterone system (RAAS) in any form of CKD **(Fig. 26.2C)**. Systemic hypertension is associated with loss of glomerular autoregulation, leading to intraglomerular hypertension that causes increased filtration pressure, glomerular injury, and proteinuria. Proteinuria triggers vasoactive signaling with release of angiotensin-II, aldosterone and endothelin-I, as well as proinflammatory signaling. Downstream signaling further mediates inflammation, epithelial mesenchymal transformation, and fibrosis **(Fig. 26.2C)**. Fibrosis may be initiated by (*i*) interstitial inflammatory cells that mediate healing and injury; (*ii*) interstitial myofibroblasts, derived from kidney stroma (fibroblasts and pericytes), that generate extracellular matrix proteins; (*iii*) tubular epithelial cells, in response to acute tubular injury; and (*iv*) loss of interstitial capillary integrity, leading to hypoxia, oxidant stress, and consequent injury and fibrosis **(Figs. 26.2A to C)**. The pathways illustrated in **Figures 26.2A to C** are potential targets for interventions aimed at retarding progression of CKD.

Risk Factors for Chronic Kidney Disease Progression

Even without additional kidney injury, most forms of advanced CKD show decline in eGFR over time. However, the rate of decline in GFR ("GFR slope") varies among individuals and diseases. Important factors that are associated with CKD progression in childhood include: (*i*) *Etiology of CKD*: Glomerular diseases progress rapidly compared to CAKUT, which are associated with slight gain in eGFR in the first 2 years of life, steady GFR through childhood and steep decline during puberty; (*ii*) *baseline eGFR*: The lower the eGFR, the steeper the GFR slope; (*iii*) *Age at onset*: Diagnosis of advanced CKD in infancy or early childhood is associated with high risk of ESKD in childhood; (*iv*) *puberty*: Rapid decline in GFR is observed during adolescence, possibly

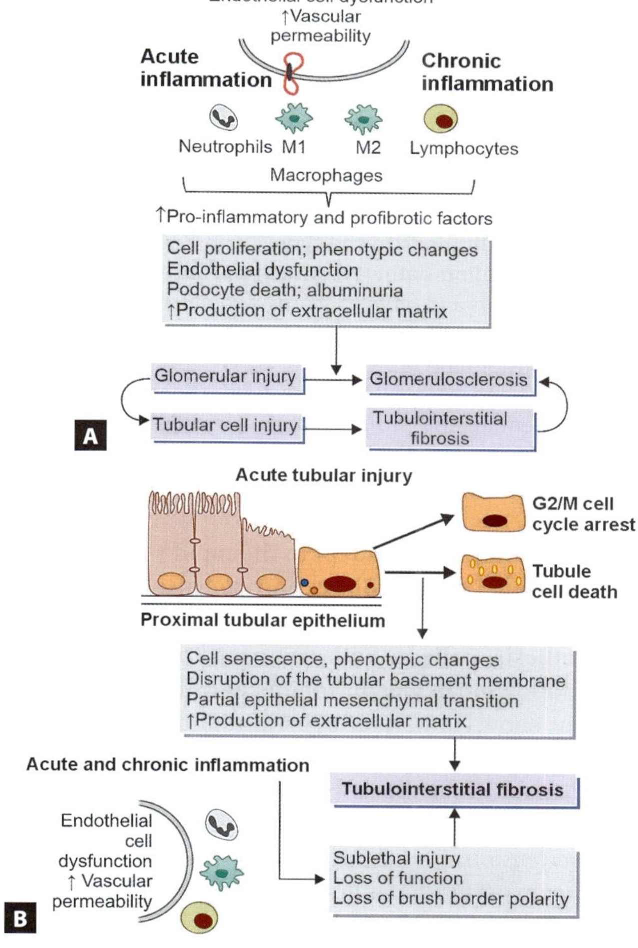

Contd...

Contd...

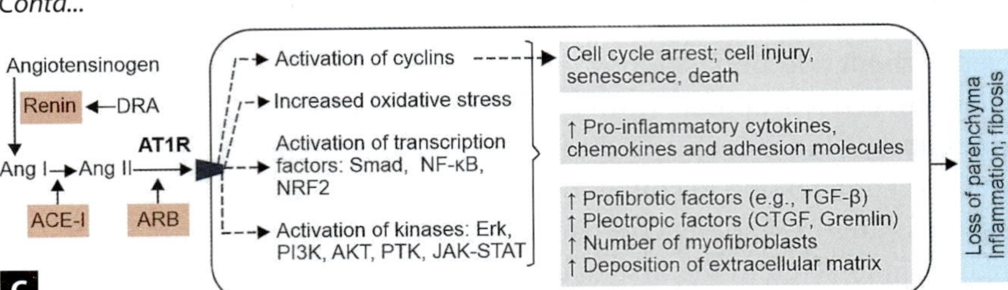

Figs. 26.2A to C: Pathophysiology of progression of chronic kidney disease (CKD). (A) Glomerular injury and fibrosis. Glomerular injury is associated with the recruitment of inflammatory cells, leading to characteristic cytokine secretion patterns of acute and chronic inflammation. Tubular cell injury and interstitial fibrosis follow, through diverse mechanisms, this induces glomerulosclerosis *via* proinflammatory and profibrotic cytokines; (B) Acute kidney injury (AKI) to CKD transition. Tubular epithelial cells are acutely sensitive to hypoxia and hypoperfusion since their cellular functions are dependent on mitochondrial ATP. Acute tubular injury is followed by either cell death due to apoptosis and regulated necrosis, or sublethal injury, leading to partial epithelial mesenchymal transition with loss of tight junctions and/or polarity, and G2/M cell cycle arrest. Stressed and injured tubular cells secrete inflammatory mediators that mediate further tubular injury. Disruption of the tubular basement membrane by activated matrix metalloproteinases contributes to tubulointerstitial fibrosis; (C) Persistent renin–angiotensin–aldosterone system (RAS) activation leads to progressive CKD. Angiotensin II (Ang II) binds to the type 1 Ang II receptor (AT1R) to activate various intracellular signaling pathways, which produce reactive oxygen species, activate transcription factors and protein kinases, and dysregulate cell growth through cyclins. Proinflammatory and profibrotic factors promote inflammation and fibrosis. Ang II upregulates transforming growth factor β1 (TGFβ1, which induces epithelial–mesenchymal transition and extracellular matrix production); connective tissue growth factor (CTGF) and Gremlin, and proinflammatory mediators. RAS blockade using angiotensin-converting enzyme inhibitor (ACEI), angiotensin receptor blocker (ARBs), or direct renin antagonists (DRA) slow progression of proteinuric CKD

because diseased kidneys fail to adapt to the rapid somatic growth through glomerular and tubular hypertrophy, and because of the negative effect of increased levels of sex steroids; (*v*) *low nephron endowment*: According to Brenner hypothesis, patients with decreased nephron number, such as in premature and low birth weight infants and those born with a solitary functional kidney, show glomerular hyperfiltration that results in secondary FSGS and progressive nephron loss; (*vi*) *albuminuria or proteinuria*: Data from seven pediatric CKD cohorts confirms findings of adult cohorts that the presence of albuminuria or proteinuria significantly increases the risk of ESKD; (*vii*) *Hypertension*: Data from two large pediatric cohorts each have demonstrated that hypertension is an independent risk factor for progression of CKD (NAPRTCS and CKiD), and that strict control of blood pressure is associated with slower decline in GFR (ESCAPE and CKiD). Less consistent risk factors include genetic predisposition, male sex, Afro-American race/ethnicity, dyslipidemia, anemia, metabolic acidosis, hyperuricemia, and obesity.

Risk Prediction

Various risk prediction equations have been validated for predicting risk of ESKD in adults with CKD G3–G5, the most widely used of which is the Kidney failure Risk Equation (KFRE, **Annexure 26.1; p 673**). In adults, the KDIGO advises that patients with a 5-year kidney failure risk of 3–5% should be referred to nephrology, those with a 2-year kidney failure risk of >10% are initiated on multidisciplinary care, and those with 2-year kidney failure risk of >40% are educated regarding options of modality for KRT to allow timely planning of placement of vascular access or peritoneal dialysis catheter or planning for live-related transplantation. Further, disease-specific risk prediction equations, e.g., for immunoglobulin A (IgA) nephropathy and autosomal dominant polycystic kidney disease, guide specific management. However, risk prediction equations developed for adults are not validated in children with CKD. Two pediatric CKD risk prediction equations derived from the Caucasian CKiD and ESCAPE cohorts, based on age, sex, glomerular or nonglomerular etiology, eGFR, hypertension, and/or proteinuria, are available at **Annexures 26.2 and 26.3 (p 673)** respectively. These require validation across ethnicities and etiologies.

SYSTEMIC FEATURES

Patients with CKD G3–G5 usually present with anorexia, not thriving well, growth retardation, anemia, hypertension, and bone deformities. These are discussed below.

Malnutrition

Lack of weight gain and slowing of linear growth are the most common findings in children with CKD. Malnutrition in CKD is multifactorial, caused by anorexia, nausea or vomiting due to uremia or gastritis, altered taste, and appropriate or inappropriate dietary restrictions. Children with advanced CKD often require restriction of dietary salt, phosphate, and/or potassium. Salt restriction makes food unpalatable, phosphate restriction inadvertently limits protein intake, and potassium restriction limits food choices. Protein restriction, while recommended for adults with CKD, is inadvisable in children, in whom evidence does not support its role in retarding CKD progression and might contribute to growth failure. Maintenance dialysis, particularly chronic peritoneal dialysis, is associated with significant loss of proteins.

Growth Retardation

One-third to two-thirds of patients with ESKD have short adult height. Age at onset of CKD and severity of CKD are the chief determinants of stature. Suppression of growth during two periods: (*i*) Infancy and (*ii*) puberty, appears to be most relevant to adult height. Normal children usually achieve one-third of their adult stature by the end of second year of life. In this period, linear growth is chiefly determined by nutrition. Malnutrition in CKD is caused by anorexia, frequent vomiting, increased catabolism, and increased losses of water and electrolytes, particularly in young children with obstructive uropathy and renal dysplasia.

Metabolic acidosis and inflammatory cytokines suppress the secretion of growth hormone (GH) from the pituitary and reduce GH receptor expression, leading to GH insensitivity **(Fig. 26.3)**. Growth plate senescence, caused by decreased proliferation of the progenitor chondrocytes in the resting zone, leads to slowing of linear growth throughout childhood. Due to retarded skeletal maturation, the height age and bone age lag behind the chronological age. The decline in height velocity is disproportionately more in the 2–3 years preceding puberty. The onset of puberty and the pubertal growth spurt are delayed by 2–2.5 years, although it occurs at the appropriate bone age **(Fig. 26.3)**. As compared to normal children, the growth spurt in children with CKD is both brief and less intense. High levels of parathormone (PTH) may destroy the growth plate architecture and may cause slipped capital femoral epiphysis or metaphyseal fractures. Conversely, patients with suppressed PTH levels (adynamic bone disease) show stunting since PTH stimulates the expression of vitamin D receptor and synthesis of insulin-like growth factor 1 (IGF-1) in the growth plate.

Other factors contributing to growth failure in CKD are metabolic acidosis, anemia, and salt wasting. Anemia might inhibit growth through anorexia, myocardial dysfunction, and reduced oxygen delivery to cartilage. Fluid and electrolyte losses in patients with renal dysplasia and tubular diseases, and prolonged use of corticosteroids in glomerular diseases also contribute to growth failure.

Mineral and Bone Disease

Kidneys participate in the homeostasis of calcium and phosphorus **(Fig. 26.4)**. Renal 1-α hydroxylase converts 25-dihydroxyvitamin D_3 into 1,25-dihydroxyvitamin D_3 (calcitriol) in response to hypocalcemia or PTH, which in turn promotes intestinal calcium and phosphate absorption, renal calcium and phosphorus reabsorption, and bone mineralization. Fibroblast growth factor 23 (FGF23), a hormone released from bones in response to high serum phosphate, PTH or 1,25-dihydroxyvitamin D_3, enhances urinary

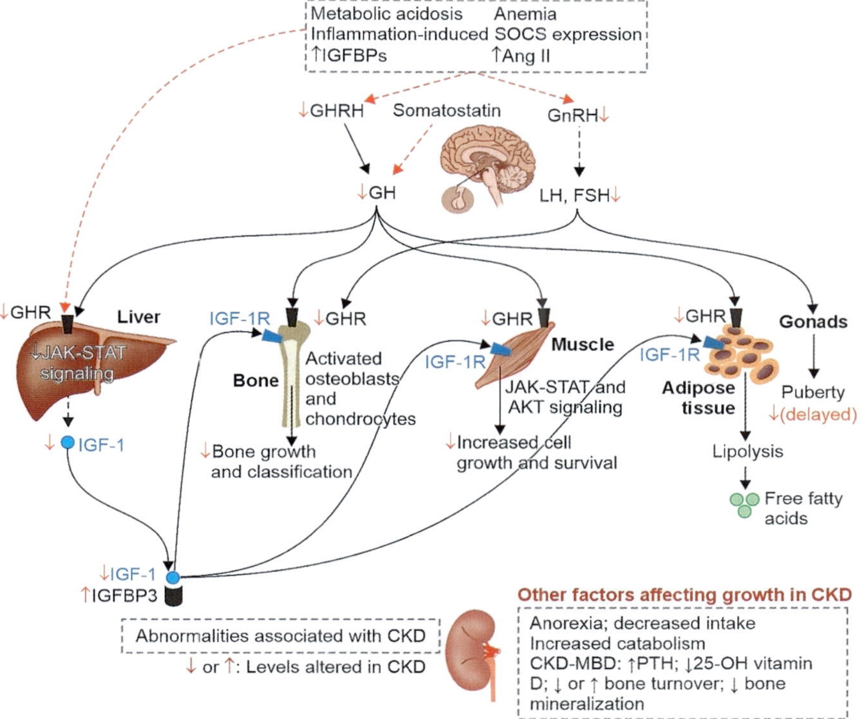

Fig. 26.3: Factors regulating growth and the impact of chronic kidney disease (CKD). Growth hormone (GH) and insulin-like growth factor 1 (IGF-1) are the key determinants of bone growth and ossification, muscle growth and survival and fat metabolism. Patients with CKD are in a state of GH insensitivity, the hallmark of which is a deficiency of functional IGF-1, due to reduced (↓) GH receptor (GHR) expression in target organs and altered GHR signaling through the Janus kinase (JAK) 2 signal transducer and activator of transcription (STAT) 5 pathway. This is chiefly secondary to increased expression of suppressor of cytokine signaling (SOCS), induced by inflammation, and excessive synthesis of IGF binding proteins (IGFBPs). Uremia also reduces the release of hypothalamic growth hormone-releasing hormone (GHRH) and gonadotropin-releasing hormone (GnRH), associated with inhibition by angiotensin II (Ang II). Decreased levels of luteinizing hormone (LH) and follicle-stimulating hormone (FSH) cause hypogonadism and delayed and reduced pubertal growth spurt. AKT: PI3K-Akt signaling pathway, comprised of phosphatidylinositol 3-kinase (PI3K) and protein kinase B (Akt). MBD: mineral bone disease; PTH: parathyroid hormone

excretion of phosphorus by downregulating luminal surface expression of sodium-dependent phosphate cotransporters, NaPi2a and NaPi2c, as does PTH. FGF23 also suppresses 1-α hydroxylase and stimulates 24-hydroxylase to downregulate 1,25-dihydroxyvitamin D_3 (calcitriol) **(Fig. 26.4)**.

The CKD-mineral bone disease (MBD) is a systemic disorder of mineral and bone metabolism in CKD that is characterized by one or more of the following—(*i*) abnormal calcium, phosphorus, PTH, or vitamin D

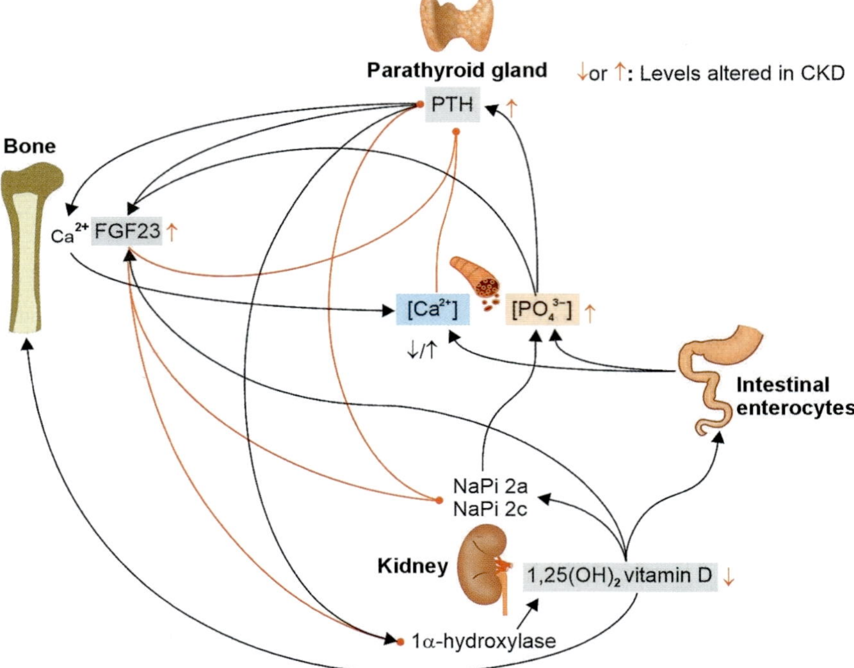

Fig. 26.4: Roles of parathyroid hormone (PTH), 1,25-dihydroxyvitamin D, and fibroblast growth factor 23 (FGF23) in regulating calcium and phosphorus balance. Arrows (↓,↑) indicate how levels are altered in mineral bone disease associated with chronic kidney disease (CKD-MBD). Black and red lines indicate stimulation and inhibition, respectively

metabolism; (*ii*) abnormal bone histology, linear growth, or strength; and (*iii*) vascular or other soft tissue calcification. The term "renal osteodystrophy" refers to histological abnormalities on bone biopsy.

The first biochemical change in patients with CKD G2–G3 is increased levels of FGF23, likely in response to episodic hyperphosphatemia due to reduced urinary phosphate excretion. As GFR declines, frank hyperphosphatemia is observed, which stimulates increased synthesis and secretion of PTH from parathyroid glands, termed secondary hyperparathyroidism. Increased levels of FGF23 inhibit synthesis of 1,25-dihydroxyvitamin D_3 to cause hypocalcemia, which further stimulates PTH release. Vitamin D deficiency, common in patients with CKD due to dietary restrictions, decreased outdoor activity, and increased catabolism and proteinuria, also contributes to secondary hyperparathyroidism. Despite secondary hyperparathyroidism and elevated FGF23, serum phosphate levels remain elevated at low GFR. Prolonged stimulation causes parathyroid gland hyperplasia, which may uncommonly be complicated by parathyroid gland adenoma, termed tertiary hyperparathyroidism.

Elevated circulating PTH leads to bone demineralization. Bone remodeling affects bone strength, while alterations in the growth plate cartilage cause failure of linear growth. Secondary hyperparathyroidism results in osteitis fibrosis cystica, bone resorption, fractures, and deformities. Additional deficiency of 1,25-dihydroxyvitamin D_3 leads to rickets or osteomalacia. Metabolic acidosis also contributes to impaired bone mineralization. Adynamic lesions (low turnover disease) may occur following oversuppression of PTH by therapy with 1,25-dihydroxyvitamin D_3, or excessive use of aluminum-containing phosphate binders.

Vascular calcifications and left ventricular hypertrophy are associated with elevated FGF23 levels and mediated by osteoblast-like transformation of arterial medial smooth muscle cells, along with loss of vascular elasticity, possibly due to decreased expression of Klotho, the coreceptor for FGF23. The risk of vascular calcifications increases with hypercalcemia, hyperphosphatemia, elevated levels of calcium-phosphorus product, and use of high doses of calcium and 25-hydroxyvitamin D.

Clinical features of CKD-MBD vary by the age at onset of CKD, CKD stage, and its duration. Infants and young children present with rickets, manifest as rachitic rosary, wrist widening, Harrison sulcus, and genu varum, often associated with hypotonia and delayed dentition and motor development. Older children present with genu valgum, femoral and wrist deformities, and rarely, slipped epiphyses. Rare findings, seen in advanced CKD, include scoliosis, vertebral compression fractures, thoracic deformities, avascular necrosis of the femoral head, and pathologic fractures of long bones.

Anemia

Anemia of CKD, usually seen in CKD G3–G4, might be the first presentation of CKD. Typical symptoms are pallor, easy fatigability, and reduced exercise tolerance. Peripheral blood film shows normocytic normochromic red cells, with or without microcytic hypochromic red cells, suggesting iron deficiency. If performed, bone marrow aspirate shows decreased or normal erythroid to myeloid ratio. Anemia impairs neurocognitive function and worsens quality of life. Cardiovascular adaptations in response to anemia lead to left ventricular hypertrophy and dilatation and myocardial ischemia, which predispose to cardiovascular morbidity and mortality and progressive CKD.

Anemia in CKD is multifactorial, arising from true and functional iron deficiency and from reduced erythropoietin production. **Figure 26.5** illustrates iron handling in health and CKD and mechanisms of anemia of CKD. Iron deficiency in advanced CKD results from reduced intake and enteral absorption of iron, and increased losses. "Functional" iron deficiency is mediated by increased levels of hepcidin, produced by the liver in response to inflammation and sequestration of iron stores. Hepcidin reduces dietary absorption of iron, while reduced erythropoietin production leads to impaired bone marrow responsiveness and utilization of iron. Hypoxia or iron deficiency induce production of hypoxia-inducible factors (HIFs) that stimulate erythropoietin production by kidneys, as well as mobilize iron from the gut and body stores **(Fig. 26.5)**. HIF-prolyl-hydroxylase inhibitors

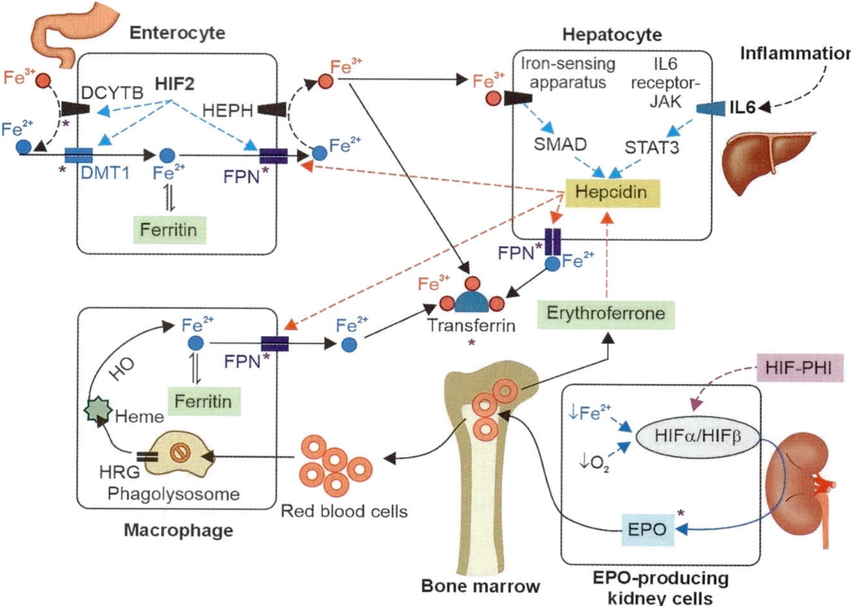

Fig. 26.5: Iron homeostasis and the pathophysiology of anemia in chronic kidney disease. Macrophages in the reticuloendothelial system recycle iron (Fe) from senescent red blood cells (RBCs) through heme oxygenase (HO) to release ferrous (Fe^{2+}) iron which exits the cell through ferroportin (FPN). A smaller amount of body iron is contributed by dietary absorption and other body stores, e.g., in liver. Intracellularly, iron is stored as ferritin, while plasma iron is bound to transferrin. Hepcidin, a hormone produced by the liver in response to iron and inflammation, prevents iron overload and limits iron availability to pathogens. Hepcidin controls systemic iron homeostasis chiefly by inducing degradation of the iron exporter FPN to reduce iron entry into plasma from dietary sources and body stores. In the kidney, low oxygen (O_2) and low iron conditions stimulate the production of HIFs. HIFs are transcription activators that regulate the production of erythropoietin (EPO) in the kidney, ferrireductase (DCYTB), FPN and divalent metal transporter 1 (DMT1) in the duodenum, and the plasma iron carrier transferrin, as indicated by purple asterisk (*). Binding of oxygen to proline hydroxylases ('oxygen sensors') induces the proteasomal degradation of HIF-1α. In hypoxia or iron deficiency, HIF-1α translocates to the nucleus, and together with HIF-1β, binds to a hypoxia responsive element on DNA to transcribe target genes. HIF-PHIs are drugs that upregulate hypoxia-inducible factors (HIFs) similar to hypoxia. In the bone marrow, EPO induces erythroid progenitor cells to produce erythroferrone, which suppresses hepcidin. Red interrupted lines indicate inhibition. DCYTB: duodenal cytochrome B; HEPH: hephaestin; HRG: heme transporter HRG1; JAK: Janus kinase; PHI: prolyl-hydroxylase inhibitor; SMAD: suppressor of mothers against decapentaplegic proteins

(HIF-PHI) achieve the same result as hypoxia to ameliorate functional iron deficiency. Apart from stimulating erythropoiesis, erythropoietin induces production of erythroferrone, which suppresses hepcidin. While erythropoiesis stimulating agents (ESAs) correct erythropoietin deficiency, they might worsen functional iron deficiency by creating an iron demand in excess of its supply. Other factors contributing to anemia of CKD include shortened red cell survival, direct bone marrow suppression by uremic toxins, folate deficiency, gastrointestinal blood loss due to uremic gastritis and/or platelet dysfunction, and aluminum toxicity from aluminum-containing antacids.

Metabolic Acidosis and Dyselectrolytemia

Metabolic acidosis in CKD results from decrease in proximal bicarbonate reabsorption and ammoniagenesis and distal acidification and titratable acid excretion. Hyperkalemia reflects impaired distal tubular excretion of potassium, despite elevated aldosterone levels. These abnormalities begin to manifest in CKD G3–G4. Patients with obstructive uropathy and tubulointerstitial disease develop acidosis and hyperkalemia earlier, as part of type IV renal tubular acidosis. Hyperkalemia is worsened by the use of RAS inhibitors (RASi) and potassium-sparing diuretics. Metabolic acidosis contributes to protein catabolism and bone demineralization, thus worsening growth failure.

Hypertension

Hypertension, observed in 20–80% of children with CKD G2–G5, results from RAS upregulation in many etiologies of CKD, especially those with glomerular involvement. It is an important modifiable risk factor for CKD progression and cardiovascular outcomes. The diagnosis, staging, and management of hypertension in CKD are discussed in **Chapter 25**.

Metabolic Syndrome

With increasing prevalence of pediatric obesity, the combination of visceral obesity and dyslipidemia, termed metabolic syndrome or syndrome X, is increasingly recognized. Metabolic syndrome results from an imbalance between dietary energy intake and expenditure, and increases the risks of hypertension, cardiovascular morbidity and mortality, and progression of CKD in native kidneys and allografts. In children older than 10 years, the International Diabetes Federation defines metabolic syndrome as follows—(*i*) *Obligatory criterion*: Central obesity, defined as waist circumference ≥ 90th percentile or above adult cut-off (≥94 cm in men and ≥80 cm in women); and (*ii*) *any two* of the following—(*a*) raised triglycerides ≥150 mg/dL or specific treatment; (*b*) reduced HDL cholesterol <40 mg/dL (<50 mg/dL in girls >16-year-old) or specific treatment; (*c*) hypertension or specific treatment; or (*d*) impaired fasting glycemia, defined as fasting plasma glucose ≥100 mg/dL or diagnosed type 2 diabetes. Metabolic syndrome should be considered in obese children aged 6–10 years in presence of a family history of metabolic syndrome, type 2 diabetes mellitus, dyslipidemia, cardiovascular disease, hypertension, and/or obesity.

The prevalence of metabolic syndrome is higher in children with CKD than in healthy children but lower than in adults with CKD. The highest prevalence is seen post-transplantation, and in children from developed countries or urban areas of developing economies like India. The most common metabolic abnormalities are hypertriglyceridemia, and post-transplantation, new-onset diabetes. The key pathophysiological feature is insulin resistance, which leads to increased hepatic synthesis of fatty acids and triglycerides, reduced inhibition of adipose tissue lipolysis, and reduced glucose uptake by skeletal muscles. Oxidative stress, leptin resistance, adiposity-induced inflammation, endothelial dysfunction, and angiotensin II-induced sympathetic nervous system activation play significant roles, modulated by altered metabolism of appetite-regulating hormones such as leptin, ghrelin, obestatin, and adiponectin in CKD. Obesity worsens progression of CKD by increasing single-nephron GFR, leading to hyperfiltration and microalbuminuria. The histological features of obesity-related glomerulopathy include glomerulomegaly, segmental sclerosis and arteriolosclerosis, with podocyte hypertrophy, focal foot process effacement, and podocytopenia.

CARDIOVASCULAR COMPLICATIONS

Clinically evident cardiovascular disease is noted in advanced CKD, chiefly during dialysis, and includes three features—(*i*) *Atherosclerotic arterial injury:* Endothelial injury leads to focal atherosclerotic plaques in large- and medium-sized arteries, usually in presence of dyslipidemia and insulin resistance; (*ii*) *Uremic arteriosclerosis:* Diffuse calcifications and calcified plaques are formed in medial layer of arteries in patients with advanced CKD and secondary hyperparathyroidism following osteoblastic transformation of medial vascular smooth muscle cells, which cause increased carotid intima media thickness and vessel wall stiffness; (*iii*) *Uremic cardiomyopathy:* Diffuse intermyocardiocyte fibrosis in patients with advanced CKD leads to diastolic dysfunction. Left ventricular hypertrophy affects 20–30% of children with CKD G2–G4 and 80–90% of those on maintenance dialysis.

Neurological Abnormalities

Infants and young children with moderate CKD are particularly susceptible to encephalopathy due to uremia. Neurological manifestations include hypotonia, delayed motor development, seizures (associated with hypertension, hypocalcemia, hyponatremia, or azotemia), truncal ataxia, and other signs of cerebellar dysfunction. Older children may present with seizures, uremic encephalopathy, and occasionally, peripheral neuropathy or severe proximal muscle weakness.

Miscellaneous

Anorexia, fatigue, increased sleep, poor school performance, platelet dysfunction, and depressed cell mediated immunity are common in CKD G3–G5. Uncommonly, patients present with severe uremia, including itching, acidotic breathing, congestive cardiac failure, pulmonary edema, pericarditis, and gastric ulcers.

DIAGNOSTIC EVALUATION AND MONITORING

A detailed history should be taken for features that suggest renal disease. Obstructive uropathy and tubulointerstitial disorders such as nephronophthisis are characterized by early onset of polyuria and polydipsia. A history of kidney disease in the family provides clues to etiology and pattern of inheritance. Clinical examination should include measurement of blood pressure and evaluation of growth, pubertal developmental and nutritional status. Anemia and features of rickets should be looked for and psychological and intellectual functions assessed.

Several methods have been proposed for estimating GFR in children (see Chapter 2). While accurate measurement of GFR is possible using plasma clearance of diethylenetriaminepentaacetic acid (DTPA), ethylenediaminetetraacetic acid (EDTA), iothalamate, or iohexol, such precise determinations are not necessary. The most used method for estimation of GFR is the modified Schwartz equation, as follows

eGFR = $k \times$ height/serum creatinine, where $k = 0.413$, height is in centimeters, and serum creatinine is in mg/dL.

Where possible, creatinine should be measured by an enzymatic method. The assay should have minimal bias compared with isotope-dilution mass spectrometry (IDMS), and the value should be rounded to the nearest 100th of a whole number when reporting in conventional units (mg/dL). Serum creatinine-based eGFR might be less accurate than cystatin-based GFR estimates at low kidney function (particularly in preterm and very low birth weight neonates), extremes of body habitus, and in specific conditions (sarcopenia and spinal cord injuries) (see Chapter 2). Where feasible, in these settings, the eGFR is derived using equations based on both analytes (Chapter 2). Further, the assays used to measure serum creatinine and cystatin C should have calibration traceable to the international standard reference materials.

Table 26.1 indicates the cut-offs to determine albuminuria categories in the CGA classification. The terminology focuses on albuminuria (preferably as albumin creatinine ratio (ACR) on a 24-hr urine collection) rather than proteinuria, unlike in children, where it is conventional to report proteinuria, as protein creatinine ratio (PCR) on a first morning spot urine specimen. For children, the KDIGO 2024 guidelines advise that the following measurements be performed on an early morning urine specimen, and used in a descending order of preference—(*i*) both urine PCR and urine ACR; (*ii*) reagent strip urinalysis for total protein and albumin with automated reading, or (*iii*) reagent strip urinalysis for total protein and for albumin with manual reading. The urine samples for albumin measurement should be analyzed fresh or stored at 4°C for up to 7 days (but not frozen at –20°C), and that laboratories should report ACR to one decimal place, whether mg/mmol or mg/g.

Box 26.2 lists the evaluations necessary to determine the etiology and severity of CKD, including complications. As discussed previously, chronicity is established by history, physical examination and review of past records of serum and urine biochemistry, imaging, and histopathological findings. Ultrasonography is useful for examining renal size, anomalies, and obstruction. Urinalysis detects hematuria, pyuria, and red or white cell casts, while serum and urine electrolytes assess renal tubular function. Ultrasound assesses kidney structure including shape, size, symmetry, and evidence of obstruction. Nuclear imaging has limited role in advanced stages of CKD but may be useful in diagnosis of reflux nephropathy or pelviureteric junction obstruction in early stages. Similarly, kidney histology is not useful in advanced CKD where nonspecific extensive scarring is expected.

Genetic testing has emerged as a valuable tool for etiological evaluation in patients with family history of CKD as well as CKD of unknown etiology. A KDIGO consensus document recommends considering genetic testing in the following settings: (*i*) High prevalence of monogenic etiology within the clinical category (e.g., cystic kidney diseases); (*ii*) early age at onset of CKD (e.g., in utero or infancy); (*iii*) syndromic or multisystem features [e.g., features suggesting Alport syndrome, hepatocyte nuclear factor 1β (HNF1β)-related kidney disease, Denys–Drash or Frasier syndrome); (*iv*) consanguinity; (*v*) high possibility of identifying a condition amenable to targeted treatment (e.g., Fabry disease, primary hyperoxaluria, and defects in coenzyme Q pathway causing nephrotic syndrome), or to nonspecific renoprotective strategies (e.g., Alport syndrome); and (*vi*) CKD or ESKD of unknown etiology when kidney biopsy would not be informative due to advanced disease. Further, genetic testing facilitates reproductive counseling to allow decisions on prenatal genetic testing based on findings in the index patient. In certain conditions, genetic test results guide screening for extrarenal manifestations (e.g., diabetes in HNF1β-related kidney disease; intracranial aneurysms in *PKD1* or *PKD2* defects; gonadoblastoma or Wilms' tumor in WT1-related

BOX 26.2: Evaluation at presentation with chronic kidney disease

Disease severity and complications
History and physical examination
Anthropometry standard deviation scores
Clinic and ambulatory blood pressure for type and stage of hypertension
Retinoscopy, cardiovascular examination for hypertensive target-organ damage
Hemogram; peripheral smear
Blood urea, creatinine, uric acid; electrolytes; pH, bicarbonate
Calcium, phosphorus, alkaline phosphatase; parathormone; 25-hydroxyvitamin D
Total protein, albumin; transaminases
Serum iron, ferritin, transferrin saturation, total iron binding capacity
Fasting lipid profile, fasting sugar, HbA1c
Urinalysis; first morning spot protein to creatinine ratio or 24-hr sample for proteinuria (mg/m^2)
Chest radiograph; electrocardiogram; echocardiography
Radiograph of left wrist, knees: Bone age, rickets, osteomalacia, osteitis fibrosa cystica

Etiology
History and physical examination
Urinalysis; 24-hr urine protein, creatinine
Ultrasonography for kidney, ureters, and bladder

Suspected congenital anomalies of the kidney and urinary tract
Micturating cystourethrography
MR urography, if complex anatomy
Radionuclide studies, if indicated: DTPA or MAG-3 scintigraphy, DMSA renal scan

Suspected tubulointerstitial disease
Kidney biopsy (in selected cases)
Next generation sequencing (in selected cases)**(Annexure 9.9, p 845)**

Suspected glomerular disease
Complement C3; antinuclear antibodies, and antibodies to double stranded DNA
Antineutrophil cytoplasmic antibody (ELISA)
Hepatitis B surface antigen; hepatitis C antibody; and HIV antibody
Kidney biopsy
Eye; ear examination
Next-generation sequencing (in selected cases)
Unknown etiology: Consider kidney biopsy; next generation sequencing

ELISA: enzyme-linked immunosorbent assay; HIV: human immunodeficiency virus

nephrotic syndrome). Finally, depending on the etiology, genetic testing may be useful when preparing for kidney transplantation to—(*i*) detect conditions at risk of recurrence after kidney transplantation (e.g., atypical hemolytic uremic syndrome due to monogenic defects in complement regulation; primary hyperoxaluria type 1; and adenine phosphoribosyl transferase deficiency); (*ii*) rule out monogenic cause, which facilitates counseling about risk of, and monitoring for or management of, disease recurrence (e.g., nonmonogenic steroid resistant nephrotic syndrome); and (*iii*) enable appropriate donor selection for live-related transplantation by avoiding donors sharing the pathogenic defect (e.g., mothers of boys with X-linked Alport syndrome; live relatives with shared implicated allele in autosomal dominant polycystic or tubulointerstitial kidney disease). **Annexure 9.9 (p 845)** provides a list of genes prioritized when sequencing patients with unknown CKD.

Common complications of CKD are described above. These are more likely in patients with CKD G3–G5. Blood levels of urea, pH, bicarbonate, electrolytes, creatinine, calcium, phosphate, alkaline phosphatase, proteins, fasting levels of triglycerides and cholesterol, 25-OH vitamin-D, PTH, and iron studies are useful in assessing complications at baseline and periodically thereafter **(Box 26.2)**.

MANAGEMENT

Management of CKD comprises management specific to etiology, measures to retard progression of CKD, monitoring for and management of complications, and preparation for long-term KRT in those at high risk of ESKD. Timely and appropriate management of specific entities, such as severe CAKUT (posterior urethral valves, high-grade vesicoureteric reflux) and glomerular diseases is essential to arrest progression to advanced CKD. Nonspecific aspects of management of CKD are discussed below.

Retarding Progression of CKD

Hypertension and proteinuria are the two most important modifiable risk factors that independently predict progression of CKD. Current therapeutic strategies to prevent progression of CKD, summarized in **Table 26.3**, aim at optimizing blood pressure control and reducing urinary protein excretion. Reduction in proteinuria to <300 mg/m^2/day, and intensified blood pressure control, aiming for target blood pressure between 50th and 75th percentile for all patients and around 50th percentile for patients with proteinuria, are both shown to retard CKD progression in children as well as adults with CKD.

Conventional RASi are antiproteinuric and antihypertensive, and retard CKD progression through multiple mechanisms, including decrease in intraglomerular pressure and reduced induction of inflammatory pathways, thus reducing glomerular hypertrophy, glomerulosclerosis, tubulointerstitial inflammation, and fibrosis **(Fig. 26.2C)**. Angiotensin-converting enzyme inhibitors (ACEi), particularly ramipril or enalapril, and angiotensin receptor blockers (ARBs), such as losartan, are the most studied and preferred in children with CKD. Dosing considerations are as advised for hypertension (see Chapter 25). While aliskiren, a direct renin inhibitor, is approved for use as an antihypertensive in children >6-year-old, its efficacy in reducing proteinuria or retarding progression is not established.

TABLE 26.3: Medications that prevent progression of chronic kidney disease (CKD) and renin–angiotensin–aldosterone system inhibitors (RASi)

Medication	*Examples*	*Site or mechanism of action*	*Effects; comments*	*Approved for children*
RASi: ACE-i	Enalapril, ramipril, and lisinopril	Inhibit angiotensin-converting enzyme to prevent formation of angiotensin II	Lower blood pressure; reduce proteinuria; slow slope of decline of estimated glomerular filtration rate (eGFR)	Yes
RASi: ARB	Losartan, telmisartan, Olmesartan, and candesartan	Inhibit angiotensin II receptor to prevent actions of angiotensin II	Lower blood pressure; reduce proteinuria; slow eGFR slope	Yes
RASi: DRA	Aliskiren	Directly inhibit plasma renin activity to prevent formation of angiotensin I	Lower blood pressure and reduce proteinuria	Yes
RASi: sMRA	Eplerenone and spironolactone	Inhibit mineralocorticoid receptor selectively (eplerenone) or nonspecifically (spironolactone)	Reduce proteinuria and blood pressure; reduce eGFR and increase the risk of hyperkalemia and AKI when added to ACEI/ARB; risk of gynecomastia	No
RASi: nsMRA	Finerenone	More selective, nonsteroidal inhibitor of the mineralocorticoid receptor	Reduce proteinuria and blood pressure and slow eGFR slope; better anti-inflammatory and antifibrotic effects; minimal hyperkalemia and in eGFR lower decline vs. MRA	No
ET-Ai	Atrasentan	Potent, selective inhibitor of endothelin type A; antifibrotic and anti-inflammatory effects	Reduces proteinuria in diabetes; being examined in IgA nephropathy and other CKD	No
DEARA (ARB + ET-Ai)	Sparsentan	Dual inhibitor of endothelin receptor type A and angiotensin II receptor	More effective than conventional RASi in reducing proteinuria and slowing progression of CKD in IgA nephropathy and FSGS	No
NEPi: ARNi	Sacubitril/valsartan	*Neprilysin inhibitor* enhances the activity of natriuretic peptide systems; angiotensin receptor blockade	Natriuresis, diuresis; lowers blood pressure; prevents and reverses cardiovascular remodeling; lower risk of AKI and similar risk of chronic renal events and hyperkalemia as ACEi or ARB	No
SGLT2i	Dapagliflozin, empagliflozin, and canagliflozin	Inhibit sodium–glucose like transporter 2	Natriuresis, diuresis; lower blood pressure; activates tubuloglomerular feedback to reduce glomerular hyperfiltration	No

ACEi: angiotensin-converting enzyme inhibitor; AKI: acute kidney injury; ARB: angiotensin II receptor blocker; ARNi: angiotensin receptor neprilysin inhibitor; DEARA: dual endothelin angiotensin receptor antagonist; DRA: direct renin antagonist; ET-Ai: endothelin receptor type A inhibitor/antagonist; FSGS: focal segmental glomerulosclerosis; NEPi: neprilysin inhibitor; SGLT2i: sodium–glucose like transporter 2 inhibitor; sMRA: steroidal mineralocorticoid receptor antagonist

Several therapeutic strategies that have been examined for their renoprotective effects in adults with CKD have not been tested adequately in children. While conventional RASi that focus in glomerular hemodynamics, mineralocorticoid receptor antagonists (MRA) additionally target inflammation and fibrosis mediated by MR overactivation **(Table 26.3)**. At equinatriuretic doses, the nonsteroidal selective MRA, finerenone, has more anti-inflammatory and antifibrotic effects on kidneys and myocardium and lower risk of hyperkalemia than the steroidal selective MRA, eplerenone. Based on evidence of its role in retarding CKD progression and enabling cardioprotection, finerenone is recommended in adults with CKD and type 2 diabetes. Neprilysin inhibitor (NEPi) and, particularly, angiotensin receptor neprilysin inhibitor (ARNi), enhance the activity of natriuretic peptide systems, leading to natriuresis, diuresis, and RASi, which are beneficial in adults with chronic heart failure and CKD. Sparsentan is a single-molecule dual endothelin angiotensin receptor antagonist (DEARA), is an emerging therapeutic option for proteinuric CKD such as IgA nephropathy and FSGS that reduces proteinuria and stabilizes the GFR slope. Meta-analysis of studies in adult patients with CKD with or without diabetes show that inhibitors of sodium–glucose like transporter 2 inhibitors (SGLT2i), such as dapagliflozin and empagliflozin, induce natriuresis, reduce proteinuria, and stabilize the GFR slope. Nonhypercalcemic doses of vitamin D analogs (paricalcitol and calcitriol) are shown to reduce proteinuria through immunomodulatory and antifibrotic effects and downregulation of RAS; however, their efficacy in retarding CKD progression was not established, and guidelines for adults with CKD do not suggest their use for proteinuria reduction.

Box 26.3 highlights important considerations when prescribing RASi and similar agents. Small nonprogressive increase in serum creatinine after initiating therapy with these agents might reflect hemodynamic changes rather than CKD progression. Patients must be counseled to avoid RASi on "sick" days **(Box 26.3)**. Meta-analyses recommend against dual blockade of RAAS (e.g., combinations of ACEI and ARB) in view of significant adverse events (hyperkalemia, hypotension, and nephrotoxicity).

Studies argue against reduction of dietary protein intake in children since this has not been shown to retard CKD progression, and might result in malnutrition and growth retardation. Other strategies proposed to prevent progression of CKD have included adequate management of anemia and prevention and management of dyslipidemia or metabolic acidosis.

Nutrition, Fluid, and Electrolytes

Protein energy malnutrition is common in children with CKD and contributes to growth failure. Attention to nutrition is particularly critical in infants and young children in whom growth depends chiefly on nutrition. **Box 26.4**

BOX 26.3: Considerations on therapy with inhibitors of renin–angiotensin–aldosterone system inhibitor (RASi)[1]

Monitor serum creatinine, potassium, and bicarbonate at initiation; 2–4 weeks following initiation or change in dose of RASi therapy; and at every routine visit (q2–4 months)
Up titrate RASi to the maximally tolerated, evidence-based dose
Avoid using combinations of RASi (high risk of hyperkalemia and AKI)
On "sick" days and before elective surgery, withhold RASi, and the following concomitant medications, if any: diuretics, NSAIDs, SGLT2i, sulfonylureas, and metformin

Anticipate, prevent, and manage hyperkalemia
Do not initiate RASi therapy at serum potassium >5.0 mEq/L
Monitor serum potassium at each visit and after every dose change
Advise to avoid juices; counsel about dietary sources of potassium (see end of box)
Continuously review concomitant medications for hyperkalemia potential
Prevent and treat metabolic acidosis (reduce intake of animal protein; use oral bicarbonate)
If mild (5.0–5.5 mEq/L) to moderate (5.5–6 mEq/L) hyperkalemia persists despite above measures, acts stepwise as follows, while monitoring serum potassium—(*i*) prescribe diuretics &/or K^+ binders; (*ii*) reduce the dose of RASi; and (*iii*) discontinue RASi
If hyperkalemia is severe (>6 mEq/L): Withhold RASi; evaluate eGFR, potassium, and bicarbonate to decide on re-initiation of therapy, with or without K^+-binder

Anticipate, prevent, and manage acute kidney injury (AKI)
Do not initiate RASi therapy at eGFR ≤20 mL/min/1.73 m^2
Monitor serum creatinine and eGFR at each visit and after every dose change
Accept rise in serum creatinine by ≤30% (if eGFR >20 mL/min/1.73 m^2) as appropriate hemodynamic response
If serum creatinine increases by >30% and <100%—(*i*) reduce RASi dose to half or temporarily withhold; (*ii*) exclude or manage reversible causes (e.g., hypovolemia due to febrile illness, gastroenteritis, recurrent vomiting, or use of diuretics; concomitant therapy with SGLT2i, NSAID, MRA, another RASi, and nephrotoxic antibiotic); (*iii*) monitor kidney function over 1–2 weeks: If AKI resolves, resume RASi at half the original dose, and monitor kidney function over 1–4 weeks
If serum creatinine increases by >100%: temporarily hold the RASi; conduct measures (*ii*) and (*iii*) as above

Withholding or reducing RASi is expected to worsen heart failure, if concomitantly present

Dietary considerations in management of hyperkalemia
Eat balanced diet with plenty of fruits, vegetables, whole grains, and legumes; reduce intake of animal meat (higher acid load and K^+ bioavailability than plant-based diets)
Limit ultra-processed foods; additives, preservatives; juices; dried food items (high K^+ content); avoid salt substitutes; and supplements with high K^+ content
Double boil food items and discard the cooking water
Treat constipation to increase gastrointestinal K^+ excretion; increase intake of dietary fiber; ensure adequate water intake; use laxatives that are safe in CKD

[1]Applicable to angiotensin converting enzyme inhibitor (ACE-i); angiotensin II receptor blocker (ARB); angiotensin receptor neprilysin inhibitor (ARNi; sacubitril/valsartan); direct renin antagonist (DRA; aliskiren); non-steroidal selective mineralocorticoid receptor antagonist (nsMRA; finerenone) and steroidal MRA (sMRA; eplerenone; spironolactone)
1ARNi, certain nsMRA (e.g., drospirenone) and nsMRA (e.g., finerenone) are not yet approved for use in children
CKD: chronic kidney disease; eGFR: estimated glomerular filtration rate; SGLT2i: sodium–glucose like transporter 2 inhibitor; NSAID: nonsteroidal anti-inflammatory drug

BOX 26.4: Assessment of nutrition status in children with chronic kidney disease (CKD)

Measure weight (all), height (≥2-year-old; ambulatory) or length (<2-year-old or unable to stand); head circumference (<3-year-old)

Use euvolemic (dry) weight for nutritional assessment; estimate dry weight if edema present (e.g., patients on dialysis; with nephrotic syndrome)

Calculate weight-for-length in children <5-year-old and body mass index (BMI) in children >5-year-old

- Plot measurements (weight; length/height; weight-for-length/height or BMI; and head circumference) serially on centile growth charts: Use WHO growth charts up to 5 years; IAP charts thereafter

Calculate z-scores [standard deviation scores (SDS)] to complement growth chart plots

- Use height age to determining BMI SDS if the height is <3rd centile, provided the child has not reached their adult height
- Calculate height/length velocity SDS over ≥6-month; use trend to guide decisions

Calculate midparental height and plot the value as a centile to estimate growth potential

Where applicable, use disorder- or genetic condition-specific growth charts

For premature infants, plot anthropometry according to gestation as well as chronological age up to 1-year-old if born at 32–37 weeks' gestation, and up to 2-year-old if born at <32 weeks' gestation

Monitor growth parameters regularly in children with CKD: More close monitoring is required in young children, advanced CKD, comorbidities, risk factors for poor growth, and those not meeting nutritional and growth targets. Monitor q 2–8 weeks in infants; q 1–3 months in children 1–3 years old, and q 3–6 months in older children

Source: Nelms CL, et al. 2021

outlines key principles of anthropometric assessment of children with CKD. Infants and children with polyuria, severe malnutrition, growth failure, and dialysis dependence require more frequent assessment of growth and nutritional status.

Box 26.5 provides guidance for the prescription of nutrition in children with CKD based on clinical practice recommendations of the Pediatric Renal Nutrition Taskforce (PRNT). **Table 26.4** provides suggested dietary intake (SDI) of calories, proteins, and minerals for children with CKD, based on guidelines by the PRNT. Protein intake is not restricted in children with CKD. Children with malnutrition require additional calories to allow catch-up growth. In patients in whom the energy requirements are not met with oral intake, supplemental nutritional support is considered in form of nasogastric tube or gastrostomy feeds **(Box 26.5)**. Infants and young children particularly benefit from nighttime tube feeds. Formulas that are high in calories and low in phosphorus are preferred. Patients with fluid restrictions due to advanced CKD should receive calorie-dense foods. In patients with risk factors for cardiovascular disease and dyslipidemia, diets high in polyunsaturated fats such as corn oil, medium chain triglyceride

BOX 26.5: Principles of oral and enteral nutrition in children with chronic kidney disease (CKD) stages 2–5D

Energy requirements

Prescribe energy (calories) to meet the needs of healthy children of the same age **(Table 26.6)**

In patients with suboptimal weight gain and linear growth, prescribe energy at the higher end of the suggested dietary intake (SDI), to promote optimal growth

In overweight or obese children, adjust energy intake to achieve appropriate weight gain, without compromising nutrition and height gain

In patients on peritoneal dialysis with excess weight gain, take into account calories from dialysate glucose content

Protein requirements

Prescribe protein intake at the upper end of the SDI, to promote optimal growth **(Table 26.6)**

Do not provide less protein than the lower end of the range ("minimum safe amount")

For children on dialysis, prescribe protein intake higher than the SDI for age by ≥0.15–0.3 g/kg/day for children on peritoneal dialysis and ≥0.1 g/kg/day for those on hemodialysis **(Table 28.7)**

For children with persistently high blood urea, reduce protein intake toward the lower end of the SDI, after excluding other causes of high blood urea

Nutritional prescription

Breastfeeding is the preferred method for providing energy to young infants with CKD

Add whey-dominant infant formula when breastfeeding or expressed breastmilk is not available in adequate amounts to meet nutrient needs of young infants

Fortify breastmilk and/or formula milk if energy needs are not met or when feeds require to be made nutrient-dense because of fluid restriction.

Concentrate feeds using dietary supplements in a graded manner to maximize acceptance and tolerance. Consider adding energy modules to formula milk to reach the following goals:

Infants: Add to infant formula, which has ~7 g carbohydrate + ~3.5 g fat per dL

<6 months old: Glucose polymer 3–5 g to get ~10–12 g carbohydrates per dL

6–12 months old: Glucose polymer 5–8 g to get ~12–15 g carbohydrate per dL

<12 months old: Fat emulsion (50% fat content) 3–5 mL to get ~5–6 g fat per dL

Child >1 year: Add to pediatric formula, which has ~12 g carbohydrate + ~4.5 g fat per dL

Glucose polymer 8–18 g to get ~20–30 g carbohydrate per dL

Fat emulsion (50% fat content) 9 mL to get 9 g fat per dL

Introduce solid foods as recommended for healthy infants, progressing in textures and content according to the infant's cues and oral motor skills

Ensure a healthy, balanced diet through childhood, with the same variety of food choices as for healthy children, taking into account possible dietary limitations

Prefer oral feeding, whenever possible: Ensure oral stimulation, even if oral intake is limited, to prevent food aversion

Intervene promptly if weight centile deteriorates or is found to be below 3rd centile

Initiate oral nutritional supplements in patients with inadequate dietary intake, after managing medically any correctable causes of reduced intake (e.g., gastroesophageal reflux, vomiting, metabolic acidosis, volume overload, and inadequate dialysis)

Initiate supplemental or exclusive enteral tube feeding in patients who are unable to meet their nutritional requirements orally

Intradialytic parenteral nutrition may not provide additional advantage over enteral feeding

Source: Shaw V, et al. 2020.

oil, and complex carbohydrates are preferred, such that saturated fats comprise <10% of calories. The dietary intake of calcium and phosphorus is assessed and the diet modified based on the child's age, CKD stage, and trends in serum calcium, phosphorus, and PTH. Similar to KDOQI guidance for adults, the PRNT suggests that the total calcium intake from diet and medications, including phosphate binders, should not exceed twice the SDI in children with CKD G2–G5D **(Table 26.4)**. Infants with CKD and those with hypocalcemia, rickets or osteomalacia might receive a higher calcium intake under careful monitoring. Most infant formulas provide at least 50–60 mg calcium per 100 kCal and have a calcium to phosphorus ratio of 1.1–2.0. The PRNT suggests that the dietary phosphorus intake of children with CKD should be within the SDI for age, without compromising protein intake **(Table 26.4)**. The latter is a concern since phosphorus content of food items is related to their protein content; usually any food with 1 g of protein contains 10–12 mg of phosphorus. Foods rich in phosphorus include milk and its products, meat, chicken, nuts, and whole grains. Processed foods contain readily absorbed inorganic phosphorus, e.g., canned meat, dried beans and peas, dairy or bakery products, colas, and flavored drinks. Egg white and vegetable proteins have low phosphate to protein ratio. Boiling and prolonged soaking variably reduce the phosphorus content of food. Children with CKD G3–G5 and persistent hyperparathyroidism with or without hyperphosphatemia require dietary phosphorus restriction to the lower limit of the SDI (corresponding to the KDOQI recommendation of 80% of dietary reference intake).

Vitamins, folic acid, copper, and zinc are supplemented at recommended dietary allowances in children with CKD. While water soluble vitamins are removed in dialysis, supplementation with multivitamin preparations should be guided by micronutrient levels, where feasible. Excess use of vitamin A is associated with hypercalcemia, anemia, and hyperlipidemia, while that of vitamin C might promote oxalate deposition in kidneys, which worsens kidney function. Folic acid supplementation is recommended at GFR <40 mL/min/1.73 m^2 to prevent hyperhomocysteinemia. Patients on peritoneal dialysis require supplemental vitamin C, folic acid, and pyridoxine to offset dialysis losses.

All children with CKD do not require salt or water restriction. Patients with salt-losing nephropathies and polyuria require free water and salt supplementation to prevent chronic intravascular volume depletion and to promote optimal growth. The water and salt intake requires to be ensured during febrile illness or gastroenteritis. In contrast, in patients with CKD and elevated blood pressure or hypertension, the salt intake should be limited to the age-based recommended daily intake, i.e., 110 mg at 0–6 months, 370 mg at 7 months–3 years, 1,000 mg at 4–8 years, 1,200 mg at 9–13 years and 1,500 mg in older children and adults. Patients with advanced CKD require

TABLE 26.4: Suggested dietary intake (SDI) in children with CKD2-5D

Age, months	*Calories, kcal/kg/day*[1]		*Protein, g/kg/day*[1]	*Protein, g/day*	*Calcium, mg/day*	*Phosphate, mg/day*
0 to <1	93–107		1.52–2.5	8–12	220	120
1–2	93–120		1.4–1.8	8–12	220	120
3–4	82–98		1.3–1.52	8–13	220	120
5–11	72–82		1.1–1.52	9–15	330–540	275–420
12–23	72–120		0.9–1.4	11–14	450–700	250–500
Age, years	*Calories, kcal/kg/day*[1]		*Protein, g/kg/day*[2]	*Protein, g/day*	*Calcium, mg/day*	*Phosphate, mg/day*
	Boys	*Girls*				
2 to <3	81–95	79–92	0.9–1.05	11–15	450–700	250–500
3 to <4	80–82	76–77	0.9–1.05	13–15	450–700	250–500
4–6	67–93	64–90	0.85–0.95	16–22	700–1,000	440–800
7–8	60–77	56–75	0.9–0.95	19–28	700–1,000	440–800
9–10	55–69	49–63	0.9–0.95	26–40	700–1,000	440–800
11–12	48–63	43–57	0.9–0.95	34–42	900–1,300	640–1,250
13–14	44–63	39–50	0.8–0.9	34–50	900–1,300	640–1,250
15–17	40–55	36–46	0.8–0.9	52–65 (boys); 45–49 (girls)	900–1,300	640–1,250

[1] For children with poor growth, refer to the SDI for height age (the age that corresponds to their height when plotted at the 50th centile on a growth chart)

[2] Assuming low physical activity level

Source: Pediatric Renal Nutrition Taskforce guidelines, 2020–2023

restriction of fluids to match less than the urine output or, in anuric children, the volume removed during dialysis. Fluid content of food items must be kept in mind when calculating fluid intakes.

Hyperkalemia is a concern in patients with low eGFR and while on therapy with RASi. Food items rich in potassium (mausami, oranges, almonds, and green vegetables), fruit juices, and salt substitutes with high potassium content should be avoided. Patients with persistent hyperkalemia might require therapy with potassium exchange resins. Rarely, hypokalemia may occur due to excessive use of diuretics, which requires management with oral or intravenous (IV) supplementation of potassium chloride.

Growth

Growth failure in CKD is multifactorial, as discussed earlier (**Fig. 26.3**). Nutritional deficiency and metabolic acidosis should be corrected by adequate prescription of calories, proteins, and base. Patients with polyuria benefit from salt and water supplementation. Optimal nutritional management often leads to catch-up growth in infants even with severe CKD.

Children with CKD with persistent growth failure should receive therapy with recombinant human GH (rhGH) therapy. **Box 26.6** enunciates key principles in prescription and monitoring of rhGH therapy. Rickets and hyperparathyroidism should be managed appropriately before initiating therapy with rhGH. Therapy with rhGH increases production of IGF-I in the liver and growth plate and improves its bioavailability. Most children treated with rhGH show catch-up growth. A meta-analysis of 15 studies on children with CKD found that rhGH, given in a dose of 28 IU/m^2/week for 1 year, was associated with height velocity 3.9 cm/year higher than untreated patients, leading to increase in height by 0.8 standard deviation scores (SDS).

Beyond the first few months, transplantation is associated with increase in height SDS, compared to no change in height SDS while on dialysis. This is particularly true for prepubertal children, particularly if <6-year-old. Children who continue to grow poorly despite successful kidney transplantation benefit from rhGH treatment. Patients who are transplanted during adolescence might show a suboptimal pubertal growth spurt, which may be optimized by the use of rhGH therapy. The high cost of rhGH and inconvenience of daily subcutaneous dosing precludes its wider use. Side effects include hyperglycemia, hypertension, enhanced skeletal maturation, and pseudotumor cerebri.

Chronic Kidney Disease Mineral Bone Disease

Monitoring for development of CKD-MBD should begin in CKD G2. Target values for serum phosphate, calcium, PTH, and the calcium phosphorus product vary with the age of the child and the stage of kidney disease **(Table 26.5)**. The European Renal Association–European Dialysis and

BOX 26.6: Therapy with recombinant human growth hormone in CKD

Indication

Persistent short stature: Height for age < 3rd percentile [<–1.88 standard deviation score (SDS)], with height velocity <25th percentile (<–2 SDS), calculated over ≥6 months

Prerequisites

Adequate caloric and protein intake

Presence of growth potential: Based on genetic height potential (calculated by parental height),[1] prepubertal status, and open epiphysis (assessed at left wrist)

Serum bicarbonate >20 mEq/L; sodium >135 mEq/L

Hemoglobin level 10–11 g/dL

Serum phosphorus <5.5 mg/dL

Parathormone between two and three times normal

If post-transplantation: >1 year after transplant, with stable GFR, and lack of spontaneous catch-up growth[2]

Contraindications

Uncontrolled diabetes

Severe osteodystrophy with PTH >500 ng/mL

Active malignancy; critical illness

Post-transplant patients with >1 episode of rejection

Dose: 0.045–0.05 mg/kg/day (4 IU/m^2/day, 30 IU/m^2/week, or 1 IU/kg/week); daily evening, subcutaneously

Monitoring

Baseline and q 3–6 months

Height, weight, and height velocity; sexual maturity rating

Calcium, phosphorus, alkaline phosphatase, parathyroid hormone, and 25(OH) vitamin D

Creatinine, eGFR, electrolytes, bicarbonate, hemoglobin, and albumin

Glucose (fasting) and glycosylated hemoglobin

Fundus examination for papilledema

Baseline and annually

Adequacy of response (adequate if growth velocity >2 cm/year over baseline)

Thyroid stimulating hormone and free T3

If available, insulin-like growth factor 1 (to assess compliance)

Radiograph of left wrist for bone age (Tanner Whitehouse 2 method); radiograph of pelvis

Adverse effects

Hyperglycemia

Worsened mineral bone disease

Avascular necrosis of hip; slipped capital femoral epiphysis

Pseudotumor cerebri

Modification of dose

Consider dose reduction by 50% when the height goal is achieved based on midparental height.

Carefully consider dose increment (up to double the dose) if response is inadequate (height velocity <2 cm/year above baseline), despite compliance and ruling out other contributing factors.

Contd...

Contd...

Indications for therapy discontinuation
Closed epiphyses; accelerated bone maturation
Development of neoplasia
Hypersensitivity to recombinant growth hormone
Increased intracranial pressure
Severe hyperparathyroidism (PTH >400 pg/mL in CKD 2–4; >900 pg/mL in CKD 5)
Unexplained decline in eGFR
Kidney transplantation
Growth potential (target height or percentile) achieved

[1]Adult height prediction methods should not be applied to children with CKD; use either of following formula:
Tanner's formula: [(Father's height + mother's height)/2] + 6.5 cm (for boys), or –6.5 cm (for girls)
Molinari formula: [(Father's height + mother's height)/2] + 10.2 cm (for boys), or –2.6 cm (for girls)
[2]Height velocity >75th centile for sex and age; seen more often with steroid-free than conventional immunosuppression
CKD: chronic kidney disease; eGFR: estimated glomerular filtration rate; PTH: parathyroid hormone

TABLE 26.5: Target ranges for blood biochemical parameters in children with chronic kidney disease (CKD)

	Calcium, mg/dL	*Phosphorus, mg/dL*	*Calcium phosphorus product*	*Parathyroid hormone, pg/mL*	*Alkaline phosphatase, mg/dL*
Age 1–12 years:					
CKD 2–3	9–10.2	4–6	<65	35–70	100–450
CKD 4	9–10.2	4–6	<65	70–110	100–450
CKD 5, dialysis	8.8–9.7	4–6	<65	200–300	100–450
Age >12 years:					
CKD 2–3	8.8–10.2	2.5–4.5	<55	35–70	40–180
CKD 4	8.8–10.2	2.5–4.5	<55	70–110	40–180
CKD 5, dialysis	8.8–9.7	3.5–5.5	<55	200–300	40–180

Transplant Association (ERA-EDTA) clinical practice guidelines for bone evaluation in children advise that these parameters are monitored 3-6 monthly in children with CKD G2–G3, 1–3 monthly in CKD G4-G5, and more frequently across stages in younger children. Treatment decisions should be guided by trends, rather than single values.

Key aspects of management are discussed below. Hyperphosphatemia is managed with dietary phosphorus intake restriction, and use of calcium-based followed by noncalcium-based binders **(Table 26.6)**. Hyperparathyroidism usually responds to control of hyperphosphatemia and correction of hypovitaminosis D. In advanced CKD, hypovitaminosis D merits treatment with native 25-hydroxyvitamin D preparations followed by activated vitamin D. **Table 26.7** summarizes the guidelines for management of various biochemical abnormalities.

Management of Hyperphosphatemia

Control of serum phosphorus level is the most important measure in the management of secondary hyperparathyroidism in CKD. Adequate control of serum phosphorus levels prevents rise in FGF23, secondary hyperparathyroidism, and vascular calcifications. Principles of dietary phosphorus restriction are detailed earlier. Dietary phosphate restriction to the upper limit of SDI is advised while ensuring adequate intake of protein.

Calcium-containing phosphate binders, such as calcium carbonate and calcium acetate, are prescribed when dietary restriction fails to control serum phosphorus within the normal range **(Table 26.6)**. The usual starting dose is 30–60 mg/kg/day of elemental calcium, taken with each meal. When taken on empty stomach, calcium salts act as a source of calcium. Given the concerns of progressive vascular calcifications associated with a positive calcium balance and hypercalcemia, the total intake of elemental calcium, from diet and calcium-based binders, should not exceed twice the SDI for age. If there is hypercalcemia, or serum PTH drops to <150 pg/dL while on dialysis, calcium-based binders are discontinued and a noncalcium binder prescribed. Although the KDIGO guidelines emphasize restricting doses of calcium-based phosphate binders across all severities of CKD in adults, for children, the choice of phosphate-lowering treatment is guided by serum calcium.

Calcium-free phosphate binders effectively maintain normal phosphate levels without risking hypercalcemia and vascular calcifications. Sevelamer hydrochloride and sevelamer carbonate are noncalcium, nonabsorbable cationic polymers that bind phosphate through ion exchange and improves blood cholesterol levels. Sevelamer carbonate is preferred to the hydrochloride preparation which might cause hyperchloremic metabolic acidosis. Both preparations reduce blood levels of cholesterol.

Four noncalcium-based binders approved for use in adult CKD patients await testing and approval in children with CKD. These agents are more potent and impose lower pill burden than sevelamer and calcium-based binders. Lanthanum carbonate, a noncalcium heavy metal binder, is not approved for use in children due to concerns of consequences of tissue accumulation. Sucroferric oxyhydroxide and ferric citrate are iron-based ligand exchangers that are approved for treatment of hyperphosphatemia

TABLE 26.6: Oral agents for management of hyperphosphatemia

Product; strengths	*Mechanism*	*% calcium (Ca) content; % Ca absorbed*[1]	*Phosphorus (P) binding per tablet*	*Pills to bind 100 mg P*	*P bound per Ca absorbed (mg: mg)*	*Dose (with meals)*	*Advantage; disadvantages; and comments*
Calcium carbonate 250, 500, and 1,250 mg	Forms insoluble P complex in the gut	40; 20–30	39 mg per 1 g	5 of 500 mg	1:8	1–2 tablets thrice a day	Inexpensive; effective Hypercalcemia; vascular calcification; gastrointestinal (GI) symptoms (nausea, vomiting, diarrhea, and constipation) Binds at low pH (avoid with H_2 blockers/ proton pump inhibitors)
Calcium acetate 667 mg	Forms insoluble P complex in the gut lumen	25; 20–22	45 mg per 1 g	13	1:3	2–4 tablets thrice a day	Less hypercalcemia (less calcium absorbed for similar phosphorus binding as $CaCO_3$); soluble over wide pH GI symptoms; hypercalcemia
Sevelamer carbonate 400, 800, and 1,200 mg	Anion exchange resin	0; 0	21 mg per 800 mg	3 of 1,200 mg	1:0	1–2 tablets thrice a day	Reduces cholesterol and uric acid; anti-inflammatory action GI symptoms (bloating); expensive

Contd...

Contd...

Product; strengths	***Mechanism***	***% calcium (Ca) content; % Ca absorbed***[1]	***Phosphorus (P) binding per tablet***	***Pills to bind 100 mg P***	***P bound per Ca absorbed (mg: mg)***	***Dose (with meals)***	***Advantage; disadvantages; and comments***
Lanthanum carbonate 250, 500, 750, and 1,000 mg[2]	Forms insoluble P complex in the gut	0, 0	135 mg per 1 g	1 of 750 mg	1:0	1–2 tablets thrice a day	Lower tablet requirement, better compliance; no hypercalcemia GI symptoms; headache, dizziness, myalgia, hypotension; not recommended in children due to accumulation in epiphyses Advise to chew rather than swallow
Sucroferric oxyhydroxide 500 mg (iron, 100 mg)[2]	Ligand exchanger; iron-based	0; 0	130 or 390 per 500 mg	<1	1:0	1 tablet 2–3 times daily	Potent; works across wide pH range; low pill burden Expensive; GI symptoms; stool discoloration Advise to chew rather than swallow
Ferric citrate 1 g (iron, 210 mg)[2]	Binds to dietary phosphorus	0; 0	20 or 46 mg per 1 g	3–5	1:0	1–2 tablets thrice a day	GI symptoms (diarrhea and nausea); discoloration of stool; and hyperkalemia
Tenapanor 5 mg, 30 mg, 50 mg[2]	Phosphate absorption inhibitor[3]	0; 0	NA	<1	1:0	1 tablet (30 mg) twice daily	Calcium-free, nonmetal compound; small tablet size; low pill burden; and less need for other binders GI symptoms (diarrhea; diverticular perforation, colitis)

[1]When taken with food
[2]Not approved for use in children
[3]Inhibits sodium/hydrogen exchanger isoform 3, and secondarily, the sodium phosphate cotransporter 2b (NaPi2b)

TABLE 26.7: Management strategies in patients with CKD and mineral bone disease

Blood levels				*Management*
Calcium	*Phosphorus*	*Parathyroid hormone, PTH*	*25 (OH) vitamin D*	
Normal	Normal	Normal	Normal	None
Low	Normal	Normal	<30 ng/mL	Supplement calcium; treat with high doses of cholecalciferol followed by recommended daily allowances of vitamin D
			>30 ng/mL	Supplement calcium; consider use of calcitriol or alfacalcidol
Normal/low	Normal	High	<30 ng/mL	*CKD stage 2–5D:* Treat with cholecalciferol followed by recommended daily allowances
				If PTH persistently high; no hypercalcemia or hyperphosphatemia: Add active vitamin D[1]
			>30 ng/mL	Restrict dietary phosphate to daily recommended intake
				If PTH persistently high; no hypercalcemia or hyperphosphatemia: Add active vitamin D[1]
Normal	High	Normal or high	–	Restrict dietary PO_4 to 80% of daily recommended intake; withhold vitamin D or analog
				If persistently high phosphate: Use oral phosphate binder
				Patients with CKD 5: Initiate dialysis

Contd...

Contd...

Blood levels				*Management*
Calcium	***Phosphorus***	***Parathyroid hormone, PTH***	***25 (OH) vitamin D***	
Normal/high	Normal/high	High	–	Measures as mentioned above
				Consider use of newer vitamin D analog, e.g., doxercalciferol, oxacalcitriol, and paricalcitol
Normal/high	Normal/high	Very high (>500 pg/mL)	–	Use newer vitamin D analog
				Consider cinacalcet
				Consider subtotal parathyroidectomy
Normal/high	Normal/high	Low	–	Withhold calcium-based binders and vitamin D
				CKD5D: Use low calcium containing dialysate

[1]Options: (1) Calcitriol: Daily dose, by weight if <3-year-old: 10–15 ng/kg/day (maximum 30 ng/kg/day); older children: 0.25–0.5 µg/day; intermittent oral or IV dose: 35 ng/kg twice weekly, or titrated to PTH and given thrice weekly: PTH 300–500 pg/mL: 0.0075 µg/kg (maximum 0.25 µg/day); 500–1,000 pg/mL: 0.015 µg/kg (maximum 0.5 µg/day); >1,000 pg/mL: 0.025 µg/kg (maximum 1 µg/day); (2) α-calcidiol: Dose 10–30 ng/kg/daily, weight-based, as follows: <10 kg: 0.25 µg twice a week; 10–20 kg: 0.25 µg on alternate days; >20 kg: 0.25 µg daily; while on dialysis; (3) Paricalcitol: Initial dose based on PTH: PTH <500 pg/mL: 0.04 µg/kg; PTH ≥500 pg/mL: 0.08 µg/kg; (4) Doxercalciferol: Oral dose thrice a week, titrated to keep PTH at 300–400 pg/mL and calcium 8.4–10.2 mg/dL

in adults with CKD. Therapy is reported to be associated with increased iron stores, decreased IV iron and ESA usage, and sustained hemoglobin levels compared to other binders. However, gastrointestinal adverse events are frequent. Both calcium and ferric citrate might increase the risk of aluminum toxicity, by enhancing aluminum absorption. Tenapanor, originally marketed for irritable bowel syndrome, has been repurposed as an inhibitor of intestinal phosphate absorption. However, gastrointestinal adverse events are dose limiting. Aluminum hydroxide is no longer used as a phosphate binder since aluminum might cause neurological dysfunction and adynamic bone disease. Other agents that have been used as phosphate binders include nicotinamide (metabolite of nicotinic acid; reduces gut phosphate absorption; increases serum high-density lipoprotein cholesterol), colestilan (nonmetallic nonabsorbable anion exchange resin; binds bile acids and phosphorus; also lowers serum low-density lipoprotein cholesterol), and chitosan (chewing gum; absorbs salivary phosphorus).

The phosphate binding capacities of the above medications vary **(Table 26.6)**. Patients with refractory hyperphosphatemia and CKD G5 should be considered for initiation of dialysis. Intermittent hemodialysis and chronic ambulatory peritoneal dialysis remove 2.3–2.6 g and 2.0–2.2 g of phosphate, respectively, per week. Extended and nocturnal hemodialysis (≥5 and ~8 h/ session, respectively) provide higher phosphate clearance (3.0–3.6 g and 4.5–4.9 g/week, respectively).

Administration of Vitamin D

If the levels of PTH remain elevated despite control of serum phosphorus levels, vitamin D deficiency should be ruled out. Blood levels of 25-hydroxyvitamin D_3 <30 ng/mL indicate insufficiency and <20 ng/mL suggest deficiency. The European Society for Paediatric Nephrology (ESPN) CKD-MBD clinical practice guidelines suggest using native vitamin D (e.g., ergocalciferol and cholecalciferol) supplements to treat vitamin D insufficiency or deficiency in children with CKD G2–G5D, and to prevent or treat secondary hyperparathyroidism in children with CKD G2–G3. Active vitamin D analogs (e.g., alfacalcidol, calcitriol, paricalcitol, and doxercalciferol) should not be used to treat vitamin D deficiency.

Cholecalciferol preparations are preferred as they are available as pharmaceutical grade products; nonpharmaceutical, over the counter, and ergocalcirol products are relatively unreliable. Infants should receive 600 IU/day during the intensive replacement phase to correct deficiency over 4–12 weeks, followed by 400 IU/day as maintenance dose. In older children, the dose during the intensive phase is guided by the 25-hydroxyvitamin D level—children with severe deficiency (25-hydroxyvitamin D <5 ng/mL) may be administered 8,000 IU/day, those with levels of 5–20 ng/mL receive 4,000 IU/day and those with insufficiency receive 2,000 IU/day. Less frequent administration of doses in weekly manner is acceptable, but mega-dose ("stoss") vitamin D therapy is not recommended. In the maintenance phase, patients receive a dose of 1,000–2,000 IU/day, varying by CKD stage. Levels of serum and urinary calcium and 25-hydroxyvitamin D should be monitored to avoid toxicity. Supplementation must be discontinued at 25-hydroxyvitamin D level exceeding 48 ng/mL. Symptomatic vitamin D toxicity, observed at 25-hydroxyvitamin D levels exceeding 100 ng/dL, is associated with hypercalcemia, hypercalciuria, and suppressed PTH.

Therapy with active vitamin D analogs is required in patients in whom hyperparathyroidism persists despite normal 25-hydroxyvitamin D levels, provided they do not have hypercalcemia and/or hyperphosphatemia. Based on recent studies in children, ESPN guidelines provide a choice among the available vitamin D analogs when treating children with CKD G2–G5D. Vitamin D analogs are initiated in the lowest dose to achieve target PTH concentrations and maintain normocalcemia (see footnote of **Table 26.6**). Subsequently, the dose is titrated based on trends in serum levels of calcium, phosphate, and PTH. Therapy is withheld if blood PTH levels are suppressed or hypercalcemia or hyperphosphatemia are observed. Daily oral calcitriol is safe, effective, and well-tolerated in children with CKD G2–G5D. High-dose intermittent oral or IV calcitriol carries risk of adynamic bone disease. Active vitamin D analogs such as paricalcitol and doxercalciferol carry lower risk of hypercalcemia than conventional active vitamin D preparations, and may be preferred in patients with persistent hyperparathyroidism despite normal to high calcium levels and normal phosphorus levels.

All forms of active vitamin D can induce increase in circulating FGF23 concentrations, which might impact cardiovascular health. Recent KDIGO guidelines no longer recommend routine use of calcitriol or its analogs in adults with CKD G3a–G5 because of risk of hypercalcemia and lack of benefit in altering left ventricular mass index and systolic function; their use is reserved for patients with CKD G4–G5 and severe progressive hyperparathyroidism. However, guidelines for children suggest that calcitriol and vitamin D analogs may be considered to maintain serum calcium levels in the age-appropriate normal range.

Management of Hypercalcemia

In patients with persistent hypercalcemia, calcium supplements are discontinued, followed by cessation of calcium-based phosphorus binders and native and active vitamin D. In patients on dialysis, a low calcium dialysate is preferred. Persistently elevated PTH levels despite hypercalcemia suggest tertiary hyperparathyroidism; a calcimimetic, such as cinacalcet, may be indicated. Rarely, immobilized patients have hypercalcemia with normal PTH level; here, short-term therapy with bisphosphonate may be considered.

Hypervitaminosis A may induce hypercalcemia, particularly in children on dialysis.

Calcimimetic Agents

Calcimimetics, such as cinacalcet and etelcalcetide, are small organic molecules that allosterically activate the calcium-sensing receptor on parathyroid cells, thereby diminishing PTH secretion. This decreases the calcium-phosphorus product and retards progressive parathyroid gland hyperplasia. Therapy requires close monitoring for hypocalcemia and is reserved for normocalcemic patients in whom hyperparathyroidism persists despite other medical measures. The safety of cinacalcet is not established in children. A meta-analysis of case studies shows significant risk of hypocalcemia. Further, interference with growth is of concern since the calcium-sensing receptor is also expressed on the growth plate.

Parathyroidectomy

Patients with tertiary hyperparathyroidism (serum PTH >800 pg/mL, hypercalcemia, and hyperphosphatemia) require subtotal parathyroidectomy or total parathyroidectomy with autotransplantation. Parathyroidectomy is also indicated in patients with high PTH levels and progressive and debilitating hyperparathyroid bone disease, refractory pruritus, progressive extraskeletal calcification or calciphylaxis, and otherwise unexplained myopathy.

Orthopedic Surgery

Patients with severe bony deformities may require orthopedic interventions, but these should follow correction of secondary hyperparathyroidism. It is recommended that lower limb angular deformity should be surgically corrected if the deformity is progressive or severe (as defined by interference with gait, or by the presence of a mechanical axis deviation of >10° between the femur and tibia). Symptomatic proximal femoral slipped epiphyses should be surgically stabilized if target values for PTH are not achieved within 3 months of the diagnosis.

Additional Evaluations

The KDIGO guidelines suggest assessing bone mineral density in adults with CKD G3a–G5D, MBD, and/or osteoporosis risk factors. However, ERA-EDTA guidelines do not recommend dual X-ray absorptiometry (DXA) in children for lack of normative data. They recommend plain radiograph in settings of bone pain or deformities, suspected fractures or slipped epiphyses, and to assess bone age. Bone biopsy is suggested to evaluate bone turnover, mineralization, and volume in adult patients with pathological ("fragility") fractures and before antiresorptive or other therapies for osteoporosis. In children, biopsy is reserved for patients with severe bone deformity or pain, low energy fracture, and persistent hypercalcemia or hypophosphatemia despite optimizing treatment. Screening for valvular and vascular calcifications in patients with CKD G3–G5D requires echocardiography and lateral abdominal radiograph. Ultrasonography for carotid intima medial thickness is limited by observer expertise, lack of wide availability, and technical limitations in children.

Anemia

Evaluation

The KDIGO guidelines endorse the WHO thresholds of hemoglobin to diagnose anemia in children. Anemia is diagnosed if hemoglobin concentration is <11.0 g/dL at 0.5–5 years, <11.5 g/dL at 5–12 years and <12.0 g/dL at 12–15 years; in older patients, anemia is the presence of hemoglobin <13.0 g/dL in boys and <12.0 g/dL in girls. Anemia should be prevented by ensuring adequate intake of iron and folic acid and management of metabolic acidosis and hyperparathyroidism. Patients should be screened for anemia at least annually in patients with CKD G3a–G3b and 6 monthly in patients with CKD G4–G5.

Useful initial tests when evaluating for cause of anemia include: (*i*) complete blood count, including hemoglobin concentration, red cell indices, white blood cell count, and differential and platelet count; (*ii*) absolute reticulocyte count; (*iii*) serum iron studies (ferritin, iron, and transferrin saturation); and (*iv*) serum vitamin B_{12} and folate levels. Inadequate iron supply, the most common etiology of anemia in CKD, is distinguished into two categories that indicate pathophysiology and guide the management. *Absolute iron deficiency* is a deficit of total body iron, leading to reduced levels of both circulating and stored iron. *Functional iron deficiency* is defined as a deficiency of circulating iron that limits erythropoiesis despite normal or elevated body iron stores. **Table 26.8** lists markers of iron status that may enable this discrimination. Reticulocyte hemoglobin indicates response to iron within 3–4 days of initiating therapy. Percentage of hypochromic red cells reflects average iron availability in the last 2–3 months. Hepcidin levels do not consistently distinguish absolute from functional iron deficiency or determine ESA responsiveness. Serum ferritin and transferrin saturation remain the most consistent markers to discriminate iron deficient and replete states.

Approach to Management

Flowchart 26.1 summarizes an approach to management of anemia. The mainstay of management is iron supplementation and ESAs. Therapy is titrated to keep hemoglobin levels above threshold and below 12 g/dL. Blood transfusions are avoided to prevent sensitization.

TABLE 26.8: Markers of iron deficiency in anemia of chronic kidney disease

Investigation	*Measure*	*Status in iron deficiency*	*Sensitivity; specificity*	*Limitations*
Ferritin	Serum ferritin, ng/dL	<100 ng/dL in CKD 2-5ND; <200 ng/dL in CKD-5D	*CKD 2-5ND:* 35%; 78% *CKD5D:* 41%; 100%	Acute phase reactant; unreliable in inflammation
Transferrin saturation (TSat)	Percentage of serum iron bound to transferrin	<20%	63%; 80%	Levels affected by malnutrition and inflammation
Hypochromic red blood cells (HRC), %	Proportion of red blood cells with reduced hemoglobin concentration	Does not reflect iron stores; suggests its reduced utilization	>6%: 82%; 95%	Levels should be measured within 6 hr of sample collection
Reticulocyte hemoglobin content (CHr)	Absolute hemoglobin content of reticulocytes, pg	Does not reflect iron stores; suggests its reduced utilization	<29 pg: 57%; 93%	Level varies with maturation of reticulocytes
Hepcidin	Blood level of hepcidin	Increased	Limited data	Levels unreliable in inflammation
Soluble transferrin receptor (sTfR)	Serum level of transferrin receptors	Increased	>1.5 mg/L: 81%; 71%	Levels increase with erythropoietin therapy

D: on dialysis ND: not on dialysis

Flowchart 26.1: Evaluation and management of anemia of CKD. While absolute iron deficiency is managed with oral iron, many patients, particularly those receiving hemodialysis (HD), require parenteral administration of iron. Functional iron deficiency, referring to the inability to synthesize erythropoietin or utilize body iron stores effectively, is managed by additional use of erythropoiesis stimulating agents (regular or pegylated erythropoietin, darbepoetin). Daprodustat is the only hypoxia inducible factor-prolyl hydroxylase inhibitor (HIF-PHI) approved for the management of anemia of CKD in adult patients. PD: peritoneal dialysis; TIBC: total iron binding capacity; TSH: thyroid-stimulating hormone

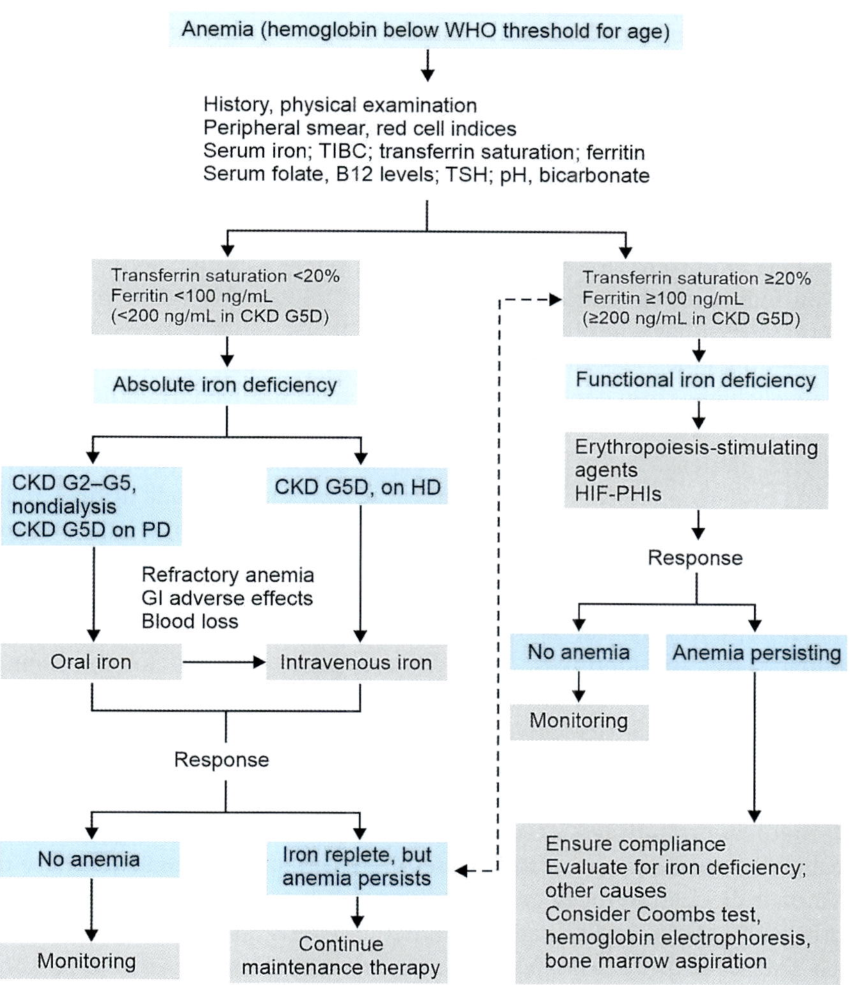

Therapy for Iron Deficiency

Therapy with oral iron is initiated in patients with serum ferritin ≤100 ng/mL (≤200 ng/mL in CKD G5D) or transferrin saturation ≤20%. **Table 26.9** provides options of iron therapy. Ferrous iron is administered orally at a dose of 2–3 mg/ kg/day, on empty stomach (or an hour after meals) in one to two doses, with juice or water. Ferric iron preparations are given in a dose of 3–5 mg/kg/day, in one or two doses, with meals, juice, or water. Oral iron is inexpensive and readily available; however, gastrointestinal discomfort often limits compliance. Studies in adult subjects suggest that switching to an alternate-day schedule might reduce gastrointestinal adverse effects while providing iron supplementation at equivalent or improved efficacy; the latter is attributed to avoidance of the physiological peak of hepcidin, which increases fractional iron absorption. Alternate day therapy has not been tested in children with CKD.

Simultaneously, adequate dietary intake of iron should be ensured. The best food source of iron is "heme iron", present in high concentrations in animal sources with a bioavailability of about 20%. Most vegetarian food sources have nonheme iron, with a bioavailability of 5%. Legumes (e.g., lentils, chickpeas, and white or soya beans), wheat bran, and nuts have relatively higher iron content. Iron absorption is improved by adding acid to food, e.g., ascorbic acid (orange, lemon, or grapefruit juice), other sources (apples, grapes, lemons, pears, and raspberries). Tannins (coffee, tea, and wine), oxalate (spinach, rhubarb, and cacao), phosphate (soda drinks), milk proteins, and egg white inhibit the absorption of nonheme iron. Except for iron-based binders, oral phosphate binders inhibit gastrointestinal absorption of iron.

Therapy with IV iron is indicated in children who continue to be iron deficient due to blood loss, cannot tolerate oral iron, are noncompliant, or are on hemodialysis. The chief benefits of IV iron therapy are assured compliance, avoidance of adverse effects (bad taste, gastrointestinal effects), and the bypassing of the intestinal mucosal barrier, which ensures a better hemoglobin response than with oral therapy. Iron sucrose is the most used IV medication, administered once a week to achieve iron-replete state. Available preparations and their doses are listed in **Table 26.9**. The dose of IV iron is dictated by the degree of anemia and status of iron stores (Ganzoni formula; **Table 26.9**). For patients on hemodialysis, the dose is given in the last half hour of hemodialysis session. Infusion reactions, ranging from chills, to hypotension, dyspnea and rarely, anaphylaxis, are most common with high molecular weight iron dextran (1% cases), less common with iron sucrose and low molecular weight iron dextrans, and uncommon with ferric gluconate, ferric carboxymaltose, and iron isomaltoside preparations. Recent "optimized" formulations (e.g., ferric carboxymaltose) allow delivery of an optimal dose of iron through fewer infusions and in shorter infusion time.

TABLE 26.9: Iron preparations used in patients with anemia of chronic kidney disease (CKD)[1]

Oral preparation	*Indian brands*	*Tablet or syrup strength*	*Elemental iron (%)*	*Dose in anemia, mg/kg/day*
Ferrous sulfate	Feosol; Generic	200 mg; 325 mg	65 mg (33; 20)	2–3
Ferric maltol	Accrufer capsules	30 mg	30 mg (100)	3–5
Ferrous fumarate	Autrin, Vitcofol capsules Nid-XT syrup	300 mg NA	98.6 mg (33) 100 mg/5 mL	2–3
Ferrous gluconate	Gynae Cvp RB Tone syrup	~500 mg 130 mg per 5 mL	67 mg (12) 15 mg/5 mL (12)	2–3
Liposomal iron pyrophosphate	Softeron, Fevirich, Ferisome	635 mg	30 mg (5)	3–5
Heme iron polypeptide	Lupiheme	835 mg	12 mg (1)	2–3
Not commented upon (KDIGO 2021)				
Colloidal iron	Tonoferon syrup Tonoferon pediatric syrup	NA NA	250 mg 80 mg	2–3
Ferric pyrophosphate	Vitcofol-Hb capsules	500 mg	30 mg (6)	3–5
Ferrous ascorbate	Autrin-XT, Feronia XT	NA	100 mg	2–3
Ferrous sulfate + ascorbic acid	Generic	200 mg	105 mg	2–3
Ferrous feredetate	Redihealth, Lexifer tablet Redihealth, Irex syrup	231 mg 231 mg per 5 mL	33 mg (14) 33 mg/5 mL	2–3
Carbonyl iron	Fefol-Z, Cofol-Z Imax forte, FE-3	50 mg 100 mg	50 mg (100) 100 mg (100)	2–3

Contd...

Contd...

Intravenous preparation[2]	*Indian (foreign) brands*	*Usual (max.) single dose; doses/week; weekly dose*	*Dilution; concentration; infusion time [in adults]*	*Elemental iron, mg/mL*	*IV iron dose guide in children (Ganzoni formula)*
Iron sucrose; similar (≥2-year-old)	Imax S, Flagfer	0.5 (7) mg/kg (NA); 3; 500 mg	In normal saline (round off to higher 100; i.e., <100 mg in 100 mL, 200–300 mg in 300 mL); ~1 mg/mL; 30–90 minutes (15–30 mins)	20	Cumulative total dose = Total iron deficiency, mg = Body weight, kg × (target Hb – measured Hb, g/dL) × 2.4 + iron stores, mg
LMW iron dextran[2]	NA (Cosmofer, INFeD)	5–10 (20) mg/kg; 3; 100 mg	*Undiluted:* 50 mg/mL; 1 mL/min [20 mins (EMA); >60 mins (FDA)]; diluted in 250–1,000 mL saline: 1–6 hr	50	Weight, kg: <35 / ≥35 Target Hb, g/dL: 13 / 15 Iron stores: 15 mg/kg / 500 mg
Ferric carboxymaltose (≥1-year-old)	Larinject; FeReload; NeFCM; Ferium	15 (20) mg/kg; 1; 1,000 mg (1,500 mg in 2 weeks)	In normal saline; 2–5 mg/mL; >15 mins [7.5 mins (FDA), 15 mins (EMA)]	50	
Sodium ferric gluconate (>6-year-old)	NA (Ferrlecit)	1.5 mg/kg (125 mg); 3; NA	25 mL normal saline; max. 5 mg/mL; 60 mins [10 mins (FDA)]	12.5	

Contd...

Contd...

Intravenous preparation[2]	*Indian (foreign) brands*	*Usual (max.) single dose; doses/week; weekly dose*	*Dilution; concentration; infusion time [in adults]*	*Elemental iron, mg/mL*	*IV iron dose guide in children (Ganzoni formula)*
Iron isomaltoside/ ferric derisomaltose (>18-year-old)	Isofer	20 mg/kg; 1; 1,000 mg	In normal saline; 1 mg/mL; ≥20 minutes [250 mg/min (EMA)]	100	
Ferumoxytol (>18-year-old)	NA (Rienso, Feraheme)	510 mg; 1; 1,020 mg	In 50–200 mL normal saline or 5% dextrose; ≥15 minutes [15 minutes (FDA)]	30	

[1]Sucroferric oxyhydroxide and ferric citrate are not included, since they are not recommended as iron supplements (elemental iron is poorly absorbed)
[2]Conventional iron dextran is no longer used due to high risk of adverse effects (1% incidence of severe acute reactions, e.g., anaphylaxis, respiratory arrest or hypotension)
(EMA: European Medial Association; FDA: Federal Drug Authority, USA; Hb: hemoglobin; IV: intravenous; KDIGO: kidney diseases improving global outcomes)
Source:
1. Babitt JL, et al. 2021
2. Mattiello V, et al. 2020
3. National Blood Authority, Australia. Paediatric and Neonatal Iron Deficiency Anaemia Guide. Available from *https://blood.gov.au/system/files/Corrected-Paed-and-Neonatal-IDA-Guide-dosing-for-iron-polymaltose.pdf* [last accessed June 2024].]

Iron status should be reassessed every 3–6 months, and more frequently when initiating or increasing ESA dose, following blood loss, and to document response to a course of IV iron. If iron deficiency persists despite IV administration, patients should be assessed for a source of active blood loss. An increase in ferritin level accompanied by decrease in transferrin saturation and hemoglobin suggests inflammation-mediated reticuloendothelial blockade.

Erythropoiesis-stimulating Agents

Table 26.10 lists options of therapy with recombinant human EPO (rhEPO) and its long-acting analogs. Therapy is initiated in iron-replete patients in whom alternative causes of anemia have been excluded (**Flowchart 26.1**).

Recombinant human EPO: Therapy is initiated at 50–150 IU/kg/week in two to three divided doses IV or subcutaneously and targeted to hemoglobin rise by 0.5–2 g/dL per month. While the IV route is painless and ensures compliance in children on maintenance hemodialysis, the required dose is usually 25–33% higher than the subcutaneous dose. Younger children require higher doses (~275–350 U/kg/week) compared to older children (~200–250 U/kg/week). Similar to adult patients with CKD, the maintenance dose is titrated based on monthly hemoglobin values to maintain it between 11 and 12 g/dL, since higher hemoglobin targets in adults are associated with increased risk of hypertension, stroke, vascular access thrombosis, serious cardiovascular events, and mortality. rhEPO is avoided in patients with history of stroke and in active malignancy. When the hemoglobin approaches 11.5 g/dL or if the hemoglobin increases by >1.0 g/dL in any 2-week period, the ESA dose is reduced by 25%, and therapy is withheld if the hemoglobin continues to increase. Therapy is reinitiated at a lower dose once hemoglobin drops below 11 g/dL.

The frequency of ESA administration depends on considerations of efficacy, convenience, and comfort. Initial therapy with short-acting rhEPO (epoetin α, β) is administered 2–3 times/week; once anemia is corrected, therapy may be switched to once a week; however, twice a week maintenance therapy is more effective than one a week therapy, since the latter is associated with large fluctuations in blood EPO levels.

Novel erythropoietic stimulatory proteins (NESPs): Darbepoetin-α has emerged as the ESA of choice in children as well as adults with anemia of CKD. This long-acting protein has extrasialic acid residues that stabilize the protein *in vivo*, providing a twofold to threefold longer half-life as compared to rhEPO. Hence, the medication may be administered at 1–4 weeks intervals with improved adherence and effective correction of anemia **(Table 26.10)**. Continuous erythropoietin receptor activators (CERA)

TABLE 26.10: Erythropoiesis-stimulating agents and hypoxia-inducible factor-prolyl hydroxylase inhibitors approved for use in anemia of CKD

	Description (brands); molecular weight, kDa	*Bioavailable, %*	*Half-life, hour (route)*	*Dose*	*Dosing interval*
Erythropoiesis-stimulating agents (ESA)					
Epoetin alpha	Unmodified rhEPO or short-acting ESA (Epogen); 32–40	30–36	8.8 (IV) 24.2 (SC)	Initial: 100–200 U/kg/week Maintenance: 60–600 U/kg/week	Two to three times per week
Epoetin beta	Unmodified rhEPO or short-acting ESA (NeoRecormon); 32–40	23–42	6.8 (IV) 19.4 (SC)	40 U/kg/wk (IV) 20 U/kg/wk (SC)	Two to three times per week
Darbepoetin alpha	Long-acting ESA (Aranesp; Darbenef; Darbatitor; Cresp); 40	37	25 (IV) 49 (SC)	0.45 mg/kg (SC, IV) 0.75 mg/kg (SC)	Every week Every 2 weeks
Methoxy polyethylene glycol epoetin beta	Long-acting ESA (Mircera); 60	47–52	133 (IV) 137 (SC)	0.6 mg/kg (SC, IV) 1.2 mg/kg (SC)[1]	Every 2 weeks[1] Every 4 weeks[1]
***Hypoxia-inducible factor-prolyl hydroxylase inhibitors*[2]**		***Oral dose in adults***			***Frequency***
Daprodustat		2–4 mg (if ESA naïve); 1–4 mg (if switch from ESA)			Daily
Enarodustat		2 mg (ESA naïve or treated)			Daily
Molidustat		25 mg (ESA naïve); 25 or 50 mg (ESA naïve or treated)			Daily
Desidustat		100 mg (ESA naïve)			Thrice a week
Roxadustat		50, 70, or 100 mg (ESA-naïve); 70 or 100 mg (ESA-treated)			Thrice a week
Vadadustat		300 mg; then 150, 450, or 600 mg (ESA-naive or ESA-treated)			Daily

[1]Dosing q2 week in CKD G2–G5 nondialysis and CKD G5D; q4 week only if CKD G2–G5 nondialysis

[2]Have not yet been approved for use in children; only daprodustat is approved for use in adults on hemodialysis

IV: intravenous; rhEPO: recombinant human erythropoietin; SC: subcutaneous; wk: week

such as methoxypolyethylene glycol-epoetin-β (e.g., MIRCERA®) have a different receptor-binding activity than other ESA, which allows continuous stimulation of erythropoiesis. Further, the agent has a prolonged half-life. These factors allow once-monthly dosing in patients with anemia of CKD. CERAs have not been tested adequately in children.

Erythropoiesis-stimulating Agent Hyporesponsiveness

Patients in whom there is no increase in hemoglobin concentration from baseline after the first month of ESA treatment on weight-based dosing, or after treatment with stable doses of ESA, require repeated increases in ESA doses beyond the dose at which they had been stable, are considered ESA hyporesponsive. These patients are evaluated for alternative causes of unsatisfactory response, including iron, folate and carnitine deficiency, non-adherence, chronic infections, inflammation and oxidative stress, chronic blood loss, secondary hyperparathyroidism, hypothyroidism, use of RASi, and underdialysis.

Pure red cell aplasia secondary to neutralizing antibodies against erythropoietin should be suspected in cases of sudden and severe hyporesponsiveness (sudden rapid decrease in hemoglobin by 0.5–1 g/dL each week or need for 1–2 transfusions per week) associated with normal leukocyte and platelet counts and low absolute reticulocyte count (<10,000/mL). The diagnosis is confirmed by demonstrating neutralizing antibodies against erythropoietin and absence of parvovirus infection. Immunosuppression and/or administration of peginesatide, a synthetic, peptide-based erythropoietin-receptor agonist, might be helpful.

Hypoxia-inducible Factors Prolyl-hydroxylase Inhibitors

This new class of agents for the therapy of anemia of CKD work by stabilizing the HIF complex and stimulating endogenous erythropoietin production, improving iron mobilization to the bone marrow, and improve its utilization for erythropoiesis **(Fig. 26.5)**. Thus, HIF-PHIs correct functional iron deficiency associated with chronic inflammation, in CKD and other indications. Large randomized controlled trials have shown that HIF-PHIs are superior to placebo and not inferior to ESAs in increasing and maintaining hemoglobin concentration among adult patients with CKD, whether on or not on dialysis. Their oral dosing is a major advantage over ESAs, which makes them more convenient, acceptable, and feasible than parenteral administration of ESA. Of six agents that have been tested, only daprodustat has received FDA approval for use in adult patients with CKD-5D. Use in children is not recommended as studies on safety and efficacy in anemia of CKD in children are awaited.

Other Measures

Guidelines recommend against using androgens, vitamin C, vitamin D, vitamin E, folic acid, L-carnitine, or pentoxifylline to manage anemia of CKD. With availability of ESA, patients with CKD do not require repeated transfusions, which carry risks of chronic viral infections, allergic reactions, anaphylaxis, and sensitization to human lymphocyte antigens. Packed cells are reserved for (*i*) acute severe hemorrhage with blood loss >25–30% of blood volume; (*ii*) need for rapid correction of anemia perioperatively, at hemoglobin < 6.5 g/dL; (*iii*) severe anemia in ESA-hyporesponsive patients. The role of immunosuppression in reducing risk of sensitization is unclear.

SUPPORTIVE CARE IN CHRONIC KIDNEY DISEASE

Metabolic Acidosis

Maintenance of acid-base balance is particularly required in infants and young children, in whom persistent metabolic acidosis contributes to failure to thrive, bone demineralization, and hyperkalemia. Patients with serum bicarbonate <15 mEq/L should receive oral supplementation with sodium bicarbonate at 2–3 mEq/kg of bicarbonate. Therapy is subsequently titrated to maintain serum bicarbonate concentration of 18–22 mEq/L. Options for bicarbonate replacement are provided in **Annexure 5**.

Bleeding Diathesis

Patients may show platelet dysfunction with increased risk of bleeding, especially following surgical and invasive procedures. Dialysis, blood transfusions, dDAVP infusion, and oral contraceptives correct this dysfunction. The role of dDAVP (1–3 μg/kg, given IV as an infusion or as intranasal spray, 30 minutes before renal biopsy or operative procedures) in correcting bleeding time is unclear.

Hypertension

Hypertension is a common complication of CKD and should be controlled using a combination of lifestyle measures and pharmacotherapy (see **Chapter 25**). Guidelines recommend that therapy for hypertension in children with CKD be started when the blood pressure is consistently above the 90th percentile for age, sex, and height. The American Academy of Pediatrics guidelines recommend that blood pressure be lowered to achieve mean ambulatory blood pressure ≤50th centile for age, sex, and height, unless achieving these targets is limited by signs or symptoms of hypotension. The European Society of Hypertension guidelines recommend blood pressure target below the 50th centile in the presence of proteinuria and below the 75th centile in the absence of proteinuria.

Regardless of the presence of proteinuria, ACEI and ARB are preferred antihypertensive agents in patients with GFR >30 mL/min/1.73 m^2. Other options include calcium channel blockers, prazosin, clonidine, and alpha and beta-blockers. Calcium channel blockers are useful and safe agents; however, agents of the dihydropyridine class (amlodipine) do not reduce proteinuria and may cause pedal edema. Beta-blockers (atenolol and metoprolol) reduce sympathetic tone and decreases renin production, which might be useful in retarding CKD progression. Diuretics are useful in patients with fluid overload. Most patients require more than one drug to control blood pressure adequately. ACEI and ARB combinations are avoided due to significant risk of adverse effects.

Medication Management in Chronic Kidney Disease

Modification of Drug Doses

Pharmacokinetics of many medications are altered in CKD. While the most well-described consequence is reduced renal clearance of drugs which are principally eliminated by the kidneys, drug absorption, distribution, transport, and metabolism might also be affected. Therefore, doses of many medications need to be adjusted for low eGFR to avoid medication toxicity. While the loading dose is usually unchanged, maintenance dosing often requires adjustments such as dose reduction, lengthening the dosing interval, or both. Where appropriate and feasible, serum drug concentrations are used to monitor bioavailability and potential for toxicity. Multiple online or electronic calculators are available to assist in dosing decisions. **Annexure 7** provides a list of common medications with advice for modified dosing at low eGFR.

Avoidance of Nephrotoxic Medications

Medications with nephrotoxic metabolites should be avoided in patients with CKD. Patients should be counseled against indiscriminate use of over-the-counter medications, especially painkillers and proton-pump inhibitors. Where unavoidable, the least nephrotoxic agents should be used. Common examples of common nephrotoxic medications, which have non-nephrotoxic alternatives, include: (*i*) *Analgesics* [nonsteroidal anti-inflammatory drug (NSAID): Reduce GFR, may cause allergic interstitial nephritis (AIN)]; (*ii*) antimicrobials: (*a*) aminoglycosides [cause acute tubular necrosis (ATN)], (*b*) vancomycin (ATN, possibly, AIN), (*c*) sulfamethoxazole-trimethoprim (AIN, ATN, crystalluria, and inhibition of tubular creatinine secretion); (*iii*) *proton pump inhibitors* (AKI and CKD due to AIN and tubulointerstitial nephritis, TIN); (*iv*) warfarin (glomerular hemorrhage, ATN, and vascular calcification); and (*v*) *lithium* (nephrogenic diabetes insipidus, chronic TIN). If patients with CKD are prescribed medications with potential nephrotoxicity or renally cleared medications with narrow therapeutic window, one should monitor closely the eGFR, serum electrolytes, any parameters specifically altered by the concerned medication, and where appropriate and feasible, drug levels (trough or area under the curve). Complementary and alternative medications and dietary supplements should be avoided; if used, their potential toxicities should be considered as their safety in patients with CKD is not established. The use of oral phosphate-containing bowel preparations is avoided in patients with GFR <60 mL/min/1.73 m^2 to avoid phosphate overload.

Prevention of Radiocontrast-associated AKI

In patients with low GFR planned for imaging with radiocontrast injection, the risk of contrast-associated AKI should be weighed against the diagnostic value and therapeutic implications of the investigation. Risk factors for radiocontrast-associated AKI include: (*i*) Acutely or chronically low GFR (<45 or <30 mL/min/1.73 m^2, with or without other risk factors, respectively); (*ii*) hypovolemia; (*iii*) concomitant nephrotoxic medications; (*iv*) diabetes mellitus; (*v*) use of high-osmolar contrast; (*vi*) large volume of contrast; (*vii*) serial contrast procedures; and (*viii*) intra-arterial procedures. For at-risk patients requiring radiocontrast administration, guidelines recommend (*i*) oral or IV hydration, (*ii*) use of the minimum volume of radiocontrast, (*iii*) preference of iso-osmolar or low-osmolality contrast, and (*iv*) where feasible, discontinuation of therapy with RASi, metformin, potentially nephrotoxic medications (e.g., NSAIDs, diuretics, aminoglycosides, amphotericin, platins, zoledronate, and methotrexate) 48-hr prior to the procedure. There is no proven role for therapy with N-acetylcysteine, ascorbic acid, furosemide, dopamine, fenoldopam, or calcium channel blockers in preventing radiocontrast-associated AKI.

Preventing Nephrogenic Systemic Fibrosis

While gadolinium chelates used during magnetic resonance (MR) imaging were reported to cause nephrogenic systemic fibrosis (NSF), this entity has been rarely reported since 2012, possibly because of worldwide reduction in use of American College of Radiology (ACR) group I gadolinium-based contrast agents (gadodiamide, gadopentetate dimeglumine, and gadoversetamide). Patients with CKD G4–G5 who require MR contrast imaging should be offered ACR group II and III gadolinium-based contrast agents (gadobenate dimeglumine, gadobutrol, gadoteridol, gadoterate meglumine, and gadoxetate disodium) to minimize their risk of developing NSF. However, the newer linear and macrocyclic gadolinium preparations are expensive, and their availability is limited in low-resource settings. None of the gadolinium-based contrast media are licensed for use in infants. While the risk of NSF in children is unclear, it is likely lower than in adults.

Prevention of Acute Kidney Injury

All patients with CKD are at increased risk of AKI and should be managed to prevent risk of AKI during intercurrent illness, and when undergoing procedures that increase the risk of AKI or drug toxicity, as discussed above. Common illnesses that predispose to hypovolemia or dehydration leading to AKI include acute febrile illnesses, diarrhea, vomiting, and urinary tract infection. Other settings of AKI in patients with CKD are uncontrolled hypertension and urinary tract obstruction. Medications such as RASi (ACEI, ARBs, and MRAs), SGLT2i, diuretics, NSAIDs, and metformin should be discontinued (*i*) on sick days (diarrhea, vomiting, high grade fever, or other settings of low oral intake during which dehydration or hypovolemia may occur); (*ii*) in the 48–72 hr prior to elective surgery; and (*iii*) during the acute management of medication-associated adverse effects, as a precautionary measure to prevent complications. In these settings, AKI and dyselectrolytemias should be actively looked for, promptly recognized, and corrected **(Box 26.3)**.

Immunization

Patients with advanced CKD, especially if on dialysis, and those receiving immunosuppression (e.g., for glomerular disease, following kidney transplantation) are at significant risk of common and opportunistic infections, many of which are vaccine-preventable. Vaccination in patients with CKD is often delayed or missed due to lack of awareness, low coverage of routine immunization in underserved areas, noninclusion of useful vaccines in national immunization program, avoidance of live vaccines while on immunosuppression, and parental concern around safety of vaccination in ill child. Further, seroprotection against hepatitis B and other pathogens may wane through childhood, particularly if immunosuppressed.

It is recommended that children with CKD receive catch-up immunization to complete routine vaccination and certain additional vaccines which are particularly important in patients on immunosuppression or those planned for kidney transplantation. **Table 26.11** lists recommended and contraindicated vaccines and dosing schedules. Killed and subunit vaccines have acceptable efficacy and safety in children with CKD and following transplantation, but their immunogenicity, as measured by antibody titers, is inconsistent, particularly for patients on immunosuppression or dialysis. Hence, the benefits and risks of booster doses require to be individualized and are preferably guided by antibody titers. Vaccination against hepatitis B is particularly relevant since dialysis and recurrent hospitalizations in advanced CKD expose patients to blood-borne pathogens. Experts advocate the use of double doses of the vaccine (20 μg instead of 10 μg) in an accelerated schedule, and regular monitoring of anti-HBs antibody titers to ensure continued protection **(Table 26.11)**.

TABLE 26.11: Vaccination advice for patients with chronic kidney disease in preparation for kidney replacement therapy and transplantation

Vaccine	*Type*	*Schedule*
Hepatitis B	Recombinant DNA	0, 1 and 6 months; or 0, 1, and 2 months;[1] prefer using double the usual dose (i.e., 1 mL) Confirm seroprotective titer (>10 mIU/mL)
Hepatitis A	Killed; live attenuated	Either two doses (killed vaccine) 6 months apart; or single dose (live vaccine)
Pneumococcal	Conjugate and polysaccharide	1–3 dose of conjugate vaccine[2] followed by one dose of the polysaccharide vaccine 8 weeks later
Human papilloma virus	Killed	Children >9 years: 0, 2, and 6 months
Varicella[3]	Live attenuated	Two doses, administered ≥4 weeks (preferably 12-week) apart Avoid for 1 month if administered blood product or tuberculin test; last dose given ≥4 weeks prior to transplant
Measles, mumps and rubella (MMR)[3]	Live attenuated	One dose; two doses ≥4 weeks apart if only one dose given previously at <1 year of age Ensure that the last dose is given ≥4 weeks prior to transplant
Influenza	Killed vaccine	One dose; repeat annually (before and after transplantation)
TdaP	Killed vaccine	Single dose
Td or TT	Killed vaccine	Booster every 5 years after transplantation
Typhoid	Conjugate	Single dose
Hemophilus influenza B (Hib)	Conjugate	Age 6–26 weeks: Three doses a month apart; two boosters at 7–11 and 15–24 months; age 6–12 months: Two doses a month apart; one booster at 15–24 months; age 12–15 months: One dose followed by one booster at 18–24 months; 16–60 months: One booster dose; no catch-up immunization beyond 5 years
Meningococcal	Conjugate	*Age >1 year:* One dose
Can be used, if indicated, after transplant		All the above vaccines, except live vaccines Japanese encephalitis; injectable polio; and rabies
Contraindicated after transplantation		Bacillus Calmette-Guérin (BCG); live-attenuated influenza; MMR; oral poliovirus; rotavirus; smallpox; oral typhoid; varicella; and yellow fever

[1]Accelerated schedule preferred if kidney replacement therapy imminent; repeat a dose after 12 months to sustain immunity; monitor titers to ensure continued seroprotection

[2]*Advice for conjugate vaccine:* (i) If not previously immunized: Age 6–26 weeks: three doses a month apart and one booster at 7–11 months; 7–11 months: Two doses a month apart and one booster after 8 weeks; 12–23 months: two doses 8 weeks apart; >24 months: Two doses 1 month apart; (ii) If previously received immunization as advised at <24 months and currently > 2 years old: One dose

[3]MMR preferred to MR; MMR-V vaccine is licensed for use only during 2–12 years age

Td tetanus: low dose diphtheria; TdaP: tetanus: low dose diphtheria, acellular pertussis; TT: tetanus toxoid

If vaccination is necessary following transplantation, doses of nonlive vaccines may be delayed to 6–12 months after transplantation to avoid the period of intense immunosuppression and ensure higher rates of seroprotection. However, the influenza vaccine should be given annually before the peak season, regardless of timing post-transplant. Despite a small risk of human leukocyte antigen (HLA) sensitization with certain vaccines, available data does not suggest an increased risk of rejection. All live vaccines are contraindicated after renal transplantation and while on significant immunosuppression. Immunosuppressed patients who are not immunized or incompletely immunized prior to transplantation remain at risk for varicella, measles, mumps, and rubella. Hence, wherever feasible, live vaccines should be administered before immunosuppression, e.g., prior to transplantation. As immunogenicity is greater before transplantation, immunization with nonlive vaccines is also preferred during this period. Immunosuppressed patients exposed to pathogens against which they lack protection might require postexposure prophylaxis, e.g., varicella. Close contacts and household members of children with CKD should complete age-appropriate vaccination schedules to increase the child's indirect protection.

Counseling and Education

It is important to discuss with the parents' issues pertaining to the child's illness at every stage of CKD, including the etiology, severity, options of management, and the risks of disease progression. The child should be encouraged to participate in age-appropriate activities and attend regular school. Beginning from CKD G3, care providers should be counseled regarding available options for KRT to allow them to discuss adequately and arrive at a counseled decision in the best interests of the child and the family. The KDIGO advises that patients with a kidney failure risk of >40% or eGFR of <15 mL/min per 1.73 m^2 should be referred to centers with expertise for placement of vascular access for long-term hemodialysis; alternatively, they may be considered for placement of catheter for peritoneal dialysis or prepared for preemptive kidney transplantation.

Transition of Care

Adolescents and young adults should be transitioned to adult care during times of medical and social stability, where possible. Many pediatric-onset kidney diseases are stable through childhood and at risk of progression to advanced CKD in early adulthood. "Emerging adulthood" is a vulnerable age with high risk of nonadherence to medications and instructions, and major lifestyle and dietary changes, which might predispose to a high risk for adverse outcomes.

Preparation for transfer should begin during pediatric care, ideally as early as 11–14 years of age. Various checklists have been developed to assess the readiness of young people and guide preparation for transfer of care. In preparation for transfer, young people should be seen by the pediatric nephrologist alone for at least part of each visit. Caregivers or significant others should be included in initial patient visits to the "adult" nephrologist, with permission of the patient. Transfer of care should always be accompanied by a comprehensive written summary of the history, examination, and investigations over the period of the child's illness. In addition, a verbal handover should be provided by the pediatric to "adult" nephrologist, which includes an assessment of cognitive ability and social support. Where feasible, complete transition to regular adult care should be preceded by a period of joint pediatric-adult care or young adult care.

Annexure 26.1: Online calculator for Kidney Failure Risk Equation (KFRE) in Adults with CKD https://kidneyfailurerisk.com *Scan the QR code below or type the following link in browser window:*	
Annexure 26.2: Online calculator for Risk of Progression to ESKD in Children with CKD https://www.kidney.org/pediatric-chronic-kidney-disease-risk-calculator *Scan the QR code below or type the following link in browser window:*	
Annexure 26.3: Online calculator for Estimating Time to Progression to ESKD in Children with CKD https://form.jotform.com/81565256783164 *Scan the QR code below or type the following link in browser window:*	

BIBLIOGRAPHY

Definitions, Epidemiology, Risk Factors

1. Harada R, Hamasaki Y, Okuda Y, et al. Epidemiology of pediatric chronic kidney disease/kidney failure: Learning from registries and cohort studies. Pediatr Nephrol. 2022;37:1215-29.
2. Kidney Disease: Improving Global Outcomes (KDIGO) CKD Work Group. KDIGO 2024 Clinical Practice Guideline for the Evaluation and Management of Chronic Kidney Disease. Kidney Int. 2024;105:S117-S314.
3. Panzarino V, Lesser J, Cassani FA. Pediatric chronic kidney disease. Adv Pediatr. 2022;69:123-32.
4. VanSickle JS, Warady BA. Chronic kidney disease in children. Pediatr Clin North Am. 2022;69:1239-54.

Progression of Chronic Kidney Disease

1. Alshahrani S. Renin-angiotensin-aldosterone pathway modulators in chronic kidney disease: A comparative review. Front Pharmacol. 2023;14:1101068.
2. Baran W, Krzemińska J, Szlagor M, et al. Mineralocorticoid receptor antagonists-Use in chronic kidney disease. Int J Mol Sci. 2021;22:9995.
3. Chou YH, Chu TS, Lin SL. Role of renin-angiotensin system in acute kidney injury-chronic kidney disease transition. Nephrology (Carlton). 2018;23 Suppl 4:121-5.
4. Chung EY, Ruospo M, Natale P, et al. Aldosterone antagonists in addition to renin angiotensin system antagonists for preventing the progression of chronic kidney disease. Cochrane Database Syst Rev. 2020;10:CD007004.
5. Gan L, Lyu X, Yang X, et al. Application of angiotensin receptor-neprilysin inhibitor in chronic kidney disease patients: Chinese Expert Consensus. Front Med (Lausanne). 2022;9:877237.
6. Padda IS, Mahtani AU, Parmar M. Sodium-glucose transport protein 2 (SGLT2) inhibitors. Treasure Island (FL): StatPearls Publishing; 2024.
7. Ruiz-Ortega M, Rayego-Mateos S, Lamas S, et al. Targeting the progression of chronic kidney disease. Nat Rev Nephrol. 2020;16:269-88.

Nutrition and Growth

1. Drube J, Wan M, Bonthuis M, et al.; European Society for Paediatric Nephrology Chronic Kidney Disease Mineral and Bone Disorders, Dialysis, and Transplantation Working Groups. Clinical practice recommendations for growth hormone treatment in children with chronic kidney disease. Nat Rev Nephrol. 2019;15:577-89.
2. Nelms CL, Shaw V, Greenbaum LA, et al. Assessment of nutritional status in children with kidney diseases-Clinical practice recommendations from the Pediatric Renal Nutrition Taskforce. Pediatr Nephrol. 2021;36:995-1010.
3. Rees L, Shaw V, Qizalbash L, et al.; Pediatric Renal Nutrition Taskforce. Delivery of a nutritional prescription by enteral tube feeding in children with chronic kidney disease stages 2-5 and on dialysis-clinical practice recommendations from the Pediatric Renal Nutrition Taskforce. Pediatr Nephrol. 2021;36:187-204.
4. Shaw V, Polderman N, Renken-Terhaerdt J, et al. Energy and protein requirements for children with CKD stages 2-5 and on dialysis-clinical practice recommendations from the Pediatric Renal Nutrition Taskforce. Pediatr Nephrol. 2020;35:519-31.

Mineral Bone Disease

1. Bacchetta J, Schmitt CP, Bakkaloglu SA, et al. Diagnosis and management of mineral and bone disorders in infants with CKD: Clinical practice points from the ESPN CKD-MBD and Dialysis working groups and the Pediatric Renal Nutrition Taskforce. Pediatr Nephrol. 2023;38:3163-81.
2. Chan S, Au K, Francis RS, et al. Phosphate binders in patients with chronic kidney disease. Aust Prescr. 2017;40:10-4.
3. Hanudel MR, Salusky IB. Treatment of pediatric chronic kidney disease-Mineral and bone disorder. Curr Osteoporos Rep. 2017;15:198-206.

4. Hu L, Napoletano A, Provenzano M, et al. Mineral bone disorders in kidney disease patients: The ever-current topic. Int J Mol Sci. 2022;23:12223.
5. Lalayiannis AD, Crabtree NJ, Fewtrell M, et al. Assessing bone mineralisation in children with chronic kidney disease: what clinical and research tools are available? Pediatr Nephrol. 2020;35:937-57.
6. McAlister L, Pugh P, Greenbaum L, et al. The dietary management of calcium and phosphate in children with CKD stages 2-5 and on dialysis-clinical practice recommendation from the Pediatric Renal Nutrition Taskforce. Pediatr Nephrol. 2020;35:501-18.
7. Santos F, Díaz-Anadón L, Ordóñez FA, et al. Bone disease in CKD in children. Calcif Tissue Int. 2021;108:423-38.
8. Shroff R, Wan M, Nagler EV, et al.; European Society for Paediatric Nephrology Chronic Kidney Disease Mineral and Bone Disorders and Dialysis Working Groups. Clinical practice recommendations for treatment with active vitamin D analogues in children with chronic kidney disease Stages 2-5 and on dialysis. Nephrol Dial Transplant. 2017;32:1114-27.

Anemia

1. Atkinson MA, Warady BA. Anemia in chronic kidney disease. Pediatr Nephrol. 2018;33:227-38.
2. Babitt JL, Eisenga MF, Haase VH, et al.; Conference Participants. Controversies in optimal anemia management: Conclusions from a Kidney Disease: Improving Global Outcomes (KDIGO) Conference. Kidney Int. 2021;99:1280-95.
3. Bruce G, Schulga P, Reynolds BC. Use of erythropoiesis-stimulating agents in children with chronic kidney disease: A systematic review. Clin Kidney J. 2022;15:1483-505.
4. Chung EY, Palmer SC, Saglimbene VM, et al. Erythropoiesis-stimulating agents for anaemia in adults with chronic kidney disease: A network meta-analysis. Cochrane Database Syst Rev. 2023;2:CD010590.
5. Guedes M, Robinson BM, Obrador G, et al. Management of anemia in nondialysis chronic kidney disease: Current recommendations, real-world practice, and patient perspectives. Kidney. 2020;1:855-62.
6. Hanna RM, Streja E, Kalantar-Zadeh K. Burden of anemia in chronic kidney disease: Beyond erythropoietin. Adv Ther. 2021;38:52-75.
7. Ku E, Del Vecchio L, Eckardt KU, et al.; for Conference Participants. Novel anemia therapies in chronic kidney disease: Conclusions from a Kidney Disease: Improving Global Outcomes (KDIGO) Controversies Conference. Kidney Int. 2023;104:655-80.
8. Mattiello V, Schmugge M, Hengartner H, et al.; SPOG Pediatric Hematology Working Group. Diagnosis and management of iron deficiency in children with or without anemia: consensus recommendations of the SPOG Pediatric Hematology Working Group. Eur J Pediatr. 2020;179:527-45.
9. Mikhail A, Brown C, Williams JA, et al. Renal association clinical practice guideline on Anaemia of Chronic Kidney Disease. BMC Nephrol. 2017;18:345.
10. Natale P, Palmer SC, Jaure A, et al. Hypoxia-inducible factor stabilisers for the anaemia of chronic kidney disease. Cochrane Database Syst Rev. 2022;8:CD013751.
11. Patino E, Akchurin O. Erythropoiesis-independent effects of iron in chronic kidney disease. Pediatr Nephrol. 2022;37:777-88.

Other Aspects

1. Bakkaloğlu SA, Özdemir Atikel Y, Paglialonga F, et al. Vaccination practices in pediatric dialysis patients across Europe. A European Pediatric Dialysis Working Group and European Society for Pediatric Nephrology Dialysis Working Group study. Nephron. 2018;138:280-6.
2. Banerjee S, Dissanayake PV, Abeyagunawardena AS. Vaccinations in children on immunosuppressive medications for renal disease. Pediatr Nephrol. 2016;31:7-48.
3. Costello J. Immunization recommendations for pediatric patients with chronic kidney disease, nephrotic syndrome, and renal transplants: A literature review and quality improvement project. Nephrol Nurs J. 2019;46:413-45.
4. Damianaki A, Polychronopoulou E, Wuerzner G, et al. New aspects in the management of hypertension in patients with chronic kidney disease not on renal replacement therapy. High Blood Press Cardiovasc Prev. 2022;29:125-35.

Chronic Hemodialysis

Priyanka Khandelwal, Rukshana Shroff

Modalities for chronic dialysis include extracorporeal dialysis modalities or peritoneal dialysis (PD) (automated or continuous ambulatory peritoneal dialysis). Extracorporeal chronic dialysis modalities will be discussed in this chapter and include in-center hemodialysis (HD) or hemodiafiltration (HDF), and home HD. Advances in technology has made HD feasible in patients of all ages including infants, and to be delivered in patients' homes. Safe and effective delivery of application of HD for clinical practice requires knowledge of the components of an appropriate HD prescription, close monitoring for complications, clinical judgment and close collaboration between physicians and dialysis staff. The goals of providing dialysis include achieving normal growth and psychosocial development, and to minimize interference to education and social life.

CHOICE OF DIALYSIS MODALITY

The primary initial choice of kidney replacement therapy in children with end stage kidney disease (ESKD) is preemptive transplantation due to the superior survival and quality of life.

In case preemptive transplantation is not feasible, home dialysis therapies are most compatible with children's schooling and social life. While PD is the most commonly available home dialysis modality, many pediatric centers are now offering home HD. There are international variations in the selection of dialysis modality with PD being twice as common than HD in Europe, whereas the ratio is reversed in Asia and the US. Overall, ~30–50% children begin dialysis by HD. There is no evidence that morbidity or transplant outcomes in children and adolescents vary based on the initial dialysis method. Both HD and PD have relative pros and cons, and the choice of method should be tailored to the healthcare system and the informed decision of the patient. A recent meta-analysis in adults showed that urgent-start PD may reduce the incidence of catheter-related bacteremia compared to HD initiated with a central vascular catheter. Lack of vascular access is the only absolute contraindication for HD, especially in infants in whom vascular access can be difficult to achieve and maintain. Patients who have experienced PD technique failure, intra-abdominal pathology, or with social difficulties that prevent them from undergoing PD may find HD to be a more appropriate option.

When to Start Dialysis?

In the absence of symptomatic uremia, volume overload, or growth failure refractory to medical therapy, there is no absolute cut-off of glomerular filtration rate (GFR) suggested for dialysis start. The timing of initiation of dialysis is guided by a composite assessment of a patient's physical and psychosocial wellbeing, fluid status, growth, level of kidney function, and biochemical abnormalities. Pediatric registries from Europe and the United States show that the median estimated glomerular filtration rate (eGFR) at the time of starting dialysis is approximately 8 mL/min/1.73 m^2. Prospective data from large international registries show that clinical outcomes are not better in patients starting dialysis early. While young children with congenital anomalies of the kidney and urinary tract can have stable kidney function and adequate urine output for many years, symptoms of uremia typically begin as the GFR drops below 15 mL/min/1.73 m^2. It is advised to use formulae (based on eGFR, proteinuria, and diagnosis) to prognosticate progression to ESKD and plan initiation of dialysis when eGFR is <15–20 mL/min per 1.73 m^2.

SOLUTE CLEARANCE BY HEMODIALYSIS AND HEMODIAFILTRATION

The principle of HD relies on the transport of molecules across semipermeable membranes in aqueous solutions: solute transfer (clearance) occurs through varying combinations of diffusion and convection, while ultrafiltration (UF) is the removal of water. The concepts of diffusion and convection are further elaborated in **Figures 27.1A and B**. Diffusive clearance during HD removes intravascular solutes more rapidly than intracellular solutes. With ongoing changes in the concentration gradient with the diffusive process, intracellular solutes gradually move to the intravascular space, and are removed. As opposed to solute clearance driven chiefly by diffusion in HD, HDF utilizes a combination of diffusive and convective solute transport across a highly permeable membrane. Convective transport achieves the clearance of middle and large molecular weight solutes by utilizing high UF rates. The classification of uremic solutes based on their molecular weights, and their method of removal during HD are presented in **Table 27.1**.

HEMODIALYSIS MACHINE, BLOOD AND DIALYSATE CIRCUITS

The semipermeable membrane of the dialyzer separates the blood circuit and the dialysate circuit **(Fig. 27.2)**. A concentration gradient is maintained between blood and the dialysate circuits operating in opposite directions, also known as countercurrent flow.

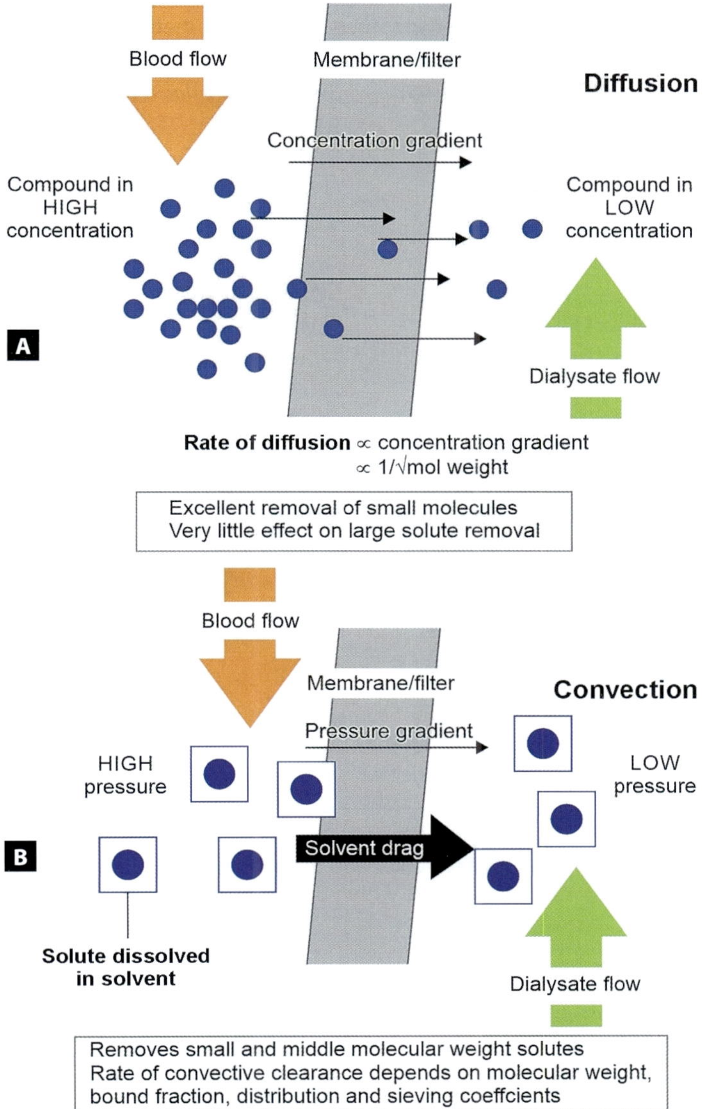

Figs. 27.1A and B: (A) Diffusion is the movement of solutes down their concentration gradient across a semipermeable membrane. Smaller molecules diffuse more quickly than larger molecules—molecules larger than the membrane pore size are restricted from moving; (B) Convection describes molecular movement across a semipermeable membrane under the force of pressure—the net pressure vector pushes water, with dissolved solutes, across the membrane. All molecules move across the membrane at an equal rate. Ultrafiltration describes the movement of the water under transmembrane pressure applied to the dialyzer. Ultrafiltration and convection always occur simultaneously

TABLE 27.1: Classification of uremic solutes and primary method of removal during dialysis

Solute	*Molecular weight (kilodalton)*	*Solute (molecular weight)*	*Removal during dialysis*
Small solutes	<500	Urea (60), creatinine (113)	Diffusion
Middle molecules	300–5000	Vitamin B_{12} (1355)	Diffusion, convection
Low molecular weight proteins	5000–50000	β2-microglobulin (11800)	Diffusion, convection
Large proteins	>50000	Albumin (60000)	Convection

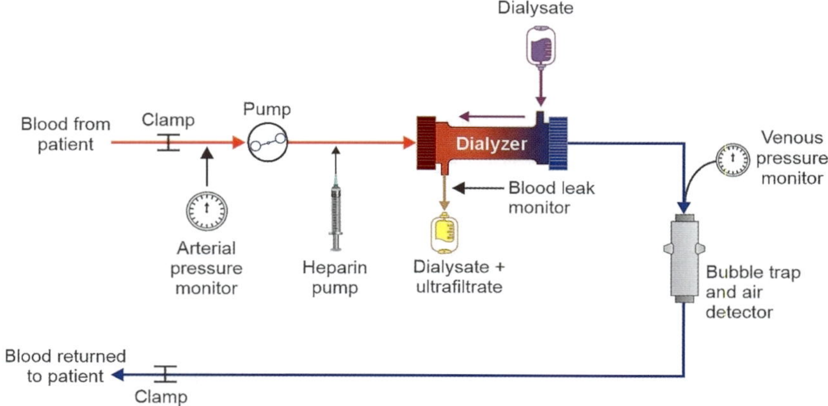

Fig. 27.2: Blood and dialysate circuits, and the countercurrent flow of blood and dialysate within the dialyzer

Blood Circuit

The blood circuit comprises of tubes that carry blood from the patient to the dialyzer (through arterial or "red" lines) and return blood back (venous or "blue" lines)**(Fig. 27.2)**. The pressure in the blood tubes is monitored between the blood pump and the dialyzer (arterial segment), and at the air detector and venous bubble trap (venous segment). Arterial or venous pressure alarms indicate problems with vascular access. The ideal arterial pressure range is between 150 and 200 mm Hg. Low arterial or venous pressure alarms signify insufficient blood flow to the blood pump, usually due to poor vascular access position. A high venous pressure alarm indicates blood flow obstruction in the venous limb, due to blood clot formation, poor access position, or fistula stenosis. As a safety measure, blood pump stops, and the tubes are clamped when an alarm is triggered.

Dialysate Circuit

The dialysate circuit includes systems to generate, test, and deliver dialysate fluid to the dialyzer. A blood leak detector is present just after the dialyzer to identify any blood leakage into the dialysate due to rupture of the dialyzer fibers. Contemporary machines can produce on-line dialysate by blending dialysis-grade water with specified amounts of electrolytes and bicarbonate during the HD session.

Pediatric HD machines should be able to function at low blood flow rates, utilize tubing with varying blood volumes, and maintain accurate UF control, so that they can be used even in infants. Automated volumetric UF systems precisely monitor transmembrane pressure (TMP) across dialysis membranes and enable accurate fluid removal. It is essential to carefully assess the patient's volume status, particularly in young children, due to the inherent level of inaccuracy in UF. Several options are now available for continuous on-line monitoring of changes in hematocrit and blood volume (blood viscosity), urea clearance, blood pressure and pulse, and oxygen saturation. Modern machines have the capability to support both HD and HDF and are appropriate for children whose body weight is above 10–17 kg.

Hemodialyzers

A capillary (hollow fiber) configuration of hemodialyzer achieves the maximal membrane surface area, with relatively low fill volume and compliance. This configuration of each capillary tube, where blood flows within capillary tubes and dialysate bathes the exterior of tubes, represents a semipermeable membrane that allows diffusion, convection, and UF. The dialyzer surface area (which determines the mass transfer area coefficient, K_0A, and solute permeability of the membrane) determines the diffusive solute clearance. The effectiveness of the dialyzer membrane to ultrafiltrate fluid is described by the UF coefficient (K_{UF}), which is the volume of UF per unit time, divided by the pressure gradient across the dialysis membrane **(Table 27.2)**.

Dialysate

The machine prepares dialysate with the addition of prescribed amounts of electrolytes including sodium, chloride, potassium, bicarbonate, calcium, magnesium, and dextrose to purified water during the dialysis session. The levels of these electrolytes can be adjusted within set limits; the standard dialysate composition settings are shown in **Table 27.3**. Prior to delivery to the dialyzer, the dialysate is warmed. The standard dialysate flow rate is 500 mL/min, but can range between 300 and 800 mL/min.

TABLE 27.2: Characteristics of dialyzers for pediatric hemodialysis

Characteristic	*Options*	*Considerations*
Surface area	0.2–2.5 m^2	A greater capacity for clearance and ultrafiltration can be achieved with a larger surface area but requires high blood flow
Priming volume	18–140 mL	Particularly consider for small patients along with tubing set volume
Membrane material	Cellulosic, modified cellulose, artificial	Modified cellulose allows greater biocompatibility; further with artificial (plastic) membranes
Sterilization	Ethylene oxide (ETO), gamma irradiation, steam, electron beam	Allergic reactions associated with ETO; fewer reactions with gamma irradiation and steam
Flux	Low flux, high flux	High flux dialyzers are more permeable (larger pores) and therefore allow better clearance of middle molecules and higher ultrafiltration
Clearance (K_D for urea, mL/min, at blood flow of 200 mL/min)	K_oA urea 170–1700 mL/min	Depends on membrane material, flux and surface area
Ultrafiltration capability (K_{UF} mL/h/mm Hg)	K_{UF} 7–111 mL/h/mm Hg	Depends on membrane material, flux and surface area

TABLE 27.3: Standard composition of dialysate for hemodialysis

Component	*Dialysis fluid concentration*
Sodium	137–144 mEq/L
Potassium	0–4 mEq/L
Chloride	98–112 mEq/L
Bicarbonate	27–40 mEq/L
Calcium	5–7 mEq/L
Magnesium	0.61–2.43 mEq/L
Glucose	0–198 mg/dL

Water

A water treatment unit is required for converting municipal water supply to a quality suitable for production of dialysate. The unit is equipped with filters to eliminate particulate matter, activated carbon to remove chlorine and chloramines, and water softeners to eliminate calcium and magnesium.

Finally, the softened water is further purified by a reverse osmosis unit to obtain water for dialysis.

VASCULAR ACCESS

A well-functioning vascular access is a lifeline for patients on dialysis. Types of vascular access available are arteriovenous fistulas (AVFs), arteriovenous grafts (AVGs), and central venous catheters. Experts recommend that children requiring chronic HD should begin with an AVF where appropriate. Pediatric studies on AVFs have demonstrated superior patency rates often lasting up to 4 years from creation, reduced need for a new access at a different location, and lower access-related infection rate compared to central venous lines. However, central venous lines remain the predominant type of vascular access used in children, due to the perceived ease of access creation.

Central Venous Line

A cuffed line that is tunneled subcutaneously is preferred for very young children, and in patients where dialysis is expected to be short, i.e., before transplantation or transitioning to PD. The selection of the catheter type and size, as well as the location of insertion is individualized **(Table 27.4)**. The internal jugular veins are the preferred option; the subclavian and femoral routes are associated with increased vessel stenosis and infection, respectively. Lines are inserted, using ultrasound guidance, in the internal jugular vein so that the tip is in the right atrium.

Arteriovenous Fistulas

The AVF can be created at different locations such as wrist (radiocephalic, radiobasilic), elbow (brachiocephalic), or by basilic vein transposition to form a brachiobasilic fistula. While distal vessels of the nondominant arm are preferred, however for the best chance of success, larger vessels with intraluminal venous diameter greater than 3 mm are suggested to be used. Patency of central vessels should be confirmed by upper limb venography

TABLE 27.4: Temporary and tunneled hemodialysis central venous lines

Patient weight	*Temporary central lines*	*Tunneled central lines*
<10 kg	6.5 Fr, 10 cm	8 Fr, 18 cm (double lumen)
10–20 kg	8.0 Fr, 10 cm	10 Fr, 15 cm (split); 8 Fr, 18 cm (double lumen)
10–20 kg	8.0 Fr, 12.5 cm	10 Fr, 18 cm (split); 14.5 Fr, 13 cm (double lumen)
20–30 kg	11 Fr, 12.5 cm	14 Fr, 24 cm; 14.5 Fr, 19 cm (double lumen)
>30 kg	11 Fr, 15 cm	14 Fr, 24 cm; 14.5 Fr, 23 cm (double lumen)

in patients with a history of previous central venous lines since ultrasound examination cannot easily visualize veins under the clavicle, and therefore may be misleading. It generally takes 8–10 weeks for AVFs to mature, and they can be cannulated by the rope-ladder or button-hole technique.

Grafts and Shunts

These techniques are infrequently used in children. A graft is an artificial connection between an artery and vein under the skin, which can be accessed with a needle. Alternatively, the connection can be brought out externally (known as a shunt) and disconnected to attach to dialysis lines. However, similar to AVF, grafts and shunts are also susceptible to clotting and stenosis, especially at the anastomosis site.

PRESCRIBING HEMODIALYSIS

Dialysis Adequacy

Dialysis adequacy is defined for the purpose of understanding the optimal dialysis regime and prescription that maximizes favorable patient outcomes and reduces morbidity and mortality. While calculation of dialysis adequacy is based on urea clearance, adequacy should also be assessed by careful clinical assessment, which includes growth, nutrition, cardiac function, bone health, and quality of life.

While urea reduction ratio (URR) is the simplest method to assess dialysis adequacy, it is not recommended as the primary measure of dialysis.

$$\text{URR} = \frac{\text{Predialysis urea} - \text{Postdialysis urea}}{\text{Predialysis urea}} \times 100\%$$

The standard measure of HD dose is estimated by urea clearance during a dialysis session standardized by total body water (which reflects the urea distribution volume): Kt/V.

Where, K is the urea clearance of the dialyzer; t is treatment time; and V is volume of distribution [0.6 × body weight (kg)].

Urea is primarily eliminated from the extracellular space during dialysis. However, its movement from the intracellular space to the intravascular compartment is slower, resulting in a variation in levels between the two compartments, which lasts for about an hour after dialysis. Therefore, assessments of dialysis adequacy may be classified as either "single pool" or "double pool"; the single pool (spKt/V) method assumes that a delayed postdialysis sample is not required.

$$\text{spKt/V} = \text{-Log n} \, (\text{R} - 0.008\text{t}) + (4\text{-}3.5 \, \text{R}) \, \text{UF/BW}$$

where, R is the ratio of the predialysis to postdialysis urea, t is the time of dialysis in hours, UF is ultrafiltration volume in L, and BW is body weight in kg.

Equilibrated (eKt/V) formulae to correct for postdialysis urea rebound include:

$$eKt/V = spKt/V - (0.6 \times spKt/V/T) + 0.03, \text{ for arteriovenous access}$$

$$eKt/V = spKt/V - (0.47 \times spKt/V/T) + 0.02, \text{ for venovenous access}$$

For patients receiving almost daily or intensified dialysis regimens, or for those who require additional sessions for UF occasionally, formulae to estimate the Kt/V averaged over the entire week, known as standardized (stdKt/V), are more helpful.

Urea kinetic modeling allows estimation of the urea generation rate. The major advantage of this particularly in children is that the normalized protein catabolic rate (nPCR), an estimate of dietary protein intake, can then be calculated.

Guidelines recommend targeting dialysis dose to achieve a minimum eKt/V of 1.2 for thrice weekly patients, or a standardized Kt/V of 2.2 for those on augmented schedules **(Table 27.5)**. The dialysis dose requires to be monitored on a monthly basis. Studies in the adult dialysis population have shown that longer treatment times (>4–4.5 hr) with or without a higher Kt/V, are associated with a lower risk of death, and is the rationale for intensified dialysis programs (more frequent and/or more prolonged dialysis sessions).

Components of Dialysis Prescription

Blood Flow Rate and Dialysis Flow Rate

The rate of blood flow (Q_B) plays a crucial role in determining solute clearance by enabling maximum diffusion and convection; the vascular access determines the maximum achievable Q_B. Wider bore central vein lines and AVF allow higher Q_B. The Q_B should be up to body weight (kg) × 5–8 mL/min. Dialysis fluid flow rate (Q_D) should be 1.5–2 times Q_B.

TABLE 27.5: Published guidelines for hemodialysis adequacy

Guideline	*Age group*	*Urea clearance*	*Other*
KDOQI	Adult	Minimum spKt/V of 1.2 Target spKt/V of 1.4	Minimum URR ~65% Target URR ~70%
European guidelines	Adults	eKt/V >1.2 spKt/V of 1.4	Double-pool urea kinetics preferred
KDOQI	Children	spKt/V >1.4	Assess nutrition by normalized protein catabolic rate (nPCR) Optimize ultrafiltration
European guidelines	Children	eKt/V ≥1.2–1.4	Assess nutrition (nPCR) Monitor growth and cardiac function

eKt/V: equilibrated Kt/V; KDOQI: National Kidney Foundation's Kidney Disease Outcomes Quality Initiative; spKt/V: single pool Kt/V; URR: urea reduction ratio

Dialyzer

When choosing a dialyzer, the surface area and priming volume should be taken into consideration **(Table 27.6)**. It is recommended that the dialyzer membrane surface area should be 0.75–1 times the patient's body surface area. In conventional HD, a small pore size low flux membrane is typically used for removing solutes mainly through diffusion. In contrast, high efficiency HD involves the rapid elimination of small solutes such as potassium and urea through diffusion, which can be achieved by using a low flux membrane with a high efficiency (K_0A) or a larger surface area membrane and high blood flow (Q_B). However, since conventional HD relies on solute clearance primarily through diffusion, it has limitations in clearing middle-sized molecules that are better eliminated through convection (HDF, as explained in the following text).

Extracorporeal Circuit

When selecting the tubings and hemodialyzer, it is important to consider the ability of a child to tolerate 8–10% of their total blood volume (TBV), which

TABLE 27.6: Dialyzer and tubings with extracorporeal priming volumes

Dialyzers	*Company*	*Surface area (m^2)*	*Volume (mL)*
FX Paed	Fresenius	0.2	18
Sureflux 03L	Nipro	0.3	25
Sureflux 05E	Nipro	0.5	35
FX40	Fresenius	0.6	32
Sureflux 07E	Nipro	0.7	45
Sureflux 09E	Nipro	0.9	55
FX50	Fresenius	1.0	53
Sureflux 11E	Nipro	1.1	65
Sureflux 13E	Nipro	1.3	78
FX60	Fresenius	1.4	74
FX80	Fresenius	1.8	95
Tubings			
Neonatal	Gambro	-	33
Pediatric	Gambro	-	85
Adult	Gambro	-	132
Paed AV set ONLINEplusBVM	Fresenius	-	111
Paed SN set ONLINEplusBVM	Fresenius	-	142
Adult HDF	Gambro	-	151
Adult AV set + BVM	Fresenius	-	192

is estimated to be about 80 mL/kg of their dry weight in the extracorporeal circuit **(Table 27.6)**. The lines are then filled (primed) with saline. However, for very young children, even the smallest circuit may exceed the safe extracorporeal volume. In such cases, it is necessary to prime the circuit with blood. One of the key limitations of this approach is the potential risk of sensitization with repeated blood primes, especially before transplantation in small infants. This risk is one of the reasons why PD may be a more suitable option for infants.

Estimate Dry Weight and Fluid Removal

Dry weight is the post-HD weight below which the child will become symptomatically hypotensive. Achieving the dry weight should be the goal of UF. The amount of fluid that can be safely removed from each child varies, but it is recommended to begin with 10–13 mL/kg/h, and no >5–8% of the body weight should be removed in a single session. Monthly clinical assessment of fluid status, dry weight, and dietary needs are necessary, and should be done more frequently for very young children. Along with clinical assessment, body composition analysis is a useful tool to objectively determine dry weight.

Managing adequate UF is difficult in patients with significant volume overload (interdialytic weight gain >8%), poor vascular tone (critically ill, sepsis), and cardiac dysfunction (risk for myocardial hypoperfusion), and in young children due to small intravascular volume. Careful bedside monitoring by using noninvasive blood volume monitors (monitor circulating blood volume by changes in hematocrit) can help in safe achievement of dry weight. Regular assessment of UF tolerance, using extended times to avoid excessive UF rates is required.

Frequency of Sessions

Conventional HD is done typically for 4 hr every three times a week. There is emerging evidence of augmented dialysis schedules in children. Several reports in children have shown that intensified dialysis is associated with improvement in height velocity, blood pressure, and enhanced control of levels of phosphate and parathyroid hormone (PTH). Guidelines suggest augmented schedules for patients with chronic fluid overload and cardiac dysfunction or for infants whose liquid diet entails relatively large UF volumes.

Anticoagulation

Heparin is the most common anticoagulant used during HD to prevent the circuit from clotting. It can be administered through the arterial side of the circuit continuously at a rate of 5–50 units/kg/h throughout the session. Some units opt for low molecular weight heparin, such as dalteparin, which is given as a bolus dose of 1 mg/kg at dialysis session start.

COMPLICATIONS OF HEMODIALYSIS

Intradialytic Hypotension

Hypotension is an important complication of HD. Children are particularly susceptible since a significant proportion of their circulating blood volume may be within the extracorporeal circuit. Therefore, any factor causing tachycardia can decrease diastolic ventricular filling, leading to hypotension. Hypotension can also be caused by various factors such as excessive UF requirements, high salt and water intake, or the use of antihypertensive agents. Pathophysiology of intradialytic hypotension is multifactorial and involves reduced plasma refilling; uremic environment predisposing to ineffective venoconstriction, inadequate metabolic stress response, and lower myocardial contractile reserve; and blood and dialyzer membrane inflammatory reactions.

Symptoms of hypotension include nausea, vomiting, itching, pains, and cramps. Repeated intradialytic hypotension can result in recurring episodes of ischemia, which can accelerate the decline in residual renal function, cause multiorgan ischemic injury and myocardial stunning (a reversible, regional, and left ventricular dysfunction). In children undergoing conventional HD, the degree of myocardial stunning often correlates with UF rate and changes in intradialytic blood pressure.

Immediate stepwise action includes: (*i*) Temporary suspension of UF; (*ii*) Isotonic fluid bolus (5 mL/kg); and (*iii*) Early discontinuation of dialysis. Reassessment of the dry weight is necessary to evaluate if the target UF has been overestimated. Similarly, daily salt intake and fluid allowance should be evaluated as they could be higher than necessary, necessitating excess fluid removal. Measures to improve hemodynamic stability are: (*i*) Withholding antihypertensive medications on dialysis days; (*ii*) Avoiding food during dialysis; (*iii*) Using noninvasive blood volume monitors to measure changes in relative blood volume during dialysis in real time. The first hour's steep gradient of the relative blood volume curve can predict hemodynamic decompensation; (*iv*) Adjusting dialysate characteristics such as decreasing sodium concentration, cooling it to at least 0.5°C below the patient temperature, use of bicarbonate buffers, adjusting dialysate calcium and potassium to avoid intradialytic hypocalcemia and large changes in potassium; and (*v*) Use of midodrine or switching to HDF or augmented dialysis in refractory patients.

Disequilibrium

Dialysis disequilibrium occurs when plasma urea decreases more rapidly than intracellular urea in brain cells, resulting in the movement of water into brain cells through osmosis. Patients who have high blood urea level at the start of dialysis are at high risk of developing this condition. The symptoms of dialysis disequilibrium can vary and may include headache, nausea, dizziness, disorientation, seizures, and coma. To prevent this condition, it is recommended to keep the URR below 50% during the first few dialysis treatments for patients initiating chronic dialysis. Although the symptoms usually resolve on their own, severe cases of dialysis disequilibrium can be treated with intravenous mannitol.

Fever and Infection

Differential diagnosis of catheter-related bloodstream infection must be kept in patients on HD who present with fever, especially if in the presence of an indwelling central venous catheter. While not all febrile HD patients will have a serious infection, it is crucial to maintain a low threshold for obtaining cultures and administering antibiotics until the results of blood cultures are obtained.

Water-related Complications

The water system of a dialysis unit can become contaminated by either microbes or biochemical contaminants, which can have catastrophic consequences for multiple patients simultaneously. For instance, if chloramine, a by-product of chlorine, is not adequately removed from the dialysis water, it can cause severe hemolytic reactions and even lead to death. Thus, it is essential to frequently monitor the entire dialysis water system as per recommended guidelines to maintain rigorous safety standards.

Intradialytic Cramping

Intradialytic cramping is a common complication of HD, that is typically associated with high UF rates, electrolyte imbalances, and eating during dialysis. If a patient experiences cramping during a dialysis session, appropriate management of these causes is necessary.

Elevated Blood Pressure

Patients who have long-term high blood pressure should slowly decrease their desired weight and restrict their consumption of salt in their diet. If blood pressure continues to be high despite limiting salt intake and attempting to improve the removal of excess total body water, it may suggest that the hypertension is caused by renin in patients with native kidneys. In such situations, angiotensin converting enzyme inhibitors may be beneficial as an adjunct to sodium and volume control.

Hemorrhage

If the blood circuit tubing set is disconnected from the vascular access, the patient may face the risk of rapid exsanguination. However, in this scenario, the blood pump is automatically stopped, and an alarm is triggered. The more common scenario is when the blood circuit becomes clotted, which can prevent the return of blood in the extracorporeal circuit to the patient. If the patient experiences symptoms, they may require volume expansion with crystalloid or, in severe cases, blood transfusion.

Other rare complications are hemolysis, air embolism, anaphylaxis, and other long-term complications including dialysis related amyloidosis, carnitine deficiency, and hyperhomocysteinemia.

Vascular Access-related Infection

Catheter-related infections may be within the catheter itself, at the exit site or in the subcutaneous tunnel. Bacterial eradication becomes difficult when biofilm develops within the catheter. Catheter-related sepsis can present with rigors soon after starting dialysis, fever with raised C-reactive protein (CRP), or as septic shock. Several factors increase the risk of catheter infection, including contamination of the hub, infection at the exit site and/or tunnel, failure of aseptic technique, frequent need to access the catheter during dialysis, long duration of use, immunosuppression, hypoalbuminemia, diabetes, and colonization with *Staphylococcus aureus* in the nasal and cutaneous regions. By reducing clot formation, administering postdialysis heparin or alteplase into the line decreases the risk of infection. An algorithm for the treatment of catheter-related infections is depicted in **Flowchart 27.1**.

Blood-borne Viruses

Patients and staff in HD units face the risk of infection with blood-borne viruses, including hepatitis B, hepatitis C, and human immunodeficiency virus (HIV). These viruses can spread through percutaneous exposure to infected blood or other fluids, droplets, or contaminated equipment. To prevent transmission, universal precautions must be followed for all patients. After each use, the entire dialysis circuit should be decontaminated using heat or chemical disinfection. External surfaces should be wiped between patients with a chlorine-based disinfectant. Hepatitis B immunization is necessary for all staff and patients, and antibody titers checked periodically to ensure immunity. Although screening for hepatitis C or HIV is not mandatory, many units choose to perform it. Hepatitis C and HIV can spread nosocomially, so patients who test positive should be kept in a separate room, but a dedicated machine is not required. Patients should be tested for hepatitis C antibody every 3 months and for HIV annually.

HEMODIAFILTRATION

Hemodiafiltration is a dialysis technique that uses both diffusive and conductive removal of solutes. To achieve this, at least 20% of the blood volume

Flowchart 27.1: Approach to the management of catheter-related bloodstream infection. CRP: C-reactive protein; CVC: central venous catheter; ECHO: echocardiography; HD: hemodialysis; IV: intravenous

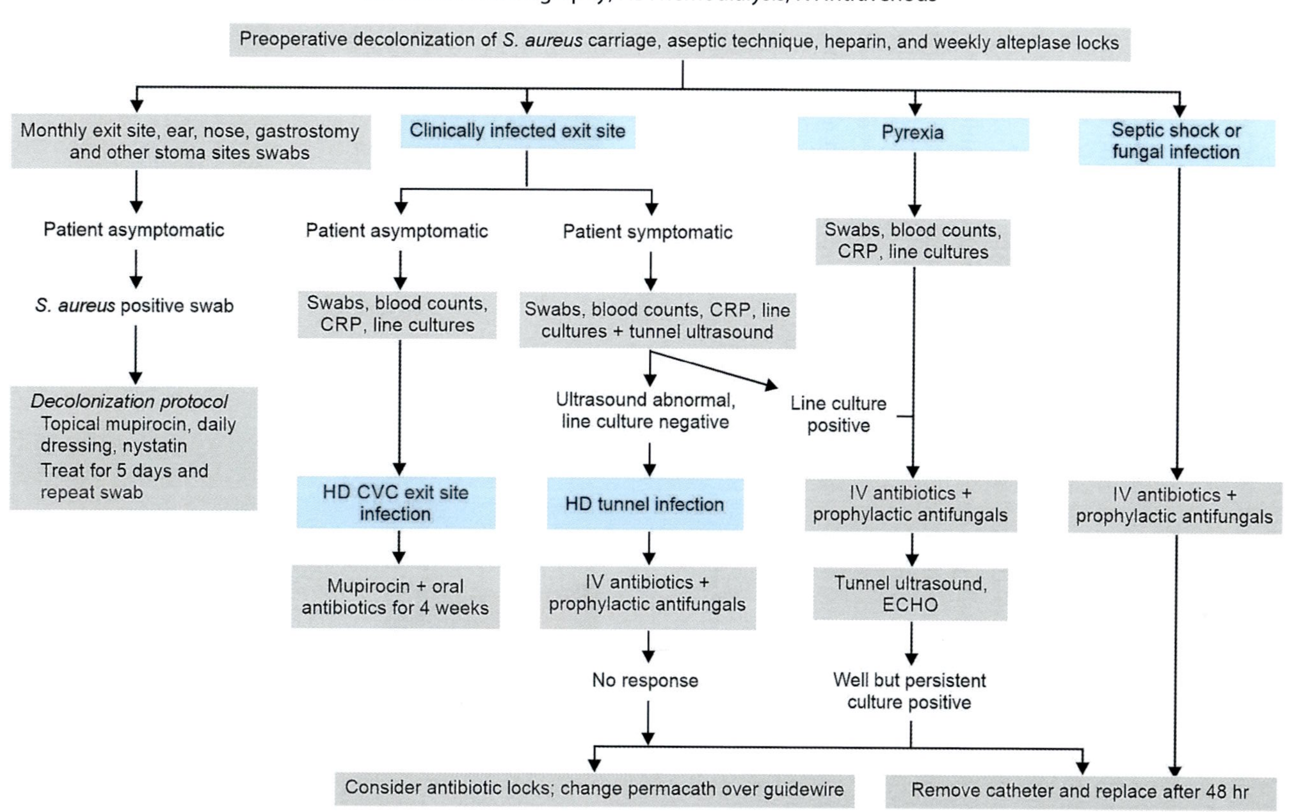

processed through a high-flux dialyzer is ultrafiltered. Sterile substitution fluid, generated on-line, is used to maintain fluid balance. Therefore, the HDF process requires (*i*) ultrapure water for the generation of substitution fluid, (*ii*) a high-flux dialyzer, and (*iii*) a dialysis machine that permits accurate UF regulation **(Fig. 27.3)**.

The "substitution fluid" is an isosmotic fluid that is employed to replace the excess ultrafiltered fluid. This fluid is created on-line by filtering dialysis fluid through filters that retain bacteria and endotoxins and is then infused into the patient's bloodstream. Sterile, nonpyrogenic ultrapure water is crucial for on-line HDF and is recommended to have <0.1 colony-forming unit/mL of bacteria and <0.03 unit/mL of endotoxin.

HDF uses highly permeable membranes that are suitable for removing middle-molecular-weight and protein-bound uremic retention solutes more effectively than conventional low- or high-flux HD. In practice, the K_{UF} (UF coefficient) should be high enough to allow for a convective flow of 2 mL/min/kg body weight in postdilution HDF. Membranes with a K_{UF} of 20 mL/min/mm Hg or greater are used for postdilution HDF.

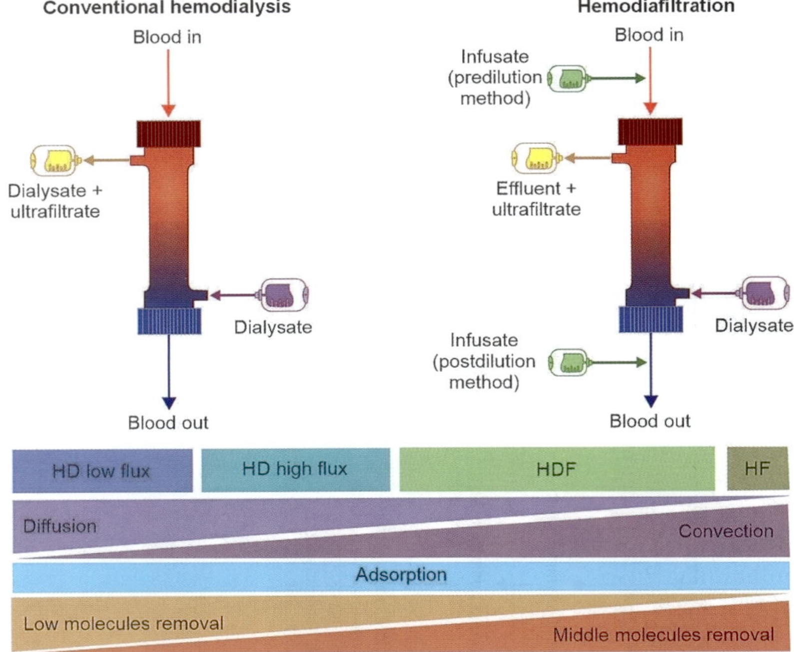

Fig. 27.3: Hemodialysis (HD) and hemodiafiltration (HDF) circuits and their mechanisms of clearance by diffusion alone (HD) compared to a combination of diffusion and convection (HDF). The term infusate refers to substitution fluid (see text)

Convective Volume

The convective volume is the sum of the net desired UF volume and the amount of substitution fluid infused. A high convective blood volume plays an important role in improving long-term survival in patients undergoing HDF. In the HDF, Hearts, and Height (3H) study, children achieved median convection volumes of 13.4 L/m^2 comparable to the average of 23 L/ 1.73 m^2 per session in adult studies. Modern HDF machines can achieve an UF volume of 30–35% of the TBV, resulting in optimal clearance.

Modes

HDF can be applied as "predilution HDF" where the substitution fluid is returned to the blood before the dialyzer or "postdilution" where the substitution fluid is returned to the blood after the dialyzer. Filtration fraction is defined as the ratio of UF rate to plasma water flow rate. If the filtration fraction is high during postdilution mode, it can lead to hemoconcentration and result in the deposition of plasma proteins on the surface of the membrane. This, in turn, can block the membrane pores and increase the TMP, leading to reduced clearance and potentially causing clotting. Therefore, UF rate is regulated in proportion to the actual Q_B or guided by TMP in order to restrict the filtration fraction to a range of 20–25%. Predilution mode is not limited by hemoconcentration, but due to decreased dialysis efficiency the convective volumes need to be 2–3 times higher than postdilution mode. Predilution mode with high volumes of substitution fluid, may be suitable for patients with low achievable blood flow rates. The principles of HD and HDF and solute clearance by both techniques are shown in **Figure 27.3**.

The components of a HDF prescription are shown in **Table 27.7**. Nowadays, most new dialysis machines have the ability to perform both HD and HDF. These machines are appropriate for children weighing a minimum of 12–17 kg and come with a low extracorporeal volume pediatric circuit.

Advantages of Hemodiafiltration over Conventional Hemodialysis

HDF has several advantages in comparison to traditional HD. It enhances the efficiency of dialysis, which allows the elimination of toxins having a broad molecular weight range. HDF also improves hemodynamic stability, reduces inflammation by using "ultrapure" dialysate and increases the elimination of inflammatory cytokines. Randomized controlled trials involving adults have shown that patients on HDF have a survival rate that is approximately 30% higher than those on conventional HD. Moreover, in these randomized trials, HDF has been shown to reduce cardiovascular mortality when higher convection volumes (>17–20 L) were used. The adult multicenter CONVINCE (Comparison of high-dose HDF with high-flux HD) trial comparing

TABLE 27.7: Components of hemodiafiltration (HDF) prescription

Dialyzer	High-flux membrane K_{UF} >20 mL/h/mm Hg transmembrane pressure/m^2; sieving coefficient for β2-microglobulin >0.6; surface area equal to patient's body surface area
Extracorporeal circuit	Volume <10 mL/kg body weight
Blood flow rate	5–8 mL/min/kg; increase from 100 mL/min in initial HDF sessions, by 10 mL/min per week, up to 200–250 mL/m^2/min
Dialysate flow	Twice the blood flow rate
Replacement fluid	Generated on-line Ultrapure (<0.1 colony-forming unit/mL; <0.03 endotoxin unit/mL) Microbiologic purity (bacterial count, endotoxin level) determined q 3 months; chemical composition q 6–12 months
Convective flow	Sum of desired ultrafiltration volume and replacement fluid *Postdilution HDF:* Convective flow ~30% blood flow; risk of filter clotting. Typically decreases over dialysis sessions, in order to maintain TMP <300 mm Hg *Predilution HDF:* Convective flow is 100% of blood flow. This can be done despite the dilution of the blood impacting negatively on urea clearance Clearance of β2-microglobulin, phosphate, and protein-bound toxins is optimized
Dialysate	Produced on-line; composition similar to that used in conventional HD Dialysate sodium level lower than conventional HD. Sodium and UF profiling helps correct fluid and sodium overload, and maintain hemodynamic stability and dialysis tolerance
Anticoagulation	Continuous heparin infusion; single dose low-molecular weight heparin

high-flux HD to high-dose on-line HDF (≥23 L/session in postdilution mode), showed ~25% lower risk of death in the HDF group.

The 3H study compared the cardiovascular risk profile, growth and nutritional status, and health-related quality of life in children receiving HDF compared to conventional HD. Children receiving daily HDF had improved blood pressure, better hemodynamic stability and cardiovascular outcomes, reduced inflammatory markers, and lower β2-microglobulin. There was impressive catch-up growth with projected final height approaching target midparental height. Children treated with HDF had lower frequency and severity of headaches, dizziness and cramps on dialysis, reduction in postdialysis recovery time, and improved school attendance and physical activity. HDF was considered safe, with no reduction in serum albumin and no difference in rate of change of residual kidney function.

HOME HEMODIALYSIS

Patients can receive their dialysis treatments at home instead of having to go to a hospital through home HD. Home HD is characterized by augmented HD prescriptions that include longer or more frequent dialysis sessions. These regimens are categorized based on the timing (daytime or overnight), frequency (alternate days or 4–7 times per week), and length of treatment (hours per session). Families opt for home HD due to the flexibility it provides in scheduling treatments around their own schedules. To qualify for home HD, a patient must be medically stable, have a suitable weight, committed caregivers, a well-functioning vascular access, and appropriate accommodation. Home HD machines must be able to produce large volumes of high-quality dialysate, requiring home water conversions. However, the NxStage System One™ (NxStage Medical, Lawrence, MA) is a portable home HD machine that does not require any home water modifications. Premixed dialysis fluid is available for home patients in sterile, 5 L bags with various fluid compositions.

To ensure the success of a home HD program, it is important to prioritize safety as the central focus. A team of experts from various disciplines, including a HD nurse, dialysis biomechanical engineer, nephrologist, dietitian, pharmacist, and social worker, should be recruited to provide support for home HD families. It is also crucial to establish a clear remote support system for the family, enabling them to access immediate assistance at any time. In-depth caregiver training and education is essential, and patients should make regular visits to the clinic while staying in touch with the home HD nurse specialist between appointments.

The home HD prescriptions can offer greater dialysis doses and allow for lower UF rates. This can lead to various benefits including reduced use of antihypertensive medications, lower incidence of left ventricular hypertrophy, better control of anemia, reduced erythropoietin dose, less use of phosphate binders, and improved nutrition. Patients undergoing home HD report an enhanced quality of life. Although the available data for children is limited, the results of home HD treatment are consistent with those observed in adults.

LONG-TERM OUTCOME

Children on dialysis still experience a mortality rate that is approximately 30% higher than age-matched children having no kidney disease, despite the advancements in biocompatible and high-flux dialysis membranes, UF controlled machines, and improved supportive management. Around 50% of all deaths in these children are caused by cardiovascular disease and infections. The primary challenge for pediatric nephrologists is to enhance the long-term outcome for these children. Managing metabolic abnormalities and promptly addressing fluid overload and cardiac dysfunction is critical. Research is necessary to determine the advantages of more frequent or intensified dialysis and the prevention of cardiovascular disease. Preemptive kidney transplantation is currently the best option for children, as it bypasses dialysis altogether.

Technical advances as well as improvements in medical and nursing skills now allows us to safely perform chronic HD treatment even in the youngest children. The benefits of intensified HD with extended hours, home HD as well as in-centre HDF with improved outcomes compared to conventional HD regimens has been shown in children. Nevertheless, children on dialysis have a significant burden of cardiovascular risk factors, and all efforts must continue to improve HD technology and patient care.

BIBLIOGRAPHY

1. Almeida BM, Moreno DH, Vasconcelos V, et al. Interventions for treating catheter-related bloodstream infections in people receiving maintenance hemodialysis. Cochrane Database Syst Rev. 2022;4:CD013554.
2. Ashby D, Borman N, Burton J, et al. Renal Association Clinical Practice Guideline on Hemodialysis. BMC Nephrol. 2019;20:379.
3. Blankestijn PJ, Vernooij RWM, Hockham C, et al. Effect of hemodiafiltration or hemodialysis on mortality in kidney failure. N Engl J Med. 2023;389:700-9.
4. Bonthuis M, Vidal E, Bjerre A, et al. Ten-year trends in epidemiology and outcomes of pediatric kidney replacement therapy in Europe: data from the ESPN/ERA-EDTA Registry. Pediatr Nephrol. 2021;36:2337-48.
5. Borzych-Duzalka D, Shroff R, Ariceta G, et al. Vascular access choice, complications, and outcomes in children on maintenance hemodialysis: Findings from International Pediatric Hemodialysis Network (IPHN) Registry. Am J Kidney Dis. 2019;74:193-202.
6. Claudel SE, Miles LA, Murea M. Anticoagulation in hemodialysis: A narrative review. Semin Dial. 2021;34:103-15.
7. Crane CR, Garimella PS, Heinze G. Predicting pediatric kidney disease progression-are 3 variables all you need? Kidney Int. 2023;104:885-7.
8. de Zan F, Schmitt CP, Shroff R. Hemodiafiltration in the pediatric population. Semin Dial. 2022;35:427-30.
9. Grewal MK, Mehta A, Chakraborty R, et al. Nocturnal home hemodialysis in children: Advantages, implementation, and barriers. Semin Dial. 2020;33:109-19.
10. Harambat J, van Stralen KJ, Kim JJ, et al. Epidemiology of chronic kidney disease in children. Pediatr Nephrol. 2012;27:363-73.
11. Haroon S, Davenport A. Hemodialysis at home: review of current dialysis machines. Expert Rev Med Devices. 2018;15:337-47.
12. Hothi DK, Shroff R, Laskin B. Pediatric hemodialysis prescription, complications, and future directions. In: Geary DF, Schaefer F, (Eds). Pediatric Kidney Disease. Berlin, Heidelberg: Springer; 2021. pp. 1725-65.
13. Hothi DK, Stronach L, Sinnott K. Home hemodialysis in children. Hemodial Int. 2016;20:349-57.
14. Htay H, Johnson DW, Craig JC, et al. Urgent-start peritoneal dialysis versus hemodialysis for people with chronic kidney disease. Cochrane Database Syst Rev. 2021;1:CD012899.

15. Kumbar L, Yee J. Current concepts in hemodialysis vascular access infections. Adv Chronic Kidney Dis. 2019;26:16-22.
16. Lang T, Zawada AM, Theis L, et al. Hemodiafiltration: Technical and medical insights. Bioengineering (Basel). 2023;10:145.
17. Nehus E, Mitsnefes MM. When to initiate dialysis in children and adolescents: Is waiting worthwhile? Am J Kidney Dis. 2019;73:762-4.
18. Ranchin B, Schmitt CP, Warady B, et al. Devices for long-term hemodialysis in small children-a plea for action. Kidney Int. 2023;103:1038-40.
19. Ronco C, Clark WR. Hemodialysis membranes. Nat Rev Nephrol. 2018;14:394-410.
20. Shroff R, Calder F, Bakkaloglu S, et al. Vascular access in children requiring maintenance hemodialysis: a consensus document by the European Society for Pediatric Nephrology Dialysis Working Group. Nephrol Dial Transplant. 2019;34:1746-65.
21. Shroff R, Ledermann S. Long-term outcome of chronic dialysis in children. Pediatr Nephrol. 2009;24:463-74.
22. Shroff R, Smith C, Ranchin B, et al. Effects of hemodiafiltration versus conventional hemodialysis in children with ESKD: The HDF, Heart and Height Study. J Am Soc Nephrol. 2019;30:678-91.
23. Tattersall JE, Ward RA; EUDIAL group. Online hemodiafiltration: definition, dose quantification and safety revisited. Nephrol Dial Transplant. 2013;28:542-50.
24. United States Renal Data System. 2022 USRDS Annual Data Report: Epidemiology of kidney disease in the United States. National Institutes of Health, National Institute of Diabetes and Digestive and Kidney Diseases, Bethesda, MD, 2022.

Chronic Peritoneal Dialysis

Soumita Bagchi

INTRODUCTION

Peritoneal dialysis (PD) is the most preferred modality for kidney replacement therapy (KRT) in children with end-stage kidney disease (ESKD) when transplantation is not an immediate option. Although PD does not have a survival advantage over hemodialysis (HD), it offers the children and families better quality of life, greater independence, and self-reliance. PD does not require vascular access, which may be difficult in young children and infants. Compared to HD, the technical ease of PD and lack of requirement for elaborate equipment, infrastructure, and trained staff, make it ideal for remote areas. Cost–utility analysis studies comparing maintenance HD and PD in adults show that both direct and indirect costs are lower for PD. In developing countries, where cost considerations and resource availability determine access and utilization of therapy, PD may be the ideal form of KRT for children with ESKD.

Chronic PD became the therapy of choice in children with ESKD in certain centers with the introduction of the permanent "Tenckhoff" catheter and continuous ambulatory peritoneal dialysis (CAPD) by Oreopoulos in 1968. The first use of CAPD in children was reported from Toronto in 1978, enabling treatment of very young infants with ESKD, thus extending the option of KRT to a patient population considered too young for chronic treatment.

PHYSIOLOGY OF PERITONEAL DIALYSIS

The PD system can be considered as nature's version of a capillary kidney **(Fig. 28.1)** comprising of three key components: The peritoneal capillaries (blood compartment), peritoneal membrane (akin to the dialyzer membrane used in HD), and the PD fluid in the peritoneal cavity (dialysate compartment). The dialysate compartment includes the dialysis solution and peritoneal access (PD catheter). The dialysis fluid is instilled in the peritoneal cavity through the PD catheter. Contrary to HD where hydrostatic pressure is the main driving force for ultrafiltration, PD primarily depends on osmotic pressure created by the hypertonic dialysate. The hypertonicity and the osmotic pressure can be modified using PD fluids with differing concentrations of dextrose or icodextrin.

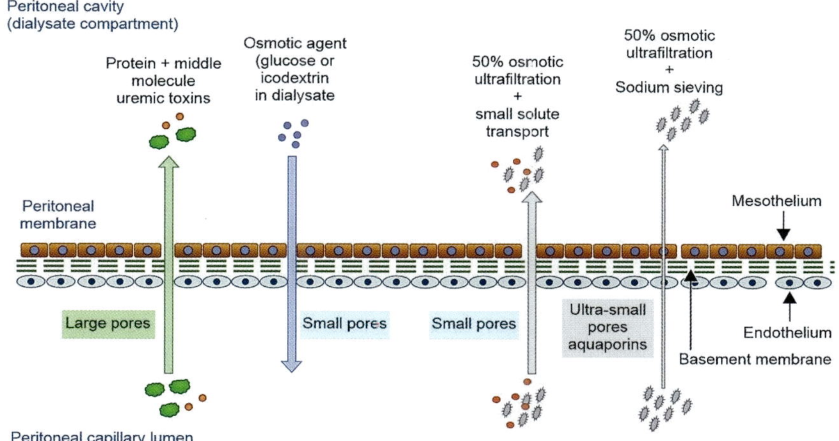

Fig. 28.1: Physiology of peritoneal dialysis

The peritoneal membrane serves as the primary interface between blood and the dialysate compartment **(Fig. 28.1)**. It consists of a monolayer of mesothelial cells, basement membrane, interstitial tissue, and a network of capillaries and lymphatics. The parietal peritoneum is more important in transport as only 25–30% of the visceral peritoneum is in contact with the peritoneal fluid. Children have disproportionately larger peritoneal surface area compared to adults. While 10% of the cardiac output goes to the mesentery, in absence of direct measures of blood flow (Q_b), the contribution of peritoneal blood flow to solute and fluid exchange is unknown.

The movement of solutes across the peritoneal membrane is bidirectional. Small solutes like urea, creatinine, and potassium diffuse from the peritoneal microcirculation into the dialysate while glucose is transported from the dialysate into the peritoneal capillaries causing loss of the osmotic gradient over time. The rate of solute movement is determined by its concentration gradient as well as the peritoneal vascularity.

Three-Pore Model of Peritoneal Transport

The three-pore model explains water and solute transport across the peritoneal membrane, which is a partially restrictive barrier. It is postulated to occur through three types of channels in peritoneal capillaries, i.e., large, small, and ultra-small pores **(Fig. 28.1 and Table 28.1)**. The large pores permit almost nonrestrictive convective mass transport of large molecules (proteins and middle molecular weight toxins) facilitated by the transcapillary hydrostatic pressure gradient. The small paracellular pores allow diffusion of low-molecular-weight compounds (e.g., urea and creatinine). The ultra-small or transcellular pores termed aquaporins, are localized in peritoneal capillaries and mesothelial cells. They are permeable to water but impermeable to most

TABLE 28.1: Three-pore model of peritoneal dialysis (PD)

	Large pores	*Small pores*	*Ultra-small pores*
Location	Interendothelial gaps and/or fused vesicles	Paracellular; in interendothelial junctions	Transcellular aquaporins in endothelium and mesothelium[1]
Size (radius)	250 Å (25 nm)	40–55 Å (4.7 nm)	<6 Å (0.4 nm)
Relative number	0.0001	1	2,000
Solute and water transport	Large or middle molecular weight compounds (proteins and toxins)	Small solutes and water	Water (impermeable to solutes, leading to sodium sieving)[1]
Type of transport	Convection	Diffusion	Diffusion
Proportion of LpS[2]	5–10%	90–95%	1–2%

[1]Aquaporin-1 is permeable only to water; aquaporin-3 is permeable to water and small molecules (glycerol and urea)
[2]LpS refers to total peritoneal ultrafiltration coefficient, which is the measure of total pore surface area available for diffusion of small solutes

solutes including sodium ions (Na^+), which prevents their movement across the barrier (termed sieving). The small and ultra-small pores each contribute to 50% of the ultrafiltration (UF) that occurs during one hypertonic exchange.

PERITONEAL ACCESS

A single lumen silicon PD catheter is inserted in the peritoneal cavity through the anterior abdominal wall. The tip of the catheter should rest in the true pelvis. The intraperitoneal segment is located between the visceral and parietal peritoneum; it then traverses the rectus abdominis where it is anchored by a Dacron cuff and then tunneled subcutaneously to the site where it exits the abdominal wall. It should have an appropriate length without creating unnatural bend or kink that can compromise its function. The deep cuff should be within the medial or lateral border of the rectus sheath and the subcutaneous cuff approximately 2 cm from the exit site. A lateral or downward-pointing exit site, away from the diaper or belt lines, is preferred to an upward pointing exit site, to avoid infection. A titanium adaptor is attached to the exiting end of the catheter, which is then connected to a transfer set that can be replaced if there is any contamination without replacing the entire catheter.

Variations in the catheter design are defined by the intraperitoneal segment (straight, coiled, and T-fluted), subcutaneous segment (prefabricated 90° or

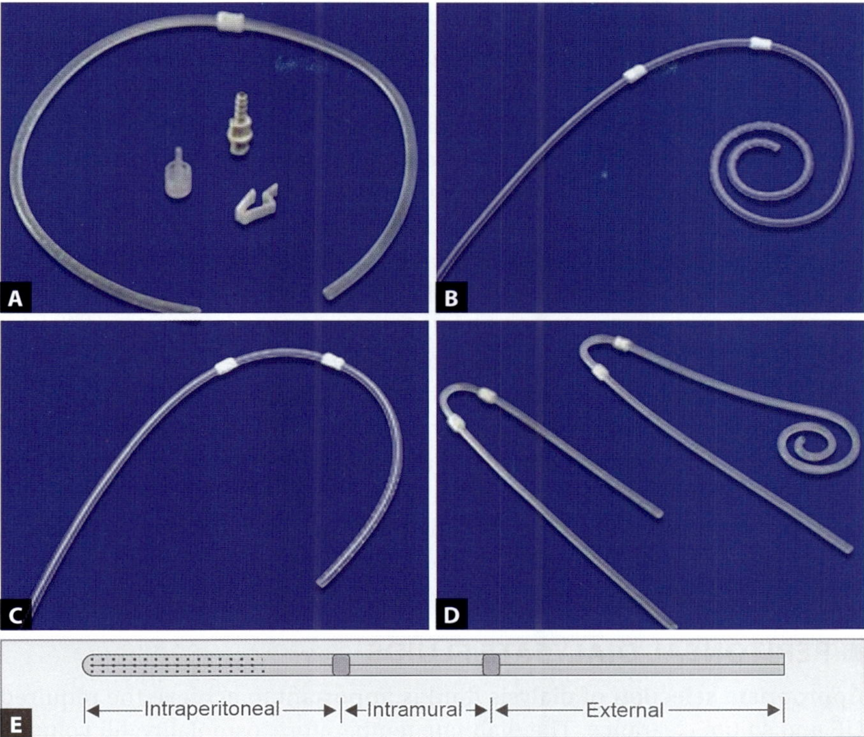

Figs. 28.2A to E: Tenckhoff catheters for peritoneal dialysis. (A) Soft straight catheter with single cuff; (B) Two-cuff catheter with straight intercuff segment and coiled tip; (C) Two-cuff catheter with straight intercuff segment and straight tip; (D) Two cuff catheter with preformed intercuff bend (swan neck) and straight (left) or coiled (right) tip; and (E) I Line diagram indicates segments of a two-cuff catheter.

150° bend or straight), the number and shape of the cuffs (single or double cuff, elongated, and bead or flange configuration), and the adaptors (plastic or titanium) **(Figs. 28.2A to E)**.

The catheter is placed though open or laparoscopic techniques. Although the laparoscopic technique takes longer operative time, laparoscopically implanted catheters have higher rates of catheter survival and fewer episodes of catheter migration or malfunction, dialysate leakage, and exit-site infection. Using either technique, catheter implantation can be done by an experienced surgeon or a nephrologist. Ideally, the catheter should be used 2 weeks after placement to allow the internal cuff to heal with pericuff fibrosis, which reduces the risk of mechanical complications like dialysate leakage. In the absence of life-threatening complications, "urgent-start" PD can be initiated less than 2 weeks after insertion of PD catheter in patients with significant uremic symptoms using small dialysate volumes which is increased subsequently.

Special Considerations in Children

Omentectomy should be performed in children during placement to minimize catheter malfunction due to obstruction of drainage. Catheter placement requires precautions in children with comorbidities, for example, structural abnormalities that require abdominal surgeries, in particular, placement of stomas and ventriculoperitoneal shunt.

Contraindications to placement of PD catheter are listed in **Box 28.1**. The PD catheter exit site should be placed as far as possible from as ostomy site to reduce risk of contamination and peritonitis. In case of a gastrostomy tube, the PD catheter exit site should ideally be placed either contralateral to the site of a current or potential gastrostomy tube or in the parasternal region. Whenever possible, the PD catheter should be placed either simultaneously or after placement of a gastrostomy tube to avoid contamination of the peritoneum from gastric contents. If a gastrostomy tube placement occurs after PD catheter insertion, use of an open surgical procedure is preferred over laparoscopic placement. Broad-spectrum antibiotic and antifungal prophylaxis is recommended in the perioperative period. PD is withheld for 24 hr or longer after gastrostomy placement if it is clinically safe to do so.

PERITONEAL DIALYSATE FLUIDS

Appropriate selection of dialysis fluid is important to achieve the required UF and solute clearance. The dialysate temperature, osmolality, fill volume, and dwell time impact the diffuse and convective transport in PD. The components of commonly used PD solutions are shown in **Table 28.2**.

Osmotic Agent

Dextrose-based solutions: Dextrose-based solutions are most widely used. The solutions contain dextrose in varying concentrations to create

BOX 28.1: Contraindications to initiation of chronic peritoneal dialysis (PD)

Absolute contraindications

Abdominal wall defects; e.g., omphalocele
Bladder exstrophy
Diaphragmatic hernia; pleuroperitoneal shunt
Damaged peritoneal membrane; e.g., postoperative adhesions and scarring

Relative contraindications

Massive organomegaly
Presence of ileostomy/colostomy
Presence of ventriculoperitoneal shunt
Lack of appropriate hygienic living conditions
Lack of caregiver/financial support to sustain home dialysis
Impending abdominal surgery
Morbid obesity
Cognitive or physical disability

TABLE 28.2: Composition of peritoneal dialysis fluids available in India

Brand name (Baxter Inc.)		***Dianeal***		***Extraneal***
Dextrose (g/dL or %)	1.5	2.5	4.25	Icodextrin (equivalent to 7.5)
Osmolarity (mOsm/L)	346	396	485	284
Sodium (mEq/L)	132	132	132	133
Chloride (mEq/L)	96	96	96	96
Calcium (mEq/L)*	3.5	3.5	3.5	3.5
Magnesium (mEq/L)	0.5	0.5	0.5	0.5
L-Lactate (mEq/L)	40	40	40	40
pH	5.2 (4–6.5)	5.2 (4–6.5)	5.2 (4–6.5)	5–6
Bag size (in Liter)	2, 5	2, 5	2, 5	2, 2.5

*2.5 mEq/L in low calcium solutions

osmotic gradients to drive UF and convective solute removal **(Table 28.2)**. Current recommendations for children include using the lowest dextrose concentration to achieve euvolemia. The osmotic gradient is lost due to the rapid and variable absorption of glucose and so these fluids fail to achieve adequate UF during long dwells and in patients with high peritoneal transport rates. Glucose absorption also tends to worsen hyperglycemia, anorexia, dyslipidemia, and cause oxidative stress. Long-term exposure to the conventionally used PD solutions with high glucose and lactate, low pH, high osmolarity, and high level of glucose degradation products (GDP) causes peritoneal membrane hypervascularization and fibrosis leading to deterioration in solute transport and UF capacity and impaired peritoneal host defense. Dextrose-based PD solutions should be stored in cool areas, as heat exposure can generate GDP. The pH is kept low to prevent caramelization during heat sterilization; however, this generates toxic GDP.

Biocompatible solutions: Biocompatible solutions were developed to reduce GDP generation. This was achieved by using dual-chamber bag system to allow storing the glucose solution at a lower pH separate from the rest of the PD solution components. Admixing of dextrose with the rest of the components is done by breaking the dividing septum within the bag to create a low GDP solution. This ensures that integrity of the peritoneum is maintained for a longer period. These fluids are more expensive and not available in low-resource settings.

Icodextrin: Icodextrin is a mixture of high-molecular-weight, water-soluble glucose polymers with an average molecular weight of 16,200 Da. The macromolecules have high reflection coefficient and create colloidal osmotic pressure resulting in fluid movement across the small and large capillary pores. Sodium removal is higher with icodextrin-based fluids as, being isosmotic, it does not activate aquaporin-associated sodium sieving. Icodextrin remains for prolonged period in peritoneal cavity and is absorbed slowly by the lymphatics. So, due to its osmotic effect, 7.5% icodextrin solution can achieve sustained UF, unlike dextrose solutions. This is ideal for long dwells in automated peritoneal dialysis (APD) or CAPD and in children with volume overload due to insufficient UF. Currently, it is licensed to be used for only one dwell per day due to insufficient information on the potential toxicity of its low-molecular-weight metabolites. Recent reports suggest that twice daily icodextrin exchanges are overall safe and associated with lower glucose load and higher UF.

Amino acids (AA) PD solutions: These contain AA as the osmotic agent to reduce glucose exposure and provide nutritional supplementation. The 1.1% AA solution is equivalent to 1.5% dextrose solution in osmotic efficiency. AA also cause peritoneal vasodilation, thus increasing peritoneal microcirculatory area, which contributes to UF and solute clearance. However, they increase blood urea nitrogen and may worsen metabolic acidosis. While it is suggested that AA solutions may be indicated in malnourished children, enteral nutrition should be preferred.

Buffer

Peritoneal dialysis solutions contain lactate or lactate/bicarbonate buffer. The former has a low pH which causes long-term damage to the peritoneal membrane. Lactate also requires conversion to bicarbonate in the liver and can cause abdominal pain during the inflow of dialysate. Lactate/bicarbonate buffered PD solutions are superior as they have a more neutral pH of 7.4, which decreases production of toxic GDP during sterilization and storage of dialysate fluids. They are more effective in correcting metabolic acidosis, cause less inflow pain, and have less protein loss.

PERITONEAL DIALYSIS TECHNIQUE

Peritoneal dialysis is performed by instilling the dialysate fluid into the peritoneal cavity through the PD catheter. After a predetermined time period this fluid is drained, and fresh fluid is introduced. This may be done manually (CAPD) or using a cycler (APD) **(Fig. 28.3)**. In CAPD, which is more frequently used, dialysate fluid exchanges are done manually 3–4 times per day, with the dwell time for each exchange being 6–8 hr.

The cycler ensures automated fill of a predetermined volume of dialysate and its removal from the peritoneal cavity after a programmed dwell time. The use of a cycler reduces caregiver workload, improves adherence to prescription and reduced risk of touch contamination, which decreases risk of peritonitis. However, systematic reviews do not show significant differences

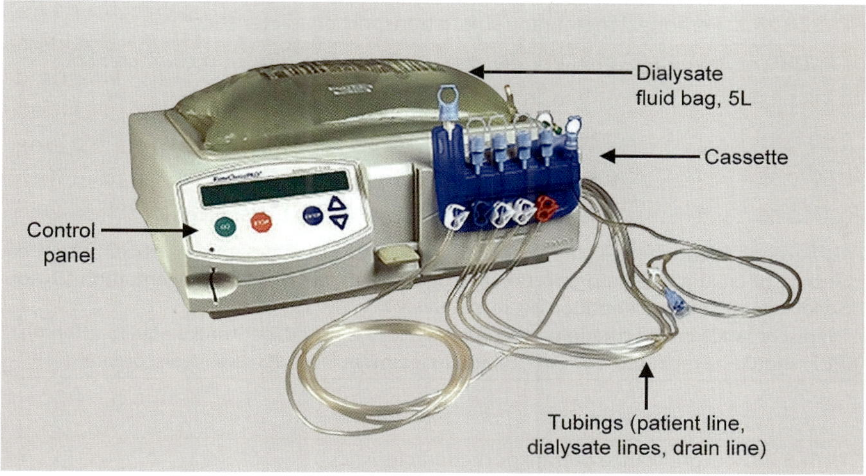

Fig. 28.3: Cycler for automated peritoneal dialysis (PD)

in terms of clinical outcomes such as mortality, risk of peritonitis, mechanical complications, technique failure, or hospital admissions in patients receiving CAPD or APD.

Peritoneal Membrane Transport Capacity

The solute and fluid movement across the peritoneal membrane varies among patients and the PD prescription needs to be tailored accordingly. Membrane transport characteristics should be evaluated at ~1 month after initiating PD, every 6–12 months thereafter, and following an episode of severe peritonitis or any major illness. Various tests are used to determine the peritoneal membrane status, including the peritoneal equilibration test (PET), dialysis adequacy and transport test (DATT), accelerated peritoneal examination (APEX), and software-based programs.

Peritoneal Equilibration Test

First described by Twardowski in 1987, it is the most widely used peritoneal function test because of its standardization, simplicity, and use in diagnostic and prognostic purposes. Urea and creatinine dialysis to plasma (D/P) ratios and dialysate glucose concentration at 2 and 4 hr compared to initial dialysate concentration (D/D_0) are calculated at 2 and 4 hr after a dwell of 1,100 m^2 of 2.5% dextrose PD solution. Patients are categorized into four groups based on solute movement across the peritoneal membrane: high, high average, low average, and low transporters **(Table 28.3)**. The terms "high" and "low" refer to the amount of transported molecules and not the speed of transport of solutes across the membrane. **Table 28.4** informs on the interpretation of the transport characteristics derived from PET.

TABLE 28.3: Peritoneal membrane solute transport characteristics*

4 hr D/P creatinine	*4 hr D/D_0 glucose*	*Peritoneal transport characteristic***
0.81–1.03	0.12–0.26	High (fast) transporter
0.65–0.81	0.26–0.38	High-average transporter
0.50–0.65	0.38–0.49	Low-average transporter
0.34–0.50	0.49–0.61	Low (slow) transporter

*Time-dependent changes during peritoneal dialysis in dialysate (D) concentration of glucose or creatinine as a proportion of original dialysate glucose concentration (D_0) or plasma creatinine concentration (P), respectively

**If discordance in D/P creatinine and D/D_0 glucose is noted, peritoneal equilibration test (PET) should be repeated; consider clinical assessment if results remain discordant

TABLE 28.4: Significance of transport characteristics

	High	*Low*
Physiology	Large effective peritoneal surface area or intrinsically high membrane permeability	Small effective peritoneal surface area or low membrane permeability
Clearance of solutes	Rapid and complete equilibration for urea; high dialysate to plasma (D/P) creatinine	Slow and incomplete equilibration of solutes; low D/P creatinine
Ultrafiltration	Early dissipation of osmotic gradient leading to low ratio of or 4 hour dialysate glucose to baseline glucose (D/D0) low net ultrafiltration	Sustained osmotic gradient with high D/D0 glucose; satisfactory net ultrafiltration
Protein losses	High dialysate protein; low serum albumin	Low dialysate protein; normal serum albumin
Implications for therapy	Use frequent short dwells, for example, with automated peritoneal dialysis (APD) cycler	Use large volume dwells for prolonged durations

Patients with high average and low average transporter status have characteristics intermediate to the two categories shown

Though the rapid night exchanges or shorter dwell times for each exchange in APD may result in variations in the PET, studies have shown that the results are still valid for APD patients. The drawback of PET is that it focuses only on small-solute transport and does not give information on UF, convection, and diffusion.

Variations of the traditional PET include the short PET, fast PET, and the modified PET. The fast PET uses only the 4-hour creatinine and glucose values while the short PET uses only the results obtained at 2 hr, which makes them less labor intensive and more suitable for children.

The modified PET uses 4.25% dextrose PD solution during the 4-hour PET and is indicated in evaluation of suspected UF failure. A net UF <400 mL during the 4-hour test despite maximal osmotic stimulus is evidence that the UF capacity of the peritoneal membrane has decreased to the extent inadequate for volume control, which becomes an indication to switch to HD. Net UF greater than 400 mL indicates that the membrane itself remains responsive to osmotic challenge. This information is useful to determine if the patient presenting with chronic volume overload has true *membrane failure* (UF <400 mL) or is overloaded from other mechanisms, such as excessive salt and fluid intake.

Dialysis Adequacy and Transport Test

Dialysis adequacy and transport test is a simple test that only requires a single blood test in the morning of the following day to determine the plasma creatinine, and 10 mL aliquot of the pooled 24-hr CAPD dialysate. The 24-hour D/P creatinine is used to determine transport status. There is reasonable correlation between PET and DATT in determining peritoneal transport status.

Accelerated Peritoneal Examination Time

Accelerated peritoneal examination (APEX) time is defined by the crossing point of the urea and glucose equilibration curves obtained from a standardized PET. It is proposed as the optimal dwell time for UF capacity. Modification of dwell time impacts dialysis efficacy, in terms of UF and solute clearances.

Software-based Programs

Computer programs, provided by dialysis manufacturers, for example, PD-Adequest (Baxter Healthcare) and PatientOnLine (Fresenius Medical), model peritoneal clearance and UF based on the law of mass conservation. PD-Adequest version 2 is based on the three-pore model of the peritoneal membrane. It requires estimation of total body water (TBW) (V), D/P creatinine, dwell volume, and dextrose concentration (%). PatientOnLine uses the parameter FT50, which refers to the time needed to obtain a saturation of 50%, equivalent of D/P creatinine 0.5. Different prescriptions are generated, and the regimen that meets the required clearance and UF targets with the least disruption in lifestyle or comfort is chosen.

INITIATION OF PERITONEAL DIALYSIS

A key factor in facilitating transition to dialysis is patient and family education. The patient and the family should be prepared for the realities of chronic dialysis long before the actual initiation. Different dialysis modalities, the choice of PD regimen whether CAPD or APD, placement of catheter, timing and initiation of PD training, timing of dialysis initiation, initial dialysis prescription, delivery and storage of supplies, impact of therapy on their daily life, and careful attention to hygiene, should be discussed. Adherence to treatment protocols is emphasized.

Timing of Peritoneal Dialysis Initiation

The timing of initiation of PD in children is not absolute. It is suggested that dialysis should be initiated in children at an estimated glomerular filtration rate (GFR) of <10 mL/min/1.73 m^2 or when the child has persistent uremic symptoms not improving with medications and/or dietary management. The decision to commence dialysis is based on a combination of clinical and laboratory parameters. Clinical indications include persistent nausea and vomiting, fluid overload refractory to diuretics, hypertension poorly responsive to antihypertensive medications, pericarditis, pleuritis, uremic encephalopathy, neuropathy, and bleeding diathesis attributable to uremia. Persistent metabolic disturbances such as hyperkalemia, metabolic acidosis, hypercalcemia, hypocalcemia and hyperphosphatemia might also require initiation of dialysis. In children, other considerations such as psychosocial well-being, nutritional status, and growth failure are important, rather than the absolute value of the GFR alone.

PERITONEAL DIALYSIS PRESCRIPTION

The PD prescription should be individualized based on child's age, body size, nutritional status, membrane transport status, required small solute and fluid removal, and residual kidney function. It should also accommodate the psychosocial needs of the patient and family members, for example, schooling of the child and the working hours of the parents. Essential components of PD prescription include the fill volume, dwell time, and dialysate composition. Patients with significant residual kidney function (RKF) may not need large volumes or numerous exchanges. The initial PD prescription is empiric and is subsequently modified after 4 weeks based on clinical and laboratory parameters and PET results.

Fill Volume

The initial fill volume following insertion of a PD catheter should be low to prevent leakage of dialysate. **Table 28.5** outlines a protocol for increasing the fill volumes and number of exchanges following Tenckhoff catheter insertion in children and infants. The maximum allowed volume per exchange is 1,200 mL/m^2 (or 50 mL/kg in infants). Rapid in-and-out exchanges for a total of five exchanges should be done after insertion of the PD catheter. Subsequently, hourly exchanges are done for 24–48 hr or until the effluent is clear.

TABLE 28.5: Protocol for increasing the fill volumes post Tenckhoff catheter insertion in children and infants

Time following insertion	*Fill (exchange) volume' mL/m² (mL/kg, in infants)*	
	Children and adolescents	*Infants*
Day 1	300	200 (10)
Day 4	500	300 (15)
Day 8	800	400 (20)
Day 10	900	500 (25)
Week 2	1,000	600 (30)
Week 3	1,100	700 (35)
Week 4	1,200	800 (40)

The duration of PD and number of exchanges should be adjusted according to the recommended fill volume based on the number of days after insertion of PD catheter. A rule of thumb for the number of cycles required is the total fluid volume (T) calculated based on the recommended maximum dialysis volume (mL/m^2) divided by the fill volume recommended for the post-operative day.

Although the surface area of the peritoneal membrane in infants is relatively larger than in adults, the membrane transport capacity is uniform across various ages and similar to adults. So, scaling the fill volume by body surface area (BSA) instead of body weight maintains the relation between the dialysate volume and peritoneal membrane area. This avoids inadvertently prescribing too small a volume, which can lead to rapid solute equilibration and inadequate clearances and UF. Conversely, too large a fill volume increases the intraperitoneal pressure which reduces dialysis efficiency due to enhanced lymphatic uptake, and may be associated with discomfort, abdominal pain, dyspnea, hernia, gastroesophageal reflux, and hydrothorax.

The volume can be adjusted according to patient's tolerance and need for solute and fluid removal. The fill volume in a CAPD regimen of 4 exchanges per day should start with 300–500 mL/m^2/exchange (200 mL/m^2/exchange in infants), slowly increasing to 800–1,000 mL/m^2 for daytime exchanges and 1,000–1,200 mL/m^2 for nighttime exchanges. In patients managed by APD, targeted individual nocturnal fill volume is 900–1,200 mL/m^2 for patients >2 years, and 600–800 mL/m^2 for children <2 years. The daytime fill volume is generally 50% of the nighttime volume. In infants <2 years old, 800 mL/m^2 (30–50 mL/kg/body weight) is taken as the maximum allowed fill volume; however, this should be determined based on the volume tolerated. The bedside intraperitoneal pressure may be monitored, with the upper limit being 18 cm water.

Dwell Time

Dwell time is determined mainly by the peritoneal membrane transport status. Generally, high transporters will benefit from shorter dwell times on the automated cycler, while low transporters will do well with prolonged dwell times on the cycler or might require CAPD **(Table 28.4)**. Long dwells allow for a better middle molecule clearance and additional sodium removal, while short dwell times increase UL and urea clearance. The length of dwell times also depends on the PD modality. In CAPD, loss of the osmotic gradient due to solute equilibration during long dwells results in ineffective UF. The dwell time may be shortened to less than 4 hr in children who have high solute transport rates. In APD, the dwell time may be individualized based on the APEX time, which corresponds to the point at which the D/P urea and D/D_0 glucose equilibration curves cross in PET and is considered the ideal duration for an APD cycle.

Dialysate Composition

Utmost care is taken to avoid unnecessary exposure to higher dextrose concentrations to reach UF targets. The use of icodextrin may be considered in patients with increased UF requirement. Biocompatible solutions are preferred for improved long-term outcomes. The role of AA solutions remains unclear.

Dialysis Regimen

Automated peritoneal dialysis is widely used in children in high income countries but its use may be limited elsewhere, due to lack of availability and cost constraints. The types of PD regimens are outlined in **Fig. 28.4 and Table 28.6**. These can be further individualized according to the patient's requirements.

In tidal PD, which is the most complex regimen, the rate of outflow is not linear. Outflow is highest at the beginning of the drain time and declines to a point when a critical intraperitoneal volume is reached. Tidal PD is more effective especially when the concept of UF efficiency, i.e., the glucose metabolic cost of UF in milliliters for every grams of glucose absorbed, and the capacity for dialytic removal of phosphate, are taken into consideration. About 10% of all home PD regimens for children in developed countries use some form of tidal PD.

High-Quality Goal-Directed Peritoneal Dialysis

Simplistically, adequate PD refers to dialysis which is enough to reduce the burden of uremic symptoms in a patient with ESKD. In the past, Kt/V_{urea} was a surrogate marker for dialysis adequacy, which was targeted to

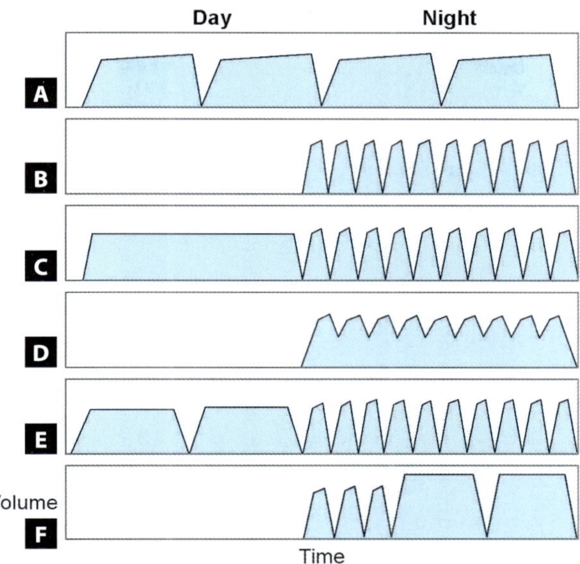

Figs. 28.4A to F: Peritoneal dialysis modalities. (A) represents continuous ambulatory peritoneal dialysis (CAPD); (B) represents automated peritoneal dialysis (APD) which is nocturnal intermittent (NIPD); (C) represents continuous cycling (CCPD); (D) shows tidal PD; (E) illustrates continuous optimized PD; and (F) shows adapted PD

achieve targeting weekly Kt/V_{urea} ≥1.7 (where Kt is the sum of the peritoneal clearance and residual kidney clearance in liters). There has been a shift in this approach with recent guidelines by the International Society for Peritoneal Dialysis (ISPD) advocating "goal-directed" therapy focused on patient well-being rather than just removal of toxins. The ISPD suggests that the fundamentals for prescribing and evaluating the delivery of "high-quality PD" to children should be same as for adults. The PD prescription should be tailored to meet the medical, mental, social, and financial requirements of the child and the family, and based on shared decision making involving all these stakeholders, with realistic goals. The prescription should consider the available resources and the lifestyle and wishes of the child as well as the family members involved in their care. The RKF should be monitored regularly, with an aim to preserve it as long as possible. Multiple assessments should be performed regularly to determine the quality of life, nutrition and volume status, and clearance of solutes with dialysis. Children with poor prognosis due to other comorbidities may benefit from a reduced dialysis prescription which reduces the treatment burden.

Monitoring of Patients on Peritoneal Dialysis

Peritoneal dialysis may be delivered in multiple ways and there is no optimal dose. The prescription is based on discussions with the child, family members, and treating team with realistic goals to: (*i*) maintain the quality of life and

TABLE 28.6: Types of regimens for peritoneal dialysis (PD)

Type	*Peritoneal dialysis (PD) exchanges*	*Characteristics; comments*
Continuous ambulatory PD (CAPD)	Fluid exchange (instillation and drainage) are performed manually by the patient/caregiver 3–4 times a day **(Fig. 28.4A)**	Most commonly used
Automated PD (APD)	The fluid exchange is done by a mechanical device (cycler)	Usually achieves higher solute and fluid removal than CAPD Reduces burden of care on careprovider; allows patient to sleep through the procedure
Nocturnal intermittent PD (NIPD)	APD during the night, usually as 6–8 exchanges over 8–10 hr; no exchanges ("dry") through the day **(Fig. 28.4B)**	Child allowed normal activities through the day Lower risk of: (*i*) glucose absorption from dialysate; (*ii*) losses of amino acids and protein; (*iii*) peritoneal membrane exposure to glucose; and (*iv*) hernias Lack of a daytime dwell limits solute clearance; hence suitable chiefly in patients with residual renal function
Continuous cycling PD (CCPD)	After completing APD cycles during the night, one dwell of PD fluid (50–100% of the nocturnal dwell volume) is left in the peritoneal cavity by the cycler the following morning; this remains till the next APD cycle at night **(Fig. 28.4C)**	Superior solute and ultrafiltration compared to NIPD
Tidal peritoneal dialysis	Similar to CCPD, but with some volume of dialysate left intraperitoneally between cycles instead of draining the peritoneal cavity completely at the end of each cycle **(Fig. 28.4D)**. The partially drained volumes are replaced by fresh dialysate to restore the initial infusion volume with each cycle. The entire dialysate volume is drained at the end of the session	Constant contact maintained between dialysate and the peritoneal membrane improves solute clearance
Continuous optimized PD	CCPD with an additional daytime exchange **(Fig. 28.4E)**, which may be done manually, if required	Maximizes solute clearance and ultrafiltration
Adapted PD	Sequentially uses shorter- and longer-dwell exchanges with smaller and larger fill volumes, respectively **(Fig. 28.4F)**	Provides more effective dialysis; not possible with current APD options in India

enable children to achieve their goals to the extent possible, for example, attending school, playing with friends, and spending time with family; (ii) minimize symptoms and treatment burden; and (iii) maintain high-quality care. It is important to consider the resource limitations in low-and-middle-income countries in deciding the feasibility of the targets of treatment.

Patient Reported Outcome Measures

The child's perception of their well-being, including symptom burden and the impact of treatment on lifestyle and mental health, should be periodically evaluated. The dialysis prescription may be modified based on these assessments to improve the quality of life of the child and the caregiver(s). Increase in dialysis dose may be indicated in children with failure to thrive.

Modification of PD Prescription

The dialysis prescription is modified based on PET results. Fill volumes, rather than dialysate dextrose concentration, should be optimized to improve UF. For children on APD who show high solute transport, the dwell time is shortened with minimal day dwell volumes. In low solute transporters, a long day dwell is recommended for those on APD and an overnight dwell for those on CAPD. Using icodextrin, for long dwell in APD or the overnight dwell in CAPD, also improves UF. However, use of icodextrin should be avoided for emergent volume overload as its UF rate is slower than 4.25% dextrose.

Volume Status

The PD prescription should ensure that the peritoneal UF combined with the residual urine output are adequate to ensure euvolemia. The European APD Outcome Study suggested that peritoneal UF may be more important than peritoneal small-solute clearance. Hypertension, left ventricular hypertrophy, and other cardiac abnormalities are recognized complications arising from inadequate salt and volume control. Regular monitoring of the volume status and dry weight based on clinical examination, UF volume, weight, blood pressure, and sodium intake are important, though currently there is no evidence to target a specific blood pressure in these patients. Objective measurement of the fluid status using bioimpedance spectroscopy may be used. Common causes of overhydration should be addressed in patients with hypervolemia **(Flowchart 28.1)**.

Solute Clearance

Small-solute clearance should be estimated regularly using weekly Kt/V_{urea} or creatinine clearance to assess the amount of dialysis provided, which may be used to guide the dialysis prescription. A total minimum weekly Kt/V_{urea} of

Flowchart 28.1: Causes and management of overhydration in chronic peritoneal dialysis (PD)
*Sodium sieving refers to the disproportionate loss of water, compared to sodium, into the effluent, due to aquaporin-mediated water transport
**Avoid hypovolemia, dehydration, and use of nephrotoxic medications and radiocontrast; use angiotensin converting enzyme inhibitors or angiotensin receptor blockers to retard rate of decline of kidney function (while monitoring carefully for hyperkalemia, hypotension, and acute kidney injury)
PET: peritoneal equilibration test; RKF residual kidney function

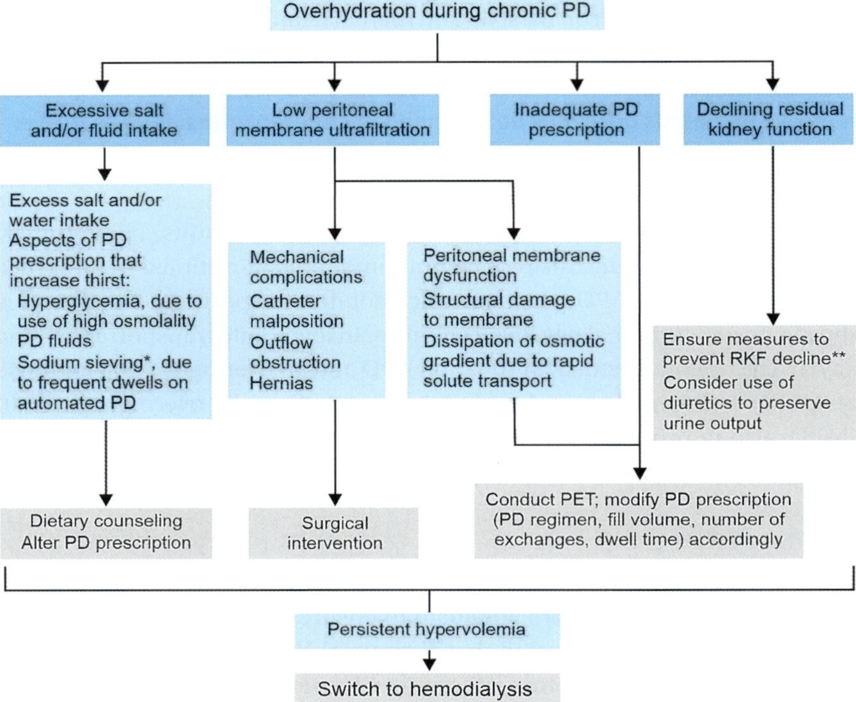

1.7 should be targeted. However, if the child's symptoms and volume status are controlled and nutrition is adequate, the PD prescription is not changed solely to increase the solute clearance. This is based on the observation that there is no evidence of an association between failure to achieve optimal solute clearance, i.e., dialysis adequacy, arbitrarily defined as Kt/V_{urea} ≥1.7, and core PD outcomes of PD infection, cardiovascular disease, mortality, PD failure, and life participation. If the child remains symptomatic despite Kt/V_{urea} ≥1.7, an increase in dialysis dose can be considered after excluding nondialysis related contributory factors. As dietary protein intake is greater in infants and children, higher Kt/V_{urea} is required to prevent progressive uremia.

Estimating small-solute clearance on PD: Measurement of total solute clearance (delivered PD dose plus residual kidney function) is recommended every 3–4 months. Peritoneal and renal contributions in patients with residual renal function (urine volume >300 mL, or GFR greater than 1 mL/min/1.73 m^2) are measured. Testing should include 24-hour urine collection and 24-hour effluent test for urea and creatinine clearance.

A quantified dose of PD is expressed as the total weekly urea clearance (Kt/V_{urea}) and weekly creatinine clearance (Cl_{cr}). Creatinine clearance is usually normalized for BSA and expressed as mL/min/1.73 m^2. The renal component should be considered when calculating both the clearances. The total weekly Kt/V_{urea} is calculated as shown below.

$$\text{Weekly Kt/V} = [D_{urea} \times V_D + (U_{urea} \times V_u)/P_{urea} \times V] \times 7$$

Where D_{urea}, U_{urea}, P_{urea} are the dialysate, urinary, and plasma concentrations of urea, respectively, and V_D and V_u are the 24-hour dialysate and urine volume, V is the urea distribution volume (TBW), and Kt is the sum of the peritoneal clearance and residual kidney clearance in liters.

The Mellits and Cheek formula, based on height and weight, is the most commonly used formula for the calculation of V. However, this was established in healthy populations and overestimates TBW in children receiving PD. A more accurate gender-specific prediction of TBW equation was based on heavy water (^2H_2O or D_2O) dilution in dialysis patients, as follows:

$$\textit{Males: } \text{TBW} = 0.010 \times (\text{height} \times \text{weight})^{0.68} - (0.37 \times \text{weight})$$

$$\textit{Females: } \text{TBW} = 0.14 \times (\text{height} \times \text{weight})^{0.64} - (0.35 \times \text{weight})$$

A simplified (Gehan and George) equation uses BSA to calculate TBW:

$$\textit{Male: } \text{TBW} = 20.88 \times \text{BSA} - 4.29$$

$$\textit{Female: } \text{TBW} = 16.92 \times \text{BSA} - 1.81$$

Preservation of RKF

The RKF outweighs peritoneal clearance in influencing long-term outcomes. Studies in adult patients on PD have shown that the residual kidney component of the total Kt/V_{urea} has greater impact on survival than the peritoneal component. RKF is calculated as the GFR by determining the average of the clearance of urea and creatinine as follows:

$$\text{RKF} = [(U_{cr} \times V_u/P_{cr}) + (U_{urea} \times V_u/P_{urea})]/2$$

Where, U_{cr} and P_{cr} are the urinary and plasma concentration of creatinine, U_{urea} and P_{urea} are the urinary and plasma concentration of urea, and V_u is the 24-hour urine volume. RKF is considered significant if urine volume >100 mL/day and urine Kt/V_{urea} is greater than 0.1/week.

Incremental Peritoneal Dialysis

The feasibility of the dialysis schedule is based on availability of family members involved in care. This is especially important in regions where resource constraints may limit optimal dialysis delivery. Patient may be initiated on chronic PD at a low dose, which is then progressively increased with decline in RKF. This helps the child to adapt to the procedure, improving adherence.

The advantages of incremental PD include: (*i*) A lower initial cost of care; (*ii*) better quality of life, with improved attendance at school and more time to spend with friends and family; (*iii*) higher adherence to dialysis prescription; (*iv*) lower risk of peritonitis due to fewer connections; and (*v*) lower exposure to glucose, which reduces risks of damage to peritoneum, hyperglycemia and dyslipidemia, and preserves RKF. On the other hand, incremental PD: (*i*) Requires frequent monitoring of RKF; (*ii*) is associated with risk of uremic symptoms and failure to thrive, due to decreased solute clearance; (*iii*) has high risk of fluid overload, due to lower UF; which lead to lower patient survival; and (*iv*) carries reasonably high risk of nonadherence when dialysis prescription is intensified. Hence, if prescribed, incremental PD should be supplemented with intensive medical monitoring and dietary support.

Nutritional Management

Regular evaluation of the appetite and laboratory parameters, such a serum sodium, potassium, bicarbonate, albumin, calcium, and phosphate, is essential to assess nutritional status. Adequate dietary protein intake should be emphasized, along with restriction of sodium, potassium, and phosphate. In children on dialysis, recommendations for dietary protein are 100% of the dietary reference intake for age and ideal body weight, plus an allowance for dialytic protein and AA losses **(Table 28.7)**. While on PD, the daily peritoneal protein losses decrease with age across childhood from an average of 0.28 g/kg in the 1st year of life to <0.1 g/kg in adolescents. Peritoneal AA losses add

TABLE 28.7: Recommended daily dietary protein intake (Pediatric Renal Nutrition Taskforce, 2020)

Age	*Suggested dietary intake (g/kg/day)*	*Additional intake during chronic dialysis (g/kg)*
0–6 months	1.3–1.8; <1 months: 1.5–2.5	0.28
7–12 months	0.9–1.3	0.28
1–3 years	0.9–1.05	0.1–0.28
4–13 years	0.85–0.95	0.1–0.28
14–18 years	0.8–0.9	0.1

Source: Shaw et al, 2020

approximately one-third to the nitrogen lost with protein, resulting in a total additional dietary protein requirement ranging from 0.15–0.35 g/kg/day, depending on the patient's age.

Supplemental nutritional support should be considered when a child is not growing normally or fails to consume the reference dietary intake for protein and/or energy. Enteral feeding may be needed to optimize nutrition and growth, especially in young infants, and is used to administer medications such as sodium chloride supplements in anuric infants with high UF losses since salt depletion is known to retard growth.

Hypokalemia and hypoalbuminemia are associated with adverse outcomes. Dietary and/or oral potassium supplements are required in patients with hypokalemia. Dietary changes, phosphate binders, and modification of the dialysis prescription are required to manage hyperphosphatemia. In patients on APD, increasing the dwell time of exchanges and switching from nocturnal intermittent peritoneal dialysis (NIPD) to continuous cycling peritoneal dialysis (CCPD) with long day dwell, may be required to achieve normal phosphate. Interventions to correct hypoalbuminemia, besides diet modification, are not beneficial.

COMPLICATIONS OF PERITONEAL DIALYSIS

Infectious and noninfectious complications may occur in PD **(Box 28.2)**.

Noninfectious Complications

Malfunction of the PD catheter is a common noninfectious complication, which presents as inflow, outflow, or a two-way obstruction. *Inflow obstruction*

BOX 28.2: Complications of chronic peritoneal dialysis (PD)

Noninfectious complications
Catheter-related
Decreased flow
Inflow or drainage pain
Dialysate leak
Complications caused by increased intraperitoneal pressure
Back pain
Hernia
Hydrothorax
Metabolic
Hyperglycemia
Dyslipidemia
Metabolic syndrome
Hypokalemia
Encapsulating peritoneal sclerosis
Infectious complications
Peritonitis
Exit-site or tunnel infections

may be due to mechanical blockage such as clamps or kinks in transfer set, tubing or catheter or intraluminal fibrin or clots. *Outflow obstruction* may be due to intraluminal mechanical blockage of catheter, constipation, extrinsic bladder compression due to urinary retention, catheter tip migration, and catheter entrapment by omentum or adhesions. The treatment of mechanical obstruction depends upon its cause. A radiograph of the abdomen is performed to visualize the catheter position. If the obstruction is due to constipation, it should be treated. In case of fibrin-related obstruction, heparin is added to each dialysate exchange in a concentration of 500–1,000 U/L. Alternatively, urokinase or recombinant tissue plasminogen activator (tPA) can be used. If noninvasive measures fail, surgical replacement, either by laparoscopy or open surgery, is required.

Increased intraperitoneal pressure due to dialysate fluid may cause back pain, hernias, leaks (hydrothorax and pleuroperitoneal leaks), and local edema. Gastrointestinal problems such as *gastroesophageal reflux* and *delayed gastric emptying*, may occur, especially in infants. *Pleural effusion* (*hydrothorax*) in a patient with no other signs fluid overload should prompt a search for pleuroperitoneal communications. Seepage of peritoneal fluid can lead to abdominal wall, peri-catheter, or genital *edema*. Contrast CT scan may be useful in diagnosing dialysate leaks. Decreasing the fill volume or performing PD in the supine position are effective in relieving back pain.

Metabolic complications are common in chronic PD. Systemic absorption of glucose leads to hyperglycemia, dyslipidemia, metabolic syndrome, and weight gain. Hypokalemia may occur as PD fluid does not contain any potassium. *Encapsulating peritoneal sclerosis* is a rare but serious complication seen in patients on PD for a prolonged time period, characterized by chronic inflammation and thickening of the peritoneum, leading to bowel obstruction and formation of a pathognomonic fibrotic cocoon.

Constipation is a common problem in patients on PD. Fecal loading predisposes to fluid overload and peritonitis by interfering with the effluent outflow. The PD catheter might get displaced from the pelvis into the upper abdomen. Management of constipation involves pharmacotherapy along with counseling for a balanced diet with sufficient fiber, adequate fluid intake, and regular physical activity, targeting passing of at least two stools per day. Lactulose is preferred over other agents due to the risk of adverse effects with polyethylene glycol (hyperphosphatemia, salt and water retention, and hyperkalemia) and magnesium salts (hypermagnesemia, hypophosphatemia, and secondary hypocalcemia). Stimulant laxatives, such as *Senna*, sodium picosulfate, and bisacodyl, appear to be safe but have not been studied adequately in children with chronic kidney disease (CKD). While enemas may be used to allow fecal disimpaction in the short term, their chronic use is not recommended. In particular, sodium phosphate enema carries high risk of hypernatremia and hyperphosphatemia.

Infectious Complications

Table 28.8 lists important definitions used for infections associated with peritoneal dialysis. The ISPD has updated their guidelines for the prevention, diagnosis, and therapy of dialysis-associated peritonitis and catheter-related infections in 2022 and 2023.

Exit-site and Tunnel Infections

The diagnosis of exit-site or tunnel infection is usually clinical and is considered whenever there is a change in appearance of the healthy exit site, with erythema, edema, induration, or tenderness over the exit site or subcutaneous pathway. The latter is often associated with a pericatheter fluid collection, demonstrated by ultrasound. These infections often occur soon after catheter insertion. Measures shown to prevent catheter-insertion-associated (as well as later) infections include: (*i*) prophylactic antibiotics administration immediately before catheter insertion; (*ii*) use of nasal antibiotic prophylaxis in those known to be nasal carriers of *Staphylococcus aureus* (detected on screening prior to PD catheter insertion); (*iii*) use of a laparoscopic technique in preference to open surgical placement; (*iv*) leaving intact the exit-site dressing for 7 days after PD catheter insertion, unless it is soiled; (*v*) attention to site of placement of exit-site stoma, to avoid trauma, allow cleaning and prevent soiling (discussed earlier); and (*vi*) rigorous training in the care of exit sites.

The ISPD recommends daily topical application of antibiotic cream or ointment (mupirocin or gentamicin) to the catheter exit site to prevent catheter-related infection. The exit site should be cleansed at least twice weekly and every time after a shower or vigorous exercise. PD catheter exit-site care should be continued even if PD has been interrupted or discontinued if the catheter is in place. A dressing cover over the exit site is not mandatory after exit-site care and topical antibiotic application. The PD catheter should be immobilized (using a waist belt, protective bag, or securing the transfer set to the abdomen by adhesive tape) to avoid traction injury of the exit site.

The diagnosis of exit-site and tunnel infections is based on swab culture results. Following clinical examination, swab culture and Gram stain, and/or (if tunnel infection is suspected) ultrasound for the tunnel, oral antibiotic therapy is begun. Empiric therapy should ensure coverage against *Staphylococcus aureus*, such as a first-generation cephalosporin or anti-staphylococcal penicillin, for example, amoxicillin/clavulanic acid, cephalexin, cloxacillin or dicloxacillin. If there is history of infection or colonization with methicillin-resistant *S. aureus* (MRSA) or *Pseudomonas* species, vancomycin (or clindamycin, if known to be susceptible) or antipseudomonal antibiotic, respectively, are preferred. Antibiotics are later adjusted according to results of culture and antibiotic susceptibility.

TABLE 28.8: Definitions of catheter-related infections associated with peritoneal dialysis (PD), based on ISPD 2022 and 2023 updates

Infection	*Definition*
Exit-site infection[1#]	Purulent discharge with or without erythema of the skin at the catheter and skin interface; further classified by the etiology (organism identified on culture of exit-site swab) or as culture-negative[2] and considered 'PD catheter insertion-related' if occurring ≤30 days of insertion
Tunnel infection	Clinical inflammation (erythema, swelling, tenderness, or induration) with or without ultrasound evidence of fluid collection anywhere along the catheter tunnel; considered 'PD catheter insertion-related' if occurring ≤30 days of insertion
Refractory catheter-related infection[3]	Failure to respond after 2 weeks of effective antibiotic therapy and appropriately intensified exit-site care, or 3 weeks for infection due to *Pseudomonas* species
Peritonitis[1@]	Presence of ≥2 of the following: (*i*) clinical features consistent with peritonitis, i.e., abdominal pain and/or cloudy dialysis effluent; (*ii*) dialysis effluent white cell count >100/mL or $>0.1 \times 10^9$ per L (after a dwell time of at least 2 hr), with >50% polymorphonuclear leukocytes (PMN); and (*iii*) positive dialysis effluent culture. Further classified by the etiology (organism identified on culture of effluent) or as culture-negative[2]; and according to the timeline[4]
Catheter-related peritonitis	Peritonitis in temporal conjunction (≤3 months) with an exit-site or tunnel infection attributable to the same organism, or with one site sterile (in the context of antibiotic exposure)
Enteric peritonitis	Peritonitis arising from an intestinal source following inflammation and perforation or ischemia of intra-abdominal organs; if culture negative, classify as enteric peritonitis rather than as culture-negative peritonitis
Refractory peritonitis	A peritonitis episode in which the effluent fails to clear (persistently cloudy bags or persistent dialysis effluent leukocyte count $>100 \times 10^9$/L) despite 5 days of appropriate antibiotics
Relapsing peritonitis	A peritonitis episode that occurs ≤4 weeks of completion of therapy for an earlier episode attributable to the same organism, or one sterile episode
Repeat peritonitis	A peritonitis episode that occurs >4 weeks after completion of therapy for an earlier episode attributable to the same organism
Recurrent peritonitis	A peritonitis episode that occurs ≤4 weeks of completion of therapy for an earlier episode, but attributable to a different organism
Medical cure	Complete resolution of peritonitis together with NONE of the following: Relapsing or recurrent peritonitis, catheter removal, transfer to hemodialysis for ≥30 days or death

[1]A center's [#]rate of exit-site infections and [@]peritonitis should each be ≤0.4 episodes per year at risk; #the proportion of PD catheter insertion-related infections should be <5% of all catheters; and [@]the proportion of patients free of peritonitis should be >80% per year at risk

[2]Culture-negative infections are caused by recent antibiotic use, suboptimal sample collection or culture, or infection with slow growing atypical organism (e.g., mycobacteria and fungus). A center's culture-negative rate should be <15% of all peritonitis episodes

[3]Infection-related catheter removal is defined as catheter removal due to catheter-related infection unresponsive to appropriate antibiotic therapy or surgical salvage procedure

[4]Further classified as pre-PD (occurring after PD catheter insertion and before commencement of PD), PD-related (occurring after the first day of PD training or PD treatment in hospital or at home, up till when PD is continued), and PD catheter insertion-related (occurring within 30 days of PD catheter insertion)

While most infections are treated for 7–10 days, to a maximum of 2 weeks, *Pseudomonas* infection requires 3 weeks of therapy with an appropriate antimicrobial. In patients with inadequate response, a second agent can be added, for example, oral rifampin for *S. aureus* and a second antipseudomonal drug for *Pseudomonas* infection. Patients with refractory infection or concomitant peritonitis require removal of the catheter.

Peritonitis

This is the most common cause of hospitalization among children on PD and the most important reason for change to HD. The frequency of peritonitis varies across centers. According to ISPD guidelines, the peritonitis rate in a PD program should not exceed 0.4 episodes/patient/year and >80% of patients should be free of peritonitis at any given time. Most episodes of peritonitis are bacterial, chiefly due to *S. aureus* or gram-negative bacteria. The worldwide incidence of gram-negative peritonitis is increasing, while ~30% cases have culture-negative peritonitis. Patients with Gram-negative or fungal peritonitis also show high risk of mortality.

The child's prolonged reliance on PD makes it imperative to address strategies for prevention and treatment of PD-associated infections. PD exchange technique and knowledge of patients and care providers should be regularly reassessed and updated, with an emphasis on direct inspection of practice of PD exchange. PD retraining is recommended following: (*i*) prolonged hospitalization, (*ii*) peritonitis and/or catheter infection, (*iii*) change of care provider or change in his/her vision or mental acuity, (*iv*) change to another PD regimen, or (*v*) other interruption in PD (e.g., shift to and from HD).

Other measures to prevent peritonitis include the use of prophylactic antibiotics at the time of catheter placement, and during invasive procedures such as gastrostomy placement, and proper hand hygiene. Early detection and treatment of exit-site and tunnel infections should be emphasized during training as important means of decreasing the risk of peritonitis. The ISPD recommends IV antibiotics prior to PD catheter insertion, colonoscopies, and invasive gynecologic procedures, ensuring coverage for the *Enterobacteriaceae* family as well as gram-positive organisms found on the skin flora in PD catheter insertion, anaerobes in colonoscopies, and common organisms from the urogenital flora in gynecologic procedures. The ISPD also recommends oral amoxicillin prior to dental procedures, but not before an upper endoscopy. The Pediatric Renal Nutrition Taskforce (PRNT), but not the ISPD, recommend antibiotic prophylaxis before gastrostomy.

Touch contamination is an important risk factor for peritonitis. Patients on PD should be instructed to immediately seek advice from their dialysis center if the sterility of PD exchange has been breached. The ISPD recommends

BOX 28.3: Method of collection of peritoneal dialysis effluent for suspected peritonitis

Equipment and supplies: (*i*) Face mask; (*ii*) gloves; (*iii*) sterile sample bag or two sterile vials for sample collection; (*iv*) blood culture bottle(s); (*v*) minicap (impregnated with povidone-iodine); (*vi*) 50 mL syringe and 20-gauge needle; (*vii*) swab with 2% chlorhexidine or 70% alcohol; (*viii*) effluent sample bag

Wear face mask; perform hand hygiene

Collect specimens as follows:

Intermittent PD

Obtain specimens during a drain cycle
Carefully remove spike from drainage bag
Clean spike with chlorhexidine or alcohol swab for 1 minute and let it dry
Open drainage roller clamp and collect 60 mL effluent directly into the sterile vial
Aseptically reinsert drainage spike into drainage bag
Open roller clamp and continue with drain cycle

Continuous cyclic PD

Obtain specimens during initial drain (drain 1)
Close clamp on sample bag
Connect bag to the short line that forms a "Y" on the drain line (sample line)
Save caps in empty sterile sample bag package
Position bag below the level of the drain line
After draining for 2 minutes, open clamps
When the sample bag is full, close both clamps
Disconnect sample bag and recap sample line (or cover with sterile gauze)

Chronic ambulatory PD

Perform CAPD (twin bag) according to protocol
Clean injection port of drain bag with chlorhexidine or alcohol swab for 1 minute and let it dry
Withdraw 60 mL effluent from drain bag using needle and syringe

Sample processing

Blood culture bottle(s) are preferred for bacterial culture of PD effluent
Transfer sample from sample bag or sterile vial into culture bottle, as follows:

- Pour 10 mL of specimen into a second vial for cell count and Gram stain
- Specimens for culture:
  - Transfer 5–10 mL sample into one each of aerobic and nonaerobic blood culture bottle or rapid blood-culture bottle kits (e.g., BACTEC)
  - Alternatively, centrifuge 50 mL of PD effluent at 3,000 g for 15 min, resuspend the sediment in 3–5 mL supernatant, and inoculate it on solid culture or standard blood-culture media

Ensure that sample arrives in microbiology laboratory within 6 hr
In case of delay, incubate inoculated culture bottles at 37°C (do not refrigerate)

Culture conditions and media

Incubate under aerobic, microaerophilic and anaerobic environments
Use appropriate fungal media; incubate under two temperatures (room temperature and 35–37°C)

CAPD: continuous ambulatory peritoneal dialysis; PD: peritoneal dialysis

antibiotic prophylaxis after "wet contamination", i.e., contamination with an open system, for example, leaks from dialysate bags, leaks or breaks in tubing proximal to the tubing clamp, and breach of aseptic technique or touch contamination of the connection during a PD exchange. Following collection of PD effluent for cell count and culture **(Box 28.3)**, a single dose of intraperitoneal cefazolin is administered intraperitoneally. Prophylaxis is not required for "dry contamination", i.e., contamination outside a closed PD system, such as disconnection distal to a closed clamp.

Other modifiable risk factors for peritonitis are avoidance of hypokalemia, restricted use of histamine type-2 receptor antagonists, and adequate management of constipation. To prevent fungal peritonitis, the ISPD suggests prescribing antifungal prophylaxis whenever PD patients receive an antibiotic course, regardless of its indication.

Flowchart 28.2: Management of patients presenting with clinical features of peritoneal dialysis (PD) peritonitis. [1]Intraperitoneal (IP) route is preferred, unless the patient has features of systemic sepsis, and/or the required antibiotics are not compatible with or stable in peritoneal fluid. APD: automated peritoneal dialysis; CAPD: continuous ambulatory peritoneal dialysis; IP: intraperitoneal; PD: peritoneal dialysis

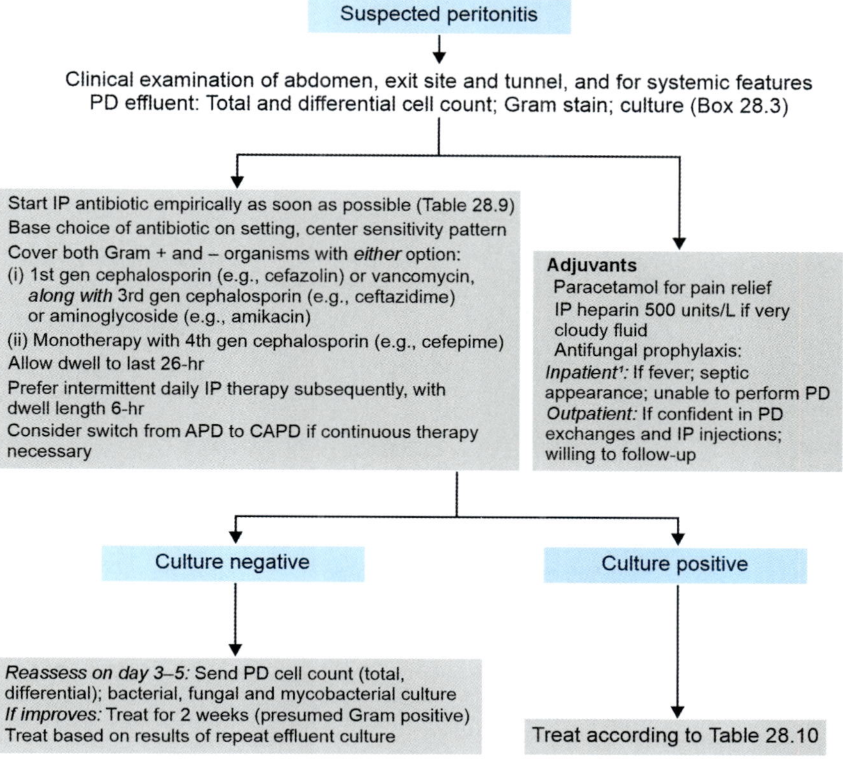

TABLE 28.9: Dosage of intraperitoneal antibiotics for treatment of peritonitis

	Continuous therapy (all exchanges)[1]		*Intermittent therapy*[1]
	Loading dose	***Maintenance dose***	***One exchange daily, for ≥6 hr***
Aminoglycosides[2]			
Amikacin	Not advised	Not advised	2 mg/kg q 24 h
Gentamicin	Not advised	Not advised	0.6 mg/kg q 24 h
Netilmicin	Not advised	Not advised	0.6 mg/kg q 24 h
Tobramycin	Not advised	Not advised	0.6 mg/kg q 24 h
Cephalosporins[3]			
Cefazolin	500 mg/L	125 mg/L	15 mg/kg q 24 h (long dwell) 20 mg/kg q 24 h (short dwell)
Cefepime	500 mg/L	125 mg/L	1 g (~15 mg/kg) q 24 h
Cefoperazone	500 mg/L	62.5–125 mg/L	No data
Cefotaxime	No data	No data	500–1,000 mg (~30 mg/kg) q 24 h
Ceftazidime	500 mg/L	125 mg/L	1–1.5g (long dwell) 20 mg/kg q 24 h (short dwell)
Ceftriaxone	No data	No data	1 g q 24 h
Glycopeptides[3]			
Vancomycin	20–25 mg/kg	25 mg/L	15–30 mg/kg q 5–7 days (CAPD) 15 mg/kg q 4 days (APD)
Teicoplanin	400 mg/bag	20 mg/L	15 mg/kg q 5 days
Penicillins[2]			
Penicillin G	50,000 U/L	25,000 U/L	No data
Amoxicillin	No data	150 mg/L	No data
Ampicillin[4]	No data	125 mg/L	4 g q 24 h
Ampicillin/ sulbactam[4]	1 g/500 mg	133.3 mg/66.7 mg	4 g q 24 h
Piperacillin/ tazobactam	4 g/500 mg	1 g/125 mg	No data
Ticarcillin/ clavulanic acid	3 g/200 mg	300 mg/20 mg/L	No data

Contd...

Contd...

	Continuous therapy (all exchanges)[1]		*Intermittent therapy*[1]
	Loading dose	*Maintenance dose*	*One exchange daily, for ≥6 hr*
Other antibiotics			
Aztreonam Meropenem	500 mg/L No data	250 mg/L 125 mg/L	2 g q 24 h 500 mg q 24 h (long dwell in APD) 1 g q 24 h (short dwell in CAPD)
Ciprofloxacin	No data	50 mg/L	No data
Ofloxacin	200 mg	25 mg/L	No data
Clindamycin	No data	600 mg/bag	No data
Imipenem/ cilastatin	250 mg/L	50 mg/L	500 mg in alternate exchanges
Daptomycin	100 mg/L	20 mg/L	300 mg q 24 h
Fosfomycin	No data	No data	4 g q 24 h
Polymyxin B	No data	300,000 U (30 mg)/bag	No data
Quinupristin/ dalfopristin[5]	No data	No data	25 mg/L in alternate exchanges
Antifungals[6]			
Fluconazole	No data	No data	150–200 mg q 1-2 days
Voriconazole	No data	No data	2.5 mg/kg q 24 h

[1]Daily intermittent therapy is preferred to continuous therapy. Intermittent therapy includes one dose given once daily in the long dwell, unless otherwise specified. In continuous therapy, the exchange with the loading dose should dwell for 3–6 hr; all subsequent exchanges should contain the maintenance dose

[2]Aminoglycosides should not be added to the same exchange as penicillin. Prolonged daily therapy with aminoglycosides should be avoided. Adjunctive oral N-acetylcysteine therapy might prevent aminoglycoside associated ototoxicity

[3]Vancomycin and ceftazidime are compatible within a dialysis solution, but incompatible when mixed in the same syringe. Patients with residual kidney function require drug level monitoring to guide dosing

[4]Not recommended for treatment of enterococcal peritonitis

[5]Given in conjunction with 500 mg intravenous twice daily

[6]Oral therapy is preferred to intraperitoneal (IP) dosing

Source: Li et al, 2022

The diagnosis of peritonitis is considered when the patient presents with cloudy peritoneal effluent, with or without fever and abdominal pain **(Table 28.8)**. **Box 28.3** shows the method for collection of effluent to investigate for peritonitis. Peritoneal effluent leukocyte count greater than 100 cells/mm^3 with at least 50% being neutrophils is presumed to indicate the diagnosis,

TABLE 28.10: Organism-specific management of peritonitis based on results of culture and sensitivity pattern

Organism	*Actions—Choice of intraperitoneal (IP) antibiotic*	*Therapy duration, if improved by day 5*[1]
Staphylococcus aureus	Discontinue gram-negative cover *If methicillin resistant Staphylococcus aureus (MRSA):* Switch to vancomycin	21 days
Streptococcus sp.	Discontinue gram-negative cover *If allergic or refractory to cefazolin:* Switch to vancomycin	14 days
Other gram-positive	Discontinue gram-negative cover *If coagulase-negative Staphylococcus (CONS):* Consider retraining for peritoneal dialysis (PD) technique *If CONS and biofilm:* Consider IP urokinase; simultaneous removal and replacement of catheter *If Corynebacterium jeikeium:* Switch to vancomycin	14 days
Enterococcus sp.	*Ampicillin sensitive:* Treat with oral amoxicillin[2] *Ampicillin resistant:* Treat with IP vancomycin *Vancomycin resistant:* Treat with IP daptomycin or oral/intravenous (IV) linezolid[3] *Polymicrobial:* Consider additional antibiotics; early catheter removal	21 days
Pseudomonas sp.	*Treat with two antibiotics with different mechanisms of action to which the organism is sensitive:* IP ceftazidime or cefepime and IP aminoglycoside or oral ciprofloxacin *If concomitant exit-site and tunnel infection:* Remove catheter	21 days
Acinetobacter sp.	Treat with IP aminoglycoside and a sulbactam-containing agent (beta-lactam/beta-lactamase inhibitor combination; including sulbactam); other options include oral ciprofloxacin; oral trimethoprim–sulfamethoxazole; IP meropenem (or other carbapenem, except ertapenem) *If carbapenem-resistant Acinetobacter baumannii (CRAB):* Treat with IP aminoglycoside or IP colistin with/without ampicillin/sulbactam	21 days

Contd...

Contd...

Organism	***Actions—Choice of intraperitoneal (IP) antibiotic***	***Therapy duration, if improved by day 5[1]***
Stenotrophomonas maltophilia	Treat with two different classes of antibiotics, including oral trimethoprim–sulfamethoxazole	21 days
Enteric gram-negative bacteria	*Resistance not specified:* IP ceftazidime or IP cefepime or oral ciprofloxacin *Extended spectrum beta lactamase (ESBL) producing:* IP meropenem; if susceptible, oral ciprofloxacin *AmpC beta-lactamase producing[4]:* IP cefepime, IP meropenem or oral ciprofloxacin *Carbapenemase producing Enterobacterales (CPE):* Based on expert advice	21 days
Polymicrobial[5]	*Surgical peritonitis (mixed Gram positive and negative):* Consider oral metronidazole with IP vancomycin and IP ceftazidime or IP aminoglycoside; or monotherapy with IP carbapenem or piperacillin/tazobactam Consider CT abdomen, laparotomy, and catheter removal *Gram positive:* Consider touch contamination; treat by sensitivity; consider PD catheter removal if infected	21 days
Fungal peritonitis	Immediate catheter removal Treat with an appropriate antifungal agent	≥14 days after catheter removal

[1]Reassessment is done clinically and based on total and differential PD effluent cell count. In refractory cases, catheter is removed and treatment is continued for 14 days
[2]Not preferred in polymicrobial enterococcal peritonitis and not recommended for *Enterococcus faecium*
[3]Intraperitoneal (IP) teicoplanin is an option if sensitivity is confirmed
[4]Include *Serratia*, *Providencia*, indole-positive *Proteus*, *Citrobacter freundii* and *Enterobacter* species
[5]Often present with hypotension, sepsis, lactic acidosis or elevated dialysis effluent amylase level; usually indicate intra-abdominal pathology
AmpC chromosomally coded ampicillin hydrolyzing molecular class c beta-lactamase

and should be treated with antibiotics, until antibiotic sensitivity patterns are available. **Flowchart 28.2** provides an approach to management of peritonitis.

Current guidelines for empiric treatment include intraperitoneal administration of either cefepime monotherapy, or the combination of cefazolin and ceftazidime, or an aminoglycoside **(Flowchart 28.2)**. In centers

BOX 28.4: Indications for catheter removal

After exit-site or tunnel infection
Lack of clinical improvement in 2 weeks
Incomplete resolution of infection after 4 weeks
Concomitant peritonitis due to the same organism (especially *Staphylococcus aureus* and *Pseudomonas aeruginosa*)

After peritonitis
Absolute
Refractory bacterial peritonitis
Fungal peritonitis
Concomitant exit-site or tunnel infection[1]

Relative
Recurrent, repeat or relapsing peritonitis
Repeatedly relapsing or refractory exit-site or tunnel infections (including *P. aeruginosa*)
Infection with *Mycobacterium spp.*
Peritonitis by multiple enteric organisms (e.g., intra-abdominal abscess or surgical peritonitis)

[1]Consider simultaneous catheter removal and replacement, except if there is involvement of the deep Dacron cuff with concurrent peritonitis

where rates of MRSA exceed 10%, addition of an intraperitoneal glycopeptide (vancomycin and teicoplanin) to cefepime or ceftazidime is recommended. **Table 28.9** provides doses of intraperitoneal antibiotics for management of peritonitis. **Table 28.10** details guidance on management of peritonitis based on the organisms cultured. **Box 28.4** lists the indications for removal of PD catheter, which is usually in the context of infections.

Eosinophilic peritonitis is relatively common in young children and infants, but is poorly understood and therefore, underdiagnosed. The etiology is unclear but is believed to result from hypersensitivity of the peritoneum to component of the dialysis system (tubing, dialysate bags and dialysate, and air in the peritoneum) or intraperitoneal medications. Most patients are asymptomatic with cloudy dialysate. Diagnosis is made when a cloudy dialysate has >100 leukocytes per mm^3 with eosinophils >10%, negative cultures, with or without peripheral eosinophilia. In most cases, the condition resolves after removal of the inciting agent(s). Other agents used are intraperitoneal heparin or hydrocortisone, oral ketotifen or diphenhydramine, and low-dose prednisolone.

BIBLIOGRAPHY

1. Abdijalil G, Shuijuan S. Laparoscopic versus open-surgery catheter placement in peritoneal dialysis patients: A meta-analysis of outcomes. Indian J Nephrol. 2022;32:8-15.

2. Auguste BL, Bargman JM. Peritoneal dialysis prescription and adequacy in clinical practice: Core curriculum 2023. Am J Kidney Dis. 2023;81:100-09.
3. Bello AK, Okpechi IG, Osman MA, et al. Epidemiology of peritoneal dialysis outcomes. Nat Rev Nephrol. 2022;18:779-93.
4. Briggs VR, Jacques RM, Fotheringham J, et al. Catheter insertion techniques for improving catheter function and clinical outcomes in peritoneal dialysis patients. Cochrane Database Syst Rev. 2023;2:CD012478.
5. Butani L, Haddad M, Joseph M. Tidal continuous cycling peritoneal dialysis in children. Pediatr Nephrol. 2023;38:3955-61.
6. Chow KM, Li PK, Cho Y, et al. ISPD Catheter-related Infection Recommendations: 2023 Update. Perit Dial Int. 2023;43:201-19.
7. Fischbach M, Warady BA. Peritoneal dialysis prescription in children: Bedside principles for optimal practice. Pediatr Nephrol. 2009;24:1633-42.
8. Hagen SM, Lafranca JA, Ijzermans JN, et al. A systematic review and meta-analysis of the influence of peritoneal dialysis catheter type on complication rate and catheter survival. Kidney Int. 2014;85:920-32.
9. Haggerty SP, Kumar SS, Collings AT, et al. SAGES peritoneal dialysis access guideline update 2023. Surg Endosc. 2024;38(1):1-23.
10. Hataya H. Current state of peritoneal dialysis in children. Contrib Nephrol. 2018;196:129-34.
11. Hsueh L, Hu SL, Shah AD. Periprocedural peritonitis prophylaxis: A summary of the microbiology and the role of systemic antimicrobials. Kidney Dis (Basel). 2021;7:90-9.
12. Kim JK, Lolas M, Keefe DT, et al. Omental procedures during peritoneal dialysis insertion: A systematic review and meta-analysis. World J Surg. 2022;46:1183-95.
13. Li PK, Chow KM, Cho Y, et al. ISPD peritonitis guideline recommendations: 2022 update on prevention and treatment. Perit Dial Int. 2022;42:110-53.
14. Manera KE, Johnson DW, Craig JC, et al; SONG-PD Workshop Investigators. Establishing a Core Outcome Set for Peritoneal Dialysis: Report of the SONG-PD (Standardized Outcomes in Nephrology-Peritoneal Dialysis) Consensus Workshop. Am J Kidney Dis. 2020;75:404-12.
15. Marie E, Navallas M, Harvey E, et al. Imaging of peritoneal dialysis complications in children. Radiographics. 2022;42:559-78.
16. Morelle J, Sow A, Fustin CA, et al. Mechanisms of crystalloid versus colloid osmosis across the peritoneal membrane. J Am Soc Nephrol. 2018;29:1875-86.
17. Ng JK, Chan GC, Li PK. Icodextrin in peritoneal dialysis: Implications on clinical practice and survival outcome. Kidney360. 2022;3:793-5.
18. Niang A, Iyengar A, Luyckx VA. Hemodialysis versus peritoneal dialysis in resource-limited settings. Curr Opin Nephrol Hypertens. 2018;27:463-71.
19. Rees L, Shaw V, Qizalbash L, et al; Pediatric Renal Nutrition Taskforce. Delivery of a nutritional prescription by enteral tube feeding in children with chronic kidney disease stages 2–5 and on dialysis-clinical practice recommendations from the Pediatric Renal Nutrition Taskforce. Pediatr Nephrol. 2021;36:187-204.
20. Shaw V, Polderman N, Renken-Terhaerdt J, et al. Energy and protein requirements for children with CKD stages 2–5 and on dialysis-clinical practice recommendations from the Pediatric Renal Nutrition Taskforce. Pediatr Nephrol. 2020;35:519-31.

21. Shen JI, Cho Y, Manera KE, et al; SONG-PD Infection Workshop Investigators. Establishing a core outcome measure for peritoneal dialysis-related peritonitis: A Standardized Outcomes in Nephrology-Peritoneal Dialysis Consensus Workshop Report. Kidney Int Rep. 2022;7:1737-44.
22. Teitelbaum I, Glickman J, Neu A, et al. KDOQI US Commentary on the 2020 ISPD Practice Recommendations for prescribing high-quality goal-directed peritoneal dialysis. Am J Kidney Dis. 2021;77:157-71.
23. Teitelbaum I. Peritoneal dialysis. N Engl J Med. 2021;385:1786-95.
24. Wan M, King L, Baugh N, et al. Gutted: Constipation in children with chronic kidney disease and on dialysis. Pediatr Nephrol. 2023;38:3581-96.
25. Warady BA, Schaefer F, Bagga A, et al. Prescribing peritoneal dialysis for high-quality care in children. Perit Dial Int. 2020;40:333-40.

CHAPTER

29

Renal Transplantation

Asha Moudgil, Stanley C Jordan, Arvind Bagga

INTRODUCTION

Kidney transplantation is the treatment of choice in most children with end-stage kidney failure (ESKF). Chronic kidney disease (CKD) causes several metabolic derangements that lead to undernutrition, growth retardation, anemia, mineral bone disease, and neurodevelopmental and pubertal delay. These abnormalities are particularly marked in infants and young children and increase with duration and severity of CKD. When estimated glomerular filtration rate (GFR) falls below 10–15 mL/min/1.73 m^2, kidney replacement therapy is required to sustain life. Kidney replacement therapy includes chronic dialysis (hemodialysis or peritoneal dialysis), or transplantation. Chronic dialysis is life sustaining but is inferior to transplantation and should be considered a bridge to transplantation in children. Kidney transplantation offers survival advantage, decreased hospitalization rate, and improved quality-of-life compared to chronic dialysis. However, it is still an imperfect therapy burdened by ongoing CKD, limited long-term graft survival (approximately 10–15 years), dependence on and side effects of immunosuppressive medications, and increased risk for infections and malignancy due to chronic suppression of the immune system.

Until a few decades ago, the success of transplantation was limited in the pediatric age group, particularly in infants and young children, because of technical difficulties, high incidence of vascular thrombosis, and allograft rejection. Advances in surgical and urologic techniques have made it possible to transplant young children once they attain a weight of about 10 kg. Availability of potent immunosuppressive medications and ability to use them effectively in children, and the ability to monitor, prevent, and treat bacterial, fungal, and viral infections has improved transplant outcomes. Infants and young children have better long-term graft survival compared with adolescents and young adults.

Preemptive transplantation offers better long-term allograft survival, and psychological and financial benefits compared with transplant performed after a period of dialysis. Additionally, preemptive transplantation may offer advantages in developing countries where providing chronic dialysis therapy could be expensive and challenging. In children with ESKF, attempts should be made to perform preemptive transplantation if a suitable donor is available.

INDICATIONS AND CONTRAINDICATIONS

Children are excellent candidates for kidney transplantation due to lack of significant comorbidities. Contraindications to kidney transplant include presence of acute infection, untreated malignancy, child with multiple comorbidities that include advance organ disease other than kidney, and progressive neurological illness. While human immunodeficiency virus (HIV) infection was considered an absolute contraindication to transplantation, selected patients have undergone successful transplantation. Patients with treated malignancies should wait for 2–5 years, depending upon the nature of malignancy, before they are considered for transplantation. Children with primary hyperoxaluria, methylmalonic aciduria, autosomal recessive polycystic kidney disease or nephronophthisis (with significant hepatic fibrosis and portal hypertension), and some children with atypical hemolytic uremic syndrome (aHUS) benefit from combined liver and kidney transplant. Chronic infection with hepatitis C infection is not an absolute contraindication, but these children need careful evaluation of liver histology and may benefit from treatment with sofosbuvir before and following kidney transplantation. In the presence of advanced liver disease, combined liver and kidney transplant may be performed.

Nonadherence to therapy and inadequate family support system is an important barrier to successful transplantation, particularly in adolescents. Children with multiple congenital anomalies and severe mental retardation pose an ethical dilemma. A multidisciplinary team should evaluate the option of transplantation in these children with input from ethicists and from parents. In developing countries, socioeconomic factors should be carefully considered before committing infants and children to transplantation, in light of financial constraints of life-long immunosuppressive medications and other follow-up care.

IMMUNOLOGY OF TRANSPLANTATION

There are several immunologic barriers to successful transplantation. These include incompatibility of blood group and major histocompatibility [human leukocyte antigen (HLA)] antigens and presence of anti-HLA antibodies, antibodies to minor HLA antigens [major histocompatibility complex (MHC) class I polypeptide-related sequence A and B—MICA and MICB], and antiendothelial, antiangiotensin receptor, and antivimentin antibodies. Among these, anti-HLA antibodies are most important.

Blood Group

ABO compatibility between donor and recipient was once considered a prerequisite for successful transplantation. ABO blood group antigens are expressed on the endothelial cells and are targets for naturally occurring hemagglutinin antibodies. These antibodies bind to the blood group antigens expressed on the endothelium, activate the complement system, and attract neutrophils and platelets resulting in thrombosis and irreversible graft loss. The same rules that govern blood transfusion apply to solid organ transplantation. Subjects with O blood group are universal donors and those with AB blood group are universal recipients.

Transplants may be performed across blood group barriers, after immunoadsorption or plasmapheresis, infusion of intravenous immunoglobulin (IVIG), and/or treatment with anti-CD20 monoclonal antibody rituximab. While data in children is limited, long-term outcomes of ABO incompatible transplantation (ABO-iKT) are highly satisfactory in adult patients. Patients receiving ABO-incompatible transplant are at risk of increased immunosuppression.

Rh matching is generally not a requirement for successful transplantation. Occasionally, antibodies to minor blood group antigens (anti-JKa antibodies) have been thought to play a role in acute rejection (AR). Screening for these antibodies is not routine practice.

Human Leukocyte Antigens

Genetic difference between individuals is recognized by differences in the composition of major histocompatibility complex antigens, also known as HLA antigens, expressed on the surface of all nucleated cells. The genes encoding these antigens are present on short arm of chromosome 6. Based on their structural differences, HLA antigens are divided into class I (A, B, and C), and class II (DR, DQ, and DP). HLA class I antigens are present on all nucleated cells; red blood cells lack HLA antigens. HLA class II antigens are present on antigen-presenting cells (APCs), including macrophages, dendritic, endothelial, and B-cells. T lymphocytes, tubular epithelial, and endothelial cells increase expression of class II molecules on stimulation with cytokines, such as interferon gamma (IFN-γ).

Histocompatibility genes are extremely polymorphic and are expressed as codominant alleles. Each individual inherits one haplotype from each parent. Siblings can be complete HLA matched, one haplotype matched or completely mismatched, depending upon the recombination of their haplotypes. The great degree of polymorphism makes complete HLA matching between two random individuals a rare event. The term *HLA mismatches* is used to define the number of nonshared HLA antigens between the donor and recipient. This may differ from number of HLA matches because of inability to characterize some HLA antigens or because of inheritance of two copies of same HLA allele. *HLA mismatches determine the strength of immunologic reaction in the recipient.* While the extent of HLA mismatching has an impact on long-term allograft survival, availability of potent immunosuppressive therapy has attenuated the effect of HLA mismatching on short-term allograft survival. Recently, DQ and DP antigens mismatches between donor and recipients have been identified to play an important role in the development of *de novo* donor-specific antibodies after transplant.

Anti-HLA Antibodies

Anti-HLA antibodies directed against foreign HLA antigens can be present in the recipient serum at the time of transplantation. Due to the extreme polymorphic nature of HLA molecules amongst individuals, exposure to the blood or tissues of another person can elicit these anti-HLA antibodies. Kidney transplant recipients can, therefore, develop anti-HLA antibodies following sensitization events that include blood transfusions, previous transplants, pregnancies, and rarely infections. Anti-HLA antibodies can bind to HLA antigens expressed on the allograft endothelium, and cause hyper-AR of the allograft resulting in immediate graft loss. These antibodies are particularly deleterious if they are directed at HLA class I antigens and are complement binding.

Testing for anti-HLA antibodies includes testing recipient's serum against a panel of donor HLA antigens, in a test termed panel reactive antibody (PRA). Testing for PRA can be performed by lymphocytotoxicity assay, ELISA, or flow cytometry in the increasing order of sensitivity for detection of anti-HLA antibodies. The antibodies to specific HLA antigens can be characterized by flow cytometry or Luminex technology using single antigen beads. In recipients with anti-HLA antibodies directed at specific HLA antigens, transplant from donors with these HLA antigens should be avoided. PRA testing also provides an idea of the robustness of immune response.

Highly sensitized individuals are likely to experience AR episodes even when unacceptable antigens are avoided. It is extremely difficult to find compatible organs for highly sensitized patients. In recent years, these individuals have been successfully transplanted by using desensitization protocols using IVIG, rituximab, and plasmapheresis.

Transplant centers need to develop an infrastructure of an advanced HLA laboratory, plasmapheresis unit, and kidney histopathology services before considering ABO or HLA incompatible transplantation. Living donor exchange programs between incompatible donor-recipient pairs are becoming popular for transplant recipients with positive cross match against their respective donors. These exchange programs can help find either cross match negative donors or the donors against which these recipients are less sensitized. This strategy allows to transplant these highly sensitized patients without desensitization if flow cross match is negative and recipient has no donor-specific antibodies (DSAs) or with less intense desensitization.

Biology of Allograft Rejection

The physical process of reimplanting and reperfusion of organs for transplantation initiates injury and stress responses. Cells of recipient innate immune system can recognize these markers of tissue injury resulting in upregulation of the genes involved in inflammatory responses. There is increased production of the proinflammatory cytokines including interleukin (IL)-1, IL-6, and tumor necrosis factor (TNF), type I IFN, chemokines, and adhesion molecules by endothelial cells that trigger the release of antigens from the graft. These donor antigens are taken up by APCs (macrophages, dendritic cells, and B lymphocytes) of either donor (direct pathway) or recipient origin (indirect pathway). APCs process donor antigens into small peptides that are presented on their cell surface in association with either HLA class I or II molecules. These allopeptides are presented to the recipient T lymphocytes, which are primarily responsible for orchestrating allograft rejection. CD4+ T lymphocytes recognize HLA class II-associated allopeptides, while CD8+ T lymphocytes recognize HLA class I-associated allopeptides. Direct pathway of antigen presentation plays an important role early after transplantation whereas indirect pathways play a more prominent role later.

The immune response to allopeptides occurs in a sequence of three signals **(Fig. 29.1)**. Signal I is the interaction between APCs presenting allopeptides and T cell receptor of CD4+ cells (signal 1 or antigenic signal). Signal II is the costimulatory signal provided by several molecules. Costimulatory molecules belong to two families—the B7 family, characterized by the T-cell costimulatory molecules CD28 and CD152 (CTLA-4) that interacts with CD80 and CD86 on APCs, and the TNF/TNF receptor (TNFR) family, of which the prototype receptor-ligand pair are CD40 and CD154 (CD40L). When the lymphocytes receive both antigenic and costimulatory signals, there is an activation of several enzymes followed by increase in cytosolic calcium. Calcium binds to calcineurin that activates nuclear factor activating transcription (NFAT), which is translocated to the nucleus and promotes synthesis of cytokines such as IL-2 and IFN-γ. IL-2 stimulates T lymphocytes through the IL-2 receptor (signal III), which stimulate a series of enzymatic reactions that eventually drive the cell cycle division resulting in clonal expansion and differentiation of graft reactive CD4+ lymphocytes. Prior to the cell division, T cells have *de novo* synthesis of purine and pyrimidine nucleotides. If T lymphocytes receive only signal I but not signal II, they undergo apoptotic cell death.

Stimulated CD4+ T lymphocytes also provide help to CD8+ cells or cytotoxic T cells. CD8+ T cells cause death of the allograft cells through secreted granzyme, perforins, and Fas/FasL cytolytic pathways. IL-2 enhances synthesis of other cytokine genes such as IL-3, IL-4, IL-5, IL-6, IL-9,

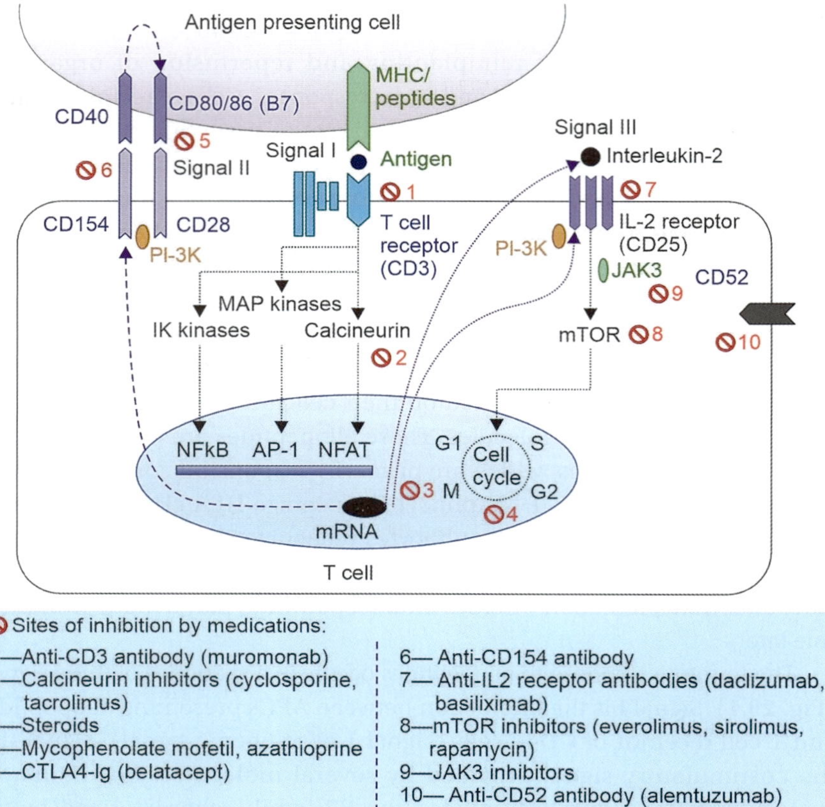

Fig. 29.1: Three-signal model of T-cell activation, and the mechanisms of action of various immunosuppressive drugs. Signal 1 involves the antigen-presenting cell (macrophage and dendritic cell) presenting the foreign antigen to the T lymphocyte, thereby activating the T-cell receptor, which relays signals through the CD3 complex, a transduction apparatus. Signal 2 is a nonantigen-specific costimulatory signal that involves the binding of the B7 molecule on the antigen presenting cell to CD28 on the T cell. The two signals 1 and 2 activate signal transduction pathways, namely the calcium–calcineurin pathway, mitogen-activated protein (MAP) kinases, and the nuclear factor-κB (NF-κB) pathway. These in turn lead to increased mRNA expression of interleukin-2 (IL-2), which binds to its receptor (IL-2R) (signal 3) to activate the cell cycle. Signal 3 activation requires the enzyme mammalian target of rapamycin (mTOR) for cell proliferation. Various drugs act on different cellular signals and achieve immunosuppression by several mechanisms, indicated in stop sign and numerical code, detailed in the inset

IL-17, and TNF-α. IL-3, IL-4, IL-5, and IL-6 stimulate B cells to form DSAs that bind complement resulting in acute and chronic antibody-mediated rejection. IL-9 stimulates mast cells and IL-17 stimulates neutrophils. In addition, these cytokines also facilitate activation of macrophages and other inflammatory cells including platelets, which add an inflammatory and destructive component to the antigen-specific destruction. Allografts-containing disparate HLA antigens generate a stronger signal I and are likely to experience rejection as compared to those more closely related to the recipient HLA.

IMMUNOSUPPRESSIVE THERAPY

The objective of immunosuppressive therapy is to prevent allograft rejection while avoiding excessive immunosuppression that can result in increased risk of infections and malignancy. Unfortunately, there are no validated markers for adequacy of immunosuppression. Immunosuppressive therapy is intense at the onset, because of the high risk of AR in the first weeks and months post-transplantation. Immunosuppressive drugs are divided into biologic and pharmacologic agents. Biologic agents are primarily targeted at cell surface molecules and include polyclonal and monoclonal antibodies. Polyclonal antibodies include antithymocyte globulin raised in horse (ATG) and rabbit (thymoglobulin). Thymoglobulin is preferred over ATG due to its increased potency. Monoclonal antibodies include anti-IL-2R antibody (basiliximab), anti CD52 antibody (alemtuzumab, also known as Campath-1H). Belatacept, is a costimulatory blocking fusion protein, composed of the F_c fragment of human IgG1 linked to the extracellular domain of CTLA4-Ig. Pharmacologic agents include cyclosporine (CsA), tacrolimus, mycophenolate mofetil (MMF), azathioprine, sirolimus (rapamycin), and corticosteroids (prednisone, prednisolone, and methylprednisolone).

Of the current medications, thymoglobulin, alemtuzumab, and basiliximab are used for induction. Induction therapy is used in high-risk patients (highly sensitized, retransplants, and patients with delayed graft function), and in steroid withdrawal protocols. Since infants and young children mount relatively strong immune reactors and have faster clearance of immunosuppressive drugs, they benefit from induction therapies. Most centers use basiliximab for induction in standard-risk children because of ease of administration and low side effects profile. Induction with thymoglobulin or alemtuzumab is reserved for high-risk transplant recipients and in steroid withdrawal protocols. In the US, most children get thymoglobulin for induction regardless of risk status of these children indicating practice pattern rather than risk-based strategy.

Belatacept is approved for use in Epstein-Barr virus (EBV) + adults by the United States Food and Drug Administration (US FDA). It has potential benefits due to lack of nephrotoxicity or neurotoxicity and might replace chronic calcineurin inhibitor (CNI) therapy. The medication should not be used in EBV naïve individuals, as they might be at higher risk for the post-transplant lymphoproliferative disorder (PTLD). Studies with belatacept and thymoglobulin induction show promise for development of CNI-free and steroid-free protocols. Major concerns with belatacept use include higher risk of early rejection in the CNI-free environment, and increased risk of infections, including CMV, EBV, and polyoma BK nephropathy.

Cyclosporine (CsA), tacrolimus, prednisone, azathioprine, MMF, and sirolimus are used for maintenance immunosuppression. Most centers use a combination of CNI (CsA and tacrolimus), antiproliferative agents (azathioprine, MMF, or sirolimus), and prednisone. Steroid avoidance or withdrawal protocols are being used often, and are associated with improved growth, less weight gain, and decreased incidence of posttransplant hyperlipidemia, diabetes mellitus, and hypertension. Many children on steroid withdrawal protocols develop leukopenia often necessitating either the adjustment of concomitant medications (valganciclovir and sulfamethoxazole-trimethoprim) or use of GCSF. An increased incidence of AR and allograft fibrosis has been noted in some adult studies. Long-term graft survival data using steroid-free protocols is limited.

Immunologic markers for adequate immunosuppression are lacking. Monitoring of mRNA transcripts of genes for granzyme B and perforin (found in activated cytotoxic T lymphocytes), and the T-cell regulatory protein FOXP3 and mRNA levels of CXCL10, the gene that encodes IFN-γ inducible protein 10 (IP10), associated with acute cellular rejection, has become commercially available. Sensitivity of these tests ranges from 88 to 100%, and specificity from 75 to 95%. In the last few years, routine post-transplant monitoring by measuring cell-free DNA in the peripheral blood for an early diagnosis of AR has become highly prevalent in adults. The data in children is emerging. In most clinical settings, the adequacy of immunosuppression is based on clinical monitoring for signs of AR and infections.

Mechanism of Action of Immunosuppressive Drugs

The targets for immunosuppressive drugs are shown in **Figure 29.1**. Polyclonal antibodies (thymoglobulin) have antibodies against several T-cell surface antigens and cause extensive T-cell depletion. Anti-IL-2R antibodies bind to the α-chain of IL-2 receptor (CD25), making it unavailable for IL-2 binding and subsequent cell division, thus blocking signal III. Alemtuzumab targets CD52 present on the surface of mature T and B lymphocytes. Belatacept blocks costimulation or signal II by binding to CTLA-4 with high affinity.

Corticosteroids act primarily on APC and inhibit their ability to produce IL-1 and other cytokines. Many cytokine genes, including IL-2, have a glucocorticoid response element in the 5' regulatory region that serves as a target for corticosteroid and intracellular glucocorticoid receptor complex. Binding of this complex with the glucocorticoid response element blocks transcription of cytokines. High-dose methylprednisolone causes lympholysis; hence, it is used for treatment of AR. CsA and tacrolimus bind to cyclophilin and tacrolimus-binding proteins (FKBP-13), respectively, and inhibit the activity of the enzyme, calcineurin. This prevents the translocation of NFAT to the nucleus, thus blocking production of IL-2 and other cytokines. Azathioprine and MMF inhibit purine synthesis required for cell division. Sirolimus (rapamycin) acts on target of rapamycin (TOR), thus blocking the ability of cells to enter the cell cycle.

Each transplant center should develop detailed treatment protocols based on local experience, strategies for tapering immunosuppression, and treatment of AR. Physicians taking care of transplant recipients should familiarize themselves with the action of various drugs including drug interactions **(Table 29.1)**, dosages, and side effects. Center-specific strategies for monitoring, prevention, and treatment of infections should be defined and made available. When immunosuppression is augmented, particular attention is paid to anti-infective measures.

PRETRANSPLANT EVALUATION OF THE RECIPIENT

Pretransplant evaluation is aimed to ensure and enhance patient's suitability as a transplant candidate.

Cause of End-stage Kidney Failure

The cause for ESKF should be determined if possible. The potential for recurrence of some conditions, such as focal segmental glomerulosclerosis (FSGS), aHUS, C3 glomerulopathy, primary hyperoxaluria, and lupus nephritis, is considered and strategies developed to monitor for recurrence and treatment. The primary diagnosis also has implications for donor selection, e.g., mothers with the same change in *COL4A5* should not donate to their sons with X-linked Alport syndrome, since they are themselves at risk of CKD.

Screening for Infections

Recipients should be screened for HIV, hepatitis B and C, *Cytomegalovirus* (CMV), EBV, varicella, and tuberculosis. Children should receive all age-appropriate immunizations including hepatitis A and B, measles-rubella, varicella, pneumococcal, meningococcal, human papilloma virus (HPV) and severe acute respiratory syndrome coronavirus 2 (SARS-CoV2) vaccines early in the course of CKD, as response to vaccination is suboptimal in the advanced stages of CKD and after transplantation. Live viral vaccines are contraindicated after transplant. Annual vaccination against influenza is recommended.

Blood Group, HLA Typing, and anti-HLA Antibodies

The HLA typing is done by DNA technology. Anti-HLA antibodies are measured by flow cytometry and Luminex technology.

Cross Match

Each recipient is cross matched with the prospective living or deceased donor prior to transplantation. For cross matching, recipient's serum is tested against donor T and B cells to detect any preformed antibodies. Conventional cross matching is done by lymphocytotoxicity [complement-dependent cytotoxicity (CDC)] assay. Autoantibodies can give a false positive test on lymphocytotoxicity assay. Pretreatment of serum with dithiothreitol that breaks S-S bonds in IgM autoantibodies differentiates between auto- and alloantibodies. A strongly positive T-cell cross match after dithiothreitol treatment is a contraindication to transplantation. In recent years, the sensitivity of cross match has increased many-fold by antihuman globulin enhanced CDC, enzyme-linked immunosorbent assay (ELISA), and flow cytometry techniques. These tests are especially useful for retransplants and highly sensitized individuals.

Surgical and Urologic Evaluation

In children with congenital and urologic problems (responsible for 40% of ESKF), evaluation of the lower urinary tract is crucial. Evaluation by an experienced pediatric urologist is, therefore, desirable. Bladder and urethra should be evaluated by ultrasonography, micturating cystourethrography, and urodynamic studies, if indicated. Urinalysis and culture are necessary. Some children may require bladder augmentation or reconstruction prior to transplantation. Children with abnormal lower urinary tract may need creation of Mitrofanoff conduit for intermittent catheterization of bladder, or creation of ileal or colonic conduits for urine drainage. Persistently abnormal functioning of the bladder is responsible for transplant failure in majority of the patients with urogenital abnormalities.

Most bladder reconstruction procedures are done prior to transplantation. Some children might require nephrectomy(ies) for chronic infection of the kidneys, severe nephrotic syndrome, polycystic kidneys, intractable hypertension, or nephrolithiasis. Nephrectomies can be done earlier or at the time of transplantation. Patients with history of umbilical venous or femoral venous catheterizations and renal venous thrombosis would need imaging of inferior vena cava by magnetic resonance imaging (MRI) to identify any vascular abnormalities ahead of transplant surgery.

Evaluation for Hypercoagulability

Since renal vascular thrombosis is an important cause of immediate graft loss in children, they should be evaluated for appropriately, including anticardiolipin antibodies, levels of factor VIII and homocysteine, activity of protein S, C and anti-thrombin III, and for mutations in methyltetrahydrofolate reductase, prothrombin, and factor V Leiden genes. Additional tests including measurement of lipoprotein A and plasminogen activator inhibitor type-1 polymorphism, and antibodies to lupus anticoagulant and β-2 glycoprotein antibodies may be indicated in patients at high risk of thrombosis.

Nutrition and Gastrointestinal Evaluation

Growth and nutrition should be optimized, as malnutrition and obesity are risk factors for post-transplant complications. Infants and young children with CKD are at risk for growth failure and malnutrition due to excessive loss of fluids and electrolytes, poor appetite, metabolic acidosis, gastroesophageal reflux, and delayed gastric motility. These children may benefit from sodium chloride and water supplementation, correction of metabolic acidosis, supplemental feeding via nasogastric tubes, G-tube feeding, and Nissen fundoplication. Additionally, treatment with recombinant growth hormone may be needed to optimize growth.

Psychosocial Evaluation

The child and family's ability to comply with immunosuppression and complex medical therapy and to cope with chronic illness should be evaluated, as *nonadherence* is the single most important cause of graft failure, particularly in adolescents. In developing countries, advance financial planning and provision for long-term care should be made.

Other Evaluations

Cardiac, pulmonary, dental, and other evaluations may be needed depending upon comorbidities. Good dental care is an integral part of CKD management.

DONOR EVALUATION

Transplant donors can be either living related (parents or siblings older than 18 years), unrelated (a person with significant emotional bond with the child), altruistic, or deceased donors. An independent physician not familiar with the child's needs should evaluate living donors to ensure that they are medically suitable to donate a kidney. Donor work-up includes evaluation of medical history, physical examination, determination of blood group and HLA typing, measurement of liver, and kidney function tests including urinalysis and 24-hr urine protein estimation, screening for infections (HIV, hepatitis B and C, syphilis, tuberculosis, and other infections relevant to the geographic area), age-appropriate screening for malignancies, and evaluation of cardiac status. Once medically cleared, renal anatomy is defined by ultrasound. Renal vascular anatomy is determined by contrast angiography, spiral CT scan with contrast, or by MR angiography. Living donors should also undergo psychological testing to ensure their emotional suitability to be a donor, and ethical practices in donation. Living donor (related and unrelated) allografts have a longer half-life compared to those obtained from deceased donors. This is thought to be secondary to relatively healthy organs, and elimination of cold ischemia time that increases the risk for AR.

Desired requirements for a transplant are a compatible blood group, a negative cross match and absence of DSAs. While HLA matching is not a requirement, HLA identical grafts have a longer half-life compared to those that are less well matched. The practice of "transplant tourism" where patients go to other countries to purchase organs from unknown living donors has been condemned by the Transplant Societies in the Declaration of Istanbul, 2008.

TRANSPLANT PROCEDURE

A kidney from a living donor can be procured by open donor nephrectomy or by a laparoscopic procedure. Advantages of open donor nephrectomy include long-track record of safety, retroperitoneal approach with less potential for trauma to abdominal organs, minimal warm ischemia time, immediate graft function, and shorter operation time. Disadvantages include long surgical scar, occasionally persistent postoperative pain and abdominal wall hernia. Laparoscopic procedures have become almost universal due to increased expertise with the procedure and decrease in the need for analgesia, and shorter hospital stay and recovery time for the donors. Disadvantages include higher potential for delayed graft function, longer operative time, shorter renal vessels, and added expense of specialized instruments. Short-term graft outcomes are comparable.

In children who weigh > 20 kg, the allograft is placed in the iliac fossa; renal artery and vein are connected to the child's common or external iliac artery and vein respectively as end to side anastomosis. In infants and young children < 20 kg, the kidney is placed higher up in the abdomen in the retroperitoneum. Renal artery and vein of the allograft are connected to the side of the aorta and inferior vena cava close to the bifurcation **(Fig. 29.2)**. When a kidney is obtained from a deceased donor, the renal artery is removed along with aortic cuff to provide a larger surface area for anastomosis. A kidney with multiple renal vessels from a living donor is at a higher risk for arterial and venous thrombosis and should be avoided, particularly in infants and young children with lower systemic blood pressure. Meticulous attention is required for vascular anastomosis to limit allograft loss secondary to renal arterial and venous thrombosis. The ureter is anastomosed to the bladder using ureteroneocystostomy, or sometimes the native ureter or urinary conduit. Attention is paid to preserve the arterial supply to the lower segment of the ureter; interruption of blood supply results in ischemia, ureteral obstruction, and/or urinary leaks.

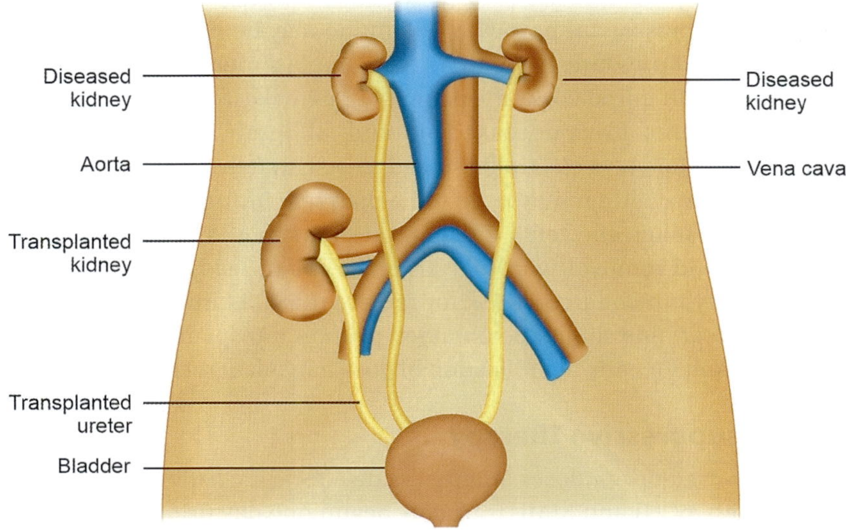

Fig. 29.2: Position of the transplanted kidney in the body

PREOPERATIVE, INTRAOPERATIVE, AND POST-TRANSPLANT MANAGEMENT

Fluid and Electrolytes

Preoperatively, some children need to be dialyzed to optimize fluid and electrolytes, particularly if receiving an organ from a deceased donor that may not have immediate function. Preoperatively, most children do not need IV fluids except if they are polyuric. Normal saline, Ringer lactate, and 5% albumin are given intraoperatively and postoperatively to maintain intraoperative systolic blood pressure higher than 100–110 mm Hg. If needed, dopamine infusion should be given to maintain blood pressure. Adult kidney can occupy 250 mL of volume that may represent a large percentage of total blood volume in an infant or small child. Central venous pressure should be maintained between 10 and 15 cm water prior to removal of aortic cross clamps to ensure good blood flow to the allograft.

In living-related transplants, the allograft kidney begins making urine almost immediately. Brisk diuresis is usually seen immediately after transplant. Fluids (normal saline, dextrose normal saline, and Ringer lactate) are usually replaced volume to volume, based on previous hour urine output, for the first 2 days. Further adjustments in fluid therapy are made based on assessment of fluid balance and blood levels of electrolytes and glucose. Blood levels of creatinine, electrolytes, calcium, magnesium, and phosphorus should be monitored every 8–12 hr. Central venous pressure should be maintained between 5 and 10 cm of water and systolic blood pressure above

100–110 mm Hg to ensure adequate perfusion to the allograft. In young infants and children, pressor support with dopamine may be needed to maintain adequate blood pressure. After 48 hr, urine replacement with intravenous fluids is gradually curtailed, as the patient's oral intake increases.

In transplants from deceased donors, allograft may not function immediately. Fluid and electrolytes need to be carefully monitored in such situation. Some children may need to be dialyzed during this period based on their fluid status and renal function. Attempt should be made to avoid aggressive fluid removal with dialysis since it can lead to acute tubular necrosis (ATN). In children at risk for recurrent FSGS, urinalysis and urine protein to creatinine should be obtained prior to transplant and then daily post-transplant for early identification of post-transplant recurrence.

Immunosuppressive Therapy

Commonly used drugs, doses and their side effects are listed in **Table 29.1**. Therapy with a CNI and MMF is usually begun one day prior to transplant. Induction dose of basiliximab is administered preoperatively and repeated on day 4. In high-risk transplants (patients with high PRA, retransplants and where delayed graft function is anticipated), thymoglobulin is given intraoperatively. IV methylprednisolone (10–15 mg/kg) is given perioperatively.

Postoperatively, these children get a combination of tacrolimus (or CsA), MMF (or azathioprine) and prednisone. Patients getting thymoglobulin induction may get three to seven doses depending upon the allograft function. Steroids are tapered and by the end of 3 months, the dose of prednisone is 0.1 mg/kg/day. In steroid withdrawal protocols, steroids are used typically for 5–7 days in tapering doses and then stopped. Since daclizumab is no longer available, most children on steroid withdrawal protocols are receiving induction with either thymoglobulin or alemtuzumab.

Approximately, 60% children across the US are receiving steroid-free (avoidance or withdrawal) protocols. Children on steroid-free protocols are more likely to have improved growth velocity, decreased risk of hypertension, diabetes, and dyslipidemia. At our center, we prefer steroid-based protocols in children at high risk for rejection (retransplants, highly sensitized and those with delayed graft function) or disease recurrence (native kidney disease primary FSGS, glomerulonephritis, or vasculitis), and in those who need steroids for reasons unrelated to transplant.

Anti-infective Prophylaxis

Antibiotics, based on unit policies, are given for 5–7 days. Therapy with oral valganciclovir is given for 3–6 months for CMV prophylaxis. Nystatin and cotrimoxazole are used to prevent fungal infections and *Pneumocystis carinii*

TABLE 29.1: Immunosuppressive drugs, dose, and side effects

Medication	*Dose*	*Side effects*
Polyclonal antibodies	Thymoglobulin 1.5 mg/kg/day, duration 5–7 days	Fever, chills, leukopenia, thrombocytopenia, and anaphylaxis
Anti-interleukin 2 receptor antagonist	Basiliximab <35 kg: 10 mg; >35 kg: 20 mg; two doses on days 0 and 4	Minimal; same as placebo
Methylprednisolone Prednisone	10 mg/kg IV (day 0) 2 mg/kg/day; 0.5 mg/kg/day by 2 weeks; 0.1–0.15 mg/kg/day by 3 months; continue in low doses	Fluid retention, infections, hypertension, acne, cushingoid features, hyperglycemia, growth suppression, osteoporosis, mood changes, and cataract
Cyclosporine A (CsA)	6–8 mg/kg/day at onset; adjust by levels Target 2-hr postdose: 0–1 months 1500–2000 ng/mL; 1–3 months 1300–1500 ng/mL; 4–6 months 1100 ng/mL; 7–12 months 900 ng/mL; later 800 ng/mL	Hirsutism, nephrotoxicity, hypertension, tremors, and gum hyperplasia
Tacrolimus	0.2–0.3 mg/kg/day, adjust by levels Target 12-hr postdose (trough): 0–2 months 10–12 ng/mL; 3–12 months 5–10 ng/mL; 6–12 months 5–8 ng/mL; and subsequently, 4–6 ng/mL in those with no AR	Nephrotoxicity, tremors, diabetes mellitus, diarrhea, and alopecia
Azathioprine	2 mg/kg/day	Myelosuppression and hepatotoxicity
Mycophenolate mofetil	1,200 mg/m²/day; decrease to 600 mg/m² in tacrolimus-based protocol once adequate tacrolimus trough levels achieved	Myelosuppression, abdominal pain, diarrhea; weight loss; and viral warts
Everolimus	0.8 mg/m² twice daily with CsA; 2 mg/m² twice daily with tacrolimus; adjust to target trough of 3–8 µg/L if used with calcineurin inhibitor (CNI), and 6–10 µg/L if without CNI	Hypertriglyceridemia; high cholesterol; pneumonia; anemia; lymphocele; delayed wound healing; and proteinuria
Sirolimus	Loading dose 6 mg/day, followed by 2–5 mg/day in children >40 kg 3 mg/m²/dose as loading dose followed by 1 mg/m²/dose in children <40 kg. Long-term goal trough 6–8 µg/L	Same as those of everolimus

pneumonia, respectively. Nystatin is given for 6–8 weeks and cotrimoxazole for 6 months. Cotrimoxazole also serves as prophylaxis for urinary tract infections. The duration of anti-infective prophylaxis depends upon recipient risk factors, intensity of immunosuppression, and therapy for episodes of AR. Children with bladder reconstructions are at higher risk for urinary tract infections, and benefit from cotrimoxazole prophylaxis.

Monitoring

Close monitoring of renal function is required since the risk of AR is highest in the first 3 months. Differential diagnosis of graft dysfunction is shown in **Table 29.2**. In addition, patients are monitored for drug levels of CNI which have very narrow therapeutic range. One must be very mindful of drug interactions as many drugs used concomitantly can increase or decrease levels of CNI **(Table 29.3)** that has the potential to cause AR or CNI toxicity. Additionally, patients should be monitored for side effects of medications, viral and bacterial infections, growth and nutrition, malignancy, dyslipidemia, metabolic, and cardiovascular complications. The frequency of monitoring decreases with time as the risk of rejection and infection decreases.

TABLE 29.2: Differential diagnosis of post-transplant graft dysfunction

Acute increase in serum creatinine (by 20% or >0.3 mg/dL above baseline)	Acute rejection Acute cyclosporine (CsA), tacrolimus nephrotoxicity Dehydration Urinary obstruction, urinary leak, and pyelonephritis
Slow increase in serum creatinine (creatinine creep)	Chronic allograft rejection Chronic CsA, tacrolimus nephrotoxicity Urinary tract obstruction (organic, functional, and bladder dysfunction) Interstitial fibrosis and tubular atrophy Recurrent or *de novo* glomerulonephritis BK virus nephropathy Renal artery stenosis
Hypertension	Side effects of steroids, CsA, or tacrolimus Acute rejection Interstitial fibrosis and tubular atrophy Recurrent and *de novo* glomerulonephritis Renal artery stenosis Diseased native kidneys
Proteinuria	Acute rejection Recurrent and *de novo* glomerulonephritis Interstitial fibrosis and tubular atrophy

TABLE 29.3: Significant drug interactions with calcineurin inhibitors

Increase drug trough levels	*Decrease drug trough levels*
Inhibition of CYP3A metabolism and/or P-gp efflux Amiodarone *Antiretroviral therapy boosting agents:* Ritonavir and cobicistat *Azole antifungals:* Fluconazole, posaconazole, and voriconazole *HIV protease inhibitors:* Atazanavir, nelfinavir, saquinavir Macrolide antibiotics, except azithromycin Nondihydropyridine calcium channel blockers *Direct acting antiviral:* Ombitasvir-paritaprevir-ritonavir, with/without dasabuvir Grapefruit juice	Induction of CYP3A metabolism and/or P-gp efflux *Antiseizure agents:* Carbamazepine, oxcarbazepine; phenytoin, fosphenytoin, phenobarbital, and primidone Enzalutamide Nafcillin *Rifamycin:* Rifabutin, rifampin, and rifapentine St. John's wort

COMPLICATIONS OF TRANSPLANTATION

Delayed Allograft Function

Delayed allograft function (DGF) refers to transplant that fails to function after blood flow through the allograft is established. DGF is much more common in organs transplanted from deceased donors, particularly those with prolonged cold ischemia time. Other causes of DGF include hyperacute allograft rejection **(Figs. 29.3A to E)**, acute renal arterial or venous thrombosis, ATN (due to prolonged warm or cold ischemia time, use of vasoconstrictor drugs in the donor, or hypotension in the donor and recipient), and rarely thrombotic microangiopathy. Urinary obstruction due to blood clots, urine leakage, and obstructed Foley catheter may also present as DGF or acute deterioration of graft function.

Management of primary DGF should be prompt because of the risk of allograft loss. After excluding urinary obstruction, ultrasound with Doppler study and nuclear renal scans are performed. If renal blood flow is adequate and excretory function is lagging, it is generally thought to be due to ATN. Urinary leak can be demonstrated by nuclear renal scans. Surgical exploration and intraoperative biopsy may be needed if etiology is thought to be vascular thrombosis or is undetermined. ATN is managed conservatively. CNI and other nephrotoxic drugs should be avoided. Alternate immunosuppressive drugs such as anti-IL-2R antibodies, ATG, or thymoglobulin may be used. Repeated allograft biopsies may be necessary to assess the viability of the graft if function remains poor. If graft is nonviable, allograft nephrectomy should be performed.

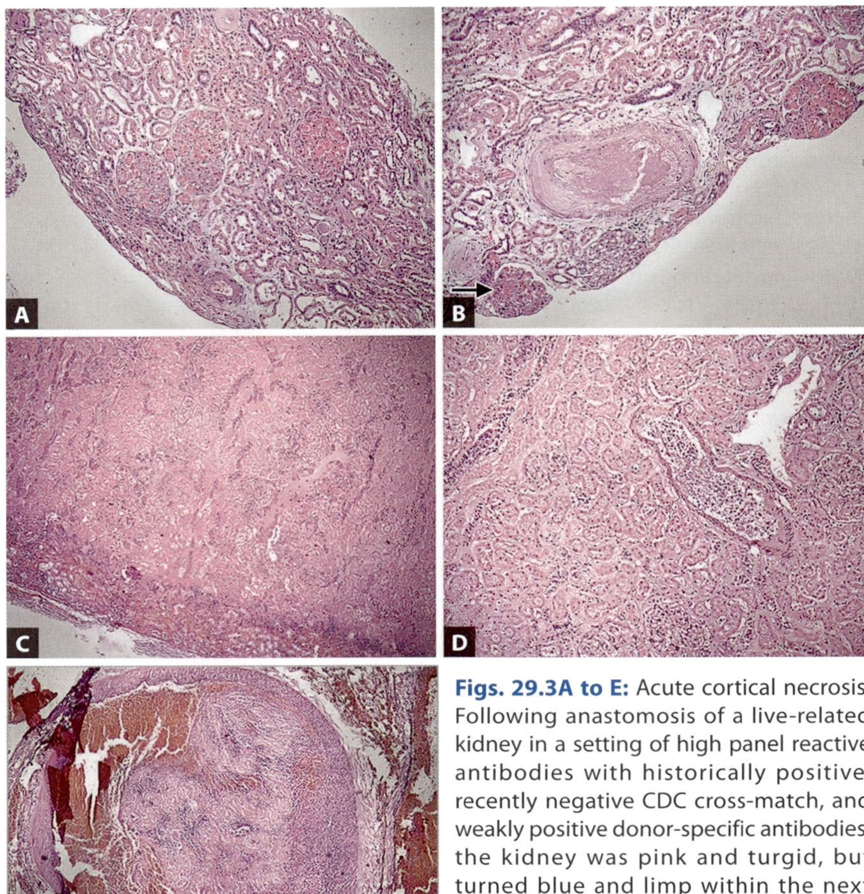

Figs. 29.3A to E: Acute cortical necrosis. Following anastomosis of a live-related kidney in a setting of high panel reactive antibodies with historically positive, recently negative CDC cross-match, and weakly positive donor-specific antibodies, the kidney was pink and turgid, but turned blue and limp within the next 3–4 minutes. Light microscopy images of an on-table allograft biopsy revealed (A) extensive mesangiolysis and diffuse acute tubular injury (hematoxylin and eosin, 40X); accompanied by (B) glomerular intracapillary thrombi (arrow) and luminal occlusion by thrombus in medium size artery in a viable area, suggesting hyperacute rejection (hematoxylin and eosin, 40X). (C to E) Light microscopy images of allograft nephrectomy, performed on day 1 postoperatively, confirm diffuse acute cortical necrosis and graft arterial thrombosis at the hilum (hematoxylin and eosin, 100X). *Courtesy:* Dr Geetika Singh, Department of Pathology, AIIMS, New Delhi

Surgical Complications

Lymphocele, perirenal serous fluid, or blood collections are the most common surgical complications encountered. Usually, no definite therapy is needed. If the fluid collection is significant or is causing pressure on the transplant kidney, percutaneous aspiration may be needed. Large lymphoceles may require injection of sclerosing agents or drainage into the peritoneum. Urinary leaks are uncommon because of the current practice of using lower doses of steroids, and a closer attention to urologic surgical techniques. Urinary obstruction at the ureterovesical junction (UVJ) may be a manifestation of ureteral ischemia, CMV or BK virus infection, or rejection. Ureteral stents may be used for prevention and treatment of UVJ obstruction.

Vascular complications include renal arterial and venous thrombosis. These are particularly common in infants and small children because of small size of the vessels. Attention to technical details and prevention of postoperative dehydration and hypotension helps to prevent these complications. Renal arterial thrombosis usually results in allograft loss unless complication is recognized in the operating room and anastomosis is revised. Renal venous thrombosis may respond to surgical exploration, thrombectomy, and use of anticoagulation. Low-dose heparin may be needed if the child has an underlying hypercoagulable state.

Allograft Rejection

Allograft rejection can be hyperacute rejection (HAR), AR or chronic rejection (CR). HAR occurs within minutes of perfusing the allograft. Sometimes, it can manifest as primary nonfunction of the graft. HAR occurs due to preformed antibodies to the ABO and HLA antigens. The incidence of HAR has decreased significantly in recent years due to availability of sensitive tests for PRA, cross-matching, and identification of antibodies to specific HLA antigens with avoidance of donors carrying these antigens. It is more common in retransplants and in patients with high PRA and is usually not amenable to therapy.

Acute rejection usually occurs within first 3 months of transplantation. AR occurring within 1 week of transplantation is known as *accelerated AR* and has a relatively poor outcome. The incidence of AR has decreased significantly (to <10%) due to availability of potent immunosuppressive drugs. Early diagnosis and treatment of AR are most important for both short- and long-term successful outcome. AR occurring after many months of transplantation is usually related to nonadherence to therapy and is called *late AR*. Sometimes, it can be triggered by an episode of infection, particularly viral infection. Clinical features of AR include fever, oliguria, hypertension, proteinuria, and graft tenderness. However, with current immunosuppressive medications, clinical features of rejection are rarely seen unless the patient is nonadherent. Increased coefficient of variation of tacrolimus level may serve as an objective marker for nonadherence. More commonly, children present with an increase in serum creatinine level on routine blood monitoring. Whenever there is increase in blood creatinine level, the differential diagnosis includes dehydration, CsA or tacrolimus toxicity, urinary obstruction, and AR **(Table 29.2)**.

The diagnosis of AR is made by examining core biopsy of the transplant kidney which is graded according to Banff classification **(Box 29.1)**. Histologically,

BOX 29.1: Diagnosis of acute allograft rejection using Banff classification

Acute T-cell mediated rejection (TCMR)
Ia: >25% interstitial inflammation with moderate tubulitis (t2)
Ib: >25% interstitial inflammation with severe tubulitis (t3)
IIa: Mild-to-moderate intimal arteritis (v1)
IIb: Severe intimal arteritis (v2)
III: Transmural arteritis and/or fibrinoid necrosis (v3)

Acute antibody-mediated rejection (ABMR)
It should fulfill all three criteria

1. Histological evidence of tissue injury
   i. Acute tubular injury
   ii. Microvascular inflammation (g >0 and/or ptc >0)
   iii. Arteritis (v >0)
   iv. Thrombotic microangiopathy without an apparent cause
2. Evidence of current/recent antibody interaction with endothelium
   v. Positive C4d staining of peritubular capillaries
   vi. Moderate microvascular inflammation (g + ptc ≥2)
   vii. Increased expression of endothelial gene transcripts in biopsy tissue
3. Serology evidence of donor specific antibodies (DSA)
   viii. Positive C4d staining/presence of ABMR-associated gene transcripts may substitute for DSA

i0: No inflammation or in <10% of unscarred cortical parenchyma; i1: Inflammation in 10–25% of unscarred cortical parenchyma; i2: Inflammation in 26–50% of unscarred cortical parenchyma; i3: Inflammation in >50% of unscarred cortical parenchyma
t0: No mononuclear cells in tubules or single focus of tubulitis only: t1: Foci with 1–4 mononuclear cells/tubular cross section (or 10 tubular cells): t2: 5–10 Mononuclear cells; t3: Foci with >10 mononuclear cells/tubular cross section or the presence of ≥ 2 areas of tubular basement membrane destruction accompanied by i2/i3 inflammation and t2 elsewhere
G: glomerulitis: none (g0), segmental or global glomerulitis in 75% of glomeruli (g3); PTC: peritubular capillaries: at least 1 leukocyte in ≥10% of cortical PTC but 10 leukocytes in most severely involved PTC (ptc3)

AR is T-cell mediated or acute antibody-mediated (AMR) rejection. In case of T-cell rejection, renal biopsy shows interstitial infiltration with lymphocytes and evidence of tubulitis **(Figs. 29.4A to F)**. AMR is recognized as distinct entity that occurs with or without a component of T-cell rejection. AMR is common in highly sensitized individuals, retransplants and in transplants performed across positive cross match and blood group barriers. Clinical features of AMR are similar but histologic features include presence of neutrophils and monocytes in peritubular and glomerular capillaries **(Figs. 29.5A to C)**. Immunofluorescence shows deposits of C4d in peritubular capillaries **(Fig. 29.5D)**. However, C4d deposition may be focal or absent in many cases of AMR. Electron microscopy shows thickened glomerular basement membrane suggesting early transplant glomerulopathy **(Figs. 29.6A to E)**. Antibodies to donor HLA class I and II antigens are present in roughly 90% of patients with C4d deposition and graft dysfunction.

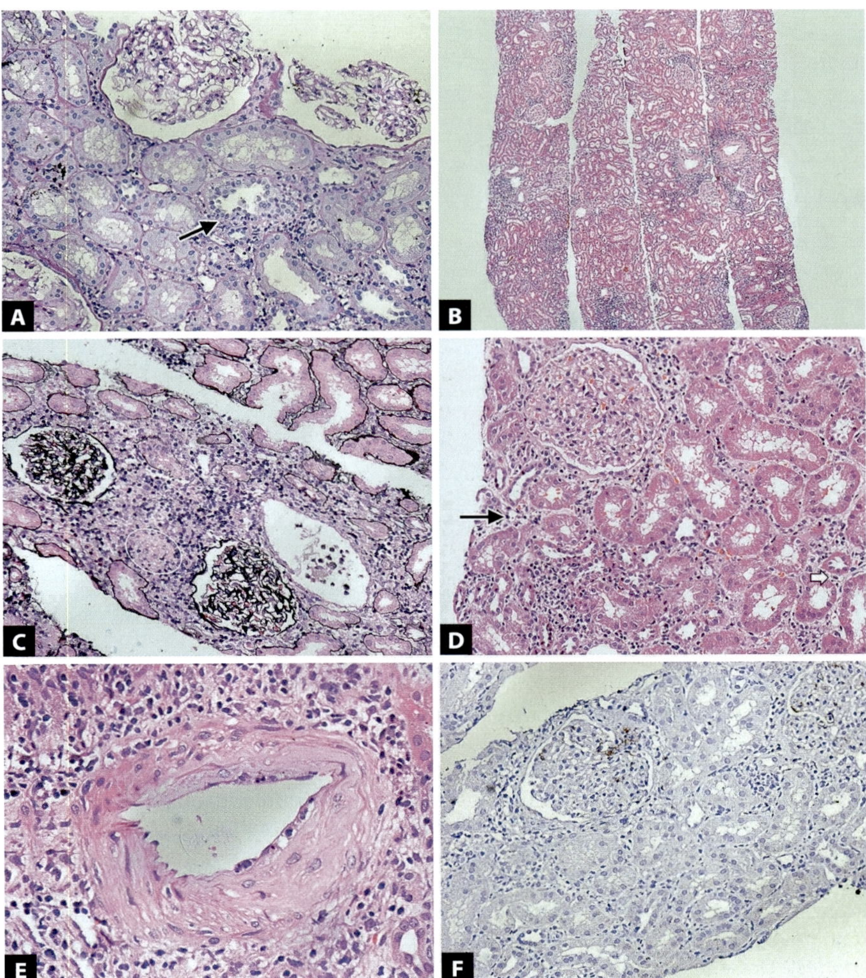

Figs. 29.4A to F: Acute T cell mediated rejection. (A) Focal interstitial infiltrates involving 10–25% of the biopsied cortex (i1) with a focus of moderate tubulitis (arrow), defined as 4–10 lymphocytes in a cross-section of a tubule (t2); this classifies as borderline (suspicious for) acute T cell mediated rejection (periodic acid Schiff, 200X). (B) With infiltrates involving approximately 30% of the four biopsy cores, this case is classified as i2. Note the surrounding interstitial edema and acute tubular injury. No significant tubulointerstitial chronicity is seen (hematoxylin and eosin, 40X). (C) At higher power there is evidence of severe tubulitis with evidence of tubular destruction (white oval) which would classify as t3 (silver methenamine, 100X). (D) In other areas, milder tubulitis is noted. The glomeruli do not show evidence of glomerulitis and the peritubular capillaries, marked with arrows, are either dilated and empty or contain 1–2 leukocytes (ptc1) (hematoxylin and eosin, 200X). (E) One of the arteries in the case showed evidence of mild intimal arteritis (v1) (hematoxylin and eosin, 400X). (F) Immunohistochemistry performed for C4d is negative in the peritubular capillaries (C4d, 200X) and therefore, this case would classify as acute T-cell mediated rejection, Banff IIA. *Courtesy:* Dr Geetika Singh, Department of Pathology, AIIMS, New Delhi

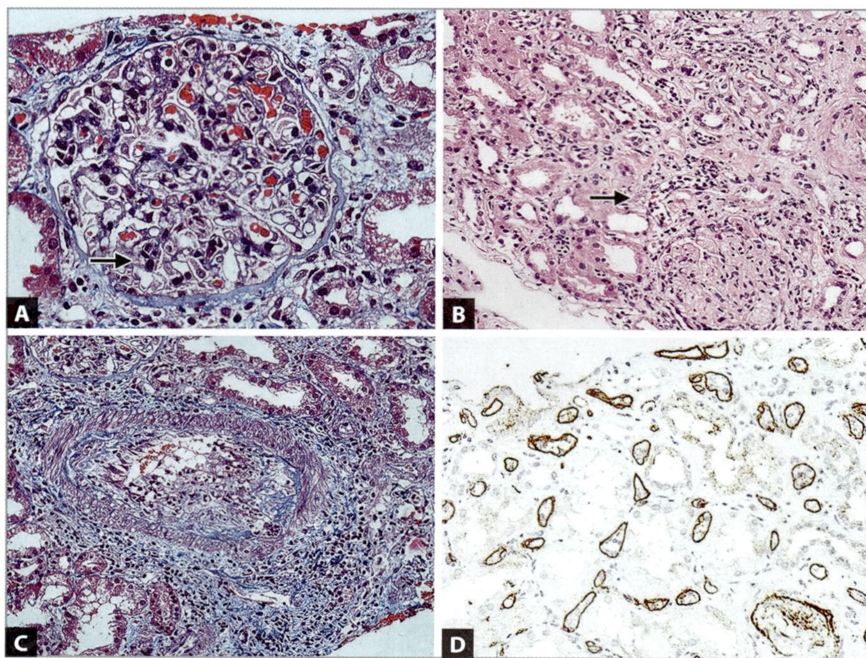

Figs. 29.5A to D: Active antibody-mediated rejection (ABMR): (A) Note the glomerulitis. A capillary loop filled with leukocytes, resulting in luminal occlusion, is marked with an arrow (Masson's trichrome, 400X); (B) At lower power, severe peritubular capillaritis can be appreciated, with more than 10 leukocytes in worst affected areas (ptc3) (hematoxylin and eosin, 100X). Glomerulitis and peritubular capillaritis constitute microvascular inflammation, which is the hallmark of active ABMR; (C) Intimal arteritis may also be part of ABMR. The image depicts severe intimal arteritis (v2), though complete transmural infiltration and fibrinoid necrosis are not seen (Masson's trichrome, 100X); (D) Immunohistochemistry for C4d shows linear capillary wall staining of peritubular capillaries involving >50% of biopsied cortex (C4d3) (C4d, 200X).
Courtesy: Dr Geetika Singh, Department of Pathology, AIIMS, New Delhi

Acute rejection is treated with IV methylprednisolone (10–15 mg/kg per day for 3 days). In steroid resistant AR, thymoglobulin (1.5 mg/kg/day) for five to seven doses, or rarely, alemtuzumab (0.3–0.4 mg/kg single dose) can be used. In case of AMR, additional therapies with IVIG, rituximab, and plasmapheresis are needed.

Chronic allograft rejection denotes a slow, progressive deterioration of allograft function caused mostly by chronic active antibody-mediated rejection (CABMR). Additionally, chronic active T-cell mediated rejection (CATCMR) may also coexist in many patients. Many of these children have DSA and occasionally show the presence of non-HLA antibodies. CABMR is very difficult to treat, and some success has been made by using a combination of IVIG and rituximab. Early results with tocilizumab use are emerging in treating IVIG and rituximab resistant CABMR.

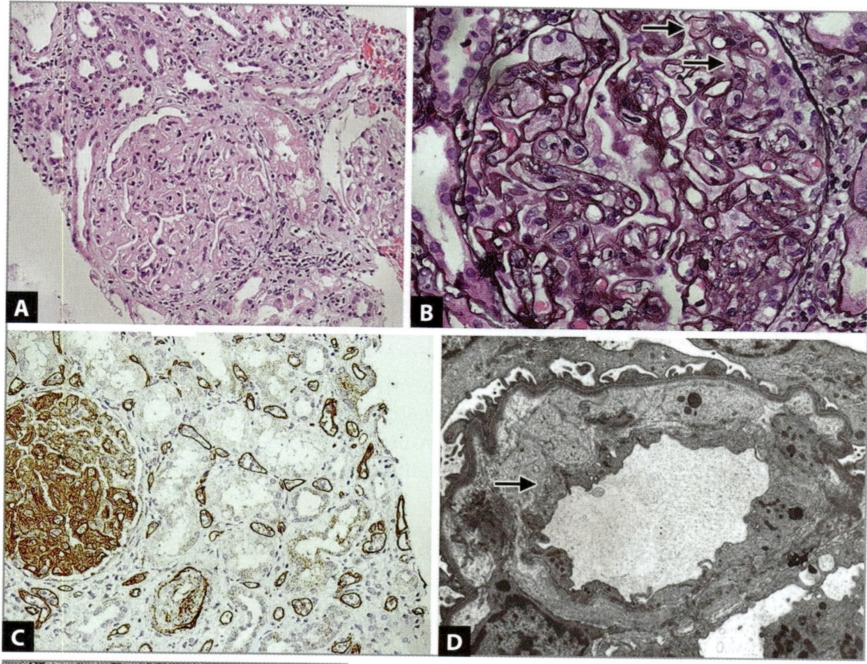

Figs. 29.6A to E: Chronic active antibody-mediated rejection: (A) The glomerular capillary walls appear remodeled along with presence of numerous leukocytes and luminal occlusion suggestive of transplant glomerulopathy with glomerulitis. Note the surrounding peritubular capillaritis (hematoxylin and eosin, 200X); (B) Transplant glomerulopathy is confirmed on silver methenamine stain, where double contouring of the glomerular basement membrane (GBM) is apparent (arrows) and involves 25–50% of the capillary loops of the worst affected glomerulus, classified as cg2 (silver methenamine, 400X); (C) Antibody interaction is confirmed with positive immunohistochemistry for C4d (c4d3) (C4d, 100X); (D) On transmission, electron microscopy reduplication of the GBM is confirmed. The neobasement membrane material is marked with arrow. Note the endothelial fenestral fusion and accumulation of subendothelial electron lucent material (Uranyl acetate/lead citrate 25000x); (E) Peritubular capillary basement membrane shows multilamellation (arrow) of >seven layers (ptcml1) (uranyl acetate/lead citrate 35,000x). *Courtesy:* Dr Geetika Singh, Department of Pathology, AIIMS, New Delhi

Infections

Infectious complications after transplantation usually follow a predictable pattern. In the first month after transplant, infectious complications are related to technical and mechanical problems and include wound infections, urinary tract infections, pyelonephritis **(Figs. 29.7A and B)**, pneumonia, and

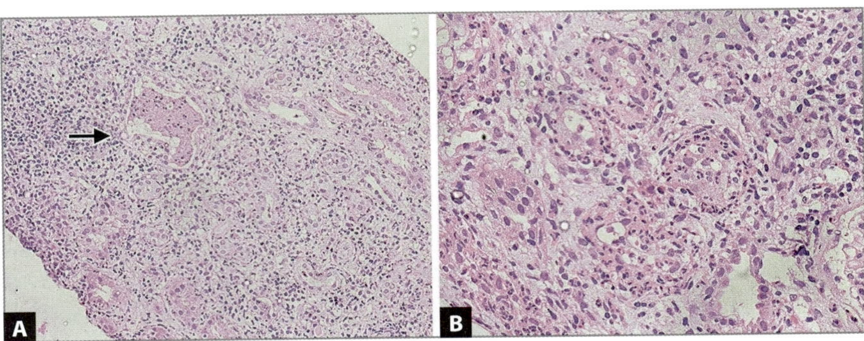

Figs. 29.7A and B: Acute pyelonephritis of the allograft: (A) The graft biopsy shows severe interstitial inflammation rich in neutrophils with an occasional white blood cell-granular intratubular cast (arrow) (hematoxylin and eosin, 100X); (B) On higher power, severe neutrophilic tubulitis can be appreciated (hematoxylin and eosin, 200X). *Courtesy:* Dr Geetika Singh, Department of Pathology, AIIMS, New Delhi

fungal infections. Between 1- and 6-month post-transplant, infections include CMV, EBV, *Pneumocystis pneumonia* (PCP), herpes simplex virus (HSV), varicella-zoster, and fungal infections. Parvovirus B19 infection can present as aplastic anemia. CMV and EBV infections can be primary infections in viral naïve recipients or may represent reactivation of these viruses under immunosuppression **(Table 29.4)**. Polyoma BK virus and adenovirus may cause hemorrhagic cystitis and interstitial nephritis resulting in an increase in creatinine; the features may mimic AR. The diagnosis is made by urine polymerase chain reaction (PCR) for adenovirus and blood PCR for BKV. Histologic examination shows nuclear atypia, focal viral inclusions in the tubular epithelium, and positive immunoperoxidase staining with antibodies to SV40 in BKV nephropathy **(Figs. 29.8A to D)**. Routine use of antiviral, antibacterial, antifungal and PCP prophylaxis, careful monitoring of viral infections by PCR, and attempts to avoid over immunosuppression has decreased the incidence, morbidity, and mortality related to infections.

After 6 months of transplantation, the patterns of infections in patients on stable maintenance immunosuppression and with good allograft function are like that seen in the general population. Patients who develop opportunistic infection > 6 months post-transplant are generally those who have higher serum creatinine, are receiving higher doses of maintenance steroids or have had recurrent rejection episodes requiring intensification of immunosuppression. Hepatitis B and C infections may become a problem in long-term survivors of kidney transplants. This may be secondary to reactivation of these viruses in the recipient or infection acquired in the peritransplant period. Tuberculosis is a serious problem in developing countries due to high risk of exposure and an immunocompromised state. Recently, deaths due to West Nile virus, rabies, and coccidioidomycosis have

TABLE 29.4: Viral infections after transplantation

Infection	*Incidence; timing*	*Risk factors*	*Clinical features*	*Diagnosis*	*Histopathology*	*Prevention; surveillance*	*Therapy*
Cytomegalovirus (CMV)	6–40%; 0–6 months, or after end of prophylaxis	D+/R- > D+/R+ status	Leukopenia, thrombocytopenia; high transaminases; fever, myalgia; pneumonitis; and colitis	CMV DNA PCR (quantitative)* in serum/blood, bronchoalveolar lavage, and colon biopsy	Intranuclear and cytoplasmic viral inclusions; CMV immunostaining; EM: 150 nm particles	Oral valganciclovir prophylaxis for 3–6 months; blood CMV PCR q3 months for first year	Reduce immuno-suppression; valganciclovir; ganciclovir for life-threatening disease
Polyoma BK virus	1–6%	Immune suppression; ureteric stent; antibody induction	Asymptomatic; allograft dysfunction; BK virus nephropathy (BKVAN)	BK virus PCR* in urine and blood (former more sensitive); kidney biopsy**	Tubulointerstitial nephritis; viral inclusions in epithelial cells; SV40 staining	Urine PCR q1–3 months in first 2 years; less frequently later	Reduce immuno-suppression; IVIG; leflunomide; cidofovir
Epstein Barr virus (EBV)	50–80% if R-;PTLD 1–4%	D+/R- status; immune suppression; ATG induction	Asymptomatic; malaise; fever; lymphadenopathy; cytopenia; PTLD	EBV DNA PCR in blood	Lymphopro-liferative disease	PCR q1–3 months for first year; after rejection therapy; close surveillance if D+/R-	Reduce immuno-suppression; rituximab; chemotherapy
Parvovirus B19	0–12%; usually first year	Immune suppression	Acute, chronic anemia;*** pancytopenia; graft dysfunction; flu-like symptoms	Blood parvovirus PCR; B19-specific IgM	Collapsing glomerulopathy; thrombotic microangiopathy	None	Reduce immuno-suppression; IVIG

*Termed quantitative nucleic acid amplification test, qNAT
**Indicated if allograft dysfunction, urine PCR ≥ 10^7 copies/mL, or plasma PCR ≥ 10^4 copies/mL
***Findings include normocytic, normochromic anemia with severe reticulocytopenia and bone marrow showing decreased erythroid precursors and giant pronormoblasts with cytoplasmic vacuoles and intranuclear inclusions
D: donor; EM: electron microscopy; IVIG: intravenous immunoglobulin; PCR: polymerase chain reaction; PTLD: post-transplant lymphoproliferative disease; R: recipient

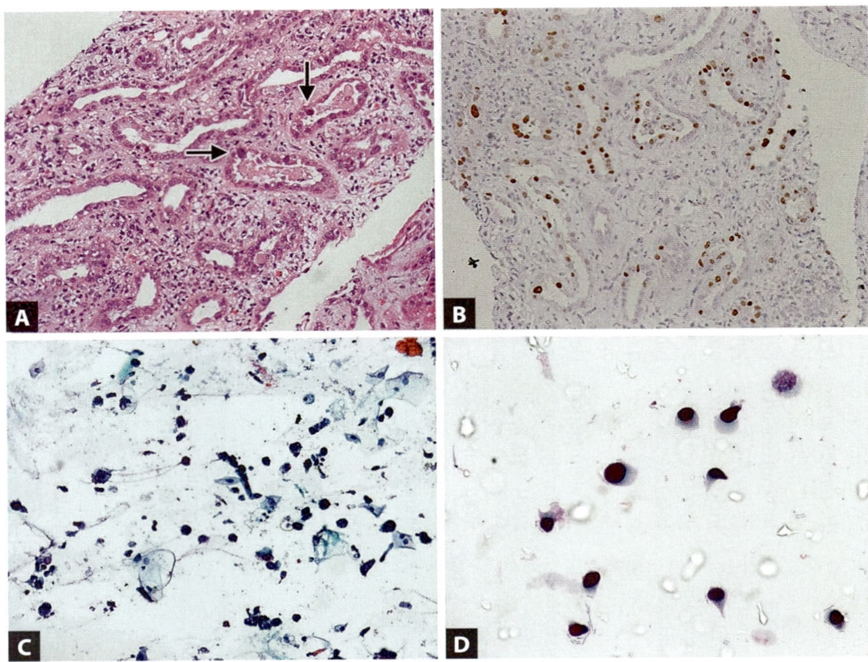

Fig. 29.8A to D: Polyoma virus nephropathy: (A) Few of the tubules show smudgy homogeneous basophilic intranuclear inclusions (arrows), classically seen in BK polyoma virus infection. There is associated severe acute tubular injury, marked interstitial edema, inflammation and tubulitis (hematoxylin and eosin, 200X); (B) Simian vacuolating virus 40 T antigen (SV40T) immunohistochemistry confirms the polyoma virus infection and would classify as pvl3 (>10% infected tubular epithelial cells) (SV40T, 100X); (C) A screening tool is the urinary sediment examination stained with Papanicolaou (PAP) stain where numerous "decoy" cells are noted, which demonstrates dark smudgy nuclei reminiscent of a high-grade urothelial malignancy. Note the dirty background with casts suggesting upper urinary tract infection, i.e., polyoma virus nephropathy (PAP, 100X); (D) Presence of decoy cells in a clean background may represent bladder reactivation and shedding of the virus without nephropathy; correlation with levels of viruria and viremia along with kidney function is indicated (PAP, 200X). *Courtesy:* Dr Geetika Singh, Department of Pathology, AIIMS, New Delhi

been reported in transplant recipients of organs from deceased donors. These infections may be fatal in the immunosuppressed recipient. A high index of suspicion for infections prevalent in the community and prompt treatment is necessary.

Appropriate immunization is an important means to prevent vaccine preventable infections in the recipient. Attempts should be made to vaccinate children early in the course of kidney failure as response to vaccines is blunted in advanced CKD. Influenza, pneumococcal, meningococcal, and HPV vaccines should be administered. Family members, close contacts, and healthcare workers should be appropriately vaccinated. After transplant, the child and the family members should receive influenza vaccine on yearly basis. Pneumococcal and hepatitis B vaccines are repeated if immunity has waned.

Hypertension

Hypertension in early post-transplant period may be secondary to fluid overload, high-dose steroids, AR, and high-dose CsA or tacrolimus. Chronic hypertension may be related to the presence of diseased native kidneys, side effect of medications such as CsA, tacrolimus and prednisone, acute and chronic rejection, recurrent glomerulonephritis, and renal artery stenosis.

Home blood pressure and ambulatory blood pressure monitoring may help in adequate management. Control of hypertension is important to prolong life of the allograft and reduce cardiovascular morbidity. Hypertension is managed with low sodium diet and antihypertensive medications. Calcium channel blockers are useful in the early post-transplant period because of their ability to counteract the vasoconstriction induced by CsA and tacrolimus. Angiotensin-converting-enzyme (ACE) inhibitors are effective on long-term management of hypertension and in prolonging the life of the allograft through inhibition of transforming growth factor-β expression. Renal artery stenosis may be treated by percutaneous transluminal angioplasty or surgical correction.

Recurrence of Primary Disease in the Allograft

Several diseases that cause ESKF in the native kidneys have potential to recur in the allograft. These include FSGS, atypical HUS, dense deposit disease, immunoglobulin A (IgA) nephropathy, membranous nephropathy, granulomatosis with polyangiitis (GPA) and lupus nephritis **(Table 29.5)**. Patients with FSGS may develop severe proteinuria within hours of transplantation **(Figs. 29.9A to F)**, and ultimately show allograft failure. Intensive plasmapheresis, and therapy with high-dose CNI and rituximab and lipid apheresis are successful in salvaging these allografts. Recurrence of atypical HUS may be treated with plasma exchanges and eculizumab. Recurrent IgA nephropathy, lupus nephritis, and GPA usually do not cause allograft failure **(Table 29.5)**.

De Novo Glomerulonephritis

These include membranous glomerulonephritis, IgA nephropathy, FSGS, and collapsing glomerulopathy. Rarely, antiglomerular basement membrane disease may occur in patients with Alport syndrome **(Table 29.5)**.

TABLE 29.5: Recurrent and de novo disease after kidney transplantation

Condition	*Pathogenesis*	*Frequency*	*Risk of graft loss*	*Risk factor*	*Therapy or prevention*
Atypical hemolytic uremic syndrome	Variants in alternate pathway genes; factor H antibodies	80%	40–60%	Significant variants; family history; low C3 at transplantation	Plasma exchange Eculizumab Kidney and liver transplant
Focal segmental glomerulosclerosis	Circulating factors	20–30%	~50%	Initial steroid sensitivity; previous recurrence; no significant genetic variants	Plasmapheresis, immunoadsorption, LDL apheresis High-dose calcineurin inhibitors (CNI) Rituximab Obinutuzumab
C3 glomerulopathy	Dysregulation of the alternate complement pathway	30–70%	10–40%	Younger age; crescents on initial biopsy; dense deposit disease; low C3 at transplant; monoclonal gammopathy	Plasmapheresis Eculizumab; corticosteroids
IgA nephropathy	Deficient IgA glycosylation; dysregulation of classic complement pathway	15–50%	3–30%	Young age; steroid avoidance; nonuse of induction therapy; crescentic nephropathy; high levels of IgA before, or galactose-deficient (Gd) IgA1 after transplant	CNI, steroids Basiliximab induction Pretransplant tonsillectomy
Membranous nephropathy	Antibodies to glomerular antigens **(*see* Chapter 13)**	3–70%	~30%	Presence (and titer) of anti-PLA2R autoantibody pre-transplant	CNI with steroids and rituximab; alkylating agents; and bortezomib
Primary hyperoxaluria type 1	Oxalate deposits	>80%	80–100%	Pathogenic *AGXT* mutation	Liver-kidney transplant Lumasiran if isolated kidney transplant
Alport syndrome; monogenic nephrotic syndrome	Nephritis due to antibodies generated against the antigen lacking in native kidneys (COL4A5, nephrin, or podocin); not true recurrence	3–5%	Unclear	Truncating mutation resulting in absence of protein in native kidneys	Plasmapheresis Steroids; rituximab; and alkylating agent

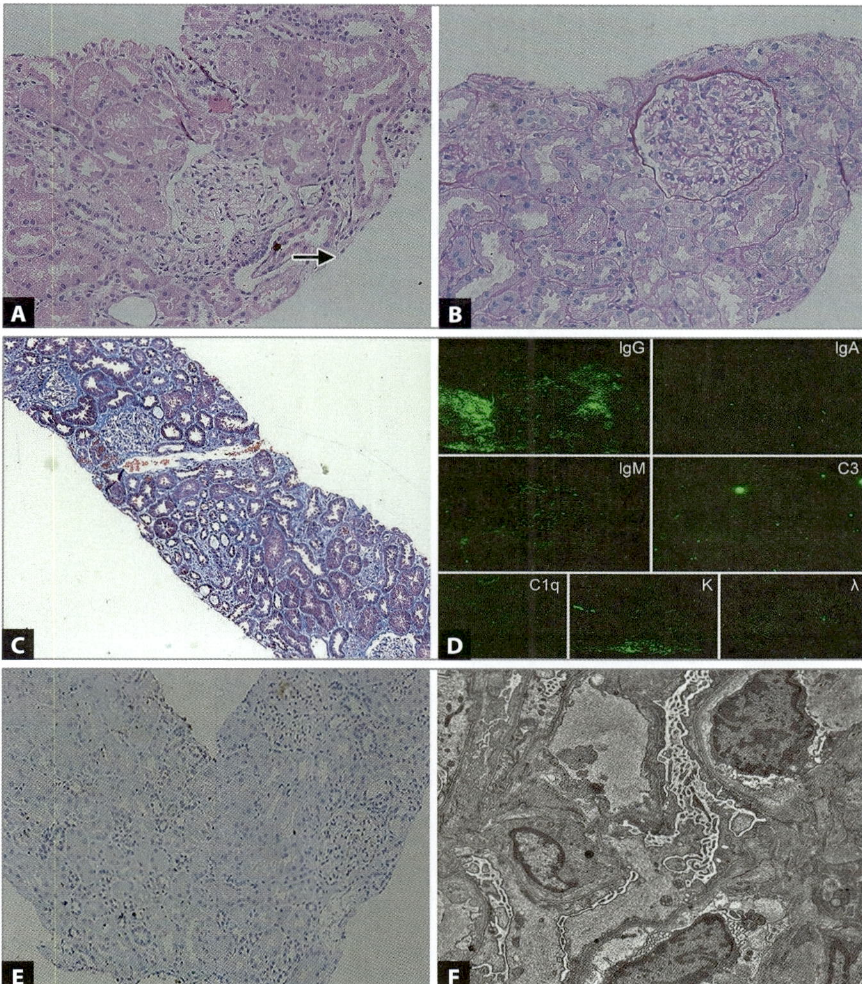

Figs. 29.9A to F: A 15-year-old boy with native kidney disease of steroid-resistant focal segmental glomerulosclerosis (FSGS), nonresponsive to immunosuppression, underwent live-related kidney transplantation. Nephrotic range proteinuria recurred within 6 hr, followed by delayed graft function. Allograft biopsy was done. (A to C) Light microscopy images show histologically unremarkable glomeruli with acute tubular injury on (A) hematoxylin and eosin (40X); (B) periodic acid Schiff (40X); and (C) Masson's trichome (10X) stains. (D) Immunofluorescence microscopy was negative for IgG, IgA, IgM, C3, kappa (κ), and lambda (λ). (E) There was no C4d deposition on glomeruli or peritubular vessels. (F) Electron microscopy showed diffuse podocyte foot process effacement, without any electron dense deposits or changes in morphology of glomerular basement membrane (Uranyl acetate; 3000 X). *Courtesy:* Dr Geetika Singh, Department of Pathology, AIIMS, New Delhi

Side Effects of Medications

In long-term survivors of allografts, the side effects of medications are very important **(Table 29.1 and Fig. 29.10)**. Cosmetic side effects are a reason for nonadherence and delayed episodes of AR in teenagers.

Delayed Acute Rejection

Delayed episodes of AR occur after 6–12 months of transplantation. The most common cause of delayed AR is nonadherence with immunosuppressive medications. Medical nonadherence is prevalent in 40–50% of the pediatric

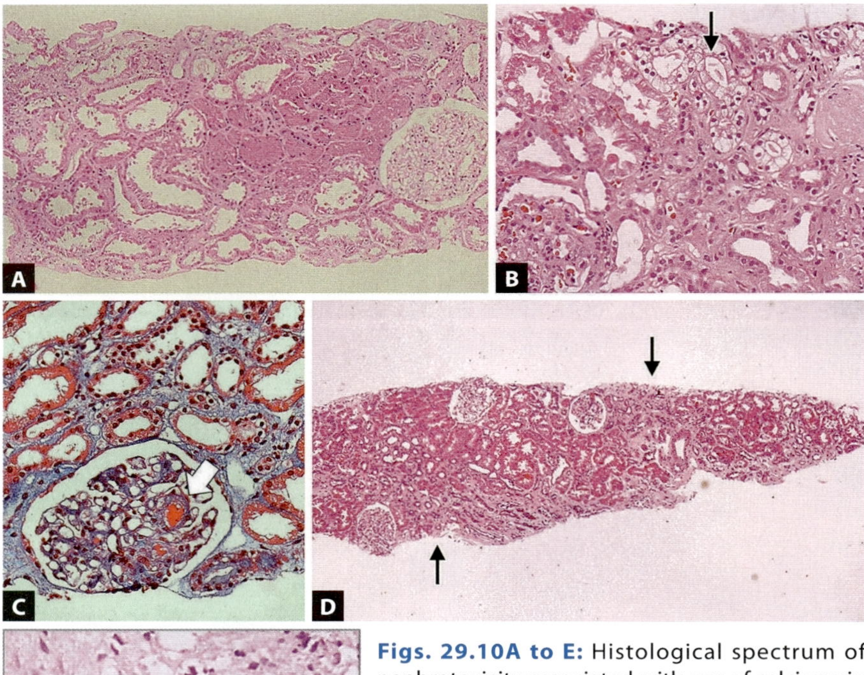

Figs. 29.10A to E: Histological spectrum of nephrotoxicity associated with use of calcineurin inhibitors (CNI): (A) Acute tubular injury, a feature of acute CNI toxicity, characterized by shedding and flattening of the tubular epithelium, is noted on the left side (hematoxylin and eosin, 40X); (B) Focal isometric vacuolization (arrow) is an additional nonspecific finding (hematoxylin and eosin, 100X); (C) Thrombotic microangiopathy, a rare finding, is indicated by a white arrow pointing to a fresh fibrin thrombus within a glomerulus (Masson's trichrome, 100X); (D) Striped pattern of fibrosis, reflecting the chronic vascular toxicity of CNI, is noted in arrows (hematoxylin and eosin, 10X); (E) Classical peripheral nodular hyalinosis in an arteriole is marked with a black circle (hematoxylin and eosin, 400X). *Courtesy:* Dr Geetika Singh, Department of Pathology, AIIMS, New Delhi

recipients and leads to allograft failure in 25%. Majority of these children with delayed AR have emergence of de novo DSA. Viral infections, aggressive weaning of immunosuppressive medications in response to viral infections may also trigger DSA development. These episodes of late AR characterized by presence of CABMR with or without CATCMR are less amenable to treatment and have a deleterious effect on the allograft.

Chronic Allograft Dysfunction

Even though the risk of AR has substantially decreased, the half-life of allografts has not changed much. Chronic allograft dysfunction leads to allograft failure and return of patients to dialysis. Causes include immune factors (episodes of AR and CABMR) and nonimmune factors (peritransplant injuries, DGF, CNI nephrotoxicity, renovascular stenosis, hypertension, hyperglycemia, hyperlipidemia, donor and recipient size mismatch, donor age, BK virus nephropathy, CMV and adenoviral infections, recurrent pyelonephritis, abnormal lower urinary tract, and recurrent and de novo glomerular lesions).

Development of DSAs and chronic CNI nephrotoxicity **(Figs. 29.10A to E)** are the two most important causes of graft failure. Interstitial fibrosis with tubular atrophy may present as worsening hypertension, proteinuria, and slow rise in creatinine. There is no specific therapy; use of an ACE inhibitor might prolong allograft life. Treatment of DSAs with plasma exchanges, IVIG, and rituximab is often useful. Reduction of CNI-based therapies may be considered if there is evidence of nephrotoxicity.

Malignancy

The risk of malignancy is increased with the intensity and duration of immunosuppression. The chief malignancy observed in children is posttransplant lymphoproliferative disease (PTLD) that occurs more commonly due to primary EBV infection in EBV seronegative recipients of EBV positive allografts **(Figs. 29.11A to K)**. Other sources of EBV infection include perioperative use of blood or community acquisition of infection. The incidence of PTLD is approximately 1–2%; risk is highest in the first year, with a second peak after 7 years. Close monitoring for EBV replication by PCR and reduction of immunosuppressive therapy may prevent some of these complications. The role of IVIG and rituximab in children with high viral load in preventing PTLD is not well established.

Use of sunscreen with SPF ≥30 is recommended to prevent skin cancers. HPV vaccination helps prevent genital warts and cervical malignancies. Ultrasound screening of native kidneys should be done periodically for malignancies though frequency of monitoring is not established. Over time, incidence of common cancers occurring in the general population increase by several fold and therefore careful follow-up is recommended. By then, most children are not under the care of pediatric nephrologists.

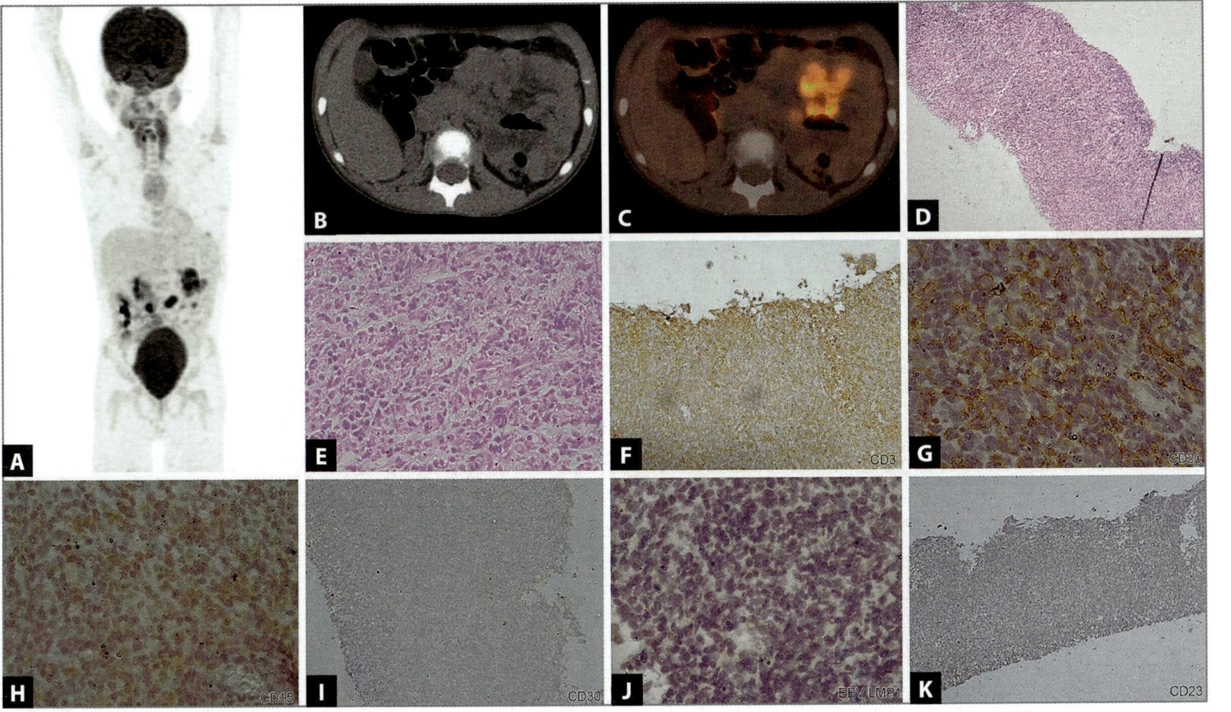

Figs. 29.11A to K: Post-transplant lymphoproliferative disease (PTLD) in a 10-year-old boy presenting with abdominal pain and weight loss. On positron emission tomography (PET), (A) the maximum intensity projection image revealed increased metabolic activity in the left upper abdomen, while (B) axial CT and (C) fused PET/CT images showed metabolically active soft tissue thickening with nodular lesions involving the jejunum. (D and E) Light microscopy of specimens of jejunal biopsy indicated a polymorphous population of histiocytes, small lymphocytes, occasional plasma cells, and few large cells (hematoxylin and eosin, D: 10X, E: 100X). (F to K) Immunohistochemistry revealed that the (F) background cells were positive for CD3; and the large cells were (G) positive for CD20 and negative for (F) CD3, (H) CD15, (I) CD30, and (J) late membrane protein 1 of Epstein–Barr virus (EBV-LMP1); (K) CD23 staining showed loss of dendritic cell network. These findings were consistent with EBV-negative, polymorphic type of PTLD.
Courtesy: Dr Nishikant Damle, Department of Nuclear Medicine, and Dr Saumya Ranjan Mallick, Department of Pathology, AIIMS, New Delhi

Miscellaneous Complications

Hematologic Complications

These include anemia, erythrocytosis, and rarely leukopenia and thrombocytopenia. Anemia after transplant may be related to bone marrow suppression due to drugs (MMF, azathioprine, CsA, tacrolimus, ganciclovir, valganciclovir, and cotrimoxazole) or due to viral infections. Incidence of hematologic complications is higher in patients on steroid-free protocols. Aplastic anemia can occur due to parvovirus B19 and CMV infections. Hemolytic anemia may occur due to recurrent or acquired HUS (secondary to drugs, infections, or hypertension). Post-transplant erythrocytosis (hematocrit > 51%) is a rare complication and may be seen in children with retained native kidneys, post-transplant diabetes, renal artery stenosis, and preserved GFR. Therapy is with ACE inhibitors, theophylline, and rarely, phlebotomy. Neutropenia and thrombocytopenia are rare and often due to side effects of medications, viral infections, or residual hyperparathyroidism.

Metabolic Complications

Metabolic complications in the post-transplant period include hypomagnesemia, hypophosphatemia, hypercalcemia, hyperkalemia, renal tubular acidosis, and dyslipidemia. Hypomagnesemia occurs due to renal tubular wasting because of CsA, tacrolimus, or diuretic use and responds to oral magnesium therapy. Hypophosphatemia may occur due to residual secondary hyperparathyroidism, elevated levels of fibroblast growth factor-23 and nutritional vitamin D deficiency. Supplementation with vitamin D and phosphorus is required. Hypercalcemia may occur due to secondary hyperparathyroidism that can take up to 12 months to resolve. Calcimimetic agents may be used to correct hypercalcemia; sometimes parathyroidectomy is indicated.

Hyperkalemia and renal tubular acidosis may be a feature of CsA or tacrolimus toxicity, AR, urinary obstruction, or use of ACE inhibitors and cotrimoxazole. Dyslipidemia can occur secondary to use of steroids, CsA, tacrolimus, and sirolimus. About 50% of patients treated with sirolimus show elevated cholesterol and triglycerides. Dyslipidemia is an important contributor to cardiovascular morbidity and mortality and may contribute to functional deterioration of the graft.

Growth Retardation

Growth retardation may be a problem after transplantation. Growth is better in patients with satisfactory allograft function, those receiving minimal or no steroids (prednisone < 6 mg/m^2/day), and patients transplanted at an early age. Still, many children do not show catch-up growth to achieve full potential for height. Growth hormone and insulin-like growth factor levels are normal or increased. Some of these children benefit from recombinant growth hormone therapy. Although treatment with growth hormone can lead to insulin resistance and aggravation of hyperglycemia, the incidence of AR is not increased. However, close monitoring of serum creatinine levels is desired in the few weeks after initiation of growth hormone treatment.

Excessive Weight Gain and Diabetes Mellitus

Excessive weight gain and its consequences are important in transplant recipients. Excessive weight gain may be responsible for sleep apnea, nocturnal enuresis, hypertension, glucose intolerance, and dyslipidemia. About 5% children develop post-transplant diabetes mellitus. The risk is higher with the use of tacrolimus. Other risk factors include family history of diabetes, excessive weight gain, and use of high-dose steroids. Strict control of diabetes is required for long-term patient and graft survival.

Osteopenia and Reduced Bone Mass

Factors contributing to osteopenia and reduced bone mass include renal osteodystrophy, residual hyperparathyroidism, use of corticosteroids, vitamin D deficiency, and prolonged hypophosphatemia. Adequate intake of calcium, phosphorus, and vitamin D helps reduce bone loss.

TRANSITION OF CARE

A systematic transition of children to adult care is necessary for success of the allograft. Analysis of the adolescent readiness skills including psychosocial evaluation, financial planning, health knowledge, and self-management skills should be undertaken and a close communication with adult providers should be maintained until smooth transition occurs.

Renal transplantation is rewarding, since it transforms chronically ill children into near normal with improvement in nutrition, growth, neurodevelopment, and quality of life, but at the price of using immunosuppressive medications. Challenges include prevention and treatment of late AR, emergence of *de novo* DSA, finding reliable noninvasive immune monitoring tools, decreasing cardiovascular morbidity and mortality in long-term survivors, dealing with organ shortage, improving adherence in adolescents, psychosocial rehabilitation of children and their families, and achieving the elusive goal of tolerance. Until such time when transplantation can be maintained without use of immunosuppression, a multidisciplinary, integrated, and diligent approach addressing each aspect of posttransplant care is required to maximize outcomes in these children.

BIBLIOGRAPHY

Recipient and Donor Preparation

1. Chandar J, Chen L, Defreitas M, et al. Donor considerations in pediatric kidney transplantation. Pediatr Nephrol. 2021;36:245-57.
2. Etesami K, Hogen R, Lestz R. Pediatric kidney transplantation, A technical update. Curr Opin Organ Transplant. 2021;26:356-59.
3. Iyengar A, McCulloch MI. Pediatric kidney transplantation in under-resourced regions: A panoramic view. Pediatr Nephrol. 2022;37:745-55.
4. Kute VB, Rela M, Gulati S, et al. Current scenarios of pediatric transplants of kidney, liver, heart, and lung in India: Systematic review and meta-analysis. Exp Clin Transplant. 2022;20:1058-68.
5. Palmer B, Kropp B. Urologic evaluation and management of pediatric kidney transplant patients. Urol Clin North Am. 2018;45:561-9.
6. Pereira LDNG, Nogueira PCK. Non-standard criteria donors in pediatric kidney transplantation. Pediatr Transplant. 2019;23:e13452.
7. Torricelli FCM, Watanabe A, Piovesan AC, et al. Urologic issues in pediatric transplant recipients. Transl Androl Urol. 2019;8:134-40.

Immunosuppression

1. Ahlenstiel-Grunow T, Pape L. Novel ways to monitor immunosuppression in pediatric kidney transplant recipients-underlying concepts and emerging data. Mol Cell Pediatr. 2021;8:8.
2. Balani SS, Jensen CJ, Kouri AM, et al. Induction and maintenance immunosuppression in pediatric kidney transplantation: Advances and controversies. Pediatr Transplant. 2021;25:e14077.
3. Haasova M, Snowsill T, Jones-Hughes T, et al. Immunosuppressive therapy for kidney transplantation in children and adolescents: Systematic review and economic evaluation. Health Technol Assess. 2016; 20:1-324.
4. Kizilbash SJ, Jensen CJ, Kouri AM, et al. Steroid avoidance/withdrawal and maintenance immunosuppression in pediatric kidney transplantation. Pediatr Transplant. 2022;26:e14189.
5. Liverman R, Chandran MM, Crowther B. Considerations, and controversies of pharmacologic management of pediatric kidney transplant recipient. Pharmacotherapy. 2021;41:77-102.
6. Pape L. State-of-the-art immunosuppression protocols for pediatric renal transplant recipients. Pediatr Nephrol. 2019;34:187-94.
7. Verghese PS. Pediatric kidney transplantation. Pediatr Res. 2017;81:259-64.
8. Yeo WS, Ng QX. Biomarkers of immune tolerance in kidney transplantation: An overview. Pediatr Nephrol. 2022;37:489-98.

Post-transplant Infections

1. Agrawal A, Ison MG, Danziger-Isakov L. Long-term infectious complications of kidney transplantation. Clin J Am Soc Nephrol. 2022;17:286-95.
2. Allen UD, Preiksaitis JK; AST Infectious Diseases Community of Practice. Post-transplant lymphoproliferative disorders, Epstein-Barr virus infection, and disease in solid organ transplantation: Guidelines from the American Society

of Transplantation Infectious Diseases Community of Practice. Clin Transplant. 2019;33:e13652.
3. Epperson K, Crane C, Ingulli E. Prevention, diagnosis, and management of donor derived infections in pediatric kidney transplant recipients. Front Pediatr. 2023;11:1167069.
4. Goldman JD, Julian K. Urinary tract infections in solid organ transplant recipients: Guidelines from the American Society of Transplantation Infectious Diseases Community of Practice. Clin Transpl. 2019;33:e13507.
5. Haidar G, Boeckh M, Singh N. Cytomegalovirus infection in solid organ and hematopoietic cell transplantation: State of the evidence. J Infect Dis. 2020;221:S23-31.
6. Levi S, Davidovits M, Alfandari H, et al. EBV, CMV and BK viral infections in pediatric kidney transplantation: Frequency, risk factors, treatment, and outcomes. Pediatr Transplant. 2022;26:e14199.
7. Scaggs Huang FA, Danziger-Isakov L. Infectious disease risks in pediatric renal transplantation. Pediatr Nephrol. 2019;34:1155-66.
8. Subramanian AK, Theodoropoulos NM. *Mycobacterium tuberculosis* infections in solid organ transplantation: Guidelines from the infectious diseases community of practice of the American Society of Transplantation. Clin Transplant. 2019;33:e13513.

Acute and Chronic Rejection

1. Ehlayel A, Simms KJA, Ashoor IF. Emerging monitoring technologies in kidney transplantation. Pediatr Nephrol. 2021;36:3077-87.
2. Fernandez HE, Foster BJ. Long-term care of the pediatric kidney transplant recipient. Clin J Am Soc Nephrol. 2022;17:296-304.
3. Hart A, Singh D, Brown SJ, et al. Incidence, risk factors, treatment, and consequences of antibody-mediated kidney transplant rejection: A systematic review. Clin Transplant. 2021;35:e14320.
4. Lefaucheur C, Louis K, Morris AB, et al. Clinical recommendations for posttransplant assessment of anti-HLA donor-specific antibodies: A sensitization in transplantation: Assessment of risk consensus document. Am J Transplant. 2023;23:115-32.

Recurrent Diseases

1. Al Shamsi HR, Shaheen I, Aziz D. Management of recurrent focal segmental glomerulosclerosis (FSGS) post renal transplantation. Transplant Rev (Orlando). 2022;36:100675.
2. Alawieh R, Boonpheng B, Blosser CD. Recurrence of glomerulonephritis after kidney transplant. Nephrol Dial Transplant. 2022;37:2090-2.
3. AlZabali S, AlBatati S, Rahim K, et al. A multicenter study evaluating the discontinuation of eculizumab therapy in children with atypical hemolytic uremic syndrome. Children (Basel). 2022;9:1734.
4. Cody E, Hooper DK. Kidney transplantation in pediatric patients with rheumatologic disorders. Curr Opin Pediatr. 2022;34:234-40.
5. Gonzalez Suarez ML, Thongprayoon C, et al. Outcomes of kidney transplant patients with atypical hemolytic uremic syndrome treated with eculizumab: Systematic review and meta-analysis. J Clin Med. 2019;8:919.

6. Knotek M, Novak R, Jaklin-Kekez A, et al. Combined liver-kidney transplantation for rare diseases. World J Hepatol. 2020;12:722-37.
7. Raina R, Jothi S, Haffner D, et al. Post-transplant recurrence of FSGS. Kidney Int. 2023;105:450-63.

Miscellaneous

1. Ashoor IF, Dharnidharka VR. Non-immunologic allograft loss in pediatric kidney transplant recipients. Pediatr Nephrol. 2019;34:211-22.
2. Bobrowski AE. School and sports participation post-transplant. Pediatr Transplant. 2021;25:e13791.
3. Bock ME, Wall L, Dobrec C, et al. Management of dyslipidemia in pediatric renal transplant recipients. Pediatr Nephrol 2021;36:51-63.
4. Cohen E, Korah M, Callender G, et al. Metabolic disorders with kidney transplant. Clin J Am Soc Nephrol. 2020;15:732-42.
5. Drube J, Wan M, Bonthuis M, et al; European Society for Pediatric Nephrology Chronic Kidney Disease Mineral and Bone Disorders, Dialysis and Transplantation Working Groups. Clinical practice recommendations for growth hormone treatment in children with chronic kidney disease. Nat Rev Nephrol. 2019;15:577-89.
6. Fox TG, Nailescu C. Vaccinations in pediatric kidney transplant recipients. Pediatr Nephrol. 2019;34:579-91.
7. Fulchiero R, Amaral S. Post-transplant lymphoproliferative disease after pediatric kidney transplant. Front Pediatr. 2022;10:1087864
8. Garro R, Warshaw B, Felner E. New-onset diabetes after kidney transplant in children. Pediatr Nephrol. 2015;30:405-16.
9. Hamdani G, Mitsnefes MM. Hypertension in pediatric solid organ transplant recipients. Curr Hypertens Rep. 2023;25:51-60.
10. Kouri A, Balani S, Kizilbash S. Anemia in pediatric kidney transplant recipients: Etiologies and management. Front Pediatr. 2022;10:929504.
11. Matsuda-Abedini M, Marks SD, Foster BJ. Transition of young adult kidney transplant recipients. Pediatr Nephrol. 2023;38:383-90.
12. Seeman T, Myette RL, Feber J. Hypertension in pediatric kidney transplantation. Pediatr Transplant. 2023;27:e14522.
13. Singer P. Post-transplant education for kidney recipients and their caregivers. Pediatr Nephrol 2023;38:2033-42.

Malignant Disorders

Arvind Bagga, Aditi Sinha

WILMS TUMOR

Wilms tumor is the most common pediatric abdominal cancer. Although most cases are sporadic, about 1% patients have one or more family members with the tumor. Wilms tumor is associated with loss of function mutations of several tumor suppressor genes, including *WT1, TP53, FWT1,* and *FWT2,* and mutations at the *WT2* gene locus (11p15.5). Conditions associated with development of Wilms tumor include WAGR (Wilms tumor, aniridia, genitourinary malformations, and a range of mental disabilities), Denys-Drash and Beckwith-Wiedemann syndromes **(Table 30.1)**. Kidney tumor surveillance is through screening ultrasound examinations every 3–6 months during childhood. Familial Wilms tumor is associated with mutations in *BRCA2* or *TP53* (Li-Fraumeni syndrome).

Clinical Features

The mean age at diagnosis is around 3 years; 95% are diagnosed before 10 years of age. The tumor is bilateral in 5–7% cases, more commonly in girls. Patients with bilateral disease and associated congenital abnormalities (aniridia and genitourinary abnormalities) are diagnosed at an earlier age. The usual presentation is with an abdominal mass, often noted by the mother or during incidental examination. Fever, abdominal pain, and gross hematuria are occasionally present. Hypertension may be detected in 25–30% of patients but is rarely severe.

Diagnosis

Ultrasonography provides diagnostic information. Multicystic renal dysplasia and hydronephrosis can be readily excluded. The size of tumor, normalcy of the opposite kidney, and patency of inferior vena cava are evaluated. A chest X-ray is done to detect pulmonary metastasis. Computed tomography (CT) scan shows definitive details and involvement of contiguous structures and distant metastasis **(Figs. 3.16 and 3.17)**. Cytogenetic studies should be done for 1p and 16q deletion. Bilateral Wilms tumor alters the treatment significantly, therefore the status of the contralateral kidney should be determined.

TABLE 30.1: Heritable syndromes associated with increased risk of Wilms tumor (WT)

Syndrome	*Locus*	*Genetic lesion*	*Phenotype*	*Risk of WT*
WAGR	11p13	11p13 deletion encompassing *WT1*	Aniridia, cryptorchidism, ambiguous genitalia, mental delay and late-onset kidney failure	~50%
Denys–Drash	11p13	Point mutation in zinc-finger region of *WT1* exon 8 or 9	Early-onset nephrotic syndrome (diffuse mesangial sclerosis) and male pseudohermaphroditism	75–90%
Frasier	11p13	Point mutation in *WT1* intron 9 donor splice site	Ambiguous genitalia, streak gonads, focal segmental glomerulosclerosis and diffuse mesangial sclerosis	Case reports
Beckwith–Wiedemann	11p15	Dysregulation of imprinted genes including *IGF2* and *H19*	Overgrowth syndrome; organomegaly, large for date, macroglossia, omphalocele, hemihypertrophy, ear pits and creases, and neonatal hypoglycemia	5–15%
Simpson–Golabi–Behmel	Xq26.2	*GPC3* mutations/deletions	Overgrowth syndrome; visceral and skeletal abnormalities, heart defects and psychomotor impairment	~3%
Li–Fraumeni	17p13	Heterozygous *TP53* mutations	Familial predisposition to cancer	Low
Fanconi anemia D1	13q12	Biallelic *BRCA2/FANCD1* mutations Genome instability disease	Short stature, radial ray defects, bone marrow failure; variable features (one-third patients have normal appearance)	20–40%
Bloom	15q26	Biallelic *BLM* mutations; genome instability disease	Short stature, photosensitivity, microcephaly, insulin resistance, and immunodeficiency	3%
Perlman	2q37	Biallelic inactivating variants *DIS3L2*	Prenatal overgrowth, facial dysmorphism, developmental delay, cryptorchidism and renal dysplasia	~60%
Trisomy 18 (Edward)	18q11.2–q23	Complete trisomy 18 (95%); mosaic trisomy 18 (5%)	Cardiac anomalies; dysmorphic features, clenched hands, rocker-bottom feet	Case reports
Mulibrey nanism	17q22–q23	Biallelic *TRIM37* mutations	Growth deficiency, cardiomyopathy, characteristic facies and type 2 diabetes	~6–8%

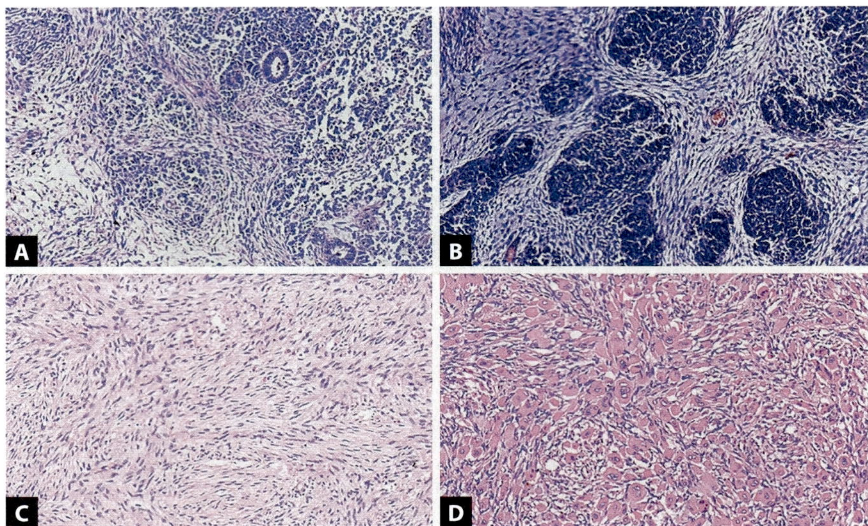

Figs. 301A to D: Histological findings in Wilms tumor. (A) Triphasic Wilms tumor with blastemal, stromal, and epithelial components; (B) Expansile nodules of undifferentiated malignant small round blue cells, in which blastema is separated by spindle-shaped stromal cells; (C) Cellular stromal component with spindle-shaped cells; (D) Rhabdomyoblastic differentiation, seen frequently following chemotherapy. (Hematoxylin and eosin, 10X).
Courtesy: Dr Aanchal Kakkar, Department of Pathology, AIIMS, New Delhi

90% of Wilms tumor show a favorable histology, with triphasic pattern of blastemal, epithelial, and stromal tissues **(Figs. 301A to D)**. Unfavorable histology includes much higher degrees of anaplasia, or loss of heterozygosity at 1p and 16q loci; these patients have unsatisfactory response to therapy. Other renal cell tumors are rare and are differentiated from Wilms tumor based on tissue histology.

Treatment

Several multicenter cooperative groups have laid down guidelines for staging **(Table 30.2)**, histological classification and therapy of Wilms tumor. Multimodal therapeutic regimens that combine surgical excision, chemotherapy, and radiation therapy have resulted in improved outcomes. For patients with stages I and II, total surgical excision of the tumor is initially carried out. This is followed by chemotherapy with vincristine and dactinomycin. Patients <2 years of age with stage I disease, favorable histology, and tumor weighing less than 550 g may not require adjuvant chemotherapy.

In case of stage III and stage IV tumors, primary surgical resection is followed by triple chemotherapy (vincristine, dactinomycin, and doxorubicin). Radiation therapy is given for involved lymph nodes, peritoneal contamination, or areas with metastasis. Patients with bilateral Wilms

TABLE 30.2: Staging of Wilms tumor (International Society of Pediatric Oncology)

Stage	*Features*
I	Tumor limited to kidney and completely excisable
II	Tumor extends beyond kidney, but completely excisable; regional extension into perirenal soft tissues and infiltration of surface vessels
III	Tumor not completely excisable; nonhematogenous spread confined to abdomen Involvement of lymph nodes; peritoneal contamination with tumor implants on peritoneal surface
IV	Hematogenous metastases involving lungs, liver, bones, and brain
V	Bilateral renal involvement at diagnosis

tumor (stage V) are initially managed with chemotherapy followed by renal parenchyma sparing resection.

The risk of tumor recurrence is dependent on its histology. Recurrent disease develops in 15% patients with favorable histology and in 50% of those with anaplastic features, usually within 2 years of initial diagnosis. Although salvage therapy has improved survival rates, the post-relapse 3- and 5-year survival rates are lower at 50–60%. Long-term follow-up is necessary for survivors for ongoing surveillance for tumor recurrence and late treatment related complications.

Outcome

Survival rates have dramatically improved in patients with Wilms tumor to the current 5-year overall survival rate of 80–90%. The prognosis is related to the stage of the tumor at diagnosis and its histological type. Extensive metastases, anaplastic tumor, and loss of heterozygosity at 1p, 1q, 11p15, and 16q, or presence of *TP53* indicate an unsatisfactory prognosis. Post-treatment survival at 2 years varies from 95–100% for stage I to 60% for grade IV tumors. Bilateral Wilms tumor has a less aggressive course than unilateral neoplasm.

OTHER KIDNEY TUMORS IN CHILDHOOD

Mesoblastic Nephroma

Mesoblastic nephroma is a rare benign tumor seen during the neonatal period and early infancy. Patients may show hypertension and hypercalcemia. Local invasion may occur but metastases are rare. Following surgical removal, the prognosis is excellent.

Clear Cell Sarcoma

Clear cell sarcoma is the second most common pediatric kidney tumor with less favorable prognosis than Wilms tumor. Bone is a common metastatic site.

Histologic appearance is distinctive with cords and nests of pale-stained tumor cells with abundant extracellular matrix.

Renal Cell Carcinoma

Renal cell carcinoma is rare in childhood, the median age of occurrence in children being 12 years. Adolescent boys may show chromosomal translocation at Xp11.2. Symptoms include abdominal pain, weight loss, fever, and hematuria. An abdominal mass may be palpable in 60% patients. Radical nephrectomy with lymphadenectomy is the treatment of choice. The 2 year survival ranges from 50 to 60%.

Rhabdomyosarcoma

Rhabdomyosarcoma of bladder is occasionally seen in children. The presenting features are usually those of obstruction and urinary retention. Hematuria is rare in children. The diagnosis is made on micturating cystourethrogram and CT scan. Radical cystectomy, chemotherapy, and radiation therapy are undertaken.

BENIGN RENAL TUMORS ASSOCIATED WITH SYSTEMIC DISEASE

Angiomyolipomas

Renal angiomyolipoma (AML) is an uncommon benign renal mesenchymal tumor, seen twice as often in girls as boys. This mesenchymal neoplasm is considered to be derived from perivascular epithelioid cells; hence it is also termed PEComa. As the name suggests, it has three components in variable proportions: Abnormal blood vessels, special spindle cells, and mature adipocytes. While usually sporadic, almost 20% of cases are associated with tuberous sclerosis complex (TSC), and rarely, sporadic lymphangioleiomyomatosis (LAM). Conversely, 55–90% of cases of TSC and 30–50% of those with LAM develop AML. Syndromic AML tend to be multifocal and bilateral. The diagnosis is suspected on ultrasonography and confirmed on magnetic resonance imaging (MRI) or CT. Uncommon cases of fat-poor AML require special imaging, such as chemical shift MRI, to distinguish them from renal cell carcinoma.

Small asymptomatic AML require only active surveillance. However, given the risk of life-threatening hemorrhage, lesions larger than 3 cm are treated with inhibitors of mammalian target of rapamycin (mTOR) such as everolimus (4.5 mg/m^2 given once daily empty stomach) or sirolimus. Refractory cases, particularly symptomatic lesions, might require radical or partial nephrectomy, selective arterial embolization, cryoablation or radiofrequency ablation.

ONCONEPHROLOGY

Nephrotoxicity Associated with Anticancer Therapies

While better understanding of immunobiology and use of targeted therapies has resulted in improved outcomes, there is increasing recognition of short- and long-term complications of cancer and antineoplastic therapies. Onconephrology is an expanding subspecialty that focuses on the intersection between hematology/oncology and nephrology, including incidence and mechanisms of drug toxicities. Various kidney-related adverse events are described, especially for targeted, immuno- and cell-based therapies. **Table 30.3** describes the chief features, including the pathogenic mechanisms of acute kidney injury (AKI), electrolyte imbalance, and hypertension associated with chemotherapeutic agents.

Tumor Lysis Syndrome

Tumor lysis syndrome (TLS) refers to metabolic derangements caused by the massive and abrupt release of cellular contents into the blood, following rapid lysis of malignant cells. While mostly observed following the initiation of cytotoxic chemotherapy for hematological malignancies (acute lymphoblastic leukemia, Burkitt lymphoma, other high-grade non-Hodkin lymphoma, and acute myeloid leukemia), TLS may also occur spontaneously, and in other malignancies with rapid proliferation, large tumor burden, or high sensitivity to cytotoxic therapy. Chief metabolic abnormalities include hyperuricemia, hyperkalemia, hyperphosphatemia, hypocalcemia, and AKI associated with uric acid or calcium phosphate crystals in kidney tubules. Clinical features, usually observed within 12–72 hr of initiating cytoreductive therapy, include nausea, vomiting, diarrhea, anorexia, lethargy, edema, fluid overload, hematuria, congestive heart failure, cardiac dysrhythmias, seizures, muscle cramps, tetany, syncope, and sudden death.

Conventionally, the Cairo–Bishop criteria have been used for the diagnosis and staging of TLS **(Table 30.4)**. Risk factors for development of TLS include:

- *Tumor type:* Burkitt lymphoma, lymphoblastic lymphoma, B-cell lymphoma, diffuse large-cell lymphoma, acute lymphoblastic leukemia, and solid tumors with high proliferative rates and rapid response to therapy.
- *Tumor burden or extent of disease:* Tumor bulk >10 cm, lactate dehydrogenase more than twice the upper limit of normal, and total leukocyte count >25,000/µL
- Preexisting kidney failure or oliguria
- Baseline serum uric acid >7.5 mg/dL
- Effective and rapid cytoreductive therapy

TABLE 30.3: Nephrotoxicity associated with chemotherapeutic agents

Syndrome; Effect/lesion	*Class of drugs*
Acute kidney injury	
Acute tubular necrosis (ATN)	*ALK inhibitors:* Crizotinib, lorlatinib, alectinib *Alkylating agent:* Ifosfamide *Antimetabolite:* Methotrexate, pemetrexed *BCR-ABL tyrosine kinase inhibitors:* Imatinib, dasatinib *BRAF inhibitors:* Vemurafenib, dabrafenib *BTK inhibitors:* Ibrutinib *mTOR inhibitors:* Everolimus *PD-1 inhibitors:* Pembrolizumab, cemiplimab, nivolumab *PDL-1 inhibitors:* Atezolizumab, avelumab, and durvalumab *Platinum-based chemotherapy:* Cisplatin, carboplatin, and oxaliplatin *Tyrosine kinase inhibitors:* Sorafenib, sunitinib, and axitinib *VEGF inhibitors:* Bevacizumab
Thrombotic microangiopathy	*Antitumor antibiotics:* Mitomycin C *Antimetabolite:* Gemcitabine *BCR-ABL tyrosine kinase inhibitors:* Imatinib, dasatinib *Protease inhibitors:* Bortezomib, carfilzomib *Tyrosine kinase inhibitors:* Sorafenib, sunitinib, axitinib *VEGF-A monoclonal antibody:* Bevacizumab
Granulomatous interstitial nephritis	*Immune checkpoint inhibitors targeting CTLA4:* Ipilimumab, nivolumab
Cytokine release syndrome	*CAR-T therapy:* Axicabtagene ciloleucel, idecabtagene vicleucel, brexucabtagene autoleucel, tisagenlecleucel
Crystal nephropathy	*Antimetabolite:* Methotrexate
Tumor lysis syndrome (TLS)	*CAR-T therapy:* Axicabtagene ciloleucel, idecabtagene vicleucel, tisagenlecleucel *Inhibitors targeting CTLA4:* Ipilimumab, nivolumab
Hematuria	
Hemorrhagic cystitis	Cyclophosphamide, nitrosoureas
Electrolyte abnormalities	
Fanconi syndrome, hypokalemia, hypophosphatemia	*Alkylating agent:* Ifosfamide *Antimetabolite:* Pemetrexed *Inhibitors targeting CTLA4:* Ipilimumab, nivolumab *Platinum-based:* Cisplatin, carboplatin
Distal RTA	*Inhibitors targeting CTLA4:* Ipilimumab, nivolumab
Hypomagnesemia	*EFGR monoclonal antibodies:* Cetuximab and panitumumab *Platinum-based:* Cisplatin > carboplatin, oxaliplatin
Hyponatremia	*CAR-T therapy:* Axicabtagene ciloleucel, idecabtagene vicleucel, brexucabtagene autoleucel, tisagenlecleucel *Inhibitors targeting CTLA4:* Ipilimumab, nivolumab *XPO inhibitor:* Selinexor
Hypokalemia	*CAR-T therapy:* Axicabtagene ciloleucel, idecabtagene vicleucel, brexucabtagene autoleucel, and tisagenlecleucel *Inhibitors targeting CTLA4:* Ipilimumab and nivolumab
Hypocalcemia	*CAR-T therapy:* Axicabtagene ciloleucel, idecabtagene vicleucel, brexucabtagene autoleucel, tisagenlecleucel *Inhibitors targeting CTLA4:* Ipilimumab, nivolumab
Hypercalcemia	*Inhibitors targeting CTLA4:* Ipilimumab, nivolumab

Contd...

Contd...

Syndrome; Effect/lesion	***Class of drugs***
Hypophosphatemia, hyperphosphatemia	*CAR-T therapy:* Axicabtagene ciloleucel, idecabtagene vicleucel, brexucabtagene autoleucel, tisagenlecleucel *Inhibitors targeting CTLA4:* Ipilimumab, nivolumab
Nephrogenic diabetes insipidus	*Alkylating agent:* Ifosfamide *Antimetabolite:* Pemetrexed *Platinum-based:* Cisplatin, carboplatin
Syndrome of inappropriate diuresis	*Alkylating agent:* Melphalan *Inhibitors targeting CTLA4:* Ipilimumab, nivolumab
Abnormal urinalysis	
Podocytopathy with proteinuria or glomerulonephritis	*ALK inhibitors:* Crizotinib, lorlatinib, alectinib *Inhibitors targeting CTLA4:* Ipilimumab, nivolumab *mTOR inhibitors:* Everolimus *PD-1 inhibitors:* Pembrolizumab, cemiplimab, nivolumab *Tyrosine kinase inhibitors:* Sorafenib, sunitinib, axitinib *VEGF-A antibody:* Bevacizumab *VEGFR2 antibody:* Ramucirumab *VEGF-Trap (fusion protein):* Aflibercept
Hypertension	
Antimetabolite: Gemcitabine *Antitumor antibiotics:* Mitomycin C *BTK inhibitors:* Ibrutinib *Protease inhibitors:* Bortezomib, carfilzomib *Tyrosine kinase inhibitors:* Sorafenib, axitinib, apatinib, pazopanib, lenvatinib, cabozantinib, nintedanib, regorafenib, vandetanib *VEGF-A VEGFR2 antibodies:* Bevacizumab; ramucirumab *VEGF-Trap (fusion protein):* Aflibercept	
Kidney cysts	
ALK inhibitors: Crizotinib, lorlatinib, alectinib	

The management of the disorder centers around its prevention and monitoring in high-risk settings, with timely intervention. Aggressive hydration (2–3 L/m^2/d or 200 mL/kg/day if <10 kg) is the key to management and ensures adequate urinary flow (80–100 mL/m^2/h or 4–6 mL/kg/h). Diuretics might be used but are contraindicated in patients with hypovolemia or urate-induced obstructive uropathy. Intravenous or oral sodium bicarbonate are no longer recommended to alkalinize the urine, particularly if allopurinol or rasburicase are used.

Allopurinol (50–100 mg/m^2 or 3.3 mg/kg every 8-hr) competitively inhibits xanthine oxidase to block production of uric acid. However, therapy with allopurinol is less effective and has delayed response. Further, it carries risks of hypersensitivity (fever and rash), acute obstructive uropathy (due to deposition of xanthine crystals), reduced clearance of chemotherapeutic agents utilizing the purine pathway (6-mercaptopurine and azathioprine), reduced clearance of high-dose methotrexate in presence of AKI, and intense myelosuppression when used alongside cyclophosphamide. Rasburicase or recombinant urate oxidase (0.1–0.2 mg/kg once daily IV) is more effective

TABLE 30.4: Cairo–Bishop definition and grading of tumor lysis syndrome (TLS)

Definition			
Laboratory TLS	Simultaneous presence of ≥2 of the following abnormalities, within 3 days before or 7 days after cytotoxic therapy: • Uric acid ≥8 mg/dL or ≥25% increase from baseline • Potassium ≥6.0 mEq/L or ≥25% increase from baseline • Phosphorus ≥6.5 mg/dL (for children) or ≥25% increase from baseline • Calcium ≤7.0 mg/dL or ≥25% decrease from baseline		
Clinical TLS	The presence of laboratory TLS in addition to one or more of the following significant clinical complications: (*i*) Acute kidney injury; (*ii*) cardiac arrhythmias or sudden death, and (*iii*) seizures		
Staging			
Laboratory	Absent or present		
Clinical	Maximal grade of any of the following manifestations*		
Grade	Creatinine**	Cardiac arrhythmia	Seizure
0	<1.5 times ULN	None	None
1	1.5 times ULN	Intervention not indicated	–
2	>1.5–3.0 times ULN	Nonurgent medical intervention indicated	One brief, generalized seizure; well controlled seizures, or infrequent focal motor seizures
3	>3.0–6.0 times ULN	Symptomatic and incompletely controlled medically, or controlled with device (e.g., defibrillator)	Seizure with consciousnes; altered; poorly controlled seizure disorder; generalized seizures despite therapy
4	>6.0 times ULN	Life-threatening (e.g., arrhythmia associated with heart failure, hypotension, syncope and shock)	Prolonged, repetitive or difficult to control seizures (status epilepticus and intractable epilepsy)
5	Death	Death	Death

ULN: upper limit of normal
*Not directly or probably attributable to therapeutic agent(s)
**Normal reference level by age: 1 year–<12 years: 0.7 mg/dL; ≥12–<16 years: 1.0 mg/dL; ≥16-year-old girl: 1.2 mg/dL; ≥16-years-old boy: 1.3 mg/dL

and better tolerated than allopurinol. Patients at high risk of TLS should receive rasburicase along with vigorous hydration. Patients at intermediate risk should undergo hydration and receive either allopurinol or one dose of rasburicase. Those at low risk of TLS can be monitored without intervention.

TABLE 30.5: Renal paraneoplastic syndromes

Syndrome	*Symptoms*	*Etiopathogenesis*	*Underlying tumor*	*Additional findings*	*Management*
Hypercalcemia	Muscle weakness, hypertonia, lethargy, nausea, vomiting, hypertension, bradycardia, and renal failure	Tumor production of parathyroid hormone related protein (PTHrP); less often vitamin D	Mesoblastic nephroma; lymphoma; renal cell carcinoma	Low/normal parathyroid hormone; elevated PTHrP	Normal saline; loop diuretics; prednisone; bisphosphonates; hemodialysis
Syndrome of inappropriate diuresis	Gait disturbances, headache, nausea, fatigue, muscle cramps, anorexia, confusion, lethargy, seizures, respiratory depression and coma	Tumor production of antidiuretic hormone	Astrocytoma; medulloblastoma; choroid plexus papilloma; neuroblastoma; lymphoma; Ewing sarcoma; ovarian teratoma; thymoma	Low serum osmolality; euvolemia; normal creatinine	Fluid restriction; adequate salt intake; hypertonic (3%) saline; demeclocycline; tolvaptan; conivaptan
Rickets; tumor-induced osteomalacia	Bone pain, muscle weakness, pathological fractures, and bony deformities	Tumor production of FGF-23	Phosphaturic mesenchymal tumor	Low serum phosphorus; low 1,25$(OH)_2$ D	Supplements of phosphorus; calcitriol; tumor resection
Nephrotic syndrome	Edema	Undefined cytokines in minimal change disease; nephritogenic target antigen in membranous nephropathy	*Minimal change:* Hodgkin lymphoma, thymoma *Membranous nephropathy:* Solid tumors	Nephrotic proteinuria; hypoalbuminemia	Manage underlying malignancy; fluid and salt restriction; diuretics

Hemodialysis is initiated if hyperkalemia, hyperphosphatemia or hypocalcemia are severe or refractory to conventional measures.

Paraneoplastic Renal Syndromes

Paraneoplastic syndrome is a group of symptoms that develops when substances released by certain malignant cells disrupt the normal function of another, often surrounding, tissue. The condition is suspected in the presence of the following characteristics: (*i*) Absence of a defined etiology for the syndrome, (*ii*) chronological relationship between diagnosis of the syndrome and the malignancy, (*iii*) clinical and histological remission after complete surgical removal or chemotherapy, and (*iv*) worsening of symptoms due to tumor residue or relapse. Paraneoplastic renal syndromes are conditions that affect tubular and glomerular function by electrolyte imbalance, hormone-producing tumors, or deposition of antigen-antibody complexes. Common paraneoplastic syndromes that affect kidney function include: hypercalcemia in malignancies, syndrome of inappropriate antidiuresis, TLS, renin-producing tumors, and paraneoplastic glomerulopathies, such as minimal change disease **(Table 30.5)**.

BIBLIOGRAPHY

1. Aldrink JH, Heaton TE, Dasgupta R, et al. American Pediatric Surgical Association Cancer Committee. Update on Wilms tumor. J Pediatr Surg. 2019;54:390-7.
2. Almazedi B, Stubbs C. Renal angiomyolipoma: From imaging to intervention. Clin Radiol. 2024;79:25-32.
3. Bacchetta J, Juillard L, Cochat P, et al. Paraneoplastic glomerular diseases and malignancies. Crit Rev Oncol Hematol. 2009;70:39-58.
4. Blosser CD, Portuguese AJ, Santana C, et al. Transplant onconephrology: An update. Semin Nephrol. 2022;42:151348.
5. Bonilla M, Gudsoorkar P, Wanchoo R, et al. Onconephrology 2022: An Update. Kidney360. 2023;4:258-71.
6. Coiffier B, Altman A, Pui CH, et al. Guidelines for the management of pediatric and adult tumor lysis syndrome. J Clin Oncol. 2008;26:2767-78.
7. Flum AS, Hamoui N, Said MA, et al. Update on the diagnosis and management of renal angiomyolipoma. J Urol. 2016;195:834-46.
8. Gupta S, Cortazar FB, Riella LV, et al. Immune checkpoint inhibitor nephrotoxicity: Update 2020. Kidney360. 2023;4:258-71.
9. Jan de Beur SM, Minisola S, Xia WB, et al. Global guidance for the recognition, diagnosis, and management of tumor-induced osteomalacia. J Intern Med. 2023;293:309-28.
10. Nelson MV, van den Heuvel-Eibrink MM, Graf N, Dome JS. New approaches to risk stratification for Wilms tumor. Curr Opin Pediatr. 2021;33:40-8.
11. Pater L, Melchior P, Rübe C, et al. Wilms tumor. Pediatr Blood Cancer. 2021;68 Suppl 2:e28257.

CHAPTER 31

Diseases of the Newborn

Arvind Bagga, Jitendra Meena

The physiology of the developing kidney and specific metabolic features of a newborn are altered by various pathologic conditions. Disease affecting the kidney may be inherited or congenital or related to certain key events occurring in the intrauterine or perinatal periods. Consequently, the practice of neonatal nephrology has features quite distinct from "classic" pediatric nephrology.

NORMAL RENAL FUNCTION

The principal function of the fetal kidney is to maintain adequate amount of fluid in the amniotic cavity. A normal volume of amniotic fluid, mostly consisting of fetal urine, is necessary for fetal lung growth and allows the fetus to exercise its joints and muscles. Severe fetal oliguria may be associated with pulmonary hypoplasia, joint contractures, and other postural deformities. Fetal fluid and electrolyte homeostasis is maintained by the placenta and maternal renal function. Even the anephric fetus is born with normal serum biochemistry, but dies of respiratory failure (secondary to pulmonary hypoplasia) before developing renal insufficiency. After birth, the neonatal kidney must adapt rapidly to conserve water, excrete waste products of metabolism, and regulate acid-base and electrolyte balance. Fortunately, the kidneys of the healthy, term infant can perform these roles with remarkable efficiency.

Renal Blood Flow and Glomerular Filtration

Renal vascular resistance in the fetus is high, and the kidneys receive only 2–4% of cardiac output compared with 15–18% in the newborn and 20–25% in the adult. The effective ultrafiltration pressure is low, only a few mm Hg, and ultrafiltration coefficient is small. Compensatory mechanisms (increase in prostaglandins and nitric oxide) enable dilatation of afferent arterioles and constriction of efferent arterioles.

Glomerular filtration begins by 9–12 weeks of gestation, initiating formation of urine and contributing to the amniotic fluid. Transition from the fetal to newborn state causes a sudden rise in glomerular filtration rate (GFR). This is chiefly due to an increase in the blood flow to the outer renal cortex and thus an increase in the number of functioning nephrons providing a greater glomerular capillary surface area for filtration. Angiotensin II and prostaglandins, which are present in abundant concentration, play a key role in increasing GFR following birth. The former causes vasoconstriction of efferent arterioles, increasing glomerular pressure. Prostaglandins cause vasodilation of afferent arterioles. There also occurs a decrease in blood levels of vasoactive substances, such as catecholamines and angiotensin. The GFR is low at birth (20–40 mL/min/1.73 m^2 in the first 3 days in the term infant), more so in the premature infant (10–15 mL/min/1.73 m^2). GFR values double (35–45 mL/min/1.73 m^2) at the end of 2 weeks, but do not reach adult levels before 2 years of life. Maturation of glomeruli is usually slow in preterm neonates, and may take up to 8 years to reach adult level GFR. Premature infants experience rapid rise in GFR at 34–36 postconceptual age correlating with completion of nephrogenesis at same age.

The serum creatinine level is high at birth, reflecting maternal values. These levels may rise during the first few days, more so in very premature infants, because of passive creatinine reabsorption through leaky immature tubules, but decrease to 0.5–0.6 mg/dL by the end of the second week. Reference values for serum creatinine have been published for children below 1 year of age **(Table 31.1)**.

TABLE 31.1: Normal values of serum creatinine (mg/dL) in infancy

Age	*Median*	*10th centile*	*90th centile*
Day 1	0.62	0.49	0.79
Day 2	0.53	0.41	0.68
Day 3	0.48	0.37	0.61
Day 4	0.44	0.35	0.57
Day 5	0.42	0.33	0.54
Day 6	0.41	0.32	0.52
Day 7	0.38	0.31	0.50
Week 2	0.35	0.27	0.45
Week 3	0.32	0.25	0.41
Week 4	0.28	0.23	0.36
Month 2	0.25	0.19	0.33
Month 3	0.23	0.18	0.29
Months 4–6	0.23	0.18	0.29
Months 7–9	0.23	0.18	0.29
Months 10–12	0.24	0.19	0.31

Source: Boer DP, et al. 2010.

Tubular Function

During the first week of life, tubular function follows a pattern similar to GFR, but at a still lower level. A pronounced difference between prenatal and postnatal tubular function is in the rate of absorption of filtered sodium. Fractional excretion of sodium (FENa) is a measure of the ability to reabsorb sodium; at birth this is <2%. In the fetus at midgestation, FENa is high and may exceed 10%. Associated with the low sodium reabsorption, is limited bicarbonate reabsorption and, consequently, reduced hydrogen ion excretion. Term babies respond appropriately to an acid load, but the renal threshold for bicarbonate is lower than in older infants and the usual serum bicarbonate concentration is about 20 mEq/L. Serum bicarbonate concentration is even lower in preterm infants up to 15 mEq/L, chiefly due to immature tubular acidification in the proximal tubules. There is a considerable increase in bicarbonate reabsorption in the postnatal period, chiefly contributed by sodium hydrogen anion exchanger (NHE3) and H^+-ATPase activity. The pH of urine of a newborn is inappropriately high for the degree of acidosis.

As in adults, dibasic sodium phosphate and ammonia buffer the hydrogen ion excretion that is not balanced by bicarbonate reabsorption. In artificially fed babies, because of the higher phosphorus intake, phosphate excretion is higher. Since the dibasic phosphate can buffer hydrogen ions, the artificially fed baby has a better capacity to counteract acidosis. This compensates for the greater acid load imposed by artificial feeds compared to breast milk. Although the fetus produces urine with an osmolality <180 mOsm/kg, it can reduce free water clearance in response to maternal dehydration, or if there is decrease in net transplacental fluid transport. The reduction in urine output and amniotic fluid volume can be detected by ultrasound.

An important challenge during early postnatal life relates to conserving water. During fetal life, water is available in abundance, while after birth, the infant receives little fluid for several days and, thereafter, a relatively fixed intake of 120–150 mL/kg/day. If the concentrating capacity does not improve swiftly, the infant will enter a state of hypertonic dehydration in response to minor reductions in fluid intake or increase in fluid loss. In the mature kidney, urine concentration depends upon medullary hypertonicity, which may exceed 1,000 mOsm/kg. Water absorption from the tubule into the hypertonic medulla is controlled by the permeability of the tubular membrane to water, which is increased in the presence of antidiuretic hormone (ADH). The main factor preventing urine concentration in neonates is the relatively low tonicity of the medullary interstitium, providing a poor osmotic gradient across the tubular membrane. Thus, even in the presence of ADH, the highest urine osmolality is 350 mOsm/kg. There is rapid increase in the concentrations of urea and sodium in the renal medulla after birth that is paralleled by increasing ability to concentrate urine to 650 mOsm/kg by 1 week, and 900 mOsm/kg by 1 month of age. The newborn can dilute his urine to a minimum of 50 mOsm/kg much like the older child, but the absolute time taken to excrete a given water load is longer in the infant.

Plasma Osmolality

Changes in plasma osmolality during the first few days of life are related to the type of feeds. If the feeds are concentrated, the plasma osmolality rises, indicating that the capacity of the kidneys to concentrate urine is limited. Therefore, delayed feeding and diluted or concentrated feeds are potentially harmful; breastfeeding is the best option.

Renal function continues to improve during the first 2 years of life. At the end of this period, various parameters of renal function approach adult values, if corrected to standard surface area. *Structural maturation parallels functional maturation.*

Adequacy of Kidney Function in the Neonate

Kidney function is subnormal by adult standards, but adequate for the needs because neonates produce proportionately much less urea than do adults. This is partly because the solute content of human milk is low, but mainly because neonates grow rapidly (proteins and other nutrients are incorporated into tissue building), and produce less waste products of metabolism. The effect of growth in reducing the demands placed on the kidney has led to growth being referred to as the "third kidney". However, if an infant is given a high protein diet, the kidney function may prove inadequate. This is likely in the premature infants in whom the kidney is particularly incompetent to handle high osmolal load. Since kidneys can achieve only a limited concentration, a large volume of water will be lost with the solutes. This would result in dehydration and azotemia if the infant is on an insufficient water intake, especially in high ambient temperatures.

Kidney Function in Preterm Infants

With advances in neonatal care and survival of premature infants, problems associated with immature kidney function have become more apparent. Infants with greatest handicaps are those born at >30 weeks of gestation and weighing below 1,500 g. Nephrogenesis is not completed until about 34–36 weeks of gestation, hence this process in preterms is completed during extrauterine life while being exposed to suboptimal environment for nephrogenesis. Before 34 weeks, blood flow to the renal cortex is low. Consequently, the GFR of very low birth weight (VLBW) infants is <25% of that in the term infant when adjusted for surface area. Reference values for GFR (mL/min/1.73 m^2) in preterm infants (27–31 weeks of gestation) are 8–30 on day 7, 11–33 on day 14, 12–35 on day 21, and 15–38 on day 28.

The rapid postnatal increase in GFR observed in term infants is not seen in the VLBW baby. Serum creatinine levels are higher and take several weeks to stabilize and reflect the true GFR.

Sepsis, hypoxia, hypotension, patent ductus arteriosus, mechanical ventilation, acidosis, exposure to nephrotoxic medications, and catabolism impose burdens in the sick infant. As a result, sick VLBW infants show high urea and creatinine concentrations despite adequate hydration. Indomethacin and high-dose dopamine may further reduce the GFR. Dexamethasone, used for therapy of bronchopulmonary dysplasia, has a catabolic effect and may result in increased levels of blood urea. Low GFR requires dose adjustment of most prescribed drugs and careful monitoring for drug toxicity.

Tubular Function in Very Low Birth Weight Babies

Urinary sodium losses are high, with FENa ~2–6%. Unless sodium concentrations are monitored carefully and appropriate replacement given, hyponatremia may occur. Increased urinary losses of sodium prevent normal growth rates from being achieved unless the dietary sodium intake is adequate. The problem of hyponatremia is aggravated by excessive water intake. Breast milk contains insufficient sodium for many growing VLBW babies and often needs supplementation. Serum potassium concentrations rise in the first 24–72 hr in premature infants, due to its shift from the intracellular to extracellular space; the increase being proportional to the degree of immaturity.

The concentrating capacity of the VLBW kidney limits the maximum urine osmolality to 300 mOsm/kg; hypertonic dehydration may thus develop if excess fluid losses occur. Large insensible water loss through poorly keratinized immature skin is a major predisposing factor. Careful balancing of fluid and electrolyte intake, guided by the results of laboratory tests, is necessary for maintaining electrolyte homeostasis.

Plasma calcium levels fall after birth, being lowest at 24–48 hr, and clinically significant hypocalcemia may develop in very premature infants, asphyxiated babies and infants of diabetic mothers. Calcium excretion through kidneys is greater in VLBW babies than in more mature infants, which predisposes them to both inadequate bone mineralization and nephrocalcinosis. Hypercalciuria is aggravated by the use of frusemide. Bone mineral content can be improved by close attention to the supply of phosphate and the ratio of calcium to phosphate in the diet. As long as calcium and phosphate are incorporated into bone at a satisfactory rate, renal losses are minimized.

Maintaining normal acid-base balance is a problem for the VLBW infant. The renal threshold for bicarbonate is low; hence, the value for plasma bicarbonate in VLBW babies is between 15 and 20 mEq/L. The capacity of the kidney to produce ammonia and titratable acid is also limited. Lactic acidosis due to tissue hypoxia and hypercarbia following respiratory insufficiency worsens the acidosis.

Effect of Intrauterine Growth Restriction

Nephrogenesis requires a balance of many factors that can be disturbed by intrauterine growth restriction (IUGR), leading to a low nephron endowment. Since nephrogenesis goes on till 32–36 weeks of gestation, early onset growth restriction affects both branching morphogenesis and nephrogenesis. Late onset (asymmetric) IUGR only affects nephrogenesis. Infant born with asymmetric IUGR can have almost 30–35% fewer nephrons compared to their healthy counterparts. The compensatory hyperfiltration in the remaining nephrons results in glomerular and systemic hypertension. The hyperfiltration is attributed to several factors, including the renin–angiotensin system (RAS), insulin-like growth factor (IGF-1) and nitric oxide. Data from human and animal studies suggest that IUGR results in faltering of the IGF-1 axis and an inhibited RAS. Hyperfiltration makes the kidney more vulnerable during additional kidney disease and is associated with glomerular damage and kidney failure. IUGR is associated with various diseases in adulthood, such as hypertension, cardiovascular disease, insulin resistance, and end-stage renal disease. Use of RAS inhibitors may prevent compensatory glomerular hyperfiltration and result in adverse long-term outcomes.

ASSESSMENT OF KIDNEY FUNCTION

Fetal urine production occurs between 9 and 10 weeks of gestation. The urine is hypotonic relative to fetal serum due to selective absorption of sodium and chloride in excess of free water. Before 16 weeks, the kidneys contribute little to the amniotic fluid, thereafter fetal urine is the major component of amniotic fluid. On sonography, normal kidneys become visible by 15–17 weeks. After 20 weeks, the kidneys have distinct architecture their growth can be estimated based on kidney length. Normal standards of kidney length at various gestational ages are available. *The length of the fetal kidney in mm or twice its anteroposterior diameter (APD) in mm approximates the fetal age in weeks.* Fetal bladder, detected along with the kidneys, is initially empty. If over a period the bladder is not seen, an abnormality should be suspected. The maximum bladder volume at term is about 40 mL and the fetus appears to void on an hourly cycle. Amniotic fluid volume is a good indicator of renal function and increasing oligohydramnios is associated with pulmonary hypoplasia and poor postnatal outcome.

About 92% of neonates pass urine within the first 48 hr. A healthy infant excretes 15–30 mL/kg/day urine on the first 2 days and 25–120 mL/kg/day during the next 4 weeks, depending upon solute intake. Urine volume <1 mL/kg/hr is oliguria. Formal evaluation of kidney function can be done

TABLE 31.2: Normal range of renal functions

	Preterm		*Term infants*		*1 year*
	First 3 days	*0–3 days*	*2 weeks*	*8 weeks*	
Urine output, mL/kg/day	15–75	20–75	25–120	80–130	40–100
Peak urine osmolality, mOsm/kg	400–500	500–600	700–800	1,000–1,200	1,200–1,400
Glomerular filtration rate, mL/min/1.73 m^2	10–15	15–20	35–45	75–80	90–110

relatively early during the first month of life. **Table 31.2** lists the normal range of renal functions. After the first week of life, when the initial decline from the maternal serum creatinine concentration is complete, the neonatal creatinine correlates with GFR. The fall in serum creatinine is slower in premature infants. Blood urea level is a function of metabolic state, protein load and changes in extracellular volume and is a poor indicator of GFR.

The FENa in the term newborn is normally <2% and may be higher (2–6%) in preterm infants. However, values of FENa overlap in newborns with and without acute kidney injury (AKI), which limits its usefulness compared to older children and adults. Urinary calcium excretion is estimated in terms of spot calcium to creatinine ratio. The ratio is greater in infants than in older children or adults, and is higher in preterm than in term infants. Urine osmolality can be measured following intranasal administration of desmopressin (DDAVP). Urine pH changes in response to plasma bicarbonate concentration and urinary acidification can be assessed.

ACUTE KIDNEY INJURY

Acute kidney injury is defined by a sudden decline in function resulting in inability of kidneys to maintain fluid and electrolyte homeostasis. AKI has replaced the term acute renal failure (ARF) with emphasis on early detection and prevention. AKI is commonly diagnosed, since survival of sick, low birth weight infants is increasing. The incidence of AKI in neonatal intensive care units (NICUs) is approximately 30%, the highest burden being observed in early preterm and asphyxiated term infants. Despite better management, the mortality in neonates (~30%) with AKI is high compared to older children (~10%).

A lack of universally accepted definition of AKI limited our ability to compare studies, predict clinical course and improve outcomes. In 2004, a working definition of AKI was proposed comprising of the risk, injury, failure, loss, and end-stage renal disease (RIFLE). This classification, extensively studied in critically ill adult populations, showed that AKI has an independent impact upon survival. In 2007, the Acute Kidney Injury

Network (AKIN) proposed a staging system, which uses mild AKI (stage 1), moderate AKI (stage 2), and severe AKI (stage 3) that develops over 48 hr, in a way similar to the risk, injury, and failure categories of RIFLE criteria. In 2012, the Kidney Diseases: Improving Global Outcomes (KDIGO) clinical practice guidelines workgroup published a definition that combined aspects of RIFLE and AKIN. Modifications to the KDIGO definition have been made in a proposed neonatal AKI definition **(Table 31.3)**. Urine output <0.5 mL/kg/hr is not a sensitive marker of AKI in neonates; output <1.0 mL/kg/hr has been proposed.

Causes

The etiology of neonatal can be categorized into three subgroups. First and most common is impaired perfusion of kidneys including hypoxemia, hypovolemia, and hypotension. Intrinsic kidney and postrenal cause of AKI are less common in neonates, unlike older children. Perinatal hypoxemia, associated with birth asphyxia or respiratory distress syndrome, accounts for most cases of prerenal AKI **(Box 31.1)**. AKI occurs in 40–50% of neonates with perinatal asphyxia. Neonates with late deceleration of fetal heart rate, 5-minute Apgar score <4 and base deficit >15 mEq/L at 1 hr after birth are at risk of developing AKI. Another important cause is hypovolemia (secondary to dehydration, intraventricular hemorrhage, and heart disease) and intravascular volume depletion following surgery for cardiac and other congenital defects. Hypovolemia might follow insensible losses (use of phototherapy, radiant warmers), twin-to-twin transfusions, and placental hemorrhage. Neonates may show hypernatremic dehydration and AKI due to delayed initiation of breastfeeding, lack of additional fluid intake, and exposure to excessive heat. AKI may occur following surgery for congenital heart disease. Neonates with patent ductus arteriosus are at risk of AKI due to the primary disease, and nephrotoxicity caused by therapeutic agents such as indomethacin.

TABLE 31.3: Proposed classification for neonatal acute kidney injury

Stage	*Serum creatinine (SCr)*	*Urine output*
0	No change in SCr or increase by <0.3 mg/dL	>1 mL/kg/hr
1	SCr increase by ≥0.3 mg/dL within 48-hr or SCr increase to ≥1.5–1.9 × reference SCr[a] within 7 days	>0.5[b] and ≤1 mL/kg/hr for 24-hr
2	SCr increase to ≥2–2.9 × reference SCr[a]	>0.3 and ≤0.5 mL/kg/hr for 24-hr
3	SCr increase to ≥3 × reference SCr[a], or SCr ≥2.5 mg/dL, or receipt of dialysis	<0.3 mL/kg/hr for 24-hr

[a]Reference SCr is defined as the lowest previous serum creatinine value
[b]Some experts recommend using <1 mL/kg/hr instead of 0.5 mL/kg/hr for urine output
Source: Zappitelli M, et al. 2017

BOX 31.1: Common causes of acute kidney injury in neonates

Renal ischemia
Perinatal asphyxia
Hemorrhage and antepartum hemorrhage
Hypotension, shock, and septicemia
Congestive heart failure and persistent fetal circulation
Major surgery
Congenital heart disease
Respiratory distress syndrome
Twin-to-twin transfusion
Hemoglobinuria
Necrotizing enterocolitis

Congenital anomalies and obstruction
Polycystic kidney disease
Bilateral renal agenesis
Posterior urethral valves
Renal tubular dysgenesis
Glomerulocystic kidneys
Uric acid nephropathy

Renovascular
Renal venous thrombosis
Renal artery occlusion

Medications
Aminoglycosides
Amphotericin B
Piperacillin-tazobactam
Vancomycin
Indomethacin
Maternal angiotensin-converting enzyme (ACE) inhibitors

Acute kidney injury may be the initial manifestation of a congenital anomaly of the urinary tract. Medications in the ICU, including aminoglycosides, indomethacin, enalapril, and furosemide, might increase the risk of AKI. Use of nonsteroidal anti-inflammatory drugs (NSAIDs) or angiotensin-converting enzyme (ACE) inhibitors in the mother may lead to fetopathy in which hypotension and AKI is prominent.

Renal Venous Thrombosis

Renal vein thrombosis (RVT) can cause AKI in neonates. Predisposing factors include prematurity, maternal diabetes, perinatal asphyxia, dehydration, sepsis, cyanotic heart disease, polycythemia, *in utero* death of twin, and catheterization of umbilical veins. Protein C or S deficiency, homocystinuria, and rare hereditary diseases should be considered in the differential diagnosis. Thromboses begin in the small renal veins (interlobular and arcuate) and progressively involve the main renal vein. During early stages, there is no renal enlargement, but later a mass may be palpable.

The classic triad of symptoms, i.e., a flank mass, macroscopic hematuria, and thrombocytopenia, is present in 25% infants with RVT. Other features include microscopic hematuria, proteinuria, oligoanuria, and hypertension; microangiopathic hemolytic anemia and thrombocytopenia are present. Ultrasonography shows enlarged and echogenic kidneys; early abnormalities with interlobular thrombi appear as echogenic streaks, and later thrombi in the renal vein and inferior vena cava. Color Doppler study shows attenuation of intrarenal and renal blood flow.

In neonates with unilateral thrombosis with extension into the inferior vena cava, systemic anticoagulation with unfractionated heparin (100 IU/kg IV; 25 IU/kg/hr thereafter) or low molecular weight heparin (1 mg/kg/dose twice daily) is recommended. In the absence of renal impairment or extension into the inferior vena cava, either anticoagulation or supportive cares are acceptable approaches. Supportive care consists of maintenance of fluid and electrolyte balance and radiologic monitoring for extension of thrombus. For bilateral thrombi, either anticoagulation only or initial thrombolytic therapy with tissue plasminogen activator followed by anticoagulation is recommended. Duration of heparin therapy should be between 6 weeks and 3 months. Activated partial thromboplastin time is maintained at 1.5–2 times normal. The role of surgical thrombectomy is limited. Recanalization of the thrombus and partial return of renal blood flow usually follows, with variable loss of renal function. Bilateral renal venous thrombosis may lead to chronic kidney disease.

Renal Necrosis

The clinical features of cortical or medullary necrosis include AKI with oligoanuria and hematuria. The causes are related to hypoperfusion (severe birth asphyxia, hypovolemia, and shock). Ultrasound with Doppler is useful in evaluation and differentiation from RVT and renal artery occlusion. Cortical calcifications may be seen later. The long-term outcome is unsatisfactory. Renal recovery may occur in patients with patchy cortical necrosis.

Clinical Features

The chief feature is oliguria but, in many patients, the AKI is nonoliguric. Edema is present if excessive fluid has been administered. With progression of renal failure, hyperkalemia with cardiac arrhythmias, acidotic breathing, vomiting, and poor feeding may be present. Seizures are not uncommon, often due to hypoxia, intracranial hemorrhage, hypoglycemia, hypocalcemia, hypertension, and uremia.

Neonates with acute tubular necrosis have microscopic hematuria; the frequency of this finding is greater than in adults and older children. Proteinuria is mild. Neonates with bilateral renal agenesis or severe dysplasia have Potter facies (beaked nose, wide-set eyes with a prominent fold arising from the inner canthus, and low-set ears) and history of oligohydramnios. Those with hydronephrosis, multicystic and autosomal recessive polycystic kidneys have enlarged kidneys. RVT should be suspected in an asphyxiated or dehydrated neonate or in polycythemia. If blood pressure is high, renal artery thrombosis should be suspected. Features suggestive of urinary tract obstruction include abdominal mass, hypertension, oligoanuria or polyuria, poor urine stream, ascites, septicemia, and metabolic acidosis.

Diagnostic Evaluation

Neonates at risk of developing AKI should be closely monitored. Urine output is measured with urine collection bag or condom drainage. Up to 60% neonates with AKI secondary to asphyxia or drug toxicity can have normal urine output. Unless plasma creatinine levels are monitored, nonoliguric AKI may be missed. However, physicians should be aware that creatinine levels are high at birth (reflecting maternal creatinine) and decrease to 0.4 mg/dL over the next 2–3 weeks. Failure to achieve the expected fall in creatinine or rapid rise suggests impaired renal function. Several indices **(Table 31.4)** help differentiate functional AKI from established intrinsic kidney injury. While FENa is a reliable test, it is not useful in patients with nonoliguric AKI and in those receiving diuretics. Extremely premature neonates normally have a high FENa (>3%).

Since the incidence of AKI continues to increase, while the outcomes remain unsatisfactory, there is interest in the role of newer urine and serum biomarkers. Current standard of care functional biomarker for detection of AKI is serum creatinine but it rises late, almost 48–72 hr after initiation of kidney injury. Some promising biomarkers which may aid in early detection

TABLE 31.4: Indices used to differentiate prerenal from intrinsic acute kidney injury (AKI)

	Prerenal	*Intrinsic AKI*
Urinary sodium, mEq/L	<20	>40
Urinary osmolality, mOsm/kg	>400	<300
Blood urea to creatinine ratio	>20:1	<20:1
Urine to plasma osmolality ratio	>2	<1
Fractional excretion of sodium (FENa), %	<2	>3

$$\text{FENa \%} = \frac{\text{Urine sodium} \times \text{serum creatinine}}{\text{Serum sodium} \times \text{urine creatinine}} \times 100$$

of AKI are serum and urine neutrophil gelatinase-associated lipocalin (NGAL), urine interleukin-18 (IL-18) and kidney injury molecule-1 (KIM-1), and serum cystatin C. However, considering the diverse etiology of neonatal AKI, it is unlikely that one biomarker of kidney injury can be used for all. These biomarkers need to be used in specific clinical contexts, which require further studies before they can be incorporated in clinical care.

Initial Management

Once functional AKI is suspected, immediate treatment is essential. Fluid replacement is undertaken after excluding congestive cardiac failure and urinary tract obstruction. Central venous pressure monitoring is the ideal guide to fluid administration, but might not be readily available. About 15–20 mL/kg of isotonic saline or Ringer lactate is infused over 60–90 minutes. In tiny premature babies, 10–20 mL/kg may be given. Vital signs are monitored, and care taken to avoid overhydration. If no diuresis occurs, the same amount of fluid is again administered cautiously, unless the neonate has signs of fluid overload. If urine output is <1 mL/kg/hr after 2 hr that does not respond to administration of 1–2 mg/kg of furosemide, intrinsic renal failure is suspected and appropriate management instituted.

Infants with hypotension or congestive cardiac failure need inotropic support. This may be achieved with dopaminergic agents. The effect of these agents is dose dependent. At low doses, the medication (0.5–2 µg/kg/min) causes renal vasodilation and increases sodium and water excretion. Medium (2–6 µg/kg/min) or high (6–10 µg/kg/min) doses increase cardiac output, mean arterial blood pressure, and renal vascular resistance. Caution is needed when using dopamine in newborns. The sensitivity of α-receptors is high in premature neonates and relatively low doses of dopamine (2 µg/kg/min) result in increased systemic blood pressure. Systematic reviews fail to show a favorable effect of low-dose dopamine infusion on prevention or treatment of AKI, patient survival or outcome. Therapy with low-dose dopamine for prevention or treatment of neonatal AKI is, therefore, not recommended.

Experimental studies have established an important role for adenosine mediated vasoconstriction of the afferent arteriole in neonatal kidneys exposed to hypoxemia due to perinatal asphyxia, leading to decreased renal blood flow and GFR. Prophylactic therapy with adenosine receptor antagonist, theophylline, reduces the incidence of AKI in term neonates with severe birth asphyxia. A single dose of theophylline (5–8 mg/kg) is recommended in neonates with severe perinatal asphyxia for preventing AKI.

Tests useful in differentiating intrinsic from postrenal AKI are ultrasonography and micturating cystourethrogram (MCU). The former identifies renal agenesis or dysplasia, hydronephrosis, and distended urinary bladder. MCU helps diagnose posterior urethral valves (PUV), bladder anomalies and vesicoureteric reflux (VUR). A Doppler study is done to detect RVT.

Subsequent Management

The principles of management of AKI in neonates are similar to those for older children.

Fluid and Electrolyte Balance

Fluid administered should be limited to insensible losses (30 mL/kg per day for full term, 50–100 mL/kg per day for preterm neonates) and gastrointestinal or renal losses. Evaporative losses are reduced in the baby receiving humidified air and increased in those with fever, tachypnea, or under a radiant warmer. Fluids administered during procedures such as endotracheal tube lavage, catheter flushes, and intravenous (IV) medications should be included. Body weight is the best guide, and the neonate should be weighed every 12 hr. Blood levels of electrolytes, calcium, and phosphate should be monitored. With optimum fluid and electrolyte management, the level of serum sodium should remain normal. Hyperkalemia (potassium >6.0 mEq/L) is an important complication that needs to be managed urgently. Interventions that redistribute potassium: insulin and glucose, and nebulized salbutamol or albuterol are effective in neonates. Other beneficial interventions include elimination of potassium through exchange transfusion or peritoneal dialysis. There is limited information on the benefits of rectal or oral administration of ion exchange resins in newborns.

Systolic blood pressure >95–100 mm Hg is abnormal and needs treatment. For hypertensive crisis, sodium nitroprusside or labetalol infusion is satisfactory. Hydralazine, atenolol, and nifedipine are effective drugs for oral therapy. There is limited evidence regarding the beneficial effects of diuretics in the treatment of incipient or established fluid overload in oliguric or nonoliguric AKI. While administration of furosemide (1–2 mg/kg IV) might result in diuresis, this has no impact on the overall outcome of these patients. Therefore, the routine use of furosemide for neonates with AKI is not recommended.

Nutrition

Provision of adequate calories, proteins, and micronutrients is crucial in neonates with prolonged AKI. A protein intake of 0.6 g/kg/day (1.5 g/kg in babies on dialysis) is advised. Calories can be supplemented with lipid emulsions. Parenteral nutrition may be required. Optimizing nutrition aids in early recovery from AKI.

Kidney Support Therapy

Indications: The most common indications to initiate kidney support therapy are fluid and electrolyte imbalance such as hyperkalemia, hypernatremia, and metabolic acidosis that are refractory to medical therapy. Complications due to uremia also require kidney support therapy. Since fluid overload has been reported to increase risk of mortality, experts suggest that patients with AKI and fluid overload of 10–20% should be considered for kidney support therapy even in absence of other urgent indications.

Modalities: Peritoneal dialysis, hemodialysis, or hemofiltration are commonly used modalities. These modalities can be used either intermittently (hemodialysis) or continuously [peritoneal dialysis or continuous kidney replacement therapy (CKRT)]. Choice of modality is influenced by cost, available infrastructure, center specific expertise, patients need, and any potential contraindications.

Most neonates with AKI are treated with peritoneal dialysis, which is technically easy. The gradual fluid removal and correction of metabolic derangement by peritoneal dialysis offers an advantage in sick infants. Soft catheters that are less traumatic and less prone to fluid leaks and infections are preferred. Soft femoral venous catheters, placed using Seldinger technique, may be safely and effectively used for acute peritoneal dialysis. Chronic indwelling soft Tenckhoff peritoneal catheters, having one or two cuffs, are used if more than a few days of dialysis are expected. The procedure is begun with small volumes (10–20 mL/kg per cycle) and increased (30–40 mL/kg) as tolerated. Larger volumes increase dialysis efficiency, but may cause respiratory distress, apnea, and rarely hydrothorax. Accurate measurement of dialysate volumes is essential. Hypothermia should be avoided by warming the dialysis fluid and use of radiant warmer. Glucose concentrations in the dialysate range between 1.5 and 3.5 g/dL. High glucose concentrations augment the transmembrane osmotic gradient and facilitate ultrafiltration. Neonates should be monitored for hyperglycemia. Most dialysis fluids contain lactate, which hypoxic babies may be unable to metabolize quickly, leading to worsening acidosis. For such babies, bicarbonate dialysate is advised. Unpredictable ultrafiltration rate is the major disadvantage of peritoneal dialysis. Since many drugs are dialyzed, appropriate amounts are added to supplement the dialysate losses **(Annexure 7)**.

Relative contraindications to peritoneal dialysis include the presence of diaphragmatic hernia, pleuroperitoneal connection, necrotizing enterocolitis, bleeding diathesis, systemic hypoperfusion, recent abdominal surgery, and ventriculoperitoneal shunt. The efficacy of peritoneal dialysis may be restricted in neonates with poor cardiac output and insufficient gut perfusion. Neonates with septicemia have increased capillary permeability that permits rapid solute removal and efficient correction of hyperkalemia. Rapid glucose absorption however results in failure of ultrafiltration.

Continuous kidney replacement therapy is useful for management of neonatal AKI with severe fluid overload, and in patients with major surgical procedures, heart failure and shock, if peritoneal dialysis is not feasible. CKRT has become widely used in neonates because of technological advances. This extracorporeal blood purification therapy provides smooth and adjustable control of ultrafiltered volume and gradual correction of metabolic abnormalities.

Solute clearance occurs by provision of replacement fluid only in continuous venovenous hemofiltration (CVVH), by dialysis fluid in continuous venovenous hemodialysis (CVVHD), or by both replacement and dialysis fluid in continuous venovenous hemodiafiltration (CVVHDF). CKRT treatment requires vascular access, hemofilter, anticoagulation, and replacement and dialysate fluids. Access is through a double lumen hemodialysis catheter (7 French) placed in umbilical vein until 4–5 days of age or femoral or internal jugular vein thereafter. Blood is pumped through the hemofilter at 10–12 mL/kg/min. A hemofilter with high ultrafiltration coefficient permits efficient removal of excess fluid in the form of protein free plasma. The ultrafiltered volume is replaced by a balanced electrolyte solution. Systemic anticoagulation is necessary to avoid clotting within the circuit. Placement of an optimally sized vascular access is technically challenging. Provision of CKRT entails a significant proportion of blood volume to be pumped through the extracorporeal circuit which may lead to hypotension or hypothermia.

Until recently CKRT machines were not designed to treat small infants who require low and accurate blood flow rates (10–30 mL/min) with minimal ultrafiltration error. The Cardio-Renal Pediatric Dialysis Emergency Machine (CARPEDIEM) has been developed for provision of CKRT to infants between 2.0 and 9.9 kg. Similarly, the Newcastle Infant Dialysis and Ultrafiltration System (NIDUS) allows effective dialysis and ultrafiltration in infants weighing <8 kg. Now smaller filters with lower extracorporeal volume are available to be used in CRRT circuits such as HF20 in Prismaflex CKRT device.

Intermittent hemodialysis (HD) is an effective modality for solute clearance. Intermittent HD is used uncommonly in neonates as rapid removal of solute and fluid in short duration leads to hemodynamic instability. However, when infrastructure for CKRT is not available and peritoneal dialysis is contraindicated, intermittent HD can be done using priming to reduce the risk of hemodynamic instability.

Outcomes

A majority of neonates with AKI without associated serious complications may require only one dialysis over 48 hr and recover in the next 7–10 days. Others with sepsis, consumption coagulopathy, and anuria beyond a week might need prolonged dialysis. Some patients have renal cortical necrosis and might not regain significant renal function. In such cases, the management is guided by kidney biopsy findings and consideration of status of other organs. The mortality in neonates with oliguric AKI is 30–50%; survival of those with nonoliguric AKI is better. About 40% neonates who recover have residual renal damage manifested by structural, glomerular, or tubular abnormalities or hypertension. The outcome is related to the underlying condition, being unsatisfactory in neonates with severe congenital renal and extrarenal anomalies, disseminated intravascular coagulation, and shock.

Some neonates recovering from AKI may show initial improvement in kidney function during the first year of life. Hypoxic ischemic insults mainly affect the mature nephrons and spare the immature glomeruli. The latter may continue to develop after recovery from AKI resulting in an apparent increase in the GFR. With the passage of time, however, the growth potential of the kidneys is exhausted, and deterioration of renal function may ensue. A considerable proportion of these neonates, especially those born premature or low birth weight can develop long-term complications such as chronic kidney disease and hypertension. *Hence, all neonates with stage 2 or 3 AKI require follow-up, with periodic estimation of blood pressure, blood creatinine, and urine protein to creatinine ratio.* Ultrasound examination is advised at 6–12 months intervals to detect anatomic abnormalities and examine renal growth.

HYPERTENSION

Blood pressure increases with birth weight, gestational and postnatal age, and neonate's state of activity. The blood pressure should be obtained when the baby is sleeping and with a proper sized cuff using the auscultatory method. Noninvasive automated oscillometric method is considered quite reliable. In acutely ill neonates, blood pressure is monitored directly *via* an indwelling arterial catheter either in the radial or umbilical artery. While definitions of hypertension in early infancy are not standardized, recent studies have provided normative data that may be used to diagnose hypertension **(Table 31.5)**. Blood pressure is considered elevated if it is above the 95th percentile for neonates of similar postconception age.

Hypertension is detected in 1–2% neonates in the NICU. Renovascular and renal parenchymal disorders account for most cases **(Box 31.2)**. Umbilical artery catheterization, complicated by aortic or renal arterial thrombi, is an important cause. Other conditions include renovascular causes, congenital and acquired renal diseases, and bronchopulmonary dysplasia. Hypertension is detected on routine monitoring, but may cause congestive cardiac failure, cardiogenic shock, feeding difficulties, tachypnea, apnea, or seizures.

TABLE 31.5: Values for blood pressure after 2 weeks of age, from 26 to 44 weeks postconception age

Postconception age		***50th centile***	***95th centile***	***99th centile***
26 weeks	Systolic	55	72	77
	Diastolic	30	50	56
	Mean	38	57	63
28 weeks	Systolic	60	75	80
	Diastolic	38	50	54
	Mean	45	58	63
30 weeks	Systolic	65	80	85
	Diastolic	40	55	60
	Mean	48	63	68
32 weeks	Systolic	68	83	88
	Diastolic	40	55	60
	Mean	49	64	69
34 weeks	Systolic	70	85	90
	Diastolic	40	55	60
	Mean	50	65	70
36 weeks	Systolic	72	87	92
	Diastolic	50	65	70
	Mean	57	72	77
38 weeks	Systolic	77	92	97
	Diastolic	50	65	70
	Mean	59	74	79
40 weeks	Systolic	80	95	100
	Diastolic	50	65	70
	Mean	60	75	80
42 weeks	Systolic	85	98	102
	Diastolic	50	65	70
	Mean	62	76	81
44 weeks	Systolic	88	105	110
	Diastolic	50	68	73
	Mean	63	80	85

Source: Dionne JM, et al. 2012

Investigations

The cause of hypertension can usually be diagnosed on careful history and physical examination. Urine is examined for presence of renal parenchymal disease. Chest X-ray film and an abdominal ultrasound with

BOX 31.2: Common causes of neonatal hypertension

Renovascular
Umbilical artery catheter-associated thromboembolism
Renal artery stenosis
Renal vein thrombosis

Renal parenchymal disease
Polycystic kidney disease
Multicystic dysplastic kidney
Pelviureteric junction obstruction
Acute tubular and cortical necrosis

Cardiopulmonary
Bronchopulmonary dysplasia
Coarctation of aorta

Miscellaneous
Congenital adrenal hyperplasia
Medications: Dexamethasone, caffeine, theophylline
Wilms tumor and neuroblastoma

Doppler studies should be obtained. Other studies include blood levels of creatinine, electrolytes, pH, bicarbonate, cortisol and aldosterone, and an echocardiogram. Renal scans, MCU, and renal angiogram are performed, as indicated.

Management

Treatment depends upon severity of hypertension. Neonates with severe hypertension are managed with continuous IV infusion of sodium nitroprusside, labetalol, or nicardipine **(Table 31.6)**. Blood pressure is monitored continuously by an indwelling arterial catheter or frequent cuff readings. The rate of the infusion is adjusted to achieve the desired blood pressure; rapid reduction is avoided to prevent cerebral ischemia. It is suggested that one-third of desired blood pressure reduction should be achieved by first 6 hr and rest over the next 48–72 hr. Oral antihypertensive agents are used with less severe hypertension or when hypertension has been controlled with IV infusions. Calcium channel blockers (e.g., amlodipine) are safe agents for blood pressure control. ACE inhibitors are effective in lower doses particularly in the preterm infant, but associated with increased risk of adverse effects such AKI, hyperkalemia, and hypotension. Beta blockers are avoided in neonates with chronic lung disease. Diuretics are useful not only in reducing blood pressure but also in improving pulmonary function. Other drugs include hydralazine and minoxidil. Nifedipine should be used cautiously since it may cause rapid and transient reduction in blood pressure. Surgery, for treatment of hypertension, is indicated uncommonly.

TABLE 31.6: Medications for treatment of neonatal hypertension

Agent	*Dose*	*Route, interval*	*Comments*
Intravenous agents			
Sodium nitroprusside	0.5–6 µg/kg/min	Constant infusion	Thiocyanate toxicity with use >72 hr, and in acute kidney injury
Labetalol	0.2–1 mg/kg/dose 0.2–3 mg/kg/hr	Intravenous bolus Constant infusion	Avoid in heart failure and chronic lung disease
Nicardipine	1–3 µg/kg/min	Constant infusion	Reflex tachycardia
Hydralazine	0.15-0.6 mg/kg/dose	Every 4–6 hr	Vasodilator and tachycardia
Oral agents			
Captopril	0.1–0.5 mg/kg/dose	Thrice daily	Angiotensin-converting enzyme (ACE) inhibitor of choice for neonates
Enalapril	0.01–0.1 mg/kg/dose	Twice daily	Monitor creatinine and potassium
Hydralazine	0.3–1 mg/kg/dose; maximum 7 mg/kg/day	Thrice daily	Tachycardia and fluid retention
Amlodipine	0.1–0.3 mg/kg/dose; maximum 0.6 mg/kg/day	Once, twice daily	Less risk of sudden hypotension
Hydrochloro-thiazide	1–3 mg/kg/dose	Once daily	Monitor electrolytes
Labetalol	0.05-1.0 mg/kg/dose	Twice to thrice daily	Alpha and beta blocker
Minoxidil	0.1–0.2 mg/kg/dose	Twice daily	Potent medication

Outcomes

The outcome for most infants with hypertension is satisfactory. In most patients, blood pressure is normal by 1–2 years of life. Hypertension related to umbilical arterial catheter usually resolves with time. Neonates with renal parenchymal disease and RVT may have persistent hypertension. Hypertension can be detected after discharge; hence, guidelines recommend that in high-risk populations (low birth weight, prematurity, intrauterine growth retardation, and umbilical artery catheterization) blood pressure should be measured at each visit to hospital.

TABLE 31.7: Causes of abdominal mass

Cystic	*Solid*
Multicystic dysplastic kidney	Renal vein thrombosis
Hydronephrosis	Neuroblastoma
Autosomal recessive polycystic kidneys	Mesoblastic nephroma
Intestinal duplication	Hepatoblastoma
Hydrometrocolpos	Teratoma
Adrenal hemorrhage	
Choledochal, ovarian, omental, and pancreatic cysts	

ABDOMINAL MASS

The kidneys may normally be palpable in the first 2–3 months of life. More than 70% of abdominal masses in term neonates are related to the urogenital tract. A multicystic dysplastic kidney is the most common abdominal mass in a neonate. Hydronephrosis may occur due to pelviureteric junction (PUJ) obstruction or severe VUR. Other renal causes include autosomal recessive polycystic kidneys, RVT, mesoblastic nephroma, and congenital Wilms tumor **(Table 31.7)**. PUV may result in a large bladder and occasionally bilaterally palpable kidneys. The prune belly syndrome, almost exclusively seen in boys, is characterized by poorly developed anterior abdominal muscles, bilaterally severe VUR, and cryptorchidism. Important nonrenal conditions include ovarian and mesenteric cysts, teratomas, and hydrometrocolpos. The renal mass should be evaluated by ultrasound and if needed, by renal scintigraphy. An MCU is done to diagnose VUR and infravesical obstruction.

HEMATURIA

Gross hematuria is rare in neonates. The chief causes include hemorrhagic disease of the newborn, urinary tract obstruction, RVT, and renal cortical necrosis. Occasionally, polycystic and multicystic kidneys may be the source of bleeding. Hemangioma of the bladder, Wilms tumor, mesoblastic nephroma, and urinary tract infection (UTI) are rare causes. The high urinary concentration of uric acid in neonates may impart a reddish-pink color to the urine. The intestinal bacterium, *Serratia marcescens,* may also cause a red or pink discoloration of the diaper.

URINARY TRACT INFECTION

The incidence of UTI in the term neonate is approximately 1%, and in the preterm, 3%, both with male preponderance (male to female ratio of 5:1). During infancy, the risk is equal in boys and girls. Majority of UTI in neonates are due to gram-negative bacteria, chiefly *Escherichia coli*; *Candida albicans* infections are seen in preterm infants. Symptoms of UTI are nonspecific in neonates and young infants where a high degree of suspicion is necessary. UTI is often a part of septicemia with features such as fever, lethargy, unstable temperature, diarrhea, vomiting, seizures, shock, and persistent jaundice. Dribbling, poor urinary stream, and a palpable abdominal mass indicate an underlying urinary tract obstruction.

Diagnosis

Leukocyturia is suggestive of UTI, but not reliable for confirming the diagnosis. While combination of urine nitrite and leukocyte esterase has shown good diagnostic accuracy, their utility in neonates is limited due to short incubation period in bladder. *Urine dipsticks are not recommended for screening of UTI in neonates.* The diagnosis of UTI requires isolation of microorganisms on urine culture. Urine collection by bag is convenient, but gives unacceptably high false-positive results. Obtaining clean catch urine is difficult in neonates and reliable ways to get a satisfactory specimen include suprapubic aspiration and bladder catheterization. On clean catch specimens, a colony count of $>10^4$–10^5/mL of a single species confirms the diagnosis. For urine collected by suprapubic aspiration and urethral catheterization, colony counts of 10^3/mL and 10^4/mL, respectively are considered significant. Infants show low colony counts because of frequent voiding, since bacteria do not have enough time to multiply, or prior antibiotic therapy.

Treatment

In patients suspected to have UTI, therapy should start immediately after obtaining urine cultures. Neonates and young infants should receive parenteral antibiotics (cefotaxime or ceftriaxone) for 7–10 days. If the patient is sick or dehydrated, IV fluids are given for the first 24–48 hr. The antibiotic may be changed as per urine culture sensitivity, if there is no clinical response.

Fungal Urinary Tract Infection

Invasive infections require systemic therapy with either amphotericin B or fluconazole. Fungal balls may occasionally obstruct the pelvis or ureters, leading to hydronephrosis and anuria. In such cases, local irrigation, parenteral antifungal agents, and surgical removal of the obstruction may be needed.

Evaluation Following Urinary Tract Infection

All neonates with UTI should be investigated to detect predisposing factors and for presence of anomalies. The aim of these investigations is to identify patients at risk of kidney damage, chiefly those with VUR or urinary tract obstruction. An ultrasound examination to detect major structural anomalies should be performed. In patients with abnormal ultrasound scan (dilated pelvicalyceal system or ureter, discrepancy in kidney size), an MCU is advised to detect primary VUR. An MCU is also done promptly if distal obstruction is suspected. An ^{99m}Tc-dimercaptosuccinic acid (DMSA) scan, highly sensitive for detecting pyelonephritis or kidney scarring, is recommended 4–6 months following UTI to detect permanent kidney scarring. Antibiotic prophylaxis is recommended for neonates with primary VUR.

DISORDERS OF SODIUM METABOLISM

Aldosterone Biosynthetic Defects

The enzymes cholesterol desmolase, 3 β-hydroxysteroid dehydrogenase and 21-hydroxylase are required for synthesis of cortisol and aldosterone in the adrenal cortex. Deficiency of any of these enzymes results in lack of both aldosterone and cortisol. Reduced levels of cortisol result in loss of feedback inhibition of corticotrophin [adrenocorticotropic hormone (ACTH)] and adrenal hyperplasia. Deficiency of 21-hydroxylase is the most common inherited cause of aldosterone deficiency.

Two major forms of the disease due to 21-hydroxylase are described, virilizing, and salt-wasting types. Patients with signs only of androgen excess have the virilizing form. Female infants show varying degrees of pseudohermaphroditism, while affected males have normal or precocious sexual development. The salt-wasting form, with aldosterone deficiency, seen in 60–70% of patients, presents with hyponatremia, hyperkalemia, and moderate to severe volume depletion. Those with markedly low aldosterone may be present in the early neonatal period with dyselectrolytemia and shock. The diagnosis of 21-hydroxylase deficiency should be suspected in any newborn with genital ambiguity, salt-wasting, or hypotension.

Neonates showing dyselectrolytemia and shock require resuscitation with IV fluids and salt supplements. Long-term replacement therapy with oral hydrocortisone (20–25 mg/m^2 daily) and 9α-fludrocortisone (2–5 µg/kg daily; starting dose 0.05 to 0.1 mg, maximum 0.2 mg) is required. Amelioration of the tendency to salt-wasting may be seen with age, due to ability of the children to regulate their dietary salt intake and maturation of proximal tubular function.

Pseudohypoaldosteronism Type 1

This rare condition, characterized by lack of response to mineralocorticoids may occasionally be diagnosed in neonates. Intrauterine polyuria may cause polyhydramnios; patients have polyuria, dehydration, and weight loss. Laboratory findings are hyponatremia, hyperkalemia, acidosis, raised values of plasma renin and aldosterone, and sodium wasting. Treatment consists of oral sodium chloride supplementation that leads to expansion of extracellular fluid volume and increased delivery of sodium to the distal nephron, resulting in increased excretion of potassium. By 2 years of age, salt requirement may decrease.

Pseudohypoaldosteronism (PHA) type 1 may involve only the kidney (autosomal dominant form) or, in the generalized serious recessive disorder also affect sweat glands, salivary glands, and colon. The genetic bases for the dominant and recessive subtypes are distinct. The former involves genes encoding for the mineralocorticoid receptor, whereas the latter involves genes encoding the epithelial sodium channel (ENaC). Similar biochemical features may result from obstructive uropathy or acute pyelonephritis.

Neonatal Bartter Syndrome

Bartter syndrome is characterized by renal salt-wasting, hypokalemic metabolic alkalosis, and low to normal blood pressure. Bartter syndrome is classified into two phenotypic variants, antenatal and classical. The former is more severe, and characterized by polyhydramnios and prematurity as a consequence of fetal polyuria. Recently, a new type of X-linked inherited Bartter syndrome due to pathogenic variants in *MAGED2* has been reported. This is characterized by early-onset severe polyhydramnios and fetal polyuria leading to extreme prematurity. In most patients, the symptoms resolve within few weeks after birth, hence the X-linked form is also known as transient Bartter syndrome. While genetic testing is preferred for antenatal diagnosis, the amniotic fluid Bartter index [total protein (multiple of median) × alpha-fetoprotein (multiple of median) × 1,000] <1.2 suggests the diagnosis. Treatment of Bartter syndrome consists of indomethacin (2 mg/kg/day) , which helps in reducing polyuria, and potassium supplements (3–5 mEq/kg/day).

ANTENATAL DIAGNOSIS OF RENAL AND URINARY TRACT ANOMALIES

The recognition of congenital abnormalities in the fetus has been facilitated by ultrasonography that is now routinely performed during pregnancy. Those involving kidney and urinary tract constitute about 15% of all prenatally detected anomalies. Significant abnormalities of the kidney and urinary tract are found in 1 to 2 per 1,000 live births **(Box 31.3)**. Almost 80% neonates with prenatally detected anomalies are asymptomatic at birth.

URINARY TRACT DILATATION

Dilation of renal collecting system [urinary tract dilatation (UTD)] is the chief anomaly diagnosed on prenatal ultrasonography as early as the second trimester. It includes a spectrum of conditions affecting 1–5% of

BOX 31.3: Anomalies detected on fetal ultrasonography

Unilateral and bilateral hydronephrosis
Pelviureteric junction obstruction
Vesicoureteric reflux
Posterior urethral valves
Ureterovesical junction obstruction
Extrarenal pelvis
Ureteric dilatation and megaureter

Bright and cystic kidneys
Solitary cyst
Polycystic kidney disease
Multicystic kidney

Absent, malformed, and enlarged kidney
Renal agenesis, unilateral, or bilateral
Abnormal renal location and fusion
Hypoplastic kidney
Neuroblastoma and renal tumor

Bladder abnormalities
Persistent enlargement
Ectopic location
Diverticulum

all pregnancies. Majority of the conditions are transient without clinical significance. The management and outcome depends upon the severity, level of obstruction, and if unilateral or bilateral.

Previously hydronephrosis was defined and graded using renal pelvic APD in antenatal period, and by the Society of Fetal Urology (SFU) grading during postnatal evaluation. Currently, the urinary tract dilation (UTD) classification system is most commonly used. This single classification system, proposed in 2014 by multispecialty experts, can be used to assess hydronephrosis in antenatal and postnatal periods. As shown in **Table 31.8** and **Figures 31.1A to E**, the UTD grade of hydronephrosis is based on anteroposterior renal pelvis diameter (APRPD), calyceal dilation, kidney parenchymal thickness and appearance, and ureter and bladder abnormality. The UTD classification has shown satisfactory accuracy in predicting the need for surgery and long-term outcomes.

An APRPD of >4 mm before 28 weeks of gestation and >7 mm after 28 weeks is considered abnormal. If antenatal ultrasound scan shows only abnormal APRPD or central calyceal dilation, then it is graded as UTD A1 (low risk). Higher APRPD (>7 mm in <28 weeks and >10 mm in >28 weeks) and peripheral calyceal dilation upgrades grading to UTD A2–3 (high risk). Presence of kidney parenchymal abnormalities, ureter dilation, or abnormal bladder in combination with any abnormal APRPD upgrades classification to UTD A2–3. As per the UTD classification system, isolated ureteric dilatation even without dilated renal pelvis classified as UTD A2–3 **(Table 31.8)**.

TABLE 31.8: Risk stratification of urinary tract dilation, based on UTD classification system

	Anteroposterior renal pelvis diameter		*Calyceal dilation*	*Parenchymal thickness*	*Parenchymal appearance*	*Ureters*	*Bladder*
Prenatal	16–27 weeks	>28 weeks					
Normal	<4 mm	<7 mm	Normal	Normal	Normal	Normal	Normal
UTD A1	4–7 mm	7–10 mm	Normal	Normal	Normal	Normal	Normal
UTD A2-3*	≥7 mm	≥10 mm	Peripheral	Abnormal	Abnormal	Abnormal	Abnormal
Postnatal							
Normal	<10 mm		None	Normal	Normal	Normal	Normal
UTD P1	≥10–15 mm		Central	Normal	Normal	Normal	Normal
UTD P2	≥15 mm		Peripheral	Normal	Normal	Abnormal	Normal
UTD P3	≥10 mm		Present or absent	Abnormal	Abnormal	Normal or abnormal	Abnormal

*Also include oligohydramnios due to a genitourinary cause

Source: Nguyen HT, et al. 2014

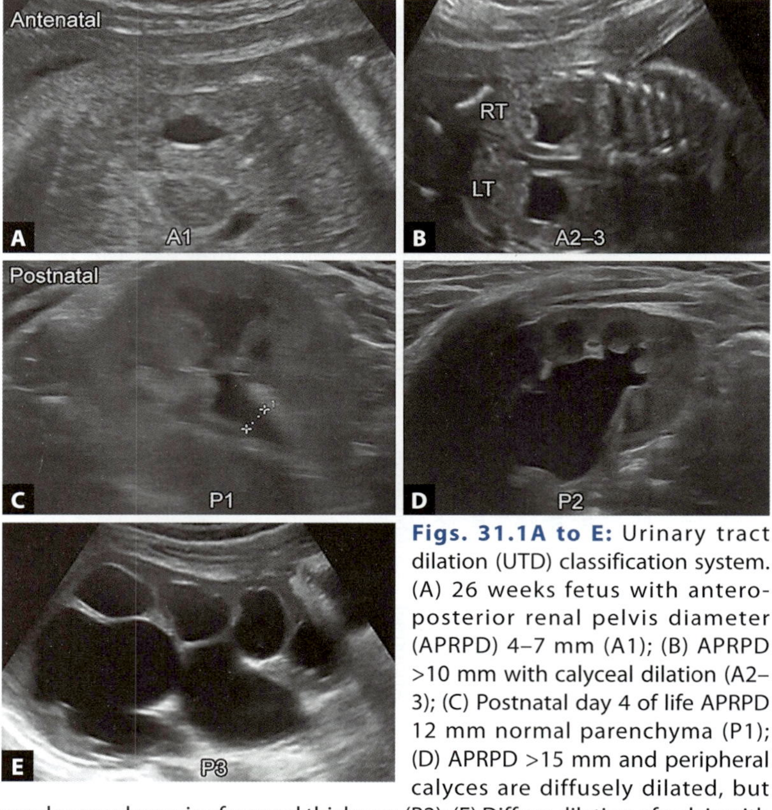

Figs. 31.1A to E: Urinary tract dilation (UTD) classification system. (A) 26 weeks fetus with anteroposterior renal pelvis diameter (APRPD) 4–7 mm (A1); (B) APRPD >10 mm with calyceal dilation (A2–3); (C) Postnatal day 4 of life APRPD 12 mm normal parenchyma (P1); (D) APRPD >15 mm and peripheral calyces are diffusely dilated, but renal parenchyma is of normal thickness (P2); (E) Diffuse dilation of pelvis with thinning of the renal parenchyma over the dilated calyces (P3)

In postnatal period, APRPD of >10 mm is considered abnormal irrespective of age. Hence, APRPD >10 mm and central calyceal dilation is classified as UTD P1. Ultrasound scan showing APRPD >15 mm or peripheral calyceal dilation is classified as UTD P2, and even those with APRPD 10–15 mm but with ureteral dilation are classified as UTD P2. Those with abnormal kidney parenchyma (echogenicity and thickness) and bladder abnormalities are classified as UTD P3.

Fetal UTD may be suggestive of trisomy 21 and other congenital malformation in fetus. Hence, its presence should prompt for focus targeted evaluation of the fetus. Presence of other congenital and/or chromosomal anomalies suggests unsatisfactory outcomes. Obstruction in the lower urinary tract, especially PUV in male infants, is carefully looked for.

Etiology of Urinary Tract Dilation

Imaging studies of prenatally detected hydronephrosis show nonobstructive transient pelvic dilatation in 40–80%, PUJ obstruction in 10–30% and VUR in 9–12%. Rarer causes include megaureter, multicystic dysplastic kidney, ureterocele, and PUV.

Management

Prenatal Intervention

Urinary tract dilation detected in early gestation can resolve or progress, hence, it is suggested that fetus with UTD A1 should be reassessed with ultrasound scan beyond 32 weeks of gestation if first scan was done earlier. Those with UTD A2–3 category should have repeat scan within 4–6 weeks. When features suggestive of PUVs are present, a rapid follow-up scan is required. Attempts have been made to bypass the lower urinary tract obstruction in cases with bilateral hydronephrosis and increasing oligohydramnios. Without prenatal intervention, the mortality is high in such cases. While fetal renal function can be assessed by examining the electrolytes in fetal bladder urine obtained by percutaneous bladder puncture, the role of this investigation is limited. Interventions that are proposed include placing a vesicoamniotic shunt and fetal corrective surgery. Following careful parental counseling, these procedures should be carried out at specialized centers. The results are often unsatisfactory.

Postnatal Management

Patients with antenatally detected hydronephrosis should be closely observed by the obstetrician. In the presence of oligohydramnios, the delivery should take place at a center having a neonatal ICU and advanced imaging facilities.

Ultrasonography should be done after birth in neonates with persistent UTD on the last antenatal scan. Infants with UTD A1 and UTD A2–3 require at least two ultrasound scans in the postnatal period beyond 48 hr, but before 4 weeks of life. A second ultrasound scan is required in the postnatal period, as the first scan may be normal in some patients. However, in neonates with suspected PUVs, oligohydramnios or severe bilateral hydronephrosis, ultrasonography is recommended within 48 hr of birth. Since distension of bladder makes pelviectasis more prominent, measurements of APD of pelvis should be taken on an empty bladder. Ultrasonography should assess for calyceal or ureteric dilation, cortical thickness, renal echogenicity and presence of cysts, and bladder wall abnormalities.

In postnatal period for UTD P1, a second ultrasound scan at 1–6 months is recommended. Similarly, for UTD P2, follow-up ultrasonography is recommended at 1–3 months of life; for infants with UTD P3, a repeat study should be done within 1 month. Since the benefits of detecting primary VUR are debated, the need for MCU is best determined by clinicians on case-by-case basis in UTD P2. MCU is recommended for all infants with UTD P3 **(Flowchart 31.1)**.

Flowchart 31.1: Approach to postnatal management of urinary tract dilation (UTD)
MCU: micturating cystourethrography; RDS: renal dynamic scan

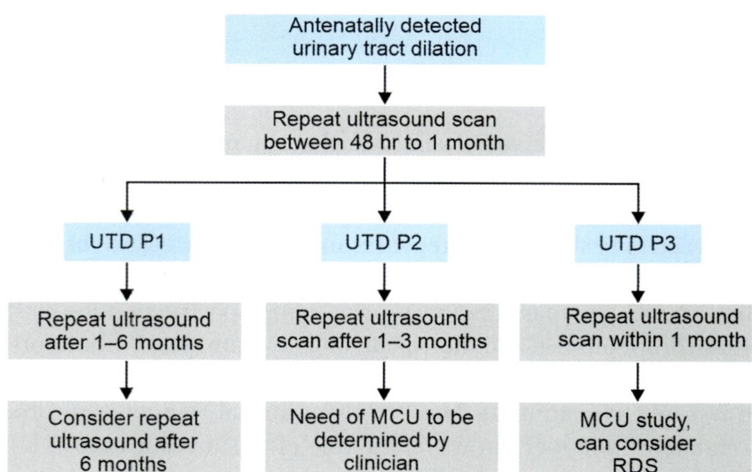

Requirement for scintigraphic (nuclear medicine) scans in UTD P2 and P3 groups is best determined by the clinician assessing the patient. Infants with UTD P3 who do not show reflux on MCU, may be considered for screening of PUJ obstruction and individual renal function. Diuretic renal scintigraphy (Tc-MAG3 and Tc-DTPA) is done at 6 weeks in these cases. The procedure and its interpretation depend upon several variables such as the hydration status, fullness of bladder, compliance of urinary system, renal function, and dose and timing of furosemide administration. An initial differential function below 35–40% in the kidney with obstructed drainage signifies impaired function.

Parents of infants with antenatal or postnatal hydronephrosis should be counseled regarding the risk of UTIs and their prompt management. Current available literature does not support routine use of antibiotic prophylaxis in all infants with UTD. Infants with high-grade vesicoureteric reflux (grade III–V) should receive antibiotic prophylaxis.

Pelviureteric Junction Obstruction

Pelviureteric junction (PUJ) obstruction is the most common cause of prenatal hydronephrosis with an incidence of ~1 in 500 live births. It is more common in boys and unilateral in 70% cases. When bilateral, it is usually asymmetrical. The obstruction is often functional due to abnormal musculature at the PUJ. Occasionally, ureteral valves, kinks in ureter, or aberrant vessel may be causative. Other renal and ureteric anomalies are often associated and should be looked for. Ultrasonography shows dilated pelvis with normal ureter and bladder. In severe PUJ obstruction, the calyces are dilated and blunted and there is thinning of parenchyma.

Vesicoureteric Reflux

About 10–15% cases of prenatally diagnosed UTD show VUR. The prevalence is higher at 20–40% in infants with bilateral hydronephrosis. Patients with high-grade VUR should receive antibiotic prophylaxis.

Ureterovesical Junction Obstruction

There is anatomic or functional obstruction at the junction. In about 10% cases the obstruction is bilateral, and boys are more often affected. There may be varying degree of true ureteric narrowing or an abnormal insertion of ureter into the bladder. Often the obstruction is functional due to abnormal musculature and increased deposition of collagen in the distal ureter that precludes normal peristalsis. Duplicated collecting system and ureterocele may be associated. Ultrasonography shows grossly dilated and tortuous ureter. The bladder is normal unless an intravesical ureterocele is present.

Posterior Urethral Valves

Posterior urethral valves (PUV) are the most common cause of lower urinary tract obstruction in boys. Ultrasonography shows bilateral hydroureteronephrosis, thickened bladder walls, and dilated posterior urethra. In severe cases, progressively increasing oligohydramnios, increased renal echogenicity, loss of corticomedullary differentiation, and subcortical cysts (suggesting renal dysplasia) are seen. A persistently dilated bladder with bilateral hydroureters is suggestive of PUV, and should be carefully investigated.

Megaureter

Normally, ureters are not seen on ultrasonography. Megaureters are dilated ureters with or without pelviectasis or caliectasis. They can be primary or secondary and refluxing or nonrefluxing. Primary megaureters result from ureterovesical junction (UVJ) obstruction, whereas secondary megaureters are caused by high-grade VUR, bladder outlet obstruction, neuropathic bladder, and prune belly syndrome.

Renal Agenesis

Failure of ureteric bud to interact with metanephric blastemal, during development, leads to renal agenesis. Unilateral renal agenesis is more common (incidence 1 in 1,000 live birth), than bilateral agenesis (1 in 3,000–4,000 pregnancies), and has more favorable prognosis. Bilateral agenesis can be detected earliest at ~12 weeks of gestation; however, it is incompatible with life. Unilateral agenesis is more common in boys; anomalies of other organ systems are associated in almost 30% children. A number of syndromes are associated and therefore a complete evaluation is necessary.

Ultrasound screening for commonly associated congenital malformation of cardiovascular, gastrointestinal, cerebral, and muscular systems is suggested in order to detect chromosomal or syndromic disorders. Pathogenic variants in *FGF20, ITA8, GFRA1,* and *GREB1L* are reported in patients with isolated renal agenesis. Oligohydramnios, pulmonary hypoplasia, and Potter syndrome are characteristic in patients with renal agenesis. Patients with unilateral renal agenesis are at risk of adverse consequences such as proteinuria, hypertension, and chronic kidney disease, hence need careful long-term follow-up.

Multicystic Dysplastic Kidney

It is characterized by noncommunicating cysts of varying sizes, absence of functioning renal parenchyma, and atresia or hypoplasia of ureter and renal artery. The anomaly is mostly unilateral, and the left side is commonly affected. However, anomalies in contralateral kidney such as VUR can be present in 40% of patients. Extrarenal malformation of gastrointestinal, central nervous, and cardiac system can be seen in 10–15%. Ultrasonography shows a large multiloculated abdominal mass with thin-walled and randomly distributed cysts. Differentiation from hydronephrosis is not difficult. Considering the low risk of long-term complications, conservative nonsurgical management is advised for most patients.

Abnormalities of the Bladder

In 90% fetuses, the bladder is normally visualized by 13 weeks. Failure of detection indicates careful scanning for kidneys and ectopic location of the bladder. A persistently enlarged bladder may be due to urethral obstruction, neuropathic bladder, and prune belly syndrome.

Kidney Tumors

Renal tumors in the newborn infant are uncommon, presenting chiefly as abdominal swelling or a palpable mass. Other symptoms include hypertension, hematuria, fever, and feed intolerance. Common neonatal tumors include congenital mesoblastic nephroma, multilocular cystic nephroma, and Wilms tumor. Malignant rhabdoid tumor is a rare but aggressive malignancy that presents in newborns and young infants and has extremely poor prognosis. Renal cell carcinoma or lymphoma is exceedingly rare in neonates.

Congenital mesoblastic nephroma is the chief kidney neoplasm during infancy. Approximately 60% patients are diagnosed before 6 months of age. Clinical features include abdominal mass, heart failure, and hypertension. Nephrectomy is curative, except for rare local recurrences and rare lung metastases. Multilocular cystic nephroma is a benign tumor that arises from metanephric blastema with histological features of immature blastema, tubules, and skeletal muscle. The prognosis is excellent with surgical removal.

Wilms tumor accounts for 90% of all kidney tumors in children. However, 80% cases are diagnosed between the ages of 1 and 5 years, making its appearance uncommon in the first year of life and rare in the neonatal period. Most Wilms tumors occur sporadically, but 15% are associated with congenital anomalies or syndromes, including congenital aniridia, hemihypertrophy, WAGR (Wilms, aniridia, genitourinary anomalies, and mental retardation) syndrome, Denys–Drash syndrome, and Beckwith–Wiedemann syndrome. Infants with Wilms tumor are treated according to standard protocols (Chapter 30).

BIBLIOGRAPHY

Kidney Function

1. Boer DP, Rijke YB, Hop WC, et al. Reference values for serum creatinine in children younger than 1 year of age. Pediatr Nephrol. 2010;25:2107-13.
2. Furgeson SB, Linas S. Mechanisms of type I and type II pseudohypoaldosteronism. J Am Soc Nephrol. 2010;21:1842-45.
3. Kelishadi R, Haghdoost AA, Jamshidi F, et al. Low birth weight or rapid catch-up growth: Which is more associated with cardiovascular disease and its risk factors in life? A systematic review and cryptanalysis. Pediatr Int Child Health. 2015;35(2):110-23.
4. Modi N. Management of fluid balance in the very immature neonate. Arch Dis Child Fetal Neonatal Ed. 2004;89:F108-11.
5. Okada T, Takahashi S, Nagano N, et al. Early postnatal alteration of body composition in preterm and small-for-gestational-age infants: implications of catch-up fat. Pediatr Res. 2015;77:136-42.
6. Schreuder M, Delemarre-van de Waal H, van Wijk A. Consequences of intrauterine growth restriction for the kidney. Kidney Blood Press Res. 2006;29:108-25.
7. Vieux R, Merdariu JM, Guillemin F. Glomerular filtration rate reference values in very preterm infants. Pediatrics. 2010;125:e1186-92.

Acute Kidney Injury

1. Coulthard MG, Crosier J, Griffiths C, et al. Hemodialysing babies weighing <8 kg with the Newcastle infant dialysis and ultrafiltration system: Comparison with peritoneal and conventional hemodialysis. Pediatr Nephrol. 2014;29:1873-81.
2. Evans RE, Peterson J, Kim JJ, et al. How to know when little kidneys are in trouble: a review of current tools for diagnosing AKI in neonates. Front Pediatr. 2023;11:1270200.
3. Gorga SM, Murphy HJ, Selewski DT. An update on neonatal and pediatric acute kidney injury. Curr Pediatr Rep. 2018;6:278-90.
4. Konrad M, Nijenhuis T, Ariceta G, et al. Diagnosis and management of Bartter syndrome: Executive summary of the consensus and recommendations from the European Rare Kidney Disease Reference Network Working Group for Tubular Disorders. Kidney Int. 2021;99:324-35.

5. Kuo J, Akison LK, Chatfield MD, et al. Serum and urinary biomarkers to predict acute kidney injury in premature infants: A systematic review and meta-analysis of diagnostic accuracy. J Nephrol. 2022;35:2001-14.
6. Moudgil A. Renal venous thrombosis in neonates. Curr Pediatr Rev. 2014;10:101-6.
7. Ronnholm KA, Holmberg C. Peritoneal dialysis in infants. Pediatr Nephrol. 2006;21:751-6.
8. Slagle C, Askenazi D, Starr M. Recent advances in kidney replacement therapy in infants: A review. Am J Kidney Dis. 2024;83:519-30.
9. Starr MC, Charlton JR, Guillet R, et al.; Neonatal Kidney Collaborative Board. Advances in neonatal acute kidney injury. Pediatrics. 2021;148:e2021051220.
10. Vemgal P, Ohlsson A. Interventions for non-oliguric hyperkalemia in preterm neonates. Cochrane Database Syst Rev. 2007;CD005257.
11. Zappitelli M, Ambalavanan N, Askenazi DJ, et al. Developing a neonatal acute kidney injury research definition: A report from the NIDDK neonatal AKI workshop. Pediatr Res. 2017;82:569-73.

Hypertension

1. Altemose K, Dionne JM. Neonatal hypertension: Concerns within and beyond the neonatal intensive care unit. Clin Exp Pediatr. 2022;65:367-76.
2. Hjorten R, Flynn JT. Neonatal hypertension. Clin Perinatol. 2022;49:27-42.
3. Kent AL, Keeskes Z, Shadbolt B, et al. Blood pressure in the first year of life in healthy infants born at term. Pediatr Nephrol. 2007;22:1743-9.
4. Zubrow AB, Hulman S, Kushner H, et al. Determinants of blood pressure in infants admitted to neonatal intensive care units: A prospective multicenter study. Philadelphia Neonatal Blood Pressure Study Group. J Perinatol. 1995;15:470-9.

Antenatally Detected Anomalies

1. Dos Santos J, Parekh RS, Piscione TD, et al. A new grading system for the management of antenatal hydronephrosis. Clin J Am Soc Nephrol. 2015;10: 1783-90.
2. La Scola C, Ammenti A, Bertulli C, et al. Management of the congenital solitary kidney: consensus recommendations of the Italian Society of Pediatric Nephrology. Pediatr Nephrol. 2022;37:2185-207.
3. Melo FF, Mak RH, Simões E Silva AC, et al. Evaluation of urinary tract dilation classification system for prediction of long-term outcomes in isolated antenatal hydronephrosis: A cohort study. J Urol. 2021;206:1022-30.
4. Nguyen HT, Benson CB, Bromley B, et al. Multidisciplinary consensus on the classification of prenatal and postnatal urinary tract dilation (UTD classification system). J Pediatr Urol. 2014;10:982-98.
5. Nulens K, Lorenzo AJ, Dos Santos J, et al. Fetal urinary tract dilation: What to tell the parents. Prenat Diagn. 2024;44:148-57.
6. Sinha A, Bagga A, Krishna A, et al. Revised guidelines on management of antenatal hydronephrosis. Indian Pediatr. 2013;50:215-31.

Annexures

Srinivasavaradan Govindarajan, Arvind Bagga

- **Annexure 1:** Nomogram for body surface area
- **Annexure 2:** Normal reference values
- **Annexure 3:** Important formulae
- **Annexure 4:** Bipolar kidney length and kidney volume
- **Annexure 5:** Alkali and electrolyte supplements
- **Annexure 6:** Tubular maximum reabsorption for phosphate
- **Annexure 7:** Drug dosage modification for impaired kidney function
- **Annexure 8:** Drugs requiring minimal dose modification in impaired kidney function
- **Annexure 9:** Gene lists for common syndromes
  - 9.1: Congenital anomalies of the kidneys and urinary tract
  - 9.2: Tubulopathies; electrolyte abnormalities
  - 9.3: Hematuria
  - 9.4: Steroid-resistant nephrotic syndrome; focal segmental glomerulosclerosis; proteinuria
  - 9.5: Thrombotic microangiopathy; hemolytic uremic syndrome
  - 9.6: Ciliopathies; cystic kidney diseases
  - 9.7: Nephrolithiasis; nephrocalcinosis
  - 9.8: Hypertension
  - 9.9: Chronic kidney disease of unknown etiology
  - 9.10: Mitochondrial diseases

Annexure 1: Nomogram for body surface area

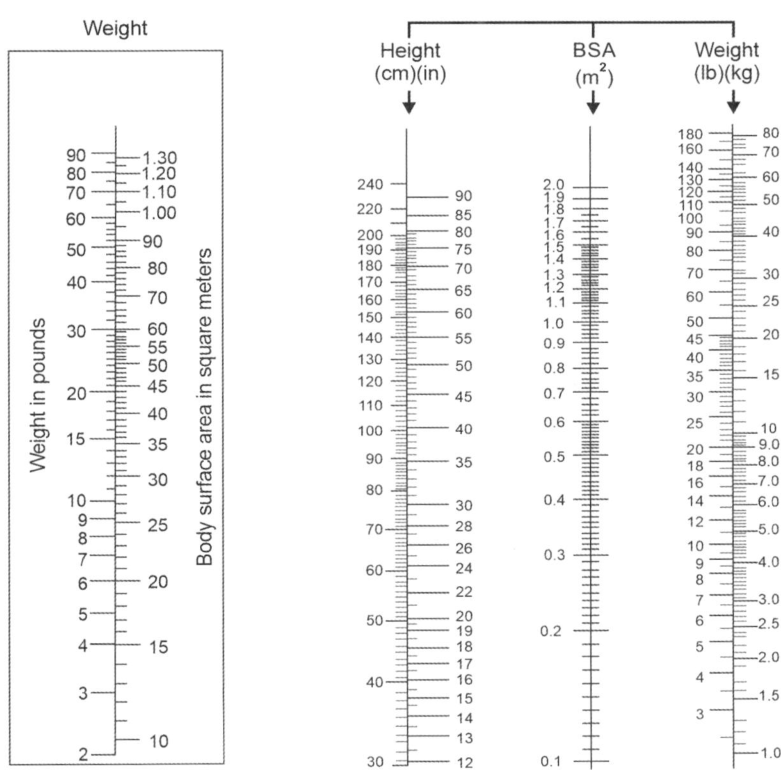

The body surface area (BSA) is indicated where a straight line connecting the height and weight intersects the BSA column

Formula for calculating BSA: $\sqrt{\dfrac{\text{Height (cm)} \times \text{Weight (kg)}}{3{,}600}}$

(Nomogram modified from data of E Boyd by CD West; from Vaughan VC and RJ McKay. Eds, Nelson Textbook of Pediatrics, 12th edn, Philadelphia: Saunders, 1983)

Annexure 2: Normal reference values

Blood or urine investigation	*Age range*	*Male*	*Female*
1,25 (OH) vitamin D3 (pg/mL) *To convert to pmol/L,* multiply by 2.4	<1 yr 1–3 yr 3–18 yr	30–181 43–140 42–95	30–181 43–140 42–95
Aldosterone (pmol/L)	<1 yr 1–5 yr 5–10 yr 10–18 yr	<2,868 <1,035 <849 <670	<3,091 <1,734 <8,40 <820
Aldosterone renin ratio	0–12 yr	>10	>10
Alkaline phosphatase (U/L)	0–15 days 15 days–1 yr 1–10 yr 10–13 yr 13–18 yr	90–273 134–518 156–369 141–460 90–400	90–273 134–518 156–369 141–460 60–280
Anti-dsDNA (IU/mL)	6–16 yr	<30	<30
Antistreptolysin O (ASO) (IU/mL)	0–6 months 6 months–1 yr 1–6 yr 6–18 yr	0 0–30 0–104 0–331	0 0–30 0–104 0–331
Calcium (mg/dL) *To convert mmol/L,* multiply by 0.25	0–1 yr 1–19 yr	8.5–10.9 9.2–10.5	8.5–10.9 9.2–10.5
Cholesterol (mg/dL) *To convert to mmol/L,* multiply by 0.0259	15 days–1 yr 1–18 yr	65–257 117–225	65–257 117–225
Complement C3 (mg/dL)	0–15 days 15 days–1 yr 1–18 yr	50–121 51–160 83–152	50–121 51–160 83–152
Complement C4 (mg/dL)	0–2 yr 3–4 yr 5–9 yr 10–18 yr	11–34 11–42 7–34 11–47	11–34 11–42 7–34 11–47
Copeptin (pmol/L)	All ages	2.4–8.6	2.4–8.6
CRP (mg/dL)	0–15 days 15 days–15 yr	3–58 1–9	3–58 1–9
Cystine (leukocyte cystine) (nmol half-cystine/mg protein)	All ages	<0.2	<0.2

Contd...

Contd...

Blood or urine investigation	***Age range***	***Male***	***Female***
Erythrocyte sedimentation rate (mm/h)	0–1 month 1 month–12 years >12 years	0–2 0–20 0–15	0–2 0–20 0–20
Ferritin (μg/dL) *To convert to pmol/L,* multiply by 22.47	4–15 days 15 days–6 months 6 months–1 year 1–5 years 5–14 years	10–72 1.4–64 0.8–18 0.5–10 1.4–7.9	10–72 1.4–64 0.8–18 0.5–10 1.4–7.9
Fibroblast growth factor 23 (FGF-23), C-terminal (RU/mL)	0–1 year 2 years 3 years 4 years 5 years 8 years 10 years 12 years 15 years	43–324 39–235 36–192 34–163 33–145 35–126 37–128 37–136 34–136	43–324 39–235 36–192 34–163 33–145 35–126 37–128 37–136 34–136
Haptoglobin (g/L)	0–15 days 15 days–1 year 1–12 years 12–18 years	0–0.1 0.1–2.2 0.1–1.6 0.1–1.8	0–0.1 0.1–2.2 0.1–1.6 0.1–1.8
Hemoglobin (g/dL)	3–5 years 6–8 years 9–10 years 11–14 years	11.4–14.3 11.5–14.3 11.8–14.7 12.4–15.7	11.4–14.3 11.5–14.3 11.8–14.7 11.9–14.8
Homocysteine, total (μmol/L)	5 days–1 year 1–7 years 7–12 years 12–18 years	2.9–10 2.8–7.6 3.4–8.5 4.7–10.4	2.9–10 2.8–7.6 3.4–8.5 4.1–12.0
Immunoglobulin G (mg/dL)	0–15 days 15 days–1 year 1–4 years 4–10 years 10–18 years	320–1407 108–702 316–1148 542–1358 658–1534	320–1407 108–702 316–1148 542–1358 658–1534
Iron (μg/dL) *To convert to μmol/L,* multiply by 0.1791	0–14 years	16–170	16–160
Lactate dehydrogenase (U/L)	0–15 days 15 days–1 year 1–10 years 10–15 years	309–1222 163–452 192–321 170–283	309–1222 163–452 192–321 157–272
Low-density lipoprotein (LDL) (mg/dL)	<18 years	<110	<110

Contd...

Contd...

Blood or urine investigation	***Age range***	***Male***	***Female***
Magnesium (mmol/L) *To convert to mg/dl,* multiply by 2.43	15 days–1 year 1–19 years	0.81–1.27 0.86–1.17	0.81–1.27 0.86–1.17
Parathyroid hormone, intact (pg/mL) *To convert to pmol/L,* multiply by 0.1053	6 days–1 year 1–9 years 9–18 years	6–88 16–63 22–87	6–88 16–63 22–87
Phosphorus (mg/dL) *To convert to mmol/L,* multiply by 0.323	0–15 days 15 days–1 year 1–5 years 5–13 years 13–16 years	5.6–10.5 4.6–8.3 4.3–6.8 3.4–6.2 3.1–4.9	5.6–10.5 4.6–8.3 4.3–6.8 3.4–6.2 3.1–4.9
Renin (pmol/mL/h)	0–3 months 3 months–5 years 6–9 years 10–18 years	4–12 2–6 1–4 0.6–2.2	4–12 2–6 1–4 0.6–2.2
Reticulocyte count (x 10^9/L)	8 months–18 years	45–110	36–100
Transferrin saturation (TSAT) %	0–1 year 1–14 years 14–18 years	4.1–59 6.5–39 10–58	4.1–59 6.5–39 5–44
Triglycerides (mg/dL) *To convert to mmol/L,* divide by 88.57	15 days–1 year 1–9 years 10–18 years	60–290 50–225 50–225	60–290 50–225 50–225
Uric acid (mg/dL)	15 days–1 year 1–12 years 12–18 years	1.6–6.3 1.8–4.8 2.6–7.6	1.6–6.3 1.8–4.9 2.6–5.9
Vitamin D3 (ng/mL) *To convert to nmol/L,* multiply by 2.5	0–1 year 1–12 years 12–18 years	11–64 17–48 12–42	11–64 17–48 12–42
Urine Investigations			
Beta-2 microglobulin to creatinine ratio, random urine (µg/g)	All ages	<300	<300
Urine beta-2 microglobulin (mg/L)	0–3 months 3 months to <2 years 2–18 years	1.9–4.7 1.3–4.5 1.2–2.3	1.9–5.8 1.3–4.5 1.2–2.3

Annexure 3: Important formulae

	Formula	Remarks
Estimated glomerular filtration rate (GFR), mL/min/1.73m^2	$GFR = \frac{k \times \text{height (cm)}}{\text{serum creatinine (mg/dL)}}$ where k = 0.413	Staging and management of chronic kidney disease
Serum anion gap, mEq/L	$Na^+ - (Cl^- + HCO_3^-)$	Normal value 6–12 mEq/L
Urine anion gap, mEq/L	$Na^+ + K^+ - Cl^-$	Index of urinary NH_4^+ excretion
Plasma osmolality, mOsm/kg	$2(Na^+) + \frac{BUN}{2.8} + \frac{glucose}{18}$ BUN: Blood urea nitrogen, mg/dL	Normal value 280–285 mOsm/kg Approximates twice plasma Na^+
Free water deficit, L	Total body water × [(sodium concentration/140) – 1]	Total body water = 0.6 × weight (kg)
Plasma volume, L	0.065 × weight (kg) × (1 – hematocrit)	Approximately 30–40 mL/kg
Urinary potassium index	Urine K^+/ (urine K^+ + urine Na^+)	Value >0.6 (60%) suggests hypovolemia
Transtubular potassium gradient (TTKG)	$\frac{\text{Urine } K^+ \times \text{plasma osmolality}}{\text{Plasma } K^+ \times \text{urine osmolality}}$	Reflects aldosterone mediated distal K^+ secretion. Normal <2.5 during hypokalemia; >7 in hyperkalemia
TmP/GFR, mg/dL	$\left[1 - \left(\frac{\text{Urine P} \times \text{serum creatinine}}{\text{Plasma P} \times \text{urine creatinine}}\right)\right] \times \text{serum P}$	Tubular maximum reabsorption of phosphate (P) corrected for GFR
Fractional excretion of sodium	$\frac{\text{Urine } Na^+ \times \text{plasma creatinine}}{\text{Plasma } Na^+ \times \text{urine creatinine}}$	<1% in volume contraction with appropriate renal Na^+ retention
Fractional excretion of magnesium	$\frac{\text{Urine } Mg^{2+} \times \text{serum creatinine}}{0.7 \times \text{plasma } Mg^{2+} \times \text{urine creatinine}}$	FeMg >4% consistent with renal magnesium wasting
Serum calcium level corrected for hypoalbuminemia, mg/dL	0.8 × (4.0 – serum albumin, g/dL) + serum calcium, mg/dL	
Change in sodium concentration following infusion of 1 L solution, mEq/L	$\frac{(\text{Infusate } Na^+ - \text{serum } Na^+)}{(\text{Total body water} + 1)}$	Infusate Na^+: Concentration of Na^+ in fluid infused
Expected bladder capacity (2–12 years of age), mL	(Age + 1) × 30	Infants: Capacity = 7 × weight (kg)

Annexure 4: Bipolar kidney length and kidney volume

Age	*Kidney length, mean (range) cm*[1,2]	*Kidney volume, mean (range) mL*[3]
1 month	5.2 (4.4–6.2)	9.9
3 months	5.6 (4.7–6.6)	12.3
6 months	6.0 (4.9–7.0)	23.8 (14–36.6)
9 months	6.3 (5.3–7.2)	
1 year	6.5 (5.5–7.7)	31.0 (26–36)
2 years	6.7 (5.6–8.0)	33.6 (22.8–51.6)
3 years	7.1 (6.7–7.6)	51.8 (42.6–61.17)
4 years	7.5 (7.2–7.8)	60.5 (50.4–70.6)
5 years	8.0 (7.5–8.4)	63.6 (56.1–71.2)
6 years	7.8 (7.4–8.3)	68.3 (59–77)
7 years	8.2 (7.7–8.6)	85.4 (75.8–95.1)
8 years	8.7 (8.1–9.3)	92.2 (80.7–103.7)
9 years	8.9 (8.5–9.4)	101.8 (83.8–119.9)
10 years	8.9 (8.4–9.4)	105 (85–123)
11 years	8.9 (8.4–9.4)	116.4 (76–140)
12 years	9.6 (9.2–10.0)	142 (122–161)
13–18 years	10.6 (9.7–10.9)	155 (135–179)

[1] For the same age, the left kidney is slightly longer and larger than the right

[2] Kidney length better correlates with statural height, regardless of sex

[3] Renal volume may be estimated by the prolate ellipsoid formula

$$V\,(\text{mL}) = L \times W \times \frac{D1 + D2}{2} \times 0.524$$

L = maximum bipolar length; W = maximum width in hilar region; D = maximum depth in the longitudinal (D1) and transverse sections (D2)

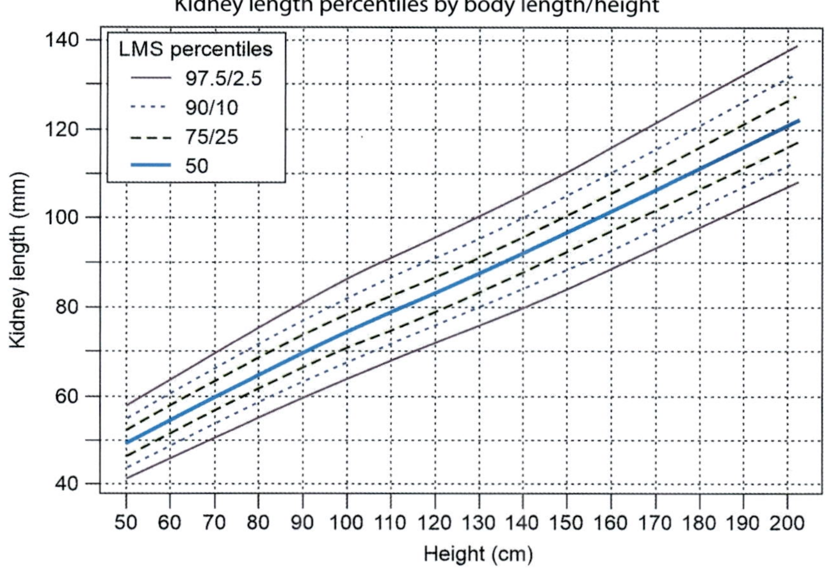

Source

1. Parks CW, et al. J Korean Med Sci. 2017;32:448-56
2. Kecler–Pietrzyk A, et al. Radiopaedia (2024). Available from https://radiopaedia.org/articles/normal-kidney-size-children
3. Dinkel E, et al. Pediatr Radiol. 1985;15:38-43
4. Obrycki L, et al. Pediatr Nephrol. 2022;37:1075-85

Annexure 5: Alkali and electrolyte supplements

Content	*Preparation*	*Constituents, per 1000 ml, sachet or tablet*	*Equivalent*
Citric acid +/- sodium or potassium citrate	Bicitra	60 g citric acid; 100 g sodium citrate	1 ml = 1 mEq base
	Shohl solution	140 g citric acid; 90 g sodium citrate	1 ml = 1 mEq base; 1 mEq Na^+
	Polycitra K; Uriliser	220 g potassium citrate; 66.8 g citric acid	1 ml = 2 mEq base; 2 mEq K^+
	Polycitra	110 g potassium citrate; 100 g sodium citrate; 66.8 g citric acid	1 ml = 2 mEq base; 1 mEq each Na^+, K^+
	Potassium citrate	1080 mg (Potrate-10 extended release)	10 mEq K^+; 3.3 mmol citrate
Potassium citrate and potassium bicarbonate	ADV7103	3660 mg sachet	24 mEq (2.61 mmol citrate; 16 mmol bicarbonate)
Sodium bicarbonate	Injection (75%)	Lifecare, Sodarc, Bicacure	1 ml = 0.9 mEq base
	Tablets	325 mg: Citragen (antacid) 500 mg: Nodosis, Nodosis-GST, Auxisoda, Sobimax, Sobisis EC 1000 mg: Nodosis DS, Sodicarb forte, Sobisis forte	325 mg = 4 mEq each of bicarbonate, Na^+ 500 mg = 5.95 mEq each of bicarbonate, Na^+ 1 g = 11.9 mEq each of bicarbonate, Na^+
	Granules	2.4 g: Nodosis 2G	2.4 g = 23.8 mEq each of bicarbonate, Na^+
	Solution	Nodosis oral suspension, 300 mL	15 ml = 11.9 mEq each of bicarbonate, Na^+
Potassium chloride	Syrup (15%)	Potklor, 100 mL	15 ml = 20 mEq each of K^+ and chloride
	Tablet (prolonged release)	Potride, Addkay, 750 mg	750 mg = 10 mEq each of K^+ and chloride
	Injection (20%)	Potklor, 15 mL	1 mL = 2 mEq each of K^+ and chloride

Contd...

Contd...

Content	*Preparation*	*Constituents, per 1000 ml, sachet or tablet*	*Equivalent*
Potassium gluconate	Tablet/capsule		465 mg = 2 mEq of K^+
Sodium or potassium phosphate +/- phosphoric acid	Solution	Joulie: 136 g dibasic sodium phosphate; 58.8 g phosphoric acid per 1 L	1 ml = 30 mg (9.66 mmol) inorganic phosphorus
	Neutral phosphate solution	Prepared by adding to 60 mL water, 1 g monobasic sodium phosphate; 3.66 g dibasic sodium phosphate	15 ml = 250 mg (8.1 mmol) inorganic phosphorus; 7.1 mEq each of sodium and potassium
	Neutral potassium phosphate sachet	K-Phos Neutral, Phospha 250 Neutral: 852 mg dibasic sodium phosphate, 155 mg monobasic potassium phosphate, 130 mg monobasic sodium phosphate monohydrate Neutra-Phos, 250 mg; Sodium, potassium, phosphorus powder concentrate (Rugby, Hargraves)	250 mg (8.1 mmol) inorganic phosphorus; 13.0 mEq sodium; and 1.1 mEq potassium 250 mg (8.1 mmol) inorganic phosphorus; 7.1 mEq each of sodium and potassium
	Sodium acid phosphate granules, effervescent tablets	Addphos, 500 mg (granules), Phosphate Sandoz, 500 mg: Sodium acid phosphate 968 mg, potassium bicarbonate 61.5 mg, sodium bicarbonate 234.5 mg	500 mg (16.1 mmol) inorganic phosphorus
	Potassium phosphate injection Potassium acid phosphate	Potphos, 15 mL: Each mL contains 224 mg monobasic potassium phosphate and 236 mg dibasic potassium phosphate K-Phos original, 500 mg	1 mL = 93 mg (3 mmol) inorganic phosphorus and 4.4. mEq potassium 500 mg = ~ 114 mg (3.7 mmol) inorganic phosphorus and 3.7 mEq potassium
Calcium carbonate	Tablet Syrup	250 mg, 500 mg, 1000 mg 250 mg per 5 mL	1000 mg = 22.3 mEq base

Contd...

Contd...

Content	*Preparation*	*Constituents, per 1000 ml, sachet or tablet*	*Equivalent*
Magnesium salts	Magnesium citrate liquid	1750 mg per 30 mL	1 ml = 100 mg (0.8 mEq) Mg^{2+}
	Magnesium hydroxide liquid	400 mg per 5 ml	1 ml = 33 mg elemental Mg^{2+}
	Magnesium oxide tablet	400 mg	400 mg = 240 mg elemental Mg^{2+}
	Magnesium gluconate tablet	500 mg	500 mg = 25 mg elemental Mg
	Magnesium chloride	535 mg	535 mg = 64 mg elemental Mg
	Magnesium lactate	500 mg	500 mg = 84 mg elemental Mg
	Magnesium orotate	500 mg	500 mg = 36 mg elemental Mg
	Magnesium aspartate	615 mg	615 mg = 61 mg elemental Mg
	Magnesium sulphate injection	50%	1 mL = 4 mEq Mg^{2+}

Annexure 6: Tubular maximum reabsorption for phosphate

The renal tubular phosphate threshold maximum per unit volume of glomerular filtrate (TmP/GFR) is the preferred method for assessment of tubular phosphate handling. In adult patients, TmP/GFR is estimated from plasma phosphate concentration and TRP, using the Walton and Bijvoet nomogram, shown below.

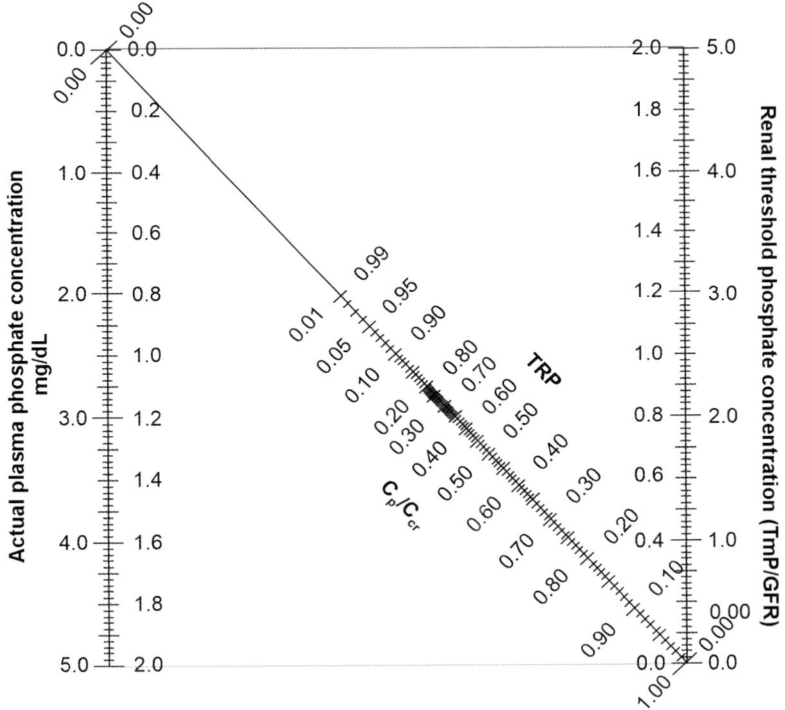

In children, TmP/GFR can be derived from tubular phosphate reabsorption, as described by Brodehl et al, as follows:

Tubular reabsorption of phosphate (TRP) =1- (Urine P x Serum Cr)/(Urine Cr x Serum P)

TmP/GFR = TRP x Serum phosphate, hence

TmP/GFR = Serum P - (Urine P x Serum Cr)/Urine Cr), where P is phosphate and Cr is creatinine. An online calculator is available at: *https://gpn.de/service/tmp-gfr-calculator/*

Normal values of TmP/GFR are relatively high throughout childhood and adolescence, with postpubertal decline to near-adult levels (2.2-4.2 mg/dl). These are shown in the Table below.

Reference Values for TmP/GFR (Brodehl's estimates)

Age	*mg/dL*
0-5 months	3.16-6.20
6-11 months	3.50-5.83
1 to 5 yr	3.25-5.52
6 to 12 yr	3.01-5.08
13 to 15 yr	2.82-5.21
≥16 yr	2.60-3.81

Reference Values for TmP/GFR, Based on TRP, using IDMS Standardized Creatinine

Age, years	*mg/dL*
1 to <3 yr	4.74 (3.50-5.94)
3 to <5 yr	4.55 (3.68-5.39)
5 to <7 yr	4.40 (3.50-5.26)
7 to <9 yr	4.33 (3.44-5.23)
9 to <11 yr	4.37 (3.53-5.17)
11 to <13 yr	4.37 (3.53-5.20)
13 to <16 yr	3.84 (2.69-4.95) / 4.15 (3.03-5.23)
16 to <19 yr	3.47 (2.38-4.52) / 3.59 (2.20-4.98)
19 to <25 yr	3.59 (2.20-4.98) / 3.59 (2.20-4.98)
25 to <35 yr	3.28 (2.29-4.30) / 3.00 (2.20-3.81)
35 to <45 yr	3.03 (2.26-3.78) / 2.97 (2.04-3.93)
45 to <55 yr	2.91 (2.17-3.68) / 2.94 (2.01-3.84)
≥55 yr	3.10 (2.23-3.99) / 3.03 (2.17-3.87)

Data presented as mean (±1.96 SD)
Data for adolescents and adults is presented separately for girls and boys (separated by /)
For phosphate, 1 mg/dl = 0.323 mmol/L; TRP tubular reabsorption of phosphate

Source

1. Stark H, et al. Nephron. 1986;44:125-8
2. Derain L, et al. Nephrol Dial Transplant. 2022;37:2150-56
3. Brodehl J. Pediatr Nephrol. 1994;8:645
4. Brodehl J, et al. Clin Nephrol. 1982;17:163-71

Annexure 7: Drug dosage modification for impaired kidney function

Dose for normal renal function		*Dose for impaired renal function based on glomerular filtration rate (GFR), mL/min/1.73 m²*			*Dose in renal replacement therapy*		
		>50	*10–50*	*<10*	*HD*	*PD*	*CKRT*
Antimicrobials							
Acyclovir Noncentral nervous system (CNS) infection	10 mg/kg/dose q8h IV	100%	eGFR 25–49: 100% q12h 10–24: 100% q24h	50% q24h	50% q24h (dose after HD)	50% q24h	100% q12–24h
Acyclovir Encephalitis, or immunocompromised	10–15 mg/kg q8h or 250–500 mg/m² q8h	100%	100% eGFR 25–49: q12h eGFR 10–24: q24h	100% q24h	100% q24h		100% q12–24h
Amikacin	7.5 mg/kg q8h IV, or 15–20 mg/kg q24h	100%	30–49: 100% q 12–18h 10–30: 100% q18–24h	100% q48–72h	67% after HD	100% q48–72h	67% q12h
Amoxicillin	25–50 mg/kg/day div q8h PO	100%	100% q8–12h	100% q24h	Dose for GFR < 10	Dose for GFR < 10	Dose for GFR >50
Amphotericin B	0.5–1.5 mg/kg/day IV over 2–6h	100%	100% q24h	100% q24–36h	Dose for GFR < 10	Dose for GFR < 10	Dose for GFR 10–50

Contd...

Contd...

Dose for normal renal function		***Dose for impaired renal function based on glomerular filtration rate (GFR), mL/min/1.73 m²***			***Dose in renal replacement therapy***		
		>50	***10–50***	***<10***	***HD***	***PD***	***CKRT***
Ampicillin	50 mg/kg q6h Meningitis/ endocarditis: 50–100 mg/kg/day q6h	100% q6h	10–29: 100% q8–12h 30-49: 100% q6h	100% q12h	Dose for GFR < 10	Dose for GFR < 10	100% q6h
Ampicillin/sulbactam	50 mg/kg (2g ampicillin) q6h	100% q6h	15–29: 100% q12h	100% q24h	100% q12–24h	100% q12–24h	100% q6h
Azithromycin	10 mg/kg/dose day 1; 5 mg/kg/dose q24h x 4 days	100% q24h	No adjustment necessary				
Aztreonam	30 mg/kg/dose q6–8h	100% q8h	10–29: 50% q8h	25% q8h	Dose for GFR < 10	Dose for GFR <10	Dose for GFR >50
Cefaclor	10–15 mg/kg/dose q8h PO	100% q8h	100% q8h	100% q8h	Dose after HD	100% q8–12h	Dose for normal renal function

Contd...

Contd...

	Dose for normal renal function	*Dose for impaired renal function based on glomerular filtration rate (GFR), mL/min/1.73 m²*			*Dose in renal replacement therapy*		
		>50	***10–50***	***<10***	***HD***	***PD***	***CKRT***
Cefazolin	16.5–50 mg/kg q8h	100% q8h	10–29: 100% q12h	100% q24h	Dose for GFR < 10	Dose for GFR < 10	100% q8h
Cefepime	50 mg/kg/dose q18h	100% q24h	*30–60:* 100% q12h *11–29:* 100% q24h	100% q48h	100% q24h Maximum: 1 g	100% q24 h–48h Maximum: 2 g	100% q8h
Cefixime	4 mg/kg/dose q12–24h PO	100% q12–24h	75% q12–24h	50% q12–24h	Dose for GFR <10	Dose for GFR <10	Dose for GFR 10–50
Cefoperazone sulbactam	20–40 mg/kg/dose each of cefoperazone and sulbactam	100% q6–12h	*15–30:* 100% q12h Maximum sulbactam 2 g	100% q12h Maximum sulbactam 1 g	Dose for GFR <10	Dose for GFR <10	NA
Cefotaxime	100–200 mg/kg/day div q6–8h IV	100%	100% q12h	100% q24h	100% q24h Dose after dialysis	ND; 100% q24h	100% q12h

Contd...

Contd...

Dose for normal renal function		*Dose for impaired renal function based on glomerular filtration rate (GFR), mL/min/1.73 m²*			*Dose in renal replacement therapy*		
		>50	*10–50*	*<10*	*HD*	*PD*	*CKRT*
Ceftazidime	50 mg/kg q8h	100% q8–12h	*30–50:* 100% q12h *10–30:* 100% q24h	100% q48h	100% q48h (dose after dialysis)	100% q48h	100% q12h
Cefuroxime sodium	25 mg/kg q8h IV	100% q8h	10–29: 100% q12h	100% q24h	Dose for GFR <10 (after HD)	Dose for GFR <10	100% q8h
Cephalexin	25–50 mg/kg/day div q6–8h PO	q8h	*30–50:* 100% q8h *10–30:* 100% q12h	100% q24h	Dose after dialysis (maximum 500 mg)	Dose for GFR <10	NA
Chloroquine	10 mg/kg/dose q24h PO for 3 days, or 4/mg/kg/dose q12h IM for 3 days	100%	100%	50% (only in prolonged use)	ND; dose for GFR <10 (only in prolonged use)	ND; dose for GFR <10 (only in prolonged use)	No adjustment

Contd...

Contd...

Dose for normal renal function		*Dose for impaired renal function based on glomerular filtration rate (GFR), mL/min/1.73 m²*			*Dose in renal replacement therapy*		
		>50	*10–50*	*<10*	*HD*	*PD*	*CKRT*
Ciprofloxacin	PO: 20 mg/kg/day, div q12h IV: 10 mg/kg/day, div q12h	100%	10–29: 100% q18h	100% q24h	100% q24h	100% q24h	100% q12h
Clarithromycin	7.5–15 mg/kg/dose q12h PO	100%	50–75% q12h	50–75% q24h	Dose after dialysis q24h	q24h	50–75% q12h
Co-amoxiclav	IV: 30 mg/kg q8h	100%	100% q12h	100% q24h	Dose after dialysis	Dose for GFR <10	Dose for GFR 10–50
Colistin	2.5–5 mg/kg/day div q6–12h	100% q8h	100% q18–24h	100% q36h	ND; dose after HD	Dose for GFR <10	
Cotrimoxazole (dose based on trimethoprim)	6–10 mg/kg/day div q12h	100% q12h	15–30: 50% q12h	<15: 25–50% q12–24h	Dose after dialysis	Dose for GFR <10	Dose for GFR 10–50

Contd...

Contd...

Dose for normal renal function		*Dose for impaired renal function based on glomerular filtration rate (GFR), mL/min/1.73 m²*			*Dose in renal replacement therapy*		
		>50	*10–50*	*<10*	*HD*	*PD*	*CKRT*
Erythromycin	10 mg/kg/dose q6h IV, PO	100%	100%	50–75%	ND; dose for GFR <10	ND; dose for GFR <10	Dose for GFR 10–50
Fluconazole	12 mg/kg stat; 6 mg/ kg q24h, IV, PO for esophageal and invasive candidiasis; 50% dose for oropharyngeal candidiasis	100%	50% q24h	50%	50% dose daily or 100% after HD	50% q48h	Dose for normal renal function
Ganciclovir	5 mg/kg q12h IV for 2–3 weeks; 5 mg/kg q24h IV	>70: 5 mg/ kg Q24h 50–69: 2.5 mg/kg q12h	25–49: 50% q24 10–24: 25% q24h	25% q48h	25% (dose after HD)	25% q48h	2.5 mg/kg q24h
Gentamicin	2–2.5 mg/kg q8h; or 5–7.5 mg/kg q24h IV	2 mg/kg q12h	30–50: 2 mg/kg q12–18h 10–30: q18–24h	2 mg/kg q48–72h	Dose for GFR <10	Dose for GFR <10	Dose for GFR >50
Imipenem–cilastatin	25 mg/kg/dose q6h IV	50% q6h	50% q8h	25% q12h	Dose after dialysis	Dose for GFR <10	Dose for GFR 10–50
Itraconazole	3–5 mg/kg/dose q12–24h PO	100%	100%	100%	ND; dose for GFR <10	ND; dose for GFR <10	ND; avoid

Contd...

Contd...

Dose for normal renal function		*Dose for impaired renal function based on glomerular filtration rate (GFR), mL/min/1.73 m^2*			*Dose in renal replacement therapy*		
		>50	*10–50*	*<10*	*HD*	*PD*	*CKRT*
Lamivudine	4 mg/kg q12h (chronic hepatitis B)	4 mg/kg q24h	2 mg/kg q24h	1 mg/kg q24h	Dose for GFR <10	Dose for GFR <10	4 mg/kg q24h
Levofloxacin	*<5 years:* 10 mg/kg q12h *>5 years:* 10 mg/kg 24h	100%	10–29: 100% q24h	100% q48h	Dose for GFR <10	Dose for GFR <10	10 mg/kg/dose q24h
Meropenem	10–20 mg/kg/dose q8h IV	100%	*30–50:* 100% q12h *10–29:* 50% q12h	50% q24h (maximum: 1 g)	Dose after dialysis	Dose for GFR <10	Dose for GFR >50
Metronidazole	10 mg/kg/dose q8 IV, PO, PR	100%	100%	4 mg/kg q6h	Dose after dialysis	Dose for GFR <10	No adjustment
Netilmicin	2–2.5 mg/kg/dose q8h IV	100%	3–4 mg/kg q12h	2 mg/kg q24h	2 mg/kg after HD	2 mg/kg q48h	Dose for GFR 10–50 and measure levels
Nitrofurantoin	5–7 mg/kg/day divided q6h PO	100%	Avoid	Avoid	Avoid	Avoid	Avoid

Contd...

Contd...

Dose for normal renal function		*Dose for impaired renal function based on glomerular filtration rate (GFR), mL/min/1.73 m²*			*Dose in renal replacement therapy*		
		>50	*10–50*	*<10*	*HD*	*PD*	*CKRT*
Ofloxacin	15 mg/kg/day divided 12h, IV, PO	100%	100% q24h	50% q24h	Dose for GFR <10	Dose for GFR <10	100%
Oseltamivir	Treatment: Age-based dose (30–75 mg) q12h, PO	100%	100% q24h	50% alternate day for maximum 5 days	50% after every dialysis	50% dose once	75 mg q24h
	Prophylaxis: Age-based dose (30–75 mg) q24h, PO	100%	100% q48h	50% every 10 days prophylaxis	50% after alternate dialysis	50% once a week	10–50
Penicillin G	100,000–250,000 U/kg/day, div q4–6h, IV, IM	q4–6h	50% q8–12h	q12–18h	Dose after dialysis	Dose for GFR <10	Dose for GFR 10–50
Penicillin V	25–50 mg/kg/day div q6–8h, PO	100%	100%	100%	Dose after dialysis	Dose for GFR <10	NA
Piperacillin	150–300 mg/kg/day, div 6–8h	100% q6–8h	100% q8h	100% q12h	Dose after dialysis	Dose for GFR <10	Dose for GFR 10–50
Piperacillin and tazobactam	As per piperacillin component	100%	30–50: 75% q6h <30: 50% q8h	50% q8h	Q12h (dose after dialysis)		Dose for GFR 10–50
Quinine	10 mg/kg/dose q8h IV 7–10 days	q8h	q8–12h	q24h	Dose after dialysis	Dose for GFR <10	Dose for GFR 10–50

Contd...

Contd...

Dose for normal renal function		*Dose for impaired renal function based on glomerular filtration rate (GFR), mL/min/1.73 m²*			*Dose in renal replacement therapy*		
		>50	*10–50*	*<10*	*HD*	*PD*	*CKRT*
Teicoplanin	10 mg/kg q12h for three doses, then 10 mg/kg 24h	100%; q24h	100% loading doses, then: 30–60: q48h or 50% <30: q72h or 33%	Dose for GFR <10	Dose for GFR < 10	Dose for GFR <10	Dose for GFR 10–50
Tetracycline	*Over 8 years:* 25–50 mg/day q6h PO	q8–12h	q12–24h	q24h	ND; dose for GFR <10	ND; dose for GFR <10	Dose for GFR 10–50
Tigecycline	Loading 1.5–2 mg/kg; 1–2 mg/kg q12h	100%	100%	100%	ND; dose for normal function	ND; dose for normal function	Dose for normal renal function
Tobramycin	2–2.5 mg/kg/dose q6–8h IV, IM	1–2 mg/kg; measure levels	50%	50%	½ full dose after HD	Dose for GFR <10	Dose for GFR 10–50; measure levels
Trimethoprim	3–4 mg/kg/dose q12h IV, PO	q12h	q18h	q24h	Dose after dialysis	q24h	q18h
Valganciclovir	450 mg/m²/day (30 mg/kg/day) for induction; q12h for maintenance	100% q24h	100% q24–48h	q48–72h	Dose after dialysis	Dose for GFR <10	Dose for GFR 10–50
Vancomycin	10–15 mg/kg q6–8h	100%	100% q24h	100% q48–72h	Dose after dialysis	Dose for GFR < 10	Dose for GFR 10–50

Contd...

Contd...

Dose for normal renal function		*Dose for impaired renal function based on glomerular filtration rate (GFR), mL/min/1.73 m²*			*Dose in renal replacement therapy*		
		>50	*10–50*	*<10*	*HD*	*PD*	*CKRT*
Voriconazole	2–12 years: 9 mg/kg q12h	100%	100%	100%	Dose after dialysis	Dose for GFR <10	Dose for GFR 10–50
Miscellaneous							
Acetaminophen	10–15 mg/kg/dose q4–6h PO	100% q4h	100% q6h	100% q8h	None	None	Dose for GFR 10–50
Acetazolamide	5–10 mg/kg/dose q6h PO	100% q6h	100% q12h	Avoid	No data	No data	Avoid
Acetylsalicylic acid	10–15 mg/kg q4–6h PO	100% q4h	100% q4–6h	Avoid	Dose after dialysis	None	Dose for GFR 10–50
Atenolol	0.5–1 mg/kg/dose PO q12–24h	100% q	100% q24h	100% q48h	½ full dose after dialysis	None	Dose for GFR 10–50
Azathioprine	1–3 mg/kg/dose q24h PO	100% q24h	75% q24h	50% q24h	50% dose after HD	50% of normal dose q12h	75% of normal dose q24h
Betamethasone	0.01–0.25 mg/kg/dose div q6–8h PO	100%	100%	100%	No data	No data	Dose for GFR 10–50

Contd...

Contd...

Dose for normal renal function		Dose for impaired renal function based on glomerular filtration rate (GFR), mL/min/1.73 m^2			Dose in renal replacement therapy		
		>50	10–50	<10	HD	PD	CKRT
Captopril	0.3–5 mg/kg/dose q8h PO	100%	75%	50%	50%	50%	75%
Cetirizine	0.25 mg/kg/dose q12–24h PO	100%	50%	25%	None	No data	NA
Chlorambucil	0.1–0.2 mg/kg/dose q24h PO	100%	100%	100%	No data		
Cyclophosphamide	Follow individual protocol	100%	100%	75%	50% after HD	75%	100%
Cyclosporine	1.5–2.5 mg/kg/dose q12h PO	100%	100%	100%	None	None	100%
Dexamethasone	0.1–0.25 mg/kg/dose q6h IV, PO	100%	100%	100%	No data	No data	Dose for GFR 10–50
Digoxin	15 µg/kg/dose stat; 5 µg/kg 6h later; then 3–5 µg/kg q12h PO	100%	30–50: 75%	25% or q48h	25% q12h or 100% q48h	None	75% q12h
Dobutamine	1–20 µg/kg/dose q6–8h PO	100%	100%	Avoid	No supplementary dose needed		No adjustment needed

Contd...

Contd...

Dose for normal renal function		Dose for impaired renal function based on glomerular filtration rate (GFR), mL/min/1.73 m^2			Dose in renal replacement therapy		
		>50	*10–50*	*<10*	*HD*	*PD*	*CKRT*
Enalapril	0.1–0.6 mg/kg/day, div q12–24h	100%	75%	25–50%	Dose for GFR < 10	Dose for GFR < 10	Dose for GFR 10–50
Enoxaparin	1.2 mg/kg/dose q12h	100%	*30–50:* 100% q12h *<30:* 100% q24h	100% q24h	Dose for GFR < 30	Dose for GFR < 30	Dose for GFR 30–50
Insulin (regular)	0.05–0.2 IU/kg/dose sc prn	100%	75%	50%	None	None	Dose for GFR 10–50
Lisinopril	0.05–0.6 mg/kg q24h PO	50%	50%	25%	25%	25%	Dose for GFR 10–50
Methyldopa	10–65 mg/kg/day div q6–12h PO	100% q8h	100% q8–12h	100% q12–24h	Dose after dialysis	None	Dose for GFR 10–50
Methylprednisolone	0.5–1 mg/kg/dose q6–24 IV, IM, PO	100%	100%	100%	Dose for normal function	No data	Dose for GFR 10–50
Metoclopramide	0.15 –0.3 mg/kg/ dose q6h IV, IM, PO	100%	75%	50%	None	No data	50–75%
Nitroprusside	0.5–10 µg/kg/min by infusion	100%	100%	100%	None	None	Dose for GFR 10–50
Omeprazole	0.4–0.8 mg/kg/dose q12–24h PO	100%	100%	100%	No data		

Contd...

Contd...

Dose for normal renal function		*Dose for impaired renal function based on glomerular filtration rate (GFR), mL/min/1.73 m^2*			*Dose in renal replacement therapy*		
		>50	*10–50*	*<10*	*HD*	*PD*	*CKRT*
Ondansetron	0.1–0.2 mg/kg/dose q6–12h PO	100%	100%	100%	No data	No data	Dose for GFR 10–50
Prazosin	5 µg/kg test; 0.025–0.1 mg/kg/dose q6h PO	100%	100%	100%	None	None	Dose for GFR 10–50
Prednisolone	2 mg/kg/dose q24h PO	100%	100%	100%	Yes	No data	Dose for GFR 10–50
Ranitidine	2–4 mg/kg q8–12h PO	75%	50%	25%	½ dose	None	Dose for GFR 10–50
Spironolactone	6.25–25 mg q12h PO	q6–12h	q12–24h	Avoid	NA	NA	Avoid
Antitubercular drugs							
Ethambutol	25 mg/kg/dose q24h PO	q24h	*>30:* No adjustment *<30:* 15–25 mg/kg thrice weekly	q48h	Dose after dialysis	Dose for GFR < 10	Dose for GFR 10–50

Contd...

Contd...

	Dose for normal renal function	*Dose for impaired renal function based on glomerular filtration rate (GFR), mL/min/1.73 m²*			*Dose in renal replacement therapy*		
		>50	*10–50*	*<10*	*HD*	*PD*	*CKRT*
Pyrazinamide	20–35 mg/kg/dose q24h PO	100%	*>30:* No adjustment *<30:* 15–25 mg/kg thrice weekly	50–100%	Dose for GFR < 10 or 25–30 mg/kg post-HD	Dose for GFR < 10	No data
Rifampin	10 mg/kg/day q24h PO	100%	100%	50–100%	ND Dose for GFR < 10	ND Dose for GFR <10	Dose for normal renal function
Streptomycin	20–30 mg/kg/dose q24h IM	7.5 mg/kg q24h	*30–50:* 7.5 mg/kg q24h *10–29:* 7.5 mg/kg q48h	7.5 mg/kg q72–96h	Dose for GFR < 10	Dose for GFR <10	Dose for GFR 10–50 and measure levels
Anticonvulsants							
Carbamazepine	2–10 mg/kg/dose q8h PO	100%	100%	75%	No adjustment required		
Phenobarbital	5 mg/kg/dose q24h IV,	100%	100%; avoid large single dose	50% q24h large single dose	Dose for GFR < 10	Dose for GFR < 10	Dose for GFR 10–50
	IM, PO						

Contd...

Contd...

Dose for normal renal function		*Dose for impaired renal function based on glomerular filtration rate (GFR), mL/min/1.73 m²*			*Dose in renal replacement therapy*		
		>50	*10–50*	*<10*	*HD#*	*PD*	*CKRT*
Clonazepam	0.05–0.2 mg/kg/d	100%	100%	75%	ND; dose for GFR < 10	Dose for GFR < 10	Dose for GFR 10–50 and measure levels
Lamotrigine	0.3 mg/kg/day for 2 weeks; 0.6 mg/kg for 2 weeks; then 4.5–7.5* mg/kg/day div q12h maintenance	100%	100%	75%	Dose for GFR < 10	Dose for GFR < 10	Dose for GFR 10–50 and measure levels
Levetiracetam	10–60 mg/kg/d, div 8h	50%	50%	50%	50% dose after dialysis	Dose for GFR < 10	Dose for GFR 10–50 and measure levels
Topiramate	3–9 mg/kg/d, div 8–12h	50%	50%	25%	Dose after dialysis	Dose for GFR < 10	Dose for GFR 10–50 and measure levels

*Dosing is higher, up to 15.6 mg/kg/day with concomitant use of enzyme inducing antiepileptic drugs, such as phenytoin, phenobarb, carbamazepine, and valproate

#Dose to be given after dialysis

Annexure 8: Drugs requiring minimal dose modification in impaired kidney function

Drug	*Dosage (mg/kg/day)*	*Frequency, route*	*Comments*
Antimicrobials			
Amphotericin B, liposomal	3–5	q24h; IV over 1–2h	If on hemodialysis, give dose after dialysis
Caspofungin	Loading 70 mg/m^2; then 50 mg/m^2	q24h; IV	
Cefoperazone	25–60 mg/kg/dose	q6–12h; IV, IM	
Ceftriaxone	50–100	q12–24h IV, IM	
Chloramphenicol	Loading 40 mg/kg; then 25 mg/kg/dose	q6h; IV, IM, PO	
Clindamycin	10–30	q6–8h; IV	
Linezolid	10 mg/kg/dose	q8h; IV, oral	
Penicillin V	25–50	q6–8h, PO	No dose modification for preexisting renal impairment
Tigecycline	Loading 1.5–2 mg/kg; then 1–2 mg/kg/dose	q12h; IV	
Voriconazole	2–12 yr: 9 mg/kg/dose	q12h; IV	
Diuretics			
Amiloride	0.2–0.6	q24h, PO	Monitor serum potassium levels
Bumetanide	0.01–0.02; maximum 0.3	q12–24h, PO	Avoid in patients allergic to sulfonamides

Contd...

Contd...

Drug	*Dosage (mg/kg/day)*	*Frequency, route*	*Comments*
Chlorthalidone	0.25–2	q24h, PO	Caution in liver and severe renal disease; may cause alkalosis, pancreatitis, hypokalemia, and hyponatremia
Hydrochlorothiazide	1–4; maximum 100 mg	q12–24h, PO	
Furosemide	1–2; maximum 8–10 IV infusion, bolus 1–2 mg/kg, then 0.1–1 mg/kg/h	q6–12h, PO/IV 24h infusion	Injection can be given orally; use with caution in hepatic disease; ototoxicity in presence of renal disease. May cause hypercalciuria, renal stones, and hypokalemic metabolic alkalosis
Metolazone	0.1–0.4	q12–24h, PO	Dyselectrolytemia, marrow suppression, and hyperuricemia. More effective than thiazides with reduced GFR
Spironolactone	1–3; maximum up to 100 mg/day	q12–24h, PO	Use with caution with ACE inhibitors, cimetidine; hyperkalemia common with GFR < 30 mL/min/1.73 m^2
Triamterene	2–4; maximum up to 300 mg/day	q8–12h, PO	
Eplerenone	50 mg/day; may increase up to 100 mg/day	q12–24h, PO	Monitor serum potassium levels. Avoid in GFR < 30 mL/min/m^2. Drug has not been studied in children < 4 years
Immunosuppressive agents			
Azathioprine	1–3	q24h, PO	Monitor white cell counts, liver functions
Abatacept	10 mg/kg/dose	2 weekly for two doses; then monthly IV	Flu-like reactions. Avoid concomitant use of anti-TNF agents, tacrolimus, and live vaccines

Contd...

Contd...

Drug	*Dosage (mg/kg/day)*	*Frequency, route*	*Comments*
Basiliximab	*<30 kg:* 10 mg *≥30 kg:* 20 mg	Two doses on day 1 and 4 of renal transplant	Anti-IL-2 receptor antibody Monitor for hypersensitivity, CBC, and renal functions
Chlorambucil	0.1–0.2	q24h, PO	Marrow suppression, seizures
Cyclophosphamide	2–3 500–750 mg/m^2	q24h, PO Single dose, IV	Monitor cell counts; use with steroids. Hemorrhagic cystitis and vomiting occur more with IV therapy
Cyclosporine	3–6	q12h, PO/IV	Monitor liver/renal functions and blood levels. Hypertension, high cholesterol; hirsutism, gum hyperplasia; and drug interactions
IV immunoglobulin	2 g/kg	3–5 days, IV	Flushing, tachycardia, chills, fever, headache, and aseptic meningitis
Levamisole	2–3	q48h, PO	Leukopenia, rash, fever; rarely seizures
Methylprednisolone	20–30	q24–48h, IV	Dilute in saline or 5% glucose; infuse over 1–2 hr
Mycophenolate mofetil	1000–1200 mg/m^2/day	q12h, PO	GI distress, diarrhea; monitor leukocyte counts
Prednisolone	1–2	q8–48h, PO	Steroid toxicity with long-term use; maximum oral dose 80 mg
Rituximab	375 mg/m^2/dose	q weekly for 2–4 doses	Monitor CBC, renal, and liver functions; CD19 counts
Tacrolimus	0.1–0.3	q12h, PO	Monitor creatinine, sugar, and blood levels; headache, seizures, and diarrhea
Miscellaneous			
Albumin	0.5–1	IV	Infuse over 1–4 hr with furosemide; watch for heart failure, hypertension
Cinacalcet	0.25; maximum 180 mg/day	OD	Used for treatment of secondary hyperparathyroidism.
Chloral hydrate	25–50 mg/kg/dose	prn; PO	Avoid in renal failure, hepatic disease

Contd...

Contd...

Drug	***Dosage (mg/kg/day)***	***Frequency, route***	***Comments***
dDAVP (desmopressin)	2–4 mcg/day 5–20 mcg/day 0.05 mg	SC/IM q12–24h Intranasal 12h, PO	For diabetes insipidus; watch for water intoxication, hyponatremia
	0.3 μg/kg	Intravenous	Prevention of bleeds; administer 30 minutes before procedure
	0.2–0.6 mg	PO	For nocturnal enuresis
Diazepam	0.04–0.2 mg/kg/dose	IV	Hypotension and respiratory depression may occur. Do not dilute in IV fluids; give no faster than 1 mg/min
Imipramine	*4–7 years:* 10–25 mg (total dose) *8–11 years:* 25–50 mg *>11 years:* 50–75 mg	Bedtime for nocturnal enuresis, PO	Do not exceed 2.5 mg/kg/day; avoid concomitant terfenadine *Side effects:* Sedation, urinary retention, constipation, dry mouth, arrhythmia
Ketamine	1–2 mg/kg (over 1–2 minutes)	prn; IV/IM	Administration of diazepam reduces emergence reactions
Midazolam	0.05–0.1 mg/kg; repeat to maximum of 0.2 mg/kg	prn; IV	Administer over 2 minutes; flumazenil is antidote for respiratory depression
Amlodipine	0.05–0.6	q24h; PO	
Warfarin	0.05–0.2	q24h; PO	
Isoniazid	10–15 mg/kg/dose	q24h; IV, IM, PO	If on hemodialysis, administer dose after dialysis
Phenytoin	5–8	q12h; PO, IV	
Valproate sodium	10–60	q8-12h; PO, IV	

Contd...

Contd...

Drug	***Dosage (mg/kg/day)***	***Frequency, route***	***Comments***
Oxybutynin	0.5–0.8 mg/kg; maximum 15 mg	q8–12h, PO	Contraindicated in GI obstruction, megacolon Dry mouth, flushing, blurry vision, constipation and heat intolerance
Tamsulosin	0.4–0.8 mg	q24h, PO	
Tolterodine	1–2 mg	q12h, PO	
Vitamin D Analogs (total dose)			
Alfacalcidol	0.25–2 μg	q24–72h, PO	Monitor calcium, phosphorus; avoid concomitant magnesium antacids Contraindicated in hypercalcemia; calcitriol most potent 1α hydroxyvitamin D_2, synthetic forms of vitamin D: Lower risk of hypercalcemia
Calcitriol	0.25–2 μg	q24–72h, PO	
Cholecalciferol	4000–40,000 IU	q24h, PO	
Doxercalciferol	2.5–5 μg/d	q24h, PO	
Phosphate and potassium binders			
Aluminum hydroxide	50–150	q6–8h, PO	10 mL provides 200 mg elemental aluminum; constipation; interferes with absorption of digoxin, INH and iron 1 g binds 50–75 mg phosphorus
Calcium carbonate	20–65	q8h, PO	Constipation, nausea, headache; hypercalcemia 1 g binds 39 mg phosphorus
Calcium acetate	1–3 tablets	q8h	667 mg has 169 mg elemental calcium; 1 g binds 45 mg phosphorus
Polystyrene sulfonate	1–3 g	q8h, PO/PR	Bowel obstruction may occur; each g resin exchanges 1–2 mEq potassium
Sevelamer	400 mg, 800 mg 2–4 tablets with meals	q8h, PO	GI side effects; metabolic acidosis with chloride preparation 400 mg tablet binds 32 mg phosphorus

The dosage modifications are approximations; each patient should be monitored for signs of drug toxicity
CBC: complete blood counts; GI: gastrointestinal

Annexure 9: Gene lists for common syndromes

Scan the QR code below or type the following link in browser window:
https://docs.google.com/spreadsheets/d/14Rdw0NAc7Go_elXABYetzrE3K3my5mlc/edit?usp=sharing&ouid=105870551856325478303&rtpof=true&sd=true

9.1: Congenital anomalies of the kidneys and urinary tract
9.2: Tubulopathies; electrolyte abnormalities
9.3: Hematuria
9.4: Steroid-resistant nephrotic syndrome; focal segmental glomerulosclerosis; proteinuria
9.5: Thrombotic microangiopathy; hemolytic uremic syndrome
9.6: Ciliopathies; cystic kidney diseases
9.7: Nephrolithiasis; nephrocalcinosis
9.8: Hypertension
9.9: Chronic kidney disease of unknown etiology
9.10: Mitochondrial diseases

Index

Page numbers followed by *b* refer to box, *f* refer to figure, *fc* refer to flowchart, and *t* refer to table.

A

B

C

D

E

F

G

I

N

O

P

Q

R

U

V

W

X

Y

Z